Paediatric surgery

Edited by **JOHN D. ATWELL** MB ChB, FRCS(Eng)

Honorary Emeritus Consultant Paediatric Surgeon, The Wessex Centre for
Paediatric Surgery, The Southampton General Hospital,
Southampton, United Kingdom

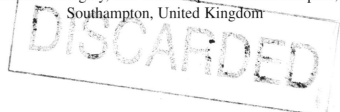

ARNOLD

A member of the Hodder Headline Group
LONDON • SYDNEY • AUCKLAND
Co-published in the USA by Oxford University Press, Inc., New York

To Sue

First published in Great Britain 1998
Arnold, a member of the Hodder Headline group,
338 Euston Road, London NW1 3BH
http: //www.arnoldpublishers.com

Co-published in the United States of America by
Oxford University Press, Inc.,
198 Madison Avenue, New York, NY 10016
Oxford is a registered trademark of Oxford University Press

Whilst the advice and information in this book is believed to be true and
accurate at the date of going to press, neither the authors nor the publisher
can accept any legal responsibility or liability for any errors or omissions that
may be made. In particular (but without limiting the generality of the preceding
disclaimer) every effort has been made to check drug dosages; however it is still
possible that errors have been missed. Furthermore, dosage schedules are constantly
being revised and new side-effects recognized. For these reasons the reader is strongly
urged to consult the drug companies' printed instructions before administering
any of the drugs recommended in this book.

British Library Cataloguing in Publication Data
A catalogue record for this book is available from the British Library

Library of Congress Cataloging-in-Publication Data
A catalog record for this book is available from the Library of Congress

ISBN 0 340 58608 7

Publisher: Annalisa Page
Project Editor: Catherine Barnes
Production Editor: James Rabson
Production Controller: Rose James

Typeset in Times 10/11pt and produced by Gray Publishing, Tunbridge Wells, Kent
Printed and bound in Great Britain by Bath Press, Avon

Contents

Contributors   ix
Foreword   xiii
Preface   xv

PART I   **General principles of care**   **1**

Chapter 1   **Causation of disease**   *J.D. Atwell*   3
Chapter 2   **Congenital causes of disease**   *C. Meijers and J.C. Molenaar*   4
Chapter 3   **Antenatal diagnosis**   *J.E.S. Scott*   11
Chapter 4   **Fetal surgery**   *M.D. Stringer*   20
Chapter 5   **Genetic counselling**   *I.K. Temple and J. Needell*   31
Chapter 6   **The child in hospital**   *J.M.S. Johnstone*   39
Chapter 7   **Nursing sick children in hospital**   *E.A. Glasper*   49
Chapter 8   **Nursing sick children in the community**   *M.A. Gow*   54
Chapter 9   **Ultrasonography**   *K.C. Dewbury*   59
Chapter 10   **Isotope renography**   *V. Batty*   67
Chapter 11   **Transport of sick infants and children**   *P.J. McHugh and M.D. Stringer*   73
Chapter 12   **Day surgery for children**   *J.D. Atwell*   80
Chapter 13   **Paediatric anaesthesia**   *P.M. Spargo and H.M. Munro*   86
Chapter 14   **Homeostasis. Fluid and electrolyte balance**   *A.G. Coran*   102
Chapter 15   **Parenteral nutrition and vascular access**   *G.P. Hosie and R.A. Wheeler*   116
Chapter 16   **Anatomy of the infant and child**   *J.A.S. Dickson*   124
Chapter 17   **Audit**   *D.C.S. Gough and J. Bruce*   137

PART II   **Neonatal surgery**   **143**

Chapter 18   **Anterior wall defects**   *P. Gornall and J.D. Atwell*   145

Chapter 19   **Congenital diaphragmatic hernia**   *D.M. Burge and M. Samuel*   153

Chapter 20   **Structural anomalies of the airway and lungs**   *D.M. Burge and M. Samuel*   170

Chapter 21   **Oesophageal atresia and tracheo-oesophageal fistula**   *S.W. Beasley*   187

Chapter 22   **Neonatal intestinal obstruction**   *J.D. Atwell*   197

Chapter 23   **Hirschsprung's disease**   *J.C. Molenaar and C. Meijers*   206

Chapter 24   **Congenital anorectal anomalies**   *N.V. Freeman*   213

Chapter 25   **Necrotizing enterocolitis**   *V.E. Boston*   226

Chapter 26   **The vitellointestinal duct**   *J.D. Atwell*   238

Chapter 27   **Biliary atresia and choledochal cyst**   *E.R. Howard and M. Davenport*   241

Chapter 28   **Hydrocephalus**   *E.P. Guazzo and J.D. Pickard*   260

Chapter 29   **Spinal dysraphism**   *J. Garfield*   270

Chapter 30   **Spina bifida**   *J.D. Atwell*   279

Chapter 31   **Ambiguous genitalia and intersex**   *I.A. Hughes and P. Malone*   290

PART III   **General surgery of infancy and childhood**   **307**

Chapter 32   **Herniae and hydroceles**   *A.E. MacKinnon*   309

Chapter 33   **The prepuce and circumcision**   *J.I. Curry and D.M. Griffiths*   320

Chapter 34   **The undescended testis**   *A. Bianchi*   327

Chapter 35   **Torsion of the testis and appendages: varicocele**   *N. Ade-Ajayi and R.A. Wheeler*   338

Chapter 36   **Infantile hypertrophic pyloric stenosis**   *P.K.H. Tam*   344

Chapter 37   **Intussusception**   *D.G. Young*   356

Chapter 38   **Gastro-oesophageal reflux in childhood**   *E.W. Fonkalsrud*   364

Chapter 39   **Acquired conditions of the anorectum and perineum**   *S.W. Beasley*   376

Chapter 40   **Inflammatory bowel disease**   *C.M. Doig*   380

Chapter 41   **Gastrointestinal duplication**   *D.M. Burge*   396

Chapter 42   **Acute abdominal pain**   *R. Surana and B. O'Donnell*   402

Chapter 43   **Recurrent abdominal pain**   *R. Surana and B. O'Donnell*   416

Chapter 44   **The gallbladder and pancreas**   *M. Davenport and E.R. Howard*   422

Chapter 45   **Constipation**   *D.M. Griffiths*   435

Chapter 46   **Portal hypertension**   *H. Rode*   442

Chapter 47   **Deformities of the chest wall**   *J.C. Molenaar*   455

Chapter 48   **Head and neck**   *D.P. Drake*   461

PART IV   **Paediatric urology**   **471**

Chapter 49	**Urinary infection: principles** *J.M. Smellie*	473
Chapter 50	**Renal failure** *S.P.A. Rigden*	484
Chapter 51	**Renal failure and growth** *P.R. Betts*	509
Chapter 52	**The genetics of congenital urological anomalies** *J.D. Atwell*	519
Chapter 53	**Double ureters and associated anomalies** *M. Horowitz and M.E. Mitchell*	531
Chapter 54	**Vesico-ureteric reflux** *J.E.S. Scott*	544
Chapter 55	**Paraureteric diverticulum** *J.D. Atwell*	552
Chapter 56	**Megaureters** *P.D.E. Mouriquand*	555
Chapter 57	**Multicystic dysplastic kidney** *D.C.S. Gough*	565
Chapter 58	**Polycystic kidneys** *E.R. Freedman and A.M.K. Rickwood*	573
Chapter 59	**Renal agenesis: ectopia and fusion** *M. Fisch and R. Hohenfellner*	582
Chapter 60	**Bladder exstrophy and epispadias complex** *P. Malone*	590
Chapter 61	**Hypospadias** *P.D.E. Mouriquand*	603
Chapter 62	**Pelviureteric junctional hydronephrosis** *T.P.V.M. de Jong and J.D. van Gool*	617
Chapter 63	**Posterior urethral valves** *D.F.M. Thomas*	626
Chapter 64	**Nocturnal enuresis** *R. Meadow*	636
Chapter 65	**Urinary and faecal incontinence** *J.P. Roberts and P. Malone*	644
Chapter 66	**Urolithiasis in children** *F.M.J. Quinn and W.G. van't Hoff*	658

PART V   **Trauma**   **667**

Chapter 67	**Reception and resuscitation of trauma patients** *R.A. Sleet*	669
Chapter 68	**Regional trauma units for children** *J.A. Haller, Jr*	676
Chapter 69	**Head injuries** *D. Lang*	681
Chapter 70	**Thoracic injuries** *S.W. Beasley*	692
Chapter 71	**Blunt trauma to the abdomen** *R.A. Brown*	696
Chapter 72	**Rupture of the urethra** *J.P. Blandy*	709
Chapter 73	**Thermal and chemical burns** *P.L. Levick*	719
Chapter 74	**Non-accidental injury: physical** *T. Stephenson*	724
Chapter 75	**Non-accidental injury: sexual abuse** *B.L. Priestley and A. Heger*	731
Chapter 76	**Causes and prevention of accidents in children** *A. MacKellar*	738

PART VI   **Miscellaneous**   **745**

Chapter 77	**Principles of transplantation** *M.T. Corbally*	747
Chapter 78	**Congenital heart disease: principles of management – medical** *B.R. Keeton*	759
Chapter 79	**Congenital heart disease: principles of management – surgical** *J.L. Monro*	766

Chapter 80   **Solid tumours of childhood**   *F.J. Rescorla and J.L. Grosfeld*   773

Chapter 81   **General principles of plastic surgery**   *B. Morgan*   790

Chapter 82   **Orthopaedic surgery**   *G.R. Taylor and N.M.P. Clarke*   800

Chapter 83   **Paediatric laparoscopic surgery**   *H.L. Tan*   825

Index   835

Contributors

N. Ade-Ajayi FRCS(I)
Research Fellow, c/o Institute of Child Health, London, UK

J.D. Atwell MB ChB, FRCS(Eng)
Honorary Emeritus Consultant Paediatric Surgeon, The Wessex Centre for Paediatric Surgery, The Southampton General Hospital, Southampton, UK

V. Batty BSc, MB BS, DMRD, FRCR, MSc(Nuc Med)
Consultant in Radiology and Nuclear Medicine, Southampton University Hospital, Southampton, UK

S.W. Beasley MB ChB(Otago), MS(Melb) FRACS
Clinical Professor of Paediatrics and Surgery, Christchurch Hospital, Christchurch, New Zealand

P.R. Betts MD, FRCP, FRCPCH
Consultant Paediatrician and Consultant Paediatric Endocrinologist, Department of Child Health, Southampton General Hospital, Southampton, UK

A. Bianchi MD, FRCS(Eng and Ed)
Consultant Paediatric Surgeon, The Royal Manchester Children's Hospital, Pendlebury, Manchester, UK

J.P. Blandy CBE, MA, DM, MCh, FRCS(Eng), FACS, FRCSI(Hon)
Emeritus Professor of Urology, University of London, London Hospital and St Peter's Hospital, London, UK

V.E. Boston MB ChB, FRCS(Eng), FRCS(I), MD
Consultant Paediatric Surgeon and Honorary Lecturer to the Department of Surgery, Queen's University of Belfast

R.A. Brown DCH(SA), FRCS(Ed), FCS(SA)
Senior Lecturer and Surgeon, Department of Paediatric Surgery, University of Cape Town and Red Cross War Memorial Children's Hospital, Rondebosch, Cape Town, South Africa

J. Bruce MB ChB, FRCS(Ed), FRACS(Paeds)
Clinical Director of Surgery and Consultant Paediatric Surgeon, Royal Manchester Children's Hospital, Pendlebury, Manchester, UK

D.M. Burge FRCS(Eng), FRCP(Lond)
Consultant Paediatric Surgeon, Wessex Centre for Paediatric Surgery, Southampton General Hospital, Southampton, UK

N.M.P. Clarke ChM, FRCS(Eng)
Consultant Orthopaedic Surgeon, Southampton General Hospital, Southampton, UK

A.G. Coran MD
Fellow at the American College of Surgeons and the American Academy of Pediatrics, Professor of Surgery, Head of the Section of Pediatric Surgery and Surgeon-in-Chief of the C.S. Mott Children's Hospital, University of Michigan, USA

M.T. Corbally MB, BCh, MCh, FRCS(I), FRCS(Paed. Surg)
Consultant Paediatric Surgeon at Our Lady's Hospital for Sick Children, Crumlin and Honorary Consultant Transplant Surgeon at St Vincent's Hospital, Dublin, Ireland

J.I. Curry MB BS, FRCS(Eng)
Specialist Registrar in Paediatric Surgery, Wessex Centre for Paediatric Surgery, Southampton General Hospital, Southampton, UK

M. Davenport ChM, FRCS (Paeds), FRCPS(Glas)
Consultant Paediatric Surgeon, Department of Paediatric Surgery, King's College Hospital, London, UK

T.P.V.M. de Jong MD
Head of Department of Paediatric Urology and Paediatric Urologist, Paediatric Renal Centre, University Children's Hospital, Utrecht, The Netherlands

K.C. Dewbury BSc, MB BS, FRCR
Consultant Radiologist and Honorary Senior Lecturer, Southampton General Hospital, Department of Clinical Radiology, Southampton, UK

J.A.S. Dickson MB ChB, FRCS(Ed & Eng)
Retired Consultant Paediatric Surgeon, Sheffield, UK

C.M. Doig MB, ChM, FRCS(Ed), FRCS(Eng)
Senior Lecturer in Paediatric Surgery, Booth Hall Children's Hospital, Blackley, Manchester, UK

D.P. Drake MA, MB, BChir, FRCS(Eng), DCH
Consultant Paediatric Surgeon and Honorary Senior Lecturer, Great Ormond Street Hospital for Children, London, UK

M. Fisch MD
Langenbeckstrabe 1, Mainz, Germany

E.W. Fonkalsrud MD
Professor and Chief of Pediatric Surgery, UCLA School of Medicine and Children's Hospital, Department of Surgery, Los Angeles, California, USA

E.R. Freedman MD, FRCS
Victoria, British Columbia, Canada

N.V. Freeman MB, BCh, FRCS(Eng) FRCS(Ed)
Head of Paediatric Surgery at the Royal Hospital and Senior Lecturer at the Sultan Qabaos University, Sultanate of Oman

J. Garfield MChir, FRCP, FRCS(Eng)
Honorary Emeritus Consultant and Neurosurgeon, Wessex Neurological Centre, Southampton General Hospital, Southampton, UK

E.A. Glasper BA, PhD, RGN, RSCN, ONC, RNT, Dip.ED, Cert.Ed
Professor of Nursing and Director of Child Health Studies, University of Southampton, School of Nursing and Midwifery, Southampton General Hospital, Southampton, UK

P. Gornall MA, MB, BChir, FRCS(Eng)
Consultant Paediatric Surgeon, Department of Paediatric Surgery, Birmingham Children's Hospital NHS Trust, Ladywood Middleway, Ladywood, Birmingham, UK

D.C.S. Gough FRCS(Eng), FRACS, DCH
Consultant Paediatric Urologist, Royal Manchester Children's Hospital, Pendlebury, Manchester, UK

M.A. Gow RGN, RSCN, DN(cert), NNEB
Manager Paediatric Community Nursing, Southampton Community Health NHS Trust, Southampton, UK

D.M. Griffiths BM, BCh, MCh(Oxon) FRCS(Eng)
Consultant Paediatric Surgeon and Senior Lecturer in Paediatric Surgery, University of Southampton, Southampton, UK

J.L. Grosfeld MD
Lafayette F. Page Professor and Chairman in the Department of Surgery, Indiana University School of Medicine and Surgeon-in-Chief and Director in the Section of Pediatric Surgery, James Whitcomb Riley Hospital for Children, Indianapolis, USA

E.P. Guazzo MB, BS, FRACS, FRCS
Neurosurgeon, North Ward Clinic, North Ward, Townsville, Australia

J.A. Haller Jr, MD
Professor of Pediatric Surgery, Pediatrics and Emergency Medicine, Division of Pediatric Surgery, Johns Hopkins Hospital, Baltimore, Maryland, USA

A. Heger MD
Director, LAC and USC Violence Intervention Program, Center for the Vulnerable Child, Los Angeles, California and Associate Professor of Clinical-Medicine, Hospital of Southern California, University of Southern California, USA

R. Hohenfellner MD
Professor of Urology, Department of Urology, University of Mainz, Mainz, Germany

M. Horowitz MD
State University of New York, Health Science Center Brooklyn, Division of Pediatric Urology, Brooklyn, New York, USA

G.P. Hosie FRCS(Ed)
Clinical Research Fellow in Paediatric Surgery, Institute of Child Health, London, UK

E.R. Howard MS, FRCS(Eng & Ed)
Professor of Paediatric Hepatobiliary Surgery, Department of Paediatric Surgery, King's College Hospital, London, UK

I.A. Hughes MA, MD, FRCP, FRCP(C), FRCPCH
Professor and Head of Department of Paediatrics, Addenbrookes Hospital, Cambridge, UK

J.M.S. Johnstone MB ChB, FRCS(Ed)
Consultant Paediatric and General Surgeon, Leicester
Royal Infirmary, Leicester, UK

**B.R. Keeton MBBS, D. Obst. RCOG, DCH, FRCP,
FRCPCH**
Consultant Paediatric Cardiologist, Wessex Cardio-
thoracic Centre, Southampton General Hospital,
Southampton, UK

P.L. Levick MS, FRCS(Ed), FRCS(Eng)
Consultant Plastic Surgeon, Priory Hospital, Birmingham, UK

D. Lang FRCS
Consultant Neurosurgeon, Department of Neuro-
surgery, Wessex Neurological Centre, Southampton
General Hospital, Southampton, UK

**A. MacKellar MB ChB, FRCS(Ed), FRACS,
FAAP(Hon)**
Emeritus Pediatric Surgeon, Princess Margaret Hospital
for Children, Perth, Western Australia, Australia

A.E. MacKinnon MB, BS, FRCS, FRCSG
Consultant Paediatric Surgeon and Honorary Clinical
Lecturer, The Sheffield Children's Hospital, Sheffield,
UK

P. Malone BSc, MCh, FRCS(I)
Consultant Paediatric Urologist, Wessex Centre for
Paediatric Surgery, Southampton General Hospital,
Southampton, UK

P.J. McHugh FRCA
Consultant Paediatric Intensivist and Anaesthetist, Paediatric Intensive Care Unit, Department of Paediatric Surgery, United Leeds Teaching Hospitals Trust, Leeds, UK

R. Meadow PCPCH, FRCP, FRCP(Ed)
Professor of Paediatrics and Child Health, Department
of Paediatrics and Child Health, St James's University
Hospital, Leeds, UK

C. Meijers MD, PhD
Medical Faculty, Sophia Childrens Hospital, Depart-
ment of Paediatric Surgery, University Hospital
Rotterdam, Rotterdam, The Netherlands

M.E. Mitchell MD
Professor and Chief of Urology, Children's Hospital
and Medical Center, Division of Pediatric Urology,
4800 Sand Point Way NE, USA

J.C. Molenaar MD, PhD
Professor of Paediatric Surgery and Chairman, Sophia
Childrens Hospital, Department of Paediatric Surgery,
Rotterdam, The Netherlands

J.L. Monro FRCS(Eng)
Consultant Cardiac Surgeon, Wessex Regional Centre
for Cardiac Surgery, Southampton General Hospital,
Southampton, UK

B. Morgan MB, FRCS, FRCOplh
Consultant Plastic Surgeon, University College London
Hospitals and Mount Vernon Hospital, Northwood, UK

P.D.E. Mouriquand MD, FEBU, FBAPU
Consultant Paediatric Urologist and Honorary Senior
Lecturer in Paediatric Urology, Department of Paediatric
Urology, Great Ormond Street Hospital, London, UK

H.M. Munro MB ChB, FRCA
Clinical Assistant Professor, University of Michigan
Medical Center, Section of Pediatric Anesthesiology,
Michigan, USA

J. Needell RGN, DipNursing, BSc(Hons)
Genetic Nurse Specialist, The Princess Anne Hospital,
Southampton, UK

**B. O'Donnell MCh, FRCS(Eng) FRCS(I), FRCS(Ed.
Hom)**
Emeritus Professor of Paediatric Surgery, Royal
College of Surgeons in Ireland and Emeritus Consultant
Paediatric Surgeon, Our Lady's Hospital for Sick
Children, Dublin, Ireland

J.D. Pickard MA, Mchir, FRCS(Eng), FRCS(Ed)
Bayer Professor of Neurosurgery, Chairman and Clinical Director of Wolfson Brain Injury Centre, Neurosurgery Unit, University of Cambridge Clinical School,
Addenbrookes Hospital, Cambridge, UK

B.L. Priestley MB, FRCP, DCH
Northwood, Middlesex, UK

F.M.J. Quinn MD, FRCS(Paed)
Consultant Paediatric Urologist, Department of Pae-
diatric Surgery, North West Armed Forces Hospital,
Tabuk, Kingdom of Saudi Arabia

F.J. Rescorla MD
Associate Professor, Department of Surgery, Section of
Pediatric Surgery, Indiana University Medical Center,
Indianapolis, USA

A.M.K. Rickwood MA, FRCS(Eng)
Consultant Paediatric Urologist, Alder Hey Children's
Hospital, Liverpool, UK

S.P.A. Rigden FRCP
Consultant Paediatric Nephrologist, Paediatric Renal
Unit, UMDS Guy's and St Thomas's Medical and
Dental Schools, London, UK

J.P. Roberts MS, FRCS(Eng & Ed) FRCS(Paed)
Consultant Paediatric Surgeon, Paediatric Surgical Unit, Sheffield Children's Hospital, Sheffield, UK

H. Rode M.Med(Chir) FCS(SA) FRCS(Ed)
Professor of Surgery (Paediatrics), Department of Paediatric Surgery, Red Cross Children's Hospital, Rondebosch, South Africa

M. Samuel MB BS, MS, DipPaed(Surgery)
Registrar and Clinical Research Fellow in Paediatric Surgery, Department of Paediatric Surgery, Southampton General Hospital, Southampton, UK

J.E.S. Scott MA, MD, FRCS(Eng), FAAP(Hon)
Honorary Senior Research Associate, University of Newcastle upon Tyne, Maternity Survey Office, Newcastle upon Tyne, UK

R.A. Sleet FRCS(Ed), FRCGP
Consultant in Charge, Accident and Emergency Department, Southampton General Hospital, Southampton, UK

J.M. Smellie MA, DM, FRCP, FRCPCH(Hon)
Emeritus Consultant Paediatrician and Senior Lecturer, Department of Paediatrics, University College Hospital, London, UK

P.M. Spargo MB BS, MRCP, FRCA
Consultant Paediatric Anaesthetist, Shackleton Department of Anaesthetics, Southampton General Hospital, Southampton, UK

T. Stephenson BSc, BM, BCh, DM, FRCP, FRCPCH
Professor of Child Health, Department of Child Health, University Hospital, Queen's Medical Centre, Nottingham, UK

M.D. Stringer BSc, MS, FRCS(Eng), FRCP, FRCPa
Consultant Paediatric Surgeon and Honorary Senior Lecturer, Department of Paediatric Surgery, United Leeds Teaching Hospitals Trust and St James's University Hospital Trust, Leeds, UK

R. Surana FRCSI
Senior Registrar, Great Ormond Street Hospital, London, UK

P.K.H. Tam MB, BS, ChM, FRCS
Professor of Paediatric Surgery, Department of Surgery, University of Hong Kong, Queen Mary Hospital, Hong Kong

H.L. Tan MB, BS, FRACS
Chief of Endosurgery, Children's Surgery Centre Pte Ltd, Gleneagles Medical Centre, Singapore

G.R. Taylor FRCS(Orth)
Consultant Orthopaedic Surgeon, Department of Orthopaedics, Southampton General Hospital, Southampton, UK

I.K. Temple FRCP
Consultant Clinical Geneticist, Princess Anne Hospital, Southampton, UK

D.F.M. Thomas MA, FRCPCH, FRCP, FRCS(Eng)
Consultant Paediatric Urologist, Department of Paediatric Surgery, St James's University Hospital, Clinical Sciences Building, Leeds, UK

J.D. van Gool MD, PhD
Paediatric Nephrologist, Paediatric Renal Center, University Hospital for Children, Utrecht, The Netherlands

W.G. van't Hoff BSc, MD, MRCP
Consultant Paediatric Nephrologist, Great Ormond Street Hospital for Children NHS Trust, London, UK

R.A. Wheeler MS, FRCS(Eng)
Consultant Paediatric and Neonatal Surgeon, Wessex Centre for Paediatric Surgery, Southampton General Hospital, Southampton, UK

D.G. Young MB ChB, FRCS(Ed & Glas) DTM&H
Professor and Head of Department of Surgical Paediatrics, Royal Hospital for Sick Children, Yorkhill NHS Trust, Glasgow, UK

Foreword

In 1935 Dr William E. Ladd, a pioneer in the field of paediatric surgery wrote, 'Undoubtedly great strides have been made in this field of surgery in the last few years and I have confidence that greater advances are soon to follow'. His prediction certainly proved true. As I reflect on the enormous changes in the 43 years since my own participation in paediatric surgery began, progress has been at a pace one could never have imagined. For example, urologic problems in children have brought to paediatric surgery many who concentrate on those problems, such as functional repair of bladder exstrophy instead of colonic diversion of the urine, re-implantation of ureters for vesicoureteral reflux, and many more. Paediatric cardiac surgery began in 1938 with division of the patent ductus arteriosus by Robert E. Gross, Ladd's successor. After complex open heart surgery began in 1954 by Walton Lillehei, progress has been made at a dizzying pace. Today, the newborn with transposition of the great vessels, which was formerly uniformly fatal, can now be cured by paediatric heart surgeons by switching the great vessels and the coronary arteries, using hypothermia and temporary cardiac arrest, with success in 98% of those babies!

This superb textbook of paediatric surgery, organized and edited by Mr John Atwell, a surgeon of great experience, is destined to find its way into the library of all who are interested in the betterment of care for infants and children afflicted by problems which require surgery. The wide range of subjects discussed in the 83 chapters, each authored by an acknowledged expert, should prove interesting and educational for physicians with different backgrounds, including the trained paediatric surgeon, the general surgeon who must also provide care for children, paediatricians, anaesthesiologists and general medical doctors. Mr Atwell is to be congratulated for his choice of subjects and the emphasis made on basic principles in caring for young patients.

The book is timely and provides an excellent look at paediatric surgery as it is currently practised. I predict that it will be a mainstay in the surgical literature for many years.

W. Hardy Hendren, MD, FACS, FRCS(I), FAAP
Chief of Surgery, Children's Hospital,
Robert E. Gross Professor of Surgery,
Harvard Medical School, Boston,
Massachussetts, USA

Preface

The aim has been to provide the principles of paediatric surgery for paediatric surgeons and trainees within the specialty. It should also be of value to the general surgeon who has the responsibility of treating children. The book covers essential care of the infant or child undergoing hospitalization for surgical treatment.

The clinical material has been subdivided into six sections: General principles of care, Neonatal surgery, General surgery of infancy and childhood, Paediatric urology, trauma and Miscellaneous, a mixed group of topics. In the first section emphasis has been placed on the overall care of the infant or child admitted to hospital, i.e. Chapter 6, Nursing care in the hospital and community (Chapters 7 and 8) and Day surgery for children (Chapter 12). The last of these and the chapter on transport of sick infants and children (Chapter 11) are organizational problems which have to be studied in order to achieve optimum care. Similarly, the establishment of trauma centres in the USA (Chapter 68) has resulted in improvement of the mortality and morbidity of injuries sustained by the accident-prone child.

There has been an increase of specialization within paediatric surgery with, for example, the appointment of paediatric urologists, neurosurgeons and oncologists. This increase in specialization has been of benefit to the patient, but one danger is that the overall care of the patient may suffer, and therefore the chapters on congenital heart disease (Chapters 78 and 79), orthopaedic surgery (Chapter 82) and plastic surgery (Chapter 81) have been included. These chapters are important to the trainee in paediatric surgery as many congenital defects are multiple and affect different systems so a broad understanding of these specialties will result in better care of the patient.

The birth of a newborn with a major congenital anomaly is a tragedy for the family. As a result parents will seek genetic advice about the risks in future pregnancies and the need for counselling (Chapter 5).

Prevention of congenital anomalies is now possible with antenatal diagnosis (Chapter 3) when a decision is made for either a termination of the pregnancy or it is allowed to proceed to term with the possibility of fetal surgery (Chapter 4) and ultrasonography (Chapter 9). There have been advances in the development of paediatric anaesthesia and intensive care (Chapters 13–15) and even more recently the development of microsurgical (Chapter 34) and laparoscopic procedures are now playing an important role in paediatric surgery (Chapter 83).

This volume does not intend to be a textbook of operative surgery, although this aspect has been covered in several of the chapters, for example, Chapter 32 on herniae and Chapter 61 on hypospadias. This has been considered reasonable as these details are fundamentally important and stress the care necessary firstly, in treating a common condition at all ages and secondly as multiple operations are available for the treatment of hypospadias and an expert opinion is required.

In conclusion one can only hope that the aims of this textbook have been achieved and that those operating on children will benefit and enjoy the text. Upon these basics they will be able to add their own personal experience and realize the importance of the multidisciplinary approach needed to achieve excellent results for their patients.

John D. Atwell

Acknowledgement

Thank you to the staff at Arnold and Gray Publishing.

PART I

General principles of care

CHAPTER 1

Causation of disease

J.D. ATWELL

Congential

(i) GENETIC: HEREDITARY

Dominant	Neurofibromatosis
Recessive	Meconium ileus, cystic fibrosis (Chapter 22)
Sex linked	Haemophilia
Chromosomal	Down's syndrome (Chapter 22)
Other	Pyloric stenosis (Chapter 36), Hirschsprung's disease (Chapter 23), renal anomalies (Chapter 53), nephroblastoma (Chapter 81)

(ii) INTRAUTERINE ENVIRONMENTAL FACTORS

Infections	Toxoplasmosis, rubella, syphilis
Vascular	Jejunoileal atresias (Chapter 22)
Deficiencies	Vitamins, folic acid, spina bifida (Chapter 30)
Failure of fusion	Spina bifida, Cleft palate and lip (Chapter 81), bladder exstrophy (Chapter 60)
Trauma	Intrauterine intervention (Chapters 3 and 4), amputations and constriction rings
Sequestrated tissue at lines of fusion	Dermoid cysts (Chapter 48), spinal dysraphism (Chapter 29)
Disordered development	Spina bifida: myelodysplasia (Chapters 29 and 30)

Acquired

(i) TRAUMA (SECTION 5)

Direct injury, e.g. stabbing, road traffic accidents

Indirect injury, e.g. falls from a height, spinal injuries

Thermal, e.g. scalds, fire, accidents in the home

Chemical, e.g. caustic soda burns, ingestion, accidents, non-accidental injury

Cold injury, e.g. hypothermia, cold injury in neonates, frostbite

Electrical, e.g. lightning, electrical burns in the house

Radiation, e.g. exposure to radiation

Poisoning, e.g. snake bites, ingestion

(ii) INFECTIONS

Acute	Bacterial, viral, parasitic
Chronic	Tuberculosis, actinomycosis, pseudo-tuberculosis

(iii) NEOPLASTIC (CHAPTER 80)

Embryonic tumours, e.g. nephroblastoma, neuroblastoma, hepatoblastoma

Sarcomas, e.g. Ewing's sarcoma

Carcinomas, e.g. thyroid carcinoma

(iv) METABOLIC: HORMONAL

Urolithiasis (Chapter 66), diabetes

(v) DEGENERATIVE

Osteoarthritis (Chapter 82), e.g. secondary to trauma or congenital defects

(vi) AUTOIMMUNE

Hashimoto's disease, autoimmune deficiency disease

CHAPTER 2

Congenital causes of disease

C. MEIJERS AND J.C. MOLENAAR

Introduction
Classification of birth defects
Associations
Syndromes
Pathogenetic classification

Special manifestations of developmental
field defects
Aetiological classification
Further reading

Introduction

From ancient times humans have been fascinated by the phenomenon of congenital abnormalities. Throughout the ages, but also in our time, the views about causes and meaning of such aberrations have been strongly determined by culture, religion and our readiness to accept scientific insights. Only a few centuries ago congenital abnormalities were often regarded as God's punishment for a wrongful life. Even in our scientific era, however, it remains advisable to pay attention to the backgrounds of human views about causes and meaning of congenital abnormalities, because the ethnic, religious and cultural diversity within societies is increasing. Only by so doing can the medical and biological aspects of congenital abnormalities discussed below be optimally applied for the benefit of patients and their relatives. It cannot be denied that even today parents with a child with congenital abnormalities often express feelings of guilt, sometimes only in covert terms. However, these are not so much imposed by prevailing, norm-setting secular or religious opinions, but rather associated with a desperate search for a cause that could have been avoided. Therefore it is obvious that patients, parents and their physicians have an interest in the knowledge of the causes of abnormalities in embryonic development.

Classification of birth defects

Over the years many different classification systems for congenital anomalies have evolved. They can be roughly distinguished into morphological, pathogenetic and aetiological systems. Which classification system is applied will usually depend on what is most practical for the user but, of course, all systems used should be consistent with current scientific insights.

For clinical purposes a proper morphological description of the anomalies is of primary importance, and this will often serve as a basis for the pathogenesis and subsequently even for the aetiology. This is why the three classification systems are discussed in this order.

In many cases the pathogenesis and aetiology remain unclear, or can be traced only by analysing the presenting anomalies in connection with the medical and obstetric history, information about family relations and the incidence of anomalies in relatives.

DYSMORPHOLOGICAL APPROACH

An accurate and complete description of the patient's anomalies is essential for a morphological classification. Careful physical examination for gross anomalies, dysmorphisms, developmental disorders and neurological function disorders is most important. Gender- and age-dependent characteristics such as height, weight, cranial circumference and other measurable body sizes should be quantified to compare with percentile curves or another suitable set of standard values. Expressing body sizes of patients in percentile values makes them comparable, and thus enables disproportions to be established. Likewise, body sizes of family members and relations can be compared. Additional diagnostic investigation such as X-ray, computerized tomography (CT) scan, magnetic resonance imaging (MRI) scan, and pathological–anatomical investigation of tissue specimens can provide valuable additional information or a more precise picture of the malformations. In cases of stillbirth or death a complete autopsy should be performed as soon as possible. A protocol adapted from Berry (1980) can be used for this purpose (Table 2.1).

Congenital anomalies can be distinguished into gross anomalies, such as cardiac defects, cleft lip or palate, or spina bifida, and dysmorphisms, such as epicanthus, protruding ears or clinodactyly. Some anomalies cannot easily be classified in one category, e.g. microtia, agenesis of the nasolacrimal duct or umbilical hernia. In our view anomalies that require reconstructive treatment, or those in which an essential embryonic structure is lacking or has undergone a structural transformation, may be counted as gross anomalies.

It is inherent to all classification systems that certain choices are arbitrary. When comparing one's own observations with those from the literature and textbooks it is essential to consider whether there are differences in definitions and, if so, to take them into account in the assessment.

Some of the frequent dysmorphisms also often manifest in the general population and thus might have relatively little meaning as an isolated presenting symptom. Most patients with Down's syndrome have a simian crease on both palms of the hand, but this is also true for around 1% of the general population. A specific combination of dysmorphisms, however, may suggest a hereditary syndrome or constitute a strong indication for the cause of other anomalies in the same patient. Moreover, the nature or degree of some dysmorphisms might be such that they are experienced as disfigurements or as annoying and may be a reason for corrective treatment.

Congenital anomalies can also be distinguished into isolated anomaly versus anomaly as a part of a syndrome, and sporadic anomaly versus familial anomaly. This global division is often used in textbooks and in practice often gives direction to additional investigation into the pathogenesis and cause of the anomaly.

Associations

For unknown reasons certain combinations of anomalies occur more frequently than might be expected on

---

Table 2.1 Routine histopathological examination of embryonic and fetal material

Embryos equal to or smaller than 35 mm CRL[a]
- Measurements of CRL, foot length, head circumference
- External examination with the use of a dissecting microscope, and description of dysmorphisms
- Photographs of whole embryo, and details when abnormal
- Serial histology of the whole embryo for examining the internal organs.

Embryos larger than 35 mm CRL and fetuses
- Measurements of weight, CRL, occipitofrontal head circumference, foot length, and others when an abnormality is suspected, e.g. inner and outer bony distance of orbits
- External examination with the use of dissecting microscope
- Photographs of whole embryo or fetus, and details when abnormal
- Description of placenta, placental weight
- X-ray (babygram)
- Internal examination with the use of a dissecting microscope
- Collection of blood (e.g. heart puncture)
- Collection of fibroblasts (sterile skin biopsy, fascia biopsy)
- Histology of internal organs
- Serial histology of abnormal organs or organ systems (e.g. heart/lung, urethra/bladder/ ureters)

Adapted from the protocol according to Berry (1980).
We acknowledge N.G. Hartwig for his permission to adapt this table from his dissertation 'Pathoembryology: developmental processes and congenital malformations' (Leiden, 1992).
[a]CRL: CRS, *see* crown–rump length.

the basis of the prevalence of each of the separate anomalies. This phenomenon is called association. Examples are the VATER (*v*ertebral malformation, *a*nal malformation, *t*racheo*e*sophageal fistula and *r*enal malformation) and VACTERL associations (VATER plus *c*ardiac and *l*imb malformation), which derive their names from the initial letters of the anomalies concerned (acronyms). In many patients not all characteristics of the VATER or VACTERL association are present. However, subcombinations also appear to occur much more frequently in a population than can be expected on the basis of each separate anomaly. Other known associations are the MURCS (*m*üllerian duct anomalies, *r*enal anomalies and *c*ervicothoracic *s*omite dysplasia), likewise a usually sporadic combination of anomalies with still unknown cause, and the CHARGE association, consisting of *c*oloboma, *h*eart defects, choanal *a*tresia, growth *r*etardation, *g*enital hypoplasia and *e*ar anomalies.

Such a morphological classification, which could also be made on the basis of epidemiological data concerning the relative prevalence of the various anomalies, does not provide an explanation of the pathogenesis or cause. Moreover, the same phenotype may result from different causes and therefore differ among individual patients. Indeed, where causes have become known, it frequently turns out to be a matter of aetiological heterogenicity. Yet the existence of such associations justifies the suspicion that these anomalies have a common aetiology or pathogenesis in at least a proportion of patients. Besides, sometimes it is possible to differentiate further the empirical recurrence risks and to look for more phenotypically homogeneous groups of anomalies in order to investigate a common aetiology and pathogenesis.

Syndromes

Certain combinations of dysmorphisms, proportional or disproportional growth disturbances, developmental disorders, neurological traits or gross anomalies are found in the population with a certain consistency and are interpreted as a syndrome. Patients with the same syndrome have in common certain clinical and genetic–epidemiological characteristics. Perhaps the best-known example is Down's syndrome. This term indicates no more than the existence of a rather large group of patients in the population who have in common a number of dysmorphisms such as brachycephaly, epicanthus, large tongue, simian crease, large gap between first and second toe, and developmental and growth retardation. Parents of an afflicted child once strikingly summarized that 'patients with the same syndrome resemble more each other than their brothers or sisters'.

Gross anomalies need not be an obligatory characteristic of the syndrome, but sometimes co-occur much more frequently than average in the population. In the case of Down's syndrome these are, in particular, duodenal atresia, cardiac defect, Hirschsprung's disease, leukaemia and at a later age Alzheimer's disease. Down's syndrome was described as a recognizable picture long before the chromosomal basis of this condition was suspected by the Dutch ophthalmologist–geneticist Waardenburg in the 1930s and could be demonstrated with cytogenic investigation in the 1950s. It is therefore only, as in the case of almost all other syndromes, a descriptive morphological typification, which in the long run has resulted in finding the underlying cause.

Pathogenetic classification

The genesis of a congenital anomaly is strongly dependent on current scientific insights. If parents with a baby with retarded development are asked for the reason for this retardation, they could simply reply that their child has Down's syndrome. Nowadays most people know that Down's syndrome is the name of a combination of visible characteristics and that an additional chromosome 21 is its cause. However, the additional chromosome 21 and thus the presence of three copies of genes on chromosome 21 in each cell of the body is a mechanism for the development of Down's syndrome, but the cause of this presence of the additional chromosome 21 is still unknown. It is known, nevertheless, that in most cases Down's syndrome can be explained by a meiotic division disorder in one of the parents, sometimes by a gonadal or somatic mosaicism due to an mitotic division disorder during the embryonic development of one of the parents, and less frequently by a *de novo* translocation or hereditary translocation of which one of the parents is the carrier. However, the causes of a meiotic division disorder in one of the parents and of the development of a translocation still require clarification.

For the pathogenetic description of congenital anomalies the following terms are used: malformation; deformation; disruption; and dysplasia.

Malformation implies that the anomaly has developed during embryogenesis. The structure involved has always been intrinsically abnormal. Examples are horseshoe kidney, organ agenesis or a severe ventricular septum defect.

Deformation means that the embryonic development in principle has been normal and has led to a normal formation, but that by virtue of external mechanical influences, in particular, deformations have occurred. A large myoma or a congenital anomaly of the uterus may result in local deformation of the fetus, which may or may not recover spontaneously after birth. A great shortage or lack of amniotic fluid restricts the embryo's freedom of movement and imposes the shape of the womb on to the embryo. If this persists long enough in a critical stage of development it may result in irreversible deformations of the embryo.

Disruption implies that embryonic or fetal development has been interfered with or has broken down, with resultant permanent residual injury of potentially normal tissues. The mechanism can be vascular, mechanical or infection. An example is the polycystic encephalopathy seen in identical twins with a common placental circulation, and notably in the twin who survives the intrauterine death of the other. It is assumed that vasoactive substances or thrombotic embolisms from the deceasing twin, by way of the common placental circulation, may cause disruptions that give rise to cerebral infarctions. Comparable mechanisms may be involved in the development of the otomandibular limb hypogenesis syndrome that from an epidemiological point of view has been associated with maternal consumption of the vasoactive substance cocaine and with an early chorionic villi biopsy for the purpose of prenatal diagnosis. In the latter case it is presumed that certain disorders in the fetoplacental blood circulation play an important role in the pathogenesis. Congenital anomaly due to intrauterine infections, e.g. microcephaly with intracerebral calcifications and blindness due to parasitic nestling in the retina (as in toxoplasmosis), is another example of exogenously induced disruptions of a basically normal embryonic and fetal development.

It is not always easy to distinguish between malformation and disruption. Moreover, it appears that anomalies that apparently seem to be malformations, such as cleft lip and spina bifida aperta, can be explained by disruptions induced experimentally in laboratory animals. The question is whether closure of the upper lip, or of the neural tube, has never taken place, or whether the defect is actually the result of a disruption of an initially already closed structure. The latter mechanism might be involved in some cases of spina bifida aperta. Furthermore, a disruption could mean that later embryonic developments are disturbed or no longer possible. It appears that chemically induced cleft lip in animal models can be primarily explained by haemorrhages that occur in regions that shortly thereafter are involved in closure of the upper lip. Certain combinations of anomalies can thus show a complex spatial and chronological (temporospatial) relationship.

Dysplasia is an abnormal development of tissues. Examples are renal dysplasia and dysplasia of (cartilaginous) bone and muscular tissue. It is a term with a broad meaning not necessarily connected with embryonic development. Bronchopulmonary dysplasia, for instance, develops as a result of high-pressure artificial ventilation with high oxygen concentrations.

In some instances it is possible to deduce, from the nature of the anomalies in combination with animal experiments, how the various anomalies are related. In this context the term *sequence* is of clinical importance.

A sequence is understood to mean that an anomaly or mechanical factor during the embryonic development of a specific organ disturbs that of other organs in a later stage, resulting in a pattern of anomalies, whereas development would have been entirely normal if the primary disturbance had not occurred. An example is the oligohydramnios sequence. The almost complete lack of amniotic fluid, for instance through agenesis of both kidneys, results in lung hypoplasia due to decreased breathing, arthrogryposis due to restriction of fetal movement and a characteristic rounding of the face (comparable to that which results from pulling a nylon stocking over one's head). The lack of amniotic fluid is a reasonable explanation for these anomalies. Likewise, experimental animal tests have revealed that comparable anomalies can be induced by artificially creating oligohydramnios at a certain stage and of a certain duration. These anomalies could be prevented or restricted by restoring the amniotic fluid compartment to its normal size at a later stage, although well before birth. Comparable indications have been obtained from observations in pregnant women who were losing amniotic fluid owing to an early rupture of the amnion, or in whom oligohydramnios was treated by creating an artificial amniotic fluid compartment by means of intra-amniotic infusion.

Circumscript areas of embryonic tissues develop into multiple and hence related morphological structures. Damage to these circumscript areas or developmental fields can result in multiple structural malformations. Application of the developmental field concept helps to explain why certain malformations occur together. Designation and understanding of developmental fields require considerable knowledge of embryology and the fates of embryonic cells. The use of the terms developmental field defect and sequence in the description of entities with multiple anomalies has apparently not clarified the pathogenesis or aetiology of many of these conditions. Implicit in the occurrence of such an entity are the notions that the component anomalies have a common aetiology, that certain of the component anomalies may have arisen from a disturbance of common precursor cells (developmental field defect), and that certain component anomalies may be secondary to preceding anomalies or mechanical forces (sequence).

An example of a developmental field defect is the caudal regression syndrome, which is characterized by underdevelopment of one or both legs (occasionally fused to a form of sirenomelia), and agenesis or hypoplasia of part of or the entire scrotum. In its most extensive form there are also lumbosacral myelomeningocele, atresia or other anomaly of the anus, disorders in the septation between rectum and vagina causing a cloaca that remains present, abnormal genitalia, vesical exstrophy with associated anomalies of ureters or kidneys, and sometimes an omphalocele. This caudal regression syndrome presents more often in boys than in girls, in monozygotic twins and in maternal diabetes (*c.* 15% of the cases are associated with diabetes mellitus of the mother during pregnancy). It is assumed that all these anomalies result from a single primary defect during the earliest stage of pregnancy, which leads to disturbance in the embryonic development of all organs in the caudal part of the embryonic axis. It is still unclear to what extent such a developmental field defect should be considered as a disruption of normal development, or as a complex malformation resulting from a defect in the expression of a gene that normally will initiate and control morphogenesis in the caudal part of the embryo.

Special manifestations of developmental field defects

A spectrum of congenital anomalies is related to the pharyngeal arch region. These include the DiGeorge syndrome, the CHARGE association, the velocardio-facial or Sphrintzen syndrome, the Treacher–Collins syndrome, the facio-auriculovertebral spectrum (Goldenhar syndrome), retinoic acid embryopathy and certain conotruncal defects. These syndromes, which seem to be related to the embryonic pharyngeal arch and the hindbrain neural crest show great clinical resemblance (Table 2.2). It is striking that, apart from in patients with the DiGeorge syndrome, microdeletions in chromosome 22q11 are also found in patients with the velocardiofacial syndrome, the CHARGE associa-tion and certain cases of familial cardiac defects. It is not yet clear whether the various conditions can be distinguished from each other by the fact that several genes in the region have been deleted or mutated and

each gene accounts for the different syndrome-specific constituent symptoms, or whether it is a matter of one gene that, provided it has been deleted or mutated, causes all of these clinical pictures and that the differences should be ascribed to variable expression of a defect in this gene.

Congenital anomalies that are almost identical to the above spontaneously presenting syndromes are also seen in retinoic acid embryopathy. Retinoic acid prob-ably acts via nuclear retinoic acid receptors that under its influence regulate the expression of several genes involved in embryonic development. The influence of the retinoic acid is modulated by cytoplasmic protein binding (cellular retinoic acid binding protein or CRABP). From *in situ* hybridization experiments it appeared that the *CRABPI* gene in time and place is particularly expressed in those parts of the embryo in which in all probability those anomalies develop that are induced by retinoic acid. The great likeness between DiGeorge syndrome and retinoic acid embryopathy suggests that the primary effect of DiGeorge syndrome must be looked for in the same area.

Aetiological classification

The aetiological classification of congenital anomalies does not differ much from that for diseases and anom-alies in general. Based on the current level of insights into the causes of congenital anomalies, a classification was made that is of practical use in hereditary counselling and prevention (Table 2.3). It should be considered in the case of diseases that present later in life and maternal factors during pregnancy, if available, have to be analysed. Furthermore, this table does not list the relative frequency of the various categories of congenital malformations. The reason is that insuffi-cient reliable data are available. Registration systems

Table 2.2 Some frequent symptoms of developmental distur-bances indicated as neurocristopathies

	1	2	3	4	5	6
Abnormal auricle	+	+	±	+	+	−
Deafness	+	−	±	+	+	−
Preauricular abnormalities	+	−	−	−	+	−
Micrognathia	+	+	+	+	+	−
Thymus aplasia	+	+	−	−	−	−
Parathyroid abnormalities	+	+	−	−	−	−
Cardiac (outflow) defects	+	+	+	+	±	+
Cerebral abnormalities	+	±	±	+	±	−
Vertebral abnormalities	+	+	−	−	+	−

1: Retinoic acid embryopathy; 2: DiGeorge syndrome; 3: Sphrintzen syndrome; 4: CHARGE association; 5: oculo-auriculo-vertebral spectrum; 6: familial cardiac outflow tract abnormality.

Table 2.3   Aetiological classification of birth defects

Cause	
Chromosomal	
Pathogenetic	Numerical prezygotic: meiotic/mitotic postzygotic: mitotic Structural *de novo*/familial
Aetiological	Hereditary (*c.* 3%), e.g. a familial translocation for which one of the parents is the carrier; or a trisomy as a result of mosaicism for that trisomy in one of the parents Known mutagenic cause (rarely demonstrable) Unknown (largest group): unknown mutagenic cause or replication error of any kind
Monogenetic	Whether or not in combination with variable expression, reduced penetrance, uniparental paternal or maternal heterodisomy or isodisomy, and genomic imprinting Autosomal dominant Autosomal recessive X-linked
Polygenic	Interaction of two or more genes

Exogenous	Nutrition
	   intoxications
	   deficiencies
	Environment
	   accidental
	   chronic
	Occupation
	   accidental
	   chronic
	Maternal diseases
	   hereditary
	   infectious
	   other
	Maternal medication
	Maternal intoxications
	   stimulants
	   narcotics

Multifactorial	Interaction between one or more genes and exogenous factors, including transplacental maternal factors
Unknown	

for congenital malformations have been in use for only a few years and do not yet cover the entire population. Besides, the classification of birth defects is subject to perpetual change owing to new insights into the molecular and genetic background of birth defects. Many birth defects that until recently were considered of multifactorial or polygenetic origin now appear to be a matter of aetiological heterogenicity, often with a range of monogenic or chromosomal causes, sometimes for one and the same clinical picture. This cannot be detected with the available genetic or epidemiological techniques, since these in particular employ a purely mathematical approach to segregation of the phenotype.

From the point of view of prevention it is highly relevant to pay attention to exogenous factors, because they can be modified in a simple way in many cases. All physicians, but especially family doctors, gynaecologists and midwives, are regularly confronted with the question of whether a maternal disease or drug therapy during pregnancy might have harmful consequences for the fetus.

Classification of birth defects can be a first step towards a better understanding of their causes and their subsequent prevention. The role of paediatric surgeons should not be underestimated in this respect. They are often the first to see patients and to describe in detail the gross abnormalities needing reconstructive treatment. A detailed description of associated anomalies and concomitant dysmorphisms is important for the documentation of the complete pattern of anomalies in the individual patient sent in for surgical treatment. From unpublished studies conducted in our department it has become clear that co-operation with a clinical geneticist is extremely important to interpret the documented symptoms into syndromes and to counsel the parents regarding future offspring. Such co-operation might pave the way for the registration of new syndromes and for better aimed molecular genetic research.

It seems unlikely that prevention of all congenital anomalies is close at hand. Families will continue to face the difficulty of having children with birth defects. Physicians will continue to face tasks of evaluating the extent of the defect, identifying the cause, planning treatment and long-term management and assisting the family members as they adapt to raising a malformed child. Scientists will continue to be challenged by the need to understand the defects that occur and to develop strategies for their management and prevention.

Further reading

Aase, J.M. 1990: *Diagnostic morphology*. New York: Plenum.

Berry, C.L. 1980: The examination of embryonic and fetal material in diagnostic histopathology laboratories. *Journal of Clinical Pathology* **33**, 317–26.

Jones, K.L. 1988: *Smith's recognizable patterns of human malformation*, 4th ed. Philadelphia: W.B. Saunders.

Larsen, W.J. 1993: *Human embryology*. New York: Churchill Livingstone.

O'Doherty, N. 1985: *Atlas of the newborn*. Hingham: MTP Press.

Stevenson, R.E., Hall, J.G. and Goodman, R.N. 1993: *Human malformations and related anomalies*. Oxford: Oxford University Press.

CHAPTER 3

Antenatal diagnosis

J.E.S. SCOTT

Introduction
The purpose of antenatal diagnosis
Techniques of antenatal diagnosis
Regional perinatal medical centres
Possible courses of action

The management of surgical abnormalities
diagnosed antenatally
Conclusion
References

Introduction

The diagnosis of congenital abnormalities in the fetus is now common and familiar practice, but it was only as recently as the mid-1980s that it began to impinge significantly on the surgical management of the newborn. Rapid and far-reaching developments in the field of ultrasound had, however, already been taking place for at least the previous 15 years, of which paediatric surgeons were regrettably unaware, and as a result an opportunity for what could have been one of the most profitable collaborative efforts in the history of medicine was lost. There is no better example of the tunnel vision from which specialists working in restricted medical fields are prone to suffer. Obstetricians and radiologists exploring the potential of ultrasound saw it only as an aid to the management of pregnancy. Even when they first realized that they were able to identify the vital organs in the fetus and observe fetal development (Robinson *et al.*, 1968), even when pathology in a fetal organ was recognized (Garrett *et al.*, 1970), and even when they started to take action on the strength of their findings (Campbell *et al.*, 1972), the message failed to get through to the professionals who were responsible for caring for the fetus after its delivery, namely the paediatric surgeons, neonatologists, cardiologists and geneticists. The obstetrician's task, however, is to carry a mother securely through her pregnancy and at the end of it to deliver her baby safely and

expeditiously into the hands of these other specialists, so it is, perhaps, not surprising that to them, ultrasound was exclusively an obstetric tool.

Greater zeal at this time on the part of the paediatric specialists to lend their knowledge and expertise in the interpretation of the ultrasound images that obstetricians were discovering and an expressed willingness to be present when examinations were being performed might have led to more rapid and certainly more harmonious progress. This failure of communication between colleagues who, although in differing specialties, were, at least, in the same profession, led to haphazard and frequently ill-informed attempts on the part of some ultrasonologists to treat congenital abnormalities in the fetus about which they had very little knowledge concerning their postnatal significance. Some of the disasters accruing from these actions reached the literature (Purkiss *et al.*, 1988).

Many of the developments in medical science have occurred more as a result of accidental discoveries than of logical thought, and the use of ultrasound in pregnancy and later in wider fields of medicine is such an example. Although it is not the only antenatal diagnostic technique it is the one that has enabled the others to be developed and is therefore the most significant. Although its use as an investigative technique in areas other than antenatal diagnosis has proved outstandingly successful (most importantly by reducing or eliminating the need for radiation in many instances), many have questioned on both scientific and ethical grounds its value in revealing, before nature intended, the hitherto secret contents of the amniotic cavity. Some authors contend that ultrasonography has little value as a means of screening for congenital malformations because of its relatively low sensitivity (Thacker, 1985; Pitkin, 1991), a contention which is supported by others (Rosendahl and Kivenen, 1989) who quoted a sensitivity figure of only 58.1%. Recently, a claim that a sensitivity rate of 85% could be achieved by scanning at 19 weeks was made (Luck, 1992) but this was hotly contested (Shirley *et al.*, 1992; Whittle, 1992; Broomhall, 1992; Bell and Lumley, 1992), a figure of 70% or even lower being suggested as more realistic. To add to the confusion over the reliability of antenatal diagnosis is the concern that has been expressed about the impact on the mother, the fetus and the family of false-positive diagnoses using ultrasound or any other screening technique (Marteau *et al.*, 1992). Many articles do not mention their occurrence and if they do, the number is questionably low. However, when correspondence and notes generated by antenatal scanning clinics are surveyed, there can be little doubt that the anxiety, apprehension and indecision that arise in the minds of radiographers, ultrasonologists and patients when an insecure antenatal finding materializes are considerable. Despite this, the scan in the eyes of the general public is now an essential step in the process of having a baby and very few, perhaps only 4–5%, refuse the offer. Furthermore, public perception has shifted the emphasis of the scan from an aid to the conduct of the pregnancy to a means of obtaining a sneak-preview of the baby. It is, therefore, essential for all who aspire to be guided in their clinical management of the newborn by the antenatal findings to be fully aware of how much or little antenatal diagnosis can achieve.

The purpose of antenatal diagnosis

From the standpoint of the obstetrician, the reasons for antenatal diagnosis are obvious. The gestational age by fetal dimension and its correlation with age by menstrual dates, the position and number of fetuses and the position of the placenta, the state of the uterus and other pelvic organs are all items of information which are essential to the satisfactory conduct of pregnancy and are routinely assimilated by ultrasonographers in all antenatal clinics. There is no need to consider these factors any further, but what is the real purpose of exploring the integrity of the fetus? Blithely casting a net to trawl for anything that might be around can produce an unpleasant surprise if a shark is caught. It is as well to know beforehand what might be revealed and how to react sensibly when the picture is not so pretty. The ultrasonographers bear the brunt of this strain as they are the first to establish hands-on contact with a

highly apprehensive individual in a defensive state of mind, who is often accompanied by an even more expectant partner. Ultrasound is 'real-time' in more ways than one, and answers to pertinent and penetrating questions are expected on the spot. The ultrasonographer, though well aware of what she or he is looking at, has neither the professional status nor legal backing to give diagnostic opinions direct to patients. Various euphemisms and circumlocutions (in good departments, agreed between doctor and radiographer beforehand) are then meted out to smooth the troubled waters until such time as a second scan can be arranged. Therefore, if the purpose of the scan is to detect fetal abnormalities (and screening of some kind is obligatory because in 80% there are no recognized risk factors), it must be done:

(i)   at the right time
(ii) with the right equipment
(iii) with immediately available on-site expert back-up for the ultrasonographer
(iv) with ready access to a regional perinatal medical centre.

These recommendations have been well described (Joint Study Group on Fetal Abnormalities, 1989). The most important point to note is that mothers should be *offered* a screening examination and that they should be made aware in advance of the limitations and implications of screening. Evidence shows that the skill with which this is done leaves much to be desired (Marteau *et al.*, 1992). Good clinics will give an explanatory leaflet to each mother at her first antenatal attendance, which she should be encouraged to read.

Techniques of antenatal diagnosis

SERUM ALPHA-FETOPROTEIN (AFP) SCREENING

AFP screening is usually offered at 16 weeks' gestation. Correct dating by ultrasound is essential. It is not a routine investigation in many clinics because resources are not available, but it should certainly be recommended in high-risk mothers, such as:

(i)   those aged 35 years or over
(ii) those who have had a fetal abnormality in a previous pregnancy or who have a poor obstetric history, such as recurrent abortion and growth retardation
(iii) those with a family history of genetic disease which can be identified by antenatal diagnostic techniques.
(iv) those with coexistent maternal disease or exposure to drugs, alcohol, heavy smoking or teratogenic medication.

The most common surgical causes of elevated serum AFP are fetal neural tube defects, abdominal wall defects, and ectopia vesicae or cloacae; closed neural tube defects may not cause an increase in serum AFP, neither may an exomphalos with an intact sac. If the level is raised a decision must then be made as to whether to proceed to amniocentesis. Some authorities claim that this can be avoided in a significant number of cases by careful ultrasound anomaly scanning (Katz *et al.*, 1991; Lindfors *et al.*, 1991; Nadel *et al.*, 1991). The surgeon should be aware of the fact that Down's syndrome can now be diagnosed by maternal serum AFP screening because in this condition the level may be below the normal value (Greenberg *et al.*, 1991). Increased accuracy has been achieved by also measuring unconjugated oestriol and human chorionic gonadotrophin levels, which may be abnormally low and high, respectively. Other factors such as fetal gestational age, maternal age and the possible presence of maternal diabetes mellitus must be taken into account before the diagnosis is conclusive (Haddow *et al.*, 1992; Wald *et al.*, 1992). The management of any antenatally diagnosed fetal abnormality potentially requiring postnatal surgical treatment will clearly be influenced by such factors.

AMNIOCENTESIS

Other invasive investigations such as cordocentesis and chorionic villous biopsy can be included in this section. There is a 0.5% fetal loss rate caused by amniocentesis which must be incorporated in the risk–benefit calculations before embarking on this procedure, and must be made clear to the mother. These tests are conducted for genetic studies, although fetal blood sampling is necessary to detect enzyme defects causing inborn errors of metabolism. From the surgeon's viewpoint, it is essential to elicit the karyotype of a fetus suspected of having an abdominal wall defect or a high intestinal obstruction: a significant number of the former has a coincident trisomy (Nadel *et al.*, 1991) and of the latter trisomy (Wald *et al.*, 1992). Genetic analyses in families at risk will also determine the presence of conditions such as congenital adrenal hyperplasia and cystic fibrosis. The former can be alleviated by antenatal treatment and it is now possible that the latter may be treatable by postnatal gene therapy.

ULTRASOUND

As already indicated, ultrasound is the most important instrument in the whole antenatal diagnostic armamentarium: it stands alone in the primary diagnosis of congenital abnormalities and is an essential component of the other diagnostic techniques mentioned above. All forms of uterine or fetal invasion need ultrasound to steer them in the correct direction. Ideally, every pregnant woman should be offered two scans, the first at approximately 16 weeks, the dating scan, and the second at 18–20 weeks, the anomaly scan.

Unfortunately, the resources available in most hospital maternity departments in the UK preclude such a programme so that the dating and anomaly scans must be amalgamated at a compromise time of 19 weeks. This allows sufficient time for action to be taken in the management of the pregnancy, so long as decisions are made quickly. If an abnormality is suspected that does not require immediate action, arrangements can be made for later scans to confirm the diagnosis and review progress.

Regional perinatal medical centres

Expertise in the antenatal recognition of congenital abnormalities and the quality of available scanning equipment varies considerably among district general hospitals. One or more centres should be available in every region to offer advice and support in diagnosis and management. They should be equipped to provide the full range of antenatal diagnostic techniques including rapid karyotyping when abnormalities are suspected in the second trimester. Another essential feature is the easy availability of experts in any fields appropriate to the abnormalities suspected in any particular fetus: the family can then be given a definitive prognosis and an opportunity to make an informed decision as to how they wish the pregnancy to be conducted. Whenever an abnormality that is likely to require immediate postnatal surgery is suspected, the mother should preferably be referred for diagnostic review and ultimately for delivery to a regional perinatal centre close to the regional neonatal surgical unit. If the diagnosis is confirmed, she should be offered an opportunity to visit the unit so that she can see where her baby will be nursed postoperatively and can interview the nursing staff.

As implied previously, developing precision techniques for accurate antenatal diagnosis is of little value unless their consequences are fully appreciated and their limitations understood. The professional directly responsible for the patient's care must be clear in his or her own mind how to react to all the information and advice that can become available and make a rational judgement on the basis of all these factors. A comment made in the early 1980s is equally appropriate today:

> Many fetal abnormalities can now be detected. Most defects are best treated after birth and prenatal diagnosis improves outcome by allowing the patient, family and physician to discuss the alternatives; to choose the optimal time, mode and place of delivery; and to prepare for optimal post-natal care. (Harrison *et al.*, 1982)

In other words, the prime purpose of antenatal diagnosis is to promote the safe delivery of a live baby whose needs can immediately be assessed and provided for.

Possible courses of action

The options will be discussed in greater detail as the various surgical abnormalities are encountered but it is worth enumerating them at this point:

(i) continue with the pregnancy
(ii) attempt prenatal treatment
(iii) terminate the pregnancy.

The latter choice is only for serious fetal abnormalities incompatible with postnatal life and for abnormalities that carry a substantial risk of serious mental and/or physical handicap. Adequate provision must be made for post-termination counselling by experienced health visitors, midwives, genetic nurses or other care workers. Furthermore, it is essential that the wishes of parents who decline the offer of termination on religious or ethical grounds should be respected. If the pregnancy goes to term they can at least hold and comfort the baby during the short time it survives.

The management of surgical abnormalities diagnosed antenatally

Data from the Northern Regional Fetal Abnormality Survey (NorCAS, 1992) covering the years 1985–1991 will be used to illustrate this section.

NEURAL TUBE DEFECTS

Of 564 cases (2/1000 births) notified to the survey, diagnostic sensitivity was 74.8% and positive predictive value 98.6%, with a prevalence of 0.53. Thus, although just over a quarter of the cases were not suspected, very few were suspected but unconfirmed. This is extremely important considering that termination of pregnancy is usually advised for anencephaly and major spina bifida. Maternal serum AFP screening combined with ultrasound can increase sensitivity to 98% and specificity to 100% (Morrow *et al.*, 1991); a good argument in favour of introducing AFP screening as a routine in all major maternity departments. AFP screening is obligatory if there is a history of neural tube defect in a previous pregnancy. There was a 40% reduction in the number of neural tube defects notified to the registry during the 7-year period, a fall which will probably continue as dietary supplementation with folate becomes more widespread. Termination is usually advised when the presence of a fetus with anencephaly or major spina bifida is suspected, with the provisos mentioned above. Fortuitously, the types of neural tube defect least likely to be suspected antenatally are the small, low, skin-covered lesions which have less serious neurological implications, meaning that the fetus would not be considered for termination.

ABDOMINAL WALL DEFECTS

Of 169 cases (0.6/1000 births) notified to the survey, diagnostic sensitivity was 65.9% and positive predictive value 93.1%, with a prevalence of 0.03. Maternal serum AFP and ultrasound are the main diagnostic tools. The results of a previous report (Walkinshaw *et al.*, 1992) suggest that diagnostic accuracy in the northern region is improving. Amniocentesis is essential for suspected abdominal wall defects to exclude chromosomal abnormalities, and AFP and acetyl cholinesterase measurements will also be made. Likewise, expert fetal cardiac Doppler examination is obligatory as concomitant serious congenital heart defects are common. If either of these problems is confirmed, termination of the pregnancy may be the best advice. If not, the family should be advised to continue the pregnancy and arrangements made for the infant to be delivered in a maternity department as near as possible to the regional neonatal surgical unit. There is evidence that this improves outcome (Stringer *et al.*, 1991), although some doubt has recently been cast on this (Stoodley *et al.*, 1993). The number of cases in this report was, however, small and the authors stated that delivery near the place of surgery was the preferred option. Labour can be induced at a time when the paediatric surgical staff are on hand and the operating facilities ready and waiting, thus avoiding an emergency operation in the middle of the night. Unfortunately, labour is often premature and rapid transfer may be necessary. Vaginal delivery should be permitted; there are no indications solely on account of the abdominal wall defect for delivery by caesarian section. The sensitivity of antenatal diagnosis for exomphalos (omphalocele) is significantly lower than for gastroschisis but emergency surgery for an intact sac is seldom necessary.

It has been suggested that antenatal dilatation of the intestinal tract in a fetus with gastroschisis is an indicator of either antenatal or intrapartum fetal distress (Crawford *et al.*, 1992), but not of poor neonatal surgical outcome. More recent work, however, indicates that there is a correlation between antenatal gut dilatation and prolonged neonatal hypoperistalsis (Langer *et al.*, 1993).

CONGENITAL DIAPHRAGMATIC HERNIA

The survey received 109 notifications of this abnormality over 7 years (0.4/1000 births). Diagnostic sensitivity was 32.3% and positive predictive value 93.9%, with a prevalence of 0.10. It is clear that under the circumstances of routine antenatal care in maternity departments of district general hospitals, congenital diaphragmatic hernia is difficult to diagnose. When it is suspected in early pregnancy (less than 25 weeks) the prognosis for postnatal survival is poor: an overall mortality of 74% has been quoted (Sharland *et al.*, 1992). Even delaying operation to allow a period of stabilization with the help of extracorporeal membrane oxygenation (ECMO) does not improve survival. (Wilson *et al.*, 1992). As with abdominal wall defects, serious coincident abnormalities are common: these include trisomy 13, 18 and 21 and many of the eponymous syndromes such as Fryns, Cornelia de Lange, Ehlers–Danlos, DiGeorge and Marfan. Congenital heart defects, quite apart from the left-sided underdevelopment which occurs as a result of the hernia itself, are also frequently seen. Thus, amniocentesis and fetal cardiac scanning must form an integral part of the diagnostic process. If any of these anomalies are discovered, termination of pregnancy is probably the best advice. Uncomplicated diaphragmatic hernia suspected in later pregnancy, and occasionally in early pregnancy (Dillon, 1992), has a slightly better prognosis (around 60% survival). These mothers should be transferred for delivery to the maternity centre nearest to the neonatal surgical unit so that surgical management can be started with minimal delay. A valid judgement on the efficacy of ECMO in promoting survival is still awaited.

INTESTINAL ABNORMALITIES

The survey registered 323 cases of assorted congenital abnormalities of the intestinal tract over 7 years (1.1/1000 births). Diagnostic sensitivity was 25.7% and positive predictive value 71.8%, with a prevalence of 0.06. Thus only one in four intestinal abnormalities are likely to be suspected antenatally: the most common are duodenal atresia and oesophageal atresia. There is a well-known association between the former and both Down's syndrome and congenital heart defects, either separately or together. Amniocentesis and fetal cardiac ultrasound examination are therefore obligatory if fetal duodenal atresia is suspected. Where the intestinal anomalies are concerned, antenatal diagnosis does not have a positive predictive value sufficiently high to induce confidence but, even so, the complicating diagnoses need to be considered in their own right and parents given the opportunity to choose whether to continue with the pregnancy. Meconium ileus is occasionally suspected because the viscous content of the intestinal tract renders it peculiarly echogenic. When there is a known family history of cystic fibrosis, a special watch for this sign should be kept during antenatal ultrasound scanning. In future, however, diagnosis will be made with the use of gene probes currently being developed.

CONGENITAL ABNORMALITIES OF THE URINARY TRACT

Urinary tract problems comprise by far the largest group of surgical abnormalities. In the 7-year period in question, 1064 cases were notified to the survey (3.75/1000 births). Sensitivity was 77.6% and positive predictive value 48%, with a prevalence 0.19. It is not possible to discuss all of the numerous types of abnormality likely to be encountered in the urinary tract, so only two will be taken as examples; hydronephrosis and posterior urethral valves.

Hydronephrosis

Uncertainty in the diagnosis of hydronephrosis in the fetus gives rise to the low positive predictive value. Dilatation of the fetal kidney is frequently seen during the second and third trimesters and may be noted for the first time during the final 4–6 weeks. This is probably due to the high urine output which is known to occur in the term mature fetus (Wladimiroff and Campbell, 1974). Many of these dilated kidneys seem to return to normal postnatally or, if they remain dilated to some extent, do not show signs of organic obstruction. Because fluid intake in the first 24–48 h of life is low, renal dilatation is likely to subside during that period whatever the cause, so postnatal scanning examinations should be delayed until the third day if possible. The following three questions immediately arise.

(a) If dilatation has disappeared, in how many infants does it return in subsequent months or years?
(b) What degree of dilatation persisting postnatally should prompt further investigation?
(c) What degree of dilatation in the fetus obligates postnatal investigation whatever the postnatal appearances?

In a study of a large number of infants whose antenatal urinary tracts were ultrasonographically normal (Paduono *et al.*, 1991), 1.8% were subsequently admitted to hospital because of urinary tract infection. Although only a few of these children had hydronephrosis, none of whom required surgery, a significant number had ureteric reflux. The published work describing follow-up investigations of babies in whom antenatal renal dilatation was present has two predominant shortcomings: the series were small and kidney measurements were not given, or if they were, there was a marked variance in their interpretation. In a series of 63 fetuses (Corteville *et al.*, 1991) hydronephrosis was found postnatally in 45. The criterion used to identify those fetuses requiring postnatal investigation was an anteroposterior renal pelvic diameter of at least 4 mm at or before 33 weeks' gestation, or at least 7 mm after 33 weeks' gestation. Other contributors, however (Callan *et al.*, 1990; Ghidini *et al.*, 1990; Mandell *et al.*, 1991), suggested a somewhat higher threshold of at least 10 mm at 30 weeks.

The reason for these differences of opinion is that, until recently, there have been no data defining the range of measurement of the normal fetal renal pelvis. These are now available (Scott *et al.*, 1995) and show that an antero-posterior dimension of 4 mm is the upper limit of normal at any gestational age. This suggests that although a fetal kidney dilated to this degree may not be obstructed, other malfunctions such as vesico-ureteric reflux (VUR) may be present. Recent work suggests that the incidence of VUR in infants who had moderate renal dilatation antenatally is of the order of 15% (Persutte *et al.*, 1997), but may be as high as 33% (Adra *et al.*, 1995).

Doubts as to which kidneys require postnatal surgery and how to identify them are widespread. An early contribution (Flake *et al.*, 1986), suggested that 'resolution of fetal hydronephrosis secondary to PUJ obstruction is rare', but this attitude is changing. In an attempt to define a measurement by which a diagnosis of significant obstruction could be made (Arnold and Rickwood, 1990), it was suggested that a kidney with a differential function exceeding 40% of total function was not in danger. The authors stated that only a modest number of infants require early surgery. It has also been suggested that surgery is seldom required before the age of 3 months and, indeed, that this is the ideal age at which to commence investigation (Ransley *et al.*, 1990). It is noteworthy, however, that 40% of the kidneys in this series were eventually operated. One of the difficulties in deducing which antenatally dilated kidneys are obstructed postnatally arises from the interpretation of radioisotope tests. In many instances it is clear that the incorrect radioisotope carrier has been employed, for instance. [99]Technetium has been bound to diethylene triamine pentacetic acid (DTPA), which measures glomerular filtration rate, instead of mercapto acetyl triglyceride (MAG3), which measures tubular secretion and urine transport. Recent opinion is divided as to the validity of these tests in ascertaining obstruction. One centre has described them as useful (Gruenewald *et al.*, 1990) and others (Gordon *et al.*, 1991; Kletscher *et al.*, 1991) as of little value.

The management of fetal renal dilatation, whether unilateral or bilateral and in the absence of a dilated bladder, cannot be said to have been settled. The majority of contributors suggest that an anteroposterior measurement of the renal pelvis of at least 10 mm at or beyond 30 weeks' gestation (Arger *et al.*, 1985; Grignon *et al.*, 1986) or an anteroposterior transpelvic to transrenal ratio of more than 0.5 (Flake *et al.*, 1986; Kleiner *et al.*, 1987) is significant. It has been shown (Scott *et al.*, 1991) that the normal reference range for the internal renal dimension in 95% of the newborn population is 5 mm, bearing in mind that the left kidney may normally be slightly larger than the right. However, any newborn whose kidneys showed significant dilatation antenatally should have an ultrasound scan postnatally at 2–3 days. If this scan is normal then it should be repeated at 3 months and ideally again at 1 year.

Posterior urethral valves

Twenty-eight cases were notified to the survey in 7 years. Diagnostic sensitivity was only 10.7% and

positive predictive value 18.8%, although this low figure must partly be influenced by the low prevalence of 0.005. It is surprising that sensitivity is so low for a condition which produces massive dilatation of both sides of the upper urinary tract and the bladder. In many instances, the significance of the ultrasound findings was not appreciated, another result of the absence of paediatric urological opinion in antenatal diagnosis. Often, however, severe oligohydramnios made visualization of the fetus difficult and in many instances there was conspicuous intrauterine growth retardation. Attempts to determine the fetal gender, which would have been extremely helpful (Scott and Renwick, 1993), were seldom made. Antenatally, the diagnosis was most frequently unsuspected, although conditions such as bladder neck obstruction, ascites and exomphalos were mentioned. Postnatally, diagnoses such as ureteric reflux, prune belly syndrome and hydrocolpos were revealed.

Obstructive uropathy, revealed in early fetal life by ultrasound scanning, initially seemed to be ideally suited to interventional treatment but, as often happens in medicine, the inclination of the uninitiated to have a go soon caused disappointment and disillusion. Attempts were made to insert tubes, catheters and other devices into fetal bladders and kidneys without any background knowledge of the physiology of the fetal urinary tract or the effects of oligohydramnios on the developing lungs. The depressing outcome described in the early papers (Farrant, 1980; Golbus *et al.*, 1982) was followed by the publication of further numerous instances of disaster. By 1986 the International Fetal Surgery Registry had recorded a survival rate for urological intervention of only 41% and mortality of 4.6%, most of the babies dying from pulmonary hypoplasia. Two years later it was shown that the survival rate in a group of fetuses with obstructive uropathy in whom no intervention was undertaken was as good as in those who did not have irremediable defects (Reuss *et al.*, 1988). A more rational approach based on fetal renal function measurements was advocated by Glick *et al.* (1985), who suggested that a level of sodium above 120 mmol/l, chloride above 100 mmol/l or osmolality above 260 mosmols/l in fetal urine were bad prognostic indicators. Furthermore, intervention after 20 weeks' gestation was unlikely to prove successful. These recommendations were supported by other workers (Nicolaides *et al.*, 1992), who suggested that urinary calcium should be measured as well as sodium.

It is now clear that a fetus with posterior urethral valves which produce a degree of obstruction sufficiently obvious to be recognized in early gestational life has a very bad prognosis (Reinberg *et al.*, 1992) and termination of such pregnancies should be offered. Of the confirmed cases registered by NorCAS, 28.6% were terminated or died, often as a result of spontaneous abortion. Attempts at antenatal intervention are not to be recommended. Early delivery at 36–38 weeks' gestation may be considered if the fetus is a reasonable size although, as previously mentioned, many suffer from intrauterine growth retardation. A long period of ventilator treatment for pulmonary hypoplasia and of peritoneal dialysis for chronic renal failure must be anticipated.

Conclusion

The contribution of antenatal diagnosis to paediatric surgery must be reviewed with a certain degree of circumspection. For some abnormalities, e.g. diaphragmatic hernia, it has actually increased treatment mortality rates because cases which would previously have been unexpected and would have died at birth are now anticipated and referred to paediatric surgical centres, where they soon die after fruitless efforts to save them. The diagnostic sensitivity for intestinal abnormalities is low and even if correctly suspected, management is not often changed as a result. Early warning of abdominal wall abnormalities has proved a significant advantage because it enables serious chromosomal and congenital heart defects to be excluded and the baby to be transferred *in utero* for delivery to a maternity department close to the regional paediatric surgical service.

Substantial confusion over correct management has been caused by the antenatal diagnosis of urological abnormalities, but light is beginning to emerge. The main advance is that babies should now be investigated soon after birth so that operative treatment, if appropriate, can be undertaken before they develop debilitating urinary infections. If surgery is deemed inappropriate at the early stage, they can be supervised through infancy and early childhood so that deteriorating renal disease can be detected. There is no doubt that more research into the characteristics and normal development of the fetal kidney is required to clarify the position with regard to the significance of different degrees of dilatation.

Serious neural tube defects can now be suspected by serum AFP screening backed up by ultrasound or amniocentesis and termination of pregnancy offered. The number of newborns requiring treatment for this condition has been dramatically reduced both as a result of this screening and through increased knowledge about the influence of preconceptual dietary intake of folate. Finally, evidence is beginning to emerge that the only contribution to outcome from routine ultrasound examination in pregnancy is as a screening technique for malformation; as it apparently neither increases the number of live births nor reduces perinatal mortality (Bucher and Schmidt, 1993). Thus there is an obligation on the part of doctors and medical staff caring for pregnant women to explain this fact clearly and not treat it as a spin-off from routine obstetric examinations.

References

Adra, A.M., Mejides, A.A., Dennaoui, M.S. and Beydoun, S.N. 1995: Fetal pyelectasis: is it always 'physiologic'. *American Journal of Obstetrics Gynecology* **173**, 1263–6.

Arger, P.H., Coleman, B.C., Mintz, M.C. *et al.* 1985: Routine fetal genitourinary tract screening. *Radiology* **156**, 485–9.

Arnold, A.J. and Rickwood, A.M. 1990: Natural history of pelviureteric obstruction detected by prenatal sonography. *British Journal of Urology* **65**, 91–6.

Bell, R. and Lumley, J. 1992: Value of routine ultrasound scanning. *British Medical Journal* **305**, 584.

Broomhall, J. 1992: Value of routine ultrasound scanning. *British Medical Journal* **305**, 584.

Bucher, H.C. and Schmidt, J.G. 1993: Does routine ultrasound scanning improve outcome in pregnancy? Meta-analysis of various outcome measures. *British Medical Journal* **307**: 13–7.

Callan, N.A., Blakemore, K., Jongsoo Park, Sanders, R.C., Jeffe, R.D. and Gearhart, J.P. 1990: Fetal genitourinary tract anomalies: evaluation, operative correction and follow up. *Obstetrics and Gynecology* **75**, 67–74.

Campbell, S., Johnstone, F.D., Holt, E.M. and May, P. 1972: Anencephaly: early ultrasonic diagnosis and active management. *Lancet* **ii**, 1226–7.

Corteville, J.E., Gray, D.L. and Crane, J.P. 1991: Congenital hydronephrosis: correlation of fetal ultrasonographic findings with infant outcome. *American Journal of Obstetrics and Gynecology* **165**, 384–8.

Crawford, R.A., Ryan, G., Wright, V.M. and Rodeck, C.H. 1992: The importance of serial biophysical assessment of fetal wellbeing in gastroschisis. *British Journal of Obstetrics and Gynaecology* **99**, 899–902.

Dillon, E. 1992: Data from the Northern Regional Fetal Abnormality Survey. Personal communication.

Farrant, P. 1980: Early ultrasound diagnosis of fetal bladder neck obstruction. *British Journal of Radiology* **53**, 506–8.

Flake, A.W., Harrison, M.R., Sauer, L., Adzick, N.S. and de Lorimier, A.A. 1986: Ureteropelvic junction obstruction in the fetus. *Journal of Pediatric Surgery* **21**, 1058–63.

Garrett, W.J., Grunwald, G. and Robinson, G.E. 1970: Prenatal diagnosis of fetal polycystic kidney by ultrasound. *Australian and New Zealand Journal of Obstetrics and Gynaecology* **10**, 7–9.

Ghidini, A., Sirtori, M., Vergani, P., Orsenigo, E., Tagliabue, P. and Parravacini, E. 1990: Ureteropelvic junction obstruction *in utero* and *ex utero*. *Obstetrics and Gynecology* **75**, 805–7.

Glick, P.L., Harrison, M.R., Golbus, M.S. *et al.* 1985: Management of the fetus with congenital hydronephrosis II: Prognostic criteria and selection for treatment. *Journal of Paediatric Surgery* **20**, 376–87.

Golbus, M.S., Harrison, M.R., Filly, R.A., Callen, P.W. and Katz, M. 1982: *In utero* treatment of urinary tract obstruction. *American Journal of Obstetrics and Gynecology* **142**, 383–8.

Gordon, I., Dhillon, H.K., Gatanash, H. and Peters, A.M. 1991: Antenatal diagnosis of pelvic hydronephrosis: assessment of renal function and drainage as a guide to management. *Journal of Nuclear Medicine* **32**, 1649–54.

Greenberg, F., Del Junco, D., Weyland, B. *et al*. 1991: The effect of gestational age on the detection rate of Down's syndrome by maternal serum alpha-fetoprotein screening. *American Journal of Obstetrics and Gynaecology* **165**, 1391–93.

Grignon, A., Filion, R., Filiatrault, D. *et al*. 1986: Urinary tract dilatation *in utero*: classification and clinical application. *Radiology* **160**, 645–7.

Gruenewald, S.M., Cohen, R.C., Antico, V.F., Farlow, D.C. and Cass, D.T. 1990: Diagnosis and treatment of antenatal uropathies. *Journal of Paediatric Child Health* **26**, 142–7.

Haddow, J.E., Palomaki, G.E., Knight, G.J. *et al*. 1992: Prenatal screening for Down's syndrome with use of maternal serum markers. *New England Journal of Medicine* **327**, 636–8.

Harrison, M.R., Filly, R.A., Golbus, M.S. *et al*. 1982: Occasional notes. Fetal treatment. *New England Journal of Medicine* **307**, 1651–2.

Joint Study Group on Fetal Abnormalities. 1989: Recognition and management of fetal abnormalities. *Archives of Disease in Childhood* **64**, 971–6.

Katz, V.L., Seeds, J.W., Albright, S.G., Lingley, L.H. and Lincoln-Boyes, B. 1991: Role of ultrasound and informed consent in the evaluation of elevated maternal serum alpha-fetoprotein. *American Journal of Perinatology* **8**, 73–6.

Kleiner, B., Callan, P.W. and Filly, R.A. 1987: Sonographic analysis of the fetus with ureteropelvic junction obstruction. *American Journal of Radiology* **148**, 359–63.

Kletscher, B., de Badiola, F. and Gonzalez, R. 1991: Outcome of hydronephrosis diagnosed antenatally. *Journal of Paediatric Surgery* **25**, 455–9.

Langer, J.C., Khanna, J., Caco, C., Dykes, E.H. and Nicolaides, K.H. 1993: Prenatal diagnosis of gastroschisis: development of objective sonographic criteria for predicting outcome. *Obstetrics and Gynecology* **81**, 53–6.

Lindfors, K.K., Gorczyca, D.P., Hanson, F.W., Tennant, F.R., McGahan, J.P. and Peterson, A.G. 1991: The roles of ultrasonography and amniocentesis in evaluation of elevated maternal serum alpha-fetoprotein. *American Journal of Obstetrics and Gynecology* **164**, 1571–5.

Luck, C.A. 1992: Value of routine ultrasound scanning at 19 weeks: a four year study of 8849 deliveries. *British Medical Journal* **304**, 1474–8.

Mandell, J., Blyth, B.R., Peters, C.A., Retik, A.B., Estroff, J.A. and Benacerraf, B.R. 1991: Structural genitourinary defects detected *in utero*. *Radiology* **178**, 193–6.

Marteau, T.M., Cook, R., Kidd, J. *et al*. 1992: The psychological effects of false-positive results in prenatal screening for fetal abnormality: a prospective study. *Prenatal Diagnosis* **12**, 205–14.

Marteau, T.M., Slack, J., Kidd, J., Shaw, R.W. 1992: Presenting a routine screening test in antenatal care: practice observed. *Public Health* **106**, 131–41.

Morrow, R.J., McNay, M.B. and Whittle, M.J. 1991: Ultrasound detection of neural tube defects in patients with elevated maternal serum alpha-fetoprotein. *Obstetrics and Gynecology* **78**, 1055–7.

Nadel, J.S., Green, J.K., Holmes, L.B., Frigoletto, F.D. Jr and Benacerraf, B.R. 1991: Absence of need for amniocentesis in patients with elevated levels of maternal serum alpha-fetoprotein and normal ultrasonographic examinations. *New England Journal of Medicine* **324**, 769–72.

Nicolaides, K.H., Cheng, H.H., Snijders, R.J. and Moniz, C.F. 1992: Fetal urine biochemistry in the assessment of obstructive uropathy. *American Journal of Obstetrics and Gynecology* **166**, 932–7.

Northern Regional Survey Steering Group. 1992: Fetal abnormality: an audit of its recognition and management. *Archives of Disease in Childhood* **67**, 770–4.

Paduano, L., Giglio, L., Bembi, B., Peratoner, L. and Benussi, G. 1991: Clinical outcome of fetal uropathy. II. Sensitivity of echography for prenatal detection of obstructive pathology. *Journal of Urology* **146**, 1097–8.

Persutte, W.H., Koyle, M., Klas, J., Ryan, C. and Hobbins, J.C. 1997: Mild pyelectasis ascertained with prenatal ultrasonography is pediatrically significant. *Ultrasound in Obstetrics and Gynecology* **10**, 12–18.

Pitkin, R.M. 1991: Screening and detection of congenital malformation. *American Journal of Obstetrics and Gynaecology* **164**, 1045–8.

Purkiss, S., Brereton, R.J., Wright, V.M. 1988: Surgical emergencies after prenatal treatment for intra-abdominal abnormality. *Lancet* **i**, 289–90.

Ransley, P.G., Dhillon, H.K., Gordon, I., Duffy, P.G., Dillon, M.J. and Barratt, T.M. 1990: The postnatal management of hydronephrosis diagnosed by prenatal ultrasound. *Journal of Urology* **144**, 584–7.

Reinberg, Y., de Castano, I. and Gonzalez, R. 1992: Prognosis for patients with prenatally diagnosed posterior urethral valves. *Journal of Urology* **148**, 125–6.

Reuss, A., Wladimiroff, J.W., Stewart, P.A. and Scholtmeijer, R.J. 1988: Non-invasive management of fetal obstructive uropathy. *Lancet* **ii**, 949–50.

Robinson, D.E., Garrett, W.J., Kossoff, G. 1968: Fetal anatomy displayed by ultrasound. *Radiology* **3**, 442–9.

Rosendahl, H. and Kivenen, S. 1989: Antenatal detection of congenital malformations by routine ultrasonography. *Obstetrics and Gynaecology* **73**, 947–51.

Scott, J.E.S., Lee, R.E.J., Hunter, E.W., Coulthard, M.G. and Matthews, J.N.S. 1991: Ultrasound screening of newborn urinary tract. *Lancet* **338**, 1571–3.

Scott, J.E.S. and Renwick, M. 1993: Urological anomalies in the Northern Region Fetal Abnormality Survey. *Archives of Disease in Childhood* **68**, 22–6.

Scott, J.E.S., Wright, B., Wilson, G., Pearson, I.A., Matthews, J.N.S. and Rose, P.G. 1995: Measuring the fetal kidney with ultrasonography. *British Journal of Urology* **76**, 769–74.

Sharland, G.K., Lockhart, S.M., Heward, A.J. and Allan, L.D. 1992: Prognosis in fetal diaphragmatic hernia. *American Journal of Obstetrics and Gynaecology* **166**, 9–13.

Shirley, I.M., Bottomley, F. and Robinson, V.P. 1992: Routine radiographer screening for fetal abnormalities by ultrasound in an unselected low risk population. *British Journal of Radiology* **65**, 583–4.

Stoodley, N., Sharma, A., Noblett, H. and James, D. 1993: Influence of place of delivery on outcome in babies with gastroschisis. *Archives of Diseases in Childhood* **68**, 321–323.

Stringer, M.D., Brereton, R.J. and Wright, V.M. 1991: Controversies in the management of gastroschisis: a study of 40 patients. *Archives of Diseases in Childhood* **66**, 34–6.

Thacker, S.B. 1985: Quality of controlled clinical trials. The case of imaging ultrasound in obstetrics: a review. *British Journal of Obstetrics and Gynaecology* **92**, 437–44.

Wald, N.J., Cuckle, H.S., Densem, J.W. and Stone, R.B. 1992: Maternal serum unconjugated oestriol and human chorionic gonadotrophin levels in pregnancies with insulin-dependent diabetes: implications for screening for Down's syndrome. *British Journal of Obstetrics and Gynaecology* **99**, 51–3.

Walkinshaw, S.A., Renwick, M., Hebisch, G. and Hey, E.N. How good is ultrasound in the detection and evaluation of anterior abdominal wall defects? *British Journal of Radiology* **65**, 298–301.

Whittle, M.J. 1992: Value of routine ultrasound scanning. *British Medical Journal* **305**, 583–4.

Wilson, J.M., Lund, D.P., Lillehei, C.W., O'Rourke, P.P. and Vacanti, J.P. 1992: Delayed repair and preoperative ECMO does not improve survival in high-risk congenital diaphragmatic hernia. *Journal of Pediatric Surgery* **27**, 368–372.

Wladimiroff, J.W., Campbell, S. 1974: Fetal urine production rates in normal and complicated pregnancy. *Lancet* **i**, 151–4.

CHAPTER 4

Fetal surgery

M.D. STRINGER

Introduction
Historical
Principles of fetal surgery
Ethical issues
Animal models
Fetal surgery organization
Congential diaghragmatic hernia
Cystic adenomatoid malformation

Fetal urinary tract obstruction
Sacrococcygeal teratoma
Other human fetal interventions
Unresolved problems and controversies
Alternative strategies
Associated developments in fetal surgery
Conclusion
References

Introduction

In recent years, major advances in maternofetal medicine, reproductive genetics and fetal imaging coupled to a better understanding of fetal pathophysiology have facilitated the development of many aspects of fetal therapy. For most major structural fetal abnormalities, parents and physicians must decide between planned delivery in a specialist centre or elective termination. A few selected life-threatening anatomical anomalies may benefit from surgical correction before birth (Table 4.1) (Adzick and Harrison, 1994).

Historical

Early studies of the human fetus were limited to careful observation (Fig. 4.1) but the advent of obstetric ultrasonography in the 1970s revolutionized our understanding. Prenatal diagnosis has become part of routine clinical practice and is largely responsible for the fetus now being regarded as a patient. During the 1980s, the feasibility of intrauterine surgery was explored in various units around the world, but principally by the Fetal Treatment Center at the University of California, San Francisco, under the direction of Harrison and colleagues. After detailed experimentation in laboratory animals, human fetal urinary tract decompression was reported by Harrison et al. (1982b), followed by the first successful in utero repair of congenital diaphragmatic hernia by Harrison et al. (1990b) and fetal lobectomy for cystic adenomatoid malformation later in the same year (Harrison et al., 1990a).

Principles of fetal surgery

Several criteria must be fulfilled before fetal surgery can be considered in clinical practice:

- a clear understanding of the pathophysiology and natural history of the condition
- the availability of accurate prenatal diagnosis and prognostic information
- the condition should have predictable life-threatening consequences
- correction of the defect in an experimental animal fetal model must be effective
- the anaesthetic, tocolytic and surgical techniques for hysterotomy and fetal surgery must not compromise either the safety or the future reproductive potential of the mother.

Table 4.1 Fetal abnormalities that may benefit from fetal surgery

Structural abnormality	Fetal intervention
Cystic adenomatoid malformation of the lung	Pulmonary lobectomy
Thoracoamniotic shunt
Sacrococcygeal teratoma	Tumour resection
Chylothorax	Thoracoamniotic shunt
Twin–twin transfusion syndrome	Fetoscopic division of placenta
Complete heart block	Percutaneous/open pacemaker
Congenital diaphragmatic hernia	Open repair of diaphragmatic hernia
Tracheal occlusion
Artificial gastroschisis
Urethral obstruction	Vesicoamniotic shunt
Fetoscopic vesicostomy
Open vesicostomy/ureterostomy
Aqueductal stenosis	Ventriculoamniotic shunt
Pulmonary/aortic valve obstruction	Percutaneous valvuloplasty

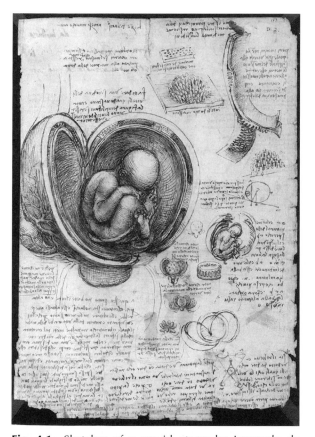

Fig. 4.1 Sketches of a gravid uterus by Leonardo da Vinci (1452–1519). With permission The Royal Collection © Her Majesty Queen Elizabeth II.

Ethical issues

The evolution of fetal surgery has brought with it complex ethical issues which are mostly concerned with the concept of the fetus as a patient and potential conflicts between the interests of the mother and those of the fetus. A pregnant woman is under no ethical obligation to confer the status of patient on her previable fetus simply because there exists a therapy that might benefit the fetus (Chervenak and McCullough, 1993). In the case of the viable fetus, fetal therapy should be recommended when the intervention is reliably judged to be beneficial to the fetus, and when the risk of disease, injury or disability to the fetus and mother are judged to be low.

Animal models

The fetal lamb model has provided much of the experimental information necessary for human fetal surgery. In the fetal lamb model of congenital diaphragmatic hernia (Fig. 4.2), a diaphragmatic defect is surgically created at 60–75 days' gestation and repaired between 100 and 120 days' gestation, and the lamb is delivered by caesarian section at term at about 140 days (Adzick *et al.*, 1985; Bealer *et al.*, 1995b). Lambs with an untreated diaphragmatic hernia have hypoplastic lungs associated with pulmonary hypertension and surfactant deficiency (Adzick *et al.*, 1985; Glick *et al.*, 1992). Fetal lambs, that have undergone prosthetic diaphragmatic repair *in utero* demonstrate improved lung function resulting in neonatal survival (Harrison *et al.*, 1980b, 1990c). The lamb model is well suited to the

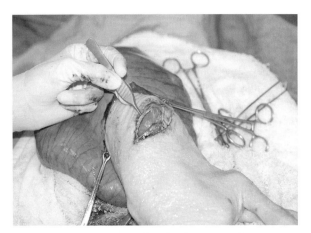

Fig. 4.2 Late creation of a diaphragmatic hernia in a fetal lamb (*c.* 120 days).

laboratory situation but the relatively quiescent bicornuate ovine uterus is a poor substitute for the human myometrium.

In contrast, the gravid primate uterus is extremely sensitive to induction of preterm labour and abortion. Before undertaking human fetal surgery, methods of anaesthesia, hysterotomy and tocolysis were further developed in primate models (Harrison *et al.*, 1982a; Esteve *et al.*, 1992). Although diaphragmatic hernia can be created in mice, rats (Nakao and Ueki, 1987; Kluth *et al.*, 1990) and rabbits (Fauza *et al.*, 1994), most researchers have continued to rely on the fetal lamb model.

Fetal surgery organization

Antenatal surgery is only possible within the context of a well-established centre for maternofetal medicine with an integrated multidisciplinary team (Howell *et al.*, 1993) (Fig. 4.3). The nurse counsellor has a critical role in patient selection, ensuring continuity of care and co-ordinating the activities of the multidisciplinary team.

TIMING

Fetal surgery should be undertaken at a stage in gestation when there is least risk to the mother and fetus and yet sufficient potential for reversal of pathological changes. Before about 18 weeks' gestation, the risk of fetal loss is prohibitive and after about 28 weeks it becomes increasingly difficult to prevent premature labour. In practice, human fetal surgery for congenital diaphragmatic hernia has been carried out between 21 and 28 weeks' gestation (Harrison *et al.*, 1990c, 1993c), fetal lobectomy for cystic adenomatoid malformation between 21 and 27 weeks' gestation (Adzick, 1993) and fetal urinary tract decompression between 18 and 24 weeks' gestation (Estes and Harrison, 1993).

EXCLUSIONS

Antenatal surgery has generally been restricted to fetuses with a normal karyotype and no other major malformation. The physical and psychological health of the mother are additional considerations. Specific exclusions apply to individual conditions and, as a result, fetal surgery is limited in practice to a highly selected group of fetuses. In fetal diaphragmatic hernia, for example, right-sided defects are excluded from repair. Furthermore, open repair of left-sided defects has usually been unsuccessful if the left lobe of the liver is in the fetal chest. This is because reduction of the liver into the abdomen compresses the ductus venosus and obstructs umbilical venous blood flow (Harrison *et al.*, 1993c). Fetuses where the umbilical vein and ductus venosus are judged by colour flow Doppler ultrasonography to be above the level of the diaphragm are now excluded from complete *in utero* repair (Adzick and Harrison, 1994).

TECHNIQUES

Perioperative maternal monitoring is achieved with a radial artery catheter, central venous pressure line, urethral catheter, electrocardiogram (ECG) and transcutaneous pulse oximeter. Prophylactic antibiotics and indomethacin are given preoperatively and anaesthesia is maintained with halogenated inhalational agents. The uterus is exposed through a low transverse abdominal incision and the position of the fetus and placenta is determined by sonography. The fetus is injected with fentanyl and pancuronium to minimize the fetal stress

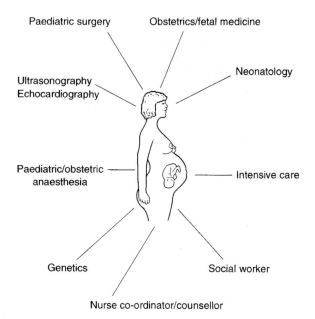

Fig. 4.3 Essential disciplines within a fetal surgery programme (reproduced with permission).

response. After aspiration of some amniotic fluid with a trocar, the hysterotomy incision is extended using specifically designed absorbable uterine staples which also provide haemostasis (Bond *et al.*, 1989). The hysterotomy is kept open with gentle, reverse-biting compression clamps (Harrison and Adzick, 1993). The fetal hand is exposed and wrapped with a miniaturized fetal pulse oximeter. A radiotelemetric device which records the fetal ECG, temperature and intrauterine pressure is then implanted subcutaneously over the fetal chest wall and retained for postoperative monitoring (Jennings *et al.*, 1993a) (Fig. 4.4). The fetus and uterus are irrigated with warm saline throughout the procedure.

In the operative repair of a fetal diaphragmatic hernia, both a thoracotomy and abdominal incision are necessary to provide adequate exposure in comparison to the standard postnatal subcostal incision (Harrison *et al.*, 1993b). The viscera are reduced from the chest and protected by soft malleable retractors passed through the subcostal incision, while the diaphragm is repaired with a patch of prosthetic material (Goretex®) via the thoracic incision. The thoracotomy is closed after instilling warm crystalloid solution into the left hemithorax and an abdominal prosthetic silo is constructed to accommodate the abdominal viscera (Fig. 4.5).

At the end of the procedure, the fetus is returned to the uterus, the amniotic fluid volume restored and the hysterotomy is closed in two layers after excising the staples from the uterine edge. Fibrin glue is applied to encourage a water-tight seal of the membranes.

POSTOPERATIVE MANAGEMENT

Maternal haemodynamics and uterine contractions are continuously monitored in an intensive care unit for at least 48 hours. Tocolytic agents are continued and the fetus is assessed both by serial sonography and using data from the radiotelemeter. A wide variety of tocolytic agents is used to subdue uterine contractions (Table 4.2).

MATERNAL MORBIDITY

Fetal surgery poses a risk to the mother as well as the fetus. The San Francisco team reported on the maternal outcome in their first 47 cases of open fetal surgery in which most of the fetuses were undergoing congenital diaphragmatic hernia repair (Longaker *et al.*, 1991; Harrison *et al.*, 1993c; Adzick and Harrison, 1994). Complications included amniotic fluid leaks occurring in five patients and requiring reoperation in two, maternal pulmonary oedema probably related to tocolytic therapy and two infective complications (pseudomembranous colitis and a wound infection). A few open fetal operations have been performed in other centres including Victoria, Australia (McMahon *et al.*, 1993), Boston and Denver, USA, and Paris, France (Esteve *et al.*, 1992), and to date no maternal deaths have been reported.

Since the midgestation hysterotomy of open fetal surgery is in the upper uterine segment, the mother is committed to future delivery by caesarian section because of the risk of uterine disruption. Two scar disruptions have been reported in subsequent pregnancies but with no serious maternal or fetal morbidity. There is no current evidence to suggest that the mother's future reproductive potential is jeopardized by fetal surgery (Longaker *et al.*, 1991).

Congenital diaphragmatic hernia

Congenital diaphragmatic hernia (CDH) is a potentially lethal anomaly with an incidence of 1 in 2000 births (Puri and Gorman, 1987). Despite optimum postnatal care, including extracorporeal membrane oxygenation, there remains a high mortality from respiratory failure due to pulmonary hypoplasia. Both the lung parenchyma and the pulmonary vascular bed are underdeveloped, probably as a result of compression of the developing lungs by herniated abdominal viscera (Harrison, 1991). Reported survival rates for CDH are notoriously variable because there is a hidden mortality occurring *in*

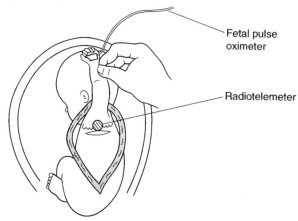

Fig. 4.4 Fetal monitoring during open surgery (reproduced with permission).

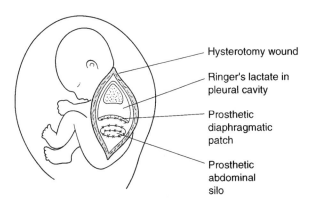

Fig. 4.5 Schematic representation of a completed fetal CDH repair (reproduced with permission).

Table 4.2   Tocolytic agents in fetal surgery (references: Scheerer and Katz, 1991; Harrison *et al.*, 1993a; Jennings *et al.*, 1993b; Norton *et al.*, 1993; Sabik *et al.*, 1993; Bealer *et al.*, 1995a)

Agent	Potential problems	Specific monitoring
Indomethacin	Constriction of fetal ductus arteriosus, tricuspid regurgitation and heart failure	Fetal echocardiography
	Fetal intracranial haemorrhage?	Fetal sonography
	Increased risk of neonatal complications	
Halogenated inhalational anaesthetics, e.g. halothane	Fetal and maternal myocardial depression	Fetal sonography
	Reduced placental perfusion	
Magnesium sulphate	Maternal pulmonary oedema	
	Arrythmias, hypocalcaemia, Respiratory depression	
Beta-sympathomimetics, e.g. ritodrine, terbutaline	Maternal pulmonary oedema	Maternal cardiovascular monitoring
	Cardiovascular and metabolic disturbances (glucose/potassium)	
Calcium channel blockers, e.g. nifedipine	Cardiovascular disturbances	
Glyceryl trinitrate	Possible effects on fetal cerebrovascular circulation and maternal vasodilatation	Fetal sonography

utero or soon after birth. A prospective study of 52 fetuses from San Francisco with isolated left-sided diaphragmatic hernia diagnosed before 25 weeks' gestation identified an overall mortality of 60%, despite optimum postnatal facilities (Harrison *et al.*, 1993a).

Sonographic studies have revealed a range of clinical severity for fetal diaphragmatic hernia, similar to that observed in the postnatal population. Fetuses with evidence of visceral herniation late in gestation or with a relatively small volume of viscera in the chest have a good outcome if delivered in specialist centres (Stringer *et al.*, 1995). More severely affected fetuses are detected early in gestation and have a larger volume of herniated viscera. If pulmonary hypoplasia associated with CDH is reversible after fetal repair, and experimental data support this (Harrison *et al.*, 1980b), it is this latter group that may benefit from prenatal surgery.

The first successful *in utero* repair of a fetal diaphragmatic hernia was reported by Harrison *et al.* (1990b) and their published experience relates to 20 fetuses selected from a total of 106 referred for treatment (Harrison *et al.*, 1993c). The CDH was successfully repaired in 11 resulting in eight live births but only four infants survived the neonatal period. Three of these subsequently required a fundoplication for gastro-oesophageal reflux and one also needed revisional diaphragmatic surgery. Experience of open fetal CDH repair at other centres has been limited and disappointing. A clinical trial is currently in progress to compare the efficacy, safety and cost-effectiveness of open repair before birth with that of optimum postnatal care (Harrison *et al.*, 1993c) but it is unlikely that the results will be favourable.

Cystic adenomatoid malformation

In common with other prenatally diagnosed structural malformations, a spectrum of disease severity is now recognized in cystic adenomatoid malformation (CAM) of the lung ranging from severe fetal disease and death through to spontaneous disappearance of the lesion (McGillivray *et al.*, 1993). The large, microcystic, echodense lesion on prenatal sonography is more often associated with serious sequelae, i.e. the development of pulmonary hypoplasia, severe mediastinal shift, cardiac compression, fetal hydrops and death. Fetal hydrops is a reliable indicator of impending fetal demise. Fetal thoracocentesis is of limited temporary value in cases with large cystic lesions but thoraco-amniotic shunts have been useful in some of these cases (Adzick, 1993). For the immature fetus (less than 32 weeks' gestation) with a CAM complicated by developing hydrops, fetal thoracotomy and lobectomy has proved to be a valuable therapy. Five of eight fetuses treated in this way demonstrated resolution of hydrops, substantial lung growth *in utero* and good quality survival (Harrison *et al.*, 1990a; Adzick, 1993).

Fetal urinary tract obstruction

Congenital anomalies of the urinary system are considered to affect more than 1 in every 1000 births. Urethral valvular obstruction accounts for a small but important proportion of these cases and is associated with the development of hydronephrosis and renal dysplasia leading to secondary oligohydramnios and potentially fatal pulmonary hypoplasia. The timing and degree of obstruction are believed to be significant determinants which can be assessed by prenatal sonography. However, posterior urethral valves associated with severe renal impairment may not always be detectable by second trimester ultrasonography (Wladimiroff *et al.*, 1985).

The concept of mitigating the effects of severe urethral obstruction by antenatal urinary tract decompression is supported by the results of studies in experimental animals (Adzick *et al.*, 1985). In clinical practice, a key issue has been the selection of appropriate cases for fetal intervention. This requires accurate anatomical and functional diagnosis and demonstration of the reversibility of impaired renal function. The scheme of management adopted by Harrison's group is summarized in Fig. 4.6. Only rarely in a fetus with obstructive uropathy is intervention appropriate. Cytogenetic anomalies and major congenital malformations of other systems must first be excluded. Renal dysplasia can be predicted by the sonographic detection of renal cortical cysts or increased renal echogenicity (Mahoney *et al.*, 1984), and although both observations are relatively specific their sensitivity is only about 50%. Poor renal function is reflected by relatively isotonic fetal urine (high concentrations of sodium, chloride, calcium and β_2-microglobulin) collected by percutaneous fetal bladder aspiration (Estes and Harrison, 1993). Fetuses with renal dysplasia and poor renal function should not undergo fetal intervention. Recently, attempts have been made to refine the anatomical diagnosis of fetal lower urinary tract obstruction by using percutaneous fibreoptic needle cystoscopy and this may lead to better case selection (Quintero *et al.*, 1995).

Decompression of the obstructed fetal urinary tract is possible by a variety of methods including percutaneous insertion of a vesicoamniotic shunt, open vesicostomy (Crombleholme *et al.*, 1988), open bilateral ureterostomies (Harrison *et al.*, 1982b) and, more recently, fetoscopic methods of urethral valve ablation or placement of a vesicoamniotic stent (Estes *et al.*, 1986; Quintero *et al.*, 1995). However, percutaneous

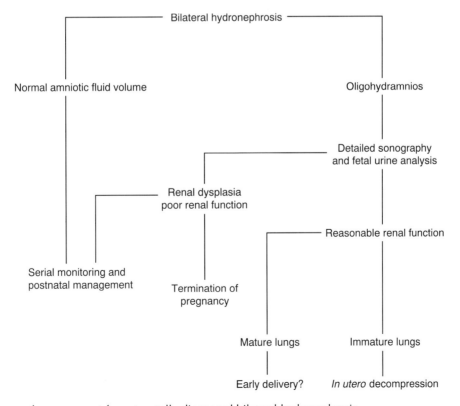

Fig. 4.6 Scheme of management for antenatally diagnosed bilateral hydronephrosis.

vesicoamniotic shunts are associated with complications in 25% or more of patients, principally shunt occlusion, displacement, abdominal wall injury, chorioamnionitis and premature birth (Manning *et al.*, 1986; Elder *et al.*, 1987; Quintero *et al.*, 1995). In 1986, the International Fetal Surgery Registry reported a procedure-related mortality of 4.6% and a survival rate of 41% in 73 fetuses undergoing catheter shunting of the urinary tract (Manning *et al.*, 1986). Nevertheless, the outcome for appropriately selected male fetuses with a posterior urethral valve was significantly better (Estes and Harrison, 1993; Holzgreve and Evans, 1993).

Open fetal surgery for urinary tract decompression has been reported in eight highly selected cases (Estes and Harrison, 1993), and amniotic fluid volume returned to normal in the four survivors, three of whom were reported to have normal renal function. Whilst decompression of the obstructed fetal lower urinary tract can restore amniotic fluid volume and prevent the development of fatal pulmonary hypoplasia, it remains uncertain as to whether fetal intervention can arrest or reverse renal dysplasia or improve long-term renal function.

Sacrococcygeal teratoma

For neonates with this rare tumour, the malignant risk is low and overall prognosis is good, albeit with potential functional disturbances due to pelvic nerve damage. The spectrum of disease in the fetus with a sacrococcygeal teratoma (SCT) is radically different, with a greater than 50% mortality (Flake, 1993). Fetal death is secondary to high-output cardiac failure due to a vascular steal by the tumour. The development of placentomegaly and fetal hydrops is hazardous to the mother but almost always fatal for the fetus. For those fetuses in whom premature delivery is not a viable option, tumour excision *in utero* may be the only useful alternative. The San Francisco group has operated on two fetuses with large SCTs and secondary heart failure; one underwent definitive tumour resection but subsequently died from prematurity and the other underwent a palliative tumour resection at 26 weeks' gestation but died postnatally at the time of further surgery (Flake, 1993).

Other human fetal interventions

In twin–twin transfusion syndrome, abnormal placental cross-circulation can jeopardize the survival of both fetuses. Fetoscopically directed laser ablation of abnormal placental vessels is a possible therapeutic approach (Delia *et al.*, 1990). Fetal cardiac interventions have included percutaneous balloon dilatation of severe aortic valvular stenosis (Maxwell *et al.*, 1991)

and insertion of a pacemaker for complete heart block (Adzick and Harrison, 1994). The role of thoraco-amniotic shunting in fetal pleural effusions/chylothorax remains controversial (Rodeck *et al.*, 1988; Holzgreve and Evans, 1993). In selected cases, this procedure may help to prevent pulmonary hypoplasia and in others, the diagnostic evaluation of the fetus may be possible only after drainage of fluid. Multicentre studies of *in utero* drainage procedures for fetal ventriculomegaly have failed to demonstrate an improved outcome (Manning *et al.*, 1986; Holzgreve and Evans, 1993), resulting in a moratorium on ventriculoamniotic shunting. This area of fetal intervention once again highlights the problems due to inaccurate diagnosis, associated major malformations, ineffective techniques and inadequate selection criteria.

Unresolved problems and controversies

Several well-recognized obstacles limit the application of human fetal surgery, as follows.

TOCOLYSIS

The inability to abolish safely those uterine contractions which seriously interfere with placental blood flow after open fetal surgery has been a major cause of fetal loss. Safer and more effective tocolytic agents are needed.

FETAL MONITORING

A reliable and safe method of establishing chronic fetal vascular access is required for fetal monitoring, resuscitation and drug therapy. Endoscopic methods of placental vessel catheterization have been developed in the primate model (Hedrick *et al.*, 1992) but have not yet proved sufficiently robust for use in humans.

PROBLEMS WITH CASE SELECTION

Fetuses with isolated CDH detected before 25 weeks' gestation, a group with a predicted mortality of 60% (Harrison *et al.*, 1993a), have traditionally been considered for fetal surgery. Excluding those with herniated liver, one may select a subgroup of fetuses with better survival chances who should not undergo fetal surgery. Better methods of risk stratification are needed. Numerous factors have been analysed (Pringle, 1991) and are summarized in Table 4.3. The most severely affected fetuses have severe pulmonary hypoplasia as estimated by the ratio of the right lung cross-sectional area to head circumference, an early gestational diagnosis and liver herniation (Metkus *et al.*, 1996), but this group is excluded from conventional *in utero* repair. As discussed previously, similar problems of case selection complicate the management of fetal lower obstructive uropathy (Holzgreve and Evans, 1993).

THE EFFICACY OF IN UTERO *SURGERY*

There is considerable evidence to support the generally accepted view that the primary defect in CDH is a failure of closure of the diaphragm and that pulmonary hypoplasia is due to pressure from herniated viscera on the developing lungs (Harrison *et al.*, 1980b; Metkus *et al.*, 1996). The mobility and type of herniated viscera, as well as the timing and degree of visceral herniation, determine the severity of pulmonary hypoplasia (Stringer *et al.*, 1995). This hypothesis has been challenged by the suggestion that pulmonary hypoplasia and the diaphragmatic defect may be part of a field defect with the passive herniation of viscera into the chest (Nakao and Ueki, 1987; Ford, 1994). If this second hypothesis was true, antenatal correction of CDH would be unlikely to induce growth and maturation of the lungs. It is not yet certain whether correction of CDH after 20 weeks' gestation in the human fetus allows sufficient improvement in pulmonary growth and function to improve survival.

In fetuses with lower tract obstructive uropathies, experimental animal evidence also supports the hypothesis that *in utero* decompression of the urinary tract may prevent ongoing renal damage (Glick *et al.*, 1987), but renal dysplasia could possibly result from a primary defect in nephrogenesis, or irreversible damage secondary to obstruction may occur very early in gestation before therapy is possible. No controlled studies of *in utero* relief of urinary tract obstruction have yet been reported.

Table 4.3 Prognostic sonographic factors in antenatally diagnosed isolated diaphragmatic hernia

Factors associated with poor prognosis:

- Gestational age <25 weeks at diagnosis
- Liver in the chest at <25 weeks' gestation
- Polyhydramnios
- Lung to thoracic ratio <0.2
- Right lung area to head circumference ratio <0.6
- Cardiac ventricular disproportion

Factors of uncertain significance:

- Fetal breathing movements
- Stomach in the chest (before 25 weeks' gestation)

References: Crawford *et al.*, 1989; Thorpe-Beeston *et al.*, 1989; Pringle, 1991; Metkus *et al.*, 1996.

THE COMORBIDITY OF FETAL SURGERY

There are undeniable but small maternal risks that must be balanced against the anticipated gains for the fetus. In addition, Bealer *et al.* (1995a) have recently reported seven cases of neurological injury after fetal surgery for CDH, an incidence of 21%. They suggest that sudden fluxes in cerebral blood flow secondary to maternal hypoxia or tocolytic therapy may have been responsible. Two of these patients had undergone the less invasive procedure of tracheal occlusion (see below).

Alternative strategies

Open fetal surgical techniques have not yet improved the overall survival of affected fetuses, with the exception of a subgroup of those with CAM lung. This is particularly disappointing in CDH and has prompted the development of the following alternative approaches.

MINIMAL ACCESS TECHNIQUES

In the fetal lamb model of CDH, tracheal obstruction prevents the normal egress of lung fluid, thereby causing expansion of the lungs with gradual reduction of the viscera back into the abdomen and improved pulmonary function at birth (Wilson *et al.*, 1993). Harrison's team have termed this procedure the PLUG (plug the lung until it grows) (Hedrick *et al.*, 1994). In fetal lambs, this produces pulmonary hyperplasia and accelerated lung maturation (Alcorn *et al.*, 1977; Wilson *et al.*, 1993; Hedrick *et al.*, 1994; DiFiore *et al.*, 1994). In humans with the analagous condition of laryngeal atresia (Fraser's syndrome), the lungs are large and hyperplastic but show delayed maturation (Wigglesworth *et al.*, 1987; Labbe *et al.*, 1992). Prenatal tracheal obstruction with either synthetic material or tracheal ligation has now been performed in human fetuses with CDH (Bealer *et al.*, 1995a) (Fig. 4.7). The first patient delivered at 30 weeks and underwent conventional CDH patch repair, but required prolonged endotracheal stenting of cervical tracheomalacia and has some evidence of neurological injury. The second patient also survived for three weeks *in utero* after insertion of the plug and was reported to have excellent postnatal lung function but died in the neonatal period with severe neurological injury.

The PLUG approach should prove much less traumatic than definitive CDH repair and, if successful, a videofetoscopic method of insertion may further reduce fetal and maternal trauma (Estes *et al.*, 1992; Deprest *et al.*, 1995a; Skarsgaard *et al.*, 1995). In practice, fetoscopic techniques have been employed in umbilical cord ligation of a parasitic, acardic twin

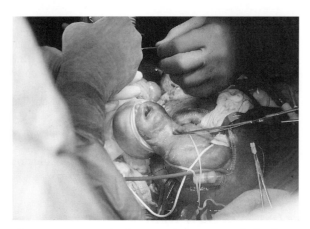

Fig. 4.7 Human fetal PLUG for congenital diaphragmatic hernia (by kind permission of Professor Michael Harrison).

(Deprest *et al.*, 1995b) and the ablation of placental communications causing the twin–twin transfusion syndrome (Ville *et al.*, 1993).

INDUCTION OF GRAFT TOLERANCE FOR POSTNATAL LUNG TRANSPLANTATION

As a result of fetal immune tolerance, *in utero* transplantation of fetal haemopoietic stem cells can lead to the development of stable long-term chimerism without graft-versus-host disease or the need for immunosuppression (Flake *et al.*, 1986; Tollraine *et al.*, 1992). This raises the possibility that a fetus with bad-risk CDH could undergo prenatal infusion of allogeneic or xenogeneic haemopoietic stem cells to induce tolerance for pulmonary transplantation after birth (West *et al.*, 1990).

CREATION OF AN ARTIFICIAL GASTROSCHISIS

The creation of an iatrogenic gastroschisis without repair of the diaphragmatic defect might decompress the fetal abdomen and lead to improved lung function. Animal experiments support this concept (Belfort *et al.*, 1994) and this technique has recently been successfully applied to the human fetus (Porreco *et al.*, 1994, 1995). Porreco *et al.* (1994) reported a 22-week fetus with isolated left-sided CDH who was treated by exteriorization of the bowel into the amniotic cavity. The baby was delivered 6 weeks later when the diaphragmatic hernia and gastroschisis were repaired but his subsequent clinical course was complicated by chronic lung disease and necrotizing enterocolitis, necessitating multiple operations. This group's second patient survived for 10 weeks *in utero* after fetal surgery but died from pneumonia in the neonatal period (Porreco *et al.*, 1995).

Associated developments in fetal surgery

The search for effective and safe fetal surgical techniques has encouraged the development of related fields of research. The spectrum and natural history of many prenatally diagnosed anatomical abnormalities have advanced dramatically in parallel with developments in fetal surgery. Fetal immune tolerance is being exploited to produce stable long-term chimerism which may have an important impact in transplant biology (Touraine *et al.*, 1992). Studies of fetal wound healing have provided unique insights into the biology of tissue repair. Surgical incisions in the fetus heal without scarring. This process is intrinsic to fetal tissue and independent of the sterile, aqueous intrauterine environment. Recent evidence suggests that the ability of human fetal skin to heal by scarless regeneration may be due to a relative lack of the cytokine transforming growth factor beta which normally promotes fibrosis (Sullivan *et al.*, 1995). This may have important implications in plastic and reconstructive surgery.

Conclusion

Despite enormous progress in our understanding of the problems and pitfalls in human fetal surgery and its therapeutic application to selected fetuses with structural anomalies, antenatal intervention for congenital diaphragmatic hernia has yet to establish itself as a practical alternative for parents and clinicians. The development of novel strategies is encouraging but until such techniques have been carefully validated, fetal surgery for human CDH should be restricted to those few centres with the necessary infrastructure and critical approach demanded by this experimental work.

References

Adzick, N.S. 1993: Fetal thoracic lesions. *Seminars in Pediatric Surgery* **2**, 103–8.

Adzick, N.S. and Harrison, M.R. 1994: Fetal surgical therapy. *Lancet* **343**, 897–902.

Adzick, N.S., Harrison, M.R., Glick, P.L. and Flake, A.W. 1985: Fetal urinary tract obstruction: Experimental pathophysiology. *Seminars in Perinatology* **9**, 79–90.

Adzick, N.S., Outwater, K.M., Harrison, M.R. *et al.* 1985: Correction of congenital diaphragmatic hernia *in utero* IV. An early gestational fetal lamb model for pulmonary vascular morphometric analysis. *Journal of Pediatric Surgery* **20**, 673–80.

Alcorn, D., Adamson, T.M., Lambert, T.F., Maloney, J.E., Ritchie, B.C. and Robinson, P.M. 1977: Morphological effects of chronic tracheal ligation and drainage in the fetal lamb lung. *Journal of Anatomy* **123**, 649–60.

Bealer, J.F., Raisanen, J., Skarsgard, E.D. *et al.* 1995a: The incidence and spectrum of neurological injury after open fetal surgery. *Journal of Pediatric Surgery* **30**, 1150–4.

Bealer, J.F., Skarsgard, E.D., Hedrick, M.H. *et al.* 1995b: The 'PLUG' odyssey: adventures in experimental fetal tracheal occlusion. *Journal of Pediatric Surgery* **30**, 361–5.

Belfort, M., Saade, G.H., Baker, B. *et al.* 1994: Does creation of a fetal gastroschisis reduce the severity of pulmonary hypoplasia in sheep with congenital diaphragmatic hernia? *American Journal of Obstetrics and Gynecology* **170**, 296(A).

Bond, S.J., Harrison, M.R., Slotnick, R.N., Anderson, J., Flake, A.W. and Adzick, N.S. 1989: Cesarean delivery and hysterotomy using an absorbable stapling device. *Obstetrics and Gynecology* **74**, 25–8.

Chervenak, F.A. and McCullough, L.B. 1993: Ethical issues in recommending and offering fetal therapy. *Western Journal of Medicine* **159**, 396–9.

Crawford, D.C., Wright, V.M., Drake, D.P. and Allan, L.D. 1989: Fetal diaphragmatic hernia: the value of fetal echocardiography in the predicton of postnatal outcome. *British Journal of Obstetrics and Gynaecology* **96**, 705–10.

Crombleholme, T.M., Harrison, M.R., Langer, J.C. *et al.* 1988: Early experience with open fetal surgery for congenital hydronephrosis. *Journal of Pediatric Surgery* **23**, 1114–21.

DeLia, J.E., Cruikshank, D.P. and Keye, W.R. 1990: Fetoscopic neodymium: YAG laser occlusion of placental vessels in severe twin–twin transfusion syndrome. *Obstetrics and Gynecology* **75**, 1046–53.

Deprest, J., Van Ballaer, P., Evrard, V., Peers, K., Van Schoubrouck, D. and Vandenberghe, K. 1995b: Leuven experience with *in utero* vascular obliteration techniques. *Ultrasound in Obstetrics and Gynecology* **6**, 23.

Deprest, J.A., Luks, F.I., Vandenberghe, K., Brosens, I.A., Lerut, T. and Van Assche, F.A. 1995a: Intra-uterine video-endoscopic creation of lower urinary tract obstruction in the fetal lamb. *American Journal of Obstetrics and Gynecology* **172**, 1422–6.

DiFiore, J.W., Fauza, D.O., Slavin, R., Peters, C.A., Fackler, J.C. and Wilson, J.M. 1994: Experimental fetal tracheal ligation reverses the structural and physiological effects of pulmonary hypoplasia in congenital diaphragmatic hernia. *Journal of Pediatric Surgery* **29**, 248–56.

Elder, J.S., Duckett, J.W. and Snyder, H.M. 1987: Intervention for fetal obstructive uropathy: has it been effective? *Lancet* **ii**, 1007–10.

Estes, J.M. and Harrison, M.R. 1993 Fetal obstructive uropathy. *Seminars in Pediatric Surgery* **2**, 129–35.

Estes, J.M., MacGillivray, T.E., Hedrick, M.H. *et al.* 1992: Fetoscopic surgery for the treatment of congenital anomalies. *Journal of Pediatric Surgery* **27**, 950–4.

Esteve, C., Toubes, F., Gaudiche, O. *et al.* 1992: Bilan de cinq années de chirurgie experimentale *in utero* pour la reparation des hernies diaphragmatiques. *Annales Francaises d'Anesthesie et de Reanimation* **11**, 193–200.

Fauza, D.O., Tannuri, U., Ayoub, A.A., Capelozzi, V.L., Saldiva, P.H. and Maksoud, J.G. 1994: Surgically produced congenital diaphragmatic hernia in fetal rabbits. *Journal of Surgery* **29**, 882–6.

Flake, A.W. 1993: Fetal sacrococcygeal teratoma. *Seminars in Pediatric Surgery* **2**, 113–20.

Flake, A.W., Harrison, M.R., Adzick, N.S. *et al.* 1986: Transplantation of fetal hematopoietic stem cells *in utero*: the creation of hematopoietic chimeras. *Science* **233**, 776–8.

Ford, W.D.A. 1994: Fetal intervention for congenital diaphragmatic hernia. *Fetal Diagnosis and Therapy* **9**, 398–408.

Glick, P.L., Harrison, M.R. and Adzick, N.S. 1987: Correction of congenital hydronephrosis *in utero*. IV. *In utero* decompression prevents renal dysplasia. *Journal of Pediatric Surgery* **19**, 649–57.

Glick, P.L., Stannard, V.A., Leach, C.L. *et al.* Pathophysiology of congenital diaphragmatic hernia II: The fetal lamb CDH model is surfactant deficient. *Journal of Pediatric Surgery* **27**, 382–8.

Harrison M.R, Adzick N.S. and Flake, A.W. 1993a: Congenital diaphragmatic hernia: an unsolved problem. *Seminars in Pediatric Surgery* **2**, 109–12.

Harrison, M.R, Langer, J.C., Adzick, N.S. *et al.* 1990c: Correction of congenital diaphragmatic hernia *in utero*. V. Initial clinical experience. *Journal of Pediatric Surgery* **25**, 47–57.

Harrison, M.R. 1991: The fetus with a diaphragmatic hernia: pathophysiology, natural history, and surgical management. In Harrison, M.R., Golbus, M.S. and Filly, R.A. (eds), *The unborn patient,* 2nd ed., Philadelphia, PA: W.B. Saunders, 295–313.

Harrison, M.R., Adzick, N.S. 1993: Fetal surgical techniques. *Seminars in Pediatric Surgery* **2**, 136–42.

Harrison, M.R., Adzick, N.S., Flake, A.W. *et al.* 1993b: The CDH two-step: a dance of necessity. *Journal of Pediatric Surgery* **28**, 813–16.

Harrison, M.R., Adzick, N.S., Flake, A.W. *et al.* 1993c: Correction of congenital diaphragmatic hernia *in utero*: VI. Hard-earned lessons. *Journal of Pediatric Surgery* **28**, 1411–18.

Harrison, M.R., Adzick, N.S., Jennings, R.W. *et al.* 1990a Antenatal intervention for congenital cystic adenomatoid malformation. *Lancet* **336**, 965–7.

Harrison, M.R., Adzick, N.S., Longaker, M.T. *et al.* 1990b Successful repair *in utero* of a fetal diaphragmatic hernia after removal of herniated viscera from the left thorax. *New England Journal of Medicine* **322**, 1582–4.

Harrison, M.R., Anderson, J., Rosen, M.A., Ross, N.A. and Hendrickx, A.G. 1982a. Fetal surgery in the primate. I. Anesthetic, surgical, and tocolytic management to maximize fetal–neonatal survival. *Journal of Pediatric Surgery* **17**, 115–22.

Harrison, M.R., Bressack, M.A. and Churg, A.M. 1980a: Correction of congenital diaphragmatic hernia *in utero*. II. Simulated correction permits fetal lung growth with survival at birth. *Surgery* **88**, 260–8.

Harrison, M.R., Golbus, M.S., Filly, R.A. *et al.* 1982b: Fetal surgery for congenital hydronephrosis. *New England Journal of Medicine* **306**, 591–3.

Harrison, M.R., Jester, J.A. and Ross, N.A. 1980b: Correction of congenital diaphragmatic hernia *in utero*. I. The model: intrathoracic balloon produces fatal pulmonary hypoplasia. *Surgery* **88**, 174–82.

Hedrick, M.H., Estes, T.M., Sullivan, K.M. *et al.* 1994: Plug the lung until it grows (PLUG): a new method to treat congenital diaphragmatic hernia *in utero*. *Journal of Pediatric Surgery* **29**, 612–17.

Hedrick, M.H., Jennings, R.W., MacGillivray, T.E. *et al.* 1992: Endoscopic catheterization of placental vessels for chronic fetal vascular access. *Surgery Forum* **43**, 504–5.

Holzgreve, W. and Evans, M.I. 1993: Nonvascular needle and shunt placements for fetal therapy. *Western Journal of Medicine* **159**, 333–40.

Howell LJ, Adzick N.S. and Harrison, M.R. 1993: The Fetal Treatment Center. *Seminars in Pediatric Surgery* **2**, 143–6.

Jennings, R.W., Adzick, N.S., Longaker, M.T., Lorenz, H.P. and Harrison, M.R. 1993a: Radiotelemetric fetal monitoring during and after open fetal operation. *Surgery, Gynecology and Obstetrics* **176**, 59–64.

Jennings, R.W., MacGillivray, T.E. and Harrison, M.R. 1993b: Nitric oxide inhibits preterm labor in the rhesus monkey. *Journal of Maternal–Fetal Medicine* **2**, 170–5.

Kluth, D., Kangah, R., Reich, P. *et al.* 1990: Nitrofen-induced diaphragmatic hernia in rats: an animal model. *Journal of Pediatric Surgery* **25**, 850–4.

Labbe, A., Dechelotte, P., Lemery, D. and Malpuech, G. 1992: Pulmonary hyperplasia in Fraser syndrome. *Pediatric Pulmonology* **14**, 131–4.

Longaker, M.T., Golbus, M.S., Filly, R.A., Rosen, M.A., Chang, S.W. and Harrison, M.R. 1991: Maternal outcome after open fetal surgery. A review of the first 17 human cases. *Journal of the American Medical Association* **265**, 737–41.

MacGillivray, T.E., Harrison, M.R., Goldstein, R.B. and Adzick, N.S. 1993: Disappearing fetal lung lesions. *Journal of Pediatric Surgery* **28**, 1321–5.

MacMahon, R.A., Yardley, R.W., Shekleton, P.A. and Renou, P.M. 1993: *In utero* repair of diaphragmatic hernia. *Journal of Paediatrics and Child Health* **29**, 393–5.

Mahony, B.S., Filly, R.A., Callen, P.W., Hricak, H., Golbus, M.S. and Harrison, M.R. 1984: Fetal renal dysplasia: sonographic evaluation. *Radiology* **152**, 143–6.

Manning, F.A., Harrison, M.R. and Rodeck, C. 1986: Catheter shunts for fetal hydronephrosis and hydrocephalus – Report of the International Fetal Surgery Registry. *New England Journal of Medicine* **315**, 336–40.

Maxwell, D., Allan, L. and Tynan, M.J. 1991: Balloon dilatation of the aortic valve in the fetus: a report of two cases. *British Heart Journal* **65**, 256–8.

Metkus, A.P., Filly, R.A., Stringer, M.D., Harrison, M.R. and Adzick, N.S. 1996: Sonographic predictors of survival in fetal diaphragmatic hernia. *Journal of Pediatric Surgery* **31**, 148–52.

Nakao, Y. and Ueki, R. 1987: Congenital diaphragmatic hernia induced by nitrofen in mice and rats: Characteristics as animal model and pathogenetic relationship between diaphragmatic hernia and lung hypoplasia. *Congenital Anomalies* **27**, 397–417.

Norton, M.E., Merrill, J., Cooper, A.B., Kulier, J.A. and Clyman, R.L. 1993: Neonatal complications after the administration of indomethacin for preterm labor. *New England Journal of Medicine* **329**, 1602–7.

Porreco, R.P., Chang, J.H.T. and Quissell, B.J. 1995: Palliative fetal surgery for diaphragmatic hernia (letter). *American Journal of Obstetrics and Gynecology* **172**, 716.

Porreco, R.P., Chang, J.H.T., Quissell, B.J. and Morgan, M.A. 1994: Palliative fetal surgery for diaphragmatic hernia. *American Journal of Obstetrics and Gynecology* **170**, 833–4.

Pringle, K.C. 1991: Fetal surgery: practical considerations and current status: where do we go from here with Bochdalek diaphragmatic hernia? In Fallis, J.C., Filler, R.M. and Lemoine, G. (eds), *Pediatric thoracic surgery*, New York: Elsevier, 333–42.

Puri, P. and Gorman, W.A. 1987: Natural history of congenital diaphragmatic hernia: implications for management. *Pediatric Surgery International* **2**, 327–30.

Quintero, R.A., Johnson, M.P., Romero, R. *et al.* 1995: *In-utero* percutaneous cystoscopy in the management of fetal lower obstructive uropathy. *Lancet* **346**, 537–40.

Rodeck, C.H., Fisk, N.M., Fraser, D.I. *et al.* 1988: Long-term *in utero* drainage of fetal hydrothorax. *New England Journal of Medicine* **319**, 1135–8.

Sabik, J.F., Assad, R.S. and Hanley, F.L. 1993: Halothane as an anesthetic for fetal surgery. *Journal of Pediatric Surgery* **28**, 542–7.

Scheerer, L.J. and Katz, M. 1991: Tocolysis for fetal intervention. In Harrison, M.R., Golbus, M. and Filly, R.A. (eds), *The unborn patient*, 2nd ed., Philadelphia, PA: W.B. Saunders, 182–8.

Skarsgard, E.D., Bealer, J.E., Meuli, M., Adzick, N.S. and Harrison, M.R. 1995: Fetal endoscopic ('Fetendo') surgery: the relationship between insufflating pressure and the fetoplacental circulation. *Journal of Pediatric Surgery* **30**, 1165–8.

Stringer, M.D., Goldstein, R.B., Filly, R.A. *et al.* 1995: Fetal diaphragmatic hernia without visceral herniation. *Journal of Pediatric Surgery* **30**, 1264–6.

Sullivan, K.M., Lorenz, H.P., Meuli, M., Lin, R.Y. and Adzick, N.S. 1995: A model of scarless human fetal wound repair is deficient in transforming growth factor beta. *Journal of Pediatric Surgery* **30**, 198–203.

Thorpe-Beeston, J.G., Gosden, C.M. and Nicolaides, K.H. 1989: Prenatal diagnosis of congenital diaphragmatic hernia: associated malformations and chromosomal defects. *Fetal Therapeutics* **4**, 21–8.

Touraine, J.L., Raudrant, D., Rebaud, A. 1992: *In utero* transplantation of stem cells in humans: immunological aspects and clinical follow-up of patients. *Bone Marrow Transplantation* **9**, 121–6.

Ville, Y., Frydman, R., Hechter, K., Ogg, D., Fernandez, H. and Nicolaides, K. 1993: Le syndrome transfuseur-transfuse, diagnostic antenatal et nouvelle approche therapeutique. *References en Gynecologie–Obstetrique* **1**, 440–6.

West, L.J., Morris, P.J. and Wood, K.J. 1994: Fetal liver haematopoietic cells and tolerance to organ allografts. *Lancet* **343**, 148–9.

Wigglesworth, J.S., Desal, R. and Hislop, A.A. 1987: Fetal lung growth in congenital laryngeal atresia. *Pediatric Pathology* **7**, 515–25.

Wilson, J.M., DiFiore, J.W. and Peters, C.A. 1993: Experimental fetal tracheal ligation prevents the pulmonary hypoplasia associated with fetal nephrectomy: possible application for congenital diaphragmatic hernia. *Journal of Pediatric Surgery* **28**, 1433–40.

Wladimiroff, J.W., Beemer, F.A., Scholtmeyer, R.J., Stewart, P.A., Spritzer, R. and Wolff, E.D. 1985: Failure to detect fetal obstructive uropathy by second trimester ultrasound. *Prenatal Diagnostics* **5**, 41–6.

CHAPTER 5

Genetic counselling

I.K. TEMPLE AND J. NEEDELL

Introduction
Approach to genetic counselling
Practical points
Mendelian risks
X-linked conditions
Mitochondrial inheritance

Empiric risks
Sporadic conditions
Counselling where there is no diagnosis
Psychological and ethical issues
Conclusions
References

Introduction

It is well recognized that many congenital malformations and childhood diseases have an underlying genetic basis. This awareness leads health professionals and patients to seek information about the genetic contribution to disease and risks to other family members and unborn children. Genetic counselling is the giving of such information.

There have been numerous definitions of genetic counselling, all of which describe it as a process of giving advice and information, but the process of counselling itself is rarely mentioned. Three aspects should be considered: the diagnosis, without which any subsequent information is insecure; the calculation or estimation of risks; and meaningful communication of information and support so that individuals or families can benefit from it.

Approach to genetic counselling

While many genetic conditions are individually rare, it is estimated that 1% of newborns have a significant single gene disorder, 1% have a microscopically visible chromosome abnormality, and 1–2% have a congenital malformation where the cause is at least partly genetic (Jacobs *et al.*, 1974; Weatherall, 1991).

Clinical geneticists aim to give families accurate information to allow them to make their own informed decision. It is generally accepted that counselling should be non-directive (Wertz and Fletcher, 1988). It is therefore not the duty of genetic counsellors to direct the lives of others. However, it is essential that families have enough pertinent information concerning the options available, to allow informed decision making. Society appears to have recognized that the right to choose whether or not to keep an affected child should be left to the parent.

Practical points

DIAGNOSIS

A clear diagnosis is essential and every effort must be made to confirm the diagnosis. This may involve requesting hospital and pathological reports from deceased relatives, examining other family members and requesting further investigations.

FAMILY HISTORY

Any health professional can take a three-generation family tree, from which invaluable information can sometimes be gained.

- Ask particularly about consanguinity. If parents are related they have more genes in common and are at increased risk of having a child with an autosomal recessive condition.
- Enquire about stillbirths, miscarriages, terminations of pregnancy and infant deaths. A good way to do this is to ask the mother to tell you the number of pregnancies she has had.
- Always obtain information from both sides of the family, even if the condition under discussion only appears to affect one branch of the family.
- Consider non-paternity.
- Dates of birth and maiden names are useful.

RISK ESTIMATION

Risks are usually given as odds, e.g. 1 in 4, or as percentages, e.g. 25%. While the numbers may be mathematically accurate the skill is in communicating their meaning to the family. Geneticists use numbers to describe risks because a numerical score is recognizable to their colleagues, but, the meaning to the patient of quoted figures varies considerably. Risk estimations of 10% or above are considered to be high risks and the responsibility of the counsellor is to allow the family to come to terms with the fact that there is a real chance that the condition could recur. Likewise, a risk of 1 in 700 may be thought by the family to be high simply because counselling has introduced for them the possibility of recurrence, which previously was not contemplated. It is important to listen carefully to preconceived health beliefs before assuming that a family will believe your interpretation of risks.

RISK ESTIMATION FOR CHROMOSOME DISORDERS

Genetic material can be visualized down a microscope when the cell is dividing (Fig. 5.1). In a human cell there are 46 chromosomes. Chromosome analysis gives an overview of a patient's genetic material but resolution is not such that individual genes can be visualized.

If a patient has a combination of congenital anomalies, particularly if there is associated mental retardation, their chromosomes should be examined. If additional or deleted chromosomal material is detected this is likely to be a significant finding as it implies the loss or gain of hundreds of genes. Some chromosomal abnormalities such as trisomy 21 (Down's syndrome), which is due to an extra chromosome 21, are chance events. The majority of parents of children with this condition have normal chromosomes and are at low risk of recurrence in a subsequent pregnancy, i.e. 0.5% for trisomy 21 alone and 1% for all major structural chromosome abnormalities (Harper, 1993) (these figures are for women under the age of 35 years). It is not understood why some children with Down's

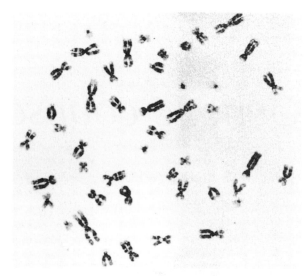

Fig. 5.1 A human karyotype.

syndrome have serious congenital malformations such as duodenal atresia and others do not. The chromosomes do not appear to differ between these groups. Duodenal atresia is 200 times more likely to occur in Down's syndrome than in the general population, and 30% of all children with duodenal atresia have Down's syndrome.

Chromosome anomalies can also occur through chromosome breakage. A reciprocal translocation occurs if chromosomes of different pairs exchange a segment of material. It is balanced if material is exchanged but not lost or gained. This is not usually associated with any clinical abnormalities, but such an individual could be at risk of having a child with an unbalanced translocation where extra or deleted material is detected. If a child with a congenital anomaly is found to have an unbalanced translocation it is important that parental chromosomes are checked because risks for future affected children may be high (Fig. 5.2).

Chromosome anomalies may also provide a clue to the genetic location of important single genes. For example, Herrera *et al.* (1986) reported a patient with mental retardation and multiple colonic polyps, with a deletion of chromosome 5q. This subsequently led to the discovery that the gene that causes familial adenomatous polyposis coli is located at 5q22.

Prenatal diagnosis is available for chromosome abnormalities as the chromosomes can be visualized in fetal tissue. The fetal cells are obtained by chorionic villus sampling or amniocentesis. It must be remembered, however, that a chromosome analysis is a test that is not specific for one particular chromosomal abnormality. For example, a test for Down's syndrome in pregnancy will reveal the entire fetal karyotype and,

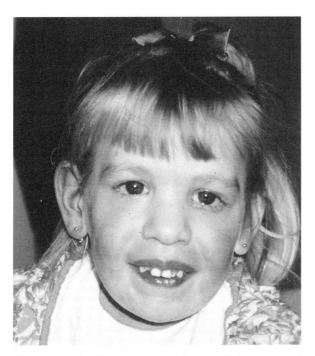

Fig. 5.2 A child born with an unbalanced chromosomal translocation. The chromosomes were examined following referral to the paediatric surgeons with a small, anteriorly placed anal opening. Additional features included developmental delay, failure to thrive and dysmorphic features. One of her parents was found to have a balanced translocation and they are therefore at risk of having further affected children in subsequent pregnancies.

Autosomal recessive

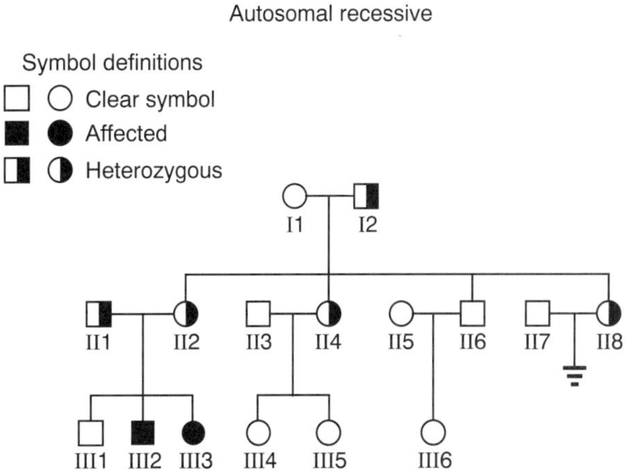

Fig. 5.3 Autosomal recessive inheritance.

while it will exclude or confirm an extra chromosome 21, it may also detect other unexpected findings such as sex chromosome abnormalities. There is concern that adequate information and preparation must be given to couples undergoing prenatal diagnosis.

Parents often find chromosome abnormalities easier to understand and accept than other types of genetic disorders. Firstly, they can often visualize the abnormality, and photographs or drawings of a patient's chromosomes can be shown to help in the explanation. Secondly, there is some public awareness of chromosomal conditions, such as Down's syndrome.

Mendelian risks

AUTOSOMAL RECESSIVE INHERITANCE

Autosomal recessive inheritance might be suspected if there are affected siblings of both genders with unaffected parents (Fig. 5.3). The condition usually only affects one sibship in a family and there is no prior family history. Disease is due to an individual inheriting two copies of a mutated gene. Parents carrying a single copy of the abnormal gene are termed carriers and carrier status is not usually associated with clinical symptoms. As a generalization, recessive diseases are often severe conditions. Carrier parents face a 25% risk of an affected child.

For many rare diseases or syndromes, the genes have not been discovered and autosomal recessive inheritance may be implied by the pattern of inheritance in the family or by consanguinity. In an unrecognized syndrome, evidence for autosomal recessive inheritance should be carefully considered, as recurrence risks are high. There are no reliable rules for the type of congenital abnormality that is likely to be inherited recessively.

In some instances it can be helpful to know that a condition is autosomal recessive. For example, the risk of an individual with an autosomal recessive condition or a sib of an affected individual having an affected child is low, as it depends on the chance of the partner being a gene carrier. The rarer the condition the lower the carrier frequency is in the population.

The case is different if the partners are related. First cousins, for example, have one-eighth of their genes in common. As a general rule, there is an increased risk of cousins having a child with a recessively inherited condition. The risk is in the order of 3% as it is estimated that humans carry at least one harmful recessive gene.

A good example of an autosomal recessive condition is cystic fibrosis (CF). It is the most common serious autosomal recessive condition in northern Europe, with a disease frequency of 1 in 2500 and a carrier frequency of 1 in 25 (Warner, 1992). Recent advances in molecular techniques now allow for an increasing number of CF gene mutations to be identified. The most common

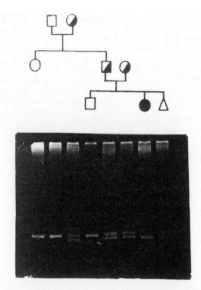

CYSTIC FIBROSIS DELTA F508

Fig. 5.4 If the DNA of an individual is extracted, amplified in one specific area and separated on an electrophoretic gel it is possible to identify the presence or absence of a specific mutation in the CF gene. This figure shows the result for the most common mutation, the delta F 508 mutation. Each track represents the family members as shown on the pedigree above. The lower two bands are the important ones to read, the upper band of which is the position of the normal CF gene and the lower band occurs when there is a mutation. The affected female has only a lower band and has a double dose of the delta F 508 mutation. The parents are both carriers and therefore have an upper and a lower band. This technology can be used for prenatal diagnosis. The last track is the fetal track which is not so clear on the diagram as less DNA was available, but it is just possible to see that the fetus is a carrier and therefore unaffected.

is a triplet base deletion causing the loss of the 508th amino acid, phenylalanine, called delta F508 (Fig. 5.4). This is responsible for 60–80% of all mutations found in northern European populations. It is found to a lesser extent in other populations. Over 200 other rare mutations have now been discovered. The isolation of the CF gene has resulted in an increased knowledge of this multiorgan disease, promising therapeutic progress and giving immense practical advantages to some families.

Parents identified as being CF carriers after the birth of their first CF child can now be offered prenatal diagnosis for subsequent pregnancies. Fetal genes in chorionic villi can be analysed in the same way as DNA (from lymphocyte). Other first-degree relatives can also be tested to determine whether they are carriers. It is

important to stress that the health of carriers is normal and they will only have an affected child if their partner is also found to be a carrier. Currently, the CF gene cannot be scanned for all mutations on a routine basis. Hence, in practice, in northern European populations, unrelated partners in northern European populations, of known carriers are screened for the 12 most common mutations (accounting for 85–90% of all mutations in a northern European population). If these are negative then their carrier risk falls from the population risk of 1 in 25 to approximately 1 in 160. This means that as a couple, the risk of having a child with CF is in the region of 1 in 640.

Direct gene analysis can also be used for diagnosis, particularly in the newborn when sweat tests are technically difficult. If a child with a meconium ileus is shown to have two mutated CF genes then there is no doubt of the diagnosis. As 85–90% of common CF mutations can be detected, it can be calculated that only 2% of individuals with CF are found to carry none of the common CF mutations in either gene. This can be a useful finding if CF is suspected clinically, as such a result clearly makes the diagnosis less likely.

Autosomal recessive inheritance can be very difficult to explain to families. The explanation that a recessive disease represents a hidden abnormality that may have lain unrecognized for generations can be met with disbelief. It is an experience of counsellors that when confronted with a recessive diagnosis, family members find the heritable concept hard to understand because there has been no evidence of the disease in the preceding generations.

AUTOSOMAL DOMINANT INHERITANCE

Affected individuals in two generations with evidence of male to male transmission suggests autosomal dominant inheritance (Fig. 5.5). Affected individuals have a single copy of a mutated gene, the other gene of

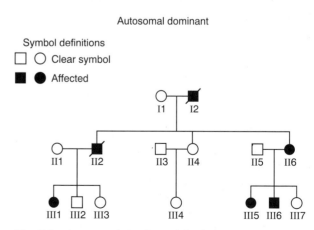

Fig. 5.5 Autosomal dominant inheritance.

the pair being normal. In dominant genetic disorders the abnormal or absent gene product of a single mutated gene has a clinical effect. However, for a condition known to be dominantly inherited there is sometimes no family history, owing to a new mutation.

Autosomal dominant conditions tend to be compatible with reproduction. The clinical features are often milder than seen in autosomal recessive conditions, and they can appear during or after childhood, as in the case of adult polycystic kidney disease. The clinical presentation is often variable both between and within families. This variability may manifest in age at onset and severity. Dominant disorders may also show lack of penetrance, with an individual having the abnormal gene but no clinical features, as in hereditary pancreatitis. Both of these problems can make it difficult to decide on clinical grounds alone whether an individual has the abnormal gene. Therefore, although an affected individual has a 50% chance of passing on the gene, the risk of having an affected child may be lower.

Familial adenomatous polyposis coli is an autosomal dominant condition and offspring of affected individuals are at 50% risk of being affected with the disease. Since the discovery of the gene for polyposis coli, it is now possible to test a relative by DNA analysis to determine whether they have the mutated gene. This involves a blood test. Individuals in which the gene mutation is found can be offered appropriate screening and treatment, thus reducing the risk of colorectal cancer developing undetected. Those members of the family who do not demonstrate the mutation can be reassured. Prior to the genetic discovery, screening had to be offered to all at risk relatives, which involved regular sigmoidoscopy or colonoscopy into late adult life, and patients would often have to make reproductive decisions before their own genetic status was clarified.

X-linked conditions

Affected males within a family with generations of unaffected intervening females suggests X-linked inheritance (Fig. 5.6). If male-to-male transmission can be demonstrated, then X-linkage can be excluded. A recessive mutation on the X chromosome will affect males as they only have one X chromosome, unlike females who will be clinically unaffected as they have two X chromosomes. Such females would be termed carriers. It is particularly important to obtain a good family history in X-linked conditions as distant relatives may be at risk.

Many counselling uncertainties revolve around determining the carrier status of the mother of a boy with an X-linked or potentially X-linked condition. Carrier status in females may be difficult to determine on clinical grounds alone, although pedigree informa-

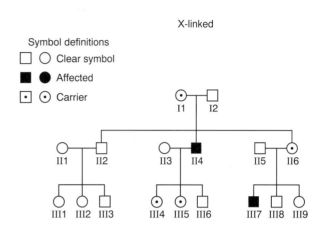

Fig. 5.6   X-linked inheritance.

tion may help. If a female has an affected son and brother, or two affected sons, or is the daughter of an affected male, she will be a carrier. It is however, more difficult to establish whether a mother is a carrier when a son is born with a known X-linked disorder and no previous family history, and this situation may represent a spontaneous mutation in the son. Sometimes females will have some clinical evidence of being a carrier; for example, carriers for Duchenne muscular dystrophy may have raised muscle creatine phosphokinase levels.

Molecular technology can now help if the gene is known, although mutations that are easy to detect in males may not be obvious in females as the normal X chromosome may mask the mutation. DNA markers used in conjunction with cytogenetic analysis (fluorescent *in situ* hybridization) are proving helpful as the two X chromosomes can be visually separated and any abnormality detected in one X chromosome. However, this technique can only be used to define the carrier status in the female relatives of boys who themselves have a known gene defect (Reid *et al.*, 1990).

If carrier detection is impossible and the X-linked condition is so severe that the boys very rarely reproduce, it has been shown that there is approximately a 2/3 risk that the mother of a single affected boy will be a carrier (Young, 1991).

Mitochondrial inheritance

The zygote receives all of its cytoplasm and thus all of its mitochondria from the ova rather than from the sperm and, hence, mitochondria are all maternally inherited. Mitochondria have genomes of their own which contain important genes. This potential mode of inheritance should not be forgotten when analysing pedigree information.

Empiric risks

In some conditions the inheritance is unknown and risk calculation is based on historical data. It is dependent on family studies and not predictable from the theoretical basis of Mendelian inheritance. It is also important to check that the data have been collected in an unbiased way and that the family that is being counselled is from a similar population.

For example, the risks for infantile hypertrophic pyloric stenosis in the general population are approximately 5 per 1000 male births and 1 per 1000 female births. However, the risks of recurrence in brothers with a male index patient is 4 per 100 (4%) and for sisters is 3%. With a female index patient the risk for brothers is 9% and for sisters 4%. These data are based on a family study of Carter and Evans (1969) who interviewed patients presenting with pyloric stenosis and found out how many sibs were subsequently affected.

Care must be taken when presenting such risks to ensure that the anomaly is isolated and not part of a syndrome following Mendelian inheritance patterns. This can be quite subtle, for example, unilateral cleft lip and palate has a recurrence risk for sibs and offspring of 4%. However, if it is associated with lip pits, which can easily be overlooked, then it is likely to be due to a single dominant gene with 50% offspring risks, the Van der Woode syndrome (Fig. 5.7).

There is a 3% risk for couples who have a child with spina bifida of having a second affected child but occasionally these risks can be altered by medical intervention. It has been shown that 4 mg daily of folic acid taken by the mother prior to conception and for 12 weeks in early pregnancy can halve this risk (MRC, 1991). It is still not clear why folic acid has this effect as the mothers are not overtly depleted of folic acid.

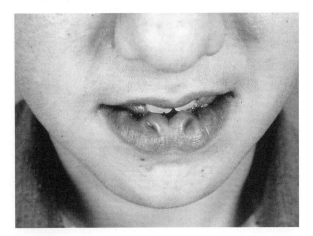

Fig. 5.7 In Van der Woode syndrome cleft lip and/or cleft palate are associated with lip pits. The lip pits are well demonstrated in this photo. This syndrome is caused by an autosomal dominant gene.

Hirschsprung's disease has empiric recurrence risks that depend particularly on the gender of the proband and sib and the length of the colonic segment involved. In rare families it appears to be autosomal dominant. Recent work has identified a gene on the long arm of chromosome 10 for familial Hirschsprung's disease (Lyonett *et al.*, 1993).

Sporadic conditions

For some congenital anomalies such as gastroschisis there is no evidence that the condition is genetic and the recurrence risk is low. The incidence of gastroschisis is increasing and there is no explanation for this.

For other conditions the genetic advice is less straightforward. Isolated tracheo-oesophageal fistula is usually a sporadic event, although not many affected children have grown old enough to have children themselves and there is a paucity of offspring data. Tracheo-oesophageal fistula may be associated with anorectal anomalies, renal, radial abnormalities and vertebral defects (VATER syndrome). Not all of the features are always present. This condition was thought to be sporadic but there have now been a few reports of affected sibs. Of these, some have been shown to have Fanconi's anaemia, an autosomal recessive condition that classically presents with varying degrees of bone marrow suppression. Additional features include low birth-weight, short stature, radial aplasia, renal abnormalities, anorectal anomalies and skin hyperpigmentation, and there are clear overlaps with the VATER association. The natural history is of infantile death or an increased incidence of acute leukaemias in survivors. Chromosome analysis to identify chromosomal damage is a diagnostic test in affected patients (Arlett and Lehmann, 1978). Clinicians should be aware of the considerable work involved for the cytogeneticists in establishing this diagnosis and the clinical dilemma is whether or not to test all individuals presenting with VATER syndrome. In our own practice, patients with a combination of features which include radial anomalies are usually tested.

Counselling patients about the cause of congenital anomalies is an expert field. Molecular biological discoveries are occurring rapidly and the best advice is to always enquire about new developments before giving a firm commitment to patients on recurrence risks.

Counselling where there is no diagnosis

This is always an uncertain situation and the experience of the geneticist may be tested considerably. If a patient has a combination of congenital anomalies that has not previously been described many cases will not be genetic. However, it is not possible to be totally reassuring about recurrence risks as the condition could represent a new recessive disorder.

Psychological and ethical issues

Genetic counselling, like many other varieties of personal counselling, addresses human attitudes, beliefs, feelings and behaviour. Important psychological issues appear to be present in every aspect of the counselling process. Whenever possible, genetic counselling is best carried out prior to pregnancy, as there is less need for haste and the family will have more time for detailed consideration. Kessler (1992) believes that genetic disorders strike to the heart of the person's 'self-system', as much of our self-image and self-esteem is expressed in the preoccupation with our own health and in producing healthy children. Though essentially an educational process, the genetic counsellor has to recognize the problems associated with providing advice and information of a personal and delicate nature. It is common for parents, following the birth of an abnormal child, to be grieving for the loss of the normal child that they expected to have. Parents of a child with any abnormality are often filled with guilt and shame. Genetic counselling provides an opportunity for parents to tell their story and obtain understanding, empathy and help.

For genetic disorders of childhood it is usual for the parents to be seen on their own. The extended family is unlikely to be present during discussions of prognosis, treatment and risks of recurrence. This can cause considerable confusion and problems of adjustment for these extended family members. The grandparents in particular should be considered, as there is often guilt and confusion on their part. They may hear reports that the problem is genetic and can feel responsible for the child's condition unless they have appropriate information and opportunity to discuss their concerns.

Counselling should always be undertaken in a quiet, secure and relaxed atmosphere. Families should be given time to express their concerns and encouraged to ask questions. Only in this way is it possible to explore a couple's attitudes to the disorder as well as their interpretation of its possible implications. The implications will inevitably concern the future of their child and possibly their own reproductive future. Following diagnosis it is important for the counsellor to recognize the speed and depth of information delivery that is appropriate. Immediately after the loss of a baby, or after the diagnosis of a serious genetic disorder, parents may simply be unable to receive or comprehend accurately detailed explanations. Knowing when and how much information to give requires considerable skill and understanding on the part of the counsellor. It is also important to recognize that not all couples will come to terms with the diagnosis of a genetic disease, despite the support of the genetic counsellor. Referral to psychologists or psychiatrists may, on occasion, be appropriate.

Communication between the genetic counsellor and individuals, parents or families is central to genetic counselling. Ensuring effectiveness involves not only trust but also a mutual understanding of the personal meaning attached to the information being given. Previously held concepts and beliefs can influence understanding and the interpretation of a genetic message. It is vital that the communicator is sensitive to this. For instance, it is not uncommon to meet a family of boys and it is not unreasonable for that family to believe they can only have boys. It can be extremely difficult to convince the family that this pattern is the result of chance and that there was an equal possibility of them having boys or girls. The same difficulties concerning beliefs and interpretation can be applied to any genetic disease within a family. It is therefore very important that the communicator is sensitive to the health beliefs of individuals and families if counselling is going to be effective.

With current molecular advances, geneticists are increasingly being forced to consider the many ethical dilemmas surrounding clinical application. Of particular concern is presymptomatic and carrier testing in childhood. Harper and Clarke (1990) suggest that there are a few areas that require consideration prior to genetic testing in childhood. For instances, how likely is it that the disorder will cause morbidity and clinical involvement in childhood? To test for a progressive and currently untreatable condition, the onset of which is generally in adult life, is currently considered unwise among most geneticists. However, when onset in childhood is evident or even likely, as in the case of congenital myotonic dystrophy, there may be sufficient reason to reach an early diagnosis. The consideration of diagnosing carrier status in children is a particular problem. Carrier status confers no health risk to that individual but will necessitate reproductive decisions for them in later life. We would oppose parental demands on the child's behalf, and prefer to postpone carrier testing until the child can make this decision when he or she is capable of informed consent.

Conclusions

A fundamental philosophy of all clinical genetic services is the need for good family management, which needs to be undertaken in conjunction with the clinical treatment of the affected individual. With the application of molecular genetics to clinical medicine and the increasing experience of geneticists in syndrome diagnosis, the demand for the service is becoming increasingly widespread. The clinical genetics service is primarily interested in providing optimal genetic counselling, ensuring that those receiving information understand it, know how to use it and are aware of their options and choices.

References

Arlett, C.F. and Lehmann, A.R. 1978: Human disorders showing increased sensitivity to the induction of genetic damage. *Annals and Reviews in Genetics* **12**, 95–1115.

Carter, C.O. and Evans, K.A. 1969: Inheritance of congenital pyloric stenosis. *Journal of Medical Genetics* **6**, 233–54.

Harper, P.S. 1993: *Practical genetic counselling*, 4th ed. Cambridge: Butterworth Heinemann, 55–68.

Harper, P.S. and Clarke, A. 1990: Should we test children for adult genetic diseases? *Lancet* **335**, 1205–6.

Herrera, L., Kakati, S., Gibas, L., Sandberg, A.A. and Pietrzak, E. 1986: Gardner syndrome in a man with an interstitial deletion of 5q. *American Journal of Medical Genetics* **25**, 473–6.

Jacobs, P.A., Lelville, M., Ratcliffe, S., Keay, A.J. and Syme, J.A. 1974: A cytogenetic study of 11,680 newborn infants. *Annals of Human Genetics* **37**, 359–76.

Kessler, S. 1992: In Evers-Kiebooms, G. (ed.), *Psychosocial aspects of genetic counselling*. March of Dimes Birth Defects Foundation, Original Article Series, **28**, 1–10.

Lyonett, S., Bolino, A., Pelet, A., Abel, L. *et al.* 1993: A gene for Hirschsprung disease maps to the proximal long arm of chromosome 10. *Nature Genetics* **4**, 346–50.

MRC Vitamin Study Research Group 1991: Prevention of neural tube defects: results of the Medical Research Council vitamin study. *Lancet* **338**, 131–7.

Reid, T., Mahler, V., Vogt, P., van Ommen, G.J.B., Cremer, T. and Cremer, M. 1990: Direct carrier detection by *in situ* suppression hybridisation with cosmid clones of the Duchenne/Becker muscular dystrophy locus. *Human Genetics* **85**, 581–6.

Warner, J.O. 1992: Cystic fibrosis. *British Medical Bulletin* **48**, 717–977.

Weatherall, D.J. 1991: *The new genetics and clinical practice*, 3rd ed. Oxford: Oxford University Press.

Wertz, B.S. and Fletcher, J.C. 1988: Attitudes of genetic counsellors: a multinational study. *American Journal of Human Genetics* **42**, 592–600.

Young, I.D. 1991: *Introduction to risk calculation in genetic counselling*. Oxford: Oxford University Press.

CHAPTER 6

The child in hospital

J.M.S. JOHNSTONE

Introduction
Foundation for change
Child-focused management
Facilities for children

Child- and family-centred care
Hospital admission
Children's rights
References

Introduction

The conditions under which children are cared for in the UK still vary widely. Many practising surgeons will have cared for a child on a Nightingale ward in an old Victorian hospital or, by contrast, in a modern purpose-built and well-staffed children's unit. Such a change is all too easily taken for granted and it is salutary to reflect on the influences that made it possible. In Victorian England, public awareness of the inequities of the Industrial Revolution were heightened by great social reformers and work of nineteenth-century authors such as Charles Dickens. Part of the response was an extensive building programme of public hospitals. Some communities were sufficiently enlightened to build hospitals for children only. Many of these remain viable and have carried a torch for the care of children to the present day. However, during the present century further improvement in children's care has been curiously uneven until the last few years when progress has accelerated exponentially. The recent change reflects a national determination to improve children's services to the highest level. Although the response has been led by health carers, it has also been driven by the demands and expectations of today's parents.

In the following chapter, child care has been interpreted broadly but where specific issues have been discussed, the emphasis is on surgery. The chapter starts by considering the foundation for change. Thereafter, the four areas listed below have been used as a framework to describe briefly current practice and suggest possible developments:

- child-focused management
- facilities for children
- child- and family-centred care
- hospital admission
- children's rights.

For those familiar with the Platt Report (Ministry of Health, 1959), it will be evident that it has been used as a base for the chapter, supported by more recent publications. It will also become apparent that high standards of care depend on adequate financial provision, suitable hospital facilities and appropriately adapted local policies. From the patient's perspective, however, the crucial point remains the interface between the child, the family and the carer. It is at this level that the intelligent application of skill and opportunity is critical, it is this level which motivates the carer, and it is from this level that many who have gone forward to contribute most to the care of children have taken their inspiration.

Foundation for change

The recent improvements in child care have been made possible by the endeavours of others who have laid the foundation for such change. Landmarks include the Platt Report (Ministry of Health, 1959), the formation of NAWCH (1963), the Court Report (Committee on Child Health Services, 1976), the United Nations Convention of Rights of the Child (UNICEF, 1989), the Welfare of Children and Young People in Hospital (Department of Health, 1991) and Children First (Audit Commission, 1991).

PLATT REPORT

In this country, the Platt Report 1959 on the *Welfare of children in hospital* was seminal to all that has followed. Within the framework of the National Health Service (NHS), the patronage of prewar years was replaced by the rights of individuals to health care. Within this new structure, the Platt Report focused attention on the physical and emotional needs of children. The report considered that the hospital environment should be open, friendly and stimulating. Hospital routine should ensure the least possible disturbance to the customary routine of the child, in contrast to the rigid discipline which was commonly enforced. Above all, the pain of separation of the child from parent was recognized and hospitals were strongly recommended to allow free visiting. Details were listed of ward design and staffing, preparation of the child for admission, reception in the ward, delivery of general care on the ward and delivery of medical treatment, the management of special groups, and advice on discharge and follow-up. Despite the recognition of the need to improve the services, progress was slow and there was little change.

NATIONAL ASSOCIATION FOR THE WELFARE OF CHILDREN IN HOSPITAL (NAWCH)

NAWCH was founded by four mothers in 1963. The mothers represented a wide group of parents concerned about the slow response to the recommendations of the Platt Report. Groups of lay and professional people were formed throughout the country to lobby hospitals and demand an improved service for children. Their Charter for Children, launched in 1984 (and endorsed by the Department of Health and all major professional bodies), set standards for the care of children in hospital (NAWCH, 1990). Since the mid-1980s, NAWCH has broadened in focus to include sick children in the community and has altered its title to Action for Sick Children. A series of quality reviews has been published, including *Setting standards for children undergoing surgery*.

COURT REPORT

The Court Report 1976 was a further outstanding landmark which looked at the broader issues of children's care including health services, social services

and education. The report advocated the need for integration of child health services: 'a child and family centred service in which skilled help is readily available and accessible; which is integrated in as much as it sees the child as a whole and as a continuously developing person'. As with the Platt Report, this widely acclaimed document made surprisingly little immediate impact on present services, largely because of indifference within the professions and resistance to change in some quarters.

THE UNITED NATIONS CONVENTION ON THE RIGHTS OF THE CHILD

Fundamental principles were expressed by Eglentyne Jebb, founder of Save the Children in 1925, when he said, 'I believe we should claim certain rights for children and labour for their universal recognition'. These words were transcribed by the League of Nations in a Declaration of Rights of the Child the following year. A second Declaration by the United Nations followed in 1959 and this was in turn finally replaced by a Convention on the Rights of the Child adopted by the United Nations Assembly in 1989. The principles of the Convention state that it should apply to all children without discrimination, that the best interests of the child are the prime consideration and that the child's views must be taken into account. Articles of the Convention are directed towards civil and political rights, provision of nutrition, health care and education, and protection from exploitation at work and physical, sexual and psychological abuse. Countries ratifying the Convention are bound by it and are obliged to report at two- and then five-yearly intervals to the Committee on the Rights of the Child to demonstrate that the provisions have been met.

WELFARE OF CHILDREN AND YOUNG PEOPLE IN HOSPITAL

The *Welfare of children and young people in hospital* was published by the Department of Health in 1991. The report was an attempt to bring together in a single publication the recommendations of numerous and diverse publications on the care of children. These views were then circulated to both health authorities and hospitals to act as guidelines in their new roles of purchaser and provider. The document became the foundation for one of the largest reviews of the care of children in hospital. The review, Children First was undertaken by the Audit Commission.

CHILDREN FIRST

The Audit Commission is responsible for auditing the National Health Service (NHS) in England and Wales. Each year, a number of health topics is researched at national level and then subject to local inspection. Children First was a report by the Commission on Children's Services. In its summary, the report observed:

- that earlier professional and government recommendations such as the Platt Report had not been implemented;
- a lack of attention of clinicians and managers to the special needs of children and their families plus a lack of senior management focus in children's service;
- a shortfall of medical and nursing staff with special skills in children's care and a lack of separate facilities for children in some hospitals;
- that the effectiveness of treatment and hospital admission was not monitored routinely or questioned.

Child-focused management

CENTRAL

Recent NHS reforms have brought profound change in both structure and style of management, which have a direct influence on children's care. Although apparently remote, there is considerable central influence on the local delivery of health care. Political and managerial direction from the Department of Health, which includes the NHS Executive, is carried through a chain of appointments from the Secretary of State to the chairpersons of local health authorities and NHS Trusts. Professional influence is expressed through the British Medical Association, the Royal Colleges and the specialty associations. The introduction of the recent NHS reforms illustrates very clearly the authority of the Secretary of State. The long-term effect of these changes on a caring profession are difficult to envisage.

LOCAL HEALTH AUTHORITY

Prior to the reforms, management was passed down in a hierarchical fashion from the Department of Health, through the regions to the health authorities, hospitals and the community. Medical influence was provided by a matching cogwheel advisory structure and decisions were based on consensus. The purpose of the reforms was to increase accountability, to create an internal market by separating the roles of purchaser and provider of health care and to increase local autonomy at hospital and community level. In this process the role of management was strengthened and the medical advisory structure displaced. Local health authorities assumed the role of purchasers with responsibility for provision and quality of services. The hospitals and the community serve to provide such services under contract and to meet specific quality and quantity standards which are subject to audit.

PROVIDER UNIT

Management within the provider unit has assumed a more vigorous profile. In general there is a senior tier of an executive supported by a medical and nurse representative. Below this most hospitals are divided into clinical directorates, which are usually consultant led but with managerial and nursing support. Depending on the size, the child health service may form a single directorate or be part of a composite body, for example, with obstetrics and gynaecology. Where possible, the single directorate is preferable because, as noted in *Children first*, poorly developed children's services may be a result of a lack of management focus. Furthermore, it is recommended by the Department of Health that a children's physician or surgeon should have a primary role in this management of a children's department. Children should receive specialist nursing services which are managed, supervised by and accountable to a senior nurse, who has RSCN or branch qualifications.

LOCAL NEEDS

In identifying local needs for children, the purchaser needs to consider the full range of services from primary health care, through health promotion and surveillance, to the care of children with special needs and disabilities, and the treatment of serious illness. Within an acute hospital, adequate facilities for children should be provided in accident and emergency, outpatients, a day unit, inpatients and neonatal care. As has been recognized by successive Secretaries of State and reinforced by the British Paediatric Association (1992), that child health services should be co-ordinated, especially at the critical interface between the acute hospital services and the community. The structural relationship between the purchaser and the provider is clearly important. An ideal model is for a purchaser to contract for children's services from a single provider, for example, as happens in Liverpool. An alternative is for a single provider to be dominant or subcontract to other units. In practice, many health authorities place contracts for children's care with separate units, so that these units, which may include the acute hospital and the community, are in competition, instead of providing a co-ordinated or 'seamless' service

Facilities for children

CHILDREN'S UNIT

In the UK the distribution of acute children's services within a hospital remains uneven. The reason for this is historical and reflects in part an earlier imbalance between central and local planning. In some major centres, a children's hospital is independent. In other centres a children's hospital may be sited within the grounds of a general hospital with the obvious advantages of sharing major resources such as pathology and imaging and convenience for students. The more common pattern, however, is that children's facilities are within a general hospital and scattered throughout the building, or that children's facilities are annexed to an adult unit. In any future planning, there should be a commitment to dedicated children's facilities and to bring those facilities together in a single area. Where for the present this is impractical then children's services should at least be managed as a single unit.

LEVEL OF SERVICES

The level of surgical services provided at a particular hospital has quite correctly been the centre of vigorous debate in recent years. The problem concerns the level of service that can safely be provided locally and the strength of the unit needed to support that level. A local service is convenient and allows for family-centred care. Furthermore, it enhances the image of the hospital within the local community and is financially attractive to the purchaser. For many families, travel to a major centre creates social, practical and financial difficulties. The pivot of the argument, however, must always be to secure the highest standard of care for the child. It is inconceivable that all children can be treated locally but it is equally impractical, even if it were desirable, for all children to be referred to a specialist centre.

To an extent the debate was clarified by the National Confidential Enquiry into Peri-operative Deaths (NCEPOD; Campling *et al.*, 1990), which found that, in general, the standard of surgical care for children was high. But, it concluded that surgeons and anaesthetists should not undertake occasional children's practice, should be competent and up-to-date and should supervise their trainees with care. In subsequent debate, arguments were made that young children were particularly at risk, so that all children under 3 or 5 years of age should be transferred to a specialist centre, whatever the surgical problem. Some paediatricians from district hospitals felt that the age limit was too stringent. They were concerned about the risks involved in transporting sick children and the loss of local expertise, which would reduce the ability to cope with local emergencies.

A consensus view has gradually crystallized that there should be two levels of service (British Paediatric Association, 1993a). At a local level, a district hospital should be competent to care for children over 5 years of age with straightforward surgical problems. To do this safely there needs to be a population of around 200 000, a suitably trained surgeon and anaesthetist, appropriate medical and nursing staff and facilities including radiology and pathology. A specialist surgical unit should be based on a regional centre or medical school. In addition to basic facilities, the unit should be supported by specialist medical, nursing and paramedical staff, a neonatal unit and a paediatric intensive care unit. It is widely accepted that care of the neonate, children with cancer, children with complex problems of the gastrointestinal tract and urinary tract and very young children should be referred to such a specialist centre. However, in practice, it is difficult to specify which children can be treated locally. Standards of care are variable and dependent on local expertise. Perhaps the more important conclusion is that surgeons do work within their own level of competence taking into account the strength of the support service.

HOSPITAL FACILITIES

In hospitals children are managed in a wide range of units: outpatients, accident and emergency, children's development centre, inpatient wards, neonatal unit, paediatric intensive care, day unit, main operating department, recovery areas and X-ray department, as well as in different specialty units. Ideally, each unit should be dedicated to the care of children and staffed appropriately. In practice, the extent to which this is achieved depends on factors such as hospital size, local policy, management focus, initiative and determination.

Inevitably some units within a hospital have to be shared with adults and in such circumstances separate provision needs to be made. Staff should be appropriately trained in the care of children and an appropriate environment can be created with the use of suitable decorations, furniture and toys. While a detailed description of the different kinds of units is beyond the scope of this chapter, brief comments have been made about outpatients, accident and emergency, day care and paediatric intensive care.

Outpatients

A visit to outpatients is for most children their first and often only hospital experience. The need for children to have a separate facility with a play area, facilities for weighing and measuring, a room for breastfeeding, suitable furnishing and easy access for handicapped children is self-evident. Although the need for separation from adults patients seem obvious, this is not always achieved. Problems arise particularly where a consultant sees too few children to justify a separate clinic, or where specialist equipment is needed which is only available on one site. In future, no doubt, pressure to provide a suitable environment for all children will come through the contracting process.

Accident and emergency department

Children make up roughly one-third of patients attending accident and emergency departments. Two groups of children are recognized. Those who present with acute trauma, and genuinely require urgent attention, and those who present with medical or surgical emergencies such as asthma, fits, and acute abdomen, etc., rather than going through the normal channels of primary health care. In certain inner-city units the latter practice is actively encouraged, and the departments are designed and staffed appropriately. In some major centres there will be a dedicated children's accident and emergency unit but in most district hospitals this is not practical. In any unit, however, it should be possible to reserve an area for children with separate waiting, prompt triage, appropriately trained staff, play facilities and examination rooms. The pattern of staffing on many mixed units is such that nurses and doctors may have little paediatric experience. Inexperienced staff may lack the expertise to recognize both serious medical illness in children, children at risk, and important psychosocial factors in childhood illness. To deal with these difficult situations each unit needs a well-rehearsed policy with ready access to support paediatric staff.

Day unit

For children, day surgery is particularly suitable because of the family structure and it is surprising that it has only reached its full potential in recent years. Day care was used extensively by Nicoll (1909) in Glasgow and continued by individual enthusiasts in the early years of the health service, but it was not until the 1970s that Atwell *et al.* (1973), amongst others, drew attention to the full advantages. More recently, the document *Just for a day* (Thornes, 1991) listed specific guidelines for day care and was widely accepted by local health authorities. Different centres report that up to 50% of children's surgery can be delivered on a day basis. Enthusiasm for day care is based both on advantage for the child and family and on perceived cost-effectiveness. Although it is widely assumed that day care is in all ways better for both children and families, there is in fact only marginal evidence of less psychological disturbance in those treated on a day basis in comparison with overnight admission (Campbell *et al.*, 1988).

Quality day care needs high standards of medical and nursing practice and an efficient organization in terms of the unit itself and integration of the unit with the primary health care services. Inevitably many units cater for both children and adults, and in such circumstances it is feasible to allocate separate sessions for children and to adjust the ward environment appropriately. The structure of the unit should be such that children awaiting surgery are separated from those recovering and parents should remain with the child throughout their time in the ward. Anaesthesia and surgery should not be delegated to juniors. Pain control using regional anaesthesia and accurate surgery will ensure a quick recovery. After discharge children should be seen the following day by a district or children's community nurse and there should be clear directions for the families to follow if complications arise.

Paediatric intensive care units

The report *The care of the critically ill child* (British Paediatric Association, 1993b) drew attention to deficiencies in the provision of intensive care for children throughout the UK. The report lists shortfalls both in facilities and in trained staff: of nearly 13 000 children cared for intensively, only half were nursed on a children's unit, a third were managed in improvised space on a children's ward and the remainder were treated on an adult unit. On the adult units only 5% of nurses were children trained, children were usually nursed on an open ward and a quarter of the children were under 1 year of age. The report recommended units of between six and eight beds based on regional centres with nursing levels of 1:6.4 whole time equivalents, an on-call consultant supported by middle-grade staff readily available and junior staff totally committed to the unit. The *ad hoc* provision of intensive care was considered unacceptable and under such circumstances children should be transferred to a recognized unit. The report provoked an immediate response by the Department of Health and funding was rapidly made available to the regions for improvement in their services. The outcome illustrates the considerable ability of central policy to influence local practice where the professional advisory bodies and the NHS executive are in accord.

Child- and family-centred care

It cannot be said too often that there are fundamental differences between the care of children and adults. Childhood is a period of growth and development, both physical and emotional. During that period the child is an integral and dependent member of a family structure. Care of the child must respect both concepts. Just as physical illness may interrupt the pattern of growth with consequences disproportionate to the original insult, so too can emotional injury, sustained either as a direct result of illness or as a consequence of management. The holistic approach to the child embraces the nature of the illness, the physical and emotional response of that child to illness, the position of the child within the context of the family and the ongoing consequences of the illness to both child and family.

Fear and anxiety in the child are engendered by the unknown, the experience of pain and separation from the family. Constant explanation, continuing reassurance and ongoing support are needed. Hospital admission, wherever possible, should either be avoided or kept short. A ward environment and routine should be such that it proximates to the normal life pattern which the child experiences at home. The ward needs to meet the needs of the child rather than imposing unfamiliar and rigid discipline. Parents are no longer seen as visitors in a children's ward, but partners in providing care for their child. They should be involved with suitable support at all stages of the hospital process. Early hospital discharge may depend on parents having the necessary skills and lifestyle to care for their sick child at home.

EMOTIONAL STRESS

The psychological and physical effects of stress associated with hospital attendance and admission are well known. Behavioural changes after discharge include eating problems, sleep disturbance, enuresis and regression of achievement levels. Physiological change is reflected in pulse, blood pressure and postoperative emesis. The various factors contributing to stress can be considered in terms of the child, the family and specific surgical procedures. Toddlers between 6 months and 3 years are particularly vulnerable. Problems can be anticipated in children with high anxiety levels (Reider and Wagner, 1975). The emotional significance of illness to the child needs careful consideration. In the young child, the response is not necessarily rational but illness may be interpreted as punishment or rejection. A confused 6-year-old is reported to have said 'God makes you sick because you are bad; but I'm not bad?' (Prugh *et al.*, 1953). Anxious parents transmit their fears and children who come from disturbed homes may react more adversely. Hospital admission is a particularly difficult period because of the complex interplay of emotions between the child and the parents, particularly as both parties may be equally distressed. Surgical procedures are especially disturbing because of fear of death, concern of disfigurement and pain and loss of control of self. High levels of anger, aggression and withdrawal have been noted after hypospadias repair compared with other comparable procedures and, in the same children, psychological disturbance has been reported in adult life compared with those who underwent appendectomy during childhood (Berg *et al.*, 1981).

Separation of the child from the parents is of special concern. Particularly in young children, separation results in disturbance of the normal attachment behaviour, causing separation anxiety. Early observers commented that the child responded to separation at first by crying and then by social regression and withdrawal. After being reunited with the parent, there may be a further period of emotional upset and difficult behaviour (Edelston, 1943). The pattern was further elaborated by describing an early period of protest followed by withdrawal and finally detachment and disinterest in the parents (Bowlby *et al.*, 1952). The changes were emotively captured on film by John Robertson, which contributed significantly to hospitals adopting a policy of free visiting and provision of overnight accommodation. Behavioural disturbance after discharge seldom lasts longer than 6 months and is not usually considered pathological. Occasionally, however, long-term consequences can be serious. A vulnerable group of children comprises those who come from a troubled family background and who may need repeated and lengthy admissions to hospital.

Considerable effort has been made to reduce the stress engendered by hospital attendance. Staff policies, hospital design and ward ambience all contribute and will be considered later. There is a series of studies with objective evidence showing that particular factors reduce stress. A supportive relationship between parent and nurse, particularly during critical periods such as admission and return from operation, seems to reduce maternal anxiety and stress levels in children (Skipper and Leonard, 1968). Films shown to parents in which a child copes successfully with distress are used widely in Britain and the USA. Children who have seen these films appear to cope better with their own anxieties. Paradoxically, for children with repeated admissions the films may sensitize and increase levels of anxiety. An analysis of 75 studies concluded that preparing children for hospital provided only a modest advantage (Saile *et al.*, 1988) but this view was challenged as it was thought that studies of preparation by coping were underrepresented (Eiser, 1988).

Hospital admission

IS ATTENDANCE NECESSARY?

A fundamental principle of child care is that hospital admission and separation from parents should be avoided. On critical review, it becomes evident that there is scope for improvement in this respect. Some children are referred for admission because of illness, which is apparently serious, when they are seen in the home. Understandably, the practitioner is unable to provide close supervision and there may be pressure from the family to refer the child to hospital. Such children may improve rapidly after a period of observation and can be discharged later the same day, thus avoiding overnight stay. Unnecessary surgical referrals can be avoided by a clear hospital policy on management of certain problems: for example, babies and toddlers with an umbilical hernia seldom need an operation before the age of 3 years and referral can be deferred until that age. Children are often brought back unnecessarily to outpatient clinics by inexperienced junior staff. Early discharge of children after surgical treatments may be feasible, providing that nursing and schooling can be brought to the home and the parents offered suitable support. Routine follow-up after minor day case surgery, for example, inguinal herniotomy, can be provided by community nursing services. These examples illustrate the importance of a close working relationship between the hospital, community and primary health care in reducing hospital attendance. Extending the role of the nurse specialist, closer co-operation between the hospital and community and strengthening the paediatric role in primary health care would add further improvement.

ADMISSION PROTOCOL

Admission to hospital is a particularly anxious time for both child and parent. However, elective admission into a good children's unit can be managed so that it becomes an acceptable adventure. Preparation can be started in outpatients, where families should have the opportunity to meet ward staff and pre-admission visits can be arranged so that the ward is familiar. Pamphlets will be distributed which describe the ward routine, provide useful information about the hospital and list personal belongings that need to be brought with the child. At the time of admission the child and family are received in a play area or at the bedside by a key nurse who provides a sense of continuity over the period of an inpatient stay. The family is introduced to the ward where the routine at home is discussed in relation to ward routine, with the child's particular likes and dislikes being recognized. Familiar objects from home such as toys and photographs can be placed at the bedside. Parents are encouraged to stay and participate in their child's care. By contrast, an emergency admission is less easy to manage. The child's natural resilience is reduced by apprehension, pain or simply feeling unwell and the parents themselves are distressed and anxious. Prompt attendance of nursing and medical staff is important so that the parents may be reassured that a diagnosis can be established and treatment started.

WARD PHILOSOPHY

It is often assumed that, to care for children in hospital, it is sufficient to follow one's natural inclination and instinct. Effective care is carefully structured and it is good practice to have a statement of policy which serves to reinforce the different elements of the structure. A simple statement of ward philosophy can be illustrated and displayed for both staff and visitors. Such a statement might recognize the child as a developing individual with a right to express his or her own ideas and feelings.

Furthermore, the child is part of a family with its own culture and individual needs and the hospital threatens this routine. In response to those needs, the ward should offer preadmission visiting, play specialists, qualified children's nurses, key nursing, school, open visiting, family routine, family partnership, individual privacy and a family environment.

OPERATION

As with adults, children approach surgery with feelings varying from relative equanimity to morbid fear. Much depends on the individual personality and family background. Young children may have no understanding of an operation and for them the experience is a sequence of events which are unfamiliar, alarming and painful. By contrast, the older child may comprehend the nature of illness and rationale of treatment, although the extent of understanding depends on age. There may be concerns about loss of consciousness, loss of body control, body image and, of course, pain. Fear of surgery may be aggravated by an earlier experience, unhelpful comments from friends or from watching television. Much can be done to allay these anxieties and both play therapists and paediatric nurses have a key role in this. Whether the surgery be elective or emergency, there normally is an opportunity to explain simply and reassuringly the forthcoming procedure to both the child and parent, to discuss how the child will feel after the operation and the care that will be needed post operatively, for example, dressings, splints, drops, catheters, drains and pain control. For children prior to elective surgery, there should be the opportunity to act out many of these procedures with a play specialist.

PLAY AND EDUCATION

The role of play in hospital is now widely recognized and guidelines can be found in *Quality Management for Children: Play in Hospital*. Play is part of childhood and contributes to intellectual, social and emotional growth. Structured and supervised play helps to create a more normal situation for the child. Not only does play distract and occupy the child, but observation during play can contribute to clinical evaluation. Children can be prepared for invasive procedures, such as catheterization or blood transfusion, by acting out the process on dolls. Play specialists have formal training and an integral role in the hospital management structure. They need their own base and should be encouraged to work widely throughout the hospital wherever children are treated.

Like play, school is part of childhood. The primary purpose of hospital schooling is to continue the child's education but in addition it provides stimulation and makes the hospital experience more normal. The Education Act 1944 empowers the local authority to provide appropriate education for all children of statutory age who would otherwise be at school. Hospitals are obliged to provide school accommodation, although the running costs are met by the local education authority. Many hospital schools have developed their role to meet the particular education needs of certain children and to provide an outreach service to the child's home, in order to bridge the gap between discharge from hospital and the child resuming normal education. Under the Education Act 1981, children with special education needs may require statutory assessment and this includes those with learning difficulties, those from disadvantaged social conditions and those with a medical condition or treatment protocol that is likely to affect their learning. Liaison with the education authority and social services may be needed in the care of such children.

ADOLESCENCE

The British Paediatric Association report on *The Needs and cares of adolescents* (1985) recommends that the age of this group is interpreted flexibly but, in general, should include those in secondary education. The reason for flexibility is evident when considering the possible differences in physical maturity and pattern of illness between an 11-year-old boy and a 15-year-old girl. Boys and girls of this age group share certain patterns of illness, but very different demands in terms of care. For this reason adolescents should be considered as a separate group and specific provision should be made for their care in both the hospital and community. The report, however, found no need for exclusive specialization in adolescent medicine.

Where possible, adolescents should be brought together as inpatients irrespective of specialty. Although they may be physically mature, their emotional needs are more akin to those of children. They should be nursed close to the children's unit or in a subunit of a children's ward. Schooling should be available, there should be opportunities for privacy and they should have their own recreation area. In spite of appearances to the opposite, adolescents are often uncertain and insecure, needing reassurance and company of their own peer group. In particular, there may be concerns about body image and sexuality. Staff should be chosen with care and it should be remembered that students and young staff are close in age to their patients and may identify with their problems or also feel threatened by the situation.

Within adolescence there are some specific areas of particular difficulty. These include emotional disturbances, anorexia nervosa, teenage pregnancy and illnesses peculiar to, or arising during adolescence. The subsequent transfer of those with chronic physical and mental handicaps to adult services needs to be handled sensitively. Provision must also be made for health advice and genetic counselling. For adolescents with continuing problems such as renal failure or paraplegia the advantage of being treated on a specialist unit may take priority over the advantage of an adolescent unit.

Children's rights

CONSENT

At its simplest, written consent must be obtained from the parent or guardian before a surgical procedure is undertaken on a child under 16 years of age. Where it is possible, in terms of understanding, the consent of the child should also be sought. Informed consent implies an explanation about the need for the operation, the alternative management options, possible complications and outcome. For more major procedures, a simple illustration is helpful and can be drawn directly into the clinical notes so as to serve as a record. However, it is important to distinguish between giving consent and the signed consent form. Consent, whether implied or written, is, of course, necessary for any medical examination, treatment or procedure.

Although consent is normally straightforward, there can be problems and the helpful *Guide to consent for examination and treatment* (NHS Management Executive, 1991) may be used for reference. While written consent must be secured for an operation, the need for signed consent for other procedures such as blood transfusion is less clear. In an emergency situation it might be necessary to move forward to operation, before consent can be obtained. Care should always be taken to confirm that parents have parental responsibility as laid down in the Children's Act 1989. This may not be the case with unmarried fathers, relatives, foster children or those at risk under court protection. Parents may refuse life-saving treatment for their child and, in such circumstances, it may be necessary to make application for a Special Issue Order under section 8 of the Children's Act 1989. A further difficulty is that a child who is judged to have adequate understanding may give, or refuse, consent to examination and treatment. However, the right to refusal is not straightforward and the courts have indicated that the right may be overriden by the consent of those with parental responsibility, when treatment is in the child's best interest.

CHILD CARE AND PROTECTION

Although individual surgeons may seldom be involved in child abuse, the possibility should not be forgotten or neglected. The key to recognition is awareness and a satisfactory explanation for trauma should always be sought and recorded. In any district the local authority and particularly the social services department is responsible for the care and protection of children at risk. The authority also discharges its responsibility through various agencies including the police, schools, community health workers, voluntary services and medical practitioners. The Child Protection Committee is a statutory body responsible to the local authority and should ensure openness and co-operation between the different agencies. Guidelines listed in the document *Working together under the Children's Act* (General Medical Council, 1991) provide a framework and draw attention to the fundamental premise that the interest of the child is paramount. There should be no delay in assessment which may be detrimental to the child. The parents should be offered every opportunity to be involved at all stages of the investigation.

Medical practitioners expressed concern about contributing fully with other agencies because of concern about confidentiality, with the result that a second document *Child protection: medical responsibilities* (General Medical Council, 1993) was published to provide guidance. Emphasis was again given to interagency co-operation with the involvement of parents and where appropriate the child himself or herself. The medical role was considered in relation to prevention, raising of awareness, investigation of related medical problems, ongoing care, treatment and attendance at the child protection conference. On the question of confidentiality; the overriding principle is to protect the child, 'because of their age and vulnerability means they cannot protect themselves'. The General Medical Council advises the medical profession and states that 'Where a doctor believes a patient may be the victim of neglect and abuse, the patient's interest is paramount and will usually require the doctor to disclose information to an appropriate responsible person or officer of a statutory agency' (General Medical Council, 1993).

At a practical level, each hospital must have a policy on how to handle suspected child abuse. A junior doctor may pursue a preliminary line of investigation but, where there is serious concern, the problem must be referred to a senior paediatrician. After further investigation social services must be involved and a child protection conference arranged. A register of children at risk should be available either through the hospital accident and emergency department or via social services.

CHILDREN FROM ETHNIC MINORITIES

A basic principle of the Children's Act 1989 is that services for children and family should take into account 'the child's religious persuasion, racial origin and cultural and linguistic background'. The Welfare of Children and Young People in Hospital advised districts and providers to be 'sensitive to the individual needs of children and families from minority groups of different ethnic, religious or cultural composition'. The purchaser is obliged to provide services to meet the needs of all the local population. In order to fulfil this obligation the needs of minority groups have to be actively identified and met. To provide a sensitive service for minority groups, it seems important that the cultural mix of the children and family is reflected amongst the hospital staff. In the past, the NHS has been described as colourblind; however, the culture of the service is founded on the tradition of the mainly white population. Inevitably there are times when the prevailing culture is assumed to be right for all and there is a failure to acknowledge the significance of particular needs of minority groups.

The services for minority groups were surveyed in *Health for all our children* (Action for Sick Children, 1993). The review lists areas of concern which included communication, staff attitudes, religious and cultural beliefs and a number of practical issues such as naming systems, food, hygiene and play facilities. It was evident that some families had little understanding of health services to the extent that they failed to realize that general practitioner services were free and that they had access to accident and emergency departments. Problems in communication relate in part to language and the need for a comprehensive interpreting service is self-evident. Attitudes of hospital staff were mainly commented upon favourably although there was a tendency to stereotype certain groups. As a result of this, individual families felt that they were less well informed about their children and consequently less able to be involved in the child's care. Religious belief and observances were not always appreciated and respected; for example, ornaments were removed unnecessarily, traditional care of children after death was not respected because of hospital protocol and private facilities for worship were not always provided. Naming systems vary widely among different groups and cause confusion both when children and relatives are addressed and in the hospital records. An individual child may not only have a family and a personal name but, also, names to indicate gender, generation and status. Moreover, the child's family name is not necessarily carried by the mother and the sequence in which names are listed vary between different cultures. Food for children was not always appropriately prepared and there was inadequate choice to allow for religious preferences. A correct feeding pattern and diet is important for child not only for nutritional reasons but so as to create a familiar environment. For most children, hygiene means a traditional soap and water scrub, but for some the time and order of washing follows religious custom. For other children moisturizing cream and light oil are a more appropriate form of cleansing. Play is a sensitive area in which there was found to be subtle misunderstanding. It is important that the selection of play equipment should reflect the cultural mix of the children.

ACKNOWLEDGMENTS

In preparing the chapter I should like to acknowledge the help and guidance of Kathy Dickenson RCN of the Children's Hospital, Leicester Royal Infirmary.

References

Action for Sick Children 1993: Health for all our children. Quality Review Series. Mary Slater.

Atwell, J.D., Burn, J.M.B., Dewar, A.K., *et al.* 1973: Paediatric day care surgery. *Lancet* **ii**, 895–6.

Audit Commission 1993: National Health Services Report No. 7. Children First: a study of hospital services. London: HMSO.

Berg, R., Svensson, J. and Astrom, G. 1981: Social and sexual adjustment of men operated for hypospadias during childhood. A controlled study. *Journal of Urology* **125**, 313–17.

Bowlby, J., Robertson, J. and Rosenbluth, D. 1952: A two year old goes to hospital. Psychoanalytical study of the child 7. New York: International Universities Press, 82–94.

British Paediatric Association 1985: Working Party on the Needs and Cares of Adolescents. London: British Paediatric Association.

British Paediatric Association 1993a: The transfer of infants and children for surgery: report of the joint working party. London: British Paediatric Association.

British Paediatric Association 1993b: Report of a Multidisciplinary Working Party on Paediatric Intensive Care. Care of Critically Ill Children. London: British Paediatric Association.

Campbell, I.R., Scaife, J.M. and Johnstone, J.M.S. 1988. Psychological effects of day care surgery compared with inpatient treatment. *Archives of Disease in Childhood* **63**, 415–417.

Campling, E.A., Devlin, H.B. and Lunn, J.N. 1990: Report of national confidential enquiry into perioperative deaths. London.

Committee on Child Health Services 1986: Fit for the future (Chairman: S.D.M. Court). London: HMSO, Cmd 6684.

Department of Health 1991: Welfare of children and young people in hospital. London: HMSO.

Edelston, H. (1943): Separation anxiety in young children: a study of hospital cases. *Genetic Psychology Monographs* **28**, 1–95.

Eiser, C. 1988: Do children benefit from psychological preparation for hospitalization? *Psychology and Health* **2**, 133–138.

General Medical Council 1991: Working together under the Children's Act 1989. London: HMSO.

General Medical Council 1993: Child protection: medical responsibilities. London: HMSO.

Ministry of Health 1959: Central Health Services Council. Committee on the Welfare of Children in Hospital. Report of the Platt Committee (Chairman: Sir Henry Platt). London: HMSO.

NAWCH (National Association for the Welfare of Children in Hospital) 1990: Setting standards for children in health care. NAWCH Quarterly Review. London: NAWCH.

NHS Management Executive 1991: Guide to consent for examination or treatment.

Nicoll, J. 1909: The surgery of infancy. *British Medical Journal* **2**, 753–4.

Prugh, D., Staub, E., Sands, H., Kirschbaum, M.S. and Lenihan, E. 1953: A study of the emotional reactions of children and families to hospitalization and illness. *American Journal of Orthopsychiatry* **23**, 70–106.

Quality management for children: play in hospital. London: Save The Children Fund.

Rieder, T. and Wagner, K.D. 1975: Reaction type and the experience of disease. *Kinderaerztl Praxis* **43**, 49–53.

Saile, H., Burgmeier, R. and Schmidt, L.R. 1988: A meta-analysis of studies on psychological preparation of children facing medical procedures. *Psychology and Health* **2**, 139–156.

Skipper, J.K. Jr and Leonard, R.C. 1968: Children, stress and hospitalization: a field experiment. *Journal of Health and Social Behaviour* **9**, 275–287.

Thornes, R. 1991: Just for the day caring for children in the health services. Children admitted to hospital for day treatment. London: NAWCH.

UNICEF 1989: Children's rights. The United Nations Convention on the Rights of the Child, Children's Rights Office. London: UNICEF.

CHAPTER 7

Nursing sick children in hospital

E.A. GLASPER

Introduction
Historical aspects of child care
Preparing children for a hospital admission
Preparation in the community
Preparing children and their families for a
hospital with written and visual material
Family information centres

Preadmission programmes
The use of anatomical dolls
Parental roles and care by parents
Trends in child health nursing
Play
Education in hospital
References

Introduction

Professional paediatric nurses working in all areas of child care are now firmly committed to the concept of family-centred care and family support. Although support of the family has been an integral part of paediatric nursing since the founding of the profession, the role of the nurse in this context has changed from a support for families to acting as a guardian to their rights of autonomy and free choice.

The traditional model of medicine was forcibly taught to nurses in a profession which since Florence Nightingale has been hierarchical with an unquestioning respect for higher rank and authority. In this context loyalty was a key virtue and criticism was not tolerated. The move towards reflective practice which characterizes modern child health nursing has facilitated a major change in the way that children and their families are cared for in hospitals and the community.

The promotion of family involvement in care since the 1960s has resulted from the increasing knowledge of the effects of a hospital admission on the welfare of the child. The growing recognition of this has caused many children's nurses to question their method of practice. Such changes in practice have come from parents wishing to become more involved with the clinical care of their own children. This presents a significant challenge for the nursing profession to become more involved in the way families are cared for in hospital. Children in the western world are regarded as innocent but vulnerable individuals and this is recognized in some societies through legislation designed to protect them. Child care is normally family orientated but when this fails the community has a statutory responsibility to act *in loco parentis* until the family can resume care of the child.

The Convention on the Rights of the Child, which was adopted by the General Assembly of the United Nations on 20 November 1989, states that 'the family', as the fundamental group of society and the natural environment for the growth and well-being of all its members and particularly children, should be protected and given assistance so that it can assume its responsibilities within the community.

The convention came into force on 2 September 1990 and on 29 September 1990 there was a gathering of world leaders at the United Nations to attend the World

Summit for children. This was the first summit supporting the rights of the child (UNICEF, 1990). This summit formed a plan of action and an agenda for the future welfare of children. It is an ambitious plan and recognizes the needs of children around the world. It should be given a high priority in the allocation of resources. The development of family-focused nursing care represents a small part of this overall strategy.

Historical aspects of child care

Over the centuries the child has been considered as either inherently evil or good, which has led to different child-rearing practices.

Lloyd de Mause (1974) in *The history of childhood* traces the changing attitudes towards children, from Rousseau who believed the child to be innocent by nature to John Wesley who believed children to be sinful and evil by nature. The altruistic stance of Rousseau had enormous influence but this did not alter child-rearing practices for the mass of the western population until the second half of the nineteenth century. In marked contrast, society fell under the influence of the puritan non-conformist Wesleyian movement. John Wesley himself was a stringent martinet and believed that children could only be saved through physical punishment and fear of the rod. Such attitudes have persisted through to the twentieth century, which is indicative of the influence of the man and his movement. The whole history of childhood is a sorry tale of institutional abuse. Solitary confinement, murder, abandonment, beatings and sexual abuse make up the web of abuse which still persists today in some parts of the world.

The emancipation of children and their families has been slow and is not yet complete. Attempts to promote the care of children in a meaningful way in the UK began in 1739 with the work of Thomas Coram, a retired sea captain who had spent most of his working life in the New World. On his return to London, he was horrified to find dying children in the gutters and rotting corpses of babies on dung heaps. Coram obtained the patronage of many influential individuals of the period and was granted a Royal Charter to open a foundling hospital in 1739, the remnants of which exist today near the site of the Hospital for Sick Children, Great Ormond Street. The Foundling Hospital was essentially a place of refuge for unwanted children, not a hospital for sick children. Besser (1977) points out that of the 15 000 children admitted during the years 1756–1760 only 4400 lived to adulthood. This high mortality rate was due to childhood infections and ignorance of the spread of disease, and was a constant reminder of the dangers of admitting children to institutions. Despite this the concept of childhood was slowly changing with the dawning of the age of philanthropy. The increase in

literacy among the population of the industrialized nations allowed authors such as Charles Dickens and Charles Kingsley to document social injustice through novels such as *Oliver Twist* and *The water babies*.

When the Hospital for Sick Children, Great Ormond Street, opened its doors for the first time on 14 February 1852, this represented a major triumph for childhood. Founded by Dr Charles West and patronized by Charles Dickens, this hospital became one of the first of many specialist hospitals to be opened in the latter half of the nineteenth century.

It should be remembered that the first children's hospitals were built and staffed in the pre-Nightingale era. The experience gained by Florence Nightingale during the Crimean War led to changes in nursing practice. The professional ethic which was the hallmark of the Nightingale model also incorporated a military ethos. Such philosophies left little place for non-professionals and parents were sadly relegated to this position. In attempting to raise its own status nursing neglected the welfare of families with children in hospital. It would be nearly 100 years before this changed. The growing professionalism of nursing gradually excluded parents from direct participation in the care of their children. This resulted in the establishment of strict visiting hours whereby parents were prohibited from visiting at times convenient to them. Thus the nursing establishment tried to protect families from the harsh realities of childhood illness in an era when childhood mortality was high. The remnants of this past history have made it difficult for many children's nurses to develop the concept of family care.

This attitude began to change after the publication of the Platt Report (Ministry of Health, 1959) and accelerated following the foundation of the National Association for the Welfare of Children in Hospital (NAWCH) in 1961 now named Action for Sick Children (ASC). This group of parents and professionals aimed for the full implementation of the Platt Report. During the 1960s and 1970s organizations such as NAWCH in the UK, Australia and the Association for the Care of Children's Health (ACCH) in North America campaigned for changes in children's hospitals such as the promotion of day surgery, residence for parents, mothers in anaesthetic rooms and free visiting of children in hospital.

Preparing children for a hospital admission

Family-centred care is now gaining universal approval and with it the concept of giving preoperative and postoperative information. The growth of surgical day care for children and shorter hospital admissions have increased the need for the preparation of families for a hospital admission. These factors and the early discharge of children from hospital have led to the development of paediatric community nursing services (Atwell and Gow, 1985; Glasper *et al.*, 1989). The arguments put forward for day care include earlier ambulation, lower costs and reduced psychological trauma (Campbell *et al.*, 1988). It is this factor more than anything else which has captured the imagination of those concerned with the welfare of children in hospital. The emotional factors concerned with a hospital admission are probably of equal importance to the family as the child's physical condition. As a result, an number of strategies have been developed, aimed at reducing stress to the child and his or her family.

Preparation in the community

Hospitalization is not an uncommon experience for many young children. Brett (1983) has indicated that preparation should begin in the classroom and feature as part of general education. The needs vary and change with the age and understanding of the child. This should be taken into consideration when planning assistance with playgroup, preschool, school, cub, brownie or church group programmes.

Families come in all shapes and sizes, good, bad and indifferent. All appear to benefit from preparation for a hospital admission. Children's nurses are well able to help in this role. The prevention of stress to the family unit is the aim of any preparatory programme whether in the classroom, community or hospital environment. As young children are susceptible to fantasy and misunderstanding, especially if separation of the child from home and family is implied.

Preparing children and their families for a hospital with written and visual material

The families of children admitted to hospital for surgery need information. Glasper and Burge (1991) discuss how patient or family information leaflets enhance the usefulness of spoken instructions. Families of children requiring surgery have the right to information, and children's nurses can assist in the production of leaflets. Specific written information is valuable in ensuring that parents understand their responsibilities before, during and following a hospital admission. The information must be easily understood and readable. Information leaflets are particularly useful in surgical settings where the use of simple anatomical line drawings can augment the text and can be highly effective in reducing the stress of a hospital admission. Many children's units send out written material with the letter of admission. This written material can play a meaningful role in communicating with the parents and child about to be admitted, with information such as facilities for parents, special diets and laundering facilities. Failure to provide adequate information is a cause of anxiety and thus the parents are less capable of providing support and security for a child during a hospital admission. In the past such information has been lacking and a cause of parental dissatisfaction (Glasper *et al.*, 1988).

Harris (1981) suggests that specific information sheets appertaining to individual operations be included in any mail-outs to parents, although this has usually been carried out at the time of the outpatient consultation. Some hospitals have produced video films or tape slide programmes to provide information to parents and their children. The effectiveness of these programmes has led to their frequent use in children's units. Films produced for television may have the effect of raising the awareness of preparing children for an admission to hospital, but are expensive to produce. Tape slide programmes are cheaper, with the added advantage that they can be easily updated. There is a number of books written for children about hospital which vary in quality. They fulfil a role as part of an overall preparatory programme for families with children about to be admitted to hospital for surgery.

Family information centres

Comprehensive family information centres that provide health information for families are being established in children's outpatient departments. Such centres of health information and promotion (CHIP) provide verbal and written advice (Glasper *et al.*, 1995). In the Hospital for Sick Children in Toronto advice is available by telephone. Such a service can provide parents with information and thus may save a visit to the hospital or family doctor (Glasper and McGrath 1993).

Preadmission programmes

In recent years many children's units, particularly surgical ones have concentrated on the development of a preadmission programme either in the outpatient department or within the hospital at a set time, usually 1 week prior to surgery. Invitations are sent out in the mail with information relating to the child's admission 1 week before being admitted. It is a challenge to children's nurses to attract families from all socioeconomic groups (Glasper and Stradling, 1989). Preadmission programmes consist of a therapeutic play session for the children, followed by a slide presentation and tour of the clinical areas including the operating department. Hospitals should allow parents to be present during the induction of anaesthesia (Glasper, 1993, 1995) and useful information about the parental role can be given during the preadmission programme. A combination of emotional support and information related to the admission appears to be an effective method of reducing preoperative anxiety in families.

The use of anatomical dolls

Preparation that involves only a verbal explanation may be wholly unsatisfactory for many children, especially those who are immature. Methods of preparation which operate at a child's level of understanding may be more suitable. Many adults use inappropriate language when explaining aspects of treatment to children. This is true of some hospital personnel who are faced with an infinite variety of children's explanations of illness. The younger preschool child often gives life to inanimate objects and this animistic trait can be adopted when discussing aspects of illness. New anatomical models have been developed specifically for use with children and families. The Zaadie Doll produced by the Zaadie Company (Lowell, MA, USA) is one such example). This is a cloth-covered rag doll of toddler-size proportions, with three layers which peel apart using velcro fastenings to expose the vital organs. This simple yet effective design facilities its use among a wide variety of age groups including adults. In many adults perceptions of their own anatomical structures is poor and inadequate. This makes the problem of explaining surgical or other procedures difficult and anatomical dolls are a useful addition of material available to prepare a child for hospital procedures. They should only be used as part of a preplanned information package and under adult supervision.

Parental roles and care by parents

Casey (1988) has used a self-care framework in describing a partnership model of paediatric nursing where care may be given by parents or others with support and teaching from the nursing staff. In direct contrast to the earlier years of paediatric nursing, the emphasis of care is now focused on the resources of the family. The parent care schemes described by Cleary *et al.* (1986) allow families to participate rather than being resident passive bystanders. Care-by-parent schemes should be embraced cautiously and never used because of staff shortages. Parents appreciate being involved in the care of their children in hospital, particularly after surgery and prior to early discharge. This allows parents to rehearse their role in preparation for nursing the child at home. The success of parental involvement in care is forcing paediatric nurses to re-examine their role in nursing sick children and has increased their educative supportive activities. This is the challenge for the future development of the profession.

Trends in child health nursing

The profound changes facing paediatric nurses is complicated by the legacy of the past with its emphasis on prescriptive care. At a time of economic austerity, it is not easy to plan for the future, but despite this paediatric nurses around the world are championing the rights of children. Many have been influential in promoting children's charters and it is not an uncommon sight in hospitals to see charters publicly displayed as standards of care which can be evaluated through quality assurance activities. One such area relates to the management of postoperative pain in childhood. The interest in patient-controlled analgesia (PCA) and the use of validated pain measurement scales is making the management of children following surgery much easier. Paediatric nurses have been at the forefront of these developments and they will continue to work in partnership with their medical colleagues as part of a multidisciplinary team supporting the family. The growth of the interface between primary and secondary care is challenging children's units to develop further the services offered by outpatient departments (Glasper, 1992; Campbell *et al.*, 1992). The children's nurses of the future will continue to be at the forefront of new innovations in the care of children in hospital.

Play

Therapeutic play is a vital component of a child's admission to hospital. Hospital play should reflect the environment in which the child is situated. This is particularly true for children admitted for surgery, who within a short period are faced with a bewildering number of strange people and machines. Young children are especially fearful of strange machines and often attribute life to inanimate objects. In view of this, strategies of play designed to facilitate coping and personal growth should be promoted by all staff whose day-to-day work brings them into contact with sick children. Increasingly, the role of play is being stressed within health care professional educational curriculae, but it often takes a back seat to the more traditional science-based subjects. The member of the multidisciplinary child health team best placed to provide play for children in hospital is the play specialist or child life worker. Such specialists are essential members of the ward team, providing the link between the child and the unfamiliar hospital environment. Play provision for children in hospital must never be considered as an afterthought when planning an admission.

Education in hospital

The provision of education for children in hospital has

now become law in the UK, following the 1993 Education Act. Previously, the educational provision for sick children was variable and depended on the hospital and local authority facilities. Now all children in hospital will benefit from the tighter legislation for education during hospital admission. Children who start school at 4 years of age will continue to receive that level of teaching whilst an inpatient. Children who do not start school until 5 years of age will not receive teaching but will continue under the supervision of the play specialist. All children involved in full-time education, up until 16 years of age, will receive a commensurate level of teaching whilst in hospital. In addition, children over the age of 16 years can expect to have education provision if they are in higher education.

References

Atwell, J.D. and Gow, M. 1985: Paediatric trained district nurse in the community. Expensive luxury or economic necessity? *British Medical Journal* **29**, 227–9.

Besser, F.S. 1977: Great Ormond Street anniversary. *Nursing Mirror* **144**(6), 60–3.

Brett, A. 1983: Preparing children for hospitalisation – a classroom teaching approach. *Journal of School Health* **5**, 561–3.

Campbell, I.R., Scaite, J.M. and Johnstone, J.M.S. 1988: Psychological effects of day case surgery compared to inpatient surgery. *Archives of Disease in Childhood.* **63**, 415–17.

Campbell, S., Glasper, E.A. and Lowson, S. 1992: Families first. The Southampton Nursing Development Unit. *Paediatric Nursing* **48**(8), 6–9.

Casey, A. 1988: A partnership with child and family. *Senior Nurse*, **8**(4), 8–9.

Cleary, J., Grayo, P., Hall, D.J., Rowlandson, P.H., Sainsbury, C.P.Q. and Davies, M.M. 1986: Parental involvement in the lives of children in hospital. *Archives of Disease in Childhood* **61**, 779–87.

Glasper, A. and Stradling, P. 1989: Preparing children for admission. *Paediatric Nursing* July, 18–20.

Glasper, E.A. 1992: Sick kids, healthy idea. *Nursing Times* **88**(20) 30–2.

Glasper, E.A. 1993: Parental pressure during anaesthesia induction in children. *Journal of the Association for the Welfare of Child Health* **19**, 1–4.

Glasper, E.A. 1995: An investigation into the effects of parental accompaniment during the induction of anaesthesia in day case children. Unpublished Ph.D. Thesis, University of Southampton. http://www.soton.ac.uk./~uossonam/papers/profag.htm

Glasper, E.A., Ball, M. and Yerrel, P. 1988: How well do we perform? Parents' perceptions of paediatric care. *Professional Nurse* Dec. 115–8.

Glasper, E.A. and Burge, D. 1991: Developing family information leaflets. *Nursing Standard* **6**(25), 24–7.

Glasper, E.A., Gow, M. and Yerrell, P. 1989: A family friend. *Nursing Times* **85**(4), 63–5.

Glasper, E.A., Lowson, S., Manger, R. and Philips, L. 1995: Developing a centre for health information and promotion. *British Journal of Nursing* **4**(12), 693–7.

Glasper, E.A. and McGrath, K. 1993: Telephone triage: extending practice. *Nursing Standard* **7**(15), 34–6.

Harris, P.J. 1981: Children in hospital. Preparation of parents and their children for a planned hospital admission. *Nursing Times* **17** (7 Oct) 44–6.

de Mause, L. (ed.) 1974: *The history of childhood, the untold story of child abuse.* London: Souvenir Press.

Ministry of Health 1959: Central Health Services Council on the Welfare of Children in Hospital. Report of the Platt Committee. London: HMSO.

UNICEF 1990: *First Call for Children. World Declaration and plan of action from the world summit for children. Convention on the Rights of the Child.* New York: UNICEF.

CHAPTER 8

Nursing sick children in the community

M.A. GOW

Introduction	Other surgical care
Day surgery	Liaison with the general practitioner
Early discharge	Conclusions
Terminal care	References
Medical care	

Introduction

Since the early 1970s there has been a change of emphasis for the nursing treatment of sick children, originally hospital based but now with community nursing to a greater extent supporting acute hospital care. Thus the nursing of the child in the home is increasingly important but for this to be carried out efficiently there is a need for the availability of specialist children's nurses, whether community or hospital based.

There is no doubt that a hospital in patient admission is traumatic to the child and the family. Even in 1877 George Armstrong stated that 'If you take a sick child from its parent you break its heart immediately'. For many years a child admitted to hospital was only allowed limited visiting by his or her parents and this led to behavioural problems on his subsequent discharge home (Douglas, 1975; Quinton and Rutter, 1976).

Thus in the modern situation for the provision of medical and surgical care for children, a hospital in-patient admission should be avoided if at all possible. Such an example is the provision of day case facilities for children requiring surgery for conditions such as circumcision, herniotomies and the correction of undescended testes (Atwell *et al.*, 1973; Atwell and Gow, 1985; NAWCH, 1991).

The special needs of such families were stated in the Platt Report (Ministry of Health, 1959) and later repeated in the Court Report (Committee on Child Health Services, 1976), both reports stating that, whenever

possible, children should be treated and looked after in their own homes. This was more recently reinforced by the report on the *Welfare of children and young people in hospital* (Department of Health, 1991).

More recently, *Homeward bound* (Audit Commision, 1992) and *Bridging the gap* (Thornes, 1993) reported on the delivery of care to children at home and suggested that there should be a more co-ordinated approach to paediatric community nursing and that increasing knowledge and information on the provision of services should be available. Thus there has been a gradual change with a shift in the balance from acute care to care in the community (Gow and Atwell, 1980; Atwell and Gow, 1985).

However, the development of a paediatric community nursing service has been a slow process. It was initially hospital based for the follow-up of both medically (Bergmann *et al.*, 1965) and surgically treated infants and children (Lawrie, 1964). In Southampton, where the service is based within the community, it was used initially for the support of children undergoing day surgical procedures (Atwell, 1978). It was some 4 years later that the service included the care of medical problems (Davis, 1982).

Southampton was not the first centre to develop a paediatric community nursing service. The first centre was in Rotherham in 1949 when several general practitioners (GPs) and two Queen's district nurses were appointed to set up a home nursing service for sick children. Progress was slow and there were only eight such services by 1974, but since the 1980s progress has been more rapid and in 1993 the directory included details of 165 generalist and specialist paediatric community nursing teams including some 55 generalist services in England. Paediatric community teams should be an integrated service with the Primary Health Care Team and the hospital paediatric service and information on their services must be readily available (Fig. 8.1 and Table 8.1).

There are financial implications in the provision of such a service and these may well be a cause of problems. Highly technical nursing was originally provided in hospitals but, with the discharge of patients home with tracheostomies and gastrostomies and after complex reconstructive procedures on the urinary tract expertise and equipment, e.g. catheters, suction tubes, must be available in the community.

Therefore, it is essential for there to be a close liaison between the hospital and the community. This means that planned discharge criteria are established, especially when this involves resources for the provision of equipment, in order for highly skilled nursing to be

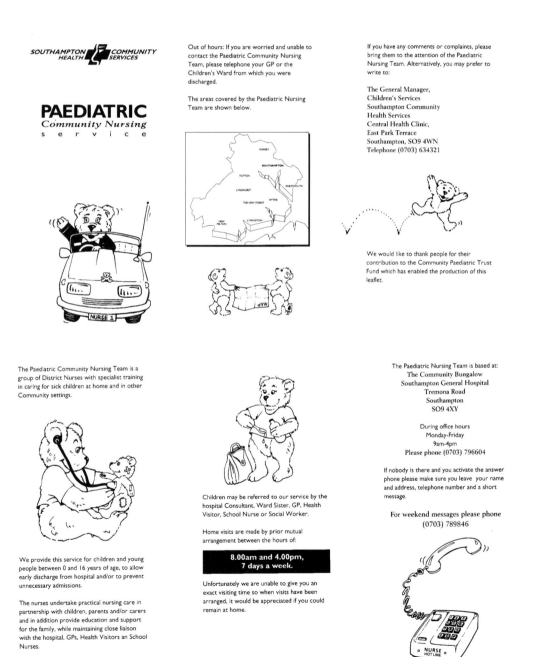

Fig. 8.1 Information available about the paediatric nursing service.

PAEDIATRIC COMMUNITY NURSING

The Role of the Paediatric Community Nurse

The role of the Paediatric Community Nurse is to provide a fully intergrated Paediatric Nursing Service that meets the nursing needs of the acute and chronically sick child at home, working with families to minimize the effects of disability and illness.

They work as part of the Primary Health Care Team, providing the interface between hospital and community.

Table 8.1 Information available about the paediatric community nursing service.

available in the home. The information required should be clearly written, and the parents and children involved must feel confident and competent. Communication between all concerned with the care of the child thus plays an important role in enabling the trust and support to the family to be maintained at a high level (Fig. 8.2).

The functions of the paediatric community nurse include the care of patients undergoing day surgery, early discharge of inpatients following medical or surgical treatment, the terminal care of children dying from malignant disease, the care of the physically handicapped, e.g. neuropathic bladder and constipation associated with spina bifida, and some mentally impaired children who may have physical problems (Fig. 8.3).

Day surgery

The success of day surgery for children depends upon careful selection of patients, availability of expert paediatric anaesthetic and surgical expertise and adequate support and nursing in the home.

The infant or child is routinely checked by a doctor from the surgical team prior to discharge and the parents are given verbal and written instructions about the necessary postoperative care and a telephone number to ring should a problem occur in the first 12 hours.

The paediatric nursing team visits every child who has had a general anaesthetic within 24 hours, in order to assess the general condition of the child, advise the family on the care required and provide reassurance to the parents. Paediatric community nurses have also been given the right to readmit a patient should they become anxious about aspects of home care or the development of complications. Thus it is essential to maintain the liaison with the GP and hospital.

Early discharge

One benefit of having an established paediatric community nurse is that the early discharge of patients following a surgical operation such as an uncomplicated appendicectomy becomes possible and part of the routine management of such patients. In practice, the majority of such patients may be discharged between 48 and 72 hours after a routine appendicectomy (Atwell, 1978).

In 1973 this policy had resulted in the average length of stay of all patients being reduced from 8.75 days (Atwell, 1978) to 4.55 days, with a financial saving at that time of some £26 000 per annum.

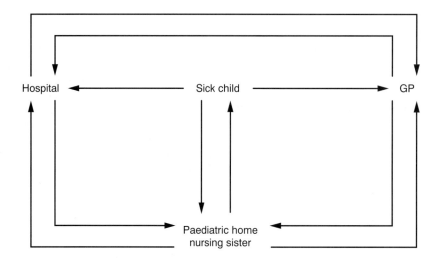

Fig. 8.2 The role of the paediatric community nurse in liaison among the GP, the hospital and the patient.

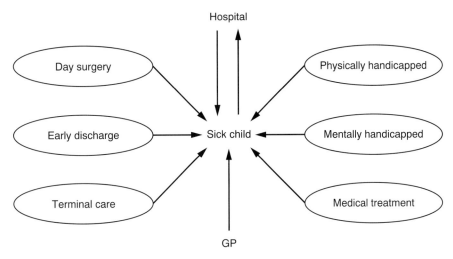

Fig. 8.3 Functions of the paediatric community nurse.

In contrast with the early discharge of patients following a Ramstedt's pyloromyotomy the financial savings are minimal as the number of patients treated annually is small. This demonstrates an important point, which is that in order to achieve worthwhile financial savings a change in policy must be made for common conditions. This would allow a better distribution of funds for the more complicated treatments which are now part of everyday surgical practice.

Terminal care

To care for the terminally ill child at home is possibly the most demanding but also the most challenging situation faced by the paediatric community nurse. The nursing care required is very variable but must meet the demands of the child and family. Such care may include the intravenous administration of platelets to prevent distressing bleeds and the adequate control of pain. Thus it can often be possible to allow a child to die peacefully in his or her own home. Such a situation is always associated with sadness but there is the privilege of being part of their overall care. Support during the bereavement process is also an essential part of care.

Medical care

Following the success of surgical care for day patients and early discharge of inpatients, by 1974 the service included medical patients. The length of stay of children in hospital with such diverse conditions as diabetes mellitus, asthma, cystic fibrosis and malignancies could be reduced. Many parents provide excellent care for their children with these chronic conditions but by

providing support to these families it is often possible to avoid a hospital admission which previously would have been a matter of course.

Other care involves the management of oxygen-dependent babies with bronchopulmonary dysplasia and the use of intravenous antibiotics to control infection, particularly in the patient with cystic fibrosis.

Other surgical care

It is now possible to nurse children safely at home with tracheostomies and gastrostomies and to provide naso-gastric feeding of infants and parenteral nutrition as well as the management of drains and stomas of varying types.

Liaison with the general practitioner

The paediatric community nursing team, as previously stated, was established originally for the care of children following day surgery. In the past, the majority of GPs relied on their practice and adults' district nurses for primary care within the community. However, with the development of more widely distributed paediatric community nursing teams they are now supplying a highly competent paediatric team and thus fewer children are requiring a hospital admission.

Conclusions

In the modern care of the surgical patient the home environment is vital and the role of the paediatric community nurse is to provide continuation of care as well as sometimes being able to prevent a hospital admission. Liaison between the GP and the hospital is an essential part of their role. Equipment and facilities must be provided so that they may achieve their aims to a rewarding and satisfactory high standard.

References

Atwell, J.D. 1978: Changing patterns in paediatric surgical care. *Annals of the Royal College of Surgeons of England* **60**, 375–83.

Atwell, J.D. and Gow, M.A. 1985: Paediatric trained district nurse in the community: expensive luxury or economic necessity? *British Medical Journal* **291**, 227–9.

Atwell, J.D., Burn, J.M.B., Dewar, A.K. and Freeman, N.V. 1973: Paediatric daycase surgery. *Lancet* **ii**, 895–7.

Audit Commission 1992: Homeward bound – a new course for community health. London: HMSO.

Bergman, A.B., Shrand, H. and Oppe, T.E. 1965: A paediatric home care programme in London – 10 years' experience. *Paediatrics* **36**, 314–21.

Committee on Child Health Services 1976: *Fit for the future.* London: HMSO.

Davis, J. 1982: The pain of separation. *Nursing Times* **78** (suppl 7).

Department of Health 1991: *Welfare of children and young people in hospital.* London: HMSO.

Douglas, J.W.B. 1975: Early hospital admissions and later disturbances of behaviour and learning. *Developmental Medicine and Child Neurology* **17**, 456–480.

Gow, M.A. and Atwell, J.D. 1980: The role of the children's nurse in the community. *Journal of Paediatric Surgery* **15**, 26–30.

Lawrie, R. 1964: Operating on children as day cases. *Lancet* **ii**, 1289–91.

Ministry of Health 1959: *The welfare of children in hospital.* London: HMSO.

National Association for the Welfare of Children in Hospital 1991: *Caring for children in the health services just for the day.* London: NAWCH.

Quinton, D. and Rutter, M. 1976: Early hospital admissions and later disturbances of behaviour: an attempted replication of Douglas's findings. *Developmental Medicine and Child Neurology* **18**, 447–59.

Royal College of Surgeons of England, Commission on the Provision of Surgical Services 1985: *Guidelines for day surgery.*

Thornes, R. 1993: *Caring for children in the health services: bridging the gap.* London: NAWCH.

CHAPTER 9

Ultrasonography

K.C. DEWBURY

Introduction
Physical principles
Diagnostic applications
Intervention

Conclusion
References
Further reading

Introduction

Ultrasound is firmly established as an important technique for tomographic imaging of soft tissue structures. It can be used to quantitate the movement of structures such as cardiac valves and, using the Doppler mode, patterns of blood flow. The soft tissue images are obtained without the need for contrast agents, although ultrasound contrast agents are now becoming available and may find a valuable role in augmenting the Doppler signal. Ultrasound used at diagnostic intensity levels does not cause damage to human tissues as far as is known. There are therefore no contraindications to the use of ultrasound but there are limitations to its use due to the mechanism by which sound penetrates tissue. There is total reflection at tissue/gas and tissue/bone interfaces. Gas-containing structures and bone cannot be imaged and may obscure deeper lying structures. This is why ultrasound is not generally useful in the head except in the neonate where the open fontanelle provides an acoustic window. When the abdomen is to be examined the bony skeleton and gas-containing viscera constitute boundaries to adequate visualization and considerable technical expertise may be required to overcome them. Fresh wounds, dressings and drainage bags may pose contact problems. Very ticklish patients may also be a challenge to examine. Ultrasound is also subject to many artefactual signals which complicate interpretation and add to the operator skill required.

Modern real-time ultrasound is a dynamic interactive examination, usually performed fairly rapidly, which is readily accepted by patients since the procedure requires only light pressure on the skin and warmed contact gel may be used. Patient preparation is minimal, with bladder filling being required for renal tract and pelvic examinations and fasting if the gallbladder is to be optimally demonstrated. The patient may otherwise be scanned as and when required, a major advantage for emergency uses. In addition mobile ultrasound systems are now widely available and may be taken to the cot or bedside. For these reasons ultrasound is an ideal imaging tool for infants and children and in recent years has become an indispensable aid to diagnosis.

Physical principles

Ultrasound is a high-frequency mechanical vibration. It is produced by a transducer of a piezoelectric material which has the property of changing thickness when a voltage is applied across it. When the transducer crystal is electrically pulsed it rings like a bell at its own resonant frequency. The piezoelectric effect is symmetrical so the transmitter can also be used as a receiver producing a small voltage when an ultrasound wave strikes it. Ultrasound is transmitted from the transducer as a longitudinal wave into the tissues. Energy from the beam is lost by absorption, and reflection is the other important tissue interaction upon which the images depend. Reflection occurs at tissue boundaries with different elasticities (acoustical impedence). The returning reflections produce a scan line of information and a large number of contiguous scan lines a tomographic slice of information. Rapid repetition of the swept images produces a moving picture in the same way as cine photography. This system is called real-time and is used in all current systems.

The Doppler principle is the basis of a method of assessment of movement by ultrasound. It depends on the shift in frequency produced in the sound wave when the source moves relative to the receiver. An ultrasound wave is transmitted into the tissue and the frequency of the echo is compared with the original. A rise in frequency is a quantitative measure of the movement of the target towards the transducer, whereas a fall in frequency indicates movement away from the transducer. Moving tissues give Doppler signals, the greatest application of which is in quantitating blood flow. Here the echoes arise from blood cells. Depth information can be obtained if the transmitted pulse is broken into short bursts, termed pulsed Doppler, which provide both imaging and Doppler information. A practical difficulty with pulsed Doppler systems is the fact that only a small area is sensitive to flow, so that a laborious search must be made if the vascular anatomy is not known. This problem is overcome with colour flow-mapped Doppler or colour Doppler which provides flow information across the whole image. The ability to demonstrate flow patterns over the entire image area is an enormous benefit where the vascular anatomy is complex. The flow information with colour Doppler is relatively crude, giving only the mean velocity, and for quantitative studies it is used as a road map to guide positioning of the pulsed Doppler gate for more detailed velocity information regarding the flow.

Diagnostic applications

As a general rule any soft tissue organ or structure that can be accessed free of bone or gas can be usefully examined by ultrasound.

NEONATAL BRAIN

The presence of the fontanelles provides ideal natural bone-free ultrasound windows for demonstration of the brain in the neonate. High-frequency sector format probes (5–7.5 MHz) with a small footprint provide the ideal transducer with which a series of sagittal and coronal sections can be obtained. The normal ventriclar system can be seen well, along with the white matter and sulci.

The two main areas for investigation of the neonatal brain are assessment of ventricular size and congenital anomalies producing structural changes, and therefore hydrocephalus, agenesis of the corpus callosum, the Dandy Walker syndrome and holoprosencephaly can all be assessed fairly reliably (Fig. 9.1). The other major application is in the diagnosis and monitoring of intra-cerebral haemorrhage and ischaemia (Harwood-Nash and Floodmark, 1982). The mean width of the lateral ventricle in the term infant is 12 mm, and the ventri-cular/hemisphere ratio is less than 30%. Haemorrhage produces a focal area of high reflectivity, which is characteristically in the region of the germinal matrix in premature infants but may be elsewhere in mature infants. More recently, the detection of contusional tears, a characteristic of child abuse, has been described (Jaspan *et al.*, 1992).

CHEST

Ultrasound is strongly reflected by air/soft tissue interfaces and so, apart from echocardiography, ultra-sound of the chest has a limited role to play and only in conjunction with other imaging techniques. Ultrasound is essentially useful in further evaluating an opacity demonstrated on the chest X-ray, showing whether this is cystic or solid and providing a little more detail about the actual structure of the opacity demonstrated. Ultrasound may be particularly useful in guiding drainage of loculated pleural effusions. The relationship of the opacity to other structures within the chest may also be demonstrated.

ABDOMEN

Abdominal scanning forms the greatest proportion of paediatric ultrasound with a vast range of indications in

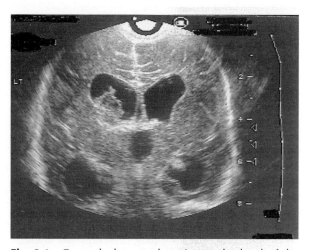

Fig. 9.1 Coronal ultrasound section at the level of the bodies of the lateral ventricles showing obvious hydro-cephalus. This is secondary to haemorrhage evidence which is seen in the left lateral ventricle.

many organs and systems within the abdomen. Ultrasound is perhaps at its most useful in answering a specific clinical question, for example: is pyloric stenosis present? The pylorus can be reliably imaged and the canal length and muscle thickness measured to give a definite answer one way or the other. However, the fact that ultrasound is non-invasive and so well tolerated by children also means that it is commonly used in a more general screening role to survey many of the intra-abdominal organs and exclude a major abnormality. Ultrasound is now the primary imaging technique in children presenting with an abdominal mass. Alongside the plain abdominal radiograph it will form the basis on which any further investigation is based. Approximately 50% of palpable abdominal masses in infants and children are renal and, as will be discussed below, this is an area where ultrasound performs particularly well.

GASTROINTESTINAL TRACT

In the gastrointestinal tract ultrasound may be used to demonstrate gastro-oesophageal reflux after feeding. The normal and mucosal layers of stomach and duodenum are visualized and any significant thickening is demonstrated, as in granulomatous disease (Gomes *et al.*, 1991).

Enteric duplication cysts of stomach or duodenum are clearly shown with ultrasound and these typically have a muscular wall helping to differentiate them from other abdominal cysts such as the choledochal cyst (Bar *et al.*, 1990). Ultrasound has become the preferred diagnostic method of infantile hypertrophic pyloric stenosis (IHPS). The usual technique is to scan the infant following a feed. The thickened pylorus is readily imaged.

The usual criteria for the diagnosis are a canal length of greater than 16 mm and a diameter of greater than 11 mm (Fig. 9.2). As in many situations the diagnosis is apparent by direct observation and measurements are hardly necessary (Davies *et al.*, 1992; Neilson and Hollman, 1994). In addition to the actual measurements the motility of the stomach and pylorus may be assessed. The superior mesenteric artery and vein normally lie in the same transverse plane, the vein to the right of the artery. In malrotation of the intestine the vein may be demonstrated to lie anterior or even to the left of the artery and this may be a useful diagnostic clue in this condition (Weinburger, *et al.,* 1992).

Ultrasound is extremely accurate in the diagnosis of intussusception. It is useful where the diagnosis is uncertain or to confirm the diagnosis prior to hydrostatic or pneumatic reductions. The typical findings on transverse section of the palpable mass are of alternating concentric rings of high and low reflectivity corresponding to the reflective mucosa and the oedematous muscle of the bowel (Verschelden *et al.*, 1992) (Fig. 9.3).

The normal appendix can rarely be imaged in children but with care the inflamed appendix may be reliably demonstrated with gentle compression scanning over the right iliac fossa. The characteristic appearances are of an oedematous blind-ending tubular structure of greater than 6 mm in diameter that does not compress. The complications of appendicitis such as a pelvic abscess or appendix abscess are usually well demonstrated with ultrasound. As in the appendix, thickened oedematous areas of bowel from many causes may also be usefully documented and this is particularly true of inflammatory bowel disease such as Crohn's disease (Puylaert, 1986; Hayden *et al.*, 1992).

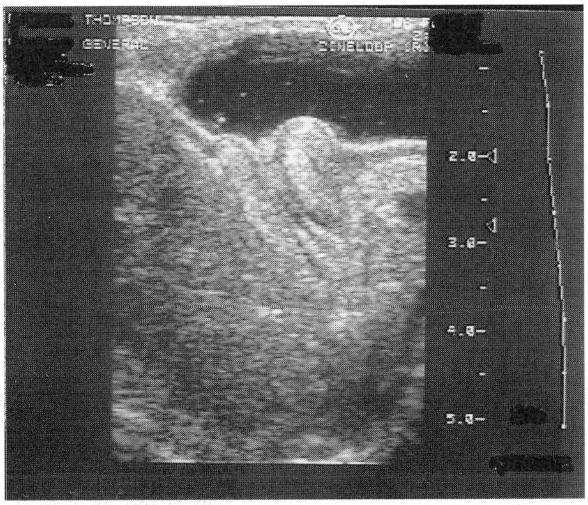

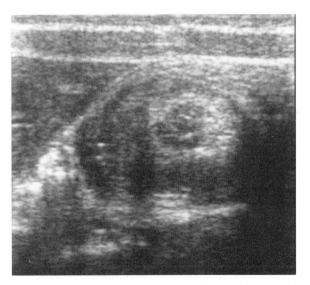

Fig. 9.2 Infantile hypertrophic pyloric stenosis. The canal length is nearly 2 cm and the diameter 14 mm. Fluid is seen in the gastric antrum.

Fig. 9.3 Ileal colic intussusception showing the typical appearances of concentric rings of high and low reflectivity.

LIVER AND BILIARY SYSTEM

The appearances of the liver and biliary system do not differ greatly from those of the adult, with ready indentification of a normal, even parenchymal reflectivity, the hepatic and portal vessels and the gallbladder.

The liver size is usually assessed by eye, with measurements playing little role. Hepatomegaly and alteration of the overall liver reflectivity are features of diffuse parenchymal liver disease. In acute hepatitis from many causes the ultrasound appearances may be normal or a diffuse poorly reflective pattern may be seen with accentuation of the periportal tracts within the liver. Apart from excluding the presence of extrahepatic biliary obstruction, ultrasound is of little clinical value in acute hepatitis. The differentiation between biliary atresia and hepatitis may be particularly difficult in the neonate. The demonstration of a normal gallbladder and common hepatic duct may be important findings in this respect. Increased reflectivity of the liver is most commonly associated with fatty infiltration. Increased reflectivity is also seen in cirrhosis and fibrosis but here the pattern is usually uneven and coarse with very nodular irregular outline to the liver. This may be a pattern seen, for example, associated with cystic fibrosis. Portal hypertension may follow intrahepatic or extrahepatic obstruction and Doppler ultrasound may be useful to sample the portal vein blood flow and to grade and follow up the portal hypertension. Collateral vessels may also be visualized.

Focal liver lesions are usually readily demonstrated, as they contrast with the surrounding normal liver tissue (Fig. 9.4). Benign focal liver lesions include cysts, abscesses, cavernous haemangiomas and adenomas. Malignant liver lesions include primary liver tumours and metastatic disease (Boechat *et al.*, 1985).

The gallbladder is identified in all normal neonates and the common hepatic duct in the majority. In older infants and children it should always be possible to identify these structures if there is adequate access.

Obstructive jaundice in childhood is ideally investigated with ultrasound. A complete and specific diagnosis is often possible. The obstruction is most likely to be associated with a choledochal abnormality including choledochal cyst and biliary calculi (Fig. 9.5).

The spleen and pancreas are readily identified in children and, as in adults, trauma, inflammation and tumour infiltration may all be assessed and followed with ultrasound.

ADRENAL GLAND

The adrenals are often more easily demonstrated in neonates and in young children than in adults, owing to their relatively large size. In neonates it is often possible to identify the cortex and medulla of the gland separately, which is very unusual in adults. The large adrenal gland of the neonate undergoes a reduction in size following birth. The vessels of the primitive adrenal cortex become distended and are prone to haemorrhage. The exact cause of haemorrhage in neonates is unknown, but stress, birth trauma anoxia and systemic disease are all implicated. Infants usually present within 2–7 days of birth. The appearances are characteristic and serial ultrasound may show resolution of the haemorrhage. Neuroblastoma is one of the most common tumours of childhood, with 80% occurring in children under 5 years of age and one-third presenting under 2 years of age. The great majority of neuroblastomas arise in the adrenal medullary tissue and are usually well demonstrated with ultrasound but must be distinguished from the other common childhood abdominal tumour, the

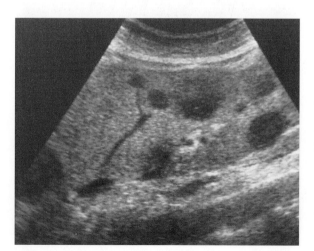

Fig. 9.4 Multiple poorly reflective liver metastases. The background liver texture shows evidence of fatty infiltration.

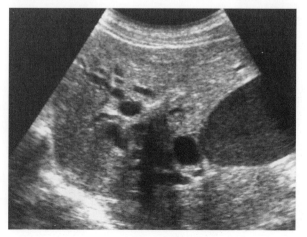

Fig. 9.5 Obstructive jaundice with evidence of intrahepatic bile duct dilatation and distension of the gallbladder secondary to a choledochal cyst.

Wilm's tumour. Neuroblastomas are typically heterogeneous with areas of high reflectivity and calcification. The margins typically are ill-defined and the tumour may often cross the midline enveloping the great vessels (Yeh, 1988).

RENAL TRACT

Ultrasound has a central role in the investigation of the renal tract, having replaced the majority of intravenous urograms (IVUs) performed in children. It now forms the basis for virtually all further imaging. The kidneys are clearly seen from the supine and the prone position, and the younger and smaller the child the more likely the prone position is to be particularly suitable for imaging and measuring the kidneys (Han and Babcock, 1985). The bladder is seen from the supine position. The size, position and axis of the kidneys are documented. The cortical thickness, the differentiation of cortex from medulla and the smoothness of the renal outlines are all demonstrated and documented.

The separation of the renal pelvis can be reliably measured, particularly in the transverse section, The size and shape of the bladder, together with the wall thickness and the lower most portion of the ureters, will usually be demonstrated. With colour Doppler the jets of urine passing from the ureteric orifices into the bladder can be demonstrated and assessed and this may be a useful observation in assessing obstruction.

Congenital renal anomalies related to the structure and position of the kidneys are usually adequately demonstrated with ultrasound. Even tiny renal cysts are sensitively demonstrated with ultrasound and, not suprisingly, ultrasound therefore plays a major role in the differentiation and classification of cystic renal disease, which includes multicystic renal dysplasia, infantile polcystic renal disease and adult type poly-

cystic renal disease as well as the renal cystic disease associated with tuberose sclerosis (Parienty *et al.*, 1981) (Fig. 9.6). Special attention is paid to the size and number of cysts, their distribution and the overall size of the kidneys. Any change or loss of corticomedullary differentiation should be noted in addition to the distension of the renal collecting system.

An increase in the reflectivity of the renal cortex is a finding corresponding with medical renal disease but ultrasound, while sensitive in the detection of this, is very non-specific. There are many causes, the most common of which is glomerulonephritis. Calcification is readily recognized on ultrasound as an area of markedly increased reflectivity often associated with distal acoustic shadowing. In the kidneys both nephrolithiasis and nephrocalcinosis show typical features (Brenbridge *et al.*, 1986) (Fig. 9.7).

Urinary tract infections are common in infants and children. It is usual for investigation to be made after the first proven urinary tract infection. The precise protocol undertaken will vary from unit to unit but ultrasound will usually be the first investigation, having a role in confirming or excluding a predisposing structural abnormality as a cause for the urinary tract infection (Ben Ami, 1984). Scarring may also be demonstrated with ultrasound but this is usually more reliably evaluated with the isotope scan.

The Wilms' tumour is the most common childhood abdominal tumour. Most are diagnosed before 5 years of age. Most present with a large palpable abdominal mass and up to one-third of patients have haematuria. Differentiation from a neuroblastoma is usually possible on the basis of the ultrasound findings. Other renal tumours are less common but are also well demonstrated with ultrasound (Cremin, 1987).

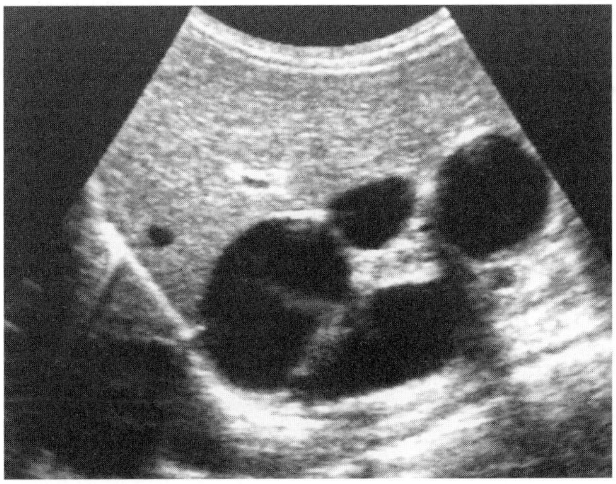

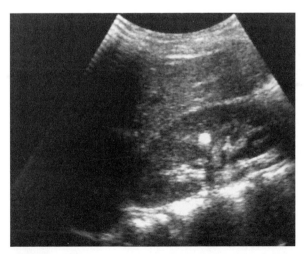

Fig. 9.6 Typical example of multicystic renal dysplasia in the neonate.

Fig. 9.7 Reflective renal calculus in the central part of the right kidney showing a little distal acoustic shadowing. There is no associated upper tract dilatation.

The full length of the ureter is not often shown with ultrasound, except when it is markedly dilated. However, the renal pelvis and calyces are reliably demonstrated, as are the lower ureters at the ureterovesical junction. The diagnosis of upper tract dilatation if readily made and documented by measuring the anteroposterior diameter of the renal pelvis in a transverse scan. This should not exceed 10 mm in an infant and in the normal situation will in practice rarely be greater than 5 mm in diameter (Tsai *et al.*, 1989).

THE PELVIS

The role of ultrasound in imaging the genital tract in infants and girls has expanded rapidly in recent years. With care, the normal uterus and ovaries, although small, can with care be demonstrated from the neonatal period onwards and so abnormalities are usually obvious (Fig. 9.8). These include ovarian cysts and tumours, and haematometra and haematocolpos at puberty. Other less common lesions within the pelvis may also be demonstrated.

SUPERFICIAL SCANNING

Over recent years there have been signficant technical improvements in high-frequency transducers which has led to greatly improved resolution for imaging structures within a few centimetres of the transducer face. This has widened the application of ultrasound for imaging organs such as the testes, thyroid and salivary glands, or any palpable superficial mass such as a branchial cyst. The normal testis and epididymis can be clearly seen, and so any textural change, mass or surrounding fluid may be demonstrated. The increasing sensitivity of colour Doppler on modern machines means that, in addition to the visualization of the testis, the blood flow to the testis may be assessed and this is

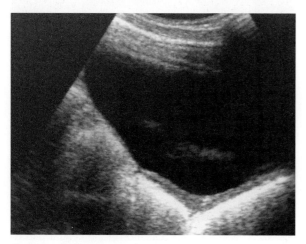

Fig. 9.8 Midline saggital section in a 3-year-old showing the typical normal appearances of the infantile uterus.

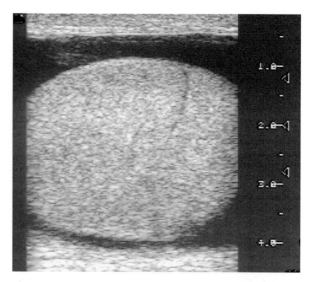

Fig. 9.9 Longitudinal scan through a normal testis in an 11-year-old boy. A tiny hydrocoele is also present.

proving to be valuable in the diagnosis of inflammatory conditions and torsion of the testis, particularly in cases where there is clinical doubt (Fig. 9.9). The texture and size of the salivary glands and the thyroid gland can be documented and the relationship of these structures to any palpable masses within the neck ascertained. Normal lymph nodes are rarely demonstrated with ultrasound; however, enlarged lymph nodes may be readily recognized.

MUSCULOSKELETAL SYSTEM

This group of applications follows directly on from the comments on the preceding paragraph. Muscles, tendons and joints may all be imaged with ultrasound. The results of trauma to muscles and tendons such as haematoma and rupture may be demonstrated, as well as the development of bursae such as the semimembranosus bursa in children (Fig. 9.10). In the neonate the hip joint is composed of cartilage. This does not show on X-rays but can be clearly seen with ultrasound. This has led to the widespread use of ultrasound in the assessment of congenital dislocation of the hip (Fig. 9.11). It may be used not only as a diagnostic test and a monitor of treatment but also as a population screening test for the detection of congenital dislocation of the hip and of hip dysplasia. In addition to demonstrating the hip itself, the detection of fluid in the hip joint is an important application for ultrasound in children. In this context it is used to assess the child with a limp. If fluid is demonstated, guided aspiration can be performed to determine whether this is infected.

VASCULAR IMAGING

Over recent years colour and spectral Doppler has

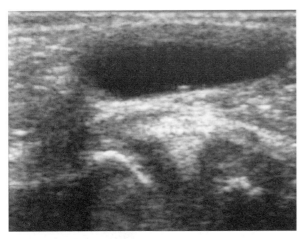

Fig. 9.10 Longitudinal scan in the popliteal fossa showing a small semimembranosus bursa.

become more widely available and the system sensitivity has increased, leading to more widespread applications. Nowhere is this more true than in echocardiology, which has now replaced many of the invasive catheter studies previously necessary to evaluate congenital heart disease. The major vessels throughout the body, such as the carotid arteries, aorta and femoral arteries, are all readily demonstrated and flow can be assessed. The velocity of flow can be measured and the degree of any stenotic lesion evaluated by measuring changes in the velocity. Major veins are also imaged and flow is assessed, which has particular applications in the diagnosis of renal vein thrombosis and deep vein thrombosis within the calf and leg veins. In organ transplants of liver and kidney a major postoperative concern is the integrity of the vascular anastomoses. Colour Doppler has proven to be the ideal first-line investigation for

assessment of the vascular supply. The ability to demonstrate the normal vascular supply to the testis, particularly in older children, has meant that ultrasound may be valuable in the assessment of torsion of the testis. This is an established role in young adults and as equipment sensitivity increases it is likely that this will assume more significance in paediatric practice. In the demonstration of tumours, Doppler ultrasound may add further information regarding the tumour vascularity in addition to allowing assessment of the tumour mass in relation to normal vascular structures. This may, for example, be particularly important in assessing the operability of neuroblastoma extending across the midline. The sensitivity of vascular assessment is now such that it is becoming feasible to image areas of infarction in, for example, the brain and kidneys. The development of ultrasound contrast agents will increase the sensitivity of Doppler still further and is likely to lead to further development of this type of application for colour Doppler.

Intervention

Ultrasound is, above all, a dynamic and interactive imaging tool and it is this aspect that is such a great asset in paediatric practice. It is also the same features that have made ultrasound a very suitable method for guiding all types of interventional procedures. Ultrasound almost provides an extension to the palpating fingers. Complex anatomy can be traced from plane to plane, providing truly three-dimensional information fairly rapidly. The tip of a biopsy needle or drainage catheter can be followed in real-time as it is inserted into a lesion (Fig. 9.12). The major groups of applications include guided biopsies of any masses that are demonstrated,

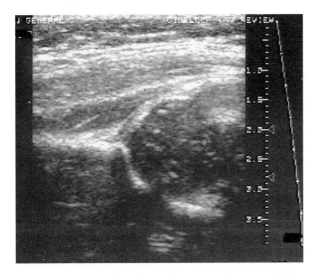

Fig. 9.11 Coronal section of a normal neonatal hip showing a normal deep acetabular cup.

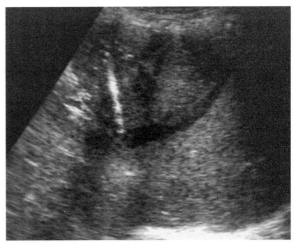

Fig. 9.12 Abscess in the right lobe of the liver into which a needle has been inserted for aspiration. Note the reflective needle track.

particularly in the liver, but in any situation where the lesion in question can be visualized. Ultrasound is routinely used as the guiding method for renal biopsy. The placement of catheters in abscesses within the liver and elsewhere in the abdomen and guidance for the placement of nephrostomy tubes are all readily and regularly undertaken using ultrasound guidance.

Conclusion

Since the mid-1980s ultrasound has become one of the most widely used diagnostic tests, and nowhere is its role more universal or important than in paediatric practice.

References

Bar, L.L., Hayden, C.K., Stansberry, S.C. and Swischuk, L.E. 1990: Enteric duplication cysts in children: are their ultrasonic wall characteristics diagnostic? *Paediatric Radiology* **20**, 326–8.

Ben Ami, T. 1984: The sonographic evaluation of urinary tract infections in children. *Seminars in Ultrasound CT MR* **5**, 19–34.

Boechat, M.A., Kangarloo, H. and Gilsanz, V. 1985: Hepatic masses in children. *Seminars in Roentgenology* **154**, 83–90.

Brenbridge, A.N., Chevalier, R.L. and Kaiser, D.I. 1986: Increased renal cortical echogenicity in paediatric renal disease: histopathologic correlations. *Journal of Clinical Ultrasound* **14**, 595–600.

Comes, H., Lallemand, A. and Lallemand, P. 1991: Ultrasound of the gastro-oesophageal junction. *Paediatric Radiology* **23**, 94–9.

Cremin, B.J. 1987: Wilms' tumour: ultrasound and changing concepts. *Clinical Radiology* **38**, 465–74.

Davies, R.P., Linke, R.J., Robinson, R.G., Smart, J.A. and Hargreave, C. 1992: Sonographic diagnosis of infantile hypertropic pyloric stenosis. *Journal of Ultrasound Medicine* **11**, 603–5.

Han, B.K. and Babcock, D.S. 1985: Sonographic measurements and appearances of normal kidneys in children *American Journal of Radiology* **145**, 611–16.

Harwood-Nash, D.C. and Floodmark, O. 1982: Diagnostic imaging of the neonatal brain: Review and protocol. *Americal Journal of Neuroradiology* **3**, 103–15.

Hayden, C.J., Jr, Kuchelmeister, J. and Lipscomb, T.S. 1992: Sonography of acute appendicitis in childhood: perforation versus non-perforation. *Journal of Ultrasound Medicine* **11**, 209–16.

Jaspan, T., Narborough, C., Punt, J.A.G. and Lowe J. 1992: Cerebral contusional tears as a marker of child abuse – detection by cranial sonography. *Paediatric Radiology* **22**, 237–45.

Neilson, D. and Hollman, A.S. 1994: The ultrasonic diagnosis of infantile hypertropic pyloric stenosis: technique of accuracy. *Clinical Radiology* **49**, 246–7.

Parienty, R.A., Pradel, J.M. and Imbert, M.C. *et al.* 1981: Computed tomography of multilocular cystic nephroma. *Radiology* **140**, 135–9.

Puylaert, J.B.C.M. 1986: Acute appendicitis: US evaluation using graded compression. *Radiology* **158**, 355–60.

Tsai, T.C., Lee, H.C. and Huang, F.Y. 1989: The size of the renal pelvis on ultrasonography in children. *Journal of Clinical Ultrasound* **17**, 647–51.

Verschelden, P., Filiatrault, D., Garel, L. *et al.* 1992: Intussusception in children: reliability of US in diagnosis – a prospective study. *Paediatric Radiology* **184**, 741–4.

Weinberger, E., Winters, W.D., Liddel, R.M., Rosenbaum, D.M. and Krauter, D. 1992: Sonographic diagnosis of intestinal malrotation in infants. *American Journal of Radiology* **159**, 825–8.

Yeh, H.C. 1988: Ultrasonography of the adrenals. *Seminars in Roentgenology* **23**, 250–8.

Further reading

Cosgrove, D., Meire, H. and Dewbury, K. (eds) 1993: *Abdominal and general ultrasound*, vols 1 and 2. Edinburgh: Churchill Livingstone.

CHAPTER 10

Isotope renography

V. BATTY

Introduction
Radionuclides
Radiopharmaceuticals
Technique

Clinical applications
Conclusions
References
Further reading

Introduction

Paediatric diagnostic imaging has developed rapidly since the 1970s. Significant advances in gamma camera and computer technology, together with the evolution of new nuclear medicine radiopharmaceuticals, have resulted in procedures that are minimally invasive, sensitive and above all safe.

Isotope renography has been at the forefront of these developments. Structural and functional data are acquired simultaneously, fulfilling a need for accurate diagnostic information not easily obtainable by other means. The active components of modern pharmaceuticals are present only in trace quantities and have no pharmacological action. They also cause no haemodynamic or osmostic effects, which is clearly advantageous in the investigation of renal disease. Furthermore, they do not provoke potentially serious allergic reactions, unlike conventional radiographic contrast media. As a result, isotope renography is a safe procedure which can be performed on severely ill children as well as premature and newborn infants.

There is an increasing public awareness of the hazards of exposure to ionizing radiation. This is of particular concern in paediatric imaging because children are significantly more sensitive than adults in this respect. It is, therefore, reassuring that the absorbed dose to the whole body and to the urinary tract for the majority of procedures is comparable with and often less than the alternative radiological examination.

Radionuclides

TECHNETIUM (Tc)

The vast majority of nuclear medicine procedures utilize ^{99m}Tc as the radionuclide tracer. It is a non-toxic and relatively pure gamma emitter with a short 6-hour half-life and no significant particulate emission. These characteristics are responsible for a relatively low radiation dose. ^{99m}Tc is widely available as an elute of sodium pertechnetate from commercial generator systems and is then readily labelled to a variety of compounds to form radiopharmaceuticals that allow specific organs, systems or disease processes to be studied.

IODINE (I)

Two radionuclides of iodine are used for imaging. ^{131}I has a long half-life and emits beta-particles. This results in a relatively high radiation dose and it is, therefore, rarely used for paediatric diagnostic imaging. ^{123}I has a half-life of 13 hours and is essentially a pure gamma emitter like technetium. However, unlike technetium, it requires a cyclotron for its production and is considerably more expensive as well as less freely available.

Radiopharmaceuticals

^{99m}Tc-DIETHYLENETRIAMINEPENTA-ACETIC ACID (^{99m}Tc-DTPA)

Following intravenous injection, ^{99m}Tc-DTPA is rapidly distributed through the extra-cellular space and excreted rapidly by glomerular filtration. Reasonable images of the renal parenchyma and collecting system images are obtained over the first few minutes of the study and quantitative analysis of the delivery, parenchymal uptake and clearance of the radiopharmaceutical provides a number of useful parameters for assessment of renal function. It is also possible to measure simultaneously the glomerular filtration rate (GFR) (Russell and Dubovsky, 1989).

ORTHO-IODO HIPPURATE (^{131}I-HIPPURAN)

^{131}I-Hippuran is rapidly excreted, predominately by tubular secretion (approximately 80%) and the remainder by glomerular filtration. This rapid clearance makes hippuran a better agent than DTPA because high-resolution images can be obtained with a lower radiation dose to the patient. It is also particularly useful in patients with impaired function, such as those with renal transplants. However, the cost and limited availability of ^{123}I restrict the use of ^{123}I-hippuran in the majority of centres.

^{99m}Tc-DIMERCAPTOSUCCINIC ACID (^{99m}Tc-DMSA)

^{99m}Tc-DMSA is initially bound to plasma proteins following intravenous injection. It has a strong affinity for the proximal convoluted tubular cells where it becomes firmly bound to sulphhydryl groups. Some 60–70% of the injected activity is found in the renal cortex within 6 hours of injection and very little is excreted in the urine. DMSA thus provides relatively high-resolution images of the renal cortex. There is also a very good correlation between the relative renal accumulation of DMSA and the effective renal plasma flow measured by other means, providing a useful measure of differential renal function.

^{99m}Tc-MERCAPTOACETYLTRIGLYCINE (^{99m}Tc-MAG-3)

^{99m}Tc-MAG-3 is a recently developed radiopharmaceutical which has similar excretion characteristics to hippuran but with the advantage of accepting a technetium label. Early studies suggest that ^{99m}Tc MAG-3 offers generally superior image quality and imaging statistics, allowing the study of renal morphology, perfusion and excretion function in a single study (Eschima and Taylor, 1992; Itoh *et al.*, 1993a).

Technique

STATIC RENOGRAPHY

Static renography or renal parenchymal imaging provides anatomical information regarding the number, size, shape and position of the kidneys as well as quantitative measure of differential function. It does not permit study of the renal collecting systems, ureters or bladder.

^{99m}Tc-DMSA is the radiopharmaceutical of choice and useful images are obtained 2 hours after intravenous administration. The child should be well hydrated and no effort should be spared to ensure that he or she is comfortable and in a calm environment. Sedation and immobilization may be required for younger children to reduce movement artefact.

Imaging is performed in the seated or supine position, depending on the age of the patient, and images are acquired routinely in the anterior, posterior and posterior-oblique projections. There are no significant side-effects or after-effects from the procedure, but it is important for parents and ward staff to remember that the urine will be radioactive for the next 24 hours or so and that some caution is required in its handling and disposal. A normal DMSA study is shown in Fig. 10.1.

DYNAMIC RENOGRAPHY

Dynamic renography adds the dimension of time to static imaging. Following a bolus injection, sequential images are obtained at 15 s intervals for 20–30 min, monitoring the delivery of tracer to the kidney, transit through the parenchyma and elimination via the pelvicalyceal system and ureter. Each of the images is stored digitally as an array of numbers and each element of the array is usually referred to as a pixel (picture element). Renogram (= time/activity) curves can then be constructed for the whole kidney and for various regions within the kidney. These data allow the derivation of useful indices of function, particularly relating to vascular supply, cortical function and drainage. Renal clearance can also be quantified during the study, either by measuring the change in activity in blood samples or by quantifying renal uptake by scintigraphy alone. The GFR and effective renal plasma flow (ERPF) can be calculated from these measurements.

The sensitivity of this technique in the assessment of the dilated upper urinary tract is considerably enhanced by challenging the kidneys with the increased urine flow produced by a diuretic. Frusemide (furosemide) in a suitable paediatric dose (0.3–0.5 mg/kg) is usually satisfactory and my personal preference is to administer this half way through the study, thus allowing the drainage characteristics of the kidneys to be observed before and after the challenge.

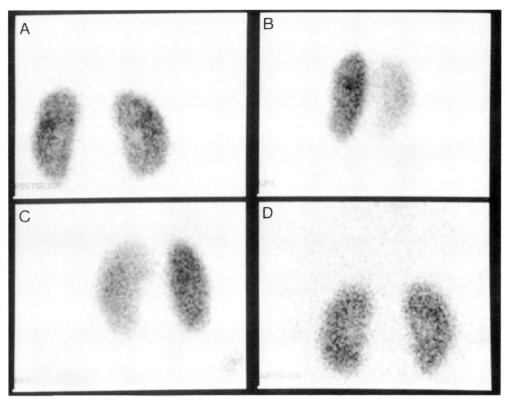

Fig. 10.1 Normal static ^{99m}Tc DMSA study. Images obtained 2.5 hours after injection: (a) posterior; (b) left posterior oblique; (c) right posterior oblique; (d) anterior. Note the normal splenic impression (curved arrow) and relatively cold hilar zone, representing the renal pelvis.

^{99m}Tc-DTPA has been the most widely used radio-pharmaceutical for dynamic renography but new compounds such as ^{99m}Tc-MAG-3 have significant advantages and will replace DTPA in the future.

Image data are acquired from the posterior projection only and the same attention to details of technique, patient comfort, immobilization and aftercare is required as for the DMSA study.

Analogue images may be obtained at the same time as digital data acquisition or may be reconstructed from the digital data when the study has been completed. Following the first pass of the bolus there is a rapid increase in activity within the renal parenchyma which peaks at about 3 min. The pelvicalyceal system usually becomes apparent between 2 and 4 min. The ureters are visualized intermittently, if at all, in the well-hydrated patient. Activity appears in the bladder at about 4 min after injection and increases throughout the study, at the same time as cortical activity declines.

Normal analogue images and renogram (= time/activity) curves are shown in Fig. 10.2.

CYSTOGRAPHY

Assessment of the bladder may be required to detect the presence of vesicoureteric reflux. This can be per-formed directly by introducing tracer into the bladder via a urethral catheter, or indirectly at the end of a standard dynamic renogram when most of the tracer has been eliminated from the kidneys. Indirect radionuclide cystography is by far the preferred method as the direct technique offers little advantage over a standard micturating cystogram performed in the X-ray department. The indirect method is non-invasive and much better tolerated by the patient. The information it provides is also likely to be more physiological. The main disadvantage is that residual activity in the kidneys may obscure minor degrees of reflux.

Clinical applications

The main indications for isotope renography are:

- obstructive uropathy
- recurrent urinary tract infection and vesicoureteric reflux
- renal vascular disease
- congenital anatomical anomalies
- evaluation of the transplanted kidney
- trauma
- investigation of renal mass lesions.

OBSTRUCTIVE UROPATHY

This is the most important and widely accepted indication for dynamic renography as upper urinary tract dilatation is a relatively frequent finding in children. Diuretic renography is extremely helpful in distinguishing those patients with true anatomical obstruction from those with other conditions that cause a dilated collecting system, such as idiopathic megaureter, baggy extrarenal pelvis, severe vesicoureteric reflux and the sequelae of previously corrected obstructive uropathy or reflux (Freeman and Blaufox, 1992).

It is important that the patient is well hydrated. In normal children or those with a dilated unobstructed system there will be a rapid response to diuretic and the pelvicalyceal system will be seen to empty properly on the analogue images. In the obstructed patient, there will be little or no response resulting in unchanged or increasing activity within the kidney on the analogue image and a rising renogram curve. The contrasting findings in dilated obstructed and unobstructed systems are shown in Fig. 10.3, which should be compared with the normal study (Fig. 10.2).

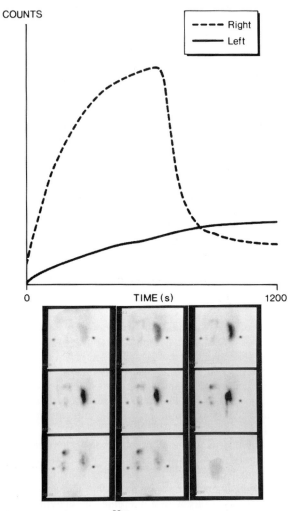

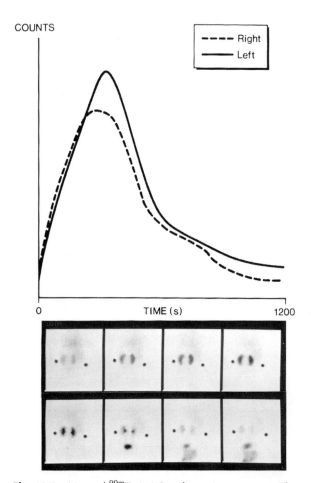

Fig. 10.2 Normal ^{99m}Tc MAG-3 dynamic renogram. The analogue images demonstrate rapid parenchymal uptake and excretion over 20 min. This is reflected in the normal shape of the renogram curves. Note activity in the heart, liver and spleen on the early images immediately after injection, and in the diaper at the end of the study.

Fig. 10.3 Abnormal ^{99m}Tc MAG-3 renogram. The right pelvicalyceal system and proximal ureter are shown and there is a good deal of retained activity on the early images. However, this clears rapidly after diuretic administration and this is reflected in a sudden change in the renogram curve. This pattern indicates dilatation without significant obstruction. Activity gradually accumulates within the left kidney over the course of the study and is still present within a hugely dilated renal pelvis 60 min after injection. This is reflected in a gradually rising renogram curve, with no response to diuretic. This is the typical pattern of severe obstruction, in this case at the pelviureteric junction.

URINARY TRACT INFECTION AND VESICOURETERIC REFLUX

Micturating cystourethrography is the established investigation for the assessment of vesicoureteric reflux. It has the advantage of good anatomical detail, but it is both unpleasant for the child and unphysiological. Direct radionuclide cystography shares some of the disadvantages of the X-ray technique, in particular, the need for urethral catheterization. Anatomical detail is relatively poor but, as with many radionuclide techniques, it is very sensitive to pathology, i.e. minor degrees of reflux. The radiation exposure is also considerably less than for micturating cystourethrography.

Indirect radionuclide cystourethrography avoids the need for urethral catheterization and is carried out as part of a routine diuretic renogram. However, it requires a good deal of patient co-operation and is unlikely to be successful in children under the age of 5 years. It is also significantly less sensitive than the direct radiological or radionuclide techniques in that reflux will only be detected during micturition and in volumes sufficient to be detected against the background of residual excreted activity in the ureters.

The effects of severe reflux and/or urinary tract infection on the renal parenchyma can be accurately assessed with a cortical study using ^{99m}Tc-DMSA. It is now generally accepted that the static DMSA renogram is a more sensitive indicator of renal scarring than either intravenous urography or ultrasonography (Verberig *et al.*, 1988) and there is also the advantage that a measure of divided function is available at the same time. An example of severe cortical scarring is shown in Fig. 10.4.

RENAL VASCULAR DISEASE

The standard diuretic renogram is frequently normal even when there is a significant degree of renal artery stenosis, because of the actions of the compensatory renin–angiotensin mechanism. There may be some decreased function by the affected kidney but this is a non-specific finding. Pharmacological challenge with captopril may temporarily interfere with the compensatory mechanism and induce significant and characteristic changes in the renogram pattern (Mann *et al.*, 1991; Itoh *et al.*, 1993b). However, this investigation is not without hazard and its place in the investigation of renovascular disease is still controversial.

Renal vein thrombosis results in typical renogram features of enlarged but non obstructed kidneys with markedly reduced function. It is seldom used as the

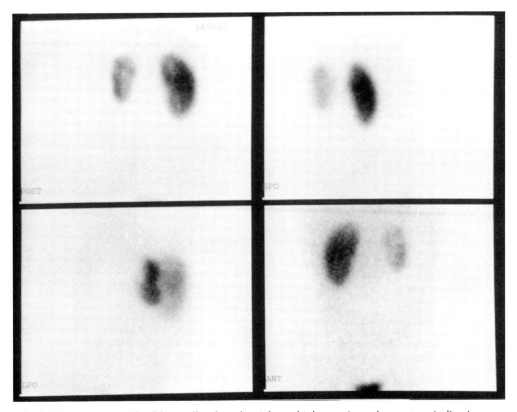

Fig. 10.4 The left kidney is considerably smaller than the right and it has an irregular contour indicating severe cortical scarring. There is also a small scar at the upper pole of the right kidney.

primary diagnostic test but may have a place in the follow up and monitoring of renal function with the development of collateral veins and recanalization of the thrombus.

CONGENITAL AND ANATOMICAL ABNORMALITIES

Congenital renal abnormalities are the most common cause of an abdominal mass in the neonate. The specific diagnosis usually requires a combination of imaging modalities. Static DMSA renography is extremely useful in identifying ectopic renal parenchyma and for assessing the differential function of renal moieties prior to surgery.

EVALUATION OF RENAL TRANSPLANTS

The sensitivity of isotope renography is a major of advantage in the follow up of transplant patients. Very small changes in function can be detected and the need for more invasive radiological procedures may be avoided. The combination of ultrasonography and renography provides an accurate diagnosis in patients with mechanical disorders of the transplant, i.e. vascular or ureteral obstruction, extravasation, reflux and perinephric collections. ^{99m}Tc-MAG-3 or ^{131}I-hippuran are the radiopharmaceuticals of choice for transplant patients because of their superior excretion and imaging characteristics in patients with impaired renal function.

Isotope renography may not provide a specific diagnosis in early parenchymal disorders due to ischaemia or rejection, but serial studies remain useful in monitoring changes in function of the at-risk kidney.

TRAUMA

Isotope renography is not a first-line investigation in renal trauma. The kidney is rarely damaged in isolation and modern cross-sectional imaging techniques allow the simultaneous evaluation of other important abdominal structures. However, a dynamic renogram may be indicated if renal injury is suspected. It provides a relatively non-invasive way of assessing renal perfusion and excretory function in the damaged kidney as well as confirming the presence of a normally functioning contralateral kidney.

INVESTIGATION OF RENAL MASS LESIONS

In general, isotope renography has been superseded by cross-sectional imaging techniques, such as ultrasound, X-ray computed tomography and magnetic resonance imaging. However, it still has a place in the investigation of renal pseudo-tumours and, in particular, lobar dysmorphism (column of Bertin).

Conclusions

Isotope renography is a sensitive, non-invasive and cost-effective investigation. It is the primary investigation of choice in many children with renal disease. The development of new radiopharmaceuticals and improved technology will increase the scope of isotope renography in the future but close co-operation between nuclear medicine physicians, radiologists and their clinical colleagues remains vital to the development of objective imaging strategies designed to solve the clinical problem.

References

Eshima, D. and Taylor, A., Jr 1992: ^{99m}Tc (mercapto-acetyl-triglycine): update on the new ^{99m}Tc renal tubular function agent. *Seminars in Nuclear Medicine* **22**, 61–73.

Freeman, L.M. and Blaufox, M.D. (eds) 1992: Well-tempered diuresis renography: its historical development, physiological and technical pitfalls and standardised technique protocol. *Seminars in Nuclear Medicine* **22**, 74–84.

Itoh, K., Tsukamoto, E., Kakizaki, H., Nonomura, K. and Furudate, M. 1993a: Comparative study of renal scintigraphy with ^{99m}Tc mercapto-acetyltriglycine and ^{123}I ortho-iodo hippurate. *Nuclear Medicine Communications* **14**, 653–7.

Itoh, K., Tsukamoto, E., Nagao, K., Nakaba, K., Kanagae, K. and Furudate, M. 1993b: Captopril renoscintigraphy with Tc-^{99}m (DTPA) in patients with suspected renovascular hypertension: prospective and retrospective evaluation. *Clinical Nuclear Medicine* **18**, 463–71.

Mann, S. L., Pickering, T.G. and Sos, T.A. *et al.* 1991: Captopril renoscintigraphy in the diagnosis of renal artery stenosis: accuracy and limitations. *American Journal of Medicine* **90**, 30–9.

Russell, C. D. and Dubovsky, E. V. 1989: Measurement of renal function with radionuclides. *Journal of Nuclear Medicine* **30**, 2053–7.

Verberig, M.R., Strudley, M.R. and Meller, S.T. 1988: ^{99m}Tc dimercapto-succinic-acid (DMSA) scan as first investigation of urinary tract infection. *Archives of Disease in Childhood* **63**, 1320–5.

Further reading

Fogelman, I. and Maisey, M. 1988: *An atlas of clinical nuclear medicine*. London: Martin Dunitz.

Slovius, L., Sty, J. and Haller, J. 1989: *Imaging of the paediatric urinary tract*. London: W.B. Saunders.

Webb, S. (ed.) 1985: *The physics of medical imaging*. Bristol: Adam Hilger.

CHAPTER 11

Transport of sick infants and children

P.J. McHUGH AND M.D. STRINGER

Introduction
Preparation for transfer
The transfer

Transport of patients with specific
surgical conditions
The receiving hospital
References

Introduction

With the development of paediatric intensive care units and the recommendation that specialist paediatric surgery is undertaken in regional centres, there has been an increasing demand for the transfer of sick infants and children for investigation and treatment (British Paediatric Association, 1993). Most children who suddenly develop a life-threatening illness or sustain severe trauma will be stabilized in their local hospital but will then require transport to a tertiary centre. Interhospital transfer may be hazardous and result in the clinical deterioration of critically ill children (Kanter et al., 1992). Transport medicine has evolved as a subspecialty, principally amongst neonatologists, anaesthetists and intensivists (Aoki and McCloskey, 1992; Jaimovich, 1996) but the essentials of optimum paediatric transport are fundamentally important to all paediatric surgeons working in tertiary centres.

Preparation for transfer

Transport of a sick child or infant needs detailed planning and careful evaluation of the potential benefits of transfer and the likely risks involved in transport. *In utero* transfer is superior to optimum postnatal transfer, particularly for very low birth weight babies and those with life-threatening neonatal surgical problems

(Lubchenco et al., 1989). For other critically ill patients, the referring unit must ensure the following (Henning, 1992):

- the airway must be fully assessed and protected by endotracheal intubation if necessary
- the child should be maximally resuscitated and stabilized prior to departure
- two reliable and secure routes of venous access should be in place
- maintenance of fluid balance, blood glucose and temperature
- adequate nasogastric tube drainage
- appropriate baseline investigations have been performed, e.g. routine blood count, electrolytes, blood group and cross-match (and maternal blood with neonates) and relevant plain radiographs
- a signed consent form authorizing any necessary surgery
- effective communication with the accepting unit or transport team and with the patient's family.

It is the responsibility of the receiving unit to advise on the best method of transport for the patient. Not all patients need the services of a specialized transport team and the configuration of the team may need to be tailored according to the type of transfer. Various authors have attempted to define a severity of illness score applicable to paediatric transport but the validity of these is uncertain (Bion et al., 1985; Pollack et al., 1988;

Kanter and Tompkins, 1989). It has been shown that it is possible to predict the need for a physician in only 72% of referrals (McCloskey and Johnson, 1990).

The transfer

The choice of transport vehicle is dictated by geography, population density and weather. In the UK most transfers are by road ambulance (Fig. 11.1) but in many countries transfer by rotor wing or fixed wing aircraft is necessary. Any vehicular transport imposes restrictions on space, access, excessive noise and vibration. Suboptimal lighting and temperature control are other considerations. The design and securing of monitoring equipment to the vehicle need to be specifically considered. Maximum patient stability must be achieved prior to departure since specialized procedures, such as endotracheal intubation, are difficult in transit. Secondary deterioration due to underlying pathology, the transfer itself or limitations of ongoing treatment must be minimized. Common reasons for secondary deterioration are inadequate circulatory and ventilatory support, inadequate monitoring, equipment failures, errors in drug administration and temperature instability (Barry and Ralston, 1994; Bennett, 1995) These prob-

lems are more likely to occur when patients are escorted by staff without adequate training and experience and when there has been little preparation for transfer (Macnab, 1991). This is one reason for the development of dedicated transport teams, which have now been shown to be effective (American Academy of Paediatrics, 1986; Gentleman *et al.*, 1993; SCCM, 1993; Edge *et al.*, 1994).

The team, comprising at least one senior doctor and an experienced sick children's nurse, is despatched to the referring unit, and assesses and stabilizes the child who is then transported under optimum conditions. On arrival, the retrieval team must obtain details of the history, investigations and previous resuscitation at the same time as making a careful but rapid assessment of the child's condition. Resuscitation is continued in preparation for the transfer and this may take several hours if maximum stability is to be achieved (Henning, 1992). Analgesia and sedation should be decided before transfer. If a retrieval service is not available, the patient should be accompanied by a senior doctor and a trained children's nurse or anaesthetic assistant familiar with advanced life-support measures. A useful checklist for transfer is detailed in Table 11.1 (Barry and Ralston, 1994; Macrae, 1994). The adult principle of 'scoop and run' is almost never necessary in paediatric practice.

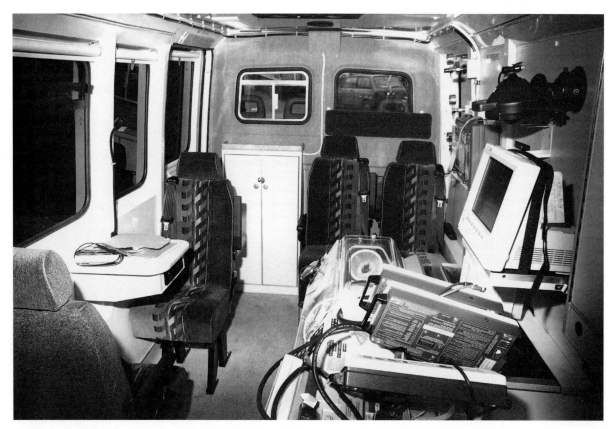

Fig. 11.1   Interior of a modern paediatric transport ambulance.

Table 11.1 Predeparture checklist for critically ill children (Barry and Ralston, 1994; Macrae, 1994)

Airway	Intubate if not secure
Check ET tube secure and correctly positioned (chest X-ray)	
Check suction equipment	
Cervical spine immobilized?	
Breathing	Note ventilator settings
Satisfactory blood gas?	
Adequate supply of oxygen for transfer	
Consider pneumothorax	
Circulation	Fully resuscitated?
Two secure intravenous cannulae	
Adequate fluids for journey? (blood, colloid, crystalloid)	
Drugs	Working weight?
Sedation/analgesia?	
Blood glucose?	
Emergency drugs available?	
Monitoring	Equipment working? Alarms set?
Spare batteries?	
Tubes	Nasogastric tube: adequate size, correctly sited, on free drainage
Urinary catheter (unconscious/sedated and diuretics)	
Arterial cannula secure?	
Chest drain secure and connected to Heimlich valve and drainage bag	
Temperature	Incubator/ambulance heating on?
Temperature monitoring in place	
Communication	Parents fully informed/consented
Aware of final destination	
Copies of notes/radiographs/charts/results	
Receiving unit informed	

Furthermore, excessive speed may risk further injury and compound the difficulties of providing ongoing care. The ambulance crew is best placed to consider optimum routes of travel.

Airway problems should be anticipated and endotracheal intubation is advisable if there is doubt. Except in patients with a basal skull fracture, significant coagulopathy, or nasal obstruction, nasotracheal intubation allows more secure fixation and causes less discomfort but it does require additional expertise. A range of airway and ventilatory equipment including self-inflating bags, masks, airways, laryngoscopes and endotracheal tubes, humidifiers, portable suction apparatus and oxygen supplies must be available. Items for vascular access should include intraosseous needles. There should be a heated transport cot or incubator (Fig. 11.2) and appropriate equipment and drugs. Hypothermia is a particular hazard in neonatal transfers and core temperature must be maintained above 35°C.

Equipment should be checked daily and on return from any journey. Oxygen cylinders, batteries and drug stocks should be fully maintained and safely stored. A selection of equipment, drugs and intravenous fluids (both crystalloid and colloid solutions) for different ages should be carried and monitors and syringe pumps should be battery operated. Full monitoring should be possible during transit. In addition to clinical assessment, this includes invasive and non-invasive measures of arterial pressure, pulse oximetry, electrocardiography (ECG), core temperature measurement and pressure transducers for central venous and intracranial pressure readouts.

Air transport poses particular problems. Acceleration and deceleration surges may have adverse effects on cardiovascular stability and intracranial pressure (Lauritzen *et al.*, 1987; Andrew *et al.*, 1990). Reductions in oxygen saturation and tensions and the expansion of gas in air-filled cavities secondary to

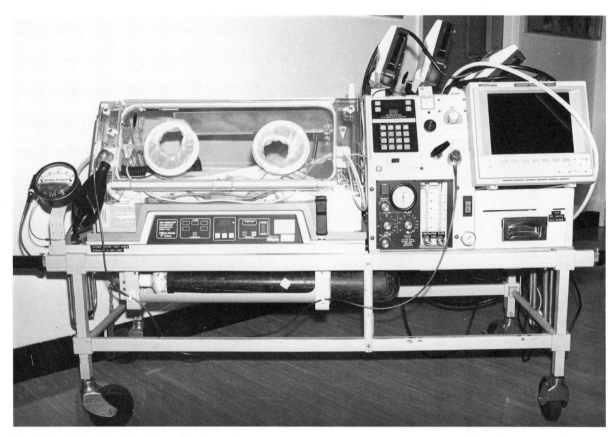

Fig. 11.2 'Trailblazer' incubator for neonatal transport.

the decrease in atmospheric pressure are additional risks. Endotracheal tube cuffs and urethral catheter balloons may be affected and should be filled with saline. Inflatable splints should be avoided and plaster casts should be split as tissue oedema can be severe. Gravity drip feed sets perform variably and infusion pumps are more efficient. Expansion of gas can be a problem in the chest, abdomen or cranial cavity. Cold and decreased humidity must be anticipated. Specific monitoring equipment may not be allowed because of interference with the aircraft's electrical systems. The pilot's decisions are paramount during the transfer.

Transport of patients with specific surgical conditions

GASTROSCHISIS

This condition imposes additional problems due to major heat and fluid loss from the exposed bowel. Temperature control and colloid replacement are essential together with adequate nasogastric tube decompression to prevent abdominal distension and pulmonary aspiration. In one retrospective study which included 31

patients transferred postnatally, complications due to inadequate nasogastric drainage, hypothermia and hypovolaemia were recorded in one-third of cases (Stringer *et al.*, 1991). Guidelines for the transport of a neonate with gastroschisis are detailed in Table 11.2 and they are largely applicable to the transfer of many other neonates requiring surgery. The exposed viscera should be gently wrapped and supported on the infant's abdomen with several layers of transparent plastic sheeting ('cling film'). This is safer than placing the infant's lower half in an intestinal bag, which does not avoid the danger of mesenteric injury or venous congestion of the unsupported, highly mobile bowel.

NECROTIZING ENTEROCOLITIS

Infants with necrotizing enterocolitis requiring transfer are usually critically ill with sepsis and shock, often associated with intestinal perforation. Aggressive resuscitation prior to departure and during transport may include colloid, blood and crystalloid infusion, intermittent positive pressure ventilation and inotropic support, correction of acidosis, sedation and paralysis, broad-spectrum antibiotics and nasogastric drainage. T-cryptantigen status must be determined prior to

Table 11.2 Guidelines for postnatal transfer in gastroschisis (Stringer *et al.*, 1991)

Early liaison with neonatal surgical unit and transport team

Adequately sited 8–10 FG nasogastric tube on free drainage with quarter hourly aspiration

Double 'cling film' wrap of the abdomen to cover and support exposed viscera

Colloid infusion (at least 20 ml/kg) followed by maintenance crystalloid requirements and replacement of nasogastric losses

Broad-spectrum prophylactic antibiotics

Meticulous temperature control in transport incubator

Consent for surgery/intramuscular vitamin K/maternal blood sample (to check for passively acquired maternal antibodies)

Rapid transport of the infant following initial resuscitation

transfusion of blood products in order to avoid potentially fatal haemolytic complications (Novak *et al.*, 1993). Insertion of an abdominal drain under local anaesthesia can be a useful temporizing measure, serving to decompress the abdomen and improve ventilation (Cheu *et al.*, 1988). This is a particularly valuable procedure in the unstable very low birthweight infant and, on occasions, may avoid the need for subsequent surgery (Ein *et al.*, 1990).

OESOPHAGEAL ATRESIA WITH TRACHEO-OESOPHAGEAL FISTULA

The well baby with oesophageal atresia and a distal tracheo-oesophageal fistula (TOF) should be transported in a slightly head up and prone position to minimize gastro-oesophageal reflux but with a Replogle tube in the upper pouch to provide continuous drainage of secretions. The infant with respiratory problems requiring endotracheal intubation and ventilation is particularly at risk and requires emergency transfer. Mechanical ventilation is relatively ineffective because of the TOF and gaseous distension of the stomach compounds the difficulties. Urgent transfer and emergency ligation of the fistula are essential (Malone *et al.*, 1990). A gastrostomy alone may be fatal.

CONGENITAL DIAPHRAGMATIC HERNIA

The infant with respiratory difficulty or poor gas exchange should be intubated and ventilated for transfer. Full sedation and paralysis will minimize the risks of barotrauma. Inotropic and volume support are frequently necessary for those presenting within hours of birth. Nasogastric drainage is mandatory. Acute deterioration may be due to a pneumothorax and equipment for intercostal drainage must be available. When facilities exist, the receiving centre should be prepared for the possibility of urgent extracorporeal membrane oxygenation (Atkinson *et al.*, 1991).

INTUSSUSCEPTION

Although relatively common, this condition can be deceptively hazardous and there is often little appreciation of the degree of decompensation that may occur in transit. Venous access should be with secure, large bore cannulae to enable the rapid transfusion of large volumes of colloid and inotropic support may be required. Nasogastric decompression and broad-spectrum antibiotics are necessary. Oxygenation, peripheral perfusion and blood glucose should be monitored frequently. An analysis of childhood deaths from intussusception demonstrated that as many as 60% of deaths were avoidable. Inadequate fluid resuscitation and hazardous transfers were contributory factors (Stringer *et al.*, 1992).

TRAUMA

Patients with multiple trauma should be triaged at the referring hospital after a primary survey. Criteria for transfer are based on (i) interhospital factors, (ii) physiological parameters such as Glasgow Coma Score, blood pressure and respiratory rate, and (iii) circumstances and mechanism of injury which predict major injury (American College of Surgeons, 1989). The airway should be secured and in cases of potential cervical spine injury, the neck must be immobilized (American College of Surgeons, 1989; Burg and Fleischer, 1993). At least two large-bore venous access routes should be established, and central venous and arterial access should be considered early. Adequate volume resuscitation is mandatory before transfer. Injuries that can be stabilized, operatively or non-operatively, by the local institution must be treated prior to transport. This may even require laparotomy for control of intra-abdominal haemorrhage. Intrathoracic bleeding should similarly be controlled. Before departure, long bone fractures should be splinted, adequate analgesia administered and tetanus and antibiotic prophylaxis given.

Criteria for transferring children with head injuries have been documented elsewhere (Gentleman *et al.*, 1993). Reviews of such children transferred to neurosurgical centres have revealed avoidable factors contributing to death or morbidity. Identified avoidable factors were found in 32% of 81 children dying from head injury in one UK health region (Sharples *et al.*, 1991). Significant problems during transfer included inadequate management of the airway and hypovolaemia due to neglected additional injuries. Head-injured patients with cerebral injury should be intubated and hyperventilated for transfer and a cervical collar applied, even if plain radiographs of the cervical spine appear normal. Other than a deteriorating or poor conscious level, reasons for endotracheal intubation include bleeding into the mouth from a skull base fracture and seizures. The guidelines of the local neurosurgical unit should be followed concerning diuretics, intravenous fluids and medications.

The receiving hospital

On receiving the patient from the transfer team, the accepting physician should ensure that the child is stable. They should then briefly review all the necessary documentation, information, and test results. The parents should be familiarized with the medical and nursing staff, and with the ward procedures. Any likely interventions should be explained, and the consent form checked and revised if necessary. Blood grouping, and crossmatching if necessary, should be organized. The records of any transfer should be retained for audit purposes and any problems encountered should be discussed with the teams involved.

There is increasing evidence to suggest that a dedicated retrieval service improves the outcome of critically ill children requiring interhospital transfer (Edge *et al.*, 1994). Various scoring systems have been devised to evaluate a transported infant's condition but they have not yet proved sufficiently robust for routine clinical practice (Hermansen *et al.*, 1988; Leslie and Stephenson, 1994).

References

American Academy of Pediatrics. 1986: Guidelines for air and ground transportation of pediatric patients. *Pediatrics* **78**, 943–50.

American College of Surgeons, 1989: Advanced Trauma Life Support Manual. Chicago, IL: American College of Surgeons.

Andrew, P., Piper, I., Deardon, N. *et al.* 1990: Secondary insults during intrahospital transport of head-injured patients. *Lancet* **335**, 330–4.

Aoki, B. and McCloskey, K. 1992: *Evaluation, stabilization and transport of the critically ill child.* St Louis, MO: Mosby Year Book.

Atkinson, J.B., Ford, E.G., Humphries, B. *et al.* 1991: The impact of extracorporeal membrane support in the treatment of congenital diaphragmatic hernia. *Journal of Pediatric Surgery* **26**, 791–3.

Barry, P.W. and Ralston, C. 1994: Adverse events occurring during interhospital transfer of the critically ill. *Archives of Disease in Childhood* **71**, 8–11.

Bennett, N.R. 1995:Transfer of the critically ill child. *Current Paediatrics* **5**, 4–9.

Bion, J.F., Edlin, S.A., Ramsay, G., McCabe, S. and Ledingham, I.M. 1985: Validation of a prognostic score in critically ill patients undergoing transport. *British Medical Journal* **291**, 432–4.

British Paediatric Association 1993: The transfer of infants and children for surgery. The Report of the Joint Working Group. British Paediatric Association.

Burg, J.M. and Fleisher, G.R. 1993: Prehospital care of the injured child. In: Eichelberger, M.R. (ed.), *Pediatric trauma.* St Louis, MO: Mosby Year Book, 99–112.

Cheu, H.W., Sukarochana, K. and Lloyd, D.A. 1988: Peritoneal drainage for necrotizing enterocolitis. *Journal of Pediatric Surgery* **23**, 557–61.

Edge, W.E., Kanter, R.K., Weigle, C.G.M. and Walsh, R.F. 1994: Reduction of morbidity in interhospital transport by specialized pediatric staff. *Critical Care Medicine* **22**, 1186–91.

Ein, S.R., Shandling, B., Wesson, D. and Filler, R.M. 1990: A 13-year experience with peritoneal drainage under local anesthesia for necrotizing enterocolitis perforation. *Journal of Pediatric Surgery* **25**, 1034–7.

Gentleman, D., Deardon, M., Midgley, S. and MacLean, D. 1993: Guidelines for the resuscitation and transport of patients with serious head injury. *British Medical Journal* **306**, 547–52.

Henning, R. 1992: Emergency transport of critically ill children: stabilisation before departure. *Medical Journal of Australia* **156**, 117–24.

Hermansen, M.C., Hasan, S., Hoppin, J. and Cunningham, M.D. 1988: A validation of a scoring system to evaluate the condition of transported very-low-birth-weight neonates. *American Journal of Perinatology* **5**, 74–8.

Jaimovich, D. 1996: *Handbook of paediatric and neonatal transport medicine.* St Louis, MO: Mosby Year Book.

Kanter, R.K. and Tompkins, J.M. 1989: Adverse events during interhospital transport: physiologic deterioration associated with pretransport severity of illness. *Pediatrics* **84**, 43–8.

Kanter, R.K., Boeing, N.M., Hannan, W.P. *et al.* 1992: Morbidity associated with interhospital transport of pediatric emergencies. *Pediatrics* **90**, 893–8.

Lauritzen, J.B., Lendorf, A., Vesterhauge, S. and Johansen, T.S. 1987: Heart rate responses to moderate linear body acceleration; clinical implications in aerodynamical evacuation. *Aviation Space Environmental Medicine* **58**, 248–51.

Leslie, A.J. and Stephenson, T.J. 1994: Audit of neonatal intensive care transport. *Archives of Disease in Childhood* **71**, F61–6.

Lubchenco, L.O., Butterfield, L.J., Delaney-Black, V., Gold-son, V., Koops, B.L. and Lazotte, D.C. 1989: Outcome of very-low-birth-weight infants: does antepartum versus neonatal referral have a better impact on mortality, morbidity, or long-term outcome? *American Journal of Obstetrics and Gynecology* **160**, 539–45.

Macnab, A.J. 1991: Optimal escort for interhospital transport of pediatric emergencies. *Journal of Trauma* **31**, 205–9.

Macrae, D.J. 1994: Paediatric intensive care transport. *Archives of Disease in Childhood* **71**, 175–8.

Malone, P.S., Kiely, E.M., Brain, A.J., Spitz, L. and Brereton, R.J. 1990: Tracheo-oesophageal fistula and pre-operative mechanical ventilation. *Australian and New Zealand Journal of Surgery* **60**, 526–7.

McCloskey, K.A. and Johnson, C. 1990: Critical care interhospital transports: predictability of the need for a paediatrician. *Paediatric Emergency Care* **6**, 89–92.

Novak, R.W., Abbott, A.E. and Klein, R.L. 1993: T-cryptanti-gen determination affects mortality in necrotizing enterocolitis. *Surgery Gynecology and Obstetrics* **176**, 368–70.

Pollack, M.M., Ruttimann, U.E. and Getson, P.R. 1988: The Paediatric Risk of Mortality (PRISM) Score. *Critical Care Medicine* **16**, 1110–16.

SCCM, ACCCM, AACCN Guidelines committee 1993: Guidelines for the transfer of critically ill patients. *Critical Care Medicine* **21**, 931–7.

Sharples, P.M., Storey, A., Aynsley-Green, A. and Eyre, J.A. 1991: Avoidable factors contributing to death of children with head injury. *British Medical Journal* **300**, 87–91.

Stringer, M.D., Brereton, R.J. and Wright, V.M. 1991: Contro-versies in the management of gastroschisis: a study of 40 patients. *Archives of Disease in Childhood* **66**, 34–6.

Stringer, M.D., Pledger, G. and Drake, D.P. 1992: Childhood deaths from intussusception in England and Wales, 1984–1989. *British Medical Journal* **304**, 737–9.

CHAPTER 12

Day surgery for children

J.D. ATWELL

Introduction
Historical
Definition
Accommodation and facilities
Selection of operations suitable for
day-case treatment

Anaesthesia for day patients
Preselection visits to a day unit
Financial implications
Postoperative care in the home
Standards for day care
Conclusions
References

Introduction

Since the 1950s there have been many changes in the practice of the specialty of paediatric surgery both in the range and in the results of surgical treatment. Advances in neonatal surgery due to improvements in paediatric anaesthesia, biochemical control with micro-methods and intensive care with the use of ventilators immediately come to mind. There have also been changes in the management of the more routine general surgical conditions, the most striking being an increase in day surgery for children.

Historical

At the turn of the century the admission of an infant or child was associated with a mortality from intercurrent infection. One of the first pioneers of day surgery was Nicol, who in 1909 reported a series of 8988 patients treated between 1899 and 1909 in the outpatient depart-ment of the Glasgow Royal Hospital for Sick Children. The series included 406 for hare lip and cleft palate, 36 for spina bifida, 18 for congenital pyloric stenosis and 220 for inguinal and umbilical hernia.

Nicol (1909) made five points about day surgery for children and his conclusions are still valid today although the reasons for his conclusions may have changed:

1. A much larger share of the operating work of a children's hospital should be handled on an out-patient basis, for the treatment of a large number of inpatients is a waste of the resources of a children's hospital or ward.
2. Patients treated in the outpatient operating theatre should be largely infants and young children because 'such young children with their wounds closed by a collodion or rubber plaster are easily carried home in their mother's arms and rest there more quietly on the whole than anywhere else'.
3. Separation of the child from the mother is harmful.
4. Preoperative skin preparation is unnecessary.
5. 'Experience of herniotomy, abdominal section and other operations in young children treated as out patients is gradually reconciling me to the view that we keep similar cases in adults too long in bed'.

Another factor which was stimulating Nicol's resolve at that early stage of his career was that he was denied the use of inpatient facilities!

The next 50 years passed with very little published material but in 1964 Lawrie reported his results on operating on young children as day cases and a year later a report appeared describing the experiences of a home care unit which was hospital based (Bergman et al., 1965).

The National Association for the Welfare of Children in Hospital (NAWCH) (now Action for Sick Children) published their charter for children and the first criterion was: 'Children shall be admitted to hospital only if the care they require cannot be equally well provided at home or on a day basis'. This along with reports by the Audit Commission (1990) and the Value for Money Unit (DHSS, 1989) has led to the expansion of facilities for day surgery in children and adults.

Definition

The following definition is used (Commission on the Provision of Surgical Services, 1985): 'Attending as a non resident patient for operative procedure and who requires some form of supervision, preparation or period of recovery involving the provision of accommodation and services'.

Originally, day case patients were admitted overnight i.e. a 24-hour stay. This is unnecessary and the current practice is to admit a patient during the day or part of the day. If an overnight stay is required the patient is then transferred to an inpatient area, i.e. he or she undergoes a formal inpatient admission.

The accurate recording of day case admissions is essential and should always be maintained separately from the inpatient statistics of a unit. It should also exclude minor operative procedures undertaken on a ambulatory basis in accident and emergency and outpatients departments.

Accommodation and facilities

There are three methods of performing day case surgery for children:

- designated children day unit (Atwell *et al*., 1973)
- use of inpatient beds for day care
- use of beds in designated adult day unit.

There can be no doubt that the first option is the ideal arrangement for children provided that there are sufficient patients. There are many advantages of such a unit, in particular that the ethos is child orientated and patients are not admitted alongside adults and are kept separate from acutely ill patients. One disadvantage is that taking day patients away from the inpatient ward leaves patients with a higher dependency in the ward, thus increasing the stress levels for the inpatient staff. A final advantage of the designated children's day unit is that the staff develop the expertise of day care, which is different from the inpatient expertise but equally rewarding.

The second option at least allows the child to be nursed in a child-orientated environment but has the disadvantages of a day case patient being nursed adjacent to an acutely ill patient, with the danger of the day patient becoming a second-class patient (CCHS,

1991). Also, the pressure on beds may lead to cancellations or undue waiting times for a bed when admitted, problems that are all avoidable in the designated children's day unit.

The third option, of admitting children to designated adult day units, has little to recommend it, as paediatricians, paediatric surgeons, nurses and managers believe that the facilities are not suitable for children. This aspect will be considered again when discussing operating facilities in a district hospital.

SIZE

The size of a children's day unit depends on the demand and its manageability. Four to ten beds are sufficient for most units and the size is in part dependent on whether investigations (endoscopy, etc.) for medical patients are admitted as well as those undergoing day surgery. Five designated day beds would allow up to 2500 admissions each year.

LOCATION

The day unit should be in close proximity to the operating theatre, thus reducing portering time. This also allows parents to accompany their children to the anaesthetic room (CCHS, 1991).

RECEPTION AREA

This is necessary for the patients and parents as an area where they may wait whilst completing admission procedures.

ANAESTHETIC ROOM

A standard anaesthetic room is required with good lighting. The risks of day case anaesthesia are no less than anaesthesia for inpatients and therefore the facilities required are comparable. It is excellent policy to allow one of the parents into the anaesthetic room with their child during induction of anaesthesia.

OPERATING THEATRE

The operating theatre is standard and the same equipment is required as for an inpatient operating theatre. The management of theatre use for day cases varies from unit to unit depending on the facilities available. The possibilities are:

1. day cases performed on routine operating lists
2. day cases mixed with adults in a specified day case theatre
3. specified lists for day cases of children in custom-designed adult day units
4. day cases in a large children's hospital which may have a designated day theatre.

Methods 1 and 4 are satisfactory, method 2 is not recommended, and the third method is used by general surgeons in district hospitals and is reasonable. It is unreasonable to mix day case children with adults unless the designed day unit has separate facilities for children and adults.

RECOVERY AREA

This is a high care area and must be suitably staffed and equipped as the management of the unconscious patient is the same whether they are recovering from minor or major surgery.

Other areas which are required are (Commission on the Provision of Surgical Services, 1992):

• day unit office
• dirty and clean utilities
• lavatories for children, parents and staff
• sister's office
• staff changing room
• storage area
• facilities for refreshments
• play area
• space for teaching (nurses and undergraduates).

Selection of operations suitable for day-case treatment

Three criteria are relevant to the choice of an operative procedure as a day case (CCHS, 1991):

1. The anaesthetic and operating time should not exceed 40 min.
2. The risk of complications from the operative procedure should be low.
3. The postoperative care at home should be manageable by the parents, possibly with the help of community nurses.

The general surgical and urological procedures suitable for day care management are seen in Table 12.1. In some centres the list has been extended to include excision of thyroglossal cysts, branchial sinuses and minor repairs of hypospadias, but many surgeons may elect to keep these patients in overnight.

Anaesthesia for day patients

The anaesthetist should be responsible for the final check on the child's fitness for operation, although prior examination and history taking has been performed by the junior medical staff. Painful procedures should be reduced to the minimum, i.e. the use of local anaesthetic creams prior to venepuncture. The anaesthetist

Table 12.1 Operations suitable for day case treatment

Inguinal hernia
Umbilical hernia
Epigastric hernia
Ligation of communicating hydrocele
Unilateral orchidopexy
Bilateral orchidopexy
Circumcision
Meatotomy
Minor revision of hypospadias
Separation of preputial adhesions
Division of tongue tie
Proctoscopy and sigmoidoscopy
Examination under anaesthesia and sphincter stretch
Manual evacuation of faeces
Excision of local skin lesions, cysts, etc.
Gastroscopy
Oesophagoscopy
Cystoscopy
Submucosal infection of Teflon for vesico-ureteric reflux
Correction of bat ears
Excision of accessory auricles and digits

has the final say on whether a parent can accompany his or her child into the anaesthetic room. This form of management is to be encouraged but it must be realized that not all anaesthetists or all parents wish to be present at this anxious time.

Adequate postoperative analgesia is needed to ensure the relief of pain (Burn, 1979; Atwell and Spargo, 1992).

Preselection visits to a day unit

It is excellent practice for a child on the waiting list for day surgery to visit the unit prior to admission. The staff and the environment then become familiar which alleviates some of the anxieties of an admission to hospital. This method of management allows the parents to familiarize themselves with their duties and responsibilities before, during and after the operative procedure.

Travel time and method of travel on discharge have to be considered. Public transport is unsuitable following a general anaesthetic and if the parents do not have their own transport, the hospital must take the responsibility for suitable transport being available (CHSS, 1991).

Financial implications

Day-case surgery is cost-effective but may also be extremely expensive. This contradictory statement needs an explanation. The cost of each patient operated on as a day case is less than the same operative procedure being performed on an inpatient. The removal of the minor surgical cases from an inpatient waiting list relieves the pressure on inpatient beds. Ideally, for the same work load some in patient beds could be closed. However, with increasing demands these 'relieved' beds are utilized fully for more major surgery, hence the increased overall costs. This situation also increases the nursing load for the inpatient staff.

Postoperative care in the home

The surgical operations undertaken as day cases are relatively free of complications. The parents are given printed sheets of the care required for their child on discharge as well as receiving preoperative advice at the time of the initial consultation and during their child's admission. This form of management should also receive the support of visits by the (home) community nurses who are trained in paediatrics. In this way the whole episode of admission, operation and postoperative care should run smoothly, with minimal disturbance to the family and the child (Atwell *et al.*, 1973; Atwell, 1978; Gow and Atwell, 1980; Atwell and Gow, 1985).

Standards for day care

The report *Just for the day* by Caring for Children in the Health Services (CCHS, 1991) list 12 quality standards for day case admissions and 42 principles underlying the establishment of a children's day programme, and as these points are so important in providing and establishing day care for children they are quoted in full.

1. QUALITY STANDARDS

(i)   The admission is planned in an integrated way to include preadmission, day of admission and post-admission care and to incorporate the concept of a planned transfer of care to primary and/or community services.

(ii) The child and parent are offered preparation both before and during the day of admission.

(iii) Specific written information is provided to ensure that parents understand their responsibilities throughout the episode.

(iv) The child is admitted to an area designated for day cases and not mixed with acutely ill inpatients.

(v)   The child is neither admitted nor treated alongside adults.

(vi) The child is cared for by identified staff specifically designated to the day case area.

(vii) Medical, nursing and all other staff are trained for, and skilled in, work with children and their families, in addition to the expertise needed for day case work.

(viii) The organization and delivery of patient care are planned specifically for day cases so that every child is likely to be discharged within the day.

(ix) The building, equipment and furnishings comply with safety standards for children.

(x)   The environment is homely and includes areas for play and other activities designed for children and young people.

(xi) Essential documentation, including communication with the primary and/or community services, is completed before each child goes home so that the after-care and follow-up consultations are not delayed.

(xii) Once care has been transferred to the home, nursing support is provided, at a doctor's request, by nurses trained in the care of sick children.

2. PRINCIPLES UNDERLYING THE ESTABLISHMENT OF A CHILDREN'S DAY PROGRAMME

Environment

1. The site of the unit, in relation to the children's inpatient facilities and the operating theatre, should be determined by local circumstances. Any conflicting requirements of anaesthetists, surgeons, paediatricians and others should be considered in terms of the best interests of the child and family.

2. The design of the unit should allow the separation of day cases from inpatients.

3. The layout of the unit should reflect the fact that children arriving for elective procedures are generally in good health and require neither a bed nor trolley in the early stages of their admission.

4. Childproof fittings, furniture, equipment and storage should be installed to reduce the likelihood of danger to active children.

5. The unit should be decorated, furnished and equipped to provide a cheerful and homely environment for children.

6. Facilities should be provided to meet the needs of parents who will be at least as numerous as the children.

7. The unit should be equipped to ensure the clinical safety of patients following a general anaesthetic. The type of equipment should depend on the facilities provided in a central recovery unit.

8. The treatment room should be fitted with appropriately sized equipment to carry out biopsies, chemotherapy, plaster work and other procedures on a day basis. If general anaesthesia is to be administered in this treatment room, it should be equipped to the standard expected in operating theatres.

9. A telephone with a direct outside line should be available for fast communication between the unit, primary and community services and patients' homes.

Staff

1. A director should be designated for the day-case services to identify the limitations, translate the objectives into policies and monitor the service.
2. A day-unit manager should be appointed to have responsibility for the day-to-day administration of the unit. This should include the number and skill mix of nursing staff and co-ordination with other departments of the hospital and the community services.
3. Nursing staff trained in the care of sick children should be specifically designated to the day-case service.
4. In children's outpatient clinic, or one in which the majority of patients are children, nurses trained in the care of sick children should be employed, because of the importance of their educational role with families.
5. Health care assistants with appropriate training should be employed to assist nurses in the day unit.
6. Medical staff should be specifically assigned to be responsible for the care of day patients.
7. Play staff should be available to provide a play service for children of all ages.
8. Clerical staff should be available to handle the large amounts of administrative and clerical work generated in a day unit.

Organization of patient care

1. The children's day unit, regardless of its location, should be part of the comprehensive children's department, sharing its philosophy.
2. An advisory committee should represent those immediately concerned and form a permanent link with the primary and/or community services.
3. The director should hold discussions with the advisory committee to determine the scope of the procedures to be undertaken on a day basis.
4. A planned systematic approach for integrated patient care should be developed covering preadmission, day of admission and after discharge. The concept of planned transfer of care should be adopted.
5. The services should be designed for ambulatory care and should not depend on attitudes and practices developed for inpatient treatment.
6. An efficient booking system should ensure that both the hospital and the family have necessary information and efficient time to enable them to make preparations.

7. An efficient system of patient management and liaison with other departments should be established, so that children admitted as day cases can normally be discharged in the day.
8. Parents should be encouraged to be present throughout the day of admission. Written information should be available to prepare them for the responsible role they undertake.
9. Guidelines should be drawn up for parents who enter the operating suite.
10. Efficient administrative and management systems should ensure that discharge notes are given to the parents before they leave the hospital and relevant information is passed to primary and/or community services.
11. Managerial and clinical audit should be a regular part of the organization and delivery of patient care. Monitoring should also include the views of parents and older children.

Outpatient and preadmission period

1. The consultant should make the decision on whether to admit the child on a day basis, in co-operation with the family; if necessary the general practitioner and community staff should be involved.
2. The staff in the outpatient clinic and the day unit should jointly ensure that parents understand their role and responsibilities and are given verbal and written information to prepare for the admission, including care after discharge.
3. A preadmission programme should be provided for children as well as preparation on the day.

On day of admission

1. The management of day-case children should reflect the fact that most are not acutely ill on arrival.
2. A parent should be enabled to be with the child and help with the care whenever the child is conscious and should be given timely, ongoing information and support.
3. Every attempt should be made to eliminate or reduce the number of painful or frightening procedures and routines while the child is conscious and to keep the admission as pleasant as possible.
4. The anaesthetist should be responsible for the final check on the child's fitness for operation.
5. Anaesthetic and analgesic techniques appropriate to day patients should be used, and adequate postoperative pain relief should be ensured.
6. Nursing staff should take responsibility for mobilizing the child and monitoring that he is ready for discharge.
7. Nursing staff should ensure that parents understand written instructions on postoperative care, are clear on what constitutes an emergency and know how to get help.

8. The anaesthetist should see all children during the recovery period, in either the central recovery area or day unit and should have agreed the criteria and delegation for discharge from the day unit to home.
9. The surgeon or a member of his team should see all children following day surgery before discharge from the day unit.

Back at home

1. Parents should know where to seek medical help for both emergency and continuing health care.
2. When the child has returned home, nursing care and/or advice should be provided for the family, as necessary.

Conclusions

There can be no doubt about the success of day case surgery for the minor to intermediate general surgical conditions of childhood. In Southampton, where a designated children's day unit was established in 1969, over 25 000 patients have been treated, all under general anaesthesia. The success of such management depends on suitable selection of patients, short anaesthetics by experienced anaesthetists, proper facilities, as for inpatients, backup facilities for in patient admission if necessary and adequate follow-up care in the community. Many of the improvements in the surgical treatment of children have followed the efforts of the group Action for Sick Children (formerly NAWCH) (Action for Sick Children, 1994).

References

Action for Sick Children 1994: Setting standards for children undergoing surgery. London: Action for Sick Children.

Atwell, J.D. 1978: Changing patterns in paediatric surgical care. *Annals of the Royal College of Surgeons of England* **60**, 375–83.

Atwell, J.D. and Gow, M. 1985: Paediatric trained district nurse in the community: expensive luxury or economic necessity? *British Medical Journal* **291**, 227–9.

Atwell, J.D. and Spargo, P.M. 1992: The provision of safe surgery for children. *Archives of Disease in Childhood* **67**, 345–9.

Atwell, J.D., Burn, J.M.B., Dewar, A.K. and Freeman, N.V. 1973: Paediatric day case surgery. *Lancet* **ii**, 895–7.

Audit Commission 1990: A short cut to better services. Day surgery in England and Wales. London: HMSO.

Bergman, A.B., Shrand, H. and Oppe, T.E. 1965: A pediatric home care program in London: ten years' experience. *Pediatrics* **36**, 314–21.

Burn, J.M.B. 1979: A blue print for day surgery. *Anaesthesia* **34**, 790–805.

Commission on the Provision of Surgical Services 1985: *Guidelines for day case surgery* Royal College of Surgeons of England.

Commission on the Provision of Surgical Services 1992: *Guidelines for day surgery* (Revised ed.) Royal College of Surgeons of England.

DHSS 1989: *Study of day surgery facilities. Report on Stage One*. Study conducted by the Value for Money Unit of the DHSS.

Gow, M. and Atwell, J.D. 1980: The role of the children's nurse in the community. *Journal of Pediatric Surgery* **15**, 26–30.

Laurie, R. 1964: Operating on children as day cases. *Lancet* **ii**, 1289–91.

National Association for the Welfare of Children in Hospital *1991: Caring for children in the health services just for the day*. London: NAWCH.

Nicol, J.H. 1909: The surgery of infancy. *British Medical Journal* **ii**, 753–7.

CHAPTER 13

Paediatric anaesthesia

P.M. SPARGO AND H.M. MUNRO

Introduction
Applied anatomy and physiology
Applied pharmacology
General principles of anaesthetic management
Principles of neonatal anaesthesia
Anaesthetic considerations for neonatal
emergencies

Anaesthetic considerations for day
case surgery
Postoperative analgesia
Removal of inhaled foreign body
Epiglottitis and croup
References
Further reading

Introduction

Advances in modern medicine and surgery since the late 1980s have led to an increase in the survival of low birth weight and preterm babies (Macfarlane *et al.*, 1988; Albermann and Botting, 1991); resulting in an increase in the number of neonates who may require surgery. The type of surgical procedure ranges from a simple hernia repair in a former preterm baby with lung disease to the correction of a major congenital abnormality such as a tracheo-oesophageal fistula. A better understanding of neonatal physiology and pharmacology, together with improvements in anaesthetic care have helped to make such surgery possible.

Neonates, infants, children and adolescents have differing anaesthetic requirements and should not simply be considered as small adults. This chapter begins with a discussion of aspects of the anatomy and physiology of neonates of importance to anaesthetists. The general principles of the anaesthetic management of children of all age groups are then outlined, followed by a more detailed discussion of the principles of anaesthesia for neonates. The concluding section deals with anaesthesia for infants and older children, with special emphasis on day case surgery and analgesic techniques. A detailed discussion on postoperative care is beyond the scope of this chapter, although the early management of children presenting with acute upper airways obstruction is briefly outlined.

Applied anatomy and physiology

RESPIRATORY SYSTEM

There are major anatomical and physiological differences between neonates and older children which become less marked with age. Anatomical features of particular importance to the anaesthetist include the large occiput, relatively small jaw and large tongue of the neonate. The larynx is situated more cephalad and anterior, and the epiglottis is proportionately larger. The trachea is short and the cricoid cartilage, which is a circular ring of cartilage, forms the narrowest part of the upper airway.

The practical implications of these differences are that tracheal intubation, a prerequisite of neonatal anaesthesia, is potentially more difficult than in the adult. The ideal position for intubation is on a flat surface with the head supported in a headring and not on a pillow as recommended in the adult. A straight bladed laryngoscope is used to lift the epiglottis and visualize the larynx. The mucosa of the cricoid cartilage may be compressed and become ischaemic with subsequent stenosis if an oversized tracheal tube is used. It is essential to ensure that there is an audible leak around the tube (at an inflation pressure of approximately 20 cm of water). Endobronchial intubation must be avoided by careful auscultation of the chest.

The work of breathing is high in the neonate owing to high airway resistance and low lung compliance. They are obligatory nose breathers and a nasogastric tube adds greatly to the airway resistance. The relatively stiff lungs and compliant chest wall predispose to intercostal and sternal recession if airway obstruction occurs. The volume of gas in the lungs after a normal expiration is termed the functional residual capacity (FRC) and acts as an important reserve of oxygen. Metabolic rate, and thus oxygen consumption, are high in neonates and infants and these, in turn, lead to an alveolar ventilation rate which is two to three times that of adults. Should airway obstruction or apnoea occur, hypoxaemia develops much more rapidly in neonates and infants, despite adequate preoxygenation.

Neonates have barrel-shaped chests with horizontally placed ribs. The 'bucket handle' effect of downward sloping ribs, seen in older age groups, is absent in neonates so that tidal volume is fixed. Increases in alveolar ventilation are achieved almost entirely by increasing respiratory rate which is thus a good monitor of impending respiratory failure. Abdominal distension impedes movement of the diaphragm, reduces lung volume and leads to basal atelectasis and intrapulmonary shunting. Inadvertent gastric distension is common after mask ventilation and an orogastric tube should always be passed to decompress the stomach.

The control of breathing in the first weeks of life differs from that in older children. The response to hypoxia is an initial but transient increase in ventilation followed by respiratory depression. Apnoeic episodes may occur in preterm babies during rapid eye movement (REM) sleep, and may be due to immaturity of respiratory control mechanisms. Excessive relaxation of upper airway musculature during sleep may also be a causative factor. Predisposing factors include hypoglycaemia, hypoxia, hyperoxia, sepsis, anaemia, hypocalcaemia and environmental temperature (Schulte, 1977; Welborn *et al.*, 1991). Preterm and former preterm babies, especially those with a history of apnoea, are at greatest risk from life-threatening postoperative apnoea. It is postulated that general anaesthesia decreases the activation threshold of various immature reflex pathways in the upper airway that cause apnoea (Kurth *et al.*, 1989).

As a result of the anatomical and physiological factors discussed above, tracheal intubation and positive pressure ventilation are considered mandatory in neonates to avoid hypoxia due to airway obstruction, hypoventilation or shunting.

CARDIOVASCULAR SYSTEM

The heart rate of neonates ranges from 100 to 170 beats per minute and decreases with age, whereas blood pressure increases with age (Table 13.1). The neonatal myocardium is relatively non-compliant and stroke volume is fixed so that cardiac output is influenced

Table 13.1 Important circulatory variables with increasing age

Age	Heart rate (beats/min)	Blood pressure Systolic (mmHg)	Diastolic
Preterm	150±20	50±3	30±2
Term	133±18	67±3	42±4
6 months	120±20	89±29	60±10
1 year	120±20	96±30	66±25
2 years	105±25	99±25	64±25
3 years	101±15	100±25	67±23
5 years	90±10	94±14	55±9
12 years	70±7	109±16	58±9

Source: Miller (1986).

mainly by changes in heart rate. Bradycardia is associated with a marked fall in cardiac output and peripheral perfusion. The parasympathetic system is easily stimulated during induction of anaesthesia and airway instrumentation. The resultant bradycardia can be prevented by the administration of atropine. Unlike adults, neonates rapidly become bradycardic in the presence of hypoxia. The treatment of hypoxia-induced bradycardia is, in the first instance, correction of hypoxia by administering 100% oxygen.

CENTRAL NERVOUS SYSTEM

Babies have well-developed neuroanatomical pathways for the transmission of noxious stimuli (Anand and Hickey, 1987). Pain assessment is difficult in neonates, and distinguishing clinically between the response to pain and the response to hunger is not easy. The humane approach is to provide appropriate analgesia while being aware that neonates have a well-documented sensitivity to the respiratory depressant effects of opioid drugs (Lloyd-Thomas, 1990).

The retina is not fully vascularized until about 42 weeks postconceptional age and hyperoxia is associated with retinal vascular injury and retinopathy of prematurity (ROP). The level and duration of elevated arterial oxygen tension are more important risk factors than the inspired oxygen concentration (Flynn *et al.*, 1992). An arterial oxygen tension above 10.7 kPa (80 mmHg) should be avoided (Flynn *et al.*, 1992), although birth weight, gestational age, sepsis, hypotension, periventricular haemorrhage and twin birth are also implicated in the pathogenesis of ROP (Duker, 1992). Pulse oximeters do not detect hyperoxia, but in the majority of patients oxygen saturations between 87 and 96% correlate with arterial oxygen tensions between 6.7 and 10.7 kPa (50 and 80 mmHg) (Ramanathan *et al.*, 1987). Hypoxia, should of course, be avoided and concerns about ROP should not preclude the adequate preoxygenation of patients before laryngoscopy and intubation.

Periventricular haemorrhage (PVH) and periventricular ischaemia are more common in preterm infants (Sinha *et al.*, 1985), but may occur rarely in full-term neonates. Autoregulation of cerebral blood flow is certainly impaired in sick preterm infants (Lou *et al.*, 1979). It has been suggested that awake intubation may predispose to PVH by causing arterial hypertension. However, there are other risk factors for the development of PVH and anaesthetic technique has yet to be directly implicated (Charlton *et al.*, 1989).

HAEMATOLOGY

The blood volume at birth is estimated to be 70–90 ml/kg depending on the degree of placental transfusion (Table 13.2). The haemoglobin at birth is approximately 17.0 ± 2 g/dl and the level drops steadily until about 3 months of age (Table 13.3). Preterm babies have a greater fall in haemoglobin which lasts longer because of lower red cell survival and decreased production. Values of less than 10.0 g/dl at any age deserve investigation although not necessarily correction (Hatch and Sumner, 1989). Fetal haemoglobin makes up 75–80% of the total, with only small amounts remaining at 6 months of age.

HEPATIC AND RENAL SYSTEMS

The hepatic enzyme systems responsible for drug metabolism are immature in the neonate. Drugs such as

Table 13.2   Estimated circulating blood volume

Age	Volume (ml/kg)
Preterm	90–100
term, newborn	80–90
3 months–1 year	75–80
3–6 years	70–75
>6 years	65–70

Source: Motoyama and Davis (1990).

Table 13.3   Normal blood values

Age	Haemoglobin (g/dl)	Haematocrit (%)
1 day	19.0	61
7 days	17.9	56
4 weeks	14.2	43
2 months	10.7	31
3 months	11.3	33
6 months	12.3	36
1 year	11.6	36
4 years	12.6	38
8 years	12.9	40
10–12 years	13.0	40

Source: Miller *et al.* (1989).

barbiturates and opioids have a prolonged effect, and drugs with toxic effects such as digoxin, chloramphenicol and gentamicin require close monitoring. The liver is unable to deal adequately with the breakdown products of haemoglobin and unconjugated hyperbilirubinaemia may occur. Babies with 'physiological' jaundice tend to be sleepy and may have apnoeic episodes. Low birth weight infants are especially prone to hypoglycaemia because of low glycogen stores and synthesis of vitamin K-dependent clotting factors is insufficient in the newborn. Neonates should receive intramuscular vitamin K before surgery.

The neonatal kidney has a low glomerular filtration rate and tubular function is poorly developed, resulting in a reduced ability to excrete either a volume or a sodium load. The ability of the neonatal kidney to concentrate urine in response to water deprivation is reduced when compared with that of adults. Adult renal function is usually achieved by 2 years of age.

TEMPERATURE REGULATION

Temperature control is less efficient in the neonate than older patients. Babies have a greater surface area to body weight ratio than adults and are less protected from heat loss by the relatively thin subcutaneous tissue layer. Heat production is primarily achieved by increased metabolic activity in brown fat stores, termed non-shivering thermogenesis. This requires the expenditure of energy and an increase in oxygen consumption, potentially worsening any existing hypoxia. There is a narrow range of environmental temperature, termed the neutral temperature range, at which oxygen consumption is minimal (Adamsons *et al.*, 1965). This is close to body temperature in newborn infants. Neonates should be nursed before and after surgery in an incubator to prevent heat loss. High operating room temperatures are uncomfortable for theatre personnel and additional methods are therefore required to maintain body temperature. These include the use of reflective blankets, radiant heat lamps and thermostatically controlled mattresses. The use of a microclimate of warm air has also been described (Nightingale and Meakin, 1986). Other methods, such as the humidification of inspired gases and the warming of intravenous fluids and surgical skin preparation, are important.

Applied pharmacology

The uptake, distribution, metabolism and elimination of drugs differ significantly in neonates when compared with adults. Neonates therefore exhibit important quantitative differences in their response to a range of drugs, which become less marked during infancy and childhood.

Total body water (TBW) constitutes 85% of body weight in the preterm baby, 80% in the neonate and 60% at 1 year of age. Extracellular water (ECW) also decreases from 50% in the preterm baby to 27% at 1 year of age. Thus, in the neonatal period, the volume of distribution of many drugs is increased. Low plasma levels of albumin and alpha-1-acid glycoprotein, and a lower affinity of these proteins for drugs, reduce drug binding in neonates and result in a greater free fraction of drug. The blood–brain barrier is relatively immature at birth so that lipid-soluble drugs rapidly enter brain tissue. Furthermore, the brain receives a greater proportion of cardiac output so that a higher brain concentration of drug may result. Immature enzyme systems in the liver mean that drug metabolism is prolonged. Drugs that rely on the kidney for excretion are eliminated more slowly in the neonate and infant due to immature kidney function. The net effect of all these differences is complex. The larger volume of distribution explains, at least in part, why a higher dose (per kilogram body weight) of some parenterally administered drugs may be required to produce a given effect in neonates. However, dose intervals may have to be increased to take account of delayed metabolism and excretion.

The potency of inhaled anaesthetic agents varies with age. The alveolar concentration required to achieve a given depth of anaesthesia is lowest in preterm babies (LeDez and Lerman, 1987) and reaches a maximum in the 1–6 month age group (Lerman *et al.*, 1983). Cardiovascular depression with resulting hypotension is a recognized adverse effect of all the volatile anaesthetic agents (Lerman *et al.*, 1983). The high alveolar ventilation of neonates, compared with adults, results in the rapid uptake of inhalational agents and a faster induction. The volatile anaesthetic agents also depress respiration in a dose-dependent manner, this being an additional reason why neonates and some infants should not be allowed to breathe spontaneously.

Neonates and infants are also more sensitive to the effects of opioids. The blood–brain barrier is more permeable than that of adults, resulting in higher brain concentrations. Immature excretory pathways, lower levels of binding proteins, increased concentrations of endogenous opioids and differences in the proportion of opioid receptors all contribute to increased sensitivity. In contrast, children may require a higher dose of morphine for pain relief compared with adults (Olkkola *et al.*, 1988).

General principles of anaesthetic management

PSYCHOLOGICAL PREPARATION

Preoperative information is vital in helping to allay the fears and concerns of parents and children. A pre-admission programme, which familiarizes patients and their family with the hospital environment, is very helpful. A guided tour and explanation of each phase of the child's care, and the opportunity for the child to play with anaesthetic equipment, may be of value. Alternatively, a photograph album illustrating each stage of the hospital stay can be produced at little cost. The preoperative visit by the surgeon and anaesthetist with an appropriate explanation of the planned procedure is very important in relieving anxiety.

PREOPERATIVE STARVATION

The purpose of preoperative starvation is to reduce the risk of pulmonary aspiration of gastric contents. A prolonged period of starvation, however, is distressing to the patient (Schreiner *et al.*, 1990), may make venous access more difficult and may predispose to hypovolaemia. Rarely, hypoglycaemia may occur.

Guidelines for preoperative fasting should vary according to the age of the patient. Modest amounts of clear fluids given 2–3 hours preoperatively have not been shown to affect gastric volume or pH significantly (Sandhar *et al.*, 1989; Splinter *et al.*, 1990). Fit children can safely be permitted modest amounts of clear fluids (water, apple juice or non-particulate fruit juice) until 3 hours before elective surgery. Healthy infants who are breast fed should be fasted for a period equal to the usual interval between feeds. Formula feeds can be given up to 6 hours before surgery with clear fluids up to 3 hours preoperatively. Some authors have recommended that the period of starvation for clear fluids need only be 2 hours (Weaver, 1993; Steward, 1995).

Drugs or illness delay gastric emptying and trauma patients have been found to have relatively high gastric volumes 8 hours after their last oral intake (Bricker *et al.*, 1989). All patients undergoing emergency surgery should be intubated to protect the airway from pulmonary aspiration and intubation is performed as part of a rapid sequence induction (also called a 'crash-induction'). Oxygen is administered for a few minutes before induction, which then begins with the intravenous administration of thiopentone and suxamethonium. Following the loss of consciousness, and virtually simultaneous onset of muscle relaxation, backward pressure on the cricoid cartilage is applied by a trained assistant. This 'cricoid pressure' prevents regurgitation of stomach contents. Manual ventilation by a facemask is avoided until the airway is secured by tracheal intubation.

CLINICAL EVALUATION AND LABORATORY INVESTIGATIONS

It is beyond the scope of this chapter to provide a detailed review of history taking and clinical examination of the paediatric patient prior to anaesthesia; however, several specific conditions that have anaesthetic implications are commonly seen in children presenting for surgery.

Anaemia

Traditionally, an adult with a haemoglobin level of less than 10 g/dl has been deemed unsuitable for anaesthesia. The risk of transmission of disease through blood transfusion has prompted a re-evaluation of 'acceptable' haemoglobin levels in patients presenting for surgery. Each case must be assessed individually. A haemoglobin level just below 10 g/dl may be acceptable in an otherwise fit child undergoing minor surgery but not in those with cardiac or respiratory disease. Unexplained anaemia should always be investigated (Hatch and Sumner, 1989).

Upper respiratory tract infection (URI)

Sore throat, runny nose, sneezing, cough and congestion are common in children and may be symptoms of an acute URI or of a chronic, non-infective disorder, such as allergic rhinitis. It is important to distinguish between the two conditions since there is good evidence of an increase in intraoperative and postoperative adverse respiratory events in children with URIs (Cohen and Cameron, 1991). Many children, however, undergo surgery to relieve chronic upper respiratory tract symptoms (myringotomy, adenoidectomy, tonsillectomy and cleft palate repair) and should not be automatically postponed. The presence of pyrexia, a productive or croupy cough, distress on deep inhalation, positive chest findings on auscultation and signs of systemic involvement are sufficient grounds to postpone surgery. A chest X-ray or white cell count may be unhelpful.

There have been isolated reports of cardiac arrest and death in children with URI undergoing anaesthesia. They have been attributed to subclinical viral myocarditis which may accompany the toxic phase of an acute viral infection (Van Der Walt, 1995).

Asthma

This is one of the most common chronic disorders of children. Preoperatively, the severity and frequency of attacks, the presence of concurrent URI, the use of bronchodilators and steroids (past or present) should be determined. Elective surgery should be deferred until the patient's condition is optimal. Bronchospasm may be exacerbated by anxiety, drugs, intubation, light anaesthesia or inadequate analgesia. Patients may benefit from sedative premedication, preoperative bronchodilator treatment and steroid therapy. Intubation (and extubation) under deep anaesthesia may abolish irritant airway reflexes and anaesthetic gases should be warmed and humidified. Histamine-releasing drugs, such as thiopentone, atracurium and morphine, may

best be avoided. Non-steroidal anti-inflammatory drugs are contraindicated. Adequate hydration, regional analgesic techniques and physiotherapy may help to prevent postoperative pulmonary complications. Airway hyperreactivity persists for some weeks following an acute asthmatic attack and elective surgery should be delayed during this period (Hal, 1994).

Heart murmurs

It is important to distinguish the innocent systolic murmur from a pathological murmur (McEwan *et al.*, 1995). An experienced physician can usually differentiate between them clinically but occasionally echocardiography (ECHO) may be required. The child with congenital heart disease (CHD) will need a recent cardiology evaluation with electrocardiography (ECG) and ECHO findings. Antibiotic prophylaxis is essential for the prevention of infective endocarditis in patients with CHD undergoing surgery or diagnostic procedures. Guidelines for the appropriate choice of antibiotics with dose schedules can be found elsewhere (McEwan *et al.*, 1995). Children with right-to-left shunts are at risk from cerebral air embolus during the administration of intravenous fluids or drugs unless bubbles are meticulously removed. A detailed discussion of the anaesthetic problems of patients with CHD undergoing non-cardiac surgery is beyond the scope of this chapter.

Epileptic seizures

Preoperative determination of the degree of control of seizures is important, together with current medications and serum anticonvulsant levels if appropriate. Some anaesthetic drugs, notably ketamine and enflurane, lower the convulsant threshold and should probably be avoided in this group of patients. Emotional stress and fluid and electrolyte disturbance may also precipitate convulsions.

Laboratory investigations

Normal healthy children undergoing minor, diagnostic or bloodless surgery do not require laboratory investigations prior to surgery (Hannallah, 1995). A haemoglobin estimation is indicated in infants under 3 months, if there is a history of anaemia or haemoglobinopathy (e.g. sickle cell disease), and before major surgery with a large anticipated blood loss. Tests of renal and hepatic function, coagulation studies, blood glucose, chest X-ray and electrocardiography are only necessary if clinically indicated.

PREMEDICATION

Neonates and infants should be premedicated with atropine (Table 13.4), primarily to prevent bradycardia during airway manipulation, but also to reduce secre-

Table 13.4 Recommended drug dosages (guidelines only)

Premedication	
Atropine	0.02 mg/kg i.v./i.m. or 0.04 mg/kg p.o.
Midazolam	0.5–0.75 mg/kg p.o. or 0.2 mg/kg i.m./i.v.
Temazepam	0.5 mg/kg p.o.
Trimeprazine	2 mg/kg p.o.
Induction agents	
Thiopentone	5–8 mg/kg i.v.
Propofol	2.5–3.5 mg/kg i.v.
Ketamine	1–2 mg/kg i.v. or 5–10 mg kg i.m.
Neuromuscular blockers	
Suxamethonium	1–2 mg/kg i.v. or 2–4 mg/kg i.m.
Atracurium	0.3–0.6 mg/kg i.v.
Vecuronium	0.1 mg/kg i.v.
Cisatracurium	0.1 mg/kg i.v.
Introperative analgesics	
Morphine	0.05–0.1 mg/kg i.v.
Fentanyl	1–2 µg/kg i.v. or 5–10 µg/kg per hour inf.
Codeine phosphate	1–1.5 mg/kg i.m. (not i.v.)
Paracetamol	10–20 mg/kg p.o./p.r.
Diclofenac	1 mg/kg p.r. (not for use in children < 12 months old)
Opioid antagonist	
Naloxone	0.01–0.1 mg/g i.v.
Antiemetics (not routinely prescribed)	
Metoclopramide	0.15–0.25 mg/kg i.v./i.m./p.o.
Droperidol	0.025–0.075 mg/kg i.v.
Ondansetron	0.1 mg/kg i.v. (up to a maximum of 4 mg)
Local anaesthetics	
Lignocaine (plain)	3 mg/kg infil. or 6 mg/kg with adrenaline
Bupivacaine (plain)	2.5 mg/kg infil. (1 ml/kg of 0.25% solution)

i.v., intravenous; i.m., intramuscular; p.o., oral; p.r., rectal; i.n., intranasal; inf., infusion; infil., infiltration.

tions. It can be given intramuscularly 30 min preoperatively, or intravenously at the time of induction. Sedative premedication is not generally necessary in this age group.

In older infants and children, premedication may be indicated to reduce anxiety and produce sedation. Anxiety as a result of separation from parents is important in children aged from about 9 months. It is now widely accepted that parental presence at the start of anaesthesia for elective surgery facilitates a smooth induction and obviates the need for premedication with sedative drugs in many patients. A distressed child may be at greater risk of laryngospasm or breathholding and a turbulent induction has potentially harmful long-term psychological effects (Eckenhoff, 1953). Patients with preoperative pain should receive analgesics, and patients with cardiac disease benefit from sedative premedication to reduce the release of endogenous catecholamines which predispose to haemodynamic distur-

bances and worsen intracardiac shunting. Uncooperative children and those undergoing multiple surgical procedures may benefit from sedative premedication. The use of local anaesthetic cream greatly facilitates an intravenous induction and a eutectic mixture of lignocaine and prilocaine (EMLA) cream applied under an occlusive dressing for at least 1 hour before induction produces dermal anaesthesia. Because of the risk of local anaesthetic toxicity, the lower age limit in the product licence is 1 year (Frayling *et al.*, 1990; Freeman *et al.*, 1993).

INDUCTION TECHNIQUES

Induction is the most hazardous and stressful period of anaesthesia for the patient. Equipment should be checked, drugs drawn up in appropriate dosage and dilution (Table 13.5), and monitors applied before induction. The most common forms of induction in paediatric

Table 13.5 Tracheal tube sizes and lengths; suction catheter sizes (guidelines only: a range of sizes should always be available)

Age	Internal diameter (mm)	Length (cm) Oral	Length (cm) Nasal	Suction catheter (French gauge)
Preterm	2.5	10	13	6
0–3 months	3.0	10.5	13.5	8
3–6 months	3.5	11	14	8
6–9 months	4.0	12	15	8
9–18 months	4.5	13	15	8
18 mths–3 years	5.0	14	16	8
3–5 years	5.5	15	17	10
5–6 years	6.0	16	19	10
6–8 years	6.5	17	21	10
8–10 years	7.0	18	22	10
10–12 years	7.5	19	22	10

General rule: uncuffed tracheal tube under 8 years of age
Quick formulae: length = age/2+ 12 cm. internal diameter = age/4 + 4.5 mm.

practice are by the intravenous or inhalational routes. Access to the circulation prior to induction is preferable, improving safety and permitting rapid loss of consciousness with an intravenous induction agent. Inhalational induction requires patient co-operation. It is important to keep the child relaxed and to maintain their confidence by constant reassurance as a mask is gently introduced. Flavour-scented face masks may be more readily accepted. Induction may be performed with the child sitting on a parent's lap with minimal monitoring applied (pulse oximeter and precordial stethoscope) until consciousness is lost. Airway obstruction may occur when pharyngeal and laryngeal tone is lost but simple manoeuvres such as chin elevation, insertion of an oral airway or continuous positive airway pressure are often all that is required to re-establish patency. Laryngospasm can be treated by gentle hand ventilation and gradual deepening of anaesthesia. Atropine and suxamethonium should be administered intravenously or intramuscularly and the trachea intubated without delay if oxygen saturation falls. Less commonly, induction can be achieved using intramuscularly or rectally administered drugs.

EQUIPMENT AND MONITORING

It is essential to have a complete range of suitable equipment for anaesthetizing neonates, infants and children safely. A range of laryngoscopes, airways and endotracheal tubes is thus essential (Fig. 13.1). Appropriate endotracheal tube sizes and lengths are given in Table 13.5.

The laryngeal mask airway (LMA) has become firmly established in anaesthetic practice and is available in different sizes for paediatric use (Table 13.6 and Fig. 13.2). It is designed to be inserted into the hypopharynx of the anaesthetized patient, affording greater airway security and convenience than the face mask (Haynes and Morton, 1993). The LMA is particularly useful in situations where intubation has traditionally been used to allow surgical access or where the anaesthetist is required to be remote. It may even be used in children in whom intubation is difficult (Markakis *et al.*, 1992). It should be remembered that the LMA does not protect against pulmonary aspiration.

The Rees modification of the Ayre's T-piece is probably the most commonly used anaesthetic breathing system in paediatric practice. It is lightweight and has a low resistance to breathing, although scavenging of expired gases is difficult. Other systems, such as the Bain or circle system are available for older children.

Standards for patient monitoring during anaesthesia include the continuous presence of the anaesthetist. There is no substitute for clinical observation. Patient colour, pulse rate and volume, skin perfusion and chest movement (depth and pattern) provide valuable information. The precordial or oesophageal stethoscope remains a simple and reliable tool. Monitoring is aimed at preventing the occurrence of life-threatening episodes such as hypoxaemia or circulatory failure. Thus, there is special emphasis on pulse oximetry in children because of the rapidity with which hypoxaemia can develop.

Table 13.6 Recommended laryngeal mask sizes (guidelines only)

Size	Patients
Size 1	Neonates and infants up to about 10 kg
Size 2	Children up to 20 kg
Size 2.5	Children 20–30 kg
Size 3	Small adults
Size 4	Normal-sized adults

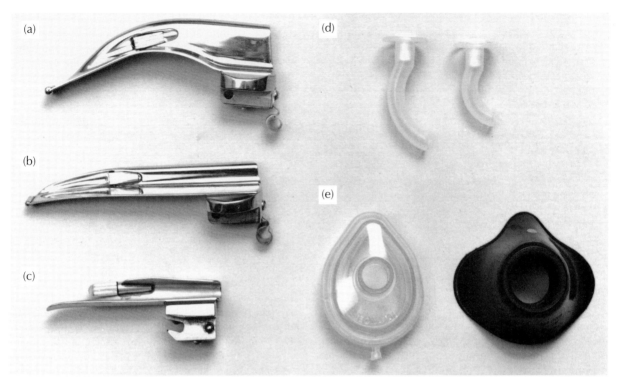

Fig. 13.1 Commonly used anaesthetic equipment: (a) Macintosh laryngoscope blade; (b) Robertshaw laryngoscope blade; (c) Wisconsin laryngoscope blade; (d) Guedel's airways; (e) Paediatric facemasks.

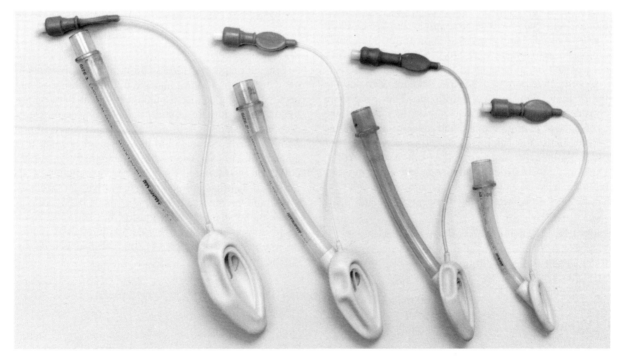

Fig. 13.2 A range of paediatric laryngeal mask airways (LMA).

Table 13.7 Intraoperative monitoring

'Essential' monitoring
  Precordial stethoscope
  Electrocardiography
  Pulse oximetry
  Non-invasive blood pressure measurement
  Inspired oxygen concentration
  Ventilator disconnect alarm
'Important' monitoring
  Core and peripheral temperature
  Capnography
  Neuromuscular function
Other monitoring
  Direct arterial pressure
  Central venous pressure
  Urine output
  Blood loss

Source: Freeman *et al.* (1994).

Temperature monitoring is regarded as essential for all but the shortest procedure because of the greater likelihood of hypothermia in children. A list of monitoring devices, with priorities for their use, is given in Table 13.7.

FLUID THERAPY

Intraoperative fluid therapy aims to replace deficits from the period of preoperative starvation, to provide maintenance fluids during surgery and to replace fluid loss caused by surgical trauma. Maintenance fluid requirements vary with age and guidelines are given in Table 13.8. The ideal composition of intravenous fluids remains controversial, with concerns about the glucose content and the avoidance of hypoglycaemia or hyperglycaemia (Welborn *et al.*, 1987). The use of hypotonic fluids may lead to hyponatraemia. The overriding consideration in preterm babies and neonates is the avoidance of hypoglycaemia, and regular intraoperative blood glucose measurements should be performed. For older children the need for glucose is less clear cut. During major surgery balanced salt solutions or albumin may be required to maintain the circulation. Tissue perfusion, heart rate, blood pressure and urine

Table 13.8 Guidelines for maintenance fluid therapy

Body weight (kg)	Rate
0–10	100 ml/kg per 24 h
11–20	1000 ml + 50 ml/kg per 24 h for each kg over 10
>20	1500 ml + 20 ml/kg per 24 h for each kg over 20

Source: Gregory (1983).

output are useful guides during replacement. Estimates of blood volume are given in Table 13.2. Blood loss should be measured as accurately as possible, and blood replacement should begin when 10% of the estimated blood volume has been lost or earlier in some cases.

Adult fluid administration devices are not suitable in paediatric practice. Precise volume chambers with microdrip administration sets and air filters minimize the risk of inadvertent fluid overload. A system incorporating a three-way stopcock allows fluid boluses via a 10 or 20 ml syringe to be given.

Principles of neonatal anaesthesia

The neonatal period is defined as the first 28 days of extrauterine life or up to 44 weeks postconceptual age (gestational plus postnatal age). Such neonates may have respiratory, cardiac and neurological abnormalities which increase the risk of even the most minor surgical procedure. A better understanding of neonatal physiology and pharmacology, improvements in anaesthetic techniques, monitoring equipment and postoperative care have allowed smaller babies to undergo more complex surgery. However, the perioperative morbidity and mortality rate still remains highest in this age group (Cohen *et al.*, 1990). Even after minor surgery, preterm infants are more prone to respiratory problems than their full term counterparts (Steward, 1992).

It is for these reasons that neonatal surgery should only be performed in specialized centres with personnel who have the appropriate training and who are able to maintain their skills.

PREOPERATIVE ASSESSMENT

Antenatal diagnosis allows the transfer of patients *in utero* to a regional unit and the optimal timing of surgery. Most surgery performed on neonates is to correct major congenital abnormalities. The purpose of preoperative assessment is to ensure that associated abnormalities, such as congenital heart disease or renal tract abnormalities, have been detected and that the patient's condition is optimal. Preoperative investigations are reviewed, instructions about preoperative starvation are given and premedication is prescribed. It is useful to check the availability of blood for transfusion, if blood loss is anticipated. Plans for postoperative care, including the need for postoperative mechanical ventilation, can be made.

INDUCTION AND MAINTENANCE OF ANAESTHESIA

Monitoring devices, which include precordial stethoscope, ECG, pulse oximetry and non-invasive blood pressure, should be applied, and intravenous access secured before starting anaesthesia. Preoxygenation is essential. Induction may be achieved intravenously or by inhalation, and tracheal intubation performed following the administration of a muscle relaxant. Awake intubation is usually reserved for situations where airway difficulties are anticipated, or when there is a need to ensure that ventilation is possible following intubation, as is the case in patients with tracheo-oesophageal fistula. Positive pressure ventilation is mandatory, either by hand with an Ayre's T-piece, or using a mechanical ventilator. Hand ventilation may detect changes in compliance more rapidly, although this has been questioned recently (Spears *et al.*, 1991). Gas flow rates and minute volumes are adjusted to produce normocapnia. An oxygen–air mixture may be preferable to oxygen–nitrous oxide. Nitrous oxide causes circulatory depression and diffuses into gas-filled spaces. It is best avoided in sick neonates or in babies with intestinal obstruction or congenital lung cysts in whom further gaseous distension of the gut or lung may be harmful. The use of volatile anaesthetic agents is safe and may even be advantageous in view of their effect on the stress response to surgery (Anand *et al.*, 1988). Intravenous opioids must be used cautiously because of the risk of respiratory depression and apnoea. Extradural analgesia has been reported in this age group but is not commonly practised (Wilson and Lloyd-Thomas, 1993). Spinal and caudal anaesthesia in awake, high-risk neonates undergoing herniotomy has been described (Mahe and Ecoffey, 1988; Gunter *et al.*, 1991; Peutrell and Hughes, 1993). After reversal of neuromuscular blockade, extubation is only performed when the patient is awake with good airway control and satisfactory respiratory effort. Supplementary oxygen is mandatory in the immediate postoperative period.

POSTOPERATIVE ANALGESIA

The need for postoperative analgesia requires individual assessment. Good nursing care and early resumption of feeding may be all that are necessary to settle the patient after minor surgery. Oral or rectal paracetamol (10 mg/kg) may sometimes be helpful (Miller *et al.*, 1976). The use of pulse oximetry and apnoea monitors adds greatly to patient safety. Systemic opioids should only be administered to spontaneously breathing neonates with extreme caution (Lloyd and Thomas, 1990). Their use may in some circumstances be an indication for postoperative ventilation.

POSTOPERATIVE APNOEA

Postoperative apnoea occurs mainly in former preterm babies (born before 37 weeks' gestation) (Welborn, 1992) but can occur, albeit rarely, in full-term babies less than 44 weeks' postconceptual age, particularly if there is a history of ventilatory problems (Cote and

Kelly, 1990). Apnoeic episodes occur more commonly in babies with a prior history of apnoea. They are usually brief and occur with greatest frequency in the first 2 hours after surgery, although they may occur up to 12 hours postoperatively (Kurth *et al.*, 1987).

When selecting otherwise healthy term infants for day surgery, a lower limit of 44–45 weeks' postconceptual age is recommended (Sims and Johnson, 1994). For preterm babies non-essential surgery should be delayed until the patient is more than 52 weeks' postconceptual age. If surgery cannot be delayed, patients less than this age should be admitted to hospital and monitored for at least 12 hours postoperatively or for 12 hours after any apnoea (Sims and Johnson, 1994). Patients with a history of apnoea or periodic breathing may be treated with theophylline or caffeine (Welborn *et al.*, 1989). Spinal anaesthesia without sedation may reduce the incidence of apnoea (Welborn *et al.*, 1990). All patients with a history of near-miss sudden infant death syndrome (SIDS) or patients with a family history of SIDS should be admitted overnight.

Anaesthetic considerations for neonatal emergencies

TRACHEO-OESOPHAGEAL FISTULA

The patient should remain prone or slightly elevated while supine to reduce the risk of aspiration prior to induction. Continuous aspiration on a sump catheter (Replogle tube) placed in the upper oesophageal pouch reduces the risk of regurgitation. As a result of the anatomical connection between trachea and oesophagus, gastric distension may occur following ventilation by face mask and some anaesthetists therefore favour awake intubation. Even following intubation it is possible to distend the stomach. This is minimized by gentle positive pressure ventilation. An intentional endobronchial intubation may be performed and the tube then slowly withdrawn while auscultating the left thorax until it is just above the carina – this method may also reduce gastric distension. It is possible inadvertently to intubate the fistula, in which case ventilation is impossible. Hand ventilation until ligation of the fistula allows early detection of major bronchial kinking due to surgical retraction. Early extubation is usually possible in these patients although postoperative ventilation may be indicated if they are small or preterm, have aspirated preoperatively, or if the oesophageal repair is under tension. Tracheomalacia may be a problem following extubation in some patients.

CONGENITAL DIAPHAGMATIC HERNIA (CDH)

Infants with CDH may present in the immediate newborn period with respiratory distress due to lung hypoplasia, increased pulmonary vascular resistance and right to left shunting. Antenatal diagnosis is now more common. Initial resuscitation involves intubation and mechanical ventilation. Mask ventilation should be avoided to prevent gastric distension. After the airway is secured, a nasogastric tube should be inserted to empty the stomach. Adequate oxygenation, hyperventilation to reduce carbon dioxide tension, and correction of acidosis help to prevent episodes of pulmonary hypertension. Minimal handling with sedation and muscle paralysis are also important. High airway pressure should be avoided to reduce the risk of pneumothorax. Surgery is delayed until the patient is stable (Charlton *et al.*, 1991; Breaux *et al.*, 1991). Other methods to reduce pulmonary vascular resistance include the use pulmonary vasodilators and extracorporeal membrane oxygenation (Charlton *et al.*, 1991).

ABDOMINAL WALL DEFECTS

Fluid loss, electrolyte imbalance and hypothermia may occur preoperatively and should be corrected prior to surgery. Raised intra-abdominal pressure following surgical closure may lead to respiratory failure and necessitate postoperative ventilation (Yaster *et al.*, 1988).

HYPERTROPHIC PYLORIC STENOSIS

Surgery should not be undertaken until rehydration is complete. Hypochloraemic alkalosis requires correction to achieve a normal bicarbonate, usually less than 25 mmol/l, and chloride greater than 95 mmol/l (Goh *et al.*, 1990). A rapid sequence induction should be performed following aspiration of the nasogastric tube. Infiltration of the wound with local anaesthetic usually provides good analgesia and avoids the need for systemic opioids (McNicol *et al.*, 1990).

INTESTINAL OBSTRUCTION/NECROTIZING ENTEROCOLITIS

Dehydration and electrolyte disturbance require correction before surgery. Increasing abdominal distension may lead to respiratory embarrassment and increase the risk of aspiration. A rapid sequence induction should be performed following aspiration of the nasogastric tube. Nitrous oxide should be avoided as it may worsen gaseous distension of the abdomen. Necrotizing enterocolitis is a disease of preterm infants and patients requiring surgery are usually already intubated and mechanically ventilated on the neonatal intensive care unit. Medical treatment includes fluid replacement, correction of acidosis and antibiotics. The anaesthetist may be involved in the transfer of the patient to the operating theatre. The endotracheal tube must be secured to prevent accidental dislodgement and respiratory and cardiovascular monitoring are essential during transfer. Intraoperatively, the maintenance of temperature, correction of fluid losses and monitoring of blood glucose are important considerations.

ANAESTHESIA IN INFANTS AND CHILDREN

Many of the considerations outlined above also apply to older children, albeit to a lesser degree. The anatomical and physiological differences discussed above are greatest in children under 3 years of age (*British Medical Journal*, 1978), becoming gradually less marked throughout childhood. This is the basis for the recommendation that specialist services for children under this age should be centralized (Atwell and Spargo, 1992). However, older children also have special needs which must be met.

Infants and children have different anaesthetic requirements. Infants are less likely than preschool children to show separation anxiety. The latter group may exhibit behavioural disturbances following discharge from hospital which can be ameliorated by good preoperative preparation (Meursing, 1989). School children have a greater understanding of events and ability to communicate but are still distressed by hospital admission and surgery. Efforts should be made to involve parents in the care of their child as separation can also be disturbing in this age group. The concerns of adolescents are different. They have worries about pain, loss of control and bodily mutilation by surgery.

Anaesthetic considerations for day case surgery

Children are particularly suited for treatment as day case patients because the majority of patients are fit, are accompanied by an adult and require minor or body surface surgery. Other advantages of day surgery include minimal family disruption, decreased risk of hospital-acquired infection and cost-effectiveness.

Surgical operations which may be performed on a day case basis are listed in Table 13.9. The duration of operation should be taken into consideration. The selection of patients suitable for day case surgery follows clinical and non-clinical principles (Thornes, 1991) and is summarized in Table 13.10. Provided close attention is paid to patient selection and the type of surgery performed, the postoperative morbidity following day surgery is low (Patel and Hannallah, 1988).

In adults undergoing day surgery, the use of modern anaesthetic agents such as propofol and sevoflurane, which have a rapid recovery profile, is becoming increasingly common. The evidence in children that these agents provide a more rapid recovery when compared with traditional agents such as thiopentone and halothane is less clear but they may have a role to

Table 13.9 Procedures suitable for day surgery

General surgery/urology	**ENT**
Hernias (inguinal, umbilical and epigastric)	Myringotomy and insertion of tubes
Communicating hydroceles	Adenotonsillectomy
Circumcision	Reduction of fractured nose
Meatotomy	Examination under anaesthesia
Separation of preputial adhesions	Laryngoscopy
Orchidopexy	Bronchoscopy
Division of tongue tie	
EUA and sigmoidoscopy	**Dental**
Cystourethroscopy	Conservation/extractions
Orthopaedics	**Oncology**
Change of plaster	Bone marrow aspiration
Removal of wires or plates	Lumbar puncture
Manipulation	Testicular biopsy
Ophthalmology	**Other**
Tear duct probing	Gastroscopy
Strabismus correction	Colonoscopy
Examination under anaesthesia	CT scan, MRI scan

Table 13.10 Selection of patients suitable for day case surgery

Clinical principles

Children having a general anaesthetic should be ASA classes 1 or 2.

ASA 1: The patient has no organic, physiological, biochemical or psychiatric disturbance. The pathological process for which the operation is to be performed is localized and does not entail a systemic disturbance.

ASA 2: Mild to moderate systemic disturbance caused by either the condition to be treated surgically or other pathophysiological processes.

Infants and children of all ages are suitable for a general anaesthetic with the exception of term neonates and former preterm babies less than 52 weeks postconceptual age. Special consideration should be given to babies who have been on ventilatory support.

Non-clinical principles

The parent must be able to cope with preprocedure instructions and with the care of the child after treatment.

The parent must agree to day treatment, following adequate information and an opportunity to discuss anxieties.

The parent must be available to stay throughout the day, although there may be exceptions for older children who attend regularly.

The parent must be able to make arrangements for the practical care of the child for a named period of time following transfer of care to home.

Facilities in the home should be taken into account.

Travel conditions and journey time should be taken into consideration. After a general anaesthetic the use of public transport is inappropriate and the hospital must take responsibility for checking that suitable transport is available.

Children with a long-term serious illness, disability or handicap whose parents are carrying out day-to-day care at home should be treated on a day basis when hospitalization is required, whenever this is appropriate and would be beneficial to the child and family.

After Thornes (1991).

play (Meakin, 1995; Lerman, 1995). Adequate post-operative analgesia is essential. The use of opioids predisposes to postoperative sedation and vomiting and they should be avoided if possible (Wilton and Burn, 1986). The use of infiltration with local anaesthetic agents, peripheral nerve blocks or caudal extradural blockade in association with general anaesthesia is common. Analgesia lasts into the postoperative period enabling a rapid recovery and early ambulation of the patient (Shandling and Stewart, 1980). Contraindications to the use of local anaesthetic techniques include infection at the site of injection, allergy to local anaesthetic agents, bleeding disorders and neurological disease. Patient age is not a limiting factor. Local anaesthetics can be administered after induction of anaesthesia by the anaesthetist, or by the surgeon after completion of surgery. A detailed description of local anaesthetic techniques is beyond the scope of this chapter and the interested reader is referred elsewhere (Arthur and McNicol, 1986; Sainte-Maurice and Schulte Steinburg, 1990). Other analgesic drugs such as paracetamol or non-steroidal anti-inflammatory agents given orally or rectally, are of great benefit.

The patient is fit for discharge when vital signs are stable, there is no bleeding and pain control is adequate. Some units recommend that the patient should be able to tolerate oral fluids and should have passed urine. Facilities for overnight admission should always be available. The incidence of postoperative nausea and vomiting varies widely and delayed vomiting is the most common cause for readmission (Baines, 1996). The use of antiemetic agents in children is not yet routine because of the fear of adverse effects but drugs such as droperidol, metoclopramide and ondansetron may be of benefit (Baines, 1986). Tracheal intubation is no longer regarded as a contraindication for day case surgery.

Postoperative analgesia

A range of analgesic methods is now available for infants and children. Analgesia for neonates has already been discussed. Pain assessment is fundamental to the provision of adequate and safe analgesia (Lloyd-Thomas and Howard, 1992). The establishment of an acute pain team for the management of the patient's analgesic requirements and for the training and education of personnel is recommended (Royal College of Surgeons, 1990).

The use of parenterally administered opioids remains the mainstay of treatment. The 'as-required' intramuscular injection is unpleasant for the patient although its acceptability can be improved by the subcutaneous placement of a cannula at the time of anaesthesia. The cannula is covered with a sterile dressing, flushed with heparinized saline and used postoperatively to administer analgesic drugs (Lavies and Wandless, 1989).

Continuous intravenous infusions of opioids have gained popularity (Lloyd-Thomas, 1990). The successful administration of continuous subcutaneous morphine infusion has also been described (McNicol, 1993). Dose recommendations for infants receiving infusions should be reduced (Lloyd-Thomas, 1990). Patient-controlled analgesia (PCA) can be used in selected children down to the age of 5 years. Patients receiving PCA require close nursing supervision and monitoring with pulse oximetry (Berde *et al.*, 1991; Gillespie and Morton, 1993). A low-dose background infusion in addition to PCA may improve the quality of analgesia without excessive sedation, especially in the immediate postoperative period (Doyle *et al.*, 1993). For children who are unable to use PCA, nurse-controlled analgesia (NCA) is a more versatile alternative to a continuous intravenous infusion (Lloyd-Thomas and Howard, 1994).

Regional anaesthetic techniques provide good analgesia when compared to the continuous intravenous infusion of opioids (Wolfe and Hughes). Orthopaedic and lower abdominal surgery are particularly suitable for lumbar extradural or continuous caudal blockade. However, the incidence of motor blockade and urinary retention is high. With few exceptions, catheter placement is performed under general anaesthesia. Thoracic epidural anaesthesia has been described in children (Tobias *et al.*, 1993).

Removal of inhaled foreign body

The removal of an inhaled foreign body is one of the most common indications for bronchoscopy in children. There may be a history of choking, coughing or cyanosis. In some cases this may have occurred days or even weeks previously. Clinical findings include decreased air entry or a fixed wheeze. A chest X-ray may reveal pulmonary collapse or, if there is a ball-valve effect, an expiratory film may show hyper-inflation on the affected side.

The principles of anaesthetic management include atropine premedication and an inhalational induction maintaining spontaneous ventilation to avoid dispersal of the foreign body. After application of local anaesthesia to the airway an endotracheal tube is inserted. This is a useful guide to the size of bronchoscope required. Muscle relaxants should be avoided. If the foreign body becomes lodged in the trachea during its removal, it should be pushed distally again to allow adequate ventilation before further attempts at its removal are made.

Epiglottitis and croup

Acute life-threatening airway obstruction in paediatric patients demands quick and decisive action by a physician skilled in paediatric airway management.

There is often no time for diagnosis, the priority being to maintain adequate oxygenation and re-establish the airway. The need for tracheal intubation is based on clinical assessment of the patient and not on arterial blood gases. A clinical croup score has been devised and may be of help (Downes and Raphaely, 1975).

Epiglottitis occurs most often in the 2–5 year old age group and is heralded by the rapid onset of pyrexia, drooling, dysphagia and respiratory distress. Typically, the child will be sitting upright and leaning forward. No attempts should be made to examine the throat, to perform any laboratory or radiological investigations, or to site an intravenous cannula. The child should be taken straight to the operating theatre accompanied by an experienced anaesthetist. An inhalational induction using increasing concentrations of halothane in 100% oxygen should be performed, and once a suitable depth of anaesthesia has been achieved, laryngoscopy is undertaken. Identification of the glottic opening may be difficult. Light pressure on the chest may reveal a bubble at the glottis, and intubation with an appropriately sized endotracheal tube can usually be achieved. A surgeon should be in theatre, scrubbed and ready to perform an emergency tracheostomy if necessary.

Laryngotracheobronchitis (LTB) or croup usually occurs in children between 6 months and 2 years old. The onset is insidious with low-grade pyrexia, croupy cough and gradual respiratory distress. Mild cases can be treated with humidifed oxygen. More severe cases can be difficult to distinguish from other causes of respiratory obstruction, and will require intubation following a similar procedure to that described for epiglottitis.

References

Adamsons, K., Gandy, G.M. and James, L.S. 1965: The influence of thermal factors upon oxygen consumption of the newborn human infant. *Journal of Pediatrics* **66**, 495–508.

Alberman, E. and Botting, B. 1991: Trends in prevalence and survival of very low birthweight infants, England and Wales: 1983–87. *Archives of Disease in Childhood* **66**, 1304–8.

Anand, K.J.S. and Hickey, P.R. 1987: Pain and its effects in the human neonate and fetus. *New England Journal of Medicine* **317**, 1321–9.

Anand, K.J.S., Sippell, W.G., Schofield, N.M. and Aynsley-Green, A. 1988: Does halothane anaesthesia decrease the metabolic and endocrine stress responses of newborn infants undergoing operation? *British Medical Journal* **296**, 668–72.

Arthur, D.S. and McNicol, L.R. 1986: Local anaesthetic techniques in paediatric surgery. *British Journal of Anaesthesia* **58**, 760–78.

Atwell, J.D. and Spargo, P.M. 1992: The provision of safe surgery for children. *Archives of Disease in Childhood* **67**, 345–9.

Baines, D. 1996: Postoperative nausea and vomiting in children. *Paediatric Anaesthesia* **6**, 7–14.

Berde, C.B., Lehn, B.M., Yee, J.D., Sethna, N.F. and Russo, D. 1991: Patient-controlled analgesia in children and adolescents: a randomized, prospective comparison with intramuscular administration of morphine for postoperative analgesia. *Journal of Pediatrics* **118**, 460–6.

Breaux, C.W., Rouse, T.M., Cain, W.S. and Georgeson, K.E. 1991: Improvement in survival of patients with congenital diaphragmatic hernia utilizing a strategy of delayed repair after medical and/or extracorporeal membrane oxygenation stabilization. *Journal of Pediatric Surgery* **26**, 333–8.

Bricker, S.R.W., McLuckie, A. and Nightingale, D.A. 1989: Gastric aspirates after trauma in children. *Anaesthesia* **44**, 721–4.

British Medical Journal 1978: Paediatric anaesthesia [leading article]. *British Medical Journal* **2**, 717.

Charlton, A.J., Bruce, J. and Davenport, M. 1991: Timing of surgery in congenital diaphragmatic hernia. *Anaesthesia* **46**, 820–3.

Charlton, A.J., Davies, J.M. and Rimmer, S. 1989: Anaesthesia and brain damage in the newborn. *Anaesthesia* **44**, 641–3.

Cohen, M.M. and Cameron, C.B. 1991: Should you cancel the operation when a child has an upper respiratory tract infection? *Anesthesia and Analgesia* **72**, 282–8.

Cohen, M.M., Cameron, C.B. and Duncan, P.G. 1990: Pediatric anesthesia morbidity and mortality in the perioperative period. *Anesthesia and Analgesia* **70**, 160–7.

Cote, C.J. and Kelly, D.H. 1990: Postoperative apnea in a full-term infant with a demonstrable respiratory pattern abnormality. *Anesthesiology* **72**, 559–61.

Downes, J.J. and Raphaely, R.C. 1975: Pediatric intensive care. *Anesthesiology* **43**, 238–50.

Doyle, E., Harper, I. and Morton, N.S. 1993: Patient-controlled analgesia with low dose background infusion after lower abdominal surgery in children. *British Journal of Anaesthesia* **71**, 818–22.

Duker, J.S. 1992: Retinopathy of prematurity. *Current Opinions in Ophthalmology* **3**, 771–5.

Eckenhoff, J.E. 1953: Relationship of anesthesia to postoperative personality changes in children. *American Journal of Diseases of Children* **86**, 587–91.

Flynn, J.T., Bancalari, E., Snyder, E.S. *et al.* 1992: A cohort study of transcutaneous oxygen tension and the incidence and severity of retinopathy of prematurity. *New England Journal of Medicine* **326**, 1050–4.

Frayling, I.M., Addison, G.M., Chattergee, K. and Meakin, G. 1990: Methaemoglobinaemia in children treated with prilocaine-lignocaine cream. *British Medical Journal* **301**, 153–4.

Freeman, J.A., Doyle, E., Tee Im, N.T. and Morton, N.S. 1993: Topical anaesthesia of the skin: a review. *Paediatric Anaesthesia* **3**, 129–38.

Freeman, N.V., Burger, D.M., Griffiths, M. and Malone, P.S. (eds) 1994: *Surgery of the newborn*. London: Churchill Livingstone, 46.

Gal, T.J. 1994: Bronchial hyperresponsiveness and anesthesia: physiologic and therapeutic perspectives. *Anesthesia and Analgesia* **78**, 559–73.

Gillespie, J.A and Morton, N.S. 1992: Patient-controlled analgesia for children: a review. *Paediatric Anaesthesia* **2**, 51–9.

Goh, D.W., Hall, S.K, Gornall, P., Buick, R.G., Green, A. and Corkery, J.J. 1990: Plasma chloride and alkalaemia in pyloric stenosis. *British Journal of Surgery* **77**, 922–3.

Gregory, G.A. 1993: *Paediatric anaesthesia*. New York: Churchill Livingstone, 474.

Gunter, J.B., Watcha, M.F., Forestner, J.E. *et al.* 1991: Caudal epidural anesthesia in conscious premature and high-risk infants. *Journal of Pediatric Surgery* **26**, 9–14.

Hannallah, R.S. 1995: Clinical review: preoperative investigations. *Paediatric Anaesthesia* **5**, 325–9.

Hatch, D.J. and Sumner, E. 1989: Neonatal physiology and anaesthesia. In Sumner, E. and Hatch, D.J. (eds), *Textbook of paediatric anaesthetic practice*. London: Baillière Tindall, 255–73.

Haynes, S.R. and Morton, N.S. 1993: The laryngeal mask airway: a review of its use in paediatric anaesthesia. *Paediatric Anaesthesia* **3**, 65–73.

Kurth, C.D., Hutchison, A.A., Caton, D.C. and Davenport, P.W. 1989: Maturation and anesthetic effects on apnoeic thresholds in lambs. *Journal of Applied Physiology* **67**, 643–7.

Kurth, C.D., Spitzer, A.R., Broennle, A.M. and Downes, J.J. 1987: Postoperative apnea in preterm infants. *Anesthesiology* **66**, 483–8.

Lavies, N.G. and Wandless, J.G. 1989: Subcutaneous morphine in children: taking the sting out of postoperative analgesia [Letter]. *Anaesthesia* **44**, 1000–1.

LeDez, K.M. and Lerman, J. 1987: The minimum alveolar concentration (MAC) of isoflurane in preterm neonates. *Anesthesiology* **67**, 301–7.

Lerman, J. 1995: Sevoflurane in pediatric anesthesia. *Anesthesia and Analgesia* **81**, S4–10.

Lerman, J., Robinson, S., Willis, M.M. and Gregory, G.A. 1983: Anesthetic requirements for halothane in young children 0–1 month and 1–6 months of age. *Anesthesiology* **59**, 421–6.

Lloyd-Thomas, A.R. 1990: Pain management in paediatric patients. *British Journal of Anaesthesia* **64**, 85–104.

Lloyd-Thomas, A.R. and Howard, R. 1992: Postoperative pain control in children. *British Medical Journal* **304**, 1174–5.

Lloyd-Thomas, A.R. and Howard, R.F. 1994: A pain service for children. *Paediatric Anaesthesia* **4**, 3–15.

Lou, H.C., Lassen, N.A. and Friis-Hansen, B. 1979: Impaired autoregulation of cerebral blood flow in the distressed newborn infant. *Journal of Pediatrics* **94**, 118–21.

Macfarlane, A., Cole, S., Johnson, A. and Botting, B. 1988: Epidemiology of birth before 28 weeks of gestation. *British Medical Bulletin* **44**, 861–93.

Mahe, V. and Ecoffey, C. 1988: Spinal anesthesia with isobaric bupivacaine in infants. *Anesthesiology* **68**, 601–3.

Markakis, D.A., Sayson, S.C. and Schreiner, M.S. 1992: Insertion of the laryngeal mask airway in awake infants with the Robin sequence. *Anesthesia and Analgesia* **75**: 822–4.

McEwan, A.I., Birch, M. and Bingham, R. 1995: Clinical review: the preoperative management of the child with a heart murmur. *Paediatric Anaesthesia* **5**, 151–6.

McNicol, L.R., Martin, C.S., Smart, N.G. and Logan, R.W. 1990: Peroperative bupivacaine for pyloromyotomy pain. *Lancet* **335**, 54–5.

McNicol, R. 1993: Postoperative analgesia in children using continuous s.c. morphine. *British Journal of Anaesthesia* **71**, 752–6.

Meakin, G. 1995: The role of propofol in paediatric anaesthetic practice. *Paediatric Anaesthesia* **5**, 147–9.

Meursing, A.E.E. 1989: Psychological effects of anaesthesia in children. *Current Opinion in Anaesthesiology* **2**, 335–8.

Miller, R.D. (ed.) 1986: *Anesthesia*, 2nd ed. New York: Churchill Livingstone, 1756.

Miller, R.D., Bachner, R. and McMillan, C. 1989: *Blood diseases of infancy and childhood*, 6th ed. St Louis, MO: Mosby, 338.

Miller, R.P., Roberts, R.J. and Fischer, L.J. 1976: Acetaminophen elimination kinetics in neonates, children and adults. *Clinical Pharmacology and Therapeutics* **19**, 284–94.

Motoyama, E.K. Davis, P.J. 1990: *Smith's anaethesia for infants and children*, 5th ed. St Louis, MO: Mosby, 338.

Nightingale, P. and Meakin, G. 1986: A new method for maintaining body temperature in children [Letter]. *Anesthesiology* **65**, 447–8.

Olkkola, K.T., Maunksela, E.L., Korpela, R. and Rosenberg, P.H. 1988: Kinetics and dynamics of postoperative intravenous morphine in children. *Clinical Pharmacology and Therapeutics* **44**, 128–36.

Patel, R.I. and Hannallah, R.S. 1988: Anesthetic complications following pediatric ambulatory surgery: a 3 yr study. *Anesthesiology* **69**, 1009–12.

Peutrell, J.M., Hughes, D.G. 1993: Epidural anaesthesia through caudal catheters for inguinal herniotomies in awake ex-premature babies. *Anaesthesia* **47**, 128–31.

Ramanathan, R., Durand, M. and Larrazabal, C. 1987: Pulse oximetry in very low birth weight infants with acute and chronic lung disease. *Pediatrics* **79**, 612–7.

Royal College of Surgeons of England and College of Anaesthetists 1990: Commission on the Provision of Surgical Services. *Report of the Working Party on Pain after Surgery*. London: HMSO.

Saint-Maurice, C. and Schulte Steinberg, O. (eds) 1990: *Regional anaesthesia in children*. Norwalk, CT: Appleton & Lange/Mediglobe.

Sandhar, B.K., Goresky, G.Y., Maltby, J.R. and Shaffer, E.A. 1989: Effect of oral liquids and ranitidine on gastric fluid volume and pH in children undergoing outpatient surgery. *Anesthesiology* **71**, 327–30.

Schreiner, M.S., Triebwasser, A. and Keon, T.P. 1990: Ingestion of liquids compared with preoperative fasting in pediatric outpatients. *Anesthesiology* **72**, 593–7.

Schulte, F.J. 1977: Apnea. *Clinics in Perinatology* **4**, 65–75.

Shandling, B. and Steward, D.J. 1980: Regional analgesia for postoperative pain in pediatric outpatient surgery. *Journal of Pediatric Surgery* **15**, 477–80.

Sims, C. and Johnson, C.M. 1994: Postoperative apnoea in infants. *Anaesthesia and Intensive Care* **22**, 40–45.

Sinha, S.K., Sims, D.G., Davies, J.M. and Chiswick, M.L. 1985: Relationship between periventricular haemorrhage and ischaemic brain lesions diagnosed by ultrasound in very pre-term infants. *Lancet* **2**, 1154–6.

Spears, R.S., Yeh, A., Fisher, D.M. and Zwass, M.S. 1991: The 'educated hand': can anesthesiologists assess changes in neonatal pulmonary compliance manually? *Anesthesiology* **75**, 693–6.

Splinter, W.M., Schaefer, J.D. and Zunder, I.H. 1990: Clear fluids three hours before surgery do not affect the gastric fluid contents of children. *Canadian Journal of Anaesthesia* **37**, 498–501.

Steward, D.J. 1982: Preterm infants are more prone to complications following minor surgery than are term infants. *Anesthesiology* **56**, 304–6.

Steward, D.J. 1995: *Manual of pediatric anesthesia.* New York: Churchill Livingstone, 71.

Thornes, R. 1991: *Just for the day. Caring for children in the health services.* Action for Sick Children.

Tobias, J.D., Lowe, S., O'Dell, N. and Holcomb, G.W. 1993: Thoracic epidural anaesthesia in infants and children. *Canadian Journal of Anaesthesia* **40**, 879–82.

Van Der Walt, J. 1995: Clinical review: anaesthesia in children with viral respiratory tract infections. *Paediatric Anaesthesia* **5**, 257–62.

Weaver, M.K. 1993: Perioperative pulmonary aspiration in children: a review. *Paediatric Anaesthesia* **3**, 333–8.

Welborn, L.E.G., Hannallah, R.S., Luban, N.L., Fink, R. and Ruttimann, U.E. 1991: Anemia and postoperative apnea in former preterm infants. *Anesthesiology* **74**, 1003–6.

Welborn, L.G. 1992: Postoperative apnoea in the former preterm infant: a review. *Paediatric Anaesthesia* **2**, 37–44.

Welborn, L.G., Hannallah, R.S., Fink, R., Ruttimann, U.E. and Hicks, J.M. 1989: High-dose caffeine supresses postoperative apnea in former preterm infants. *Anesthesiology* **71**, 347–9.

Welborn, L.G., Hannallah, R.S., McGill, W.A., Ruttimann, U.E. and Hicks, J.M. 1987: Glucose concentrations for routine intravenous infusion in pediatric outpatient surgery. *Anesthesiology* **67**, 427–30.

Welborn, L.G., Rice, U., Broadman, L. *et al.* 1990: Postoperative apnea in former preterm infants: prospective comparison of spinal and general anesthesia. *Anesthesiology* **72**, 838–42.

Wilson, P.T.J. and Lloyd-Thomas, A.R. 1993: An audit of extradural infusion analgesia in children using bupivacaine and diamorphine. *Anaesthesia* **48**, 718–23.

Wilton, N.C.T. and Burn, J.M.B. 1986: Delayed vomiting after papaveretum in paediatric outpatient surgery. *Canadian Anaesthetists Society Journal* **33**, 741–4.

Wolf, A.R. and Hughes, D. 1993: Pain relief for infants undergoing abdominal surgery: comparison of infusions of i.v. morphine and extradural bupivacaine. *British Journal of Anaesthesia* **70**, 10–6.

Yaster, M., Buck, J.R. and Dudgeon, D.L. *et al.* 1988: Hemodynamic effects of primary closure of omphalocele gastroschisis in human newborns. *Anesthesiology* **69**, 84–8.

Further reading

Hatch, D.J., Sumner, E. and Hellmann, J. 1994: *The surgical neonate: anaesthesia and intensive care.* London: Edward Arnold.

Morton, N.S. and Raine, P.A.M. 1994: *Paediatric day case surgery.* Oxford: Oxford University Press.

Peutrell, J.M. and Mather, S.J. 1996: *Regional anaesthesia for babies and children.* Oxford: Oxford University Press.

Steward, D.J. 1995: *Manual of pediatric anesthesia.* New York: Churchill Livingstone.

Sumner, E. Hatch, D.J. (eds) 1989: *Textbook of paediatric anaesthetic practice.* London: Baillière Tindall.

CHAPTER 14

Homeostasis. Fluid and electrolyte balance

A.G. CORAN

Introduction
Hormonal and metabolic response to
stress in the neonate
Hormonal response to surgery
Metabolic response to surgery
Fluid and electrolyte management
Insensible water loss
Renal water requirements

Water loss from the gastrointestinal tract
Sodium requirements
Potassium requirements
Acid–base status
Fluid and electrolyte infusion
Venous access
Intraosseous infusion
References

Introduction

Quite often the success of an operation on a child, especially an infant, is dependent on the proper metabolic management of the patient preoperatively, intraoperatively and postoperatively. This requires a thorough understanding of the normal physiology of the infant and the impact of the operative stress on that normal physiology. This chapter consists of a section on the hormonal and metabolic response to operative stress in the infant, more specifically the neonate; a discussion of fluid and electrolyte balance, requirements and management; and, finally a description of peripheral (including intraosseous) and central venous access techniques for infusion of various electrolyte solutions.

Hormonal and metabolic response to stress in the neonate

Postoperative or post-traumatic morbidity and mortality in high-risk adult patients have been correlated with and may be precipitated by the magnitude and the duration of the endocrine and metabolic response to the stressful event. Specifically, complications such as severe weight loss, cardiopulmonary insufficiency, thromboembolic disorders, gastric stress ulcers, impaired immunological function, prolonged convalescence, and even death have been related to aspects of the hormonal and metabolic response to surgical or traumatic stress (Kehiet, 1979; Moyer et al., 1981).

These hormonal and metabolic responses to stress in the adult have been the subject of laboratory and clinical investigation for the past century; however, similar responses in newborn infants are not as well documented. Metabolic complications or aberrations induced by stress may upset the delicate metabolic balance of a neonate already involved in the process of adaptation to its postnatal environment. The normal neonatal reserves of nutrients are limited, and the energy-consuming processes of rapid growth and maturation are occurring simultaneously with the additional demands produced by an operation. This difference is accentuated by experimental data that demonstrate a higher morbidity and mortality in neonates than in older children or adults subjected to similar procedures (Rackow et al., 1961; Schweiss and Pennington, 1981). Knowledge of the specific aspects of the neonatal stress response is imperative for those providing care to these infants.

Hormonal response to surgery (Table 14.1)

Suits and Bottsford (1987) outlined a neuroendocrine reflex that is set in motion by significant stress. Components of this reflex include an afferent arc, consisting of those stimuli that initiate the metabolic responses, and an efferent arc, leading to volume restoration and energy substrate production. The sequence is initiated by surgical stress affecting the neuroendocrine reflex directly through a nervous system signal to the central nervous system (CNS) and indirectly through the elaboration of catecholamines, the major mediators of

the hypermetabolic response, and adrenocorticoids, the major augmentors of this response. Components of the afferent arc involved in such a system are nociceptors, chemoreceptors and baroreceptors, all of which are capable of sending signals to the hypothalamus, where they become integrated into the physiological response observed in the stress state.

The efferent arc is described as originating in the hypothalamus, with efferent limbs travelling through the brainstem's autonomic regions and the pituitary. These brainstem autonomic areas send efferent fibres via the parasympathetic and sympathetic nervous systems to the periphery, affecting neuromuscular junctions in the circulatory system and receptors at end

Table 14.1 Hormonal response to operative stress in the adult and neonate

Hormone	Adult	Neonate
Endorphins	Actions: Modulate ACTH secretion ↑ ↑ Hypothalamic sympathetic response → ↑ catecholamine release Modulate insulin and glucagon secretion ? Immune modulation	No postoperative data ↑ After stress of delivery ? Role in septic shock
Pituitary hormones	↑ ACTH, growth hormone (GH), prolactin, vasopressin (GH → ↑ Lipolysis and FFA production → ↑ protein synthesis → ↓ insulin action)	No direct data (pharmacological administration of ACTH → ↑ Cortisol as in postop. neonates, therefore suggests ↑ ACTH postop.)
Catecholamines	↑ Epinephrine and norepinephrine – believed responsible for majority of stress-related catabolic response	Birth stress → ↑ two-fold in epinephrine and norepinephrine. Mild asphyxia → additional two-fold ↑ in norepinephrine and epinephrine ↑ Postop. ? Initiates hyperglycaemic response with ↓ insulin release and ↑ glucagon release provides substrate (peripheral tissue glycogen → lactate and pyruvate) for hepatic gluconeogenesis → ↑ minute ventilation, ↑ cardiac output. ↑ heart rate, ↑ blood pressure
Pancreatic hormones	Insulin ↓ intraoperatively; conflicting data for postoperative ↑ or ↓ ↑ Glucagon → amino acid mobilizatiton which → gluconeogenesis and new protein synthesis	↑ Insulin in term neonates. No change in preterm neonates ↓ Insulin/glucose ratio secondary to relative ↑ glucose Few data. No change until 24 h postoperatively and then ↓
Adrenocorticoids	Cortisol ↑ → Lipolysis and FFA release → amino acid mobilization from skeletal muscle → glucagon production	Age dependent ↑ – ↑ Response in older infants – Earlier peak in younger infants (< 9 days) secondary to ↓ foodstuff reserves and need for earlier precursor mobilization
Aldosterone	↑ → Volume restoration	No available data
Renin/angiotensin	3 × ↑ in renin ↑ angiotension	No available data
Antiduretic hormone	No available data	Indirect evidence of ↑
Thyroid hormone	↓ T$_3$ (active) and ↑ or T$_3$ (inactive)	No available data

organs, which stimulate the release of peripheral hormones. The pituitary response leads to increased adrenocorticotropic hormone (ACTH), vasopressin, growth hormone and prolactin release.

Neonates have well-developed neural pathways for pain (Anand and Hickey, 1987). In fact, the density of the nociceptive nerve endings in newborn skin is at least equivalent to that in adult skin. These receptors have been noted to be present throughout fetal cutaneous and mucosal surfaces by the 20th week of gestation (Valman and Pearson, 1980). Thus, the initial component of the proposed afferent arc is present early in fetal development and the capacity for initiating a stress response is present. The endocrine response of adult patients to operative and non-operative trauma is characterized mainly by a substantial decrease in the circulating concentration of the global anabolic hormone, insulin. The magnitude and duration of this response, particularly with respect to changes in the plasma concentrations of cortisol, catecholamines, glucagon, growth hormone and vasopressin, appear to be proportional to the extent of the injury. In addition, the duration of changes in the blood concentrations of some of these hormones may be prolonged in patients with postoperative complications. These hormonal changes may have profound effects on metabolic homeostasis, circulatory haemodynamics, immuno-competence, renal homeostasis, and gastrointestinal physiology. Behavioural and psychological effects on patients who are undergoing surgery are also possible. The adjustments in fuel metabolism during and after stress resulting from these hormonal changes are discussed in the following section.

The neonatal hormonal response to stress is much less well characterized. This response is predominantly catabolic, with documented elevations of catecholamine and endorphin levels. The alterations in glucagon and insulin levels in data from neonates do not parallel those from adults. Cortisol responsiveness in the neonate is also diminished in comparison with the adult. This difference may depend on maturation. Many areas of the hormonal response to operative and non-operative stress still have not been thoroughly investigated in the neonatal age group.

Metabolic response to surgery (Table 14.2)

Considerable data have accumulated that characterize the metabolic response of adults to surgery and trauma. A great deal less is known about the metabolic effects produced in neonates by major operative and non-operative stress. Metabolic studies, even on normal

Table 14.2   Metabolic response to operative stress in the adult and neonate

Metabolite	Adult	Neonate
Metabolic rate and oxygen consumption	↓ Briefly, then ↑	↓ Compared to adults (minimal change compared to age-matched controls)
Carbohydrate	↑ Hyperglycemic response ↑ Gluconeogenesis and ↓ glugose utilization	↑ Glucose 2× immediately postoperatively (less persistent ↑ than in adults) – probably secondary to glycogenlysis rather than ↑ gluconeogenesis – neonates may be unable to carry out hepatic gluconeogenesis secondary to lack of key enzyme
Protein	Negative nitrogen balance – Slight ↑ protein breakdown, dependent on severity of stress; ↑ with increased severity – ↓ Protein synthesis in extra-hepatic tissues ↑ Amino acid utilization for gluconeogenesis, acute-phase reactant synthesis and synthesis of components of healing process	↑ Nitrogen excretion, sustained up to 5 days Negative nitrogen balance 72–96 hours postoperatively. ↑ Nitrogen loss in neonates compared to older infants Muscle protein breakdown, impaired nitrogen utilization, transient ↑ nitrogen excretion ↓ (vs adult) in gluconeogenic amino acids in postoperative plasma
Fat	Adipose tissue lipolysis → Mobilization of nonesterified fatty acids and ↑ ketone body formation – Kinney (1970): 75–90% of postoperative requirements supplied by fat metabolism (10–25% by protein)	↑ Lipolysis + ketogenesis (? catecholamine stimulated) → ↑ total ketone bodies, ↑ glycerol, ↑ non-esterified fatty acids. Postoperative fat utilization exceeds rate of mobilization of free fatty acids

infants, are few, because of the limitations caused by insensitive assays, difficulties inherent in conducting prolonged observations and limited amounts of blood that can be withdrawn ethically. Postoperative treatment would be greatly improved if a thorough understanding of the metabolic consequences of stress was achieved. The evidence suggests that neonates frequently respond to trauma and stress in a manner different from that of adults or older children.

Adult patients show an increase in oxygen consumption (V_{O_2}) after trauma or surgery following a brief 'ebb' period of a depressed metabolic rate (Cuthbertson, 1942, 1959). The V_{O_2} of a full-term, normally fed, non-operated neonate increases with advancing age, until approximately the 2nd or 3rd week of life (Brandt *et al.*, 1978). Investigators have demonstrated that some postoperative newborns, predominantly those undergoing major abdominal operations, manifest a lower postoperative V_{O_2} than would be expected for their age and size. Ito *et al.* (1976) concluded that postoperative V_{O_2} in neonates is better correlated with the caloric intake than with the intensity of the operative stress. These findings are in striking contrast to the increased metabolic rate found in adults.

The purpose of the stress response is to provide energy sources to meet metabolic demands as well as to provide essential building blocks for synthetic activities occurring in the postoperative period. The hyperglycaemic response may be essential in supplying the increased glucose requirements of injured tissue (Im and Hoopes, 1970). In addition, the proteolytic component of the stress response provides the necessary amino acid components for reparative protein synthesis and production of acute-phase reactants by the liver.

The changes in metabolic patterns induced by the stress response are satisfied in part by increased lipolysis and ketogenesis to provide an alternative source of metabolic fuel for tissues, such as the brain and skeletal muscles. Additionally, the observed gluconeogenesis may aid in maintaining the glucose supply for vital organs principally dependent on glucose (Wilmore, 1981; Elliott and Albert, 1983). However, this metabolic response has also been shown to potentiate many adverse conditions in the postoperative period and to exacerbate the stress response. Examples include a hypermetabolic state with attendant elevations in V_{O_2}, energy requirements, temperature, and cardiac output and altered or impaired inflammatory or immune responsiveness.

Numerous investigators have demonstrated that adult patients exposed to severe degrees of traumatic stress are subjected to higher rates of complications, such as cardiac or pulmonary insufficiency, myocardial infarction, impaired hepatic and/or renal function, gastric stress ulcers, and sepsis. Furthermore, evidence exists to suggest that this response may be life-threatening if the induced catabolic activity remains excessive or unchecked for a prolonged period. It is possible to identify with a great degree of certainty the patients who are likely to succumb based on a single analysis of a variety of plasma-borne substrates, obtained up to 9 days prior to death (Moyer *et al.*, 1981).

Modulating or blunting the catabolic response induced by the stress state may have beneficial effects. In studies of postoperative pain management, improved pain control resulted in reduction of postoperative nitrogen loss and in shortened periods of convalescence following operation (Brandt *et al.*, 1978; Kerri-Szanto, 1973). Newborns, even those born prematurely, are capable of mounting an endocrine and a metabolic response to operative stress. Unfortunately, many of the areas for which a relatively well-characterized response exists in adults, are poorly documented in neonates. As is the case in adults, the response seems to be primarily catabolic in nature, because the combined hormonal changes include an increased release of catabolic hormones such as catecholamines, glucagon and corticosteroids, coupled with a suppression of and a peripheral resistance to the effects of the primary anabolic hormone, insulin.

The catecholamines may be the agents of primary importance in this response and, thus, may modulate the remaining components of the hormonal response to stress as well as the metabolic changes including an inhibition of insulin release, a marked hyperglycaemia and a breakdown of the neonate's stores of nutrients (carbohydrate, protein and fat). These reactions result, ultimately, in the release of glucose, non-esterified fatty acids, ketone bodies, and amino acids. Although these metabolic byproducts are necessary to meet the body's altered energy needs in a time of increased metabolic demands, a severe or prolonged response would be very detrimental to a previously ill neonate with limited reserves of nutrients and already high metabolic demands imposed by rapid growth, organ maturation and adaptation to the postnatal environment. Preliminary investigations indicate that alterations in anaesthetic technique with the addition of agents such as halothane and fentanyl may be able to decrease this catabolic response significantly (Anand, 1995; Anand and Aynsley-Green, 1985; Anand and Hickey, 1987; Anand *et al.*, 1985a, b, 1987, 1988) Modulation of the immune response may also greatly affect the postoperative catabolic response. Future developments and acquisition of more detailed knowledge of the response will allow the modification of the stress response in neonates, in order to decrease mortality and morbidity further.

Fluid and electrolyte management

Fluid and electrolyte management of neonates and infants requires a thorough understanding of the body fluid compartment changes that occur before and after birth (Fig. 14.1) (Friis-Hansen, 1954, 1957, 1961, 1971, 1983; Friis-Hansen *et al.*, 1951). During the first trimester, total body water (TBW) accounts for 95% of body weight. This percentage falls to 80% by 32 weeks' gestation, to 78% at term, and to 75% by the end of the first postnatal week. Body water then decreases slowly over the next 1–2 years to 60% of total body weight. Similarly, extracellular fluid (ECF) volume decreases from 60% of body weight during the second trimester to 45% at birth and eventually to 20% during the next 2 years. This normal physiological process is interrupted in premature neonates, who must diurese excess fetal and postnatal total body water in a relatively short period after birth. This interruption has a significant effect on the fluid and electrolyte requirements of premature infants undergoing major surgery. An expanded ECF volume in a premature infant is a potent stimulus for the release of prostacyclin E_2, which maintains the patency of a ductus arteriosus (Stevenson, 1977; Bell *et al.*, 1979, 1980a).

Renal function is related to two physiological processes: glomerular filtration and tubular excretion and reabsorption. In newborns, glomerular filtration rates are 25% of adult values, which are reached by the age of 2 years. Likewise, renal concentrating ability is significantly reduced in both premature and full-term infants. A full-term infant can maximally concentrate urine to only 500–600 mOsm/kg (vs 1200 mOsm/kg for an adult) (Aperia *et al.*, 1975, 1983) and a premature infant has even less concentrating ability (up to a maximum of 400 mOsm/kg). As a consequence, newborns tolerate dehydration poorly. Furthermore, the kidneys of newborns cannot excrete a water load as effectively as mature kidneys can. This phenomenon, combined with the low concentrating ability of the newborn's kidneys, makes fluid management very difficult. An initial fluid and electrolyte programme for newborns and infants must replace the insensible water loss, the renal water loss and the sodium and potassium losses.

Insensible water loss

Insensible water loss is a result of continuous loss of water from the respiratory tract and the skin (Doyle and Sinclair, 1982). In both full-term and premature infants, transepithelial water loss is the major component of insensible water loss (Hammarlund *et al.*, 1977) (Fig. 14.2). The stratum corneum is the major barrier to the passive diffusion of water from the superficial capillaries of the skin to the epidermal surface. Premature infants have a less developed stratum corneum than full-term infants and, therefore, experience a greater diffusion of water through the epidermal surface and a greater insensible water loss through the skin. In full-term neonates, in an environment of thermal neutrality and a humidity of 50%, total insensible water loss is

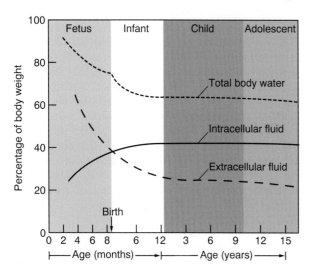

Fig. 14.1 Total body water and extracellular fluid decrease and intracellular fluid increases during gestation and infancy.

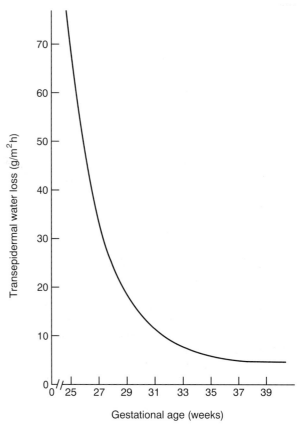

Fig. 14.2 Transepithelial water loss decreases as postnatal age increases and is directly related to gestational age.

12 ml/kg per 24 hours, of which 7 ml is lost through the skin and 5 ml through the lungs. Overhead radiant heaters and phototherapy may increase insensible water loss from skin by 50% (Oh and Karecki, 1972; Bell *et al.*, 1979, 1980b; Baumgart *et al.*, 1981; Tan and Jacob, 1981; Engel *et al.*, 1981, 1982).

Full-term babies sweat at birth if body temperature exceeds 37.5°C (99.5°F); however, the amount of water they lose by this mechanism is quite small. Respiratory water loss accounts for about one-third of total insensible water loss in full-term infants and is related to the volume of inspired air, respiratory rate, body temperature and the humidity of the expired air (Sosulki *et al.*, 1977). Premature infants of less than 36 weeks' gestation do not sweat in the first few days of life. In these infants, especially those who are born after less than 32 weeks' gestation, the respiratory water loss is less than it is in full-term infants and the transepithelial water loss is greater.

Renal water requirements

The water required for excretion of the products of catabolism is based on the renal solute load, including any exogenous solute load (Saigal and Sinclair, 1977) and on the maximal renal concentrating ability. Therefore, the volume of fluid administered must allow excretion of the entire solute load at an osmolality of 250 mOsm/kg, a level achievable by even the smallest premature infant. The solute load of the newborn is approximately 15 mOsm/kg per 24 hours during the first week of life if the infant receives only intravenous fluids, 17.5 mOsm/kg per 24 hours during the second week of life if the infant is on partial oral intake, and 30 mOsm/kg per 24 hours thereafter if the infant is maintained on formula. The amount of water required for excretion of these osmolar loads can be calculated by using the following formula:

$$H_2O \text{ requirements (ml/kg per 24 hours)}$$
$$= \frac{\text{Osmolality of solute load (mOsm/kg)}}{\text{Osmolality of urine (mOsm/kg)}} \times 1000$$

If the urine osmolality is 250 mOsm/kg, the renal water requirements are 60 ml/kg per 24 hours during the first week of life, 72 ml/kg per 24 hours during the second week of life and 84 ml/kg per 24 hours thereafter. This rate of fluid infusion will produce a urine output of approximately 2.5 ml/kg/hour. Renal water requirements are modified by a number of factors. An anabolic, growing infant has a lower solute load and, therefore, a lower water requirement. A certain amount of water is required for active growth, between 10 and 15 ml/kg per 24 hours. However, if the infant has recently undergone an operation or is otherwise stressed, a catabolic state exists and the solute load will increase. Tissue destruction secondary to trauma or surgery increases the solute load even further.

Water loss from the gastrointestinal tract

In general, water loss from the stool need not be considered in calculating water requirements as it amounts to an expenditure of only 5–10 ml/100 kcal. Infants receiving nothing through the gastrointestinal tract will have smaller losses than infants being fed orally. Short-bowel syndrome or significant diarrhoea increases the stool water loss and phototherapy doubles stool water content. Measurable water and electrolyte losses from the gastrointestinal tract or other sites should be replaced.

Sodium requirements

Sodium requirements of full-term infants average 2 mEq/kg per 24 hours; preterm infants older than 32 weeks' gestational age require 3 mEq/kg per 24 hours; and babies who are low gestational age or critically ill require 4–5 mEq/kg per 24 hours. Conditions such as intestinal obstruction and peritonitis increase sodium loss, and, therefore, increase the requirements.

Although full-term infants can retain sodium as well as adults in the face of a sodium deficit, they are unable to excrete excess sodium as effectively as adults. As a result, excessive infusion of intravenous sodium can rapidly result in hypernatraemia. The problem is exaggerated in premature infants. Sodium excretion during the last half of gestation is significant but quickly drops off after birth in full-term infants. Premature neonates excrete large amounts of sodium to complete the normal intrauterine process of sodium excretion, but this ability appears to be fixed. Premature infants are unable to respond to an excessive infusion of sodium by increasing sodium excretion, perhaps because of immaturity of the renal tubules or because of unresponsiveness of the renal tubules to aldosterone.

Potassium requirements

Potassium requirements of infants are well documented. The generally accepted requirements are 2 mEq/kg per 24 hours after the first two to three days of life. The delay in administration has been recommended because of the concern about immature renal function in the first few days of life. In fact, however, potassium requirements are significant in the first few days of life, especially after a major operation, because in the catabolic state, protein breakdown leads to nitrogen loss in the urine and a concomitant potassium loss. Thus, potassium should be administered in the first day or two of life after an operation once urine output is established.

Acid–base status

Metabolic alkalosis caused by electrolyte loss, specifically chloride, may occur with prolonged gastric suction or vomiting and is usually easily corrected by replacement of the appropriate electrolytes (e.g. with potassium chloride). Metabolic acidosis, in contrast, is usually the result of poor tissue perfusion and lactic acidosis. It is best corrected by treating the underlying cause of the poor perfusion and by temporarily administering buffers, such as sodium bicarbonate, which is usually done when the pH falls below 7.3. Standard sodium bicarbonate solutions are extremely hypertonic and should be diluted before being administered, especially in neonates. The dose can be calculated from the following formula:

$$NaHCO_2 \text{ dose (mmol)} = \frac{\text{base excess} \times \text{body weight (kg)}}{3}$$

Fluid and electrolyte infusion

The initial parenteral fluid administered to the newborn infant should be a dextrose solution that contains no electrolytes. After the first day of life, electrolytes are added to the solution. A parenteral solution that contains 25–30 mEq/l of sodium and chloride and 5–10% dextrose (D5 or D10 0.2NS) with 10–20 mEq/L of potassium will meet the objectives of maintenance fluid therapy when administered at a rate calculated from Table 14.3.

Dynamic fluid and electrolyte management requires ongoing assessment and adjustment of dextrose, electrolytes and fluid rates. Serial physical examinations should include inspection and palpation of the skin for the presence and absence of oedema, palpation of the peripheral pulses, and auscultation of the heart and lungs. In addition, the parameters of body weight, net fluid intake, urine output, blood glucose and serum sodium, chloride and potassium are useful to monitor.

EXAMPLE

A 4.2 kg male infant with an antenatal diagnosis of gastroschisis is delivered vaginally. After delivery, the infant is placed beneath a warmer and the viscera are wrapped in saline-saturated gauze and enclosed in a plastic wrap (Saran Wrap) to reduce evaporative losses. In addition, the viscera are suspended in this gauze and plastic wrap 'silo' to reduce oedema and venous congestion. A nasogastric tube is inserted and peripheral intravenous access is established. Approximate initial intravenous fluid therapy preoperatively should be 10% dextrose at a rate of 100 ml/kg per 24 hours. However, because of the sequestration of serum into the exposed, inflamed viscera and inflamed peritoneum ('third spacing'), resuscitation with colloid boluses (5% albumin, 10 ml/kg per bolus) should be initiated and given each hour prior to operation. Postoperatively, after primary closure of the defect, the infant's hydration status can be reassessed with serial physical examinations and urine output can be monitored with the aid of a urinary catheter. An appropriate urine output is 1–2 ml/kg/hour. The appropriate intravenous fluid for an infant less than 24 hours of age is 10% dextrose, with 0.2% NaCl added at 1 day of life. Potassium is added to the fluid after the infant urinates. This infant will continue to 'third space' postoperatively, sequestering fluid within the bowel wall and peritoneum, and will require repletion of the intravascular volume. The intravascular volume can be augmented, as in the preoperative phase of management, with colloid boluses. Crystalloid boluses of normal saline or lactated Ringer's solution are not used in the first day of life because of the excessive salt load delivered to the neonate.

Venous access

PERIPHERAL ACCESS

Because of anatomical variations, different cannulation sites are more appropriate in different age groups. In general, neonates' veins are easily visible because of the paucity of subcutaneous body fat. Within the first 1–2

Table 14.3 Daily fluid requirements for neonates and infants

	Weight (kg)	Volume
Premature	< 2	150 ml/kg
Neonates and infants	2–10	100 ml/kg for first 10 kg
Infants and children	10–20	1000 ml +50 ml/kg over 10 kg
Children	>20	1500 ml +20 ml/kg over 20 kg

weeks of life, cannulation of the umbilical vessels should be considered. Scalp veins are readily located and utilized in the neonate and infant. During infancy, with the development of a thick layer of fat, hand and arm veins become invisible but remain palpable. In older children, with fat redistribution, veins become superficial as in the adult (Murdoch and Bingham, 1990). The basilic and cephalic veins in the antecubital fossa are among the largest and easiest to cannulate. Deep, percutaneous antecubital venipuncture of the venae comitantes of the brachial artery may be performed in larger children. The basic anatomic principle is that major arteries are accompanied by large veins (venae comitantes). This technique is an alternative to routine superficial, percutaneous venipuncture and should be used in order to avoid a cutdown (Roseman, 1983). Dorsal veins in the hands and feet are accessible cannulation sites in infants, toddlers and older children. The superficial radial vein is well developed in adults but may be difficult to locate in the small child. The long saphenous vein may be cannulated percutaneously or accessed by surgical cutdown. The constant anatomy of the saphenous vein at the ankle (superior and anterior to the medial malleolus) makes it a logical and safe cutdown site (Zimmerman and Strauss, 1989).

Complications of peripheral venous cannulation include bleeding, thrombosis, arterial cannulation and local or, rarely, systemic sepsis, which resolves on removal of the cannula. Perivenous administration of fluid and drugs may cause tissue necrosis and sloughing. If peripheral venous cannulation is unsuccessful, central venous cannulation can be performed.

Rapid intravenous access during paediatric resuscitations is difficult. When faced with a critically ill or injured child the options for gaining access to the venous circulation include, peripheral percutaneous venous cannulation, intraosseous infusion, percutaneous central venous access or peripheral venous cutdown. Percutaneous central venous cannulation is not routinely used as the primary site of access for resuscitation in adult trauma patients and should not be used as such in pediatric trauma victims. Sites available for central venous cannulation include the femoral, internal jugular and subclavian veins. Peripheral venous cutdown can be accomplished by using either the saphenous vein at the ankle or the saphenofemoral junction.

CENTRAL ACCESS

Central venous cannulation is preferred if hypertonic, irritant or vasoconstrictor solutions are used. Dudrick *et al.* (1986) described a technique for long-term venous catheterization in infants. In 1973, Broviac *et al.* introduced a Silastic (silicone rubber) catheter that consisted of a thin intravascular segment and a thicker extravascular segment with an attached Dacron cuff to reduce dislodgement and infection.

The most popular methods of placement of indwelling central venous catheters include percutaneous venipuncture, venous cutdown and use of an extremity vein with advancement of the catheter to a central venous position (Weber *et al.*, 1983). Sites for long-term central venous access in infants, in order of preference, are the external jugular veins, the facial veins, the internal jugular veins, the saphenous veins at the groin and the subclavian veins.

External jugular vein

In neonates and infants, a cutdown may be performed using an incision placed midway between the clavicle and the ramus of the mandible, which allows access to the external jugular vein, facial vein and internal jugular vein. Dilatation of the vein may be aided by placing the patient in the Trendelenberg position or by occluding the vein with digital compression of the soft tissues above the clavicle. Each external jugular vein enters the central venous system in almost a straight line and, therefore, the catheter must make an acute angle into the subclavian vein (Cobb *et al.*, 1987). Traction of the vein laterally may permit a more direct path into the superior vena cava.

Common facial vein

The common facial vein is a large anterior tributary of the internal jugular vein that is formed by the confluence of the anterior and posterior facial veins. The common facial vein enters the internal jugular vein midway between the angle of the mandible and the clavicular head (Cobb *et al.*, 1987). A transverse skin incision is made at the midpoint of a line connecting the angle of the mandible and the hyoid bone. The incision is deepened and the common facial vein is located. To confirm the identity of the vein, the dissection is continued laterally tracing the common facial vein to where it drains into the internal jugular vein. The advantages of using this vein are twofold. Advancement of the catheter into the central venous system via the common facial vein is easily performed. This is in contrast to the difficulties commonly encountered when using the external jugular vein as an entry site. Ligation of the internal jugular vein is also obviated (Zumbro *et al.*, 1971).

Subclavian vein

The use and safety of percutaneous central lines in infants and children, using the infraclavicular subclavian approach, have been established (Groff and Ahmed, 1974; Filston and Grant, 1979; Eichelburger *et al.*, 1981; Pybus *et al.*, 1982; Gauderer *et al.*, 1982; Bonventre *et al.*, 1989). The techniques obviate the need for surgical exposure and ligation of a peripheral vein in the neck and permit repeated catheterization of central veins.

Femoral vein

Percutaneous femoral vein catheterization has been used for emergency venous access, cardiac catheterization and invasive haemodynamic monitoring. The safety and effectiveness of femoral venous catheterization have been established in preterm infants, full-term infants and children (Kanter *et al.*, 1986, 1989; Abdulla *et al.*, 1990) The palpable femoral arterial pulsation serves as a landmark for percutaneous femoral venous access. Relative contraindications to percutaneous femoral venous catheterization include malformation of the lower extremity causing potential vascular distortion, suspected anatomic interruption of the inferior vena cava, trauma involving the lower extremity, pelvis or the inferior vena cava, an abdominal mass compressing the vena cava, suspected femoral hernia, local skin or soft tissue lesion or a plan for future transfemoral cardiac catheterization (Kanter *et al.*, 1986). For long-term access, the femoral vein may be cannulated by saphenous vein cutdown at the groin.

Alternative sites

The cephalic vein is cannulated through an incision in the deltopectoral groove just below the lateral third of the clavicle (Kosloske and Klein, 1982). The catheter is then brought out through a subcutaneous tunnel on the chest wall. Axillary vein catheterization may be performed percutaneously or by cutdown. For permanent access, the axillary vein may be cannulated through an incision in the axilla, and the catheter may be brought out through a subcutaneous tunnel on the chest wall. Percutaneous placement of inferior vena caval-tunnelled Silastic catheters via the translumbar approach has been described in patients with difficult vascular access. Central venous access using the azygous system by cannulation of an intercostal vein has been described. The intercostal vein is accessed through a transverse incision made over the chosen interspace.

COMPLICATIONS

Complications of central venous access include catheter sepsis, catheter breakage, dislodgement and embolization, pneumothorax, hydrothorax, pulmonary embolus, vena caval and intracardiac catheter-tip thrombosis and vascular injury.

Sepsis is the most common serious complication of central venous catheters (Vane *et al.*, 1990). King *et al.* (1985) described criteria for catheter sepsis, which included: (1) an apparent clinical infection; (2) presence of a central venous catheter; (3) positive blood cultures; and (4) no other source of infection. It is considered optimal to remove the foreign body when infection is suspected; however, this is frequently not possible because of the continuing need to use the catheter and the limited number of central venous access sites. Catheter-related bacterial infections can be successfully treated with intravenous antibiotics in the majority of pediatric patients without catheter removal (Nahata *et al.*, 1988).

Vascular thrombosis is the result of hypercoagulability, stasis and endothelial disruption. Endothelial injury may be related to the catheter or due directly to the hyperosmolar infusate. The incidence of major venous thrombosis associated with central indwelling catheters has been reported to range from 5% to 10% (Mollitt and Golladay, 1983). Catheter-induced vena caval occlusion has been previously reported to produce few serious sequelae (Fonkalsrud *et al.*, 1982). Hydrocephalus, pulmonary lymphangiectasia, chylothorax, pulmonary embolus, endocarditis and cardiac dysfunction have been associated with catheter-induced central venous thrombosis, with the majority of these complications occurring in children less than 1 year of age. The newborn and infant are at greatest risk for thrombosis and thrombotic complications. Central venous occlusion is confirmed radiographically. Contrast injection will demonstrate central occlusion and collateralization. Ultrasound can localize thrombi and evaluate the cardiac valves for vegetations.

Propagation of caval thrombosis has been demonstrated to occur both proximally and distally. With involvement of both subclavian veins, there may be occlusion of the thoracic duct with stasis within the pleural and pulmonary lymphatics resulting in pulmonary oedema and chylothorax. Propagation of the thrombus into the right atrium may interfere with valvular competence and result in tricuspid insufficiency and/or predispose to clot disruption with resultant pulmonary embolism (Mollitt and Golladay, 1983).

Complications of placement of small percutaneous central venous catheters (Per-Q-Cath) include mechanical problems such as catheter occlusion, catheter dislodgment and perforation of the tubing. The incidence of catheter-associated sepsis is lower than that observed with larger diameter catheters (Loeff *et al.*, 1982). Mechanical complications have also included embolization of a portion of the catheter and perforation of the right atrium with a resultant pericardial effusion. Both complications may be attributed to initial improper catheter tip placement or subsequent catheter tip migration. In the former complication, inadvertent placement of the tip in the right ventricle results in weakening of the catheter due to tricuspid valve movement and ventricular contractions (Khilnani *et al.*, 1990). In the latter complication, autopsy findings have demonstrated thrombus formation at the site of the catheter contact within the heart with myosclerosis of the atrial or ventricular wall. It appears that this lesion occurs as a consequence of the constant exposure of a small area of the endocardium to hypertonic fluid (Giacoia, 1991).

Intraosseous infusion

Immediate vascular access can usually be established in adults using peripheral and central venous catheterization techniques. However, it may be extremely difficult to find venous access in infants and small children. All health care workers who have dealt with emergencies in paediatric patients, such as cardiopulmonary arrest, seizures, sepsis, dehydration, trauma and burns, are aware of the frustration of establishing intravascular access in these small patients. It is sobering that when critically reviewed, the time required to establish vascular access is often excessive. In one study, one quarter of the paediatric patients in cardiac arrest required greater than 10 min to establish intravascular access (Rossetti *et al.*, 1984). Intravascular access by cut-down, usually of the saphenous vein at the ankle, in the hands of an experienced paediatric surgeon, long accepted as the gold standard of intravenous access in children, requires more than 5 min in the hands of most surgeons (Iserson and Criss, 1986). The technique of intraosseous infusion provides another option for vascular access and has emerged as the procedure of choice in children under 6 years of age in whom immediate intravenous access cannot be established (Glaeser *et al.*, 1988).

HISTORY

Intraosseous infusion was used extensively for the parenteral administration of blood, fluids and pharmacological agents in the 1940s. Drinker and Drinker had earlier described the circulation in the bone marrow of dogs and had proposed it as a site for parenteral infusion (1916; Drinker *et al.*, 1922). Quilligan and Turkel's (1946) view of intraosseous infusion includes an international bibliography on the subject, indicating extensive use of intraosseous infusion throughout the world at that time. As better, more reliable intravascular catheters for paediatric use became available, the technique of intraosseous infusion fell into disuse. The technique was rediscovered and popularized again during the 1980s as the limitations of peripheral, central and cut-down venous access techniques in emergency situations were recognized. Intraosseous infusion is a rapid, reliable, easily taught and mastered method to provide intravascular access in children (Hodge, 1985; Rossetti *et al.*, 1985; Spivey, 1987; Fiser, 1990; Kulick and Cilley, 1990). Intraosseous infusion has now become incorporated into the advanced life support protocols taught as advanced trauma life support, advanced cardiac life support and advanced life support (American College of Surgeons, 1988; American Heart Association, 1988, 1990).

ANATOMY AND PHYSIOLOGY

During intraosseous infusion, the rich vasculature of long bones is used to transport fluids and drugs to the central circulation. Sinusoids within the marrow of long bones function as rigid conduits that do not collapse in the presence of hypovolaemia. Blood passes into the venous channels of the medulla and then leaves the bone via nutrient or emissary veins entering the general circulation (Begg, 1954). Substances injected intraosseously are found rapidly (less than 10 s) in the central circulation (Tozantis, 1940). Tibial blood flow responds to the perfusion pressure of intraosseous infusion and permits infusion at relatively rapid rates. Flows of 10 ml/min with gravity and up to 40 ml/min with 300 mmHg pressure have been demonstrated using 13-gauge needles in the long bones of calves (Shoor *et al.*, 1979). Similar flows of 11–24 ml/min have been demonstrated in hypovolemic dogs using 20-gauge needles (Hodge *et al.*, 1987). Intraosseous infusion results in equal or more rapid transport to the central circulation than peripheral intravenous drug administration during the performance of cardiopulmonary resuscitation and during hypovolaemia in animal models (Spivey *et al.*, 1985; Brickman *et al.*, 1987; Cameron *et al.*, 1989; Orwlowski *et al.*, 1990). Many substances have been administered by the intraosseous route. A catalogue of drugs and fluids has been given by the intraosseous route, both clinically and experimentally. It is not recommended that hypertonic solutions be given by the intraosseous route. Hypertonic solutions may be associated with higher risks of osteomyelitis and permanent bone changes and should be diluted prior to administration via the intraosseous route if possible (Heinild *et al.*, 1947; Wallden, 1948; Neish *et al.*, 1988). Blood samples can be obtained for biochemical analysis and bacteriology as well as type and cross-match; however, sampling may occlude the infusion needle and is not routinely performed (Ros *et al.*, 1991). Blood gas samples have values midway between arterial and venous samples, while alkaline phosphatase may be somewhat elevated (Orlowski *et al.*, 1989b). Peripheral blood haematological studies obtained shortly after intraosseous infusion must be interpreted with caution. Abnormal white blood cell counts and blood smears are found after intraosseous infusion in animals (Ros *et al.*, 1991). When drugs are administered rapidly via the intraosseous route, peak serum levels are somewhat lower than with intravenous injections (Spivey, 1987). Within minutes, the differences disappear. Serum levels of drugs administered intraosseously tend to be elevated somewhat longer than when administered intravenously. Drugs should be given in the equivalent dose used for intravenous administration and fluids should be administered at the same rate.

The recognized contraindications to intraosseous infusion include osteopetrosis and osteogenesis imperfecta. Intraosseous needles should not be placed in fractured extremities because extravasation will occur at fracture sites. Ideally, intraosseous needles should not be placed through areas of burned skin or cellulitis.

TECHNIQUE

Multiple sites have been used for intraosseous infusion, including the sternum, humerus, iliac crest, femur and tibia. However, the tibia and distal femur are the recommended sites for emergency vascular access in infants and children (Hodge, 1985; Rossetti *et al.*, 1985; Spivey, 1987; Mofensen *et al.*, 1988; Wagner and McCabe, 1988; Fiser, 1990; Kulick and Cilley, 1990). These sites are easily identified by topical landmarks and the bones are superficially located. Needles inserted in these locations traverse tissue planes devoid of important structures and the marrow cavity is relatively large. These sites are also physically removed from other resuscitative efforts such as airway management and chest compressions that may be occurring simultaneously.

The preferred site for intraosseous infusion in paediatric patients is the proximal tibia. Insertion is performed 1–3 cm below the tibial tuberosity on the flat anteromedial surface of the tibia where it is easily palpable. The needle is directed away from the growth plate (caudally) by using an entry angle 10–15° from the perpendicular. In the smallest infants, the insertion site should be only 1 cm from the tibial tuberosity.

After about 5 years of age, the proximal tibial cortex is relatively difficult to penetrate, and the distal tibia or femur are the preferred sites. The distal tibia is approached 2–3 cm above the medial malleolus posterior to the saphenous vein on the palpable flat surface of the bone. The needle is directed away from the growth plate (cranially) by angling it 10–15° from the perpendicular.

For access to the distal femur, insertion is performed on the flat anterior surface 3 cm above the external condyle. The needle is angled 10–15° from the perpendicular away from the growth plate (cranially). Another site that may be considered in children is the iliac crest. Sternal intraosseous infusion is not recommended because the sternal marrow cavity of children is small and mediastinal penetration can occur with this procedure.

Although any stiff needle can be used for intraosseous infusion, it is preferable to use a needle with an inner stylette that occludes the lumen, allowing passage into the marrow without plugging of the needle with bone. If a specialized device is unavailable, a spinal needle is an alternative in any hospital setting. Needles manufactured specifically for bone marrow entry are preferred. Both bone-marrow aspiration needles and needles made specifically for resuscitative intraosseous infusion are available. Common design features include structural rigidity, sharp removable bone-piercing stylettes that lock in place and a flange or hand grip to facilitate controlled insertion. Some devices have positioning marks to indicate depth of penetration, while others have mechanisms to control the amount of exposed shaft to help guide penetration. Eighteen- or 20-gauge needles are normally used in children less than 1 year of age, whereas larger 13- or 16-gauge needles are used in older children.

COMPLICATIONS

When used in routine practice, intraosseous access is successfully established more than 95% of the time. Placement failure may occur as much as 20% of the time when catheters are inserted under emergency conditions (Spivey, 1987).

Extravasation of fluid outside the medullary space can occur by any of several mechanisms: (1) the cortex may be incompletely penetrated with resultant administration of fluid into the subcutaneous tissue or subperiosteally; (2) the needle may penetrate both bony cortices which, in the tibia, results in infusion into the posterior compartment of the leg; (3) the puncture holes from multiple attempts can allow fluid to escape; and (4) theoretically, extravasation can also occur through nutrient vessel foramina. A recent report documents bilateral lower extremity compartment syndromes requiring bilateral fasciotomies from tibial intraosseous infusion devices (Galpin *et al.*, 1991). The exact mechanism of extravasation in this patient was unknown. An additional case of lower extremity compartment syndrome requiring amputation has been reported (Moscati and Moore, 1990). Early use of direct compartment pressure measurements when extravasation is suspected, especially in obtunded patients, is recommended.

Improper placement has also resulted in tibial fractures in infants (LaFleche *et al.*, 1989; Melker *et al.*, 1990). In an infant, 3 cm below the tibial tuberosity may be near the midshaft of the tibia. The smaller the child the closer the needle should be placed to the tibial tuberosity.

Concern that intraosseous infusion may damage the growth plate of developing bones has been investigated in pigs that underwent intraosseous infusion through needles purposefully placed through the physeal growth plate (Brickman *et al.*, 1988). Radiological assessment showed no bony abnormalities 2 and 6 months after intraosseous infusion. The tract of the needle into the bone can be seen radiographically for 4–6 weeks after needle insertion in patients. The tract is usually unrecognizable after this time (Spivey, 1987).

Post-mortem studies in patients and in a canine model have uniformly shown evidence of small bone marrow and fat emboli in the lung after intraosseous infusion (Orlowski *et al.*, 1989a). They appear to be of little clinical importance in patients. The possibility of clinically significant paradoxical emboli in patients with intracardiac right-to-left shunts must be considered.

The risk of osteomyelitis appears to be very low, with an incidence of less than 1% (Massey, 1950; Rossetti *et al.*, 1985). Osteomyelitis occurred most commonly when the intraosseous infusion device was left in place longer than 1 day or when the patient was bacteraemic. When used as an emergency procedure and left in place for less than 1 day, the risk of infection from intraosseous infusion should be minimal.

References

Abdulla, F., Dietrich, K.A. and Pramanik, A.K. 1990: Percutaneous femoral venous catheterization in preterm neonates. *Journal of Pediatrics* **117**, 788–91.

American Heart Association. 1988: *Textbook of pediatric advanced life support*. Dallas, TX: American Heart Association, 43.

American Heart Association. 1990: *Textbook of advanced cardiac life support*, 2nd ed. Dallas, TX: American Heart Association, 263.

Anand, K.J.S. 1985: Metabolic and endocrine effects of surgery and anaesthesia in the human newborn infant. D.Phil. thesis, University of Oxford.

Anand, K.J.S. and Aynsley-Green, A. 1985: Metabolic and endocrine effects of surgical ligation of patient ductus arteriosus in the human preterm neonate: are there implications for further improvement of post-operative outcome? *Modern Problems of Paediatrics* **23**, 143–57.

Anand, K.J.S. and Hickey, P.R. 1987: Pain and its effects in the human neonate and fetus. *New England Journal of Medicine* **317**, 1321–9.

Anand, K.J.S., Brown, M.J., Bloom, S.R. and Aynsley-Green, A. 1985: Studies on the hormonal regulation of fuel metabolism in the human newborn infant undergoing anaesthesia and surgery. *Hormone Research* **22**, 115–28.

Anand, K.J.S., Brown, M.J., Causon, R.C. *et al.* 1985: Can the human neonate mount an endocrine and metabolic response to surgery? *Journal of Pediatric Surgery* **20**, 41–8.

Anand, K.J.S., Sippell, W.G. and Aynsley-Green, A. Randomized trial of fentanyl anesthesia in preterm babies undergoing surgery: effects on the stress response. *Lancet* **8527**, 243–8.

Anand, K.J.S., Sippell, W.G., Schofield, N.M. and Aynsley-Green, A. 1988: Does halothane anaesthesia decrease the metabolic and endocrine stress responses of newborn infants undergoing operation? *British Medical Journal* **296**, 668–72.

Aperia, A., Broberger, O., Herin, P. *et al.* 1983: Postnatal control of water and electrolyte homeostasis in pre-term and full-term infants. *Acta Paediatrica Scandinavica* (Suppl.) **305**, 61–5.

Aperia, A., Broberger, O., Thodenius, K. *et al.* 1975: Renal control of sodium and fluid balance in newborn infants during intravenous maintenance therapy. *Acta Paediatrica Scandinavica* **64**, 725–31.

Baumgart, S., Engle, W.D., Fox, W.W. *et al.* 1981: Radiant warmer power and body size as determinants of insensible water loss in the critically ill neonate. *Pediatric Research* **15**, 1495–9.

Begeryg, A.C. 1954: Intraosseous venography of the lower limb and pelvis. *British Journal of Radiology* **27**, 318–24.

Bell, E.F., Neidich, G.A., Cashore, W.J. *et al.* 1979: Combined effect of radiant warmer and phototherapy on insensible water loss in low-birth-weight infants. *Journal of Pediatrics* **94**, 810–3.

Bell, E.F., Warburton, D., Stonestreet, B.S. *et al.* 1979: High-volume fluid intake predisposes premature infants to necrotizing enterocolitis. *Lancet* **ii**, 90.

Bell, E.F., Warburton, D., Stonestreet, B.S. *et al.* 1980: Effect of fluid administration on the development of symptomatic patent ductus arteriosus and congestive heart failure in premature infants. *New England Journal of Medicine* **302**, 598–604.

Bell, E.F., Weinstein, M.R. and Oh, W. 1980: Heat balance in premature infants: comparative effects of convectively heated incubator and radiant warmer with and without plastic heat shield. *Journal of Pediatrics* **96**, 460–5.

Bonventre, E.V., Lally, K.P., Chwals, W.L. *et al.* Percutaneous insertion of subclavian venous catheters in infants and children. *Surgery, Gynecology and Obstetrics* **169**, 203–5.

Brandt, M.R., Fernandez, A., Mordhurst, R. and Kehlet, H. 1978: Epidural analgesia improves post-operative nitrogen balance. *British Medical Journal* **1**, 1106–8.

Brickman, K.R., Rega, P. and Guinness, M. A. 1987: A comparative study of intraosseous versus peripheral intravenous infusion of diazepam and phenobarbital in dogs. *Annals of Emergency Medicine* **16**, 1141–4.

Brickman, K.R., Rega, P., Koltz, M. *et al.* 1988: Analysis of growth plate abnormalities following intraosseous infusion through the proximal tibial epiphysis in pigs. *Annals of Emergency Medicine* **17**, 121–3.

Broviac, J.W., Cole, J.J. and Scribner, B.H. 1973: A silicone rubber atrial catheter for prolonged parenteral alimentation. *Surgery, Gynecology and Obstetrics* **136**, 602–6.

Cameron, J.L., Fontanarosa, P.B. and Passalaqua, A.M. 1989: A comparative study of peripheral to central circulation delivery times between intraosseous and intravenous injection using a radionuclide technique in normovolemic and hypovolemic canines. *Journal of Emergency Medicine* **7**, 123–7.

Cobb, L.M., Vincour, C.D., Wagner, W.W. *et al.* 1987: The central venous anatomy in infants. *Surgery, Gynecology and Obstetrics* **165**, 230–4.

Cuthbertson, D.P. 1942: Post-shock metabolic response. *Lancet* **i**, 433–7.

Cuthbertson, D.P. 1959: Protein metabolism in relation to energy needs. *Metabolism* **8**, 787–808.

Doyle, L.W. and Sinclair, J.C. 1982: Insensible water loss in newborn infants. *Clinical Perinatology* **9**, 453–82.

Drinker, C.K. and Drinker, K.R. 1916: A method for maintaining an artificial circulation through the tibia of the dog with a demonstration of the vasomotor control of the marrow vessels. *American Journal of Physiology* **40**, 514–21.

Drinker, C.K., Drinker, K.R. and Lund, C.C. 1922: The circulation in the mammalian bone-marrow. *American Journal of Physiology* **62**, 1–92.

Dudrick, S.J., Groff, D.B. and Gilmore, D.W. 1968: Long term venous catheterization in infants. *Surgery, Gynecology and Obstetrics* **129**, 805–8.

Eichelberger, M.R., Rous, P.G., Hoelzer, D.J. *et al.* 1981: Percutaneous subclavian venous catheters in neonates and children. *Journal of Pediatric Surgery* **16**, 547–553.

Elliott, M. and Albert, K.G.M.M. 1983: The hormonal and metabolic response to surgery and trauma. In Kleinberger, G. and Deutsch, E. (eds), *New aspects of clinical nutrition.* Karger, 247–70.

Engel, W.D., Baumgart, S., Schwartz, J.G. *et al.* 1981: Insensible water loss in the critically ill neonate: combined effect of radiant-warmer power and phototherapy. *American Journal of Disease in Children* **135**, 516–20.

Engle, W.D., Baumgart, S., Fox, W.W. *et al.* Effect of increased radiant warmer power output on state of hydration in the critically ill neonate. *Critical Care Medicine* **10**, 673–6.

Filston, H.C. and Grant, J.P. 1979: A safer system for percutaneous subclavian venous catheterization in newborn infants. *Journal of Pediatric Surgery* **14**, 564–70.

Fiser, D.H. 1990: Intraosseous infusion. *New England Journal of Medicine* **322**, 1579–81.

Fonkalsrud, E.W., Ament, M.E., Berquist, W.E. *et al.* 1982: Occlusion of the vena cava in infants receiving central venous hyperalimentation. *Surgery, Gynecology and Obstetrics* **154**, 189–92.

Friis-Hansen, B. 1954: The extracellular fluid volume in infants and children. *Acta Paediatrica* **43**, 444–58.

Friis-Hansen, B. 1957: Changes in body water compartments during growth. *Acta Paediatrica* **207** (Suppl.), 1–57.

Friis-Hansen, B. 1961: Body water compartments in children: changes during growth and related changes in body composition. *Pediatrics* **28**, 169–81.

Friis-Hansen, B. 1971: Body composition during growth: *In vivo* measurements and biochemical data correlated to differential anatomical growth. *Pediatrics* **47**, 264–74.

Friis-Hansen, B. 1983: Water distribution in the fetus and newborn infant. *Acta Paediatrica Scandinavica* **305** (Suppl.), 7–11.

Friis-Hansen, B., Holiday, M., Stapleton, T. *et al.* 1951: Total body water in children. *Pediatrics* **7**, 321–7.

Galpin, R.D., Kronick, J.B., Willis, R.B. *et al.* 1991: Bilateral lower extremity compartment syndromes secondary to intraosseous fluid resuscitation. *Journal of Pediatric Orthopaedics* **11**, 773–6.

Gauderer, M.W., Stellato, T.A. and Izant, R.J. 1982: Broviac silastic catheter insertion in children: a simplified direct subclavian approach. *Journal of Pediatric Surgery* **17**, 580–4.

Giacoia, G. 1991: Cardiac tamponade and hydrothorax as complications of central venous parenteral nutrition in infants. *Journal of Parenteral and Enteral Nutrition* **15**, 110–3.

Glaeser, P.W., Losek, J.D., Nelson, D.B. *et al.* 1988: Pediatric intraosseous infusions: impact of vascular access time. *American Journal of Emergency Medicine* **6**, 330–2.

Groff, D.B. and Ahmed, N. 1974: Subclavian vein catheterization in the infant *Journal of Pediatric Surgery* **9**, 171–4.

Hammarlund, K., Nilsson, G.E., Oberg, P.A. *et al.* 1977: Transepidermal water loss in newborn infants: I. Relation to ambient humidity and site of measurement and estimation of total transepidermal water loss. *Acta Paediatrica Scandinavica* **66**, 553–62.

Heinild, S., Sondergaard, T. and Tudvad, F. 1947: Bone marrow infusion in childhood: experiences from a thousand infusions. *Journal of Pediatrics* **30**, 400–12.

Hodge, D. 1985: Intraosseous infusions: a review. *Pediatric Emergency Care* **1**, 215–8.

Hodge, D., Delgado-Paredes, C. and Fleisher, G. 1987: Intraosseous infusion flow rates in hypovolemic 'pediatric' dogs. *Annals of Emergency Medicine* **16**, 305–7.

Im, M.J.C. and Hoopes, J.E. 1970: Energy metabolism in healing skin wounds. *Journal of Surgical Research* **10**, 459–66.

Iserson, K.V. and Criss, E.A. 1986: Pediatric venous cutdown: utility in emergency situations. *Pediatric Emergency Care* **2**, 231–4.

Ito, T., Iyomasa, Y. and Inoue, T. 1976: Changes of the postoperative minimal oxygen consumption of the newborn. *Journal of Pediatric Surgery* **11**, 495–503.

Kanter, R.K., Gorton, J.M., Palmiervi, K. *et al.* 1989: Anatomy of femoral vessels in infants and guidelines for venous catheterization. *Pediatrics* **83**, 1020-2.

Kanter, R.K., Zimmerman, J.J., Strauss, R.H. *et al.* 1986: Central venous catheter insertion by femoral vein: safety and effectiveness for the pediatric patient. *Pediatrics* **77**, 842–7.

Kehiet, H. 1979: Stress-free anesthesia and surgery. *Acta Anesthesica Scandinavica* **23**, 503–4.

Kerri-Szanto, M. 1983: Demand analgesia. *British Journal of Anesthesia* **55**, 919–20.

Khilnani, P., Toce, S. and Reddy, R. 1990: Mechanical complications from very small percutaneous central venous Silastic catheters. *Critical Care Medicine* **18**, 1477–8.

King, D.R., Komer, M., Hoffinan, J. *et al.* 1985: Broviac catheter sepsis: the natural history of an iatrogenic infection. *Journal of Pediatric Surgery* **20**, 728–33.

Kosloske, A.M. and Klein, M.D. 1982: Techniques of central venous access for long term parenteral nutrition in infants. *Surgery, Gynecology and Obstetrics* **154**, 394–9.

Kulick, R.M. and Cilley, R.E. 1990: Intraosseous infusion: an alternative technique for emergency vascular access in children. *Pediatric Rounds* **10**, 1–5.

LaFleche, F.R., Slepin, M.J., Vargeryas, J. *et al.* 1989: Iatrogenic bilateral tibial fractures after intraosseous infusion attempts in a 3-month old *Annals of Emergency Medicine* **18**, 1099–101.

Loeff, D.S., Matlak, M.E., Black, R.E. *et al.* Insertion of a small central venous catheter in neonates and young infants. *Journal of Pediatric Surgery* **17**, 944–9.

Massey, L.W.C. 1950: Bone-marrow infusions: intratibial and intravenous routes compared. *British Medical Journal* **2**, 197–8.

Melker, R.J., Miller, G., Gearen, P. *et al.* Complications of intraosseous infusion. *Annals of Emergency Medicine* **19**, 731–2.

Mofenson, H.C., Tascone, A. and Caraccio, T.R. 1988: Guidelines for interosseous infusions [Letter]. *Journal of Emergency Medicine* **6**, 143–6.

Mollitt, D. and Golladay, E.S. 1983: Complication of TPN-catheter-induced venal caval thrombosis in children less than one year of age. *Journal of Pediatric Surgery* **18**, 462–7.

Moscati, R. and Moore, G.P. 1990: Compartment resultant amputation following intraosseous infusion [Letter]. *American Journal of Emergency Medicine* **8**, 470–1.

Moyer, E., Cerra, F., Cheiner, R., *et al.* 1981: Multiple systems organ failure. VI. Death predictors in the trauma septic state – the most critical determinants. *Journal of Trauma* **21**, 862–9.

Murdoch, L. and Bingham, R. 1990: Venous cannulation in infants and small children. *British Journal of Hospital Medicine* **44**, 405–7.

Nahata, M.C., King, D.R., Powell, D.A. *et al.* 1988: Management of catheter-related infections in pediatric patients. *Journal of Parenteral and Enteral Nutrition* **12**, 58–9.

Neish, S.R., Macon, M.G., Moore, J.W. *et al.* 1988: Intraosseous infusion of hypertonic glucose and dopamine. *American Journal of Disease in Children* **142**, 878–80.

Oh, W. and Karecki, H. 1972: Phototherapy and insensible water loss in the newborn infant. *American Journal of Disease in Children* **124**, 230–2.

Orlowski, J.P., Julius, C.J., Petras, R.E. *et al.* 1989: The safety of intraosseous infusions: risks of fat and bone marrow emboli to the lungs. *Annals of Emergency Medicine* **18**, 1062–7.

Orlowski, J.P., Porembka, D.T., Gallagher, J.M. *et al.* 1989: The bone marrow as a source of laboratory studies. *Annals of Emergency Medicine* **18**, 1348–51.

Orlowski, J.P., Porembka, D.T., Gallagher, J.M. *et al.* 1990: Comparison study of intraosseous, central intravenous, and peripheral intravenous infusions of emergency drugs. *American Journal of Disease in Children* **144**, 112–7.

Pybus, D.A., Poole, J.L. and Crawford, M.C. 1982: Subclavian venous catheterization in small children using the Seldinger technique. *Anaesthesia* **37**, 451–3.

Quilligan, J.J. and Turkel, H. 1946: Bone marrow infusion and its complications. *American Journal of Disease in Children* **71**, 457–65.

Rackow, H., Salanitre, E. and Green, L.T. 1961: Frequency of cardiac arrest associated with anesthesia in infants and children. *Pediatrics* **28**, 697–704.

Ros, S.P., McMannis, S.I., Kowal-Vern *et al.* 1991: Effect of intraosseous saline infusion on hematologic parameters. *Annals of Emergency Medicine* **20**, 243–5.

Roseman, J.M. 1983: Deep, percutaneous antecubital venipuncture: an alternative to surgical cutdown. *American Journal of Surgery* **146**, 285.

Rosetti, V.A., Thompson, B.M., Miller, J. *et al.* 1985: Intraosseous infusion: an alternative route of pediatric intravascular access. *Annals of Emergency Medicine* **14**, 885–8.

Rossetti, V., Thompson, B.M., Aprahamian, C. *et al.* 1984: Difficulty and delay in intravascular access in pediatric arrests. *Annals of Emergency Medicine* **13**, 406.

Saigal, S. and Sinclair, J.C. 1977: Urine solute excretion in growing low-birth-weight infants. *Journal of Pediatrics* **90**, 934–8.

Schweiss, J.F. and Pennington, D.G. 1981: Anesthetic management of neonates undergoing palliative operations for congenital heart defects. *Cleveland Clinic Quarterly* **48**, 153–65.

Shoor, P.M., Berryhill, R.E. and Benumof, J.L. 1979: Intraosseous infusion: pressure–flow relationship and pharmacokinetics. *Journal of Trauma* **19**, 772–4.

Sosulski, R., Polin, R.A. and Baumgart, S. 1983: Respiratory water loss and heat balance in intubated infants receiving humidified air. *Journal of Pediatrics* **103**, 307–10.

Spivey, W.H. 1987: Intraosseous infusions. *Journal of Pediatrics* **111**, 639–43.

Spivey, W.H., Lathers, C.M., Malone, R. *et al.* 1985: Comparison of intraosseous, central and peripheral routes of sodium bicarbonate administration during CPR in pigs. *Annals of Emergency Medicine* **14**, 1135–40.

Stevenson, J.G. 1977: Fluid administration in the association of patent ductus arteriosus complicating respiratory distress syndrome. *Journal of Pediatrics* **90**, 257–61.

Suits, G.S. and Bottsford, J.E. Jr 1987: The metabolic response to trauma. *Res Staff Phys* **33**, 21–9.

Tan, K.I. and Jacob, E. 1981: Effect of phototherapy on neonatal fluid and electrolyte status. *Acta Paediatrica Hungarica* **22**, 187–94.

The American College of Surgeons. 1988: *Advanced trauma life support student manual*. Chicago, IL: American College of Surgeons, 222.

Tocantis, L.M. 1940: Rapid absorption of substances injected into the bone marrow. *Proceedings of the Society of Experimental Biology and Medicine* **45**, 292–6.

Valman, H.B. and Pearson, J.F. 1980: What the foetus feels. *British Medical Journal* **280**, 233–4.

Vane, D.W., Ong, B., Rescorla, F.J. *et al.* 1990: Complications of central venous access in children. *Pediatric Surgery International* **5**, 174–8.

Wagner, M.B. and McCabe, J.B. A comparison of four techniques to establish intraosseous infusion. *Pediatric Emergency Care* **4**, 87–91.

Wallden, L. 1948: On injuries of bone and bone-marrow after intraosseous injections: an experimental investigation. *Acta Chirurgica Scandinavica* **96**, 152–62.

Weber, T.R., West, K.W. and Grosfeld, J.L. 1983: Broviac central venous catheterization in infants and children. *American Journal of Surgery* **145**, 202–4.

Wilmore, D.W. 1981: Glucose metabolism following severe injury. *Journal of Trauma* **21**, 705–7.

Zimmerman, J.J. and Strauss, R.H. 1989: History and current application of intravenous therapy in children. *Pediatric Emergency Care* **5**, 120–7.

Zumbro, G.L., Mullin, M.J. and Nelson, T.G. 1971: Catheter placement in infants needing total parenteral nutrition utilizing common facial vein. *Archives of Surgery* **102**, 71–3.

CHAPTER 15

Parenteral nutrition and vascular access

G.P. HOSIE AND R.A. WHEELER

Historical	Monitoring
Indications	Metabolic complications
Nutritional requirements	Long-term parenteral nutrition
Composition of parenteral nutrition	Vascular access
Preparation of feeds	References

Historical

Intravenous feeding has been attempted over many centuries, with honey, olive oil, milk and wine, often with disastrous results (Wretlind, 1978; Consett, 1989). The first account of complete intravenous feeding was reported in 1944, when a 5-month marasmic infant with Hirschsprung's disease was fed with an intravenous solution of 50% glucose, 10% protein hydrolysate and olive oil emulsified with lecithin. This provided 130 kcal/kg/day in a volume of 150 ml/kg per day, with the result that after 5 days 'the fat pads of the cheek had returned, the ribs were less prominent, and the general nutritional status was much improved' (Helfrick and Abelson, 1944). Further efforts to establish intravenous feeding were hampered by the instability and toxicity of the oil emulsion used, leading to its withdrawal in the early 1960s. Ethanol was used as an alternative high-energy substrate but there were difficulties with its peripheral administration, toxicity and the unpredictability of patients' requirements. However, in 1962 an emulsion of soybean oil (Intralipid) was introduced for intravenous feeding. Combined with the report in 1968 by Wilmore and Dudrick of the infusion of a hypertonic nutrient solution via a large central vein, the potential now existed for the delivery of adequate calories to be administered in an appropriate infusion volume.

Indications

As well as being neccessary for normal growth and development, adequate and appropriate nutrition plays an essential role in the recovery of children with diseases of the gastrointestinal tract. Enteral feeding, either orally or tube-assisted, should be aimed for whenever possible, but in situations where adequate nutritional support cannot be provided enterally then intravenous therapy is indicated. The establishment of parenteral feeding is part of a planned treatment programme and there are no indications for its emergency use, its use in the first 24 hours of life, its prophylactic use preoperatively or for its use for less than 5 days. The duration of therapy should be as short as possible; most indications require 5–10 days of use, although certain children, such as those with short gut, can be maintained on such therapy for months or years. Parenteral nutrition is now essential in the management of children with gastroschisis, necrotizing enterocolitis and some cases of intestinal atresia, as well as an adjunct in the care of many other conditions (Table 15.1).

Nutritional requirements

As well as energy for metabolism and activity, children require additional energy intake for growth and

Table 15.1 Indications for use of parenteral nutrition (175 patients; Great Ormond Street Children's Hospital December 1993 to June 1994)

Surgical

Oesophageal atresia/TOF	6
Short bowel	6
Necrotizing enterocolitis	24
Gastroschisis	3
Small bowel atresia	4
Duodenal atresia	1
Perforated ileal volvulus	1
Separated conjoint twin	1
Hirschsprung's disease	2
Congenital diaphragmatic hernia	3
Diaphragmatic eventration	1
Intestinal obstruction	3
Cardiac anomalies/surgery	37
Intestinal pseudo-obstruction	3
Idiopathic megacolon	1
Total	**96**

Medical

Neoplasia		43
Ulcerative colitis		1
Protracted diarrhoea		5
Failure to thrive		19
Intractable vomiting		2
Pulmonary:	Meconium aspiration	1
	ECMO	2
	Bronchiolitis	1
	Pneumonia	1
	Aspiration/GOR	1
Enteral myopathy		2
Pneumococcal meningitis		1
	Total	**79**

maturation. The basal metabolic requirement is predictable and is dependent on weight, gender and age (FAO/WHO, 1983). Energy requirements are increased during periods of nutritional stress, including the catabolic state induced by surgery. Although studies in adults suggest that severe stress does not increase energy requirements by any more than 10–15% (Baker *et al.*, 1984), children and neonates have limited stores of fat and muscle, and thus have less capacity to compensate for increased energy requirements. Surgery induces an initial catabolic state, with glycogenolysis, gluconeogenesis, lipolysis, endogenous protein breakdown and an increase in energy expenditure so that the basal metabolic rate (BMR) peaks 3 days after surgery (Winthrop *et al.*, 1987). The ensuing anabolic stage of recovery demands the adequate provision of amino acids and calories for wound healing, so that in the postoperative period a considerable increase in the blood urea nitrogen level is observed (Pinter, 1973).

Energy requirements are also increased by intercurrent sepsis, such that for every degree of pyrexia above 37°C the BMR increases by 12%, with an increase of 50% in severe sepsis.

Composition of parenteral nutrition

Any feeding regime should include calories, nitrogen, essential amino and fatty acids, minerals, vitamins and trace elements. Despite many refinements, there is still no ideal infusate; indeed, the differing needs of individual patients necessitate flexibility in the composition of the feed.

CARBOHYDRATE

Glucose is the natural energy source for red cells, the central nervous system, retina, renal medulla, skeletal muscle and intestinal mucosa. It provides the major source of calories in parenteral regimes. Glucose provides 4 kcal/g, and so the normal energy requirements of 110 kcal/kg per day in neonates, which fall to 60 kcal/kg per day in older children, could theoretically be achieved by the administration of up to 15 g/kg of glucose per day. However, there is a limit to the amount of glucose that can be directly oxidized to meet an individual's energy needs; the remaining glucose has to be converted to lipid before it can be oxidized. This inefficient process can utilize only 15% of the infused glucose calories and a more efficient regime is the provision of calories by both glucose and fat.

FAT

Providing 9 kcal/g, fat is a rich source of energy and milk-fed infants derive half their energy requirement from this source. Linoleic acid and linolenic acid are essential fatty acids for normal growth. Lipid is administered in the form of Intralipid, which consists of 54% linoleic, 26% oleic, 9% palmitic and 8% linolenic acid. The lipid is provided in the form of triglycerides, the solubility being facilitated by the addition of 1.2% egg phospholipid. The addition of 2.5% glycerol gives the emulsion an osmolality of 280 μOsm/l, rendering it isotonic with plasma and suitable for peripheral infusion. The administration of lipid overcomes the difficulty of supplying adequate calories without making the volume of the infusate excessive. There is a limit to the amount of fat that can be utilized by the body, the rate-limiting step being the ability of the endothelial lipoprotein lipase activity to metabolize the triglyceride emulsion. This limitation is more marked in preterm infants, who have a correspondingly decreased capacity to utilize lipid (Periera *et al.*, 1980). Administration of Intralipid has been implicated in the impairment of the immune system, resulting in increased susceptibility to bacterial and viral infection (Fischer *et al.,* 1980). Additionally, the presence of sepsis is known to have an inhibitory effect on lipoprotein lipase activity (Dahn, 1990; Park *et al.,* 1986), so that infants with sepsis are at a theoretical risk of lipid overload. For this reason, it has been advocated that lipid infusion is stopped in the presence of sepsis but, unfortunately, this is often the time that a child needs an increase in energy provision. The relationship of sepsis to the administration of lipid in children is still not determined and so it is our policy to continue the use of Intralipid infusion in septic children.

Lipid is administered over a period of 20 hours, leaving a 4-hour gap each day for clearance of the fat emulsion from the plasma, after which accurate serum biochemical assay can be performed.

AMINO ACIDS

The provision of amino acids is necessary to produce positive nitrogen balance. This should be achieved without toxicity (O'Neill *et al.,* 1976). If using parenteral solutions designed for adults, it is important to monitor plasma amino acid profile since certain amino acids are not fully metabolized by neonates, particularly threonine, phenylalanine, glycine and methionine (Beck, 1990; Collins *et al.,* 1991). Amino acid solutions used for neonates are designed to avoid the development of hyperaminoacidaemia and hyperbilirubinaemia (Puntis *et al.,* 1989; McIntosh and Mitchell, 1990).

As well as the eight essential amino acids, infants cannot manufacture histidine and cannot synthesize proline, cystine, cysteine, tyrosine and alanine in adequate amounts, so these should be included in infant parenteral nutrition solutions (Heird *et al.,* 1988; Beck, 1990). Unfortunately, cystine is sparingly soluble and cysteine is unstable in aqueous solution and are not included in most commercially available amino acid preparations (Sherman *et al.,* 1970). The protein hydrolysates have now been superseded by crystalline L-amino products, containing variable proportions of 15 amino acids. In order for the administered amino acids to be utilized for protein synthesis rather than energy, at least 125 kcal/g N of non-protein calories needs to be provided. Optimal nitrogen retention is achieved by providing a physiological balance of fat and carbohydrate (Nose *et al.,* 1987).

MINERALS

Before commencing intravenous feeding it is important that any electrolyte or acid–base imbalances are corrected (Candy, 1980). Once parenteral nutrition is established, normal serum levels of sodium, chloride and potassium should be easily maintained unless there are large unpredictable losses from the gastrointestinal tract (Puntis *et al.,* 1993). Maintenance intake of sodium is

3 mmol/kg per day, that of potassium is 2 mmol/kg per day. Because of immature renal function, low birth weight babies may require greater intakes of sodium to replace urinary losses, and nutritionally depleted infants may require greater potassium intake.

Infants have a high requirement for calcium. The limited solubilities of calcium and phosphate in parenteral solutions result in the inadequate provision of calcium (Koo *et al.,* 1989), such that osteopenia, rickets and collapsed vertebrae have been reported in infants on long-term total parenteral nutrition (TPN) (Koo and Tsang, 1984). This could be overcome by reducing the phosphate intake, but this can lead to hypophosphataemia. Some of the newer amino acid solutions have a lower pH, which aids the solubility of calcium.

TRACE ELEMENTS

Earlier preparations of intravenous nutritional solutions contained trace element contaminants. As the natural protein hydrolysates were replaced by purer preparations of synthetic amino acid solutions the consequences of a number of deficiencies were reported in patients on long-term parenteral nutrition. When parenteral nutrition is only supplemental or is limited to 1 or 2 weeks, then only zinc needs to be added to the infusate. If TPN continues for longer than 4 weeks, then supplementation with selenium, chromium, copper, manganese and iodine needs consideration (Green *et al.,* 1988). The situation in preterm infants is more immediate, the neonate being more susceptible to copper and zinc deficiency because of limited stores and increased requirement due to rapid growth. It has been estimated that two-thirds of the zinc and copper in the fetal body are accumulated during the last 10–12 weeks' of gestation (Widdowson *et al.,* 1974), thus unless zinc supplementation is provided, growth impairment will ensue. In the presence of renal impairment or cholestatic jaundice, the dosage of the trace elements should be reduced. There has been much debate as to whether trace elements should be provided together in prepared formulations, or should be provided as separate entities. There is certainly a rationale for the provision of zinc alone; however, for the sake of simplicity, trace elements have been administered in the form of pre-prepared formulations, the composition of which will need further review as certain of the trace elements are being implicated in the aetiology of some of the complications of parenteral nutrition administration, e.g. manganese and cholestatic jaundice (Hanbridge *et al.,* 1989).

VITAMINS

Neither the intravenous requirement of vitamins nor the minimum dose causing toxicity has been adequately defined. The lipid-soluble vitamins A, D, E and K are provided in an aqueous suspension by mixing the vitamins with a synthetic detergent such as polysorbate, in the form of Vitalipid. In our institution, this has resulted in high serum levels of vitamin A and low levels of vitamin E, and so the amount of vitamins added is being revised. The water-soluble vitamins B and C are added in the form of Solvito as required. Loss of fat-soluble vitamins due to adsorption to the walls of plastic nutrient bags and tubing (Hartline and Azchman, 1976) and to light exposure (O'Strea *et al.*, 1982) has been reported, thus it is normal practice to limit the exposure to light and the storage time of the lipid solutions.

Preparation of feeds

The provision of parenteral feeding to a sick child requires close supervision and standardization. The most appropriate way of achieving this is through a multidisciplinary team which can involve surgeon or gastroenterologist, pharmacist, biochemist, dietitian and nurse. Solutions should be prepared by the pharmacist using a sterile laminar flow system. Computer software is now available to assist in the preparation of the intravenous feeding solution specified for each patient. The nutrient solution is provided in two bags, solution 1 containing glucose, amino acids, electrolytes and trace elements and solution 2 containing lipid, fat-soluble vitamins and water-soluble vitamins. The two solutions are kept separate owing to the instability of Intralipid in the presence of electrolytes, especially divalent ions. Since Intralipid contains phosphate, calcium phosphate may precipitate if the solutions are mixed.

Monitoring

There has been little consensus as to the frequency of monitoring required for a child on parenteral nutrition, which may have led to excessive monitoring in the past. Although frequent biochemical monitoring is necessary during the early stages of parenteral nutrition, once the programme is established children may only require blood tests once or twice a month.

Initially, urine should be Clinistix tested with each voiding and if glycosuria or acetone is present, then the blood glucose measured. BM reagent strips are adequate for the detection of hypoglycaemia, but are not accurate for measuring hyperglycaemia. Weekly urea and electrolytes as well as bilirubin levels should be estimated.

If parenteral nutrition is long term, then 6-monthly measurements of aluminium (Sedman *et al.*, 1985), selenium, chromium (Moukarzel *et al.*, 1992) and manganese (Hanbridge *et al.*, 1989), as well as estimation of vitamin B_{12} and folate are required; levels of vitamins

A, E, D, B_1, B_2 and B_6 should also be measured. Because of the tendency to biliary sludging (Messing *et al.*, 1983), a 6-monthly ultrasound scan of the liver and gallbladder should be performed.

Both physiological measurement and biochemical assessments can be used to monitor the nutritional status of the child. On commencing the feeding regime an accurate fluid input/output record is maintained, and daily weight and weekly length and head circumference are recorded. For those grossly malnourished, measurement of the serum albumin and total protein will indicate the degree of nitrogen deficiency. A number of measurements of nutritional status has been devised including the triceps skinfold thickness (Frisancha, 1974), the arm muscle and arm fat areas (Burgess and Burgess, 1969), grip strength, and for infants below 3 months of age, the mid arm circumference/head circumference ratio (Sasanow *et al.*, 1986).

The presence of catheter-related sepsis is monitored by daily recording of temperature and pulse and the measurement of the white cell count and C-reactive protein, with cultures taken from the delivery line for culture as indicated.

Metabolic complications

The development of glucose intolerance in a previously stable child on parenteral nutrition may indicate occult sepsis. At the commencement of the nutrition regime the carbohydrate content is increased slowly and the appearance of glucose intolerance is managed by a reduction in the rate of infusion. The need for the addition of insulin is rare, but is exceptionally required in

Table 15.2 Metabolic complications of parenteral nutrition

Hyperglycaemia/hypoglycaemia
Hypophosphataemia
Hypokalaemia
Metabolic acidosis/alkalosis
Hyperammonaemia
Hypercholesterolaemia/phospholipaemia
Essential fatty acid deficiency
Abnormal fatty acid profile
Abnormal amino acid profile
Glucose intolerance
Osmotic diuresis
Respiratory failure
Thrombocyte and neutrophil dysfunction
Anaemia
Eosinophilia
Cholestasis:cirrhosis
Cholelithiasis

the very low birth weight preterm infant in order to maintain adequate energy intake in the presence of persistent glucose intolerance (Binder, 1989). The fear of hypoglycaemia led to the practice of tailing off parenteral nutrition at the end of a regime. In practice, hypoglycaemia is a rare occurrence in those children finishing parenteral regimes (Table 15.2).

Severely malnourished children are susceptible to hypophosphataemia when parenteral nutrition is commenced, owing to a reversal of the catabolic state. The requirement for the accumulation of intracellular potassium in this state can lead to hypokalaemia, so that up to 4 mmol/kg per day of potassium supplementation may be required.

Fatty acid deficiency becomes apparent after 2–3 weeks of fat-free TPN, especially in the newborn where the effects can be seen within days (Friedman *et al.*, 1976). If a regime does not include lipid, then essential fatty acids can be provided by the daily application of sunflower seed oil to the skin of the chest (Press *et al.*, 1974). Administration of excessive lipid can be hazardous for infants with hyperbilirubinaemia since the free fatty acids that are produced during the metabolism of fat compete with bilirubin for binding to albumin. For those infants with pulmonary disease excessive lipid may be harmful (Roulet, 1983) as fat is cleared by pulmonary macrophages and this process can hinder gas exchange in the alveoli.

Carbohydrate has a high respiratory quotient and so its metabolism results in the production of a high load of carbon dioxide, the clearance of which can be a critical burden in those infants with pre-existing pulmonary disease (Binder *et al.*, 1989). Administration of large volumes of hypertonic glucose can result in the production of an osmotic diuresis.

Because of sepsis, iron deficiency or vitamin B_{12} and folate deficiency, anaemia is a common finding in patients on parenteral nutrition.

The most serious complication of TPN administration remains cholestasis (Touloukian and Dowing, 1973; Merritt, 1980). Increases in serum levels of lactate dehydrogenase and serum glutamic oxaloacetic transaminase, as well as bilirubin, may be observed soon after commencing TPN but, these return to normal on commencing enteral feeding. If TPN is continued for long periods, the cholestasis can precipitate hepatic fibrosis, progressing to cirrhosis and liver failure. The aetiology of this is the subject of much recent investigation. The presence of sepsis (Wolf and Pohlandt, 1989), prematurity (Sandheimer *et al.*, 1978) and the absence of enterohepatic stimulation (Hughes *et al.*, 1983) have all been implicated. In addition cholestasis can lead to biliary sludging and gallstone formation (Messing *et al.*, 1983).

Long-term parenteral nutrition

Certain children, such as those with chronic pseudo-obstruction or inflammatory bowel disease, or those who end up with a short bowel, cannot sustain enteral nutrition and require long-term parenteral feeding. It is important for both the child and its family that as normal a lifestyle is achieved as soon as possible, and this can be facilitated by the provision of home parenteral nutrition, a process that requires parents who are highly motivated with appropriate social arrangements; however, if this is the case then treatment can be given at a third of the cost of hospitalization, with very low morbidity (see Table 15.3). In a recent review of ten patients on home TPN supervised by our nutrition team the major complication, catheter-related sepsis occurred, with a frequency of one episode in 476 days, with the average lifespan of the central line being 680 days. The children received the intravenous nutrition over a 12-hour period at night, and all children over the age of 5 years attended a normal school (Bissett *et al.*, 1992).

The care of patients with short bowel presents challenges to surgeon, parents and child. Term infants are born with 200 cm of small intestine, the length having increased 2.4-fold in the last trimester (Touloukian and Smith, 1983). Loss of small intestine is often the end result of surgery for mid-gut volvulus, ischaemia or necrotizing enterocolitis. The length of bowel that remains will determine whether a child can grow independent of nutritional support. The minimum required is reported as 40 cm if the ileocaecal valve is

Table 15.3 Parenteral nutrition regime

		Neonate	Child
Volume (ml/kg)		150	50
Energy (kcal/kg per day)	Peripheral	119	48
	Central	139	52
Carbohydrate (g/kg per day)	Peripheral	12.8	4.0
	Central	<18.0	5.0
Amino acids (g/kg per day)		3.0	1.40
Lipid (g/kg per day)		3.5	2

lost and 15 cm if the valve is preserved (Wilmore, 1972), although there are anecdotal reports of neonates left with as little as 7 cm of small bowel who have survived and eventually been weaned off TPN (Kiely, E.M., personal communication, 1993).

If children are to receive prolonged parenteral nutrition it is important that some attempt at oral feeding is made as soon as is possible. Considerable evidence exists that the bowel lumen needs stimulation of food for the enterohepatic circulation of bile salts and that food has a trophic effect on bowel, playing a major role in the adaptation of bowel, which undergoes dilation with villous hypertrophy and hyperplasia (Feldman *et al.*, 1976). An additional factor is that children need to develop the habit of eating. A long period without any oral intake may make it difficult for the child to learn how food should be ingested, chewed and swallowed. Such problems may be addressed by the speech therapist. Even if enteral feeding is not possible, sham feeding should be established in early infancy.

Vascular access

Long-term vascular access for a duration of more than 3–4 weeks in children has undergone major changes. The development of central venous catheters (CVC) suitable for children has encouraged this proliferation. The conventional material of silicone rubber had the disadvantage of having a high ratio of wall thickness/lumen diameter, necessitated by the relatively poor tensile strength of the rubber. The poor flow rate of CVC which had a small enough external diameter to be inserted into an infant was thus a limiting factor. Although improvements in the silicone led to long-term TPN being practicable in infancy, the penetration of the silicon molecule by lipids led to inevitable fragmentation and fracture of the catheter. The resultant multiple venous access procedures under general anaesthesia could lead to the destruction of all conventional sites of venous access, i.e. internal jugular, subclavian, saphenofemoral junction and azygous veins. The development of new materials such as polyurethane have led to marked improvement in some of these areas. With a higher tensile strength, polyurethane CVC have thin walls and thus achieve improved flow rates with much smaller external diameters. There is no lipid penetration, and thus fracture has not occurred despite prolonged *in vivo* usage (Wheeler *et al.*, 1991). The configuration of some of these CVC (Cuff Cath, Ohmeda, UK) permits a retrograde tunnelling technique, ensuring immediate and permanent fixation (Wheeler *et al.*, 1991), which has reduced the rate of CVC displacement, previously a major problem in the paediatric population, to zero. However, the relative stiffness of polyurethane has led to kinking during insertion and this may be one factor that has prevented a large-scale shift away from the use of silicone catheters in children.

The concept of completely implantable venous access reservoirs (Pegelow *et al.*, 1986) has been facilitated by the development of low profile devices suitable for small children (Vascuport, Ohmeda, UK). These have a clear advantage in that accidental (or wilful!) removal by the child is prevented and infection may be reduced. Swimming is also easier with a subcutaneous reservoir, although waterproof dressings also allow submersion in children with more conventional CVC. However, there have been some complications of prolonged use in children. They are sometimes reluctant to have the port accessed, despite the mandatory use of topical local anaesthetic creams, and non-coring cannulae have been developed to give overnight access to the port because of occasional problems with skin necrosis if the reservoir is used too frequently. Blood transfusion and the lipid component of TPN have both been implicated in reservoir blockage. The totally implantable reservoir undoubtedly has a vital role to play in the field of long-term venous access in children, but should not be considered as universally appropriate and its usage may have to be modified according to individual therapeutic requirements. Although delivery of TPN is feasible via a port, the external CVC is more suitable for long-term intravenous feeding.

Further development in extrusion techniques has allowed the introduction of 'short long lines', silicone catheters (Epicutaneocath, Vygon, UK) of 0.6 mm external diameter which are threaded via a peripherally punctured basilic or saphenous vein up to the right atrium. Although very prone to blockage and thus only suitable for continuous infusion techniques, these catheters are ideal for the neonate or infant requiring medium-term, e.g. up to 21 days, intravenous feeding (Stringer *et al.*, 1992). They have the advantage of requiring only local anaesthesia for insertion and can be performed whilst a neonate is still in the incubator, thus avoiding the heat loss and disturbance that may be involved with open procedures in theatre. There is evidence that percutaneous central venous line insertion in neonates is associated with fewer complications than those inserted surgically (Puntis *et al.*, 1987). There are further advantages in that peripheral cannulation is not associated with the potentially serious mechanical complications of internal jugular or subclavian venous access, and the percutaneous lines are cheaper and do not leave thoracic scars (Stringer *et al.*, 1992).

Complications relating to percutaneous cannulation are well recognized and may result from accidental perforation of any structures that the exploring needle may encounter. The open approach allows cannulation under direct vision, but is prone to the complications associated with mobilization of the vein and venotomy. The complications of having a CVC *in situ* are mainly of breakage, blockage, displacement and infection. Less frequently, vascular perforation and air embolus are also reported in children. Although venous thrombosis in association with the CVC is widely reported, the additional problem of chronic pulmonary thromboembolic disease has only recently been recognized as a complication of long-term TPN (Milla, P., personal communication, 1993) and has led to the addition of 1 IU per ml/kg of sodium heparin to the TPN of all children receiving TPN through a central venous catheter. The incidence of catheter-related sepsis remains static. Quantitative microbiological methods now exist for supporting the clinical diagnosis. Early recognition and treatment of sepsis may have reduced the number of CVC that have to be removed, but insistence on a scrupulous technique for catheter insertion and subsequent management by an identified team continue to be crucial. Elective replacement of 27G polyurethane CVC after a maximum of 13 days led to a reported zero rate of line sepsis complicating a series of high-risk neonates weighing less than 1200 g (Nakamura *et al.*, 1990). The principle of CVC exchange is thus combined with peripheral percutaneous central venous cannulation to minimise sepsis if the need for prolonged parenteral access is anticipated.

The techniques of venous access, the materials available for catheter manufacture and the management of complications are all evolving to allow the increasingly reliable delivery of parenteral nutrition in children.

References

Baker, J.P. *et al.* 1984: Randomised trial of TPN in critically ill patients: metabolic effects of varying glucose; lipid ratios as the energy source. *Gastroenterology* **87**, 53–9.

Beck, R. 1990: Use of a paediatric parenteral amino acid mixture in a population of extremely low birthweight neonates; frequency and spectrum of direct bilirubinaemia. *American Journal of Perinatology* **7**, 84–6.

Binder, N.D., Raschko, P.K., Benda, G.I. and Reynolds, J.W. 1989: Insulin infusion with parenteral nutrition in extremely low birth weight infants with hyperglycaemia. *Journal of Paediatrics* **114**, 273–80.

Bisset, W.M., Stapleford, P., Long, S., Chamberlain, A., Sokel, B. and Milla, P.J. 1992: Home parenteral nutrition in chronic intestinal failure. *Archives of Disease in Childhood* **67**, 109–14.

Burgess, H.S.L. and Burgess, H.P. 1969: The arm circumference as a public health index of protein calorie malnutrition of early childhood II. A modified standard for mid-upper arm circumference in young children. *Journal of Tropical Paediatrics* **15**, 189.

Candy, 1980: Parenteral nutrition in paediatric practice – a review. *Journal of Human Nutrition* **34**, 287–96.

Collins, J.N., Hooper, H., Browne, K. *et al.* 1991: A controlled trial of parenteral nutrition in extremely low birth weight infants with glucose intolerance. *Journal of Paediatrics* **118**, 929.

Consett, J.E. 1989: The origins of intravenous fluid therapy. *Lancet* **i**, 768–71.

Dahn, M.J. 1980: Alteration in the metabolism of exogenous lipid with sepsis. *Journal of Parenteral and Enteral Nutrition* **4**, 503–10.

FAO/WHO 1983: Expert Committee Report – Energy and Protein requirements. Food and Agriculture Organization of the United Nations, Rome.

Feldman, E.J., Dowling, R.H., McNaughton, J. and Peters, T.J. 1976: Effects of oral versus intravenous nutrition on intestinal adaptation after small bowel resection. *Gastroenterology* **70**, 712–19.

Fischer, G.W., Hunter, K.W., Wilson, S.R. and Mease, A.D. 1980: Diminished bacterial defences with intralipid. *Lancet* **ii**, 819–20.

Friedman, Z., Danan, A., Stahlman, M.T. *et al.* 1976: Rapid onset of essential fatty acid deficiency in the newborn. *Pediatrics* **58**, 640.

Frisancho, A.R. 1974: Triceps skinfold and upper arm muscle size norms for assessment of nutritional status. *American Journal of Clinical Nutrition* **27**, 1052–7.

Green, H.L., Hanbridge, K.M., Schanler, R. and Tsang, R.C. 1988: Guidelines for the use of vitamins, trace elements, calcium, magnesium and phosphorous in infants and children receiving total parenteral nutrition: report of the Subcommittee on Paediatric Parenteral Requirements from the Committee on Clinical Practice Issues of the American Society for Clinical Nutrition. *American Journal of Clinical Nutrition* **48**, 1324.

Hanbridge, K.M., Sokal, R.J., Fidanza, S.J. and Goodall, M.A. 1989: Plasma manganese concentrations in infants and children receiving parenteral nutrition. *Journal of Parenteral and Enteral Nutrition* **13**, 168–71.

Hartline, J.V. and Azchman, R.D. 1976: Vitamin A delivery in total parenteral nutrition solution. *Paediatrics* **58**, 448.

Heird, W.C., Hay, W., Helins, R.A. *et al.* 1988: Paediatric parenteral amino acid mixture in low birthweight infants. *Pediatrics* **81**, 41.

Helfrick, F.W. and Abelson, N.M. 1944: Intravenous feeding of a complete diet in a child. *Journal of Paediatrics* **25**, 400–5.

Hughes, C.A., Talbot, I.C., Ducker, D.A. and Harran, M.J. 1983: Total parenteral nutrition in infancy; effect on liver and suggested pathogenesis. *Gut* **24**, 241–8.

Koo, W.W.K. and Tsang, R.C. 1984: Bone metabolism in infants. *Progress in Food and Nutrition Science* **8**, 229–302.

Koo, W.W.K., Tsang, R.C., Succop, P., Krug-Wispe, S.K., Babcock, D. and Oestreich, A.E. 1989: Minimal vitamin D and high calcium and phosphorous needs of preterm infants receiving parenteral nutrition. *Journal of Paediatric Gastroenterology and Nutrition* **8**, 225–33.

McIntosh, N. and Mitchell, V. 1990: A clinical trial of two amino acid solutions in neonates. *Archives of Disease in Children* **65**, 692–9.

Merritt, R.J. 1980: Cholestasis associated with total parenteral nutrition. *Journal of Paediatric Gastroenterology and Nutrition* **5**, 9–22.

Messing, B., Bories, C., Kunstlinger, F. and Bernier, J.J. 1983: Does total parenteral nutrition induce gallbladder sludge formation and lithiasis? *Gastroenterology* **84**, 1012–19.

Moukarzel, A.A., Song, R.J., Bachman, A.L. *et al.* 1992: Excessive chromium intake in children receiving total parenteral nutrition. *Lancet* **339**, 385–8.

Nakamura, K.T., Sato, Y. and Erenberg, A. 1990: Evaluation of a percutaneously placed 27G central venous catheter in neonates weighing < 1200 g. *Journal of Parenteral and Enteral Nutrition* **14**, 295–9.

Nose, O., Tipton, J.R., Ament, M.E. and Yabuuchi, H. 1987: Effect of the energy source on changes in energy expenditure, respiratory quotient and nitrogen balance during total parenteral nutrition in children. *Paediatric Research* **21**, 538–41.

O'Strea, E.M., Greene, C.D. and Balim, J.E. 1982: Decomposition of TPN solutions exposed to phototherapy. *Journal of Paediatrics* **100**, 669–70.

O'Neill, J.A., Meng, H.C., Caldwell, M.D. and Stahlman, M.T. 1976: Metabolic evaluation of a synthetic amino acid mixture for parenteral nutrition in infants and children. *Journal of Paediatric Surgery* **11**, 979–85.

Park, W., Peust, H. and Brosicke, H. 1986: Impaired fat utilisation in parenterally fed low birthweight infants suffering from sepsis. *Journal of Parenteral and Enteral Nutrition* **10**, 627

Pegelow, C.H., Narvael, M. and Toledano, S.R. 1986: Experience with totally implantable venous device in children. *American Journal of Disease in Children* **40**, 69–71.

Pereira, G.P., Fox, W.W., Stanley, C.A., Baker, L. and Schwartz, J.G. 1980: Decreased oxygenation and hyperlipidaemia during intravenous fat infusions in premature infants. *Pediatrics* **81**: 41.

Pinter, A. 1973: Metabolic effects of anaesthesia and surgery in the newborn infant. *Zeitschift für Kinderchirgue* **12**, 149–62.

Press, M., Hartop, P.J. and Protty, C. 1974: Correction of essential fatty acid deficiency in man by cutaneous application of sunflower seed oil. *Lancet* **i**, 597–8.

Puntis, J.W.L., Ball, P.A. and Booth, I.W. 1987: Percutaneous central venous feeding lines in infants: do they perform as well as surgically positioned catheters? *Zeitschift für Kinderchirgue* **42**, 354–7.

Puntis, J.W.L., Ball, P.A., Preece, M.A., Green, A., Brown, G.A. and Booth, I.W. 1989: Egg and breast milk based nitrogen sources compared. *Archives of Disease in Children* **64**, 1472–77.

Puntis, J.W.L., Hall, S.K., Green, A., Smith, D.E., Ball, P.A. and Booth, I.W., 1993: Biochemical stability during parenteral nutrition. *Clinical Nutrition* **12**, 153–9

Roulet, M. 1983: A controlled trial of the effect of parenteral nutritional support on patients with respiratory failure and sepsis. *Clinical Nutrition* **2**, 97–105.

Sandheimer, J.M., Bryan, H., Andrews, W. and Forstner, C.G. 1978: Cholestatic tendencies in premature infants on and off parenteral nutrition. *Pediatrics* **62**, 984–9.

Sasanow, S.R., Georgieff, M.K. and Pereira, G.P. 1986: Mid-arm circumference and mid-arm/head circumference ratios: standard curves for anthropometric assessment of neonatal nutritional status. *Journal of Paediatrics* **109**, 311–15.

Sedman, A.B., Klein, G.L., Merit, R.J. *et al.* 1985: Evidence of aluminium loading in infants receiving intravenous therapy. *New England Journal of Medicine* **312**, 1337–43.

Shurman, J.A., Gaull, G.A. and Raidlia, N.C.K. 1970: Absence of cystathionase in human liver; is cystine essential? *Science* **169**, 74.

Stringer, M.D., Brereton, R.J. and Wright, V.M. 1992: Performance of percutaneous silastic central venous feeding catheters in surgical neonates. *Pediatrical Surgery International* **7**, 79–81.

Touloukian, R.J. and Dowing, S.E. 1973: Cholestasis associated with longterm parenteral hyperalimentation. *Archives of Surgery* **106**, 58.

Touloukian, R.J. and Smith, G.J.W. 1983: Normal intestinal length in preterm infants. *Journal of Paediatric Surgery* **18**, 720–3.

Wheeler, R.A. and Griffiths, D.M. 1992: Cuff Cath: an initial experience of cuffed polyurethane central venous catheters in children. *Journal of Parenteral and Enteral Nutrition* **16**, 384–5.

Wheeler, R.A., Griffiths, D.M. and Burge, D.M. 1991: The retrograde tunnel: a new method of long term paediatric CVC fixation. *Journal of Parenteral and Enteral Nutrition* **15**, 114–155.

Widdowson, E.M., Dauncey, J. and Shaw, J.C.L. 1974: Trace elements in foetal and early postnatal development. *Proceedings of the Nutrition Society* **33**, 275.

Wilmore, D.W. 1972: Factors correlating with a successful outcome following extensive intestinal resection of newborn infants. *Journal of Paediatrics* **80**, 88–95.

Wilmore, D.W. and Dudrick, S.J. 1968: Growth and development of an infant receiving all nutrients by vein. *Journal of the American Medical Association* **203**, 860–4.

Winthrop, A.L., Wesson, D.E., Penchorz, P.B., Jacobs, D.G., Heim, T. and Filler, R.M. 1987: Injury severity, whole body protein turnover and energy expenditure in paediatric trauma. *Journal of Paediatric Surgery* **22**, 534–7.

Wolf, A.and Pohlandt, F. 1989: Bacterial Infection; the main cause of acute cholestasis in newborn infants receiving short term parenteral nutrition. *Journal of Paediatric Gastroenterology and Nutrition* **8**, 297–303

Wretlind, A. 1978: Total parenteral nutrition. *Surgical Clinics of North America* **58**, 1055–70.

CHAPTER 16

Anatomy of the infant and child

J.A.S. DICKSON

Introduction and growth
Radiological changes
Respiratory system
Gastrointestinal system
Genitourinary system

Cardiovascular system
Musculoskeletal system
Central nervous system: spinal cord
References
Further reading

Introduction and growth

Why is there a place for a special chapter on paediatric anatomy? The anatomy of the child is essentially the same as that of an adult but growth affects relative sizes, and relations of structures change (Tanner, 1978). Similar changes are seen in the embryo, though to a greater extent (Tanner, 1978). The need is not simply to record the appropriate smaller sizes for tubes for use in children, e.g. endotracheal tubes, cystoscopes and endoscopes, but also to record the different positions and relations of structures.

The growth of a fetus into an adult has been well documented. Figure 16.1 shows the relative changes in body proportions during growth. The increase expressed by weight is greater than that in length, with the expansion of surface area lying in between (Table 16.1).

There is least growth of the head, and the greatest growth in the legs. These changes mean that special charts are required to assess the surface area affected in burned children (Fig. 16.2). The simple rule of nines is inadequate. The shape of the abdomen changes from wider than it is long in the newborn to longer than it is wide in the adult. Similarly, the ratio of the length from the xiphisternum to the umbilicus to that from the umbilicus to the symphysis pubis changes with the growth of the lower half of the body (Fig. 16.3). These changes have practical implications and partly explain the adult

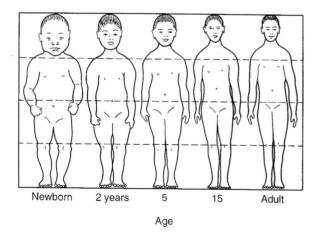

Fig. 16.1 Relative changes in proportions during growth.

Newborn   2 years   5   15   Adult

Age

Table 16.1 Growth parameters

	Weight (kg)	Length/height (cm)	Body surface area (m^2)
Birth	3.5	50	0.21
1 year	10.0	76	0.44
5 years	19.0	110	0.75
10 years	30.5	138	1.08
Adult			
Ratio of adult:			
newborn	20:1	3.5:1	8.8:1

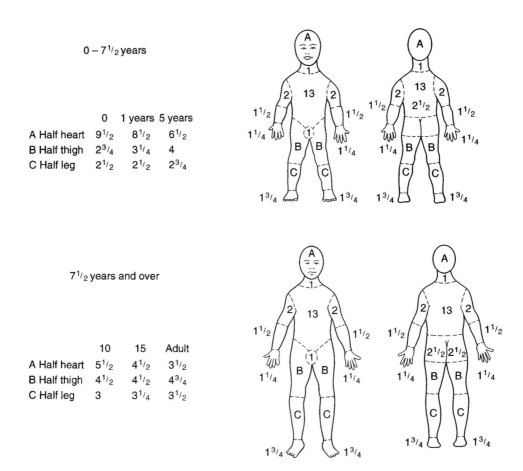

0 – 7¹⁄₂ years

	0	1 years	5 years
A Half heart	9¹⁄₂	8¹⁄₂	6¹⁄₂
B Half thigh	2³⁄₄	3¹⁄₄	4
C Half leg	2¹⁄₂	2¹⁄₂	2³⁄₄

7¹⁄₂ years and over

	10	15	Adult
A Half heart	5¹⁄₂	4¹⁄₂	3¹⁄₂
B Half thigh	4¹⁄₂	4¹⁄₂	4³⁄₄
C Half leg	3	3¹⁄₄	3¹⁄₂

Fig. 16.2   Changes in body surface area with age.

surgeon's preference for vertical midline incisions and the paediatric surgeons preference for transverse supraumbilical incisions, particularly in the infant, for conventional abdominal surgery. Abdominal scars not only lengthen with growth, they also migrate. A gastros-

tomy placed in the epigastrium in the newborn ends up as a scar over the costal margin and a transverse colostomy migrates round towards the loin (Fig. 16.4).

The fetus at birth can be described as a head, the size of which has been limited by the diameter of the birth

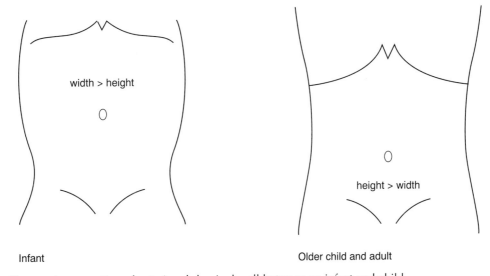

Fig. 16.3   Changes in proportion of anterior abdominal wall between an infant and child.

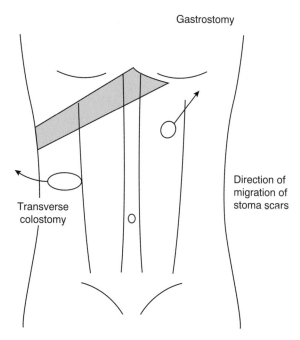

Fig. 16.4 Diagram to demonstrate migration of scars due to growth of the patient.

canal, attached to an undeveloped body. The vascular system has to develop to cope with the sudden increase in the partial pressure of oxygen of air-breathing life. The high oxygen levels are compensated for by free-radical scavengers and antioxidants. Immature capillaries are at risk from changes in blood pressure and circulation. These effects can be seen in the brain and retina, with periventricular haemorrhage in the brain

and the retinopathy of prematurity (retrolental fibroplasia). During the last 4 weeks of intrauterine growth the main deposition of fat in the subcutaneous tissues occurs. Glycogen storage in the liver increases and calcium and trace elements are deposited in the bones and liver.

Radiological changes

SKULL

The comparison of drawings of the skulls (Fig. 16.5a, b) of an adult and of a newborn (Fig. 16.6a, b) show similar changes in growth with much greater growth of the facial skeleton and mandible compared with the vault of the skull (Fig. 16.7). The skull bones themselves show a major change from the thin single table of the infant to the much thicker calvarium with well-formed diploë between the two bony layers in the adult. This is important in the performing of a burr hole as there is only one table to drill through in the infant. In Fig. 16.6 accessory suture lines, in addition to the well-known ones, are shown. These additional sutures may cause confusion with skull fractures and have been marked: on Fig. 16.6(a) the metopic suture in the middle of the frontal bone, on Fig. 16.6(b) a parietal fissure and the interparietal suture and, in the occipital bone, the mendosal suture. On the Towne's view of the skull, the midline occipital suture entering the foramen magnum and persistent membranous fissures lateral to it are more difficult to differentiate from fractures and must be diagnosed with caution (Fig. 16.8).

(a)

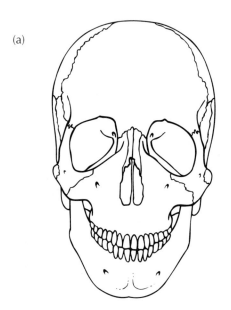

(b)

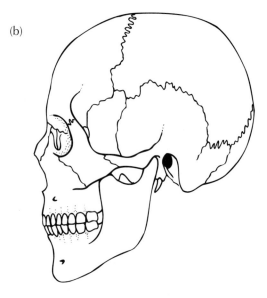

Fig. 16.5 Adult skull: note greater growth of facial bones compared to infant skull.

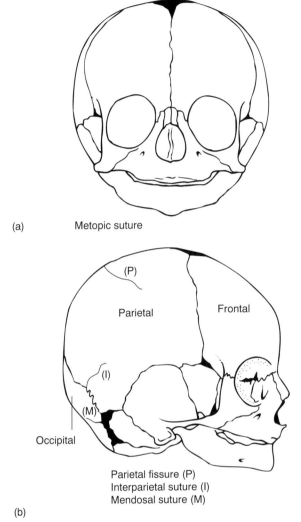

(a) Metopic suture

(P)

Parietal   Frontal

(I)

(M)

Occipital

Parietal fissure (P)
Interparietal suture (I)
Mendosal suture (M)

(b)

Fig. 16.6 Infant skull: note congenital suture lines which may be confused with fractures.

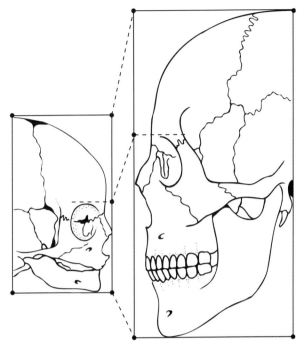

Fig. 16.7 Growth of the facial bones: comparison between a neonate and adult skull.

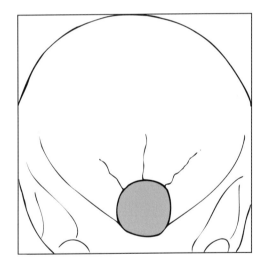

Persistent membranous fissures
Midline lineoccipital suture

Fig. 16.8 Towne's view of the skull to show midline occipital suture and persistent membrane sutures laterally.

NECK

Among the problems seen on X-rays of the soft tissues of the neck in younger children is a false appearance of displacement of the oesophagus and trachea forwards, suggesting a retropharyngeal abscess, which can occur in a crying, distressed child. The normal appearance is shown in Fig. 16.9(a), with degrees of displacement, varying with inspiration and expiration, in Fig. 16.9(b, c).

CHEST RADIOGRAPHS

The major differences in the shape of the heart and relative size of heart and chest of the adult and infant are compared: in the infant the heart lies more horizontally and occupies more of the chest (Fig. 16.10) and the upper mediastinum is filled by the thymic shadow (Fig. 16.11). The appearances of the thymus may be confusing, with the typical appearances shown in Fig. 16.11. In the older child, on deep inspiration, the heart may appear very narrow (Fig. 16.12); this can also be produced by severe hypovolaemia.

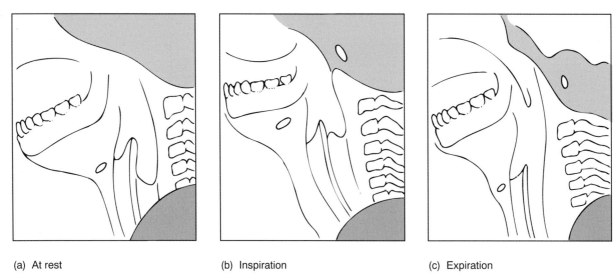

(a) At rest   (b) Inspiration   (c) Expiration

Fig. 16.9   Anterior displacement of oesophagus and trachea during inspiration and expiration: (a) at rest, (b) inspiration and (c) expiration.

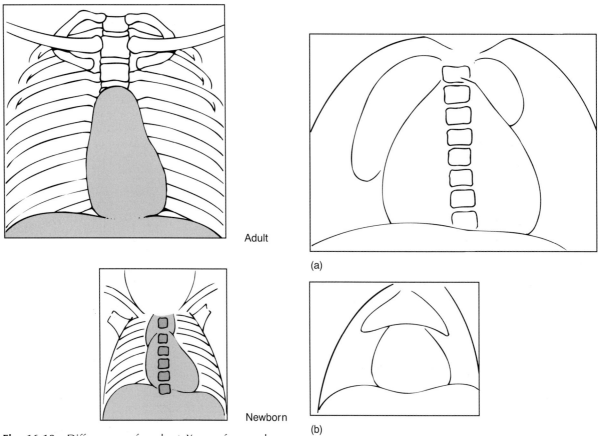

Adult

Newborn

(a)

(b)

Fig. 16.10   Differences of a chest X-ray of a newborn compared to an adult. Note the horizontal line of the heart in the newborn.

Fig. 16.11   The thymus has an obvious appearance in the infant and young child.

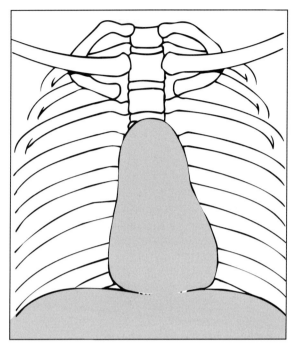 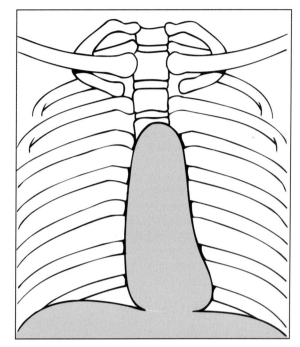

Fig. 16.12 Note the narrow heart in deep inspiration which may be normal or a sign of hypovolaemia.

ABDOMEN

In the child, unlike the adult, it is not possible to differentiate the large and small gut on its outline appearance, but the anatomical position of a loop may suggest its nature. In the sigmoid colon in particular it is often wise to confirm its identity by the use of contrast media.

Respiratory system

In the newborn the ribs are horizontally aligned, tending to lie in a position of inspiration, and their descent to the more oblique position found in later life begins after the first year of life. The adult configuration is achieved in later childhood. Thus, in the first year of life, it is not possible to increase the internal volume of the chest using the adult 'bucket handle' movement of the ribs, through the action of the intercostal muscles. Respiration depends entirely on the function of the diaphragm. Abdominal distension interferes with diaphragmatic movement and causes respiratory distress.

PLEURA

In early life the pleura strips easily from the chest wall, permitting an extrapleural approach to mediastinal structures.

UPPER AIR PASSAGES

For the first 3 months of life the newborn baby is an obligatory nose breather, owing to the tongue filling the oral cavity. This may be of value by ensuring warming and humidifying of the inspired air. The nasal passages contribute only 40–50% of the airflow resistance, compared with around 63% in the adult. This is important because of the effects on the airway of nasogastric and other tubes passed through one or both nostrils.

The infant epiglottis lies at an angle of 45° to the posterior pharyngeal wall and during growth achieves the adult position closely approximated to the base of the tongue. It is soft, cartilaginous and often folded, and

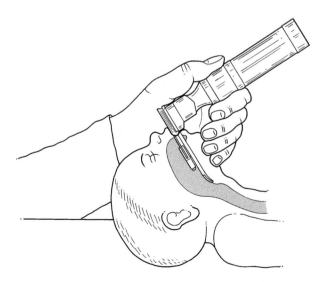

Fig. 16.13 Intubation of a neonate with a straight blade on the laryngoscope.

may be rather short. The glottis lies with its aperture inclined more anteriorly than in the adult, opposite the lower border of the fourth cervical vertebra. During growth it descends to lie in the adult position opposite the fifth and sixth vertebrae by the fourth year of life. Because of this high position, intubation is often most easily performed using a straight laryngoscope blade. In the infant, the epiglottis should be picked up with the tip of the blade (Fig. 16.13), whereas in older children the tip is passed anterior to the epiglottis into the glosso-epiglottic sulcus.

The narrowest part of an adult's airway is the glottis, but in a child, the cricoid ring is narrower. This is a complete ring of cartilage, unlike the tracheal rings below it. By the age of 10–11 years the adult configuration is achieved. The average cross-sectional area at the cricoid ring in the neonate is 28 mm^2, and 1 mm of oedema from infection or trauma will reduce this by 65%.

TRACHEA AND MAIN BRONCHI

The trachea at birth is 4 cm in length and 6 mm in diameter, whereas the average adult length is 12 cm with a width of 20 mm. The rate of growth is not linear, but spurts occur from the first few months of life to the third or fourth year and again around puberty. The trachea lies anterior to the vertebral column, but to the right of the midline: the younger the child, the more to the right. Expected endotracheal tube sizes at each age are given in Table 16.2.

The right main bronchus is shorter than the left. At birth, the bifurcation of the trachea lies opposite the third to fourth vertebrae, but as growth proceeds it descends at 6 years of life and lies at the level of the fifth, and at 12 years the sixth thoracic vertebra.

Table 16.2   Expected tube size

Age (years)	Tube size (internal diameter, mm)
Preterm	2.5–3
Newborn	3.5
3/12–9/12	4.0
9/12–2	4.5
2	5.0
3	5.0
4	5.5
5	5.5
6	6.0
7	6.0
8	6.5
9	6.5
10	7.0
11	7.0
12	7.5
13	7.5

MAIN BRONCHI

Because of the difference between the angles of the two main bronchi, it is more common for foreign bodies and other aspirated material to enter the right main bronchus and from that the upper lobe bronchus at any stage of life. This is less true in younger children, in whom the angulation is less marked and mobility and flexibility are greater.

LUNGS

Lung volume at birth is around 250 ml, whereas the adult volume is 6000 ml. The combined lung weight increases from 60 g at birth to around 750 g. Bronchial segmental development is complete before birth. Postnatal development occurs in the acinar region. New alveoli form most rapidly in the first 2 years of life. They continue to form less rapidly during the first 8 years of life and only stop forming with the cessation of growth of the chest wall.

Gastrointestinal system

ABDOMEN AND CONTENTS

The changes in overall shape of the abdomen have already been alluded to (Fig. 16.3). The liver and spleen are relatively large. The edge of the liver is normally palpable below the right costal margin in the infant and remains palpable across the epigastrium throughout childhood. A palpable spleen in a neonate may be normal.

OESOPHAGUS

The oesophageal length can be measured from the lips at endoscopy, or from the nose, using a marked catheter. On measurement, it correlates as closely with age in months as with height and body surface area. The age formula, measuring from the lips, is: oesophageal length = 21 + 0.136 × age in months, which gives the length with an accuracy of 4 ± 4.1 cm. An alternative height formula used in pH measurement is: 0.207 × height in cm + 4.61. Using this measurement a transnasal oesophageal probe should lie 2–4 cm from the oesophago-gastric junction.

In the infant, the antireflux mechanism at the lower end of the oesophagus is less competent, probably because of relatively low pressure in the 'high-pressure' lower oesophageal sphincter zone and the short length of the intra-abdominal oesophagus. These achieve more adult proportions from the second year of life.

STOMACH

The relative capacity of the stomach is greater than in the adult. A 4 kg baby takes a feed of 120 ml (equivalent to

2 litres in an adult). As a result, with crying and air swallowing, the stomach can expand to take up the greater part of the abdomen. This distension becomes even greater in upper gastrointestinal obstructions, e.g. longstanding hypertrophic pyloric stenosis or duodenal atresia or stenosis. The pylorus normally lies to the right of the midline in the epigastrium but is very mobile. The transpyloric plane of the adult, said to pass through the pylorus, lies at the lower body of L1 on an X-ray and midway between the manubrial notch and the upper border of the symphysis pubis, but has no relevance to children. Analysis of the pyloric volume in patients with infantile hypertrophic pyloric stenosis and other vomiting children has shown that the size of the pylorus correlates well with the weight of the baby (Carver *et al.*, 1987).

SMALL BOWEL

Gut function is well developed even in a preterm infant, with swallowing starting from 20 weeks, organized motor activity from 32 weeks and sucking from 35 weeks of gestation. Lymphoid tissue development follows the same pattern as elsewhere. The length of the small bowel from the duodenojejunal flexure to the ileocaecal valve in a term newborn is 250 cm (± 100 cm). The adult length quoted is 1.5 m. Growth measured in experimental animals does not occur evenly or at the same rate as growth in height. The increase in length after gut resection is generally about that to be expected from normal growth. The diameter increases markedly and the mucosa hypertrophies.

LARGE BOWEL

The caecum may be relatively high at birth and continues to descend into the right iliac fossa during growth. In the younger child the appendix is more frequently retrocaecal. The shallow pelvis means that pelvic appendicitis does not occur before the age of 5 years.

The caecum, ascending and transverse colon are supplied by the superior mesenteric artery through the ileocolic, right colic and middle colic arteries. The descending colon from the left third of the transverse colon is supplied from branches of the inferior mesenteric artery. Traditionally the weakest part in the marginal artery of the colon has been assumed to be between the sigmoid vessels and the superior rectal artery (Sudeck's point); however, the most tenuous link is actually at the junction of the superior and inferior mesenteric supply, between the ascending branch of the superior left colic and the middle colic vessels.

The anal canal, 4 cm long in the adult, is 2–3 cm long in children and should be empty on digital examination. The anus of a newborn will take a 10–12 Hegar dilator, i.e. it is 10–12 mm in diameter, narrower than an average male adult little finger, but it will usually accept its gentle insertion without damage.

Genitourinary system

BLADDER

The shallow pelvis of the newborn and young child means that the bladder is an abdominal organ, making suprapubic aspiration of urine a simple procedure, provided the bladder is palpable. The bladder capacity in millilitres can be estimated approximately from the formula: (25 × age in years) + 25 = volume in ml.

OVARIES AND UTERUS

At birth the ovaries lie on the pelvic brim and until the pelvic cavity enlarges, any increase in size from tumour or cyst formation will bring them into the abdomen as palpable or visible lumps. As the pelvic cavity enlarges, the fallopian tubes and uterus descend into it to take up the adult position by the menarche. The newborn uterus, under the influence of maternal hormones, is between 2.5 and 3.5 cm long. By 6 months, it has regressed to 80% of its size at birth, regaining its neonatal size around 5 years. Growth to adult size occurs with puberty and just prior to the menarche. Until then there is no uterine flexion.

MALE GENITALIA

The development of the penis and scrotum has been divided into five stages

1. Infantile from birth to the onset of puberty. There is a slight increase in overall size but no change in appearance.
2. The start of scrotal enlargement.
3. Further increase in scrotal size: the penis increases in length.

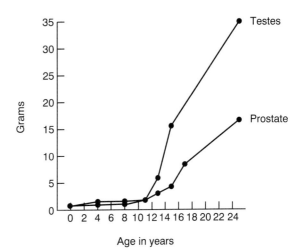

Fig. 16.14 The increase in weight of the testes and prostate which occurs during puberty.

4. Further increase in scrotal size and darkening of the scrotal skin. The penis enlarges and the glans develops.
5. The adult appearance.

TESTICULAR DEVELOPMENT

Testicular growth is minimal until the onset of puberty but then progresses rapidly, and this increase in size precedes the changes in the penis. The dramatic growth and weight of the testes and prostate at puberty are seen in Fig. 16.14.

Cardiovascular system

For the first few years of life the heart lies more horizontally than in the adult. With growth, the thorax lengthens and the heart elongates and descends to take up the adult position. The surface markings are as follows. The right margin lies to the right of the sternal edge from the second intercostal space to the junction of the sixth costal cartilage with the sternum. The left border runs obliquely from the second left intercostal space to the fourth intercostal space in the mid-clavicular or nipple line. The adult position is achieved in later childhood. The surface marking for placement of a ventriculoatrial shunt for hydrocephalus is the fourth right interspace. At birth, the foramen ovale is still valvular and is closed functionally by the increase in systemic pressure in the left atrium. In 75% of children this has fused by 12 weeks of age but in up to 25% the 'foramen' remains probe patent throughout life. The ductus arteriosus joins the left pulmonary artery to the arch of the aorta. It starts to close by muscular contraction after birth and should be obliterated to form the lig-

amenta arteriosum within a few weeks. Closure may be expedited by the prostaglandin antagonist indomethacin and delayed by the prostaglandin epoprostenol.

VASCULAR ACCESS: VENOUS

Central

Central venous access can be gained by direct puncture of the internal jugular, subclavian or femoral veins.

The internal jugular vein lies immediately deep to the sternomastoid muscle within the carotid sheath and is easily approached through the muscle (Fig. 16.15). A point 2–3 cm above the clavicle is chosen, over the medial third of the sternomastoid muscle directing the needle towards the suprasternal notch. The subclavian vein at its junction with the internal jugular may be approached from above the clavicle. The needle is introduced in the angle between the clavicular head of the sternomastoid muscle and clavicle and directed towards the sternal angle. From below, the needle is inserted 0.25–1 cm below the lower border of the clavicle just lateral to its midpoint and directed towards the upper border of the sternoclavicular joint. The lower border of the clavicle is felt and the needle is then directed just below that point, advancing slowly until the vein is entered. The femoral vein is identified lying just medial to the femoral artery which is at the mid-inguinal point just caudal to the inguinal ligament.

Peripheral

Peripheral veins are best identified by seeing and feeling them. The long saphenous vein a the ankle lies anterior to the medial malleolus of the tibia and can be palpated even when empty. In the cubital fossa the laterally placed cephalic vein is easy to cannulate but a central catheter inserted up it may be difficult to manipulate round the sharp bend where it pierces the clavipectoral fascia to join the subclavian vein. Distally, the cephalic vein may be accessible as it passes from the venous arch on the back of the hand laterally round the lower part of the radius to enter the forearm. The medial basilic vein passes directly into the axillary vein.

VASCULAR ACCESS: ARTERIAL

The radial artery is favoured because of its free communication with the ulnar artery through the superficial ulnar and deep palmar arches and its superficial position. This communication can, and probably should, be checked before cannulating it by occluding the artery by finger pressure, to see whether this affects the colour of the fingers. The artery is palpable proxi-

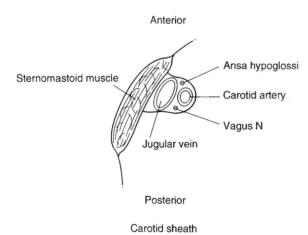

Fig. 16.15   Position of the internal jugular vein in the carotid sheath deep to the sternomastoid muscle.

mal to the wrist crease on the radius just lateral to the flexor carpi radialis tendon. When it is not palpable in very small babies it can be seen by transillumination of the wrist.

The branchial artery in the mid-upper arm lies below the skin on the triceps and brachialis muscles midway between the medial borders of the biceps and long head of the triceps muscles. It is accompanied by the median nerve. The femoral artery emerges into the thigh under the inguinal ligament at the mid-inguinal point, midway between the symphysis pubis and the anterior superior iliac spine, and is separated from the pubic bone by the psoas muscle.

The dorsalis pedis artery, the continuation of the anterior tibial artery, is palpable on the dorsum of the foot over the first intermetatarsal space midway between the malleoli, then just medial to the extensor hallucis longus tendon.

Musculoskeletal system

The times of appearance and closures of the centres of ossification of the skeleton are given in detail in standard orthopaedic and radiological texts. Primary centres are present in the long bones at birth. The timing of the appearance of the epiphyses and later centres of ossification are used to establish a child's 'bone age' and to distinguish normal epiphyseal lines from fractures (Fig. 16.16). Two methods are used for estimating the bone age, using either the bones of the wrist (Greulich and Pyle, 1959), or assessment of skeletal maturity TW2 (Tanner *et al.*, 1975).

OSSIFICATION

In the long bones, the critical 'growth plate' consists of three layers: the growth cartilage; the metaphysis, the site ossification on the growth plate and a surrounding collar of fibrous tissue; and the groove of Ranvier, seen on X-rays or the perichondral ring of La Croix which strengthens the bone by providing a bridge across the weak epiphysis. The blood supply to the bone comes from the nutrient artery to the shaft (which is an end artery), small vessels from the periosteum and anastomoses around the epiphysis. Epiphyses are mostly outside joint capsules. In the shoulder, hip and knee the epiphyseal line lies within the joint, permitting infection from the metaphysis to spread directly into it. As no vessels cross growth plates the blood supply to the head of the femur, prior to fusion at the epiphysis, is at risk. Increase in pressure within the joint will cut off the blood supply through the retinacular and central vessels, leading to death of the head. Damage to the retinacular vessels is also possible through slipping of the capital femoral epiphysis, dislocation of the hip or fracture of the femoral neck.

THE GENERAL SKELETON

The vertebral column in the neonate has only the two primary curves, thoracic and sacral, both of which are concave forwards (kyphosis). By 3 months, as the infant begins to raise its head the cervical spine becomes lordotic and lumbar lordosis appears with sitting at 6–9 months. Thus by the time the child is standing upright and walking, the adult spinal curves are established.

The venous drainage of the spine forms a series of freely interconnecting plexuses inside and outside the vertebral canal draining into the vertebral, intercostal and lumbar veins. This unvalved venous system is subject to reverse flow, explaining bloodborne infection and malignant metastases from the abdomen and pelvis affecting the vertebral bodies. The intervertebral disc develops around remnants of the notochord which have disappeared by 10 years. It is relatively large at birth and initially contains vascular channels essential for nutrition and growth, which disappear in the third decade.

NORMAL DEVELOPMENT OF THE LEG

During growth the shape and angle of the leg joints change as the child learns to bear weight and walk. What are now recognized as normal variants were previously considered to be precursors of deformity and treated with unnecessary splinting.

At birth the angle of the femoral neck with the shaft is 150°, reducing steadily to 148° at 1 year, 145° at 3 years, 138° by 9 years and 120° in the adult. Similarly, the anteversion of the neck reduces from 39° at 6 months to the adult value of 15° at 16 years.

GENU VARUM AND VALGUM

Minor degrees of genu varum (bow legs) and valgum (knock knee) are common. Genu varum is seen in infants but corrects after the child has been walking for some time. It may then go on to valgum but by the age of 6 years the legs should be straight. Genu valgum is common and is measured by the distance between the malleoli when the knees are touching. At 3–3.5 years 22% of children have a gap of greater than 5 cm yet by 7 years it persists in only 2%.

Central nervous system: spinal cord

The spinal cord develops from the ectodermal neural plate. Failure of closure to form the neural tube explains the occurrence of spina bifida, craniumbifidum and anencephaly. The floor of the fourth ventricle shows a persisting unclosed neural tube. Neural tube closure should be complete by 4 weeks into

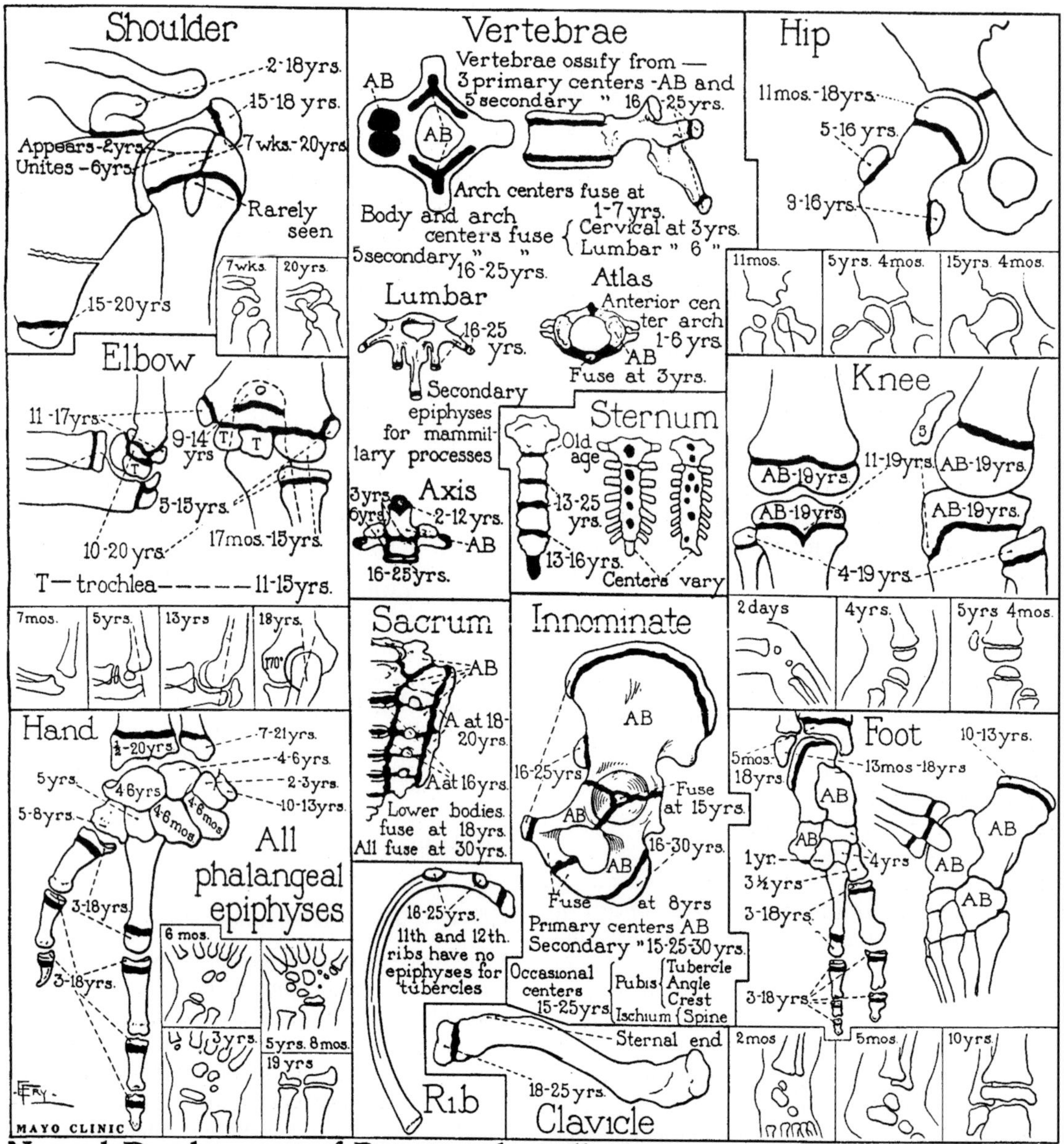

Shoulder

Appears-2yrs.
Unites –6yrs.
2-18yrs.
15-18 yrs.
7 wks.-20yrs.
Rarely seen
15-20yrs
7wks. 20yrs.

Elbow

11-17yrs.
9-14 (T) (T) yrs.
5-15yrs.
10-20yrs.
17mos.-15yrs.
T — trochlea – – – – –11-15yrs.
7mos. 5yrs. 13yrs. 18yrs. 170°

Hand

1-20yrs.
7-21yrs.
5yrs.
4-6yrs.
4·6yrs.
2-3yrs.
5-8yrs.
4·8mos.
10-13yrs.
4·8mos.
3-18yrs.
3-18yrs.
6 mos.
All phalangeal epiphyses
5yrs. 8mos. 19yrs.
FRY.
MAYO CLINIC

Vertebrae

Vertebrae ossify from — 3 primary centers -AB and 5 secondary " 16-25yrs.
AB   AB
Arch centers fuse at 1-7yrs.
Body and arch centers fuse { Cervical at 3yrs.
5 secondary " " { Lumbar " 6 "
16-25yrs.

Lumbar
16-25 yrs.
Secondary epiphyses for mammillary processes
3yrs.
Axis
6yrs. 2-12yrs. AB
16-25yrs.

Atlas
Anterior center arch 1-6 yrs.
AB
Fuse at 3yrs.

Sternum
Old age
13-25 yrs.
13-16yrs.
Centers vary

Sacrum
AB
A at 18-20yrs.
A at 16yrs.
Lower bodies fuse at 18yrs.
All fuse at 30yrs.

18-25yrs.
11th and 12th ribs have no epiphyses for tubercles
Rib
18-25yrs.

Innominate
AB
16-25yrs.
Fuse at 15yrs.
AB
16-30yrs.
AB
Fuse at 8yrs.
Primary centers AB
Secondary " 15-25-30yrs.
Occasional centers 15-25yrs.
Pubis { Tubercle Angle Crest
Ischium { Spine
Sternal end
18-25yrs.
Clavicle

Hip
11mos.-18yrs.
5-16 yrs.
9-16yrs.
11mos.   5yrs. 4mos.   15yrs. 4mos.

Knee
AB-19yrs.   11-19yrs. AB-19yrs.
AB-19yrs.   AB-19yrs.
4-19yrs.
2days   4yrs.   5yrs 4mos.

Foot
5mos.-18yrs.   13mos-18yrs.   10-13yrs.
AB   AB
AB   AB
1yr.   3½yrs.   4yrs   AB
3-18yrs.
3-18yrs.
2mos.   5mos.   10yrs.

Normal Development of Roentgenologically Important Bones and Epiphyses
JOHN D. CAMP, M. D. AND EARL I. L. CILLEY, M. D.

1. A = Appears. U = Unites.
2. The number on a tarsal or carpal bone indicates the age at which calcification is roentgenologically visible.
3. AB - Ossification visible at birth.
4. Two numbers, i.e. 16 – 25 indicate visible ossification at 16 yrs. and union at 25 yrs.
5. The number at a cartilaginous junction indicates age at which ossification occurs.
6. There is considerable normal variation at any given age

Fig. 16.16   Normal development of roentgenologically important bones and epiphyses.

gestation. The final development of the cord is not complete at birth and full myelination takes up to 2 years.

Up until birth the vertebral column steadily outgrows the spinal cord which recedes within the spinal canal. It has long been believed that this process continues throughout childhood. Advances in imaging, with ultrasound in the newborn and magnetic resonance imaging (MRI) at all ages, have made it easier to study the position of the conus (Wilson and Prince, 1989). Investigations showed that this is much more variable than was previously understood and no evidence of differential growth was found. The range for the vertebral level of the tip of the conus medullaris from 0 to 2 years was from the T12 to the L2 disc space. A termination as low as L3 was found in normal subjects at all ages and the mean position lay over the body of L1 at all ages. A criticism of these findings was that they were not serial studies but isolated in individual children. The deteriorating neural function associated with tethering of the cord by an abnormal filum terminale, lipoma of the cord or following repair of a myelomeningocele suggests that the answer is not simple. In addition, the cord may recede dramatically when a tethered filum is divided.

VENTRICULAR SYSTEM

The lateral ventricles lie within the cerebral hemisphere separated by the septum lucidum. They communicate through the foramina of Monro with the third ventricle, which lies in the midline between the thalami and communicates back through the narrowest part of the system, the cerebral aqueduct (of Sylvius), leading into the fourth ventricle, which is roofed by the cerebellum and has as its floor the hindbrain. The foramina of Magendie central and of Luschka in the lateral recesses allow cerebrospinal fluid (CSF) into the subarachnoid

space around the brain. The CSF is secreted by the choroid plexuses in the lateral, third and fourth ventricles and from the ependymal surface. It passes through the ventricular system, then over the surface of the brain, down the central canal of the spinal cord and over the surface of the cord. It is absorbed back into the bloodstream through the arachnoid granulations in the superior longitudinal (sagittal) sinus. Blockage at any point, including within the granulations or superior longitudinal sinus, causes hydrocephalus. In communicating hydrocephalus, there is free communication between the intraventricular systems and the arachnoid space around the cord. Pressure can be obtained from lumbar puncture and drainage is possible through a thecoperitoneal shunt. In non-communicating hydrocephalus, any attempt to lower the pressure around the cord may induce coning of the hindbrain into the foramen magnum and sudden death. Access to the system is easy before the anterior fontanelle is closed. A needle passed through the angle of the fontanelle vertically downwards towards the midline should hit the ventricle at 5 cm from the surface. Once the fontanelle has closed a burr hole 1–2 cm from the midline is required. The choroid plexuses in the lateral ventricle lie posterior to the foramina of Monro and an intraventricular catheter placed in the anterior horn of the lateral ventricle in front of this should not, in theory, become obstructed by the choroid plexus wrapping round it.

The cerebral veins cross the subarachnoid space from the relatively mobile cortex to drain into the rigid superior sagittal sinus. They run obliquely forwards, increasingly so posteriorly. This arrangement leaves them vulnerable to injury from rapid head movement either in a head injury or during severe shaking, leading to subdural bleeding and effusion.

INNER EAR AND INTRACRANIAL PRESSURE

The inner ear consists of two parts, the bony labyrinth within the petrous temporal bone and the membranous labyrinth, a series of communicating sacs and ducts, including the semicircular canals and the cochlea. Within the cochlea lies the scala tympani which is continuous with the subarachnoid space through the aqueduct

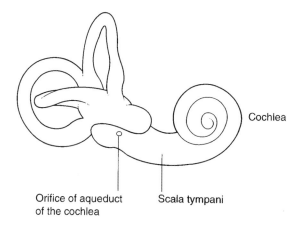

Fig. 16.17 Inner ear showing the orifice of the aqueduct of the cochlea.

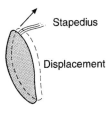

Fig. 16.18 Middle ear: alterations in intracranial pressure produces variations in the kinematics of the middle ear ossicles and thus the position of the stapes.

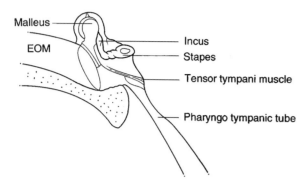

Malleus

EOM

Incus

Stapes

Tensor tympani muscle

Pharyngo tympanic tube

Fig. 16.19 In response to a loud noise there is displacement of the tympanic membrane due to the stapedial reflex contraction. The displacement is related to the perilymphatic pressure and is measurable.

of the cochlea. This minute canal, which tends to close with age, has become important as this link enables an approach to the measurement of CSF pressure through the middle ear (Fig. 16.17).

Perilymphatic pressure reflects CSF pressure when the cochlear aqueduct is patent. Changes in the perilymphatic pressure produce small but measurable variations in the kinematics of the middle ear ossicles and tympanic membrane (Fig. 16.18). Alterations in pressure influence the resting position of the stapes footplate in the oval window and consequently the degree of movement of the bones and tympanic membrane. Contraction of the stapedius muscle, which is attached by a ligament to the head of the stapes, moves the bone (Fig. 16.19). This pattern of tympanic membrane displacement during the stapedial reflex contraction, in response to loud noise, is a measure that relates to perilymphatic pressure and can be used to measure intracranial pressure.

NERVE BIOPSY

Two sites are suitable for obtaining a specimen of a peripheral nerve for neurological diagnosis. The sural nerve is easily found as it lies posterior to the lateral malleolus midway between this and the tendo achilles and alongside the small saphenous vein. Complete division of the nerve only causes anaesthesia on the lateral side of the heel and foot. This can be reduced by splitting the nerve and sending only a half thickness for biopsy. If motor fibres are required, the most distal part of the deep peroneal (anterior tibial) nerve where it lies on the dorsum of the foot, lateral to the dorsalis pedis artery, can be taken. Anaesthesia is produced only in the web space between the first and second toes and loss of power in the extensor digitorum brevis is not easily detectable.

References

Carver, R.A., Okorie, N.M., Steiner, G.M. and Dickson, J.A.S. 1987: Infantile hypertrophic pyloric stenosis – diagnosis from the pyloric muscle index. *Clinical Radiology* **138**, 625–7.

Greulich, W.W. and Pyle, S.I. 1959: *Radiographic atlas of skeletal development of the hand and wrist*, 2nd ed. Stanford, CA: Stanford University Press.

Tanner, J.M. 1978: 1. *Human growth – collected work*. Falkner, I., Tardrew, F., Mourilyan, J. (DNLM: 1. Growth; 2. Gestational Age. WS103 H918). *Human Growth* Vol. 2. *Postnatal growth* 1978. New York: Plenum Press, First published 1918.

Tanner, J.M., Whitehouse, R.H., Marshall, W.A., Healy, M.J.R. and Goldstein, H. 1975: *Assessment of skeletal maturity and prediction of adult height (TW2 method)*. New York: Academic Press.

Wilson, D.A. and Prince, J.R. 1989: MR imaging determination of the location of the normal conus medullaris throughout childhood. *American Journal of Neuroradiology* **10**, 259–62.

Further reading

Camp, J.D. and Cilley, E.I.L. 1931: Diagramatic chart showing time of appearance of various centers of ossification and period of union. *American Journal of Roentgenology* **26**, 905–6.

Keats, T. E. *Atlas of normal Roentgen variants that may simulate disease*, 6th ed. St Louis, MO: Mosby.

Michels, N.A. 1955: *Blood supply and anatomy of the upper abdominal organs*. London: Pitman.

Reid, A., Marchbanks, R.J., Bateman, D.E., Martin, A.M., Brightwell, A.P. and Pickard, J.D. 1989: Mean intracranial pressure monitoring by a non-invasive audiological technique: a pilot study. *Journal of Neurology, Neurosurgery and Psychiatry*, **52**, 610–12.

CHAPTER 17

Audit

D.C.S. GOUGH AND J. BRUCE

Introduction
What is audit?
The reasons for audit
The theory of audit
The practice of audit

The methodology of audit
What do you audit?
Is audit effective?
The future
References

The surgical staff at the Massachusetts General Hospital did this: They reorganized in such a way that each member of the staff undertook to give special study to some difficult class of cases, and in return the hospital assigned to each member all the cases of that group. The result has been that the mortality in these groups of cases showed a great improvement (E.A. Codman, 1914).

Introduction

One could be forgiven for thinking that the practice of audit in medicine was new. It is certainly fashionable, and for those hospitals in the UK wishing to continue to employ junior medical staff it is compulsory, but new it is not. Surgical audit is as old as surgery itself. In 1882 Burdett researched the mortality from amputation in 61 different cottage hospitals with a total of 553 beds and found it to be 18%. He compared this with a large series from London, Paris, Zurich, Edinburgh and Glasgow, where the mortality averaged nearly 50%, and those from Hamburg where aseptic policies were adopted, and found a mortality of 3%. Audit, comparative audit and research, we believe, all in one paper!

That paper also reflects the fact that surgeons have been primarily interested in the outcome of their intervention, and have been made personally and painfully aware of their own shortcomings. Codman noted that all results of surgical treatment that 'lack affection' might be explained by a number of factors which might involve the surgeon, the patient or the delivery of the treatment. Surgical errors may be due to lack of technical knowledge or skill, lack of surgical judgement or lack of diagnostic ability. There may be deficiencies in the structure of the health care system secondary to lack of surgical or other equipment. The patient may be in such an enfeebled condition that they were unable to stand the surgery, or suffer from an unconquerable disease. They might also refuse treatment.

Lastly, there were those calamities of surgery or those accidents and complications over which we have no known control. Codman placed audit on a systematic and scientific footing.

Systematic medical audit in the UK was, however, quite rare until 1980. What made audit fashionable was the health service reforms commencing in the early 1990s which put audit high on the political agenda and made money available for its institution. The altruistic rationale behind clinical audit lies in the improvement of quality of care given to patients. However, it would also be naive to ignore the implications of reducing the cost of medical care and increasing the cost efficiency of treatment.

What is audit?

In the *Oxford English Dictionary* the verb 'audit' is defined as making an official, systematic examination of accounts, but in modern medical parlance audit is taken to mean the systematic critical analysis of the quality of medical care, including the procedures used for diagnosis and treatment, the use of resources, and the resulting outcome and quality of life for the patient. It is a review of the care of patients based on data obtained by systematic enquiry and makes judgements about the quality of care.

There is still confusion existing in some minds as to the difference between audit and research, probably because a similar scientific method is used in both clinical research and audit. This confusion still exists and audit is sometimes thought of as some form of inferior research exercise. It has been said that research is discovering what is the right thing to do, whereas audit is intended to make sure that the right thing is done (Smith, 1992). An example of audit and research would be to state that research is the appropriate tool to establish links between cure rates in Wilms' tumour and various forms of chemotherapy or radiotherapy. When research has established clinical standards and the link between clinical care and outcome is clearly defined, then audit would assess individual performance against this standard. One could assess by audit whether the delivery of treatment in stage 3 Wilms' tumour patients in one's own institution matched the protocol that had been adopted as a national standard.

Research studies must be designed so that the results of a study are transferable into different patient populations, but audit is only designed to produce results for the patients within the project (Bull, 1993). Audit assesses the clinical care that is being given to a particular set of patients within a certain time.

The simplest and most widely known form that the systematic examination of medical accounts takes in practice is in the deaths and complications meeting. This is often combined with an analysis of workload for the unit in question and, as these data need to be collected for so many different purposes, they are relatively easy to obtain and classify.

Much of the interpretation of this sort of audit is subjective, and small groups of doctors can be forgiven for not confronting some of the issues raised by audit which might lead to confrontation with friends and colleagues with whom some form of professional relationship may be necessary for the best part of a quarter of a century. These problems with audit led to the development of criterion audit in the USA.

A topic is chosen by the audit committee and can be applied to any group of patients with characteristics held in common. An agreement is then reached on a limited number of criteria that are considered critical to the process and outcome of treatment. Medical records or audit staff collect data from the patients in the study group and those records that show deviation from the agreed criteria of diagnosis, treatment or outcome are specifically examined by clinicians. An example of a criterion audit is given later in the chapter.

As it is usually easier to identify what constitutes bad practice than to specify what constitutes good practice, other forms that audit may take are occurrence screening or critical incident reporting. This provides a way of focusing on incidents where agreement of suboptimal treatment is invariably accepted and this can encompass all aspects of the health care process and start to broaden audit into a multidisciplinary approach.

Occurrence screening can be done using hospital records and may look for information such as the occurrence of a wound infection after surgery or the development of a pressure sore whilst an inpatient. Incomplete operative consent forms, blocked catheters and falls whilst in hospital have all been deemed the subject for this type of audit.

Critical incident reporting is a form of audit that collects data on specific events in individual patients in a prospective manner. It may take the form of a study looking at patients who need reintubation after extubation following general anaesthesia and could identify reasons for this critical incident occurring and lead to prevention of this complication.

Comparative audit, as its name signifies, compares one set of audit data against another and the widespread development of computer systems allows easy access to a comparative audit service. This can show evidence of variation in clinical practice, mostly with regard to outcome. It does not, however, identify variations in input that can be useful in giving guidance in situations where there are no clear standards to adopt. This form of audit data needs to be treated with caution. Although it is relatively easy to define on paper the differences between various forms of audit and research, once one gets into the rough and tumble of day-to-day clinical practice the boundaries between audit and research are more difficult to define.

The reasons for audit

Currently, within the National Health Service (NHS), the regional health authority is responsible for ensuring that all hospitals set up a framework for medical audit in which each doctor will participate. This is done through a hospital's medical audit committee, which is responsible for ensuring that regular systematic audit takes place and providing managers with reports and results that show that effective audit is taking place. Hospital managers, in their turn, make sure that adequate resources and staff and systems are in place to perform audit and that time and money are available for training.

All hospitals within the NHS are audited by the Royal Colleges to see that there are adequate facilities for the practice of surgery and that surgeons and physicians may be trained in a professional and personal environment that allows them to work and study in a proper manner. If audit is not taking place then the accreditation of such a hospital for training would be in jeopardy. The professional enthusiasm for audit has in some sense been related to these two factors. There would, however, be no one who would deny that the systematic appraisal and examination of their own surgical accounts is something that is professionally desirable and can be effective in changing practice and improving the quality of surgery. If there's a will, then this can be the way.

The theory of audit

The theory of audit is encompassed in the following diagram of the audit cycle:

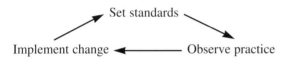

The audit cycle allows standards to be set, observed and improved. The practical nature of medical audit is a discussion between doctors on the quality of care provided as judged against agreed standards. If the agreed standards of care have not been met, then practice needs to be changed in an agreed way and feedback in the form of re-audit then completes the audit cycle (Standing Medical Advisory Committee, 1990).

Health care professionals involved in medical audit must be prepared to change, but the process of audit should be seen as educational and not punitive. Although individual doctors will participate in the meeting, confidentiality is essential and the documentation of audit meetings should be provided in an anonymous form where general conclusions and recommendations are published but specific doctors or patients are not named.

The practice of audit

It has been noted previously that effective audit can be conducted without a computer but the computer cannot compensate for inadequate method. The NHS Executive has produced clear guidelines containing the fundamental principles of audit, stating that it should be professionally led with appropriately trained and specifically appointed staff. This helps to ensure an element of objectivity and minimize bias in the performance of audit studies. It also relieves the pressure on clinicians and lessens the amount of potentially distracting time which could sap energy from clinical care. The Royal College of Physicians suggests that consultants should occupy about 1 hour per week in the practice of audit.

Audit is part of an ongoing educational process, which involves all aspects of the multidisciplinary unit, including junior and senior medical staff nursing staff and ancillary staff, with managerial involvement. We have begun to move away from medical audit into multidisciplinary audit.

Audit is an essential part of the routine clinical process. The accumulation of data and their analysis has to be a continual process and, consequently, it has to be included in normal clinical activity. Data are difficult to analyse when collected in a retrospective manner and clinicians should ensure that all audit data are recorded for collection prospectively.

Audit should lead to improvement in the quality of care of patients. Before this can come about, the setting of the basic minimum standards is necessary to provide a basis for comparison. Consequently, an extensive database of activity should be the aim in audit. The setting of standards may be, by necessity, reliant on the experience of others and on publications in medical literature or the experience of recognized experts.

Data can be collected through an individual's surgical logbook, which can record deaths or major complications. This is already done longhand and is a necessary part of each surgeon's training programme. It is examined by the appropriate specialist advisory committee in the course of the surgeons training. The ability for portable pocket computers to now accomplish this task has allowed swifter management of the data involved. The use of a Psion computer for this purpose is gaining in popularity.

Card index systems have now largely been replaced by the use of personal computers which, to be really effective, need to be linked to the hospital management system. They most frequently rely on ICD and OPCS coding for disease and procedures. The Read coding system is more cumbersome, but allows more detailed coding. There is a bewildering array of software available for the process of audit, and many departments have developed their own personal systems which, or course, have value locally but not nationally.

Returning to the audit cycle, the basic practice of audit is to:

1. set clinical objectives
2. collect the information
3. evaluate the process and outcome
4. review the objectives and clinical consequences of care, and
5. repeat the audit.

The methodology of audit

Before anyone starts an audit programme the question, 'Why are we doing this audit, and for whom are the results intended?' ought to be asked. One assumes that the audit resources are available and that there is some reliable scientific method of analysis, but the audit should be done for a specific purpose, not as an end in itself. In assessing what data need to be collected the following questions need to be asked:

- Will the data be available in a similar and comparable form from different departments?
- Will the data allow comparison with already published research or good practice?
- Will the data allow comparison before and after changes are made?
- Will the data attribute cause and effect changes on re-audit?

It is often best to start with a simple discharges and deaths meeting on a regular basis with a specific chairperson involved who may be on a rotational basis. The danger with this form of meeting is that the discussion can become repetitive and there needs to be a selection at some point of specific activity that should be audited.

It is best to start with some common condition where there are agreed standards and one can check local practice against published data. Again, the chairperson should have the selection of the topic to be audited in his or her hands, and determine whether all cases under a specific heading need to be audited. It is sometimes helpful to have statistical input. An example here would be that an acceptable recurrence rate after inguinal hernia repair might be chosen as 2%. If an apparent recurrence rate of 4% was seen in an individual hospital practice some 240 patients would need to be involved in the audit before statistical significance was reached (Evans, 1989).

Therefore, any action following audit needs to be looked at in a scientific manner and consensus decisions, if arrived at, published and disseminated throughout the hospital or department. If remedial action is called for this ought to be documented and it might require an increase in resources, training or a change in practice. There needs to be a permanent record in which the patient's identity is protected and guaranteed, and those charged with the responsibility for any information held on computer should take steps to make that system secure. All working papers for the audit should be destroyed and the anonymous conclusions and recommendations should ideally be kept to one sheet of paper, which is the permanent written record of the meeting.

What do you audit?

It was suggested initially by Sheldon (1982) that three main factors can be looked at in the health care delivery systems: the structure of health care, the process of health care and the outcome of health care. The structure of health care delivery is perhaps not so important to individual surgeons and it falls to us to look at

either the process or the outcome of healthcare delivery. Faced with a choice between good process with poor outcome and poor process with good outcome, most patients and physicians would opt for the latter (Schroeder, 1987).

Few would deny, however, that there is a link between good process and good outcome. The provision of rapid response trauma teams and major trauma centres leads through good organization, on to good practice and good teaching, which will attract good staff and subsequently a high quality of care.

Because death in paediatric surgery is not an especially sensitive indicator of the quality of care, as mortality is such a rare event, then surgical complications, the quality of outcome and the length of time necessary to deliver this outcome are probably more important to an individual surgeon. These factors should be the subject of regular audit.

To be useful, the topic chosen for audit should either be common or involve the patient in high risk or the hospital in high cost. An example of a criterion audit of this nature would be to look at children who presented to the outpatient department with a urinary tract infection. Based on scientific evidence and an appraisal of the literature, most paediatric departments will have protocols for the investigation of children with urinary infection. For instance, we suggest in our own unit that all patients under the age of 3 years presenting with a clinical symptomatic urinary infection should have an ultrasound, a DMSA scan and a micturating cystogram. A simple audit would analyse 20 consecutive patients under the age of 3 years presenting with urinary infection and ask the simple question from the hospital records, did they or did they not receive all three investigations?

In discussing the results, the question would be asked 'if not, why not?' and there must be allowable exceptions to what might apparently be deviations from protocols. The parents might refuse to have their 3-year-old daughter undergo a micturating cystogram, and if the ultrasound and DMSA scans were normal then the paediatrician may increase the degree of outpatient surveillance rather than insisting on this investigation. If it had been decided in the protocol that once all these three investigations were normal then the patient would only have one further outpatient follow-up, then we would again have allowable exceptions as to why such a patient was continuing to attend hospital.

A further subject on this audit might be that all young girls attending with lower urinary tract symptoms should be advised not to use bubble bath and that this feature should be recorded either in the record of attendance at outpatients or in the letter to the general practitioner.

The application of performance indicators is a useful tool in the development of audit. This approach was initially developed in the USA as the various funding agencies attempted to control the escalating costs of medical care as well as the great variation in treatments administered by the medical profession. In addition, with the explosion in the cost of litigation which burdened hospitals and insurance companies, scrutiny of acceptable clinical practice was undertaken. The analysis of performance indicators does not tend to identify individual clinical performances but more trends of activity. However, with the development of the newer comprehensive computerized systems, individual performances are more accessible to analysis.

Several factors have been identified that offer an indication of performance. The duration of inpatient stay is a guide to efficiency of clinical management when compared to measured levels of expected duration of stay. The levels of expectation duration can be extrapolated from data accrued from comparable centres in other regions or districts. Using the ratio of the actual versus the expected provides a standardized ratio that can be used for comparative purposes, such as individual professional activity or to compare data from different institutions. Similarly, patient turnover and throughput per bed can be measured and analysed by comparing actual and expected figures with their standardized ratios. With increasing impetus to minimize inpatient stay, a useful performance indicator is the percentage of day case surgery. Similarly, inappropriate admissions to a surgical day unit and delays in treatment can be indicated by the rate of patients who are admitted but who do not undergo surgery. Surgical factors include the period of preoperative and postoperative stay and this can also be judged against expected data. Theatre sessions per bed in the hospital and number of cases per list would imply that only minor surgery is being performed. Other mathematical indicators of activity or efficiency are waiting list statistics, including the actual numbers, the times involved, the waiting list numbers per 1000 operations and the notional days to clear the waiting list.

The performance indicators discussed above relate poorly to individual activity. Individual performance can be assessed from the clinical data available but caution is required for appropriate interpretation of individual performance. Complication rates for certain procedures should be recorded and compared to establish standards within the institution and also the accepted published literature. Recurrence of pathology, either early or late, early return to hospital after discharge, or reoperation during the inpatient stay, may all be indicators of unusual or unexpected events in treatment. Comparison between preoperative and postoperative diagnosis and delays in definitive diagnosis are also useful in identifying difficulties. It must be emphasized that there is a considerable margin for error in the interpretation of this form of audit data. The fact that some patients stay longer may simply be an indication of personal consultant practice which, none the less, may require change. However, knowledge of widely discrepant management

practices should provide the focus for debate and discussion at the appropriate audit presentation and, with intellectual discussion, change may be effected.

Is audit effective?

A good example of how effective audit can be was published by Cooper *et al.* (1978). Through a reporting of critical incidents and an overall assessment of anaesthetic working practice, the authors established those aspects of working practice that could be changed to improve safety and the quality of care. In essence this was a process audit on how care was delivered and, probably as a result of this paper, the introduction of the low-pressure alarm into a breathing circuit during ventilation was facilitated and has led to safer anaesthesia.

Audit is certainly effective in reducing costs, and may thereby indirectly benefit healthcare outcome. Perhaps, in some instances, audit does little more than reduce hospital stay. It has certainly been responsible for documenting and pushing for early hospital discharge even though in 1972 it was shown to be dangerous to stay in hospital and to be in bed after surgery (Asher, 1972)! Pressure on costs induced by audit may, therefore, have beneficial effects by reducing length of stay. To be effective for clinicians audit should concentrate on quality and not on cost. Quality equals outcome, efficiency equals process.

Little effort has gone into researching audit itself to see whether any tangible benefit ensues but there are suggestions that audit does improve care and reduce deaths and complications in general surgical patients (Gruer *et al.*, 1986).

Few of us can deny that properly conducted audit meetings are effective methods of teaching and communication and have led to significant changes in hospital practice. They have certainly increased the move to surgical specialization and an overall improvement in the standards of surgical care, both at local and at national level. There are, however, other pressures on doctors to specialize and this trend may be a feature of the age, not audit.

To be effective as an educational exercise, the lessons of previous audit meetings need to be acted upon. It is usually necessary to devote one or two audit meetings per annum to ensure that previous recommendations have been followed.

The future

There is no longer any need to look across the Atlantic Ocean to see what the future holds for those involved in medical audit. With the changes to purchasers and providers within the NHS it is quite clear that managers are becoming much more involved in the way that health care is delivered. The dialogue between hospital management, clinicians and, now more importantly, the purchasers, means that standards and quality issues are likely to be high on the agenda well before the turn of the century.

Managers are spending money on audit and they will need to see what they are getting. The burden of medical negligence claims is now falling directly on individual hospital trusts and the use of audit in risk management is likely to become more important for cost containment. We are already seeing the transfer of medical audit into clinical or multidisciplinary audit. The management is in the driving seat (Bowden and Walsh, 1991). Competition between hospitals for the 'health care business' may well reach a pitch where hospitals succeed or fail not purely on the quality of their service, but on the ability to prove their effectiveness in terms of outcome.

Purchasers (health authorities) will require audit data supporting the quality of service that they buy and expect ongoing audit to reflect the quality of service being delivered. Hospital league tables are now published widely in the national press and are the subject of considerable debate within the profession. In the USA some hospitals are forced to purchase software packages that allow standardized reporting of both cost and outcome of care.

The cost to the bureaucracy involved in the collection and collation of this form of audit data is considerable and the ability of purchasers to switch providers is limited as few have spare capacity. Where audit data show up incompetent providers it is the intention of the new market structure that these units are forced out of business by 'the market's invisible hand'. What is more likely is that individuals will be forced to retrain or the institution reform. In a limited system the fit will not only survive, but need to be created.

References

Asher, R. 1972: The dangers of going to bed. In Asher, R. (ed.), *Talking sense.* London: Pitman Medical, 119–23.

Bowden, D. and Walsh, K. 1991: When medical audit starts to count. *British Medical Journal* **303**, 101–3.

Bull, A.R. 1993: Audit and research: complimentary but distinct. *Annals of the Royal College of Surgeons of England* **75**, 308–11.

Burdett, H.C. 1882: The relative mortality after amputation of large and small hospitals, and the influence of the antiseptic system on such a mortality. *Journal of the Statistical Society*, **45**, 444–83.

Cooper, J.B., Newbowe, R.S., Long, C.D. and McPeek, B. 1978: Preventable anaesthesia mishaps: a study of human factors. *Anesthesiology* **49**, 399–406.

Evans P.A. 1989: *Surgical audit.* London: Butterworths.

Gruer R, Gordon, D.S., Gunn, A.A. and Ruckley, C.V. 1986: Audit of surgical audit *Lancet* **i**, 23–6.

Schroeder, S.A. 1987: Outcome assessment 70 years later: are we ready? *New England Journal of Medicine* **316**, 160–2.

Sheldon, M.G. 1982: *Medical audit in general practice.* Royal College of General Practitioners Occasional Paper **20**, 1–21.

Smith, R. 1992: Audit and research. *British Medical Journal* **305**, 905–6.

Standing Medical Advisory Committee 1990: *The quality of medical care* (report). London: HMSO.

PART II

Neonatal surgery

CHAPTER 18

Anterior wall defects

P. GORNALL AND J.D. ATWELL

Embryology and classification
Exomphalos: omphalocele
Repair of gastroschisis

Repair of a secondary ventral hernia
References

Embryology and classification

Failure of closure of anterior abdominal wall results in an omphalocele or gastroschisis. In the fetus the omphalocele contains the midgut on the superior mesenteric axis. The return of the midgut to the true abdomen and its rotation allow the abdominal wall to close (Fig. 18.1). This process starts at the 5-mm stage (35 days), the omphalocele increases in size to accommodate the developing intestine by the 23-mm stage (53 days) and closure of the anterior abdominal wall is complete by the 50-mm stage (90 days).

The covering membrane of the omphalocele is thin, but it thickens as the ventrolateral part is invaded by the developing myotomes and dermatomes. These structures then differentiate to form the abdominal muscles. The rectus abdominis develops in the free ventral edge and fusion of the free edges closes the abdominal cavity. The fusion occurs initially in the upper then lower and finally the central portion of the abdomen (Duhamel, 1963) (Fig. 18.2).

Failure of closure of the abdominal wall in the midline results in a series of different abdominal wall defects. Failure of the proximal fold to close results in the syndrome of Cantrell (Cantrell *et al.*, 1958) with ectopia cordis, diaphragmatic hernia and exomphalos. Failure of the distal or inferior folds to close results in bladder exstrophy and exomphalos and if the hind gut is absent the rare vesicointestinal fissure (Rickham,

1960). Failure of the free edge on the right side adjacent to the umbilical vessels, which are normally inserted, plus loss of the covering membrane results in a gastroschisis (Bernstein, 1940).

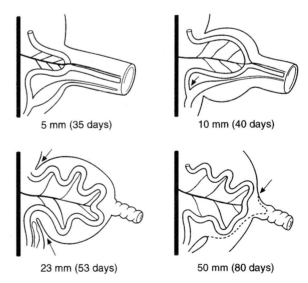

5 mm (35 days)   10 mm (40 days)

23 mm (53 days)   50 mm (80 days)

Fig. 18.1 Embryology of the closure of the anterior abdominal wall.

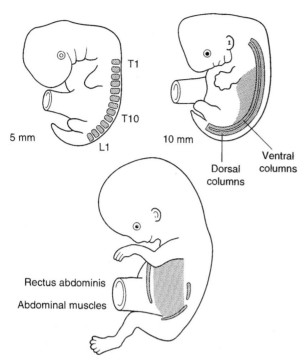

There are several different classifications for omphalocele and gastroschisis. These depend on several factors such as the size and position of the defect, the presence of a covering and the association with other congenital anomalies which may be life threatening.

A defect smaller than 2.5 cm in diameter at the umbilicus may be called a hernia into the cord or a type I non-syndrome omphalocele, whereas, a defect measuring 2.5–5.0 cm in diameter it is a type II non-syndrome omphalocele. Sometimes these two groups are classified as exomphalos minor. A defect greater than 5.0 cm in diameter is called a type III non-syndrome omphalocele or an exomphalos major (Moore, 1977) (Fig. 18.3).

Syndrome omphaloceles are fairly common and include the upper midline syndrome with sternal, diaphragmatic, pericardial and cardiac defects. The lower midline syndrome is associated with bladder exstrophy and vesicointestinal fissure. The central midline syndrome is associated with the Beckwith–Weidemann syndrome with gigantism and macroglossia.

Fig. 18.2 Diagrams to show the development of the muscles of the abdomen from the segmental myotomes.

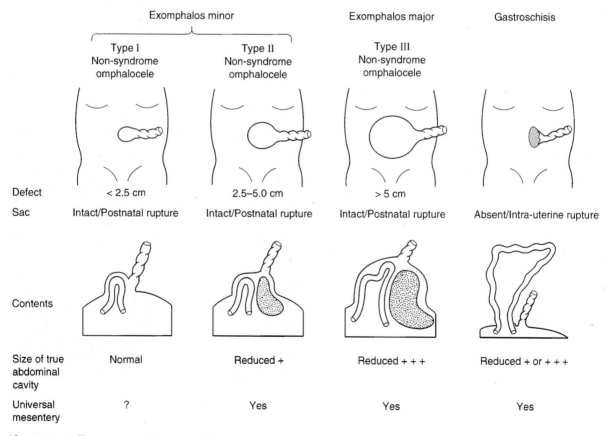

	Exomphalos minor		Exomphalos major	Gastroschisis
	Type I Non-syndrome omphalocele	Type II Non-syndrome omphalocele	Type III Non-syndrome omphalocele	
Defect	< 2.5 cm	2.5–5.0 cm	> 5 cm	
Sac	Intact/Postnatal rupture	Intact/Postnatal rupture	Intact/Postnatal rupture	Absent/Intra-uterine rupture
Contents				
Size of true abdominal cavity	Normal	Reduced +	Reduced + + +	Reduced + or + + +
Universal mesentery	?	Yes	Yes	Yes

Fig. 18.3 Different types of anterior abdominal wall defects and associated pathological findings.

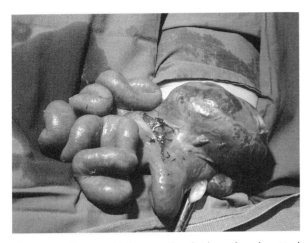

Fig. 18.4 Gastroschisis: note the thickened and matted loops of small bowel including the stomach.

In gastroschisis the sac or covering is either absent or has disappeared during intrauterine life (Fig. 18.4 and also Plate 5). With the advent of antenatal ultrasonography evidence has accumulated showing the presence of a sac which is later shown to be absent. The defect is to the right of normally inserted umbilical vessels and the abdominal viscera protrudes through the defect and is bathed in the amniotic fluid. The effect of fetal urine on extruded intestine has been studied in a number of different amniotic models (Kluck *et al.*, 1983; Phillips *et al.*, 1991). It seems likely that there is a time relationship between the length of exposure of the gut to amniotic fluid, the development and reversibility of histological changes on the surface of the intestine and, in turn, its contractility and absorptive function (Langer *et al.*, 1990; Crawford *et al.*, 1992). Whether this is the cause of the marked oedema of the intestines is debatable but the swelling results in apparent shortening of intestinal length. Other congenital defects associated with gastroschisis include a universal mesentery (Fig. 18.5) predisposing to a malrotation and intestinal atresia, usually at the level of the rim of the defect. This low incidence of associated anomalies is in marked contrast to the high incidence of serious congenital malformations associated with exomphalos major. Another difference is the statistically significant difference in birth weights, with gastroschisis cases usually weighing less than 2.25 kg, compared with birth weights of over 3.0 kg for exomphalos (Moore, 1977).

In the two decades 1970–1989, the incidence of gastroschisis was generally thought to be less than that of omphalocele, with an incidence of 1 in 12 000 live births. Evidence is now accruing that gastroschisis has become more common than omphalocele (Drongowski *et al.*, 1991). Studies in the UK suggest an incidence

for gastroschisis of 1 in 7000 live births, but with marked regional differences (Buick *et al.*, 1995). These regional variations appear to be independent of the rates of termination of pregnancies. In areas where the incidence is high figures of 1 in 5000 occur.

There are no marked differences in gender ratio or birth order, but younger mothers may be more likely to produce affected offspring (Werler *et al.*, 1992). A familial incidence has been described.

ANTENATAL DIAGNOSIS

The advent of maternal ultrasonography has brought the diagnosis of gastroschisis and exomphalos into the antenatal era for the majority of parents (Langer *et al.*, 1993). Raised levels of alpha-fetoprotein in maternal blood of mothers with a gastroschisis may be the first sign of abnormality and the diagnosis is confirmed by an ultrasound examination of the fetus. The absence or presence of the sac is easily demonstrated (Pryde *et al.*, 1994). Antenatal rupture of an exomphalos is extremely rare and thus the diagnosis of a gastroschisis can be made with confidence.

Counselling of the parents is essential. The options are to continue with the pregnancy or to recommend a therapeutic abortion. In gastroschisis the usual recommendation is to proceed to delivery because of the low incidence of other serious congenital defects. In

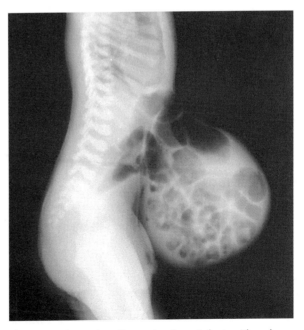

Fig. 18.5 Lateral radiograph of an infant with a large omphalocele. Note the small size of the true abdomen and the small intestine within the sac on a universal mesentery (malrotation).

exomphalos, in particular exomphalos major which has a high incidence of serious congenital anomalies, a therapeutic termination of the pregnancy is the treatment of choice.

In gastroschisis an intestinal atresia is sometimes found and therefore regular ultrasound examination of the fetal intestine is required. In a report dilated intestine was correlated to the likelihood of foetal distress (Langer *et al.*, 1990; Crawford *et al.*, 1992). The risks of prematurity have to be balanced against leaving a fetus *in utero* with dilated intestine (Bond *et al.*, 1988; Langer *et al.*, 1993; Pryde *et al.*, 1994). The extent of intestine that is not protruded before delivery and therefore less affected may be relevant. Unfortunately, ultrasound estimation of the length of extruded intestine is not very accurate.

OBSTETRIC CONSIDERATIONS

It is advisable to transfer the pregnant mother with either an exomphalos or gastroschisis to a department which is adjacent to a regional neonatal surgical unit, although this is debatable (Nicholls *et al.*, 1996). The second consideration is to decide whether the delivery should be normal or whether a caesarean section is required. Finally, it should be decided whether the delivery should be allowed to go to term or be induced as soon as lung maturity has been demonstrated (Swift *et al.*, 1992). Controlled trials to answer these questions are difficult to organize but a substantial amount of data from patients delivered vaginally has been accumulated and their results compare favourably with a comparable series delivered by caesarean section (Bethal *et al.*, 1989). In gastroschisis it is important to give clear instruction to the attending paediatricians on the management of the newborn (Bethal *et al.*, 1989). The paediatric surgical team should always be informed prior to the delivery of a known patient with either gastroschisis or an omphalocele.

Exomphalos: omphalocele

CLINICAL FEATURES

The diagnosis is immediate and visual. The treatment depends on the size of the defect and whether the sac is intact or ruptured (Fig. 18.6 and also Plate 6).

PREOPERATIVE CARE

The care of the patient with a ruptured omphalocele or gastroschisis is similar. The immediate management is to cover the defect with 'clingfilm' or a bowel bag as used by adult surgeons. This prevents the sac and/or exposed intestines from drying out and reduces heat loss. It is important to prevent traction on the mesentery, which tends to flop to one side. This can be pre-

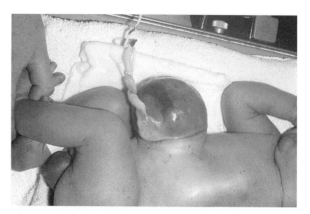

Fig. 18.6 Exomphalos major with an intact sac and the liver as a content of the sac and the umbilical vessels running over the surface of the sac.

vented either by lying the patient on their back with lateral support (sand bags) to prevent the intestine from rolling to the side or by positioning the patient on their side with the intestines lying in front. Any movement of the patient for a technical procedure must be accompanied by the correct positioning of the protruded intestines. Gastric drainage is important and a large 10 Fr. gauge nasogastric tube is passed and aspirated and left on free drainage and regular aspirations. This reduces the risk of an aspiration pneumonia.

Broad-spectrum antibiotics are prescribed to cover organisms expected to be found in the maternal genital tract and an intravenous infusion is established.

OPERATIVE REPAIR

Primary closure

This is the treatment of choice for defects less than 5.0 cm in diameter. The initial superior incision allows scissors to be inserted in the plane between the peritoneum and the amniotic membrane. The peritoneum is opened after completing the circumferential dissection. The umbilical vessels are ligated and the contents of the sac returned to the abdomen (usually only intestine in these small defects). A formal laparotomy is not necessary in defects such as a hernia into the cord. A Meckel's diverticulum with or without a congenital band to the umbilicus is excluded. The repair of the defect is then completed with non-absorbable sutures and skin closure with either subcuticular continuous or interrupted sutures.

Staged repair of exomphalos major

In the past there were two operative approaches to the management of exomphalos major, namely the Gross (1948) operation (Fig. 18.7) and the Grob (1963) technique. The objective was the same in both procedures, i.e. to obtain skin cover over the intact sac of the exomphalos. The main disadvantage of these two techniques was that a large ventral defect containing the liver still remained and a closure at a later date was still necessary. These two procedures have now been replaced by the use of a silastic bag or silo (Schuster, 1967), which has the advantage that a full primary closure of the ventral defect is achieved in the first month of life. A brief description of both of the older procedures now follows.

In the Gross operation the umbilical vessels are ligated as close as possible to the abdominal wall. The skin is then incised in the midline above and below the sac and a circumfertial incision is continued around the defect at the junction of the skin and sac. The skin is then undermined so that flaps can be approximated over the intact omphalocele. Care is taken to avoid mobilizing the skin above the costal margin, which would prevent the later moulding of the liver within the sac. It may be necessary to produce lateral relieving incisions to reduce tension on the midline sutures.

In the Grob technique the growth of skin across the sac of an omphalocele varies from patient to patient. Provided the surface of the sac is sterile the skin will grow circumferentially to cover the omphalocele, thus producing a skin-covered ventral hernia. Antibiotic sprays and 2% mercurocrome (Swift *et al.*, 1992) have been used to keep the surface of the omphalocele sterile. In large omphaloceles it takes 3–4 months for the skin to cover the defect. The use of 2% mercurochrome has been abandoned as mercury poisoning has become a recognized fatal complication.

Repair of gastroschisis

PREOPERATIVE PREPARATION

Gastric drainage, covering the defect to restrain and prevent heat loss, and the use of broad-spectrum antibiotics have already been discussed. In gastroschisis the management of the circulation is vitally important, as these patients lose fluids rapidly through the large exposed surface area of the intestine. A colloid solution is started as soon as possible and the majority of patients will require 20 ml/kg to ensure an adequate circulation as judged by fingernail bed capillary return time.

Care must be taken during induction of anaesthesia to prevent any traction on the prolapsed intestine. The intestine may be supported by using rolled-up towels against the flanks. The patient is paralysed and ventilated using an inhalation anaesthetic with air rather than nitrous oxide. Nitrous oxide tends to distend the intestine, making reduction more difficult.

Intravenous analgesia is also given, particularly at the time of stretching the abdominal wall. Central venous pressure monitoring, as well as monitoring of the ventilation pressure, is helpful.

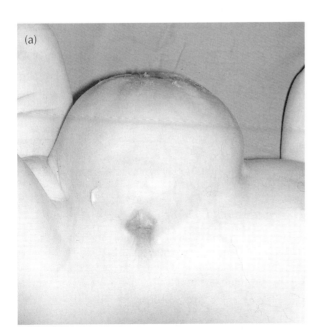
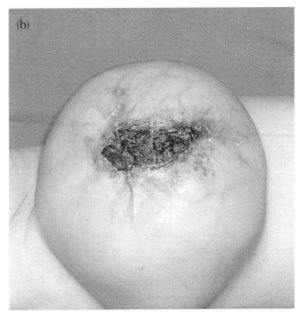

Fig. 18.7 Late stages following a Gross operation. Separation of midline skin suture was treated with mercurochrome. Note the healing lateral relieving incisions and that the primary problem of a large ventrical hernia still requires treatment.

OPERATION

Primary closure

One-stage primary closure may be achieved in up to 50% of patients. The use of postoperative ventilation may be of considerable assistance in primary closure. It is important that the intra-abdominal pressure is not too high, thus avoiding a decrease in venous return to the heart (Philston, 1983).

Two-stage repair

It is essential to exclude an associated intestinal atresia (Thomas and Atwell, 1967, Gornall, 1989, Shah and Woolley, 1991). The defect is small and is extended in the midline up to the xiphisternum. Using fingers under the lateral edges of the defect, the abdominal wall is stretched to increase the capacity of the true abdomen. The intestine is returned to the abdomen and skin closure is achieved. Postoperative ventilatory support may be necessary. The result is a small ventral hernia which can easily be closed by the extraperitoneal Maingot keel operation at a later date (Maingot, 1961).

Silastic bag or Silo

In some patients none of the above procedures will allow closure of the defect. In this situation it is necessary to produce a ventral hernia with a prosthesis fashioned from a sheet of silastic (Schuster, 1967) (Fig.

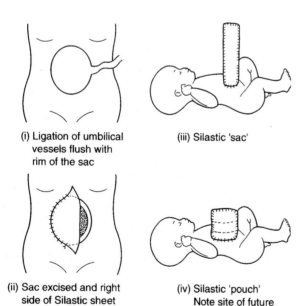

(i) Ligation of umbilical vessels flush with rim of the sac

(ii) Sac excised and right side of Silastic sheet sutured to edge of defect. Left side sutured in a similar manner

(iii) Silastic 'sac'

(iv) Silastic 'pouch' Note site of future line for graded reduction

Fig. 18.8 Staged repair of a gastroschisis or exomphalos using silastic sheet to accompany the intestines and/or the liver.

18.8). A silo may be fashioned without extending the defect, or a bag after extending the defect in the midline. The silastic is sutured with continuous 20 silk, then the two halves are sutured inferiorly and superiorly to accommodate the intestine. The bag or silo is then closed at the upper margin with a continuous suture. No attempt is made to clean the intestine, apart from inspection to exclude an associated atresia.

The capacity of the silastic bag can be reduced every 48–72 hours. The aim is for final closure to be achieved in 2 weeks, thus avoiding the potential hazard of separation of the silastic bag from the skin around the defect.

POSTOPERATIVE CARE

The aims are to prevent respiratory failure, to sustain the neonate with sufficient calories, to maintain electrolyte and fluid homeostasis, and to prevent infection. Assisted ventilation is given as required.

EARLY COMPLICATIONS

Associated anomalies

These have already been discussed, but intestinal atresia may cause a problem.

Prematurity

Patients with gastroschisis have a low birth weight but this is less common with exomphalos. The low birth weight, is probably caused by several factors, such as early delivery, intrauterine growth retardation or a combination of these factors.

Respiratory failure

This may be caused by a high intra-abdominal pressure interfering with diaphragmatic movements. Additional respiratory complications are usually associated with prematurity.

Infection

Broad-spectrum antibiotics are used to reduce the risks of infection.

Gastrointestinal complications

Prolonged ileus is a common complication and is related to the inflammatory changes in the exposed bowel. An intestinal atresia may have been missed at the time of the original closure if the intestines were matted together. An intestinal obstruction due to adhesions may occur at any time, and necrotizing enterocolitis is another possible early postoperative complication (Ein *et al.*, 1988; Oldham *et al.*, 1988; Shanbhogue *et al.*, 1991).

LATE COMPLICATIONS

Growth and development

The outlook for patients with a gastroschisis is excellent for the majority, mainly because of the low incidence of other serious congenital defects.

Ventral hernia

A ventral hernia may result from the closure as either a planned or an unexpected event. Closure is necessary at a late date using the Maingot keel operation with an extraperitoneal approach (Maingot, 1961).

Inguinal hernia

An inguinal hernia may develop, which may be primary and related to either the prematurity or raised intra-abdominal pressure at the time of closure.

Undescended testis

The prolapse of intestines through the defect may interfere with the descent of the testes, resulting in maldescent.

Repair of a secondary ventral hernia

The operation of choice is the Maingot (1961) keel operation with an extraperitoneal approach. The skin over the defect is excised leaving a fibroperitoneal fascial layer intact. Minor holes in this layer are repaired with absorbable sutures. The medial margins and anterior sheath of the rectus abdominis are exposed. The margins of the rectus abdominis are then sutured together with a continuous non-absorbable suture. This suture line is repeated to fold in the rectus to form a 'keel', thus achieving a sound repair. The skin is then closed, leaving a redivac suction drain *in situ*.

By the use of the extraperitoneal approach a postoperative ileus or dilation of the intestine due to handling is avoided.

References

Bernstein, P. 1940: Gastroschisis, a rare teratological condition in the newborn. *Archives of Pediatrics* **57**, 503–5.

Bethal, C.A., Seashore, J.H. and Toulouvian, R.J. 1989: Caesarean section does not improve outcome in gastroschisis. *Journal of Pediatric Surgery* **24**, 1–3.

Bond, S.J., Harrison, M.R., Filley, R.A., Callen, P.W., Anderson, R.A. and Golbus, M.S. 1988: Severity of intestinal damage in gastroschisis: correlation with prenatal sonographic findings. *Journal of Pediatric Surgery* **23**, 520–5.

Buick R.G., Upadhyay, V., Tan, K.H. *et al.* 1995: Is there an epidemic in gastroschisis? Paper presented at the 42nd Annual International Congress. Sheffield: British Association of Paediatric Surgeons.

Cantrell, J.R., Hailer, J.A. and Ravitch, M.M. 1958: A syndrome of congenital defects involving the abdominal wall, sternum, diaphragm, pericardium and heart. *Surgery, Gynaecology and Obstetrics* **107**, 602.

Crawford, R.A., Ryan, G., Wright, V.M. and Rodeck, C.H. 1992: The importance of serial biophysical assessment of fetal well being in gastroschisis. *British Journal of Obstetrics and Gynaecology* **99**, 899–902.

Drongowski, R.A., Smith, R.K. Jr, Coran, A.G. and Klein, M.D. 1991: Contribution of demographic and environmental factors to the etiology of gastroschisis: a hypothesis. *Fetal Diagnosis and Therapy* **6**, 14.

Duhamel, B. 1963: Embryology of exomphalos and allied malformations. *Archives of Disease in Childhood* **38**, 142–7.

Ein, S.H., Superima, R., Bagwell, C. and Wiseman, N. 1988: Ischaemic bowel after primary closure for gastroschisis. *Journal of Pediatric Surgery* **23**, 728–30.

Gornall, P. 1989: Management of intestinal atresia complicating gastroschisis. *Journal of Pediatric Surgery* **24**, 522–4.

Goulet, O.J., Revillon, Y., Jan, D. *et al.* 1991: Neonatal short bowel syndrome. *Journal of Pediatrics* **119**, 18–23.

Grob, M. 1963: Conservative treatment of exomphalos. *Archives of Disease in Childhood* **38**, 148–50.

Gross, R.E. 1948: New method for surgical treatment of large omphalocele. *Surgery* **24**, 277–92.

Kluck, P., Tibboel, D., Van Der Kamp, A.W.H. and Molenaar, J.C. 1983: The effect of fetal urine on the development of the bowel in gastroschisis. *Journal of Pediatric Surgery* **18**, 47–50.

Langer, J.C., Bell, J.G., Castillo, R.O. *et al.* 1989: Etiology of intestinal damage in gastroschisis: I. Effects of amniotic fluid exposure and bowel constriction in fetal lamb model. *Journal of Pediatric Surgery* **24**, 992–4.

Langer, J.C., Bell, J.G., Castillo, R.O. *et al.* 1990: Etiology of intestinal damage in gastroschisis: II. Timing and reversibility of histological changes, mucosal function and contractility. *Journal of Pediatric Surgery* **25**, 1122–6.

Langer, J.C., Khanna, J., Card, C., Dykes, E.H. and Nicolaides, K.H. 1993: Prenatal diagnosis of gastroschisis: development of objective sonographic criteria for predicting outcome. *Obstetrics and Gynaecology* **81**, 53–6.

Maingot, R. 1961: Operations for sliding herniae and for large incisional herniae. *British Journal of Clinical Practice* **15**, 993–6.

Moore, T.C. 1977: Gastroschisis and omphalocele: clinical differences. *Surgery* **82**, 561–8.

Nicholls, G., Upadhyay, V., Gornall, P., Buick, R.G. and Corkery, J.J. 1996: Is specialist centre delivery of gastroschisis beneficial? *Archives of Disease in Childhood* **69**, 71–2.

Oldham, K.T., Coran, A.G., Drongowski, R.A., Baker, P.J., Westley, J.R. and Polley, T.Z. Jr 1988: The development of necrotising enterolocolitis following repair of gastroschisis. A surprisingly high incidence. *Journal of Pediatric Surgery* **23**, 945–9.

Phillips, J.D., Kelly, R.E., Fonkalsrud, E.W., Mirzayan, A. and Kim, C.S. 1991: An improved model of experimental gastroschisis in fetal rabbits. *Journal of Pediatric Surgery* **26**, 784–7.

Philston, H.C. 1983: Gastroschisis: primary fascial closure. The goal for optimum management. *Annals of Surgery* **197**, 160–264.

Pryde, PG., Bardicef, M., Treadwell, M.C., Klein, M., Isada, N.B. and Evans, M.I. 1994: Gastroschisis: can antenatal ultrasound predict infant outcomes? *Obstetrics and Gynaecology* **84**, 505–10.

Rickham, P.P. 1960: Vesico-intestinal fissure. *Archives of Disease in Childhood* **35**, 97–102.

Shah, R. and Woolley, M.M. 1991: Gastroschisis and intestinal atresia. *Journal of Pediatric Surgery* **26**, 788–90.

Shanbhogue, L.K., Tam, P.K. and Lloyd, D.A. 1991: Necrotising enterocolitis following operation in the neonatal period. *British Journal of Surgery* **78**, 1045–7.

Shuster, S.R. 1967: A new method for the staged repair of large omphaloceles. *Surgery, Gynecology and Obstetrics* **125**, 837–50.

Swift, R.I., Singh, M.P., Ziderman, D.A., Silverman, M., Elder, M.A. and Elder M.G. 1992: A new regime in gastroschisis. *Journal of Pediatric Surgery* **27**, 61–3.

Thomas, D.F.M. and Atwell, J.D. 1976: The embryology and the surgical management of gastroschisis. *British Journal of Surgery* **63**, 893–7.

Werler, M.M., Mitchell, A.A. and Shapiro, S. 1992: Demographic, reproductive, medical and environmental factors in relation to gastroschisis. *Teratology* **45**, 353–60.

CHAPTER 19

Congenital diaphragmatic hernia

D.M. BURGE AND M. SAMUEL

Historical
Surgical embryology
Incidence
Pathophysiology
Associated anomalies
Clinical features
Prognosis

Antenatal management
Postnatal management
Surgical repair
Postoperative management
Morgagni hernia
Eventration of the diaphragm
References

Historical

Bonet (1679) described congenital diaphragmatic hernia (CDH) as an incidental finding in a 24-year-old man. Morgagni (1769) described various types of diaphragmatic hernias and the anterior diaphragmatic hernia which bears his name. Bochdalek (1848) described the posterolateral diaphragmatic hernia and in 1853 the clinical features of a congenital diaphragmatic hernia at presentation and the criteria leading to diagnosis were presented by Bowditch. The first successful operation for the closure of a CDH was performed in 1902 (Heidenhain, 1905) and an 18-year follow-up of this patient was reported by Aue in 1920. Gross (1946) reported a successful closure of a Bochdalek diaphragmatic hernia in a 24-hour-old neonate and in 1953 he reported a mortality of eight patients in a series of 63 children, of whom 6 were 24 hours old at surgery. Early diagnosis, appropriate resuscitation and rapid transportation has resulted in neonates reaching surgical centres who previously would have died. This has produced an apparent decrease in overall survival to about 50% in recent years (Fitzgerald, 1977; Puri and Gorman, 1984).

The association of pulmonary hypoplasia and persistent pulmonary hypertension in CDH was appreciated as early as 1819 (Korns, 1921; Campalane and Rowland, 1955). Latterly, the high mortality in CDH has been shown to be due to these factors (Areechon and

Reid, 1963; Murdock et al., 1971; Rowe and Uribe, 1971; Nair et al., 1983). Delayed surgery and preoperative stabilization have been shown to be beneficial and the timing of reduction of the hernia has been shown not to be a critical factor (Cartlidge, 1986; Charlton et al., 1991).

With increasing use of obstetric ultrasound for detection of fetal anomalies, prenatal diagnosis of CDH is now commonplace and fetal surgery is now a possibility (Bell and Ternberg, 1977; Torvar et al., 1979; Harrison et al., 1982; Benacerraf and Adzick, 1987).

Surgical embryology

NORMAL LUNG DEVELOPMENT

Fetal lung development is divided into five time bands, although these overlap. They are the embryonic phase (up to 5 weeks), the pseudoglandular phase (5–16 weeks), the canalicular phase (16–24 weeks), the saccular phase (24–36 weeks) and the alveolar phase (from 36 weeks until 3 years of age). The relative length of these phases varies greatly from species to species, which makes the results of animal experimentation in CDH difficult to transpose to humans.

The laryngotracheal groove arises as a ventral enlargement of the foregut by the third week, and grows caudally to form the primordia for the trachea. The branching pattern of the conducting system of the airway is complete by 16 weeks, but the alveolar buds, destined to produce alveoli, continue to proliferate until 24 weeks. By 25 weeks most of the future gas exchange spaces are still terminal sacs which subsequently divide to produce alveoli, a process that starts at about 28 weeks and has reached the appearance found at term by 34 weeks (Jeffrey *et al.*, 1995). Alveolar numbers continue to increase to term and beyond for some years (Dunhill, 1962). The air-spaces are lined by type 1 pneumocytes by the 26th week. By 22–24 weeks of gestation, type 2 precursor pneumocytes appear and mature into type 2 pneumocytes, destined to produce surfactant, by the 24th week (Pringle and Puri, 1989).

Lung vessel development starts at 28 days and is complete by 20 weeks. Pulmonary arterioles have thick muscular walls. This maintains pulmonary artery pressure at systemic levels in the fetus, a situation that is necessary to encourage preferential flow of oxygenated blood from the placenta through the ductus arteriosus to the rest of the body and not to the lungs. In the normal infant pulmonary vascular resistance drops rapidly after birth although the adult vascular structure is not attained until 2 years of age (Jeffrey *et al.*, 1995).

LUNG DEVELOPMENT IN DIAPHRAGMATIC HERNIA

Lung hypoplasia is more severe on the ipsilateral side, with a reduction in the number of generated bronchi (Areechon and Reid, 1963). The lungs are in the saccular phase of development, with decreased alveoli (Pringle and Puri, 1989) and an increase in the frequency of type 2 pneumocytes. There is an increase in the muscle mass in small pulmonary arteries (Naeye *et al.*, 1976), with evidence that this increase is usually in the peripheral vessels (Bohn *et al.*, 1987). These two features of hypoplasia, alveolar insufficiency and pulmonary vascular maldevelopment, combine to determine the clinical features and outcome in babies with CDH.

NORMAL DEVELOPMENT OF THE DIAPHRAGM

During week 4 of embryonic life the lateral mesenchyme splits caudally to form the pleural canals which communicate with the pericardial cavity cranially and extra-embryonic coelom laterally. The caudal portion of the pericardial sac thickens to form the septum transversum in which the liver develops. At the same time the heart rotates caudally and dorsally to occupy its embryonic position. The septum transversum forms an incomplete ventral partition between the pericardial and peritoneal cavities, leaving spaces laterally, i.e. the pleuroperitoneal canals. The lungs grow into these spaces and then the pleuroperitoneal canals close, separating the lungs from the abdomen and completing the formation of the diaphragm (Kluth *et al.*, 1993).

ABNORMAL DEVELOPMENT OF THE DIAPHRAGM (FIG 19.1)

Agenesis of the diaphragm is the most profound anomaly. It most commonly affects the left hemidiaphragm (80%) and can be bilateral (Jaznosz *et al.*, 1994; Tsang *et al.*, 1995). The most commonly encountered defect occurs posterolaterally (Bochdalek) and is probably due to the failure of closure of the pleuroperitoneal canal. The cause of such defects is unknown, although it has been suggested that hypoplasia of the lung could be the primary abnormality and the diaphragmatic hernia is secondary to this (Iritani, 1984). Lung hypoplasia is more likely due to the progressive compression of the developing lung parenchyma (Harrison *et al.*, 1980). A defect in the septum transversum results in a retrosternal hernia. This may be associated with a lower sternal defect, pericardial defect, cardiac anomalies (ventricular or atrial septal defect, vascular ring and coarctation of the aorta) and epigastric omphalocele comprising the pentalogy of Cantrell (Cantrell *et al.*, 1958). The hernia of Morgagni is located anterolateral on either side at the junction of the septum transversum and costal elements of the diaphragm. The herniated viscera are covered by a sac and usually discovered to the right or left of the midline.

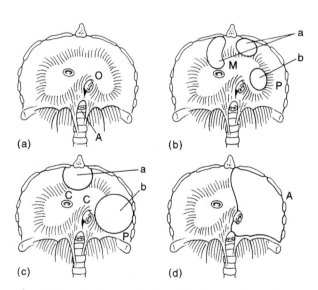

Fig. 19.1 Anatomy of the inferior surface of the diaphragm. (a) Normal diaphragm: I, inferior vena cava; O, oesophageal hiatus; A, aorta. (b) Morgagni hernia defects (M a) with a muscular defect arising from the sternum and ribs; posterolateral defect (P b). (c) Defect found in pentalogy of Cantrell (C a) associated with sternal clefting. Also shown is a large posterolateral defect (P b). (d) Agenesis in the left hemidiaphragm with absence of the aortic and oesophageal crura.

Incidence

The incidence of diaphragmatic hernia varies between 1 in 2200 to 1 in 5000 live births. One series reported an incidence of 1 in 2107 total births (Puri and Gorman, 1957) and demonstrated that the variable incidence previously reported was due in part to many babies never reaching surgical centres before they died. Females are more frequently affected than males (male/female ratio 1:1.8). CDH is considered to be sporadic although familial cases have been reported.

Pathophysiology

In order to understand the clinical features and management of infants with CDH it is necessary to understand how pulmonary hypoplasia affects lung function. As discussed above, the two main features of this hypoplasia are reduced alveolar development and abnormal pulmonary arteriole development. Although the situation is complex it is convenient to consider these two features separately. The development of spaces for gas exchange (alveoli and respiratory bronchioles) may be so severely impaired that it is impossible for the baby to become oxygenated under any circumstances other than by establishing heart–lung bypass [extracorporeal membrane oxygenation (ECMO)] within minutes of birth. Virtually all babies with such severe lung hypoplasia die.

Many babies with CDH will achieve adequate oxygenation with conventional treatment, only to deteriorate after some hours or days. These babies have demonstrated that they have sufficient lung surface area to achieve good gas exchange. In these babies it is the pulmonary arteriolar pathology that causes many of their problems. The vessels have abnormal, increased muscularization of the walls (Fig. 19.2) which means that they have a tendency to constrict. This produces reduced lung perfusion, pulmonary hypertension and shunting of desaturated blood away from the lungs via the foramen ovale, ductus arteriosus and intrapulmonary vessels (right-to-left shunt). This situation is often referred to as persistent fetal circulation (PFC) but is now more commonly termed persistent pulmonary hypertension of the newborn (PPHN). It is made worse by any stimulus that produces increased constriction of the abnormally muscularized, highly reactive arterioles. Such stimuli include pain, stress, hypothermia, acidosis, hypoxia and systemic hypotension. Much of the management of babies with CDH is aimed at minimizing this response. If the baby can be kept alive long enough, this pulmonary vascular reactivity may diminish such that these stimuli no longer produce pulmonary vasoconstriction.

Associated anomalies

Serious associated anomalies were found in 40% of liveborn babies with CDH. In those dying in the first few hours the incidence was 63% compared to only 4% of those who survived for surgery (Sweed and Puri, 1993). Cardiac and neural tube defects were the most common. Trisomy 18 and 13 are associated with CDH and usually result in stillbirth.

Clinical features

PRENATAL DIAGNOSIS

CDH is readily detected on prenatal ultrasound, usually by observing the fluid-filled stomach bubble within the chest. In the absence of this feature CDH may be missed as bowel, collapsed lung and liver have very similar textures on ultrasound. For this reason, right-sided CDH is more difficult to detect. Polyhydramnios is present in 70% of cases, appearing in the second trimester (Adzick *et al.*, 1989), and is probably due to defective fetal swallowing. Differential diagnosis prenatally includes cystic adenomatoid malformation, bronchogenic cyst, lung sequestration, cystic teratoma, neuroblastoma, thymic cyst, neuroenteric cyst and duplication cyst.

Prenatal diagnosis of CDH is a devastating event for the family. It may, however, offer some potential benefits including *in utero* transfer to an obstetric unit linked to a neonatal surgical unit, the option of termination, especially when associated with chromosomal aberration or lethal congenital anomalies, and *in utero* intervention in selected cases. The fetus with CDH should be karyotyped and a detailed search made for associated anomalies, particularly cardiac, as these may influence outcome (Sweed and Puri, 1993).

POSTNATAL DIAGNOSIS

The majority of babies with CDH will present in the first few hours of life with respiratory distress. It is now generally accepted that this symptom is due largely to pulmonary hypoplasia and that its speed of onset and response to treatment are dependent on the severity of that hypoplasia. Whilst it is the presence of the abdominal contents in the chest in fetal life that has led to the lung hypoplasia, the presence of bowel in the chest after birth contributes little to the symptoms.

The clinical features after birth vary with the severity of hypoplasia. Some babies have insufficient lung surface area for adequate gas exchange under any conditions. These babies are severely cyanosed at birth, never become pink and all die. Other babies have enough lung surface area to allow adequate oxygenation to be

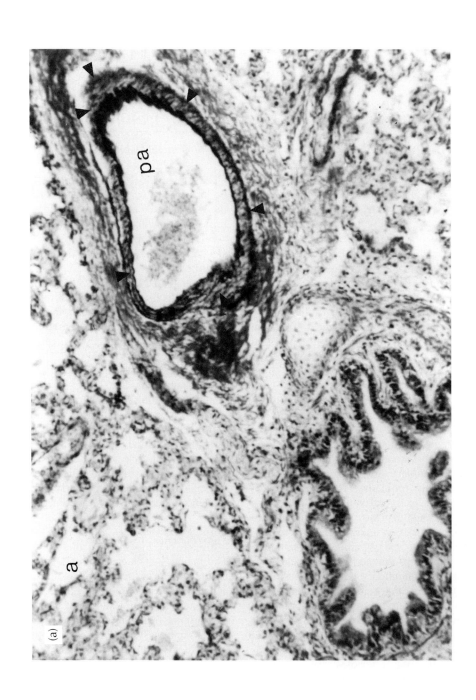

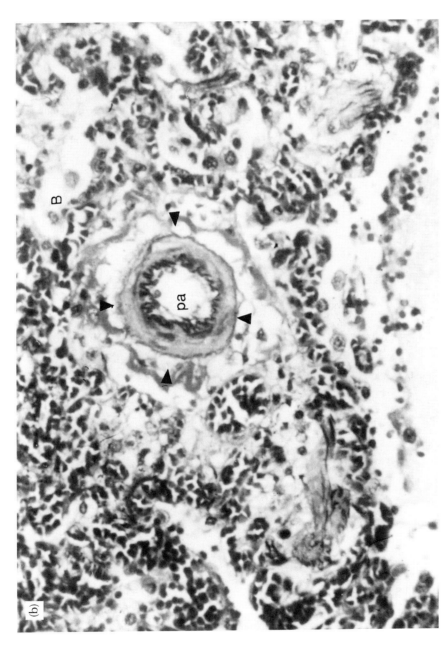

Fig. 19.2 Histopathological comparison of (a) normal lung and (b) hypoplastic lung in CDH. The pulmonary artery wall (pa) is much thicker in the hypoplastic lung. An increase in the type 2 pneumocyte is seen in the hypoplastic lung (B).

achieved, at least for a while, but still have a combination of alveolar and pulmonary vascular maldevelopment that results in a high mortality. Some infants with CDH have near-normal lung development and may present after some days, weeks or months of normal life. Prematurity significantly worsens the outcome for babies with CDH (Puri and Gorman, 1987).

Immediate presentation

Babies presenting within minutes or hours after birth have profound respiratory symptoms. Cyanosis, tachypnoea, sternal and intercostal recession, and increased respiratory effort are the cardinal symptoms. Physical examination reveals mediastinal shift, reduced breath sounds, and occasionally bowel sounds heard on auscultation of the affected side of the hemithorax. There may be an increase in the anteroposterior diameter of the chest. The apical heart beat is displaced to the side opposite the defect. The abdomen is scaphoid and associated congenital anomalies may be present.

Both plain chest and abdominal X-ray should be performed and will demonstrate air-filled loops of bowel in the chest in left-sided CDH and liver, air-filled loops in right-sided CDH, absence of the diaphragmatic margin, mediastinal shift, minimal inflation of the ipsilateral and to a lesser extent the contralateral lung, and paucity of normal intestinal gas pattern in the abdomen (Figs 19.3 and 19.4). In order to make the diagnosis of CDH on plain radiology it is essential to be able to see this abdominal feature and, ideally, a loop of bowel traversing from the abdomen into the chest. The diagnosis should never be made on the basis of a chest X-ray alone. In cases where the abdominal gas pattern looks normal it is likely that the diagnosis is not CDH. The most common condition producing this appearance is congenital cystic adenomatoid malformation of the lung (CCAM). The differential diagnosis also includes staphylococcal pneumonia with pneumatoceles, streptococcal pneumonia, agenesis of the lung, hypoplasia of the lung with an elevated diaphragm and eventration of the diaphragm. A further clue towards the diagnosis of diaphragmatic hernia is the presence of the nasogastric tube in the chest, indicative of an intrathoracic stomach. In some cases a contrast swallow is required to delineate the anatomical position of the misplaced viscera.

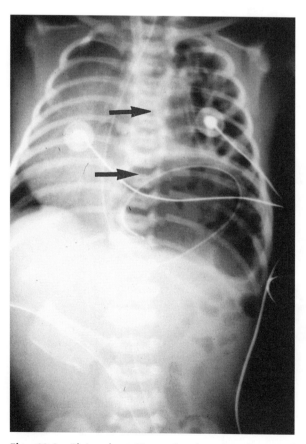

Fig. 19.3 Plain chest X-ray showing the chest and abdomen in an infant with a left-sided Bochdalek hernia. Bowel gas is seen in the left chest (arrows) with a shift of the mediastinum to the right and diminished lung volume. There is paucity of intestinal gas in the abdomen.

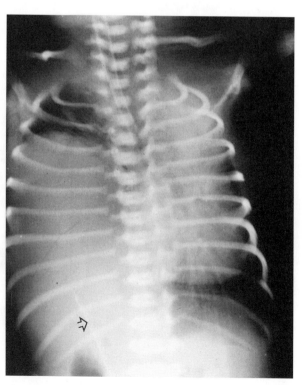

Fig. 19.4 Chest X-ray of an infant with a right-sided CDH. The liver is herniated into the right hemithorax with a shift of the mediastinum to the left. An umbilical venous catheter is seen in the liver (arrow).

Late presentation

In 10–20% of cases diaphragmatic hernia presents beyond the first few hours of life (Malone *et al.*, 1989). In general, late onset of symptoms represents better prognosis and lowered postoperative mortality. Symptoms include chest infections (acute or chronic), anorexia, failure to thrive, vomiting, acute or chronic abdominal pain and diarrhoea. Presentation may also be as an unexpected finding on chest X-ray, or acutely with volvulus and strangulation of the herniated viscera. A previously normal chest X-ray does not exclude a diaphragmatic hernia. It is possible for a small defect to plugged by liver of spleen for months or years before allowing bowel herniation during an episode of increased intra-abdominal pressure, for example during coughing with a respiratory infection. If doubt exists a barium meal is useful in making a conclusive diagnosis.

Right-sided diaphragmatic hernia

Most series in the literature report an incidence of 20% of right-sided posterolateral diaphragmatic hernia. The symptoms may be milder in infants with right-sided diaphragmatic hernia, although a higher mortality has been reported (Towokian and Markowitz, 1984).

Prognosis

The persistent high mortality associated with diaphragmatic hernia in the neonate has led to a search for clinical and laboratory criteria to distinguish between those neonates who have reversible pulmonary hypertension and those who do not, and to predict overall outcome (Norden *et al.*, 1994). Such assessments may also be used to determine at which point more aggressive forms of management (e.g. ECMO) should be instigated.

ANTENATAL PROGNOSTIC FACTORS

Early reports suggested that prenatal diagnosis of CDH before 25 weeks' gestation was, in itself, a predictor of poor outcome with a mortality of 100% (Adzick *et al.*, 1989). More recent studies suggest that, for isolated CDH (i.e. without associated chromosomal or other structural anomalies) mortality may not be any worse than that associated with postnatal diagnosis (Harrison *et al.*, 1994; Wilson *et al.*, 1994b). Ventricular disproportion in the second trimester is associated with 100% mortality while its absence is suggestive of a good prognosis (Crawford *et al.*, 1989). Polyhydramnios has been reported to be associated with poor outcome (Adzick *et al.*, 1989). The lung/thorax transverse ratio may be useful in predicting the degree of lung hypoplasia and postnatal respiratory condition (Hasgauta *et al.*, 1994). Smaller diaphragmatic hernias are associated with a better outcome. Fetal breathing characteristics may also give prognostic information (Badalian *et al.*, 1994). These different factors have recently been reviewed (Fox and Badalian, 1994).

AGE AT PRESENTATION

The later the clinical presentation the more likely it is that pulmonary function will be normal and survival assured. Presentation after 24 hours of age has been shown to be associated with 100% survival (Weiner, 1982). In the authors' institution all babies presenting after 2 hours of age over the last 15 years have survived.

ANATOMY

Survival rates of 93–100% have been reported if the stomach is in the abdomen, compared with <30% if the stomach is in the thorax (Burge *et al.*, 1989) The main value of this information is that babies with an intra-abdominal stomach will survive and this can help in planning postnatal management. Right-sided diaphragmatic hernias have a worse prognosis (Tokowian and Markowitz, 1984).

ASSOCIATED CONGENITAL ANOMALIES

All stillborns with CDH are associated with major congenital anomalies (Sweed and Puri, 1993) and there was a 63% mortality in neonates with CDH prior to surgery, of which 90% had major congenital anomalies.

LABORATORY DATA

Blood gases

Low pH and a high $PaCO_2$ are poor prognostic factors (Boix Ochoa *et al.*, 1974). Patients with low PCO_2, and a normal PO_2 have a good prognosis and respond favourably following ventilation. Measurement of the preductal and postductal arterial PaO_2 can help to predict the degree of right-to-left shunting.

Alveolar–arterial oxygen tension difference (AaDO$_2$) at FiO$_2$ of 1.00

This is calculated by the formula:

$$AaDO_2 = FiO_2 (BP - 47) - PaO_2 - PaCO_2.$$

where BP is barometric pressure. The chances of survival are minimal if the $AaDO_2$ is between 400–500 mmHg and those patients with $AaDO_2$ greater than 500 mmHg will not survive (Harrington *et al.*, 1982).

Ventilatory index (mean airway pressure × ventilatory rate)

The ventilatory index against PCO_2 2 hours prior to and 2 hours postsurgery has been studied in 58 patients.

Infants with a ventilatory index of less than 1000 survived and those with a high ventilatory index had 100% mortality (Bohn and Puri, 1980).

Oxygenation index (OI)

Babies with an OI greater than 0.4 have poor prognosis while an oxygenation ventilation index (OVI) of less than 4 predicts non-survival (Wilson *et al.*, 1991). These indices are calculated by the formulae:

$$OI = MAP \times FiO_2/PaO_2 \times 100$$

$OVI = PO_2/MAP \times$ respiratory rate $\times 100$, where MAP is mean airway pressure. The oxygenation index and the ventilatory index seem to be the most reliable of these tools in predicting mortality.

Pulmonary artery pressure

Echocardiographic measurement of pulmonary artery pressure may be able to indicate when pressures have fallen and surgery is more likely to be tolerated (Haugen *et al.*, 1991).

Antenatal management

Fetal anomaly scanning is now performed routinely at 18–20 weeks' gestation in most obstetric units in the UK. As a result, an increasing proportion of babies with CDH is detected before birth. The management of the baby and its family begins at this point. Paediatric surgeons should be involved in the counselling process as early as possible and should remain involved throughout the pregnancy. Fetal karyotyping is indicated, as is a detailed sonographic search for any other associated anomalies. If a significant chromosomal or structural abnormality is detected then termination of the pregnancy may be the most appropriate advice. If the CDH is an isolated defect the family will need to be fully informed about the mortality risk (60%; Harrison *et al.*, 1994), as well as the likely stressful postnatal course and potential for long-term morbidity if the baby survives. The stress on the family during the rest of the pregnancy and during the postnatal period of intensive care should not be underestimated. In the face of this information some families will still opt for termination for isolated CDH. If the pregnancy continues so should the surgical counselling. Parents can be offered visits to the neonatal surgical unit, contact with other families who have experienced prenatal diagnosis of CDH and accurate answers to questions specific to CDH and its management. Delivery should be planned at a centre with direct access to neonatal surgery to minimize the risks of postnatal transfer. Prenatal surgical repair of CDH is still experimental (Harrison *et al.*, 1990a, b, 1993b; Kamata *et al.*, 1992; Ford, 1994).

A dilemma arises as to the management of a baby with prenatally diagnosed CDH on delivery: should the baby be treated as if PPHN is to be expected, and thus be intubated and subjected to preventive measures, or should the baby be allowed to declare its clinical category and awaited respiratory symptoms? It is the authors' policy to carry out the former as a baby with good lungs will clearly be overventilated with ease and treatment reduced accordingly, whereas if PPHN is allowed to develop it may be hard or impossible to regain control.

Postnatal management

In cases where the CDH has not been detected prenatally preoperative management will largely be determined by the clinical condition of the baby. As described above, symptoms can vary from extreme respiratory embarrassment to mild tachypnoea. In babies with severe symptoms respiratory support will usually precede radiological diagnosis. Once the diagnosis has been made a nasogastric tube should be passed in all cases to facilitate bowel decompression and maximize lung expansion, and intravenous access obtained. Bag and mask ventilation should be avoided as it will increase gastric distention and reduce lung expansion. Subsequent management will be guided by the degree of pulmonary hypoplasia and the resulting clinical effects.

MILD RESPIRATORY SYMPTOMS

If presentation is mild and delayed beyond the first few hours of age outcome is likely to be good (see above). In these patients early surgery, within the first 24 hours or so, is appropriate. Persistent fetal circulation may develop but is usually successfully treated (see below).

SEVERE RESPIRATORY DISTRESS

Many babies present within minutes of birth with cyanosis. Their management can be very complex and should only be undertaken in centres equipped for, and experienced in, the treatment of PPHN. The reader is referred to neonatology texts on the subject. What follows is a brief outline of management methods, which can be considered under four headings.

Maximize existing alveolar function

It is clearly important to ventilate the hypoplastic lungs as efficiently as possible. This may be achieved using standard positive pressure ventilation, although the high pressures and inspired oxygen concentrations required may produce pulmonary barotrauma, interstitial emphysema and pneumothoraces in the short term, or bronchopulmonary dysplasia in the longer term (Bos *et al.*, 1993a). High-frequency oscillation ventilation has been used with some success (Paranka *et al.*, 1995) and has the theoretical advantage that the risk of pneumothorax, which is greater in hypoplastic lungs than in normal lungs, will be reduced. The use of artificial surfactant is gaining popularity. There is evidence that the lamb model of CDH is surfactant deficient (Glick *et al.*, 1992) but there is debate as to whether this is the case in the human (Scheffers *et al.*, 1994; Wilcox *et al.*, 1995). Some animal studies have failed to show any benefit from surfactant administration (Scheffers *et al.*, 1994), although others have shown a short-term benefit (Wilcox *et al.*, 1994). The results of therapeutic trials in humans are awaited.

Minimize stimulation of pulmonary vasoconstriction

As discussed above, many factors such as pain, handling, hypoxia, acidosis, cold and hypotension can induce pulmonary vasoconstriction. To minimize this, the baby is paralysed and sedated, handling should be kept to a minimum and strenuous efforts are made to maintain blood pressure and tissue perfusion. This requires invasive arterial and central venous monitoring. Inotropic support may be required (dobutamine), whilst low-dose dopamine can improve renal perfusion and acid–base balance. Alkalosis and hyperoxia both stabilize the pulmonary vasculature. Thus efforts are made to maintain PaO_2 at about 12.5 kPa and to maintain pH at 7.5 or above. This may be achieved by hypocarbia or alkali infusion. Close monitoring of PaO_2 will identify the development of PPHN and will also allow reduction of support as the baby's condition improves.

Reverse pulmonary vasoconstriction

If the above measures fail to prevent pulmonary vasoconstriction, severe right-to-left shunting will occur at the level of the ductus arteriosus, foramen ovali and intrapulmonary vessels resulting in severe hypoxia. If shunting is predominantly at ductal level, preductal and postductal PaO_2 sampling may be helpful in monitoring its progress and the effects of therapy. Reversal of PPHN can be attempted using vasodilators. Unfortunately, most do not confine their action to the pulmonary circulation but produce systemic hypotension which, in itself, may then worsen pulmonary vasoconstriction. The most commonly used vasodilators have been tolazoline and prostacycline. Whilst both can produce dramatic improvements, the latter seems more specific (Bos *et al.*, 1993b). Other agents such as magnesium sulphate have showed some success (Tolsa *et al.*, 1995) but the most promising pulmonary vasodilator is nitric oxide (Roberts *et al.*, 1992; Kinsella *et al.*, 1992). This inhaled gas has a direct relaxation effect on the pulmonary vasculature as it diffuses from the alveoli through the vessel wall to the blood. Here it is rapidly bound to haemoglobin and becomes inactive so that no systemic dilator effect is produced. Studies have shown both success (Frostell *et al.*, 1993; Kinsella *et al.*, 1993; Hennenberg *et al.*, 1995) and failure (Shah *et al.*, 1994) using nitric oxide, and larger studies are needed. Although it is a cheap and in some ways convenient therapy, its use is accompanied by significant risk to both the baby (methaemoglobinaemia, toxicity of metabolites, rebound pulmonary hypotension on withdrawal) and to staff (possible toxic effects of the gas and its metabolites nitrogen dioxide and nitric acid). Great care must be exercised in its use (Miller *et al.*, 1994).

Buying time for pulmonary vascular maturation

Most of the major problems encountered in the management of CDH are related to the pulmonary vascular abnormalities described above. These are known to improve with time. If the baby can be kept alive while this maturation process occurs then survival should improve. Two main techniques have evolved which allow this to happen to some extent. These are ECMO and delayed surgery.

Delayed surgery

Against the background of medical management, an operation is required at some point to repair the diaphragmatic defect. Clearly, the baby will not be able to breathe well without positive pressure support in the presence of paradoxical movement of the bowel in and out of the chest with each breath. The optimal timing of the operation is still debated.

Until the early 1980s immediate surgical repair of the diaphragm was thought to be mandatory. It is now generally accepted that this is inappropriate (Cartlidge *et al.*, 1986; Langer *et al.*, 1988a; Charlton *et al.*, 1991; Goh *et al.*, 1992) and, although there has never been a prospective randomized trial of sufficient size to prove it, most surgeons feel that a period of preoperative stabilization does no harm and probably confers benefit. The optimal duration of this period has not been defined. The main reasons for considering delaying surgery are as follows:

1. General: it would seem obvious that a few hours' stabilization of the baby's general condition (temperature, circulation, ventilation) to obtain optimal conditions for anaesthesia and surgery is sensible. Indeed, the baby's intensive care requirements will often diminish over this time.
2. Pulmonary vascular changes: the sensitivity of the abnormal pulmonary vasculature in CDH eventually diminishes. It would seem reasonable to delay the insult of surgery until this has happened. However, it

is not known how long this may take although there is post-mortem evidence that this may take 3 weeks or more (Beals *et al.*, 1992). This time may vary according to the severity of pulmonary hypoplasia.

3. Lung compliance: the anatomical changes that result from surgery may cause a deterioration in lung function via worsening lung compliance (Moulton *et al.*, 1991; Nakayama *et al.*, 1991). Repair of the hernia leaves a virtually empty hemithorax which cannot be filled by the hypoplastic ipsilateral lung. As the extrapulmonary air resorbs, the mediastinum is shifted towards the side of the repair, producing overexpansion of the contralateral lung which is providing most of the pulmonary function. With increasing overexpansion ventilation deteriorates. This phenomenon takes some hours to happen and may explain the 'honeymoon' effect often seen in CDH patients where lung function deteriorates after an initial stable postoperative period. One rationale for delaying surgery is to defer this process to a time when the pulmonary vasculature may be able to withstand the insult. Various manoeuvres have been tried to avert this process, such as inflating balloons in the ipsilateral thoracic cavity, but have not generally been successful.

Uncontrolled reports indicate improved survival if surgery is delayed for some days (Roberts *et al.*, 1994). One prospective randomized study has shown no benefit of prolonged stabilization (>96 hours) over early surgery (<6 hours of age) (Nio *et al.*, 1994). It is the authors' practice to allow all CDH babies a period of stabilization before surgery. If the clinical presentation has been one of respiratory symptoms after the age of 2 hours then survival is to be expected and PPHN absent or mild. Surgery can be undertaken early (within the first 2 days) and a good outcome expected. If the presentation has been early by antenatal diagnosis or respiratory distress under 2 hours of age, more prolonged medical management of PPHN is undertaken as above, with surgery being performed once the baby is in 40% FiO$_2$ or less. This protocol results in some babies dying without surgery, but they would have died anyway.

ECMO

This technique was developed from a modification of heart–lung bypass techniques used during cardiac surgery (Bartlett *et al.*, 1982). By cannulating the great vessels blood is diverted to a gas-exchange mechanism outside the body and then returned to the circulation. In this way the inability of the blood to reach the alveoli in PPHN can be circumvented. Since the early 1980s the technique has become increasingly refined and it is now used routinely in the management of CDH in the USA. However, it has been slow to become accepted in the UK and parts of Europe. One reason for this is the lack of any reliable data to demonstrate improved survival

with its use. No properly controlled prospective trials of ECMO have been produced from the USA. A recent randomized multicentre trial of ECMO in PPHN due to various conditions carried out in the UK demonstrated its benefit in PPHN in general but no benefit was demonstrated for ECMO in the management of CDH. Of 18 infants randomized to receive ECMO 14 died, compared with 17 deaths amongst the 17 infants who received conventional management (UK Collaborative ECMO Trial Group, 1996).

Even supporters of ECMO agree that it is less helpful in CDH than in other causes of PPHN such as meconium aspiration of hyaline membrane disease. This is probably because in these other conditions the disease process is producing PPHN by an effect on normal pulmonary arterioles that will recover once the underlying process has reversed. In CDH the arterioles are themselves abnormal and the process of them becoming normal may take weeks to occur, beyond the time that ECMO can be continued (Beals *et al.*, 1992).

A detailed description of the technique of ECMO is beyond the scope of this text but the basic principles will be discussed. Access to the circulation is either venoarterial (VA) or venovenous (VV). The former technique has been the most commonly used as it supports cardiac as well as lung function but the VV route offers some advantages (Heiss *et al.*, 1995), particularly preservation of the carotid artery. VA ECMO requires cannulation of the internal carotid artery and internal jugular vein. Unless heparin-bonded tubing is used the patient will need to be anticoagulated. Paralysis is discontinued and the lungs kept gently ventilated at about 10 breaths per minute with low pressure. The clinical response is often dramatic and the baby can change from being moribund to looking normal within hours. Surgery can be undertaken with the baby on ECMO (Wilson *et al.*, 1994a) or ECMO can be discontinued first (Adolph *et al.*, 1995), which may reduce the risk of haemorrhage (Vazquez and Cheu, 1994).

The selection of patients for ECMO is usually based on clinical and laboratory data. Most authors believe that patients should not be considered for ECMO if pulmonary hypoplasia is so severe that survival off ECMO will be impossible. Babies who fit into this category are those that never achieve adequate oxygenation with standard measures postnatally. However, some authors suggest that such infants should not be excluded (Newman *et al.*, 1990). It is generally accepted that babies who are very preterm or have existing intraventricular haemorrhage should not be offered ECMO because of the risks associated with anticoagulation.

Various indications for commencing ECMO in CDH have been suggested and include failure to respond to conventional treatment, AaDO$_2$ > 600 mmHg for 8 hours, OI > 40 for 3 hours, acute deterioration (pH < 7.15 and/or PaO$_2$ < 40 mmHg for 2 hours) and evidence of pulmonary damage from barotrauma. There are no absolute values for initiating ECMO and in many centres babies are being started on ECMO earlier and earlier in their management in an attempt to improve outcome. As 'conventional' methods of treatment continue to develop (e.g. nitric oxide; see above) it is possible that the need for ECMO may diminish.

Complications arising from ECMO may occur acutely as a result of mechanical problems such as vascular catheter dislodgment, or haemorrhage resulting from anticoagulation. The latter may be at the site of surgery or, more seriously, within the brain (Goodwin *et al.*, 1995). Other complications may be more long term, such as hemiplegia from ligation of the carotid artery. This complication may be reduced by reconstructive carotid surgery (Moulton *et al.*, 1991). Survivors of ECMO may be more at risk from chronic lung disease and many other complications have been reported (Nakayama *et al.*, 1991).

Surgical repair

Surgery should be undertaken as a planned procedure when that baby's condition is felt suitable (see above). Emergency surgery may be required for gastric perforation (usually due to injudicious face-mask ventilation prior to intubation) or volvulus of the intrathoracic bowel. This complication may be difficult to diagnose but should be suspected in a baby with persistent metabolic acidosis and bloody nasogastric aspirate.

The surgical technique of the repair of a CDH is diagrammatically presented in Fig. 19.5. An abdominal approach is preferred as it offers adequate exposure, ease of reduction of abdominal contents, correction of associated gastrointestinal abnormalities, when required, and ease of access to the anterior and posterior lips of the diaphragm. Although abnormal bowel position is inherent in all babies with CDH, malrotation with its serious predisposition to midgut volvulus is not often present. If the root of the bowel mesentery is narrow, predisposing to volvulus, then attempts should be made to widen it as with Ladd's procedure.

The recommended incision is a subcostal transverse muscle cutting incision. Gentle retraction of the abdominal contents will reveal the diaphragmatic defect. Reduction of the hernial contents must be done with care. If the defect is small it may be difficult to remove all the herniated viscera (e.g. the spleen) from the chest. The thoracic cavity is then inspected for evidence of a hernial sac, which is present in 20% of cases. This should be excised. The margins of the defect should then be defined. In most cases a good anterior leaf of diaphragm is present and in some the posterior rim is also obvious. In some cases there can appear to be no posterior component but in many of these a muscle rim is detected after incision over the posterior peritoneum or by dissection lateral to the ipsilateral diaphragmatic

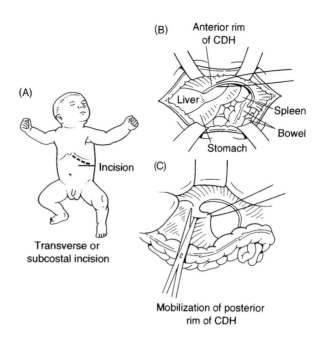

Fig. 19.5 Diagrammatic representation of the surgical repair of CDH. (A) The diaphragm is approached by a transverse incision in the left hypochondrium. (B) The posterolateral defect usually has a definite anterior leaflet. (C) The posterior rim is mobilized by incising the peritoneum at the base of the left diaphragmatic crus.

crus. The anterior and posterior rims are approximated using interrupted non-absorbable sutures. If the posterior rim is absent or, as is often the case, deficient laterally, the anterior rim can be approximated to the chest wall.

In some cases, particularly those with the most severe lung problems, the defect may be very large, with occasionally complete absence of the hemidiaphragm. In these cases, the defect can be repaired using synthetic material such as reinforced silastic, Gortex or Marlex mesh (Fig 19.6). Various muscle flap techniques have also been described (Bianchi *et al.*, 1983).

The use of chest drains is controversial. The authors do not use them unless a pulmonary air leak is present, on the basis that it will promote rapid withdrawal of air from the void around the small ipsilateral, lung resulting in overexpansion of the contralateral lung, and worsening lung compliance. The abdomen can usually be closed without tension but, if this is not possible, skin closure alone or prosthetic patch closure may be needed.

Postoperative management

All patients require standard monitoring of postoperative vital signs as for any neonatal surgical procedure.

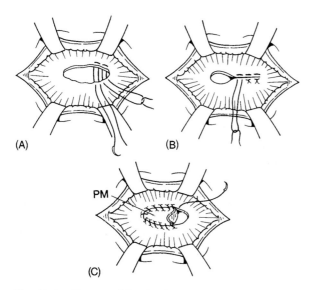

Fig. 19.6 Closure of the diaphragmatic defect. (A and B) Non-absorbable mattress sutures are used for approximation of the anteroir and posterior rim. (C) A prosthetic material (PM) is being used to facilitate closure of a large defect.

Babies who had PPHN before or at the time of surgery are likely to develop further signs of this after surgery and may deteriorate from their preoperative state despite having been quite stable prior to surgery. Some babies who did not exhibit PPHN before surgery will develop it afterwards. Therefore all these babies must be managed with great diligence.

Pneumothorax is a potential danger in these infants as hypoplastic lungs are more likely to leak than normal ones. Sudden deterioration in oxygenation status should raise the suspicion of a pneumothorax, but chest radiographs must be interpreted by someone experienced with the management of CDH prior to insertion of a chest drain. This is because the usual chest X-ray appearance after surgery in CDH can mimic a tension pneumothorax with mediastinal displacement (owing to inability of the mediastinum to centralize because of the hypoplastic contralateral lung), free air in the chest (operating theatre air filling the void around the small ipsilateral lung) and the flattened diaphragm (due to tension in the repair). If doubt exists, an intravenous cannula attached to underwater seal can be inserted to identify air under pressure.

Many other postoperative problems may arise, including pneumonia, pleural effusions, chylothorax, gross oedema from prolonged paralysis, intestinal stress ulceration, side-effects of vasodilators and renal failure. The baby with CDH and PPHN is one of the most challenging situations in neonatal intensive care.

RESULTS

Mortality figures for CDH need to be interpreted in the light of many different factors. Overall mortality figures will vary according to the proportion of high-risk patients (those presenting under 6 hours of age), the proportion with associated serious anomalies, the proportion antenatally diagnosed, and the proportion who die at referral centres before transfer can be arranged. These factors explain why mortality figures differ considerably from one report to another. In the absence of randomized trials it is difficult to determine what treatment modalities are of benefit.

Overall, the mortality for CDH is about 50%. The mortality for babies diagnosed antenatally was initially reported at 85% or more (Adzick *et al.*, 1989; Sharland *et al.*, 1992), but a more recent report has shown that for isolated CDH detected before 24 weeks gestation the mortality is 58% (Harrison *et al.*, 1994).

The influence of ECMO on mortality is hard to define. Most reports indicate improved survival compared with historical controls (Breaux *et al.*, 1992; West *et al.*, 1992) whereas other reports indicate no difference (O'Rourke *et al.*, 1991). With the advent of new pulmonary vasodilators and ventilation techniques it is likely that the question will remain unanswered.

The long-term outlook for survivors with CDH has, in the past, thought to be excellent. Respiratory function is reported as being clinically normal, although measurable changes in lung function can be detected (Frenckner and Freyschuss, 1988). However, by virtue of the fact that long-term studies will have been looking at the survivors from CDH who were treated many years ago, at a time when babies who survive now would have died, the long-term outlook for babies with high-risk CDH is likely to be different. Chronic lung disease has been reported after treatment for CDH (Bos *et al.*, 1993a) and in 60% of patients discharged after ECMO for CDH (D'Agnostino *et al.*, 1995). Other long-term problems are now being reported after ECMO (Lund *et al.*, 1994), including developmental delay, hemiplegia, fits, hearing and visual impairment, and thoracic cage deformities. Gastro-oesophageal reflux is well reported and seems to be becoming an increasing problem (Koot *et al.*, 1993; Nagaya *et al.*, 1994; Sigalet *et al.*, 1994). In a review of 60 adult survivors of CDH at a mean age of 30 years, symptoms of reflux were found in 60% (Vanamo *et al.*, 1996). In those having a barium meal, 73% had a hiatus hernia and 13% had biopsy evidence of Barrett's oesophagus. Considering that these were survivors from 30 years ago, the risks to today's survivors will be higher.

THE FUTURE

Given the poor results of conventional management and ECMO for high-risk CDH and the uniform fatality in babies with severe lung hypoplasia, a search is still being carried out for new treatment options. Fetal surgery has been undertaken, with successful repair of the diaphragm but a high mortality associated with premature labour (Harrison *et al.*, 1990a, 1993a; Jennings *et al.*, 1993) and is still being evaluated. Lung transplantation is an attractive option (Van Meurs *et al.*, 1994) Experimental studies suggest that temporary tracheal obstruction *in utero* may improve lung development (Di Fiore *et al.*, 1994; Hedrick *et al.*, 1994).

Morgagni hernia

A Morgagni hernia is a small defect in the anterior part of the sternal or the costal part of the diaphragm (Fig. 19.1). These hernias are associated with a hernial sac, a small hiatus traversed by the epigastric or internal mammary vessels, and may be on one or both sides of the diaphragm. They may remain asymptomatic for many years and are usually diagnosed on a chest X-ray taken as a result of chronic non-specific symptoms such as coughing, choking, vomiting and epigastric distress. Congenital heart defects and trisomy 21 are associated with Morgagni hernias. The defect is more often to the right and herniation of the liver, small bowel, colon, spleen and stomach are known to occur. Transabdominal repair is the preferred approach. In unusually large defects, the posterior edge of the diaphragmatic defect may be close to the phrenic nerve, favouring a thoracic approach to avoid injury to the phrenic nerve at the time of repair.

Eventration of the diaphragm

The term eventration implies that the diaphragm is present but that the muscle within it has either never formed (congenital eventration) or atrophied as a result of phrenic nerve damage (acquired eventration). Both sides of the diaphragm may be affected, although it is more common for one hemidiaphragm, usually the left, or its anterior or posterior leaf, to be affected. It has been detected in 4% of 2500 neonatal chest X-rays, although only three of these infants were symptomatic (Beck and Motsay, 1952).

Congenital eventration is not common and may be associated with various congenital malformations which may themselves have an influence on outcome (Wayne *et al.*, 1974). Bilateral congenital eventration has been reported (Elberg *et al.*, 1989) and has been detected on prenatal ultrasound (Hasegawa *et al.*, 1994).

Acquired eventration may result from birth trauma, usually from excessive stretching of the neck and the shoulder during difficult vaginal delivery, when it may be associated with brachial plexus palsy or Erb's or Klumpke's palsy. However, the most common cause is phrenic nerve injury during thoracic surgery.

PRESENTATION

The lack of diaphragmatic contraction during respiration results in paradoxical movement of the diaphragm, which will thus move up on inspiration and down on expiration. As the mediastinum in infants is very mobile, and as infants rely heavily on the abdominal phase of ventilation, the effect is to reduce lung expansion and ventilation.

Congenital eventration may result in severe pulmonary hypoplasia as in CDH and thus may be fatal. Some infants are dependent on ventilators, some have mild respiratory symptoms, some have symptoms only with respiratory infections and some remain asymptomatic. Apart from respiratory symptoms, eventration may present with abdominal pain and vomiting due to the well-recognized complication of left-sided eventration, gastric volvulus (Del Rossi *et al.*, 1993).

DIAGNOSIS

The diagnosis of eventration is made by a combination of plain radiology and ultrasound screening of the diaphragm. The diaphragm appears elevated on chest X-ray. A lateral view will identify whether the eventration is affecting the complete hemidiaphragm or only the anterior of posterior leaf. Ultrasound screening will confirm that the diaphragm is moving paradoxically and should be able to confirm, by attention to the thickness of the diaphragm, that eventration is present rather than CDH with a hernial sac.

TREATMENT AND RESULTS

Although the surgical treatment for eventration is simple, there is some controversy as to which patients require surgery and when. Patients in whom the condition is detected on incidental chest X-ray and who do not have symptoms will require no treatment. Many patients have the X-ray performed because of mild respiratory symptoms that may be transient and resolve without treatment of the eventration (Wayne *et al.*, 1974). In some patients it has been suggested that the paradoxical diaphragmatic movement predisposes to atelectasis and recurrent chest infections (Beck and Motsay, 1952). One commentator has reported that individuals who are asymptomatic for years can have a profound reaction to an otherwise potentially mild respiratory illness and therefore all eventrations should be treated (Pilling, 1974).

When the eventration is acquired as a result of surgical or birth trauma, there is a potential for complete recovery over a few weeks. In one report, 84% of infants with eventration after cardiac surgery recovered without complication (Watanabe *et al.*, 1987). Most authors advise respiratory support for 2–4 weeks. If, after this time the support cannot be weaned, the diaphragm should be plicated (Haller *et al.*, 1974; Watanabe *et al.*, 1987; Langer *et al.*, 1988). If the phrenic nerve is known to have been divided, early plication would seem prudent (Langer *et al.*, 1988).

Surgical treatment is by plication of the diaphragm. Whilst this can be undertaken from below via the abdomen, particularly on the left side, a thoracic approach is usually preferred. This enables accurate identification of the phrenic nerve so that it can be avoided in the plication is case function returns. The dome of the diaphragm is pushed down and plication performed using interrupted non-absorbable sutures so as to produce a flat diaphragm that can no longer move paradoxically.

Results of surgery are good if the underlying lung is normal and no other anomalies exist (Kizilcan *et al.*, 1993). However, congenital eventration may be associated with lung hypoplasia or various severe anomalies and chromosomal abnormalities and children with acquired eventration have often had surgery for congenital heart disease. This accounts for some authors reporting a high mortality after plication (Smith *et al.*, 1986).

References

Adolph, V., Flageole, H., Perreault, T. *et al.* 1995: Repair of congenital diaphragmatic hernia after weaning from extracorporeal membrane oxygenation. *Journal of Pediatric Surgery* 1995; **30**, 349–52.

Adzick, N.S., Vacanti, J.P., Lillehei, C.W., O'Rourke, P.P., Crone, R.K. and Wilson, J.M. 1989: Fetal diaphragmatic hernia: ultrasound diagnosis and clinical outcome in 38 cases. *Journal of Pediatric Surgery* **24**, 654–7.

Areechon, W. and Reid, L. 1963: Hypoplasia of the lung with congenital diaphragmatic hernia. *British Medical Journal* **1**, 230–3.

Aue, O. 1920: Uber angeborene zwerchfel hemien. *Deutsche Zeitschrift für Chirurgie* **108**, 14.

Badalian, S.S., Fox, H.E., Chao, C.R., Timor-Tritsch, I.E. and Stolar, C.J. 1994: Fetal breathing characteristics and post-natal outcome in cases of congenital diaphragmatic hernia. *American Journal of Obstetrics and Gynecology* **171**, 970–8.

Bartlett, R.H., Andrews, A.F., Toomasian, J.M., Haiduc, N.J. and Gazzangia, A.B. 1982: Extracorporeal membrane oxygenation of newborn respiratory failure. *Surgery* **92**, 425–33.

Beals, D.A., Schloo, B.L., Vacanti, J.P., Reid, L.M. and Wilson, J.M. 1992: Pulmonary growth and remodeling in infants with high-risk congenital diaphragmatic hernia. *Journal of Pediatric Surgery* **27**, 997–1002.

Beck, W.C. and Motsay, D.S. Eventration of the diaphragm. *Archives of Surgery* 1952; **65**, 557–63.

Bell, M.J. and Ternberg J.L. 1977: Antenatal diagnosis of diaphragmatic hernia. *Pediatrics* **60**, 738–40.

Benacerraf, B.R. and Adzick, N.S. 1987: Fetal diaphragmatic hernia: ultrasound diagnosis and clinical outcome in 19 cases. *American Journal of Obstetrics and Gynecology* **156**, 573–6.

Bianchi, A., Doig, C.M. and Cohen, S.J. 1983: The reverse latissimus dorsi flap for congenital diaphragmatic hernia repair. *Journal of Pediatric Surgery* **18**, 560–3.

Bochdalek, V.A. 1848: Eininge Betrachtungen uber die Entstehung des angeborenen Zwerchfellbruches, Als Beitrag zur pathologischen Anatomie der Hemien. *Vierteljahrsschrift Prakt Heilkunf* **3**, 89.

Bohn, D., Tamura, M., Perrin, D., Barker, G. and Rabinovitch, M. 1987: Ventilatory predictors of pulmonary hypoplasia in congenital diaphragmatic hernia, confirmed by morphologic assessment. *Journal of Pediatrics* **111**, 423–31.

Bohn, D.J. and Puri, P. (eds) 1989: Congenital diaphragmatic hernia. In *Ventilatory management of blood gas changes in congenital diaphragmatic hernia.* Basel: Karger, 76–89.

Boix Ochoa, J., Peguero, G., Seijo, G., Natal, A. and Canals, J. 1972: Acid base balance and blood gases in prognosis and therapy of congenital diaphragmatic hernia. *Journal of Pediatric Surgery* **9**, 49–57.

Bonet, T. 1697: De suffocatione. Observatio XLI. Suffocatio excitata a tenuium intestorum vulnus diaphragmatis, in thoracem ingrestu. Selpulchretum sive anatomia proctela et cadaveribus morbo denatus. Geneva.

Bos, A.P., Hussain, S.M., Hazebroek, F.W., Tibboel, D., Meradji, M. and Molenaar, J.C. 1993a: Radiographic evidence of bronchopulmonary dysplasia in high-risk congenital diaphragmatic hernia survivors. *Pediatric Pulmonology* **15**, 231-4.

Bos, A.P., Tibboel, D., Koot, V.C., Hazebroek, F.W. and Molenaar, J.C. 1993b: Persistent pulmonary hypertension in high-risk congenital diaphragmatic hernia patients: incidence and vasodilator therapy. *Journal of Pediatric Surgery* **28**, 1463–5.

Bowditch, H.I. 1853: Peculiar care of diaphragmatic hernia. *Buffalo Medical Journal* **9**, 85–95.

Breaux, C.W., Jr., Rouse, T.M., Cain, W.S. and Georgeson, K.E. 1992: Congenital diaphragmatic hernia in an era of delayed repair after medical and/or extracorporeal membrane oxygenation stabilization: a prognostic and management classification. *Journal of Pediatric Surgery* **27**, 1192–8.

Burge, D.M., Atwell, J.D. and Freeman, N.V. 1989: Could the stomach site help predict outcome in babies with left sided congenital diaphragmatic hernia diagnosed antenatally? *Journal of Pediatric Surgery* **24**, 567–9.

Campalane, R.P. and Rowland, R.H. 1955: Hypoplasia of the lung associated with congenital diaphragmatic hernia. *Annals of Surgery* **142**, 178–89.

Cantrell, J.R., Haller, J.A. and Ravitch, M.M. 1958: A syndrome of congenital defects involving the abdominal wall, sternum, diaphragm, pericardium and heart. *Surgery, Gynecology and Obstetrics* **107**, 602–14.

Cartlidge, P.H. 1986: Preoperative stabilisation in CDH. *Archives of Diseases in Childhood* 1986; **61**, 1226.

Cartlidge, P.H.T., Mann, N.P. and Kapila, L. 1986: Preoperative stabilisation in congenital diaphragmatic hernia. *Archives of Disease in Childhood* **61**, 1226–8.

Charlton, A.J., Bruce, J. and Davenport, M. 1991: Timing of surgery in congenital diaphragmatic hernia. Low mortality after pre-operative stabilisation. *Anaesthesia* **48**, 820–3.

Crawford, D.C., Wright, V.M., Drake, D.P. and Allan LD. 1989: Fetal diaphragmatic hernia: the value of fetal echocardiography in the prediction of postnatal outcome. *British Journal of Obstetrics and Gynaecology* **98**, 705–10.

D'Agostino, J.A., Bernbaum, J.C., Gerdes, M. *et al.* 1995: Outcome for infants with congenital diaphragmatic hernia requiring extracorporeal membrane oxygenation: the first year. *Journal of Pediatric Surgery* **30**, 10–15.

Del Rossi, C., Cerasoli, G., Tosi, C., De Chiara, F. and Ghinelli C. 1993: Intrathoracic gastric volvulus in an infant. *Paediatric Surgery International* **8**, 146–8.

DiFiore, J.W., Fauza, D.O., Slavin, R., Peters, C.A., Fackler, J.C. and Wilson, J.M. 1994: Experimental fetal tracheal ligation reverses the structural and physiological effects of pulmonary hypoplasia in congenital diaphragmatic hernia. *Journal of Pediatric Surgery* **29**, 248–56; Discussion 256.

Dunhill, M.S. 1962: Postnatal growth of the lung. *Thorax* **17**, 329–33.

Elberg, J.J., Brok, K.E., Pedersen, S.A. and Kock, K.E. 1989: Congenital bilateral eventration of the diaphragm in a pair of male twins. *Journal of Pediatric Surgery* **24**, 1140–1.

Fitzgerald, R.J. 1977: Congenital diaphragmatic hernia: a study of mortality factors. *Irish Journal of Medical Science* **148**, 280–4.

Ford, W.D. 1994: Fetal intervention for congenital diaphragmatic hernia. *Fetal Diagnosis and Therapy* **9**, 398–408.

Fox, H.E. and Badalian, S.S. 1994: Ultrasound prediction of fetal pulmonary hypoplasia in pregnancies complicated by oligohydramnios and in cases of congenital diaphragmatic hernia: a review. *American Journal of Perinatology* **11**, 104–8.

Frenckner, B. and Freyschuss, U. 1988: Pulmonary function after repair of congenital diaphragmatic hernia – a short review. *Paediatric Surgery International* **3**, 11–14.

Frostell, C.G., Lonnqvist, P.A., Sonesson, S.E., Gustafsson, L.E., Lohr, G. and Noack, G. 1993: Near fatal pulmonary hypertension after surgical repair of congenital diaphragmatic hernia: successful use of inhaled nitric oxide. *Anaesthesia* **48**, 679–83.

Glick, P.L., Stannard, V.A., Leach, C.L. *et al.* 1992: Pathophysiology of congenital diaphragmatic hernia II: the fetal lamb CDH model is surfactant deficient. *Journal of Pediatric Surgery* **27**, 382–7.

Goh, D.W., Drake, D.P., Brereton, R.J., Kiely, E.M. and Spitz, L. 1992: Delayed surgery for congenital diaphragmatic hernia. *British Journal of Surgery* **79**, 644–6.

Goodwin, D.A., Lally, K.P., Clark, R.H. and Null, D.M.J. 1995: Factors asociated with the development of intracranial haemorrhage in patients treated with extracorporeal membrane oxygenation. *Paediatric Surgery International* **10**, 229–32.

Gross, R.E. 1948: Congenital hernia of the diaphragm. *American Journal of Disease in Children* **71**, 579.

Gross, R.E. 1953: *Surgery in infancy and childhood.* Philadelphia, PA: W.B. Saunders.

Haller, J.A., Richards, L.R., Tepas, J.J., Rogers, M.C., Robotham, J.L., Shorter, N. and Shermeta, D.W. 1974: Management of diaphragmatic paralysis in infants with special emphasis on selection of patients for operative plication. *Journal of Pediatric Surgery* **14**, 779–85.

Harrington, J., Raphaely, R.C. and Downes, J.J. 1982: Relationship of alveolar–arterial oxygen tension difference in diaphragmatic hernia of the newborn. *Anesthesiology* 1982; **58**, 473–6.

Harrison, M.R., Adzick, N.S., Flake, A.W. and Jennings, R.W. 1993a: The CDH two-step: a dance of necessity [Review]. *Journal of Pediatric Surgery* **28**, 813–16.

Harrison, M.R., Adzick, N.S., Estes, J.M. and Howell, L.J. 1994: A prospective study of the outcome for fetuses with diaphragmatic hernia. *Journal of the American Medical Association* **271**, 382–4.

Harrison, M.R., Adzick, N.S., Flake, A.W. *et al.* 1993b: Correction of congenital diaphragmatic hernia *in utero*: VI. Hard-earned lessons. *Journal of Pediatric Surgery* **28**, 1411–17; discussion 1417.

Harrison, M.R., Adzick, N.S., Longaker, M.T. *et al.* 1990a: Successful repair *in utero* of a fetal diaphragmatic hernia after removal of herniated viscera from the left thorax. *New England Journal of Medicine* **322**, 1582–4.

Harrison, M.R., Filly, R.A. and Golbus, M.S. 1982: Fetal treatment. *New England Journal of Medicine* **307**, 1651–2.

Harrison, M.R., Jester, J.A. and Ross, N.A. 1980: Correction of congenital diaphragmatic hernia *in utero* I. The model: intrathoracic balloon produces fetal pulmonary hypoplasia. *Surgery* **88**, 174–82.

Harrison, M.R., Langer, J.C., Adzick, N.S. *et al.* 1990b: Correction of congenital diaphragmatic hernia *in utero*: V. Initial clinical experience. *Journal of Pediatric Surgery* **25**, 47–55.

Hasegauta, T., Kamata, S., Imura, K. *et al.* 1990: The use of lung–thorax transverse area ratio in the antenatal evaluation of lung hypoplasia in congenital diaphragmatic hernia. *Journal of Clinical Ultrasound* **18**, 705–9.

Hasegawa, T., Imura, K., Kubota, A. *et al.* 1994: Congenital diaphragmatic eventration detected by antenatal ultrasound: rationale for early operation. *Paediatric Surgery International* **9**, 405–6.

Haugen, S.E., Linker, D., Eik-Nes, S. *et al.* 1991: Congenital diaphragmatic hernia: determination of the optimal time for operation by echocardiographic monitoring of the pulmonary arterial pressure. *Journal of Pediatric Surgery* **26**, 560–2.

Hedrick, M.H., Estes, J.M., Sullivan, K.M. *et al.* 1994: Plug the lung until it grows (plug): a new method to treat congenital diaphragmatic hernia *in utero*. *Journal of Pediatric Surgery* **29**, 612–17.

Heidenhain, L. 1905: Geschichte eines Falles von chronischer Incarceration des Magens in einer angeharenen Zwerchfellhernie welcher durch laparotomie geheilt wurde mitan schiessenden Bemerkungen uber die Moglichkeit, das kard iacarcinom der Speiserohre zu reseciren. *Deutsche Zeitschrift für Chirurgie* **78**, 394.

Heiss, K.F., Clark, R.H., Cornish, J.O. *et al.* 1995: Preferential use of venovenous extracorporeal membrane oxygenation for congenital diaphragmatic hernia. *Journal of Pediatric Surgery* **30**, 416–19.

Henneberg, S.W., Jepsen, S., Andersen, P.K. and Pedersen, S.A. 1995: Inhalation of nitric oxide as a treatment of pulmonary hypertension in congenital diaphragmatic hernia. *Journal of Pediatric Surgery* **30**, 853–5.

Iritani, I. 1984: Experimental study on embryogenesis of congenital diaphragmatic hernia. *Anatomy and Embryology* **169**, 133–9.

Jasnosz, K.M., Hermansen, M.C., Snider, C. and Sang, K. 1994: Congenital complete absence (bilateral agenesis) of the diaphragm: a rare variant of congenital diaphragmatic hernia. *American Journal of Perinatology* **11**, 340–3.

Jeffery, P.K., Hislop, A.A., Brewis R.A.L, Corrin, B., Geddes, D.M. and Gibson, G.J. (eds) 1995: *Respiratory medicine*, 2nd ed, 1.1, Embryology and growth. London: WB Saunders, 3–21.

Jennings, R.W., Adzick, N.S., Longaker, M.T., Lorenz, H.P. and Harrison, M.R. 1993: Radiotelemetric fetal monitoring during and after open fetal operation. *Surgery, Gynecology and Obstetrics* **176**: 59–64.

Kamata, S., Hasegawa, T., Matsuo, Y., Fukuzawa, M., Imura, K. and Okada, A. 1992: Fetal diaphragmatic hernia: prenatal evaluation of lung hypoplasia and effects of immediate operation. *Paediatric Surgery International* **7**, 109–12.

Kinsella, J.P., Neish, S.R., Shaffer, E. and Abman, S.H. 1992: Low-dose inhalational nitric oxide in persistent pulmonary hypertension of the newborn. *Lancet* **340**, 819–20.

Kinsella, J.P., Neish, S.R., Ivy, D.D., Shaffer, E. and Abman, S.H. 1993: Clinical responses to prolonged treatment of persistent pulmonary hypertension of the newborn with low doses of inhaled nitric oxide. *Journal of Pediatrics* **123**, 103–8.

Kizilcan, F., Tanyel, F.C., Hiesonmez, A. and Buyukpamukeu, N. 1993: The long-term results of diaphragmatic plication. *Journal of Pediatric Surgery* **28**, 42–4.

Kluth, D., Tenbrinck, R., von Ekesparre, M. *et al.* 1993: The natural history of congenital diaphragmatic hernia and pulmonary hypoplasia in the embryo. *Journal of Pediatric Surgery* **28**, 456–62; discussion 462.

Koot, V.C., Bergmeijer, J.H., Bos, A.P. and Molenaar, J.C. 1993: Incidence and management of gastroesophageal reflux after repair of congenital diaphragmatic hernia. *Journal of Pediatric Surgery* **28**, 48–52.

Korns, H.M. 1921: The diagnosis of eventration of the diaphragm. *Archives of Internal Medicine* **28**, 192–212.

Langer, J.C., Filler, R.M., Coles, J. and Edmonds, J.F. 1988b: Plication of the diaphragm for infants and young children with phrenic nerve palsy. *Journal of Pediatric Surgery* **23**, 749–51.

Langer, J.C., Filler, R.M., Bohn, D.J. *et al.* 1988a: Timing of surgery for congenital diaphragmatic hernia: is emergency operation necessary? *Journal of Pediatric Surgery* **23**, 731–4.

Lund, D.P., Mitchell, J., Kharasch,V., Quigley, S., Kuehn, M. and Wilson, J.M. 1994: Congenital diaphragmatic hernia: the hidden morbidity. *Journal of Pediatric Surgery* **29**, 258–62; discussion 262.

Malone, P.S., Brain, A.J.L., Kiely, E.M. and Spitz, L. 1989: Congenital diaphragm defects that present late. *Archives of Diseases in Childhood* **64**, 1542–4.

Miller, O.I., Celernajer, D.S., Deanfield, J.E. and Macrae, D.J. 1994: Guidelines for the safe administration of inhaled nitric oxide. *Archives of Disease in Childhood* **70**, F47–9.

Morgagni, G.B. 1769: *Seats and causes of disease investigated by anatomy*.

Moulton, S.L., Lynch, F.P., Cornish, J.O., Bejar, R.F., Simko, A.J. and Krous, H.F. 1991: Carotid artery reconstruction following neonatal extracorporeal membrane oxygenation. *Journal of Pediatric Surgery* **26**, 794–9.

Murdock, A.I., Burrington, J.B. and Swyer, P.R. 1971: Alveolar to arterial oxygen difference and venous admixture in infants born with congenital diaphragmatic hernia. *Biology of the Neonate* **17**, 161–72.

Naeye, R.L., Shoehat, S.J., Whitman, V. and Maisels, M.J. 1976: Unsuspected pulmonary vascular abnormalities associated with diaphragmatic hernia. *Pediatrics* **58**, 902–6.

Nagaya, M., Akatsuka, H. and Kato, J. 1994: Gastroesophageal reflux occurring after repair of congenital diaphragmatic hernia. *Journal of Pediatric Surgery* **29**, 1447–51.

Nair, U.R., Entress, A. and Walker, D.R. 1983: Management of neonatal posterolateral diaphragmatic hernia. *Thorax* **38**, 254–7.

Nakayama, O.K., Motoyama, E.K. and Tagge, E.M. 1991: Effect of preoperative stabilization on respiratory system compliance and outcome in newborn infants with congenital diaphragmatic hernia. *Journal of Pediatrics* **118**, 793–9.

Newman, R.D., Anderson, K.D., Van Meurs, K., Parson, S., Loe, W. and Short, B. 1990: Extracorporeal membrane oxygenation and congenital diaphragmatic hernia: should any infant be excluded? *Journal of Pediatric Surgery* **25**, 1048–52.

Nio, M., Haase, G., Kennaugh, J., Bui, K. and Atkinson, J.B. 1994: A prospective randomized trial of delayed versus immediate repair of congenital diaphragmatic hernia. *Journal of Pediatric Surgery* **29**, 618–21.

Norden, M.A., Butt, W. and McDougall P. 1994: Predictors of survival for infants with congenital diaphragmatic hernia. *Journal of Pediatric Surgery* **29**, 1442–6.

O'Rourke, P.P., Lillehei, C.W., Crone, R.K. and Vacanti, J.P. 1991: The effect of extracorporeal membrane oxygenation on the survival of neonates with high-risk congenital diaphragmatic hernia: 45 cases from a single institution. *Journal of Pediatric Surgery* **26**, 147–52.

Paranka, M.S., Clark, R.H., Yoder, B.A. and Null, D.M., Jr 1995: Predictors of failure of high-frequency oscillatory ventilation in term infants with severe respiratory failure. *Pediatrics* **95**, 400–4.

Pilling, G.P. in discussion after Haller, J.A. *et al.* 1974: *Journal of Pediatric Surgery* **14**, 786.

Pringle, K.C. and Puri, P. (eds) 1989: *Congenital diaphragmatic hernia: Lung development in congenital diaphragmatic hernia*. Basel: Karger, 28–53.

Puri, P. and Gorman, F. 1984: Lethal non-pulmonary anomalies associated with congenital diaphragmatic hernia. *Journal Pediatric Surgery* **19**, 29–32.

Puri, P. and Gorman, W.A. 1987: Natural history of congenital diaphragmatic hernia: implications for management. *Paediatric Surgery International* **2**, 327–30.

Roberts, J.D., Polaner, D.M., Lang, P. and Zapol, W.M. 1992: Inhaled nitric oxide in persistent pulmonary hypertension of the newborn. *Lancet* **340**, 818–19.

Roberts, J.P., Burge, D.M. and Griffiths, D.M. 1994: High risk congenital diaphragmatic hernia: how long should surgery be delayed? *Paediatric Surgical International* **9**, 555–7.

Rowe, M.I. and Uribe, F.L. 1971: Diaphragmatic hernia in the newborn infant: blood gas and pH considerations. *Surgery* **70**, 758–61.

Scheffers, E.C., Ijsselstijn, H., Tenbrinck, R., Lachmann, B., de Jongste, J.C.M.J.C. and Tibboel, D. 1994: Evaluation of lung function changes before and after surfactant application during artificial ventilation in newborn rats with congenital diaphragmatic hernia. *Journal of Pediatric Surgery* **29**, 820–4.

Shah, N., Jacob, T., Exler, R. *et al.* Inhaled nitric oxide in congenital diaphragmatic hernia. *Journal of Pediatric Surgery* **29**, 1010–14; discussion 1014.

Sharland, G.K., Lockhart, S.M., Heward, A.J. and Allan, L.D. 1992: Prognosis in fetal diaphragmatic hernia. *American Journal of Obstetrics and Gynecology* **166**, 9–13.

Sigalet, D.L., Nguyen, L.T., Adolph, V., Laberge, J.M., Hong, A.R. and Guttman, F.M. 1994: Gastroesophageal reflux associated with large diaphragmatic hernias. *Journal of Pediatric Surgery* **29**, 1262–5.

Smith, C.D., Sade, R.M. Crawford, F.A. and Othersen, H.B. 1986: Diaphragmatic paralysis and eventration in infants. *Journal of Thoracic and Cardiovascular Surgery* **91**, 490–7.

Sweed, Y. and Puri, P. 1993: Congenital diaphragmatic hernia: influence of associated malformations on survival. *Archives of Disease in Childhood* **68**, 68–70.

Tolsa, J., Cotting, J., Sekarski, N., Payot, M., Micheli, J. and Calame, A. 1995: Magnesium sulphate as an alternative and safe treatment for severe persistent pulmonary hypertension of the newborn. *Archives of Disease in Childhood* **72**, F184–7.

Torvar, J.A., Nogues, A. and Echeverria J. 1979: Antenatal diagnosis of posterolateral diaphragmatic hernia. *Zeitschrift für Kinderchirurgie* **26**, 202–4.

Towokian, R.J. and Markowitz, R.I. 1984: A preoperative scoring system for risk assessment of newborns with congenital diaphragmatic hernia. *Journal of Pediatric Surgery* **19**, 252.

Tsang, T.M., Tarn, P.K., Dudley, N.E. and Stevens, J. 1995: Diaphragmatic agenesis as a distinct clinical entity. *Journal of Pediatric Surgery* **30**, 16–18.

UK Collaborative ECMO Trial Group 1996: UK collaborative randomised trial of neonatal extracorporeal membrane oxygenation. *Lancet* **348**, 75–82.

Van Meurs, K.P,. Rhine, W.D., Benitz, W.E *et al.* 1994: Lobar lung transplantation as a treatment for congenital diaphragmatic hernia. *Journal of Pediatric Surgery* **29**, 1557–60.

Vanamo, K., Rintala, R.J., Lindahi, H. and Louhimo, I. 1996: Long-term gastrointestinal morbidity in patients with congenital diaphragmatic hernia *Journal of Pediatric Surgery* **31**, 551–4.

Vazquez, W.D. and Cheu, H.W. 1994: Hemorrhagic complications and repair of congenital diaphragmatic hernias: does timing of the repair make a difference? Data from the Extracorporeal Life Support Organization. *Journal of Pediatric Surgery* **29**, 1002–5; discussion 1005.

Watanabe, T., Trussler, G., Williams, W.G., Edmonds, J.F., Coles, J.G. and Hosokawa, Y. 1987: Phrenic nerve paralysis after cardiac surgery. *Journal of Thoracic and Cardiovascular Surgery* **94**, 383–8

Wayne, E.R., Campbell, J.B., Burrington, J.D. and Davis, W.S. 1974: Eventration of the diaphragm. *Journal of Pediatric Surgery* **9**, 643–51.

Weiner, E.S. 1982: Congenital diaphragmatic hernia: new dimensions in management. *Surgery* **92**, 889–81.

West, K.W., Bengston, K., Rescorla, F.J., Engle, W.A. Grosfeld JL. Delayed surgical repair and ECMO improves survival in congenital diaphragmatic hernia. *Annals of Surgery* 1992; **218:** 454–60; discussion 480.

Wilcox, D.T., Glick, P.L,, Karamanoukian, H., Rossman, J., Morin, F.C., III and Holm, B.A. 1994: Pathophysiology of congenital diaphragmatic hernia: V. Effect of exogenous surfactant therapy on gas exchange and lung mechanics in the lamb congenital diaphragmatic hernia model. *Journal of Pediatrics* **124**, 289–93.

Wilcox, D.T., Glick, P.L., Karamanoukian, H.L., Azizkhan, R.G. and Holm, B.A. 1995: Pathophysiology of congenital diaphragmatic hernia: xii. Amniotic fluid lecithin/sphingomyelin ratio and phosphatidylglycerol concentrations do not predict surfactant status in congenital diaphragmatic hernia. *Journal of Pediatric Surgery* **30**, 410–12.

Wilson, J.M., Bower, L.K. and Lund, D.P. 1994a: Evolution of the technique of congenital diaphragmatic hernia repair on ECMO. *Journal of Pediatric Surgery* **29**, 1109–12.

Wilson, J.M., Fauza, D.O., Lund, D.P., Benacerraf, B.R. and Hendren, W.H. 1994b: Antenatal diagnosis of isolated congenital diaphragmatic hernia is not an indicator of outcome. *Journal of Pediatric Surgery* **29**, 815–19.

Wilson, J.M., Lund, D.P., Lillehei, C.W. and Vacanti J.P. 1991: Congenital diaphragmatic hernia: predictors of severity in the ECMO era. *Journal of Pediatric Surgery* **26**, 1028–33.

CHAPTER 20

Structural anomalies of the airway and lungs

D.M. BURGE AND M. SAMUEL

Upper airway anomalies
Lower airway anomalies
The lungs

The pleural cavity
References

Most of the conditions described in this chapter present with respiratory difficulty, the precise manifestation of which depends on the anatomical level of the lesion (see Table 20.1). Conditions affecting the nasal airway and pharynx tend to produce obstructive apnoea, those of the larynx inspiratory stridor and those of the trachea biphasic stridor. Lung lesions present with respiratory distress without obstructive features. All grades of severity of these features may be encountered and although many of these conditions produce mild symptoms which may be self-limiting, in their severe forms they can cause death or cerebral damage from hypoxia.

Upper airway anomalies

CHOANAL ATRESIA/STENOSIS

Choanal atresia is a congenital obstruction of the posterior nares at the level of the posterior border of the nasal septum. Although it has an incidence of about 1:10 000 the perceived incidence in the neonatal period is less than this because unilateral cases, which are more common, may not produce clinical features at birth. In 10% of cases the obstruction is only membranous but in the remainder it is bony. In some cases choanal atresia is the presenting feature of the CHARGE association: *c*oloboma of retina and/or iris, *h*eart abnormalities,

Table 20.1 Structural anomalies of the airway and lungs

Upper airway	Choanal atresia/stenosis
	Transient nasal obstruction
	Craniofacial anomalies
	Pierre Robin syndrome
	Extrinsic tumours
	Intrinsic tumours
	Macroglossia
Larynx	Laryngomalacia
	Vocal cord palsy
	Subglottic stenosis
	Haemangioma
	Laryngeal cleft
	Miscellaneous: web, cysts
Trachea and bronchi	Tracheal agenesis or stenosis
	Vascular ring
	Tracheomalacia
	Bronchomalacia
Lungs	Agenesis
	Congenital lobar emphysema (CLE)
	Congenital cystic adenomatoid malformation (CCAM)
	Pulmonary sequestration
	Bronchogenic cyst
Pleura	Chylothorax

*a*tresia choanae, *r*etardation (which may be physical and mental), *g*enital anomalies and *e*ar anomalies (Pagan *et al.*, 1981). It is important that any baby with choanal atresia is screened carefully for these other features because the associated developmental implications may be considerable.

Clinical features

Babies within the first few weeks of life are obligatory nose breathers. This explains the marked respiratory difficulty that choanal atresia can produce considering that all the baby has to do to overcome the obstruction is to open its mouth to breath. Some babies will do this readily and present with breathing difficulty with feeding only, when the mouth is otherwise occupied. Other infants present with cyanosis at rest and only become pink when they open their mouths to cry. Unilateral atresia may become apparent in the neonate if the other nostril is blocked by oedema or secretions. In most cases it presents in later childhood with unilateral nasal discharge.

Investigation

The diagnosis is usually suggested by failure to pass a suction catheter beyond the posterior nares. A simple test of nasal patency is to listen with a stethoscope at the external nares. Confirmation of the diagnosis is best achieved by someone who has seen the condition before probing the nose gently with a small metal sound. Contrast can be instilled into the nostril to obtain radiological confirmation (Fig. 20.1) but this is not usually required. Computed tomography (CT) or magnetic res-

onance imaging (MRI) should be performed in every case to clarify the bony anatomy. This not only identifies the type of atresia (bony or membranous) but also shows the bone thickness. More importantly, it will demonstrate the anatomy of the postnasal space which may be considerably narrowed in many cases. This information is essential prior to attempting surgical correction to prevent damage to adjacent structures (Crockett *et al.*, 1987).

Treatment

If the atresia is membranous simple perforation and dilatation under general anaesthesia may suffice. Bony atresia can be treated by a transnasal or transpalatal approach. The latter provides better visualization of the area to be resected but can cause palatal damage (Prescott, 1995). Most surgeons still practice the transnasal approach. The atretic area should be visualized endoscopically from in front (0° telescope) and behind (120° telescope) and the bony wall perforated and resected using a drill or forceps. Once a reasonable passage has been created it should be stented to reduce the risk of stenosis. This is best achieved using thick-walled silastic tubing passed down one nostril and up the other with a fenestration sited posteriorly (Fig. 20.2). A cross-bar of the same tubing is then placed across the two external limbs and sutured in place. This prevents inward movement of the stent. The stent is usually needed for some weeks but despite this repeated dilatations under anaesthetic may be needed in the first months.

TRANSIENT NASAL OBSTRUCTION

Nasal mucosal oedema is a common cause of nasal obstruction in the newborn. It can be distinguished from

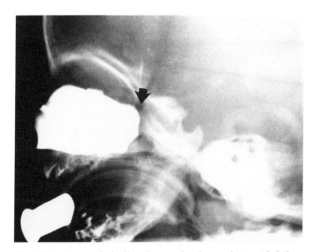

Fig. 20.1 Lateral skull radiograph of an infant with bilateral choanal atresia who has had contrast instilled into the nostrils. Whilst this investigation clearly indicates the level of the atresia at the posterior nares (arrow), it is not usually required in the assessment of children with this condition.

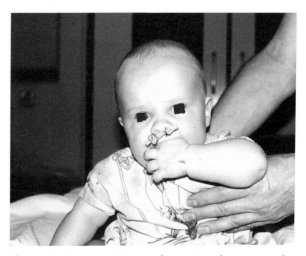

Fig. 20.2 Postoperative nasal stenting after surgery for choanal atresia.

choanal atresia by the passage of a nasopharyngeal tube. It is a transient condition. and nasal decongestants may be helpful.

CRANIOFACIAL ANOMALIES

Conditions in which there is abnormal maxillary development may be associated with posterior nares or nasopharyngeal obstruction. These include Treacher Collins', Crouzon's and Apert's syndromes.

PIERRE ROBIN SYNDROME

This condition is characterized by micrognathia, posterior displacement of the tongue (glossoptosis) and cleft palate. Babies with all three features clearly fall into the syndrome but those with some but not all features are often included. This has resulted in a wide variation in the reported incidence of the syndrome from 1:2000 to 1:10 000. The degree of micrognathia can be very severe (Fig. 20.3) and can persist into childhood, requiring mandibular surgery. It can be postulated that micrognathia is the primary defect and that posterior tongue displacement is secondary and in itself causes maldevelopment of the palate.

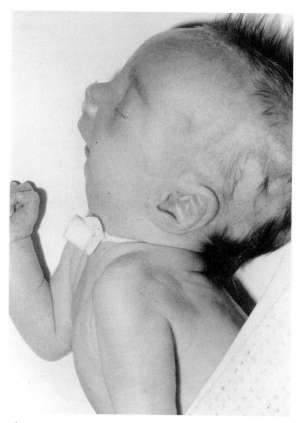

Fig. 20.3 An infant with Pierre Robin syndrome with severe micrognathia requiring tracheostomy.

Clinical features and management

Airway obstruction is caused by the tongue obstructing the hypopharynx (Benjamin and Walker, 1991). This can be profound and cause severe hypoxia. The cause of obstruction can usually be deduced because of the obvious micrognathia and, where present, the cleft palate. Confirmation that glossoptosis is the cause can usually be obtained by positioning the baby prone. This allows the tongue to fall forwards and relieves obstruction. This may indeed be all the treatment that is needed. However, in some cases this is not adequate. Passage of a nasopharyngeal tube – a standard endotracheal tube of suitable diameter passed through one nostril to a position behind the tongue and above the larynx – may produce an adequate airway, both through and alongside the tube. If this fails, intubation of the trachea may be needed but is notoriously difficult in these cases because the position of the tongue makes visualization of the larynx very difficult. In rare cases tracheostomy may be required.

Spontaneous improvement in airway obstruction gradually occurs as the child gets older. Surgery is needed for palatal repair and sometimes for mandibular lengthening later in childhood. The likely difficulty in intubation for these procedures should be brought to the attention of the anaesthetist.

HEAD AND NECK TUMOURS

Extrinsic tumours anywhere in the neck can cause respiratory obstruction, with the most common tumours being cystic hygroma, cervical teratoma (Fig. 20.4) and haemangioma. In these conditions relief of obstruction can be very difficult or even impossible. Anatomical distortion may impede both tracheal intubation and tracheostomy. In such cases the careful siting of a nasopharyngeal tube may be life-saving.

Intrinsic smaller space-occupying lesions may cause obstruction depending on their position. These include nasopharyngeal lesions (dermoid, encephalocele, rhabdomyosarcoma) and oropharyngeal or hypopharyngeal lesions (lingual thyroid, vallecular cysts, haemangioma, etc.). Cross-sectional imaging and careful endoscopy are required to establish the diagnosis.

MACROGLOSSIA

This may be secondary to a generalized disorder (e.g. hypothyroidism or Beckwith–Weidemann syndrome) or localized pathology (haemangioma or lymphangioma) or it may be an isolated abnormality. It is important to consider Beckwith–Weidemann because this may be associated with neonatal hypoglycaemia and subsequent neurological impairment which may be prevented if the diagnosis is made early. Surgical reduction of the tongue may be possible, although haemangiomatous lesions are difficult to treat.

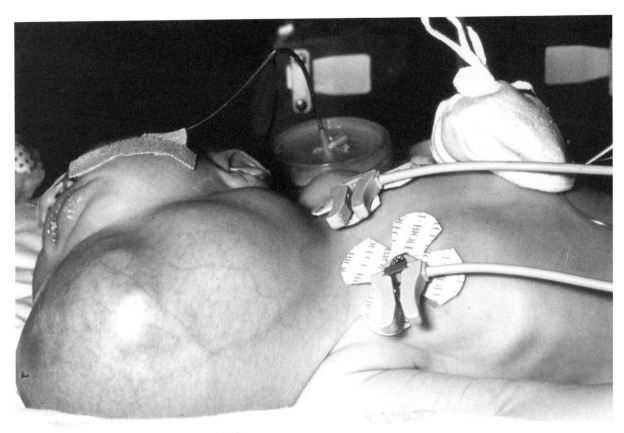

Fig. 20.4 An infant with a massive cervical teratoma.

Lower airway anomalies

LARYNX

Laryngomalacia

Clinical features

This is the most common cause of laryngeal stridor in infants. The inspiratory stridor may not be present at birth but develops over the first few days or weeks of life. It is due to inherent floppiness of the aryepiglottic folds, the cuneiform cartilages and, to some extent, the epiglottis itself, all of which are sucked into the larynx on inspiration and expelled on expiration. Classically the condition does not distress the infant despite the quite dramatic stridor that it may produce (Holinger, 1961). Although the stridor may vary in severity with crying, the cry itself is normal.

Investigation

In the past this condition has often been diagnosed without endoscopy based on the clinical features and the knowledge that it is the most common cause of these features in babies. However, there is now a greater tendency to perform endoscopy to ensure precise diag-

nosis. This approach is to be encouraged as some conditions producing laryngeal stridor can be progressive and may cause complete obstruction and death (e.g. laryngeal cysts and subglottic haemangioma). Worsening stridor in an infant is an absolute indication for endoscopy.

Endoscopy may be performed under sedation using a fine flexible bronchoscope but in many centres rigid endoscopy with general anaesthesia is used (Benjamim *et al.*, 1994). It is essential that the larynx be inspected with the child breathing spontaneously in order for the diagnosis to be made.

Management

In most cases the stridor decreases over the first 1–2 years of life, although it may worsen again temporarily with respiratory infection. In rare cases hospital admission may be required during infections but most cases require no treatment. Very severe forms may require tracheostomy.

Vocal cord palsy

Cord palsy in the neonate is usually unilateral and self-limiting. A common cause is birth trauma and as a result there may be other features of a traumatic delivery such as Erb's palsy or phrenic nerve palsy. Unilateral palsy may be so mild as to go unnoticed but, when clinically apparent, presents with a weak cry, a tendency to aspirate secretions and choking with feeds. Bilateral palsy causes severe stridor and cyanosis and, although recovery may occur in the first 6 months, tracheostomy is usually required until then. Diagnosis of unilateral cord palsy is particularly difficult and requires considerable experience of infant endoscopy.

Subglottic stenosis

This may be congenital or acquired. With improved neonatal intensive care techniques and endotracheal tube materials, acquired stenosis is now, thankfully, much less common than it was. In fact it is quite surprising how rarely it now occurs given that many small infants with chronic lung disease still undergo prolonged intubation. The narrowest point in the airway is at the level of the cricoid ring. It is at this site that acquired stenosis secondary to prolonged intubation may occur. Stenosis is suggested clinically when attempts to extubate an infant after prolonged ventilation fail and are accompanied by evidence of obstruction (stridor, sternal and subcostal recession, etc.).

In many cases extubation failure is due to a combination of subglottic oedema or stenosis and chronic lung disease. The relative importance of these may be hard to define but endoscopy is valuable in determining optimal management. If oedema alone is present, a course of steroids (which may also improve coexisting chronic lung disease) may enable subsequent extubation. Minor granulations require no treatment. Thin web stenoses can be resected by laser. More severe fibrous scarring may often be circumferential and tracheostomy with subsequent laryngoplasty and bone grafting may be needed (Cotton, 1984). More recently, surgical incision of the cricoid over the indwelling endotracheal tube without the need for tracheostomy has been described (Bagwell *et al.*, 1987; Cotton, 1991).

Congenital subglottic stenosis is rare. It usually presents with stridor but this may not be apparent at birth, presenting later during respiratory infection. The added airway narrowing produced by such infection may sufficiently compromise the airway as to make intubation necessary. As a result, further oedema occurs, making extubation difficult. Most children with congenital stenosis require no treatment and improve with age. Severe cases require tracheostomy and laryngoplasty.

Haemangioma

Subglottic haemangiomas present with stridor in infancy. As with other haemangiomas the lesion may be absent or very small at birth but may enlarge over the first few months, only to regress during the first 2–5 years. Thus stridor may not be present at birth but once

present may become increasingly severe. As this process may be quite rapid, any infant with worsening stridor requires urgent endoscopy. Diagnosis is usually possible without resort to biopsy. Cutaneous haemangiomas are present in the head and neck region in 50% of cases. Another association is with sternal clefting (Ingelvans and Debengny, 1965). Tracheostomy is usually required, followed by expectant treatment awaiting resolution or medical (steroids, radiotherapy) or surgical (laser resection, cryosurgery) treatment.

Laryngeal cleft

Congenital clefting of the larynx with or without trachea may occur alone or in combination with other anomalies such as oesophageal atresia, congenital heart disease, cleft lip and palate and genitourinary anomalies. It probably arises from incomplete separation of the foregut into the trachea and oesophagus and has been classified into four types (Benjamin and Inglis, 1987):

- type I: interarytenoid cleft
- type II: partial cricoid cleft
- type III: total cricoid cleft
- type IV: clefting extending into the trachea. Severe forms extend to the carina.

Presentation varies with the extent of clefting but includes feed aspiration, recurrent pneumonia, stridor and weak cry. Complete stage IV clefts may result in total tracheal collapse requiring intubation from birth.

The diagnosis of minor clefts is difficult and they are often missed. Laryngoscopy must include careful inspection of the posterior commissure. Surgical treatment of minor clefts is usually straightforward but gastro-oesophageal reflux must be looked for and treated if present (Hof *et al.*, 1987). Children with longer clefts require tracheostomy and major reconstruction. The prognosis for this group is poor and few children with complete tracheal clefting have survived (Donahoe and Gee, 1984).

Miscellaneous anomalies

Various types of webs and cysts can cause laryngeal obstruction and the reader is referred to Benjamin *et al.* (1994).

TRACHEA AND BRONCHI

Tracheal agenesis and stenosis

Tracheal agenesis is, fortunately, extremely rare. It comprises failure of development of the trachea, although the extent of this failure and the subsequent anatomy vary. Seven different anatomical types have been described (de Lorimier *et al.*, 1986). In the most common variety (56%) the trachea ends blindly at or just below the vocal cords and arises again from the lower oesophagus. Presentation is with immediate cyanosis, impossible endotracheal intubation but, in 80%, improvement with positive pressure ventilation via the oesophagus. No long-term survivors with this condition have been reported although various techniques have been employed which have kept the baby alive in the short term (Altman *et al.*, 1972). With this in mind accurate diagnosis must be obtained by endoscopy and the parents counselled that oesophageal ventilation may need to be discontinued and the baby allowed to die. New techniques such as lung transplantation (Cromble-holme *et al.*, 1990) or tracheal transplantation may arise for this condition and any cases in which this diagnosis is made or suspected should be discussed with a specialist paediatric ENT or thoracic surgical department.

Congenital tracheal stenosis is characterized by loss of the pars membranosa of the trachea such that the tracheal rings, which are normally horseshoe shaped, are complete circles (Landing and Dixon, 1979). This abnormality may extend to the bronchial cartilages. Although the whole of the trachea may be involved, the stenosis is more commonly confined to a section of the trachea. Presentation is with respiratory distress. This can usually be relieved by positive pressure ventilation even if the endotracheal tube will not pass through the affected area. The diagnosis is confirmed by bronchoscopy, although bronchography may be required to determine the extent of tracheal or bronchial involvement (Nakayama *et al.*, 1982). Because of the reported association with pulmonary artery slings (Gumbiner *et al.*, 1980), echocardiography should be performed. Treatment of short stenoses is by surgical resection of the stenotic segment and primary anastamosis. Up to 66% of the length of trachea can be resected in this way (Longaker *et al.*, 1990). Tracheal longitudinal incision and cartilage grafting are required for longer segments but are hazardous (Kimara *et al.*, 1982).

Vascular ring

Abnormalities of development of the major vessels near the trachea can result in compression of the trachea by a double aortic arch, pulmonary artery sling or other vessels (Marmon *et al.*, 1984). In double aortic arch one branch passes in front of the trachea and one behind. One branch is usually larger than the other. All affected infants present with stridor but this may not become apparent until a few years of age. Aortic arch abnormalities may also cause dysphagia. Pulmonary artery slings, however, are notorious for producing life-threatening obstruction which may in part be due to associated tracheal stenosis (see above). In most cases the left pulmonary arises from its partner on the right and passes between the trachea and oesophagus. Investigation

for these anomalies should include a contrast swallow and bronchoscopy. If these suggest a vascular anomaly, echocardiography and arteriography may be required. Double aortic arch is treated by division of the smaller branch. Pulmonary artery sling surgery is more complex and may involve resection of tracheal stenosis if this coexists (Jonas *et al.*, 1989).

Whether or not the innominate artery can cause symptomatic tracheal compression is debated. Although in the normal adult this vessel runs to the right of the trachea it was noticed in some infants with stridor that it ran across the trachea from left to right and was thought to be compressing the trachea in these cases (Gross and Neuhauser, 1984). Subsequent reports have shown that this course of the innominate artery is found in many normal children (Strife *et al.*, 1981). The condition certainly overlaps with tracheomalacia and is discussed below.

Tracheomalacia

This is a common cause of tracheal (biphasic) stridor. In paediatric surgical practice it is most commonly encountered in association with oesophageal atresia (OA) and tracheo-oesophageal fistula (TOF) and in its common mild form is responsible for the 'TOF cough'. However, tracheomalacia can occur either in isolation, or as a result of external tracheal compression by cysts or tumours or from long-term intubation. The primary abnormality is defective development of the tracheal cartilage rings which support the trachea during respiration. Instead of being horseshoe shaped, the rings are opened out posteriorly as well as often collapsing inwards anteriorly (Baxter and Dunbar, 1963; Wailoo and Emery, 1979).

Clinical presentation in OA is with the TOF cough, which in more severe cases is combined with stridor and 'dying spells'. In these life-threatening events the trachea collapses completely but usually reopens as the child relaxes as consciousness is lost. The diagnosis can usually be made easily on bronchoscopy under conditions that allow spontaneous respiration. In the absence of OA as an underlying explanation a search for another causative lesion (e.g. mediastinal cyst or vascular ring) should be made. Although the condition is usually self-limiting such that stridor may have ceased by a few months of life and TOF cough by a few years, severe cases will require aortopexy (Kiely, 1987; Filler *et al.*, 1992). This procedure approximates the aorta to the sternum, which has the effect of pulling the anterior wall of the trachea forwards, increasing the tracheal lumen, but is most suited for the treatment of short-segment tracheomalacia. If the whole trachea is involved tracheostomy may be required. Such severe cases may eventually improve spontaneously, allowing removal of the tracheostomy after a few years, but in others tracheal reconstruction may be required.

The same process of weakness of cartilage support may also involve the bronchi (bronchomalacia). This may be an isolated defect or may be found in conjunction with tracheomalacia. If unilateral it may present as recurrent pneumonia but if bilateral and combined with tracheomalacia it can cause serious respiratory obstruction. This may be treatable (Mair *et al.*, 1990; Kosloske, 1991) but in some cases is fatal.

The lungs

AGENESIS

This rare anomaly is a result of primary arrest of lung bud development. In about 50% of cases other anomalies coexist (cardiac lesions, vertebral and skeletal anomalies, oesophageal atresia (Hoffman *et al.*, 1989), gastrointestinal anomalies, etc.). Mortality is high in the neonatal period and usually due to the associated anomalies. In surviving infants the diagnosis is usually made on routine chest X-ray and although lobar agenesis can occur, pulmonary agenesis is more common. Although the condition requires no treatment (Sbokos and McMillan, 1977), the dramatic radiological features of mediastinal displacement in a child who has presumably had sufficient symptoms in the first place to merit X-ray usually result in further investigations being considered, the most useful being V/Q scan, bronchoscopy and bronchography.

CONGENITAL LOBAR EMPHYSEMA (CLE)

Definition

CLE is defined as an overexpansion of the alveolar spaces of a segment or lobe of a histologically normal lung. It is thought to result from cartilaginous deficiency in the tracheobronchial tree (Buntain *et al.*, 1974) which produces a check-valve type of obstruction and air-trapping within a lobe (Jones *et al.*, 1965). Compression of the adjacent lung may compromise ventilation depending on the volume occupied by the emphysematous lobe.

This condition has various aetiologies as indicated by histopathological analysis:

- intrinsic bronchial obstruction resulting from bronchomalacia or abnormal bronchial cartilage support is seen in 35–50% of patients
- congenital or post-infective alveolar septal fibrosis
- pulmonary alveolar hyperplasia or polyalveolar lobe, found in one-third of CLE patients (Hislop and Reid, 1970; Trapper *et al.*, 1980). A polyalveolar lobe is characterized by a normal number of bronchi, but the acini contain three to five times the normal number of alveoli of normal size, and a decreased number of arterial branches per unit volume of the emphysematous lobe
- extrinsic bronchial compression resulting in CLE can occur in association with an enlarged heart due to congenital cardiac anomalies (i.e. ventricular septal

defect, patent ductus arteriosus, tetralogy of Fallot and dilated atria) or aneurysmal dilatation of the major vessels, in 15% of infants (Jones *et al.*, 1965; Stanger *et al.*, 1969). Bronchogenic cysts are known to cause regional CLE from external bronchial obstruction (Stigers *et al.*, 1992)

- pulmonary hypoplasia due to diminished number of bronchial branches and abnormal small arteries
- lobar emphysema can also be an acquired disorder, particularly in preterm neonates and small-for-date infants who have been on long-term ventilation in whom bronchial obstruction may occur owing to redundant bronchial mucosa, inspissated mucus plugging the bronchus and torsion of the bronchus.

Pathophysiology

In complete bronchial obstruction, regional hyperinflation is due to a check-valve mechanism in the collateral ventilation through the alveolar pores of Kohn, the bronchoalveolar channels of Lambert or the interbronchiolar channels. In partial obstruction of the bronchus, air is allowed through during inspiration but during expiration the bronchus is completely occluded, resulting in overinflation and overexpansion of the lung, and breakdown of alveolar septae.

In polyalveolar lobes the number of bronchial branches is normal but there is an abnormal increase in the number of alveoli in each acinus, with a decrease in the number of arteries per unit volume of emphysematous lung. Infants with polyalveolar lobe present early and the condition is indistinguishable from other forms of CLE. The distribution of lung involvement is represented diagrammatically in Fig. 20.5 (Cremin and Movsowitz, 1971; Stigers *et al.*, 1992).

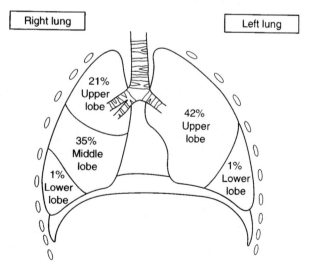

Fig. 20.5 Distribution of lobar involvement by congenital lobar emphysema (CLE). In cases where CLE is bilateral the right middle and left upper lobes are most commonly affected.

Clinical features

CLE presents dramatically within hours of birth with rapidly progressive respiratory distress in 50% of affected neonates. In other cases presentation is delayed for days or even months, but symptoms usually become apparent in the first 6 months of life (Cremin and Movsowitz, 1971). Males are three times more commonly affected than females. The earlier the onset of symptoms, the more probable the progression to life-threatening progressive pulmonary insufficiency from compression of normal adjacent lung. Tachypnoea, dyspnoea and cyanosis form the complex of symptoms, and hyper-resonance and diminished breath sounds over the affected area are the detectable physical signs. CLE has been detected on antenatal ultrasonography (Richards *et al.*, 1992).

Differential diagnosis

The differential diagnosis includes giant congenital cystic adenomatoid malformation, tension pneumothorax, atelectasis of one lung or lobe with compensatory emphysema in the other as a result of inspissated mucous plugging or torsion of the bronchus, and pneumatocele.

Investigations

The diagnosis is usually suspected on review of a chest X-ray performed because of respiratory symptoms (Fig. 20.6). Radiological features include:

- hyperlucent overexpanded lung
- herniation of the emphysematous segment into the opposite side anterior to the heart and great vessels
- wide separation of bronchovascular structures
- shift of the mediastinum
- compression and atelectasis of the adjacent lung structures depending on the magnitude of overexpansion
- depression of the ipsilateral diaphragm.

In most cases no other form of investigation is needed and indeed may delay urgently required surgery. In cases where the onset of symptoms has been gradual, a CT scan can be useful to demonstrate a causative lesion such as a bronchogenic cyst. A V/Q scan is useful in long-term follow-up and assessment of the unaffected segments of the lung and of the affected segment when conservative treatment has been adopted. Echocardiography may be used to define cardiac abnormalities, as 15% of these patients have major cardiac anomalies.

Treatment

Surgical lobectomy is the treatment of choice. Urgent surgical intervention is indicated when there is a life-threatening progressive pulmonary insufficiency from compression of adjacent lung structures. There is no role for bronchoplastic procedures. In occasional cases rapid deterioration occurs under anaesthesia due to positive pressure ventilation of the obstructed lobe with increased air-trapping. For this reason spontaneous respiration should be adopted until the chest is opened. At thoracotomy the emphysematous lobe is usually

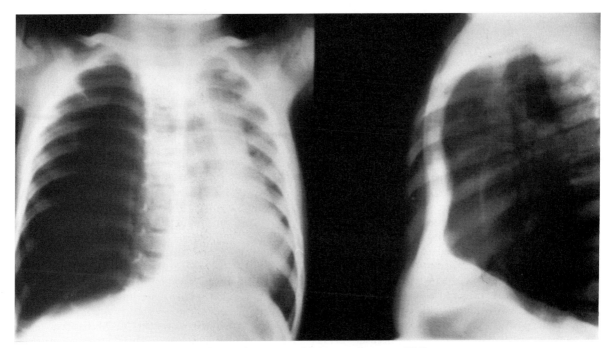

Fig. 20.6   Chest X-ray of a newborn infant with congenital lobar emphysema (CLE).

impossible to compress. This can make access to the hilum of the lung difficult, although in some cases the affected lobe can be delivered through the wound, thus improving access. Once the hilum is identified resection is usually straightforward.

Conservative management of CLE has been reported in older children (Eigen *et al.*, 1972; Man *et al.*, 1983). Selective bronchial intubation can be used in acquired forms to isolate the affected lung and thereby hasten resolution.

Results

Lobectomy is usually well tolerated provided the remaining lobes are normal. Long-term follow-up has shown no symptomatic functional impairment, although respiratory flow rates are diminished to 60–80% of normal (Eigen *et al.*, 1976). Patients who have been treated conservatively have been shown to have improved ventilation rather than an improvement in perfusion, as assessed by initial and follow-up V/Q scans (Kennedy *et al.*, 1991; Azizkhari *et al.*, 1992). Long-term evaluation of surgically and conservatively managed children has shown that the pulmonary function remained equivalent in both groups and an asymptomatic hyperlucent overdistended lobe may not impair the normal development of the remaining lung (Eigen *et al.*, 1976).

CONGENITAL CYSTIC ADENOMATOID MALFORMATION (CCAM)

This abnormality was first described in 1949 by Ch'in and Tang and, although uncommon, is being encountered more frequently as a result of prenatal ultrasound screening.

Definition

CCAM is a multicystic mass of pulmonary tissue in which there is a proliferation of bronchial structures at the expense of alveoli. In rare cases skeletal muscle may be present in the cyst walls.

Pathology and embryology

Histopathologically, there is an abnormal proliferation of mesenchymal elements and failure of maturation of bronchiolar structures. Proliferation of polypoid glandular tissue occurs at the expense of alveolar development. CCAMs communicate with the tracheobronchial tree. Air-trapping occurs secondary to lack of cartilaginous bronchi. The absence of bronchial cartilage and the high incidence of associated anomalies suggest that the prenatal insult has occurred before 31 days of gestation and the mixture of epithelial and mesenchymal structures suggests that the insult occurs after the two lung buds appear at 26–28 days (Stocker *et al.*, 1977; Miller *et al.*, 1993).

Classification

This is based on the clinical and histopathological characteristics which Stocker *et al.* (1977), delineated into three types (see also Miller *et al.*, 1980):

- type 1: single or multiple cysts over 2 cm in diameter that are lined by pseudostratified columnar epithelium. Relatively normal alveoli may be present between the cysts with contralateral mediastinal herniation.
- type 2: multiple small cysts less than 1 cm in diameter that are lined by ciliated cuboidal or columnar epithelium. Respiratory bronchioles and distended alveoli may be present between the cysts. There is a high frequency of other congenital anomalies (26%).
- type 3: a large, bulky, non-cystic lesion. Bronchiole-like structures are lined by ciliated cuboidal epithelium and separated by masses of alveolar size structures lined by non-ciliated cuboidal epithelium.

Overlap among these types is known to occur.

Clinical features

CCAM usually presents to the paediatric surgeon in one of three ways: on prenatal ultrasound, as respiratory distress in the newborn or infant, or as recurrent chest infections in later childhood. However, 25–35% of affected infants will never present to a surgeon as they are so severely affected that they are stillborn or die rapidly after birth with severe pulmonary insufficiency. This should be kept in mind when considering the management of prenatally diagnosed CCAM which is discussed below.

Neonates usually present with gradually progressive respiratory distress as the lesion enlarges postnatally due to air-trapping. The rapidity of development of symptoms depends not only on the size of the lesion but also on the degree of pulmonary hypoplasia in the rest of the ipsilateral and contralateral lung induced by *in utero* compression, which is exactly analogous to the situation occurring in congenital diaphragmatic hernia. Hyperresonance of the affected hemithorax is found with displacement of the cardiac apex.

In some cases small Stocker type 1 CCAM may be asymptomatic at birth and present as unresolving or recurrent respiratory infection in an older child (Wolf *et al.*, 1980; Nishibayashi *et al.*, 1981; Haddon and Bowen, 1991).

In 80% of patients a single lobe is involved. Any lobe can be affected. Rarely, two or more lobes are involved (Miller *et al.*, 1980) and therefore careful cross-sectional imaging of the chest should be performed if time allows. The affected lobes are not always grossly abnormal macroscopically and it is possible to resect one lobe only to find that further resection is needed a week or two later.

Malignant transformation in CCAMs has been reported in later life in the form of rhabdomyosarcoma (Murphy *et al.*, 1992), bronchioalveolar carcinoma (Weinberg *et al.*, 1980; Sheffield *et al.*, 1987) and pulmonary blastoma (Benjamin and Cahill, 1991) amongst others (Pritchard *et al.*, 1984; Benjamin and Cahill, 1991).

Associated anomalies have been reported with CCAM and include diaphragmatic hernia, jejunal atresia, prune belly syndrome and hydrocephalus.

Radiological investigations

The diagnosis of CCAM can usually be made on chest X-ray (Fig. 20.7). However, the radiological features are variable and include marked hyperlucency of the hemithorax with mediastinal and diaphragmatic displacement mimicking tension pneumothorax or congenital lobar emphysema (usually type 1 lesions), multiple smaller cysts full of air and fluid mimicking diaphragmatic hernia (type 1 or 2 lesions) or solid space-occupying mass (type 3 lesions) (Fig. 20.8). It is essential to perform an abdominal X-ray to demonstrate a normal abdominal gas pattern and exclude congenital diaphragmatic hernia. If the baby is deteriorating clinically owing to increasing air-trapping this may be the only imaging that time allows before urgent surgery. There is no place for elective delay in surgery, as in diaphragmatic hernia.

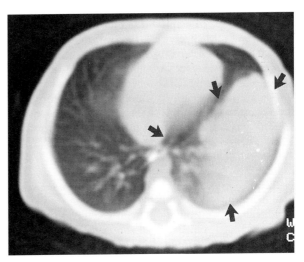

Fig. 20.8 CT scan of the chest of a newborn infant with a type 3 CCAM (arrows).

If the baby's condition allows, further imaging in the form of CT scanning is useful to determine whether more than one lobe is affected. Since there is overlap between CCAM and pulmonary sequestration an attempt should be made to determine whether there is an anomalous systemic arterial supply from, for example, the abdominal aorta. This is particularly important if the lesion appears to be affecting the lower lobe. Such vessels may be detected by Doppler ultrasound. Although MRI will also identify anomalous vessels, any procedure other than corrective surgery that might involve general anaesthesia should be avoided because positive pressure ventilation will usually increase the cyst size and worsen the baby's condition.

Management

The treatment of symptomatic CCAM is excision of the affected lobe or lobes. Fortunately, most infants with symptomatic CCAM will have fairly mild respiratory symptoms. When preoperative stabilization is required it is essential to try to avoid positive pressure ventilation as this will risk further air-trapping and can result in rapid deterioration. This also affects anaesthetic management and if possible the infant should be allowed to breath spontaneously until the chest is opened. Mobilization of the affected lobe should include careful examination to exclude an anomalous vascular supply. Whilst most CCAMs are supplied by the pulmonary circulation, some, particularly those arising from the lower lobe, are supplied systemically. If a lower lobe CCAM is found, the inferior pulmonary ligament should be inspected carefully prior to division. It is possible to avulse the often large systemic artery as it comes through the diaphragm. This vessel will then retract out of the site, usually followed by the death of the baby. Lobectomy is otherwise usually straightforward. Local segmental resection is not usually

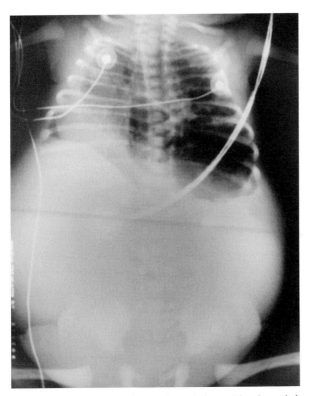

Fig. 20.7 Chest X-ray of a newborn infant with a large left lower lobe type 1 CCAM causing mediastinal and diaphragmatic displacement. The lesion had been detected prenatally. The remaining lung was severely hypoplastic and the baby died despite surgical resection of the CCAM.

required but can be employed to preserve lung tissue in bilateral cases (Mentzer *et al.*, 1992).

In most cases recovery from surgery is uneventful. However persistent fetal circulation akin to that found in congenital diaphragmatic hernia may occur, requiring aggressive treatment including extracorporeal membrane oxygenation (ECMO) (Atkinson *et al.*, 1992). Long-term outcome is normal in most cases.

Prenatal diagnosis

Detection of CCAM by prenatal ultrasound is now commonplace and has altered our knowledge of the natural history of the condition. Such knowledge is essential for prenatal counselling. It is now clear that CCAM will follow one of three courses. (1) The lesion may become so large *in utero* as to distort the heart and great vessels and produce cardiac failure which is manifested as hydrops. This will frequently result in death *in utero* (Adzick and Harrison, 1993). (2) The fetus may survive and be symptomatic at birth, as described above. (3) Perhaps most commonly (McCullagh *et al.*, 1994), the infant will be born asymptomatic. Regression of CCAMs can occur *in utero* and there are many reports of them diminishing in size or vanishing completely (Fine *et al.*, 1988; Neilson *et al.*, 1991; MacGillivray *et al.*, 1993).

Lesions producing hydrops are usually solid, Stocker type III lesions. Whilst these can rarely resolve (Neilson *et al.*, 1991), the only treatment affecting outcome after development of hydrops is fetal surgery (Adzick *et al.*, 1993). Large cystic lesions rarely cause hydrops, although they are amenable to *in utero* shunting. The role of fetal surgery in CCAM is controversial. Adzick *et al.* (1993), reported successful *in utero* resection of type 2 and 3 CCAM with reversal of fetal hydrops and good long-term outcome. However, the choice of which fetuses may benefit from intervention is difficult as even large lesions can regress spontaneously prior to delivery.

Controversy exists about the postnatal management of asymptomatic infants with CCAM. Given that regression of these lesions can occur *in utero*, then perhaps further regression can occur postnatally such that the lesion will never cause a problem. However it is often reported that recurrent and severe infections can occur in CCAMs in later life (Ravitch and Hardy, 1949; Soosay *et al.*, 1992). Perhaps even more worrying is the reported development of malignancy in CCAM (see above).

A chest X-ray of asymptomatic infants with CCAM should be conducted within hours of birth. This will often show the affected area of lung to be radiopaque owing to delayed clearance of lung fluid (Fig. 20.9a). This area will clear after 24–48 hours and subsequent X-rays may show air-filled cysts or may appear normal (Fig. 20.9b). Subtle changes are often

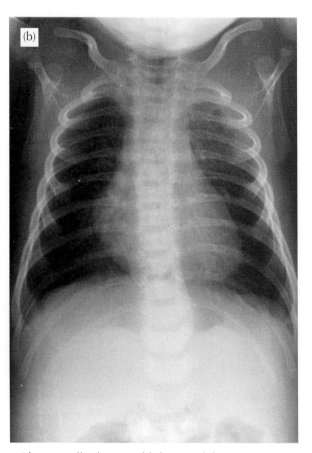

Fig. 20.9 (a) Chest X-ray taken on day 1 of life in an infant with prenatally diagnosed left upper lobe type 1 CCAM showing opacity due to delayed clearence of lung fluid; (b) Chest X-ray of the same infant on day 2 of life.

visible on close scrutiny and a CT scan will frequently show the lesion to be much more dramatic than expected (Fig. 20.10a, b). Whatever the decision made in the newborn period the lung should not be declared normal until CT or MRI has been performed. If a decision is made not to resect, long-term follow-up is essential.

PULMONARY SEQUESTRATION

Definition and clinical features

CCAM and pulmonary sequestration are known to be associated and in some cases there is an overlap of the two pathologies within the same patient (Samuel and Burge, 1996). Pulmonary sequestration is defined as a congenitally abnormal area of non-functioning lung tissue which does not communicate with the tracheo-bronchial tree and which receives its blood supply from anomalous systemic vessels. Two main types occur:

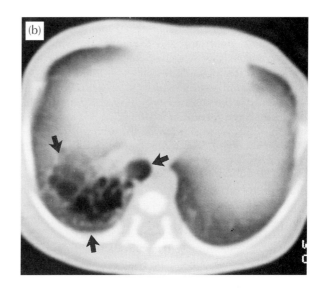

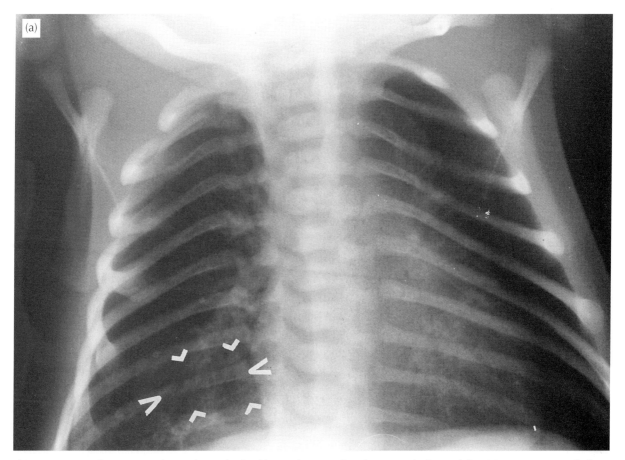

Fig. 20.10 (a) Chest X-ray of an infant who had been diagnosed as having right lower lobe CCAM on prenatal ultrasound. Although outlined with arrows, the lesion is virtually undetectable; (b) CT scan of the same infant showing clear cystic changes in the right lower lobe.

intralobar, in which the sequestrated lobe is contained within the normal lung and extralobar, in which the sequestration has its own visceral pleura and is separate from the normal pulmonary lobe.

Intralobar pulmonary sequestration (IPS) occurs predominantly in the posterior lateral basal segment of the left lower lobe. Arterial blood supply is via solitary or multiple moderate-sized vessels arising from the abdominal aorta (75%) or via arteries arising from the thoracic aorta or other abdominal vessels (25%) (Savic *et al.*, 1979; Stocker and Malczak, 1984). Venous drainage is usually into the pulmonary vein, although drainage into the hemiazygos and azygos veins occurs in one-third of the cases. IPS usually presents in older children as recurrent pneumonia, but it has been detected on prenatal ultrasonography scan and postnatal scans. Extralobar pulmonary sequestration (EPS) has been diagnosed by antenatal ultrasound scans at 19–20 weeks' gestational age (Romero *et al.*, 1982; Sauerbrei, 1991; Samuel and Burge, 1996). It is characteristically seen as a hyperechogenic mass in the posterior basal part of the left hemithorax. More often, EPS are detected during the management of infants with thoracic or cardiac anomalies. In 60% of EPS there is associated left-sided diaphragmatic hernia and there is a high incidence of other associated congenital anomalies (John *et al.*, 1989) such as CCAM, congenital cardiac anomalies, pericardial defects, pectus excavatum, bronchogenic cysts and vertebral anomalies. EPS may also occur below the diaphragm (Fig. 20.11).

Investigation

Plain radiology alone is not sufficient to make the diagnosis and some form of imaging to demonstrate the systemic arterial supply is required not only for diagnosis but also to facilitate surgery. Doppler ultrasonography scan is often able to do this and although angiography has been popular in the past, it has now been supplanted by MRI.

Treatment

The treatment of pulmonary sequestration is resection. This usually involves lobectomy for IPS, although EPS can usually be resected in isolation. Care must be taken in identifying the anomalous vessels and in securing control of these blood vessels to avoid torrential haemorrhage and operative mortality. Conservative management can be adopted following prenatal diagnosis but long-term follow-up is then indicated because of the risks of infection and possible malignancy.

BRONCHOGENIC CYST

These congenital cysts are derived from the primitive foregut and probably represent abnormal bronchial budding. They are rare but can present in adult life or be found incidentally at post-mortem (Opsahl and Berman, 1962). They can occur in the mediastinum, where they represent about 5% of mediastinal masses in children, within in the lung parenchyma, in the neck or attached to the chest wall. They vary in size from

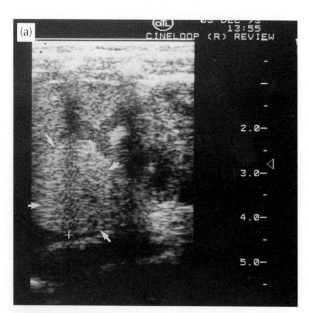
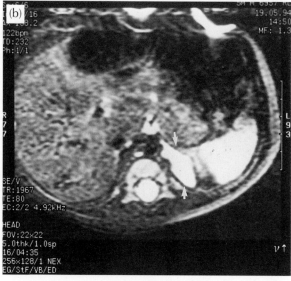

Fig. 20.11 (a) Prenatal ultrasound of a fetus with a left-sided suprarenal EPS (arrows); (b) postnatal MR scan in the same infant showing the lesion still present, although proportionally smaller. The lesion was asymptomatic but was excised at 9 months of age after the onset of respiratory symptoms (not due to the lesion) and increased parental anxiety. (Reproduced with permission from Samuel and Burge, 1996.)

2 to 10 cm in diameter and contain viscid, milky mucus although they may occasionally communicate with the airway.

Presentation is in one of four ways: as an incidental finding of a smooth mediastinal mass on chest X-ray (Fig. 20.12), as a cause of respiratory distress in infancy due to pressure on the airway, as a cause of recurrent or persistent pneumonia (when the cyst communicates with the bronchial tree), or on prenatal ultrasound scan.

Investigations should include plain radiology of the chest and cross-sectional imaging (CT or MRI) to define the exact location of the lesion and help with the differential diagnosis, particularly from solid lesions such as lymphoma and other tumours.

Treatment is by excision. This is usually very easy but may be made more difficult if the lesion is within the oesophageal or tracheal wall (Di Lorenzo *et al.*, 1989) or lung parenchyma. There is a temptation to manage asymptomatic lesions conservatively and this might be justifiable. However, in the knowledge that these lesions may become symptomatic if they enlarge and cause bronchial compression, and because sarcomatous change has been reported in such cysts (Krous and Sexauer, 1981), most authors still recommend excision.

One pitfall for the surgeon is that a bronchogenic cyst may cause bronchial compression and air-trapping in the neonate, producing a clinical presentation and radiological features identical to those in congenital lobar emphysema (Ramenovsky *et al.*, 1979). For this reason, careful inspection of the lung hilum at thoracotomy is essential prior to lobectomy for CLE.

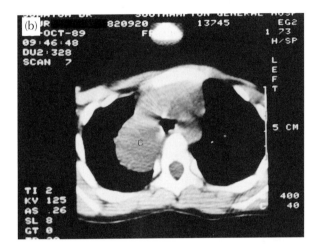

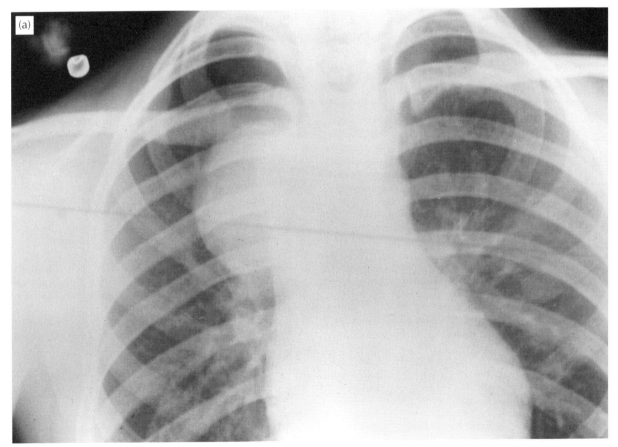

Fig. 20.12 (a) Chest X-ray showing a right-sided bronchogenic cyst; (b) CT scan of the same child showing a cyst (C).

The pleural cavity

CHYLOTHORAX

Chylothorax can occur secondarily to thoracic surgery or central venous thrombosis but it may also occur as a primary congenital phenomenon, possibly due to abnormal thoracic duct development. It is one of the causes of fetal pleural effusion and may produce sufficient fetal compromise to merit prenatal drainage (Puntis *et al.*, 1987).

Postnatal presentation is with respiratory distress with clinical and radiological features of pleural effusion. Diagnosis can be made on sampling the pleural fluid but this will only have the typical milky colour of chyle if the infant is receiving milk feeds. The diagnostic feature of the fluid is its high leucocyte content, of which 80–90% are lymphocytes (Puntis *et al.*, 1987).

Treatment involves tube drainage for around 3 weeks during which time the volume of chyle being produced should be minimized by the use of enteral feeds containing medium-chain trigyceride or by the use of parenteral nutrition. If the chyle leak persists after 3 weeks, surgical ligation of the thoracic duct leak (if it can be located) (Curci and Dibbins, 1980), pleurodesis or pleural fluid shunting (Kirkland 1965; Azizkhan *et al.*, 1983) should be undertaken. Persistence with conservative management carries a high mortality (Azizkhan *et al.*, 1983).

References

Adzick, N.S. and Harrison, M.R. 1993: Management of the fetus with a cystic adenomatoid malformation [Review]. *World Journal of Surgery* **17**, 342–9.

Adzick, N.S., Harrison, M.R., Flake, A.W., Howell, L.J., Golbus, M.S. and Filly, R.A. 1993: Fetal surgery for cystic adenomatoid malformation of the lung. *Journal of Pediatric Surgery* **28**, 806–12.

Altman, R.P., Randolph, J.G. and Shearin, R.B. 1972: Tracheal agenesis: a clinical approach. *Journal of Pediatric Surgery* **7**, 112–18.

Atkinson, J.B. Ford, E.G., Kitagawa, H., Lally, K.P. and Humphries, B. 1992: Persistent pulmonary hypertension complicating cystic adenomatoid malformation in neonates. *Journal of Pediatric Surgery* **27**, 54–6.

Azizkhan, R.G., Canfieldood, J., Alford, B.A. and Rogers, B.M. 1983: Pleuroperitoneal shunts in the management of neonatal chylothorax. *Journal of Pediatric Surgery* **18**, 842–9.

Azizkhan, R.G., Grimmer, D.L., Askin, F.B., Lacey, S.R., Merten, D.F. and Wood, R.E. 1992: Acquired lobar emphysema (overinflation): clinical and pathological evaluation of infants requiring lobectomy. *Journal of Pediatric Surgery* **27**, 1145–52.

Bagwell, C.E., Marchildon, M.B. and Pratt, L.L. 1987: Anterior cricoid split for subglottic stenosis. *Journal of Pediatric Surgery* **22**, 740–2.

Baxter, J.D. and Dunbar, J.S. 1963: Tracheomalacia. *Annals of Otology, Rhinology and Laryngology* **72**, 1013–23.

Benjamin, D.R. and Cahill, J.L. 1991: Bronchioloalveolar carcinoma of the lung and congenital cystic adenomatoid malformation. *American Journal of Clinical Pathology* **95**, 889–92.

Benjamin, B., Freeman, N.V., Burge, D.M., Griffiths, D.M. and Malone, P.S. (eds) 1994: *Surgery of the newborn*, vol. 31, Airway obstruction, Part 1: Laryngeal obstruction. Edinburgh: Churchill Livingstone, 409–24.

Benjamin, B. and Inglis, A. 1989: Minor congenital laryngeal clefts: diagnosis and classification. *Annals of Otology, Rhinology and Laryngology* **98**, 417–20.

Benjamin, B. and Walker P. 1991: Management of airway obstruction in the Pierre Robin sequence. *International Journal of Pediatric Otorhinology* **22**, 29–37.

Booth, P., Nicolaides, K.H., Greenough, A. and Gamsu, H.R. 1987: Pleuro-amniotic shunting for fetal chylothorax *Early Human Developement* **15**, 365–7.

Buntain, W.L., Isaacs, H., Payne, V.C. *et al.* 1974: Lobar emphysema, cystic adenomatoid malformation, pulmonary sequestration and bronchogenic cyst in infancy and childhood. *Journal of Pediatric Surgery* **9**, 85–93.

Ch'in, K.Y. and Tangery, M.Y. 1949: Congenital adenomatoid malformation of one lobe of a lung with general anasarca. *Archives of Pathology* **48**, 221.

Cotton, R.T. 1984: Paediatric laryngotracheal stenosis. *Journal of Pediatric Surgery* **19**, 699–704.

Cotton, R.T. 1991: Cricoid release in a preterm neonate. *Journal of Laryngology and Otology* **105**, 398.

Cremin, B.J. and Movsowitz H. 1971: Lobar emphysema in infants. *British Journal of Radiology* **44**, 692–6.

Crockett, D.M., Healy, G.B., McGill, T.J. and Friedman, E.M. 1987: Computed tomography in the evaluation of choanal atresia in infants and children. *Laryngoscope* **97**, 174–83.

Crombleholme, T.M., Adzick, N.S., Hardy, K. *et al.* 1990: Pulmonary lobar transplantation in neonatal swine: a model for treatment of congenital diaphragmatic hernia. *Journal of Pediatric Surgery* **25**, 11–18.

Curci, M.R. and Dibbins, A.W. 1980: Bilateral chylothorax in the newborn. *Journal of Pediatric Surgery* **15**, 663–5.

Di Lorenzo, M., Collin, P.P., Vaillancourt, R. and Duranceau, A. 1989: Bronchogenic cysts. *Journal of Pediatric Surgery* **24**, 988–91.

Donahoe, P.K. and Gee, P.E. 1984: Complete laryngeotracheoesophageal cleft: management and repair. *Journal of Pediatric Surgery* **19**, 143–7.

Eigen, H., Lemen, R.I. and Waring, W.W. 1976: Congenital lobar emphysema: long term evaluation of surgically and conservatively treated children. *American Review of Respiratory Disease* **113**, 823–31.

Filler, R.M., Messineo, A. and Vinograd, I. 1992: Severe tracheomalacia associated with esophageal atresia: results of surgical treatment. *Journal of Pediatric Surgery* **27**, 1136–41.

Fine, C., Adzick, N.S. and Doubilet, P.M. 1988: Decrease in size of a congenital adenomatoid malformation *in utero*. *Journal of Ultrasound in Medicine* **7**, 405–8.

Gross, R.E. and Neuhauser, E.B.D. 1948: Compression of the trachea by an anomalous innominate artery. An operation for its relief. *American Journal of Diseases in Children* **75**, 570–4.

Gumbiner, C.H., Mullins, C.E. and McNamara, D.G. 1980: Pulmonary artery sling. *American Journal of Cardiology* **45**, 311–15.

Haddon, M.J. and Bowen, A. 1991: Bronchopulmonary and neurenteric forms of foregut anomalies. Imaging for diagnosis and management. *Radiological Clinics of North America* **29**, 241–54.

Hislop, A. and Reid, L. 1970: New pathological findings in emphysema of childhood. 1. Polyalveolar lobe with emphysema. *Thorax* **25**, 682–90.

Hof, E., Hirsigery, J., Giedion, A. and Pochon, J.P. 1987: Deleterious consequences of gastroesophageal reflux in cleft larynx surgery. *Journal of Pediatric Surgery* **22**, 197–9.

Hoffman, M.A. Superina, R. and Wesson, D.E. 1989: Unilateral pulmonary agenesis with esophageal atresia and distal tracheoesophageal fistula: report of two cases. *Journal of Pediatric Surgery* **24**, 1084–5.

Holinger, P.H. 1961: Clinical aspects of congenital anomalies of the larynx, trachea, bronchi and esophagus. *Journal of Otolaryngology* **75**, 1–44.

Ingelvans, P. and Debengny, P. 1965: Sternal cleft and tracheal haemangioma. *Annals of Chirurge* **6**, 123–8.

John, P.R., Beasley, S.W. and Mayne, V. 1989: Pulmonary sequestration and related congenital disorders. A clinical–radiological review of 41 cases. *Pediatric Radiology* **20**, 4–9.

Jonas, R.A., Spevak, P.J., McGildool, T. and Castaneda, A.R. 1989: Pulmonary artery sling primary repair by tracheal resection in infancy. *Journal of Thoracic and Cardiovascular Surgery* **97**, 548–50.

Jones, J.C., Almond, C.H., Snyder, H.M. *et al.* 1965: Lobar emphysema and congenital heart disease in infancy. *Journal of Thoracic and Cardiovascular Surgery* **49**, 1–10.

Kennedy, C.D., Habibi, P., Matthew, D.J. *et al.* 1991: Lobar emphysema: long term imaging follow-up. *Radiology* **180**, 189–93.

Kiely, E.M. 1987: Management of tracheomalacia by aortopexy. *Paediatric Surgery International* **2**, 13–15.

Kimura, K., Mukohara, N., Tsugawa, C. *et al.* 1982: Tracheoplasty for congenital stenosis of the entire trachea. *Journal of Pediatric Surgery* **17**, 869–71.

Kirkland, I. 1965: Chylothorax in infancy and childhood. A method of treatment. *Archives of Disease in Childhood* **40**, 186–91.

Kosloske, A.M. 1991: Left mainstem bronchopexy for severe bronchomalacia. *Journal of Pediatric Surgery* **26**, 260–2.

Krous, H.F. and Sexauer, C.L. 1981: Embryonal rhabdomyosarcoma arising within a congenital bronchogenic cyst in a child. *Journal of Pediatric Surgery* **16**, 506–8.

Landing, B.H. and Dixon, L.G. 1979: Congenital malformations and genetic disorders of the respiratory tract. *American Review of Respiratory Diseases* **120**, 151–5.

Longaker, M.T., Harrison, M.R. and Adzick, N.S. 1990: Testing the limits of neonatal tracheal resection. *Journal of Pediatric Surgery* **25**, 790–2.

Lorimier, A.A., de, Welch, K.J., Randolph, J.G., Ravitch, M.M., O'Neill, J.A. and Rowe, M.I. (eds) 1986: *Pediatric Surgery*, 4th ed, vol. 62, *Congenital malformations and neonatal problems of the respiratory tract*. Chicago, IL: Year Book Medical Publications, 631–44.

McCullagh, M., MacConnachie, I., Garvie, D. and Dykes, E. 1994: Accuracy of prenatal diagnosis of congenital cystic adenomatoid malformation. *Archives of Disease in Childhood* **71**, F111–13.

MacGillivray, T.E., Harrison, M.R., Goldstein, R.B. and Adzick, N.S. 1993: Disappearing fetal lung lesions. *Journal of Pediatric Surgery* **28**, 1321–4.

Mair, E.A., Parsons, D.S. and Lally, K.P. 1990: Treatment of severe bronchomalacia with expanding endobronchial stents. *Archives of Otolaryngology and Head and Neck Surgery* **116**, 1087–90.

Man, D.K.W., Hamdy, M.H., Hendry, G.M.A., *et al.* Congenital lobar emphysema. *Archives of Disease in Childhood* **58**, 709–12.

Marmon, L.M., Bye, M.R., Haas, I.M,, Rohinton, K.B. and Dunn, T.M. 1984: Vascular rings and slings: long term follow up of pulmonary function. *Journal of Pediatric Surgery* **19** 683–92.

May, A.D., Barth, A.R., Yeageryer, S. *et al.* 1993: Perinatal and postnatal sonography. *Radiological Clinics of North America* **31**, 499–516.

Mentzer, S.J., Filler, R.M. and Phillips, J. 1992: Limited pulmonary resections for congenital cystic adenomatoid malformation of the lung. *Journal of Pediatric Surgery* **27**, 1410–13.

Miller, R.K., Sieber, W.K. and Yunis, E.J. 1980: Congenital cystic adenomatoid malformation of the lung: a report of 17 cases and review of the literature. *Pathological Annals* **1**, 387–407.

Murphy, J.J., Blair, G.K., Fraser, G.C. *et al.* 1992: Rhabdomyosarcoma arising within congenital pulmonary cysts: report of three cases. *Journal of Pediatric Surgery* **27**, 1364–7.

Nakayama, D.K., Harrison, M.R., de Lorimier, A.A., Brasch, R.C. and Fishman, N.H. 1982: Reconstructive surgery for obstructive lesions of the intrathoracic trachea in infants and small children. *Journal of Pediatric Surgery* **17**, 854–68.

Neilson, I.R., Russo, P., Laberge, J. *et al.* 1991: Congenital adenomatoid malformation of the lung: current management and prognosis. *Journal of Pediatric Surgery* **26**, 975–81.

Nishibayashi, S.W., Andrassy, R.I. and Wooley, M.M. 1981: Congenital cystic adenomatoid malformation: a 30 year experience. *Journal of Pediatric Surgery* **16**, 704–7.

Opsahl, T. and Berman, E.J. 1962: Bronchogenic mediastinal cysts in infants. Case report and review of the literature. *Pediatrics* **30**, 372.

Pagon, R.A., Graham, J.M., Zonana, J. and Yong, S. 1981: Coloboma, congenital heart disease and choanal atresia with multiple anomalies: CHARGE association. *Journal of Pediatrics* **99**, 223–7.

Prescott, C.A.J. 1995: Nasal obstruction in infancy. *Archives of Disease in Childhood* **72**, 287–9.

Pritchard, M.G., Brown, P.J.E. and Sterrett, G.F. 1984: Bronchioalveolar carcinoma arising in longstanding lung cysts. *Thorax* **39**, 545–459.

Puntis, J.W.L., Roberts, K.D. and Handy, D. 1987: How should chylothorax be managed? *Archives of Disease in Childhood* **62**, 593–6.

Ramenofsky, M.L., Leape, L.L. and McCauley, G.K. 1979: Bronchogenic cyst. *Journal of Pediatric Surgery* **14**, 219–24.

Raviewitch, M.M. and Hardy, J.B. 1949: Congenital cystic disease of the lung in infants and children *Archives of Surgery* **59**, 1.

Richards, D.S., Langham, M.R., Jr and Dolson, L.H. 1992: Antenatal presentation of a child with congenital lobar emphysema. *Journal of Ultrasound in Medicine* **11**, 165–8.

Romero, R., Chervenak, F.A., Kotzen, J. *et al.* 1982: Antenatal sonographic findings of extralobar pulmonary sequestration. *Journal of Ultrasound Medicine* **1**, 131–2.

Samuel, M. and Burge, D.M. 1996: Extra-lobar pulmonary sequestration. *European Journal of Pediatric Surgery* **6**, 107.

Sauerbrei, E. 1991: Lung sequestration. Duplex Doppler diagnosis at 19 weeks gestation. *Journal of Ultrasound Medicine* **10**, 101–5.

Savic, B., Birtel, F.J., Tholin, W. *et al.* 1979: Lung sequestration: report of 7 cases and review of 540 published cases. *Thorax* **34**, 96–101.

Sbokos, C.G. and McMilan, I.K.R. 1977: Agenesis of the lung. *British Journal of Diseases of the Chest* **71**, 183.

Sheffield, E.A., Addis, B.J., Corrin, B. *et al.* 1987: Epithelial hyperplasia and malignant change in congenital lung cysts. *Journal of Clinical Pathology* **40**, 612–14.

Soosay, G.N., Baudouin, S.V., Hanson, P.J. *et al.* 1992: Symptomatic cysts in otherwise normal lungs of children and adults. *Histopathology* **20**, 517–22.

Stanger, P., Lucas, R.V. and Redward, J.E. 1969: Anatomic factors causing respiratory distress in acyanotic congenital heart disease. *Pediatrics* **43**, 760.

Stigers, K.B., Woodring, J.H. and Kanga, J.F. 1992: The clinical and imaging spectrum of findings in patients with congenital lobar emphysema. *Pediatric Pulmonology* **14**, 160–70.

Stocker, J.T. and Malczak, H.T. 1984: A study of pulmonary ligament arteries: relationship to intralobar sequestration. *Chest* **86**, 611–15.

Stocker, J.T., Madewell, J.E. and Drake, R.M. 1977: Congenital cystic adenomatoid malformation of the lung. *Human Pathology* **8**, 155–77.

Strife, I.L., Baumel, A.S. and Scott Dunbar, J. 1981: Tracheal compression by the innominate artery in infancy and childhood. *Radiology* **139**, 73–5.

Trapper, D., Shuster, S., McBride, J. *et al.* 1980: Polyalveolar lobe: anatomic and physiologic parameters and their relationship to congenital lobar emphysema. *Journal of Pediatric Surgery* **15**, 931–7.

Wailoo, M.P. and Emery, I.L. 1979: The trachea in children with tracheo-oesophageal fistula. *Histopathology* **3**, 329–38.

Weinberg, A.G., Currarino,G., Moore, G.C. *et al.* 1980: Mesenchymal neoplasia and congenital pulmonary cysts. *Pediatric Radiology* **9**, 179–82.

Wolf, S.A., Hertzler, J.H. and Philippart, A.I. 1980: Cystic adenomatoid dysplasia of the lung. *Journal of Pediatric Surgery* **15**, 925–8.

CHAPTER 21

Oesophageal atresia and tracheo-oesophageal fistula

S.W. BEASLEY

Introduction
Diagnosis of oesophageal atresia
Anatomical types

Management
Tracheo-oesophageal fistula (the 'H' fistula)
Further reading

Introduction

Oesophageal atresia is a congenital abnormality in which a variable length of the midportion of the oesophagus is missing. In about 85% of affected infants there is a communication between the distal oesophagus and the trachea, called a distal tracheo-oesophageal fistula.

Diagnosis of oesophageal atresia

The diagnosis of oesophageal atresia could be established at birth if obstetric units followed the practice of routine passage (or attempted passage) of a tube into the stomach in all babies at birth. This routine is not widely practised and has the potential disadvantage to the baby of inadvertently injuring the larynx, and may induce apnoea.

Any baby drooling excessive saliva (the 'mucousy baby') should be assumed to have oesophageal atresia. The diagnosis is confirmed when a size 10 orogastric catheter cannot be passed through the mouth into the stomach. A history of maternal polyhydramnios during pregnancy in an infant born slightly prematurely heightens the suspicion of oesophageal atresia.

If, for some reason the diagnosis is not made at birth and feeding is commenced, explosive rejection of the first feed will occur, usually with cyanosis, choking and respiratory distress. This should immediately alert the clinician to the correct diagnosis. Sometimes, the infant may suffer cyanotic attacks without feeding.

Where possible the diagnosis should be made prior to feeding. Milk entering an obstructed oesophagus has a high chance of being aspirated into the lungs and causing an aspiration pneumonia. The situations in which oesophageal atresia should be suspected are summarized in Table 21.1.

If the diagnosis is suspected, an attempt should be made to insert a relatively stiff 10 English gauge orogastric catheter through the mouth into the oesophagus (Fig. 21.1). If the catheter cannot be introduced beyond 9–13 cm from the gums, the diagnosis of oesophageal

Table 21.1 When to suspect oesophageal atresia

- The baby is excessively mucousy or is drooling saliva
- There are cyanotic episodes (due to aspiration of saliva which has accumulated in the blind upper oesophageal pouch) and/or respiratory distress shortly after birth
- There is a history of maternal polyhydramnios
- There are other abnormalities, e.g. imperforate anus, radial dysplasia, which are known to occur in association with oesophageal atresia

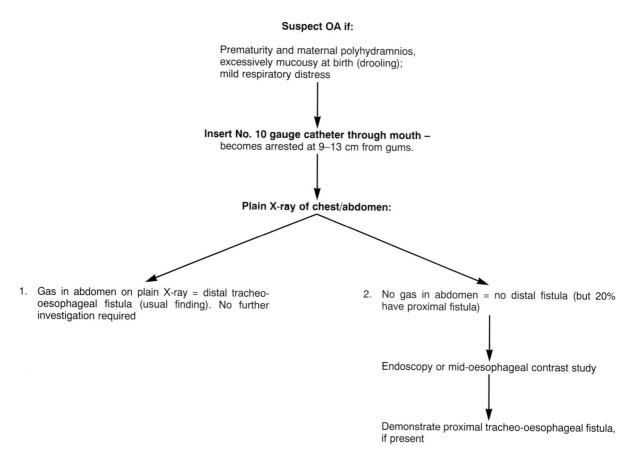

Suspect OA if:

Prematurity and maternal polyhydramnios,
excessively mucousy at birth (drooling);
mild respiratory distress

Insert No. 10 gauge catheter through mouth –
becomes arrested at 9–13 cm from gums.

Plain X-ray of chest/abdomen:

1. Gas in abdomen on plain X-ray = distal tracheo-oesophageal fistula (usual finding). No further investigation required

2. No gas in abdomen = no distal fistula (but 20% have proximal fistula)

Endoscopy or mid-oesophageal contrast study

Demonstrate proximal tracheo-oesophageal fistula, if present

Fig. 21.1 Diagnosis of oesophageal atresia.

atresia is established, and the baby should be transferred to a tertiary paediatric centre for further investigation and management. No further delineation of the anatomy is required before transfer.

A tube of smaller calibre is not used because it may curl up in the upper pouch and give a misleading impression of oesophageal continuity. Introduction of the tube through the nose should not be attempted because it may injure the nasal passages, which are small in a newborn infant. Contrast studies, if any are required, should be performed after transfer to the tertiary institution.

Anatomical types

The majority of infants with oesophageal atresia have a distal tracheo-oesophageal fistula. Therefore, gas will be present in the bowel below the diaphragm, from passage through the fistula. If there is no gas in the abdomen for longer than a few minutes after birth, the patient is unlikely to have a distal tracheo-oesophageal fistula, although in about 20% of these there will be a proximal tracheo-oesophageal fistula (Fig. 21.1).

ASSOCIATED ANOMALIES

Major associated congenital anomalies are present in about 50% of babies with oesophageal atresia. When a baby is diagnosed at birth as having oesophageal atresia it is necessary to examine the infant for one or more associated anomalies (Fig. 21.2). The commonest anomalies belong to the VATER association, and include vertebral (V), imperforate anus (A), radial aplasia (R), renal/or urinary tract abnormalities and congenital heart disease. Major chromosomal abnormalities (e.g. trisomy 13, 18 or 21) and the CHARGE association (*c*oloboma, *c*hoanal *a*tresia, congenital *h*eart disease, *g*enital anomalies and *e*ar abnormality) are encountered frequently.

Management

MEDICAL CARE BEFORE AND DURING TRANSPORT

General considerations

Handling should be kept to a minimum because excessive disturbance increases the infant's oxygen con-

? Associated abnormalities

Clinical inspection	Plain X-ray	Urine passed (prior to surgery)	Echocardiograph
Look for:	1. Vertebral: (e.g. hemivertebrae)	**Yes**: Proceed to surgery	? Duct-dependent cardiac lesion
1. Features of VATER association:	2. Rib (e.g. super-numerary; bifid or absent)	**No**: Do renal ultrasound to confirm presence of renal tissue	**No**: Repair OA
• imperforate anus • radial aplaisia • syndactyly	3. Duodenal atresia: 'double bubble'	Kidney present but ultrasound abnormality ↓	**Yes**: Commence PGE₁ infusion ↓
2. Features of chromo-somal abnormality:		MCU ± other tests as indicated after OA repair	Repair OA when infant stable
• rocker bottom feet • Downs' syndrome • If suspected, consult geneticist + chromo-somal studies			

Fig. 21.2 Investigation of associated abnormalities in oesophageal atresia.

sumption, exposes the infant to cold stress and, if unstable, may cause dramatic cardiovascular responses. Care must be exercised to avoid excessive cooling in the delivery room and during subsequent stabilization and transport. The environmental temperature required in a standard incubator in the first 6 hours of life according to birth weight is shown in Table 21.2.

Oxygen therapy

A number of infants with oesophageal atresia will have respiratory distress, either because of prematurity, other congenital abnormalities or aspiration pneumonia, or from diaphragmatic splinting caused by excessive escape of air through the distal fistula into the stomach. If no blood gas monitoring facilities are available, the infant must be kept pink at all times: it is preferable to have several hours of hyperoxia than a short period of hypoxia.

Posture

In general, the infant in transport should be nursed in the right lateral position to assist the infant in main-

Table 21.2 Incubator temperature required

Weight (g)	Incubator temperature (°C)
< 1000	35–37
1000–1500	34–36
1500–2000	33–35
200–2500	32–34
> 2500	30–31

taining a clear airway should any fluid enter the pharynx. This will also minimize regurgitation of gastric contents up the distal tracheo-oesophageal fistula, and will decrease the work of breathing and improve oxygenation. The neonate depends almost entirely on contraction of the diaphragm for effective ventilation, which is more easily accomplished in this position.

Care of the upper pouch

The upper oesophagus should be suctioned intermittently to remove accumulating saliva. This should be done at least every 10–15 min, irrespective of whether there appears to be any excessive secretions or not, and more often if necessary. Saliva may accumulate in large volumes in the upper pouch, regurgitate suddenly and be aspirated into the lungs if not sucked out. Occasionally, a distended upper pouch may compress the trachea from behind, particularly if tracheomalacia is marked.

The suction catheter should be firm but soft, such as 8 or 10 gauge. Y-suction catheters are preferred, because they enable pressure adjustment to minimize oesophageal mucosal damage.

Gentle handling

The infant should be handled gently to minimize crying, since crying tends to fill the stomach with air. This, in turn, increases the likelihood of regurgitation of gastric contents into the trachea, increases abdominal distension and impedes ventilation.

Care of associated medical problems

One-third of infants with oesophageal atresia are premature. Therefore they require attention to temperature control, oxygen therapy, and earlier fluid and dextrose solution resuscitation, to limit the problems of apnoea, respiratory distress and hypoglycaemia. The majority of infants with oesophageal atresia and respiratory distress can be managed with increased ambient oxygen concentration, but about 7% will require ventilation in transit. This presents problems if the ventilation pressures are high, since gastric distension (and rupture) may develop, making ventilation more difficult. This problem can be reduced by placing the tip of the endotracheal tube just proximal to the carina but distal to the fistula. Infants with intrauterine growth retardation are at risk of hypoglycaemia, which must be avoided.

Care of the family

The parents should be given an honest appraisal of the situation, and provided there are no associated severe congenital abnormalities, the prognosis for survival is excellent. An outline of the nature of oesophageal atresia should be given, and the parents should be informed of the transport planned and of what to expect at the tertiary institution, with details of the receiving unit, including names of the personnel who will be caring for their infant, if these are known.

The transfer of their infant can leave an enormous sense of loss in parents. It is thus of great importance for them to view, and if practicable to touch, stroke and cuddle their infant before transfer. A Polaroid photograph of the infant left with the parents is often helpful. Parents may require advice on their own travel and accommodation arrangements if they live far from the neonatal receiving unit.

SURGICAL TREATMENT

Prior to surgery, a renal ultrasound is obtained if the infant has not passed urine, because in about 3% of cases there is inadequate renal tissue for long-term survival (e.g. bilateral severely dysplastic kidneys or bilateral renal agenesis), in which situation no surgery is justified. An echocardiogram is obtained, because 25% of infants with oesophageal atresia have congenital heart disease. It is important to identify duct-dependent cardiac lesions preoperatively so that a prostaglandin E_1 infusion can commence before repair of the oesophagus. In most babies, congenital heart disease does not delay the oesophageal surgery and oesophageal repair usually takes precedence over surgery to the heart. An echocardiograph may also identify a right aortic arch and influence the surgical approach to the oesophagus.

Timing of surgery

Complete correction of the abnormality is performed as a single operation shortly after birth, following the renal ultrasound and echocardiogram. The distal tracheo-oesophageal fistula is divided and the upper oesophageal segment anastomosed to the lower segment with interrupted single-layer sutures as an end-to-end anastomosis. Postoperatively, oral feeds can be commenced on about the third day.

The operative procedure

The infant is placed in the full lateral position with the right side uppermost and a towel folded underneath the body to give lateral flexion. The right arm is raised over the head to facilitate the thoracic approach. A transverse incision is made just below and centred on the angle of the scapula and, after division of fibres of the latissimus dorsi in the line of the incision, the posterior fibres of the serratus interior are divided near their origin, as low as possible in the incision, thus preserving the muscles' innervation. The chest is entered through the fourth intercostal space and the pleura swept off the chest wall. The oesophagus is approached in this extrapleural plane, and the azygos vein is ligated and divided.

After incision of the fine endothoracic fascia of the posterior mediastinum, the lower oesophagus can be found immediately anterior to the aorta, and is highlighted by vagal fibres running along its surface. The communication of the oesophagus to the trachea is exposed. A vascular sling may be passed around the fistula where the upper part of the lower oesophageal segment joins the trachea, once the angle between the oesophagus and trachea has been dissected clear. Care is taken to avoid damage to the vagus nerves and blood supply of the oesophagus. The tracheo-oesophageal fistula is closed with 4/0 or 5/0 polyglycolic acid transfixion sutures, and divided.

The fundus of the upper oesophageal segment can be readily identified within the chest, once the anaesthetist passes a catheter into it. A stay suture, passed through its lowest part, assists its mobilization and avoids unnecessary handling of (and trauma to) the oesophagus. The upper oesophagus can be mobilized as far as the cricopharyngeus muscle, should it be necessary to make the oesophageal anastomosis without excessive tension. Once the upper segment has been mobilized, its most dependent part is opened. In many instances, the gap between the oesophageal ends is such that little mobilization is required.

The end-to-end oesophago-oesophageal anastomosis is now constructed by inserting three interrupted 5/0 polyglycolic acid sutures in the posteromedial aspect (furthest away) of the oesophagus, taking in all layers, with moderately large 'bites' of tissue. Special care must be taken to ensure that the mucosal layer of the upper pouch is included, because it tends to retract upwards out of view when the upper pouch is opened. When the three sutures have been placed, the oesophageal ends are gently apposed and the sutures tied on the mucosal surface. The orogastric tube can now be passed through the upper oesophagus into the lower segment, before completion of the anastomosis with a further four to six all-layers, interrupted sutures, with the knots tied on the outside.

Before closure, the orogastric tube is removed (unless gavage feeding is planned, as in the premature infant) and the thoracic cavity is irrigated with warm antibiotic saline solution. This fluid allows confirmation that there is no air leakage from the closed fistula with ventilation. A chest drain is not normally required, unless there is concern about the integrity of the anastomosis.

Intraoperative difficulties

Right aortic arch

This may be suspected on the plain film of the chest or by preoperative echocardiography. If diagnosed preoperatively, the operation is best performed through a left thoracotomy. If the right arch is first recognized during a right thoracotomy, it may still be possible to achieve an anastomosis from this side. An anastomosis to the right of a right arch does not usually cause compression of the oesophagus and has the advantage of being relatively easy to perform when the arch would otherwise obscure the level of the anastomosis. When an anastomosis would be difficult to construct from the right, the right thoracotomy is best closed, the infant repositioned, and a left thoracotomy performed.

Identification of lower oesophagus

The location of the lower oesophagus may not be immediately apparent, particularly if there is no distal fistula. In this situation, the vagus nerves may act as a guide to its location. They can be recognized as fine white fibres, which leave the posterolateral aspect of the trachea to sweep downwards and encompass the lower oesophagus. These fibres should not be divided or have traction applied to them during dissection of the tracheo-oesophageal junction or mobilization of the oesophagus.

Continuous oesophagus

Apparent continuity of the oesophagus at thorocotomy may lead the surgeon to believe the preoperative diagnosis to be incorrect. However, the lumen may be obstructed even though it appears intact externally. Advancement of the catheter in the upper oesophagus peroperatively by the anaesthetist will clarify the level of obstruction.

Double fistula

The surgeon should be aware of the possibility of a second (upper pouch) fistula, which may extend upwards from the oesophagus to the trachea. A proximal fistula is rare when there is a distal fistula. Clues to its presence include distension of the upper oesophagus during ventilatory inspiration and difficulty in separating the oesophagus from the trachea during upper pouch mobilization. Where routine preoperative endoscopy is performed, it can be diagnosed during bronchoscopy prior to surgery.

COMPLICATIONS

A number of problems may occur following repair of oesophageal atresia. Some, such as anastomotic leak, recurrent tracheo-oesophageal fistula and a shelf at the site of anastomosis, are the result of technical inadequacies, whereas others, such as poor oesophageal clearance and gastro-oesophageal reflux causing the late development of a stricture, reflect abnormalities more directly related to the oesophageal atresia itself.

Anastomotic leak

Leakage from an oesophageal anastomosis represents a serious complication of repair of oesophageal atresia. The likelihood of an anastomotic leak occurring depends on the type of anastomosis employed, and the extent of mobilization of the oesophagus. An interrupted, all-layers, end-to-end oesophageal anastomosis using an absorbable suture appears to have the lowest leakage and stricture rate, making it the anastomosis of choice. Leakage from an anastomosis may vary enormously in significance, from a minor radiological leak in an otherwise well infant (for which no treatment is required) to complete anastomotic disruption with mediastinitis, empyema, pneumothorax and septicaemia. Factors that contribute to anastomotic leakage include: incorrectly placed sutures, insecure sutures, excessive tension at the anastomosis, ischaemia of the oesophageal ends and sepsis. The extent of the oesophageal dissection undertaken is the balance between that dissection required to gain adequate length to avoid excessive tension at the anastomosis, and damage to the blood supply of both oesophageal ends which may occur when the oesophagus is mobilized extensively or oesophageal myotomy is performed. There is a relationship between leakage and subsequent stricture formation and recurrent tracheo-oesophageal fistula.

In most infants an anastomotic leak can be managed non-operatively. Safe total parenteral nutrition enables oral feeds to be ceased. Antibiotics are commenced and the leak will usually close spontaneously. Cervical oesophagostomy is only rarely necessary, when supportive therapy has been unsuccessful and there is ongoing difficult-to-control sepsis. A long-standing leak may require gastrostomy to allow continuation of enteral feeds.

Recurrent tracheo-oesophageal fistula

A recurrent tracheo-oesophageal fistula is a severe and potentially dangerous complication. Failure to close the fistula adequately at the time of surgery and subsequent anastomotic leak with local infection increase the chance of developing a recurrent fistula. The use of silk appears to be another predisposing factor.

The development of coughing, gagging, choking, cyanosis, apnoca, dying spells and recurrent chest infections suggests that a recurrent tracheo-oesophageal fistula has developed. The typical presentation is that of an infant who coughs and splutters with each feed. The most reliable method of confirming the diagnosis is cineradiographic tube oesophagography with the patient in the prone position. Barium is introduced through a nasogastric tube positioned in the oesophagus as the tube is gradually withdrawn. Bronchoscopy is an alternative method.

Spontaneous closure of recurrent fistulae is unlikely. Most centres wait for at least 4 weeks from the first operation before closing a recurrent fistula. A thorocotomy is performed through the original incision when the child is in optimal respiratory and general condition following a period of intravenous nutrition. The fistula is divided via a transpleural approach. Some surgeons like to pass a fine ureteric catheter through the fistula endoscopically to facilitate its localization, and some surgeons place mediastinal tissue between the ends of the divided fistula in an attempt to prevent a further recurrence.

Anastomotic stricture

Anastomotic stricture is the most common reason for further surgery to the oesophagus being required after repair of oesophageal atresia. Factors that influence the development of an oesophageal stricture include rough handling of the oesophagus at the time of repair, ischaemia of the oesophageal ends, excessive tension of the oesophageal anastomosis, the choice of suture material (e.g. silk), anastomotic leak or dehiscence, the use of a two-layer anastomosis and gastro-oesophageal reflux. Gastro-oesophageal reflux is the most common cause of late stricture development.

Patients with a stricture develop feeding difficulties and dysphagia, the onset of which may be insidious. The first symptom is often that they are slow feeders and have excessive regurgitation, with or without cyanotic episodes. Older children present with foreign body impaction of food in the oesophagus. Diagnosis is confirmed by barium swallow or endoscopy.

In patients with mild narrowing of the oesophagus, one or two dilatations may be all that is required. However, in patients with associated gastro-oesophageal reflux, it will usually be necessary to perform an anti-reflux operation (e.g. Nissen fundoplication), after which the stricture will resolve.

Motility problems

Oesophageal motility is abnormal, both before and after repair of oesophageal atresia. It is likely that vagal fibres are injured during mobilization of the oesophagus, worsening the already abnormal oesophageal motility. Oesophageal motility tends to improve gradually with age, but children with oesophageal atresia often need to drink with their meals. Abnormal oesophageal motility may contribute to oesophagitis and oesophageal stricture formation in the presence of gastro-oesophageal reflux: the fact that the oesophagus does not empty normally allows acidic gastric juice to sit in the lower oesophagus for a longer period than in patients with normal muscular action.

Oesophageal diverticulum and shelf

A pseudodiverticulum may occur following leakage from the oesophageal anastomosis. Ballooning at the site of a circular myotomy is common and may result in a diverticulum. A shelf at the site of the oesophageal anastomosis occurs when the upper oesophageal pouch has been opened eccentrically, or the end-to-end oesophageal anastomosis has not been performed with sufficient precision.

OESOPHAGEAL ATRESIA WITHOUT FISTULA

When there is no tracheo-oesophageal fistula present, there is almost always a substantial gap between the oesophageal ends. Sometimes there is virtually no lower oesophageal segment above the level of the diaphragm. Figure 21.3 provides guidelines for the management of long-gap oesophageal atresia. The absence of a fistula and long-gap oesophageal atresia may produce a number of specific surgical problems, which are described below.

Small stomach

Where there is no distal tracheo-oesophageal fistula the stomach is small, as a result of the inability of the fetus to swallow amniotic fluid or of fluid to enter the stomach through the distal fistula. The significance of this relates to the problems created by a small stomach when a gastrostomy is being fashioned so as not to compromise later gastric interposition (if required) or a subsequent antireflux operation.

Assessment of length of gap

The length of the upper segment of the oesophagus can be demonstrated by a contrast study (performed to

A. Suspect 'long gap' if:

1. Gasless abdomen on plain X-ray
2. Proximal tracheo-oesophageal fistula
3. OA and cleft palate
4. Short (i.e. high) upper pouch on plain X-ray

B. Assessment of length of cap: (under GA, using image intensifier)

- Gastrostomy and pass metal sound through gastro-oesophageal junction up into lower oesophageal segment
- Anaesthetist simultaneously passes radio-opaque tube into upper pouch

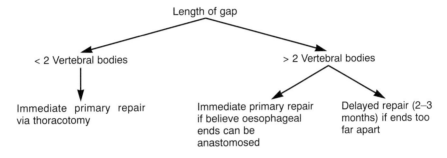

Length of gap

< 2 Vertebral bodies   > 2 Vertebral bodies

Immediate primary repair   Immediate primary repair   Delayed repair (2–3
via thoracotomy   if believe oesophageal   months) if ends too
                               ends can be   far apart
                               anastomosed

C. Manoeuvres to achieve anastomosis:

1. Full upper pouch mobilization
2. Dissection of lower segment to (or through) oesophageal hiatus
3. Myotomy: circular (spiral)
   Usually of upper pouch
   ? Lower pouch too
4. Mobilization of stomach into chest
   - through oesophageal hiatus
   - division of lesser curve (Scharli)

D. If anastomosis fails:

Cervical oesophagostomy (or regular upper pouch suction) and gastrostomy
Later oesophageal replacement at 10 kg or 1 year (or earlier if infant well)
Options:

- greater curvature tube
  – isoperistaltic gastric tube
  – reversed gastric tube
- gastric transposition
- jejunal interposition
- oesophagocoloplasty

Fig. 21.3   Management of long-gap oesophageal atresia.

exclude a proximal fistula) and confirmed at operation by the passage of a radiopaque flexible catheter through the mouth into the upper oesophagus by the anaesthetist.

The lower segment is evaluated at the time of gastrostomy by introducing a metal bougie through the gastro-oesophageal junction into the lower oesophageal segment. Gentle pressure exerted on the catheter from above, and the bougie from below, can be used to assess how closely the oesophageal segments can be approximated, as an indicator of the likelihood of early successful oesophageal anastomosis.

Timing of definitive repair

As soon as the gap appears small enough to enable primary anastomosis, or at 3 months, primary anastomosis is attempted.

The following manoeuvres may be undertaken to overcome a long gap between oesophageal ends in oesophageal atresia.

1. The upper pouch is identified and fully mobilized, avoiding damage to the trachea. The mobilization

can be extended superiorly as far as the crico-pharyngeus without compromising the blood supply to the upper oesophagus. This should always be the first manoeuvre.

2. Mobilization of the distal segment. The lower oesophagus can be identified by following the fine white fibres of the vagus nerve as they run down the posterior mediastinum. Mobilization of the lower segment can be achieved without disruption of the segmental vascular supply, which appears as a small leash of vessels from the aorta.

3. If the above manoeuvres still do not allow the oesophageal ends to be anastomosed, more exten-sive mobilization of the oesophagus through the oesophageal hiatus can be employed, to allow the intra-abdominal oesophagus to ride up into the tho-rax, with or without a portion of the stomach. This comes at the cost of producing significant gastro-oesophageal reflux, which will almost certainly require surgical correction at a later date.

4. A circular (or spiral) myotomy of the upper oesoph-agus can be performed, but this may damage the motility and vascular supply of the upper pouch, or result in later diverticulum formation. Preferably, it should be done more than 2 cm from the end, which

Table 21.3 Indications for cervical oesophagostomy

- No distal oesophagus, or an extensive gap between the oesophageal ends making an oesophageal anastomosis impossible

- Life-threatening anastomotic complications

- Long-gap oesophageal atresia where there are inade-quate facilities for prolonged upper pouch care

- A cervical oesophagostomy is very rarely required in a patient with oesophageal atresia and a distal fistula

Table 21.4 Indications for oesophageal replacement

- Oesophageal atresia without fistula where there is min-imal or no intrathoracic component to the lower oesophageal segment

- When attempted oesophageal anastomosis at thoraco-tomy proves impossible (a rare event)

- Where total anastomotic disruption with sepsis has required a cervical oesophagostomy, (even in this situ-ation, in some infants, it may still be possible to salvage the oesophagus)

Table 21.5 Selection of method of oesophageal replacement

Viscus	Stomach: antegrade tube
	retrograde tube
	transposition
	Colon
	Small bowel (jejunum)
Route	Retrosternal
	Transpleural
	Posterior mediastinal

may be difficult when the upper oesophageal seg-ment is short (as is often the case when a myotomy is required).

5. An anterior mucomuscular flap can be fashioned using the upper oesophageal segment. Viability of the flap relies on the fact that the upper oesophagus has an excellent longitudinal blood supply and is somewhat wider (more dilated) than the lower oesophagus.

6. If all of these measures fail a cervical oesophagosto-my (Table 21.3) as a prelude to subsequent oesophageal replacement, may be required (Table 21.4). A number of methods is available for achiev-ing oesophageal replacement (Table 21.5).

EXTREME PREMATURITY

In the extremely premature infant who is likely to develop or is developing severe hyaline membrane dis-ease (HMD) early division of the tracheo-oesophageal fistula by a thoracotomy, with or without simultaneous oesophageal anastomosis, depending on the condition of the infant at the time of operation, is important. The greater the difficulty in achieving adequate gaseous exchange, the more urgent the need to close the fistula. Ideally, this is done in the first 12 hours of life and before the HMD becomes fully established. Attempts to venti-late the infant until the HMD resolves before closing the fistula tend to be hazardous: to achieve adequate ventila-tion in the presence of severe HMD, high ventilatory pressures may be required over a prolonged period, and it is only effective if the airway resistance is lower than that of the fistula. If the fistula acts as a low resistance vent, ventilation becomes ineffective and the stomach distends with air, leading to gastric perforation, pneumo-peritoneum, elevation of the diaphragm with splinting, hypoxia, cardiac arrest and death. Placement of a gas-trostomy may encourage preferential passage of air through the fistula, preventing satisfactory ventilation.

Whether administration of surfactant will allow delayed division of the fistula in the extremely prema-ture infant with the potential for HMD, remains to be determined.

Tracheo-oesophageal fistula (the 'H' fistula)

Tracheo-oesophageal fistula without oesophageal atresia presents a different clinical spectrum because the oesophagus is intact and patent. It is usually included in discussion of oesophageal atresia because of its presumed common embryological origin.

A fistula passes obliquely from the trachea in a caudal direction to enter the oesophagus at a slightly lower level. Air may pass through the fistula from the trachea to the oesophagus, and oesophageal contents (e.g. saliva and gastric juice) may enter the trachea.

CLINICAL FEATURES

Maternal polyhydramnios and prematurity are uncommon, unlike in oesophageal atresia. Symptoms result from the passage of air or liquid through the fistula, and include choking and cyanotic attacks with feeds, usually relieved by gavage feeding, pneumonia abdominal distension with air. Excessive drooling is sometimes seen, secondary to irritation of the respiratory tract from the passage of saliva and milk through the fistula. Vomiting, a hoarse cry and failure to thrive are less common features.

INVESTIGATION

The objectives of further investigation are to confirm the diagnosis of a tracheo-oesophageal fistula and to establish the level of that fistula. The two methods used are radiology and endoscopy. A properly performed contrast study requires meticulous attention to detail, including recording the entire study on video. Barium introduced through a catheter placed in the mid-oesophagus will identify a fistula in a high percentage of cases. Should

Table 21.6 Summary of management of 'H' fistula

Preoperative management	Cessation of feeds Commencement of antibiotics Observation and monitoring of vital signs, particularly respiratory rate and temperature
Surgical ablation of the fistula	Cervical approach Division of fistula
Postoperative management	Inspection of vocal cords Commencement of oral feeds on day 3

diagnostic doubt persist despite an adequate mid-oesophageal radiological study, bronchoscopy should be performed. Alternatively, bronchoscopy may be the initial investigation. There is no role for oesophagoscopy (the fistula is difficult to find) or for the introduction of dyes, such as methylene blue. Both contrast radiology and endoscopy have a place in the diagnosis of tracheo-oesophageal fistulae and, with appropriate expertise, neither is clearly superior to the other.

OPERATIVE MANAGEMENT

A summary of the management of the 'H' fistula is provided in Table 21.6. The best surgical approach is usually through a supraclavicular incision on the right side, to reduce the likelihood of injury to the thoracic duct. A 2–3-cm-long incision above the clavicle, deepened through the platysma, will allow access to the fistula without the need for division of the sternomastoid muscle. The strap muscles are retracted medially and the dissection is continued anteromedial to the carotid sheath. Introduction of a naso-oesophageal tube by the anaesthetist may help to determine the exact position of the oesophagus. The trachea can be recognized by its rings. The fistula will be found in the groove between the trachea and oesophagus: it is short and runs obliquely. Damage to the recurrent laryngeal nerves, which also run between the oesophagus and trachea, must be avoided. It is not necessary to place catheter slings around the oesophagus above and below the fistula because they increase the risk of damage to the recurrent laryngeal nerves. However, a sling placed around the fistula itself may help to control it during division. Each end of the fistula is closed using 4/0 or 5/0 polyglycolic acid sutures. Drainage of the wound is not normally necessary, nor is a routine gastrostomy. The anaesthetist should inspect the vocal cords at the completion of the operation.

COMPLICATIONS

Recurrent laryngeal nerve palsy (unilateral or bilateral) and recurrence of the fistula may both occur. Leakage at the site of closure may result in mediastinitis, a recurrent fistula or oesophagocutaneous fistula. Pneumothorax, tracheal obstruction, pneumonia and postoperative aspiration have also been reported. Good surgical technique reduces the likelihood of complications.

Further reading

Beasley, S.W. 1991: Oesophageal atresia without fistula. In Beasley, S.W., Myers, N.A. and Auldist, A.W. (eds), *Oesophageal atresia*. London: Chapman & Hall Medical, 137–59.

Beasley, S.W. 1997: Esophageal atresia and tracheoesophageal fistula. In Oldham, K.T., Colombani, P.M. and Foglia, R.P. (eds), *Surgery of infants and children: scientific principles and practice*. Philadelphia, PA: Raven–Lippincott, 1021–34.

Myers, N.A. and Beasley, S.W. 1991: Diagnosis. In Beasley, S.W., Myers, N.A. and Auldist, A.W. (eds) *Oesophageal atresia*. London: Chapman & Hall Medical, 77–92.

Scharli, A.F. 1992: Esophageal reconstruction in very long atresia by elongation of the lesser curvature. *Pediatric Surgery International* **7**, 101–5.

Spitz, L. 1988: Gastric replacement of the oesophagus. In Spitz, L.V. and Nixon, H.H. (eds), *Rob and Smith's operative surgery. Paediatric surgery*, 4th ed. London: Butterworths, 142–5.

Spitz, L., Keily, E., Brereton R.I. and Drake, D. 1993: Management of esophageal atresia. *World Journal of Surgery* **17**, 296–300.

CHAPTER 22

Neonatal intestinal obstruction

J.D. ATWELL

Introduction	Jejunoileal atresia: stenosis
Duodenal atresia – stenosis – annular pancreas	Meconium ileus
Malrotation: volvulus neonatorum	References

Introduction

SURGICAL EMBRYOLOGY

The development of the intestinal tract is completed by the 10th week of intrauterine life. The intestinal tract has been subdivided into foregut, midgut and hindgut, with their respective blood supply of the coeliac axis, superior mesenteric and inferior mesenteric arteries. In the early stages the midgut consists mainly of the vitellointestinal duct. Up to the fifth week of fetal life the intestinal tract is a hollow tube but then there is a proliferation of the intestinal mucosa which appears to occlude the lumen. Whilst this is occurring the midgut is increasing in length and this, together with vacuolization of the epithelium leads to a restoration of the lumen. One theory of the causation of intestinal atresias was it resulted from a failure of the vacuolization of the intestinal epithelium (Tandler, 1902). Since then other workers have shown by serial sectioning of the fetal intestine that the lumen persists. Later workers found that vascular insufficiency to the developing fetal intestine was the prime cause of jejunoileal atresias (Louw and Barnard, 1995; Louw, 1959).

The liver and pancreas arise from two large extramural glands from the duodenum. The hepaticopancreatic bud grows ventrally into the mesentery of the duodenum and the dorsal outgrowth forms the body and tail of the pancreas with its own duct (Santorini). The ventral outgrowth divides into a hepatic and a pancreatic component, which forms the head of the pancreas with its own duct (Wirsung). Rotational effects on the long axis of the duodenum result in the bile ducts and head of the pancreas coming to lie close to the dorsal mesoduodenum. Fusion of the two outgrowths then occurs to form the adult type of pancreas. A communicating duct then joins the ducts of Santorini and Wirsung. As a result the separate opening of the duct of Santorini may either persist or disappear (Fig. 22.1).

FIXATION OF THE INTESTINE

The omphalocele closes by the 80th day of fetal life and coincides with the disappearance of the vitellointestinal duct. The abdominal cavity has been expanding before this in order to accommodate the increasing length of the developing intestine. Rotation of the intestine occurs during this time so that the intestine assumes its adult position. This rotation of the intestine on its

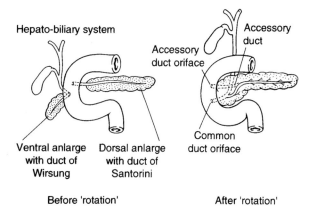

Fig. 22.1 Embryological development of the pancreas.

universal mesentery and its return from the omphalo-cele lead to zygosis of the parietal and viscerial peritoneum of the mesentery, thus attaching parts of the intestinal tract to the abdominal wall (duodenum, ascending and descending colon) (Fig. 22.2).

CLASSIFICATION OF NEONATAL INTESTINAL OBSTRUCTION

The causation of intestinal obstruction in the newborn can be classified on a positional basis (Table 22.1). Other causes of intestinal obstruction in the newborn are excluded from this classification, such as inguinal hernia, Meckel's diverticulum, intussusception and congenital bands, all of which are rare in the first 4 weeks of life, except for intestinal obstruction associated with an inguinal hernia.

GENERAL PRINCIPLES OF SURGICAL MANAGEMENT

The classical signs and symptoms of intestinal obstruction are primary, including abdominal pain, vomiting and absolute constipation, or secondary, such as dehy-dration, loss of weight, biochemical imbalance, distension, visible peristalsis, increased bowel sounds, tenderness due to peritonitis which may be associated with gangrene, and perforation of the bowel. The secondary factors, if left untreated, lead to the death of the patient (Fig. 22.3).

Variations in the pattern of presentation of intestinal obstruction depend on the level of obstruction and whether the obstruction is complete or incomplete (Atwell, 1971).

Group I

The obstruction in duodenal atresia is either above (34%) or below 66% the opening of the bile ducts. The absence of bile in the vomit with obstruction above the ampulla may lead to delay in diagnosis (Young, 1966). Vomiting occurs early in both groups, i.e. within 48 hours of birth. There may have been a history of hydramnios. Abdominal distension and visible peristal-sis is limited to the upper abdomen. The diagnosis is confirmed by a straight X-ray of the abdomen, which shows the classical double bubble.

When the obstruction is incomplete, e.g. with an annular pancreas, a perforation in a septum, or a mal-rotation or volvulus, the clinical presentation is altered. Distension is less, and vomiting may be intermittent and is either bile or non-bile stained. Distension does not occur with a volvulus of the small bowel, a fact not often understood by clinicians, and this may lead to a signifi-

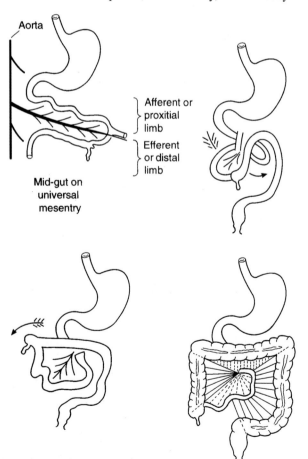

Fig. 22.2   Growth and rotation of the midgut.

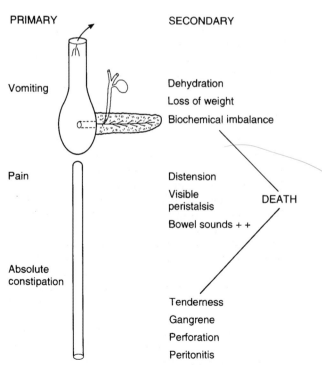

Fig. 22.3   Primary and secondary symptoms and signs of intestinal obstruction.

Table 22.1 Causes of intestinal obstruction in the newborn

Group	Obstruction	Causes
I	Duodenal	Atresia: stenosis Annular pancreas Malrotation with or without volvulus
II	Jejunoileal	Atresia: stenosis Meconium Ileus: peritonitis Volvulus neonatorum Inguinal hernia Meckel's diverticulum Congenital bands
III	Colorectal (see Chapters 23 and 24)	Hirshsprung's disease Atresia: stenosis (rare) Anorectal anomalies
IV	Idiopathic intestinal obstruction (see Chapter 25)	Meconium plug Milk plug Faecal plug Hypothyroidism Nectrotizing enterocolitis Exchange transfusion Infection Pseudo-Hirschsprung's Hypoganglionosis Hypoplastic left colon Drugs Cold injury Central nervous system anomalies

cant delay in diagnosis and to mortality (Atwell, 1971). Straight radiographs demonstrate a double bubble with gas beyond and malposition of loops of intestine. Contrast studies from either above or below may show evidence of a volvulus or malposition of the caecum.

Group II

There is seldom any delay in diagnosing jejunoileal atresias or meconium ileus. In jejunoileal atresia vomiting of bile accompanied by abdominal distension and visible peristalsis occurs early in upper small bowel obstruction but may be delayed in distal small bowel obstruction. The diagnosis is confirmed by a straight X-ray showing distended loops and fluid levels. Distension is absent in the rare septum with a perforation in the ileum and because of some stasis and alteration of the bacterial flora, the infant may present with loose stools.

Delay in diagnosing intestinal obstruction with meconium ileus with or without meconium peritonitis is unusual. Abdominal distension is often gross and may even be present at the time of delivery. Vomiting is often minimal, which contrasts markedly with the degree of abdominal distension. On rectal examination the rectum feels tight and empty. In about 60% of patients with meconium ileus there is a volvulus and in

some, when this has occurred during fetal life, there may be an associated intestinal atresia (25%). In some infants there will be a family history of fibrocystic disease. The diagnosis of fibrocystic disease may be confirmed by estimating and finding an elevated level of sodium in the sweat obtained by iontophoresis.

Group III

See Chapters 23 and 24, pages 206 and 213.

Group IV

See Chapter 25, page 226.

MANAGEMENT

Preoperative care

The principles of preoperative care are the same irrespective of the level or cause of the intestinal obstruction. Prevention of the aspiration of a vomit may be lifesaving, so a 10 Fr. gauge nasogastric tube is passed, aspirated at regular 30-min to 1-hour intervals and left on free drainage between aspirations. The degree of dehydration is assessed and replacement of fluids and electrolytes is started by the intravenous route (see

Chapters 14 and 15). Careful monitoring of the biochemical state of the patient is undertaken. Blood is sent for grouping and cross-matching. Radiographs with straight supine and erect films are often the only investigation needed to confirm a diagnosis. Contrast studies are occasionally required.

Duodenal atresia – stenosis – annular pancreas

SURGICAL PATHOLOGY

An intrinsic obstruction to the duodenum may be caused by either an atresia or stenosis, i.e. a complete or incomplete obstruction of the duodenal lumen. Another cause of obstruction is from an annular pancreas (Fig. 22.4). The level of duodenal obstruction is usually distal to the ampulla of Vater (66%) and proximal in the remainder. Extrinsic obstructions to the duodenum do occur, usually secondary to a volvulus or extrinsic bands.

With intrinsic obstructions there is a high incidence of other congenital defects, supporting the hypothesis that the obstruction occurred early in intrauterine life, which contrasts with the low incidence of congenital anomalies associated with jejunoileal atresias. Trisomy 21 is one of the most common associated anomalies (Table 22.2).

MANAGEMENT

Preoperative care

See the earlier chapter on general principles of management of neonatal intestinal obstruction.

Operation

The aim is to restore continuity of the intestine and the procedure of choice is a duodenoduodenostomy. The debatable point is whether to combine this with a gastrostomy and a transanastomotic feeding tube. A gastroenterostomy is to be avoided but a retrocolic duodenojejunostomy is a useful alternative to a duodenoduodenostomy (Fig. 22.5).

In patients with a duodenal diaphragm it is possible to miss the obstruction because of the 'windsock' effect. The duodenum must be opened and the membrane is found prolapsed distally. The membrane is excised either with cutting diathermy or by oversewing the cut edges. The duodenum is then closed transversely.

Postoperative care

The stomach is kept empty either by aspiration from the gastrostomy tube or from a 10 Fr. gauge nasogastric tube. The volume of aspirate is high and usually is within 100–150 ml per day, which must be replaced,

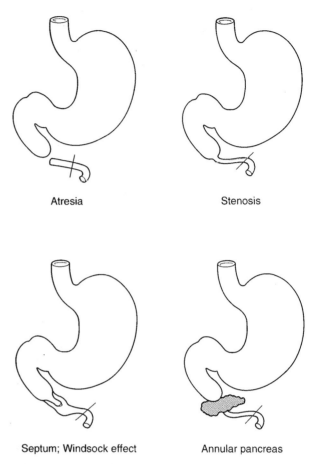

Atresia   Stenosis

Septum; Windsock effect   Annular pancreas

Fig. 22.4   Types of duodenal obstruction atresia: stenosis.

either parenterally or down the transanastomotic feeding tube. The problem with transanastomotic feeding tubes is that they tend to be returned to the stomach, thus defeating their purpose. This can be partially avoided by the slow administration of the aspirations at 1 ml/min.

Table 22.2   Associated anomalies in 40 patients with duodenal atresia and stenosis

Defect	Number
Trisomy 21	14
Anomalies of gastrointestinal tract	17
Malrotation	6
Oesophageal atresia and tracheo-oesophageal fistula	3
Anorectal atresia	1
Jejunoileal atresia	2
Meckel's diverticulum	2
Meconium peritonitis	1
Ectopic pancreas	1
Congenital bands	1
Congenital heart disease	3
Vertebral anomalies	6

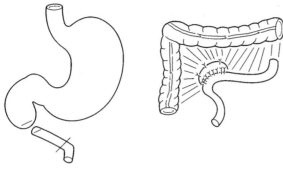

Duodenoduodenostomy	Duodenojejunostomy (retrcolic)

Fig. 22.5 Operations for duodenal obstruction.

The volume of gastric aspirations gradually decreases usually over a period of 5–10 days, although occasionally it persists for a prolonged period. As the aspirates decrease and become non-bile stained oral or tube feeds may be introduced, initially 5% dextrose, then half-strength and finally full-strength feeds. The volumes are gradually increased by 2.5–5.0 ml/hour. In the transition from partial to full feeds the aspirations are reduced from hourly to 4- or 6-hourly, or longer depending on the progress of the infant.

COMPLICATIONS

Early

- Anastomotic leak: this may result in a localized or subphrenic abscess.
- Duodenal ileus: the gross dilatation and hypertrophy of the duodenal wall proximal to the obstruction need time for recovery. During this time the onward peristaltic propulsion of intestinal contents may be ineffective, with a failure of the nasogastric aspirations to decrease.
- Stenosis: this may be intrinsic due to an inadequate anastomosis or extrinsic from adhesions or a localized abscess.
- Perforation of the bowel wall: if a transanastomotic feeding tube is used it should be polyvinyl, and feeds given this way must be given slowly.

Late

- Blind loop syndrome: chronic dilatation secondary to stenosis at the anastomosis may lead to alteration of the bacterial flora of the gut and development of a blind loop syndrome. There is an iron deficiency anaemia, failure of normal growth and complete loss of appetite. Contrast studies will confirm the diagnosis and a further laparotomy and revision and/or refashioning of the anastomosis is required.
- Associated anomalies: these conditions may complicate the postoperative course with the development of

heart failure and the need to counsel parents of the infant with trisomy 21. Other gastrointestinal tract anomalies should have been observed at the time of the original laparotomy and appropriate treatment undertaken. Renal and vertebral anomalies can be investigated with ultrasound and appropriate radiographs.

Malrotation: volvulus neonatorum

SURGICAL PATHOLOGY

The term malrotation is used to describe the condition of the failure of the intestine to undergo its anticlockwise rotation to take up the normal adult position. This usually occurs with the midgut returning from the omphalocele to the true abdominal cavity. This failure of rotation may result in intestinal obstruction from two main causes. The first and most dangerous of these is a volvulus due to the midgut being suspended on a very narrow pedicle, like a tightly gathered curtain, which is easy to twist through 360° or more. The second cause is that a condensation of parietal peritoneum (Ladd's band) may cross the duodenum and is attached to a high-lying caecum (Fig. 22.6). In some instances the gut has rotated normally but the small intestine mesentery has a narrow attachment to the posterior abdominal wall rather than the longer oblique normal attachment from the duodenojejunal junction to the right iliac fossa. The narrow attachment predisposes to a volvulus (volvulus neonatorum).

Other conditions associated with a universal mesentery (i.e. the primitive embryological state) include congenital diaphragmatic hernia, exomphalos and gastroschisis, duplication cysts of the small intestine and abdominal masses such as a right-sided severe pelviureteric junctional hydronephrosis (Fig. 22.7).

MANAGEMENT

The findings at a laparotomy vary from finding a high caecum with Ladd's band crossing the duodenum to those with a volvulus through 180°, 360° or even greater when associated with a maypole mesentery.

It is essential to deliver the intestine completely into the wound in order to determine the precise nature of malrotation present. A volvulus, if present, is usually clockwise. If there has been ischaemia the blood supply to the intestine may be compromised. If this ischaemia occurred during intrauterine life there may be associated single or multiple atresias, usually of the upper jejunum.

The volvulus is untwisted, which will improve the blood supply to the intestine if it had been threatened. Ladd's band is then divided and the duodenum mobilized so that the midgut is now on its universal mesentery, with the small intestine to the right and the caecum and large intestine to the left. No attempts are made to fix the intestine. Appendicectomy need not be performed

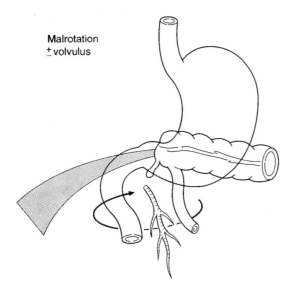

Malrotation
± volvulus

Fig. 22.6 Clinical findings with an intestinal malrotation. Note the high-lying caecum with a condensation of parietal peritoneum which may sometimes obstruct the duodenum. The vascular pedicle of the superior mesenteric vessels is narrow and is thus prone to undergo a volvulus.

but the parents of the infant or child must be informed that the appendix lies in an abnormal position so that any future inflammation should not be difficult to diagnose.

If ischaemic gut is present the above procedure may have an intestinal resection added with restoration of continuity by an end-to-end or end-to-back anastomosis. The loss of intestinal length may be severe. This is often due to delay in diagnosis and occasionally a resection is not possible. In such cases a second-look operation after 48 hours is indicated in the hope that some of the intestine will have recovered and that a more limited resection is possible.

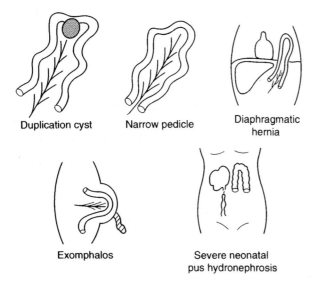

Duplication cyst   Narrow pedicle   Diaphragmatic hernia

Exomphalos   Severe neonatal pus hydronephrosis

Fig. 22.7 Conditions associated with universal mesentery.

POSTOPERATIVE CARE

A prolonged period of duodenal ileus may require nasogastric aspiration and intravenous replacement of fluid losses. Parenteral nutrition may be required, together with antibiotic cover in the complicated case. As a malrotation can present at any time from infancy to adult life there may be considerable duodenal dilatation in the older patient, with a longer postoperative spell of vomiting.

COMPLICATIONS

- Recurrent volvulus: this is an unusual complication unless a volvulus neonatorum is only untwisted and not combined with a Ladd's operation.
- Intestinal obstruction: subsequent intestinal obstruction due to adhesions is a real risk and occurs in about 10% of patients following a Ladd's operation.
- Short gut syndrome: malabsorption may be severe in those patients who have lost intestinal length from intrauterine ischaemia of the bowel or those needing a resection of the bowel for gangrene.
- Anastomotic 'leak': if a resection has been necessary a leak may occur to produce either a localized or a generalized peritonitis.

Jejunoileal atresia: stenosis

SURGICAL PATHOLOGY

There are two main theories for the aetiology of the jejunoileal atresias. The first is a failure of recanalization of the bowel following mucosal growth and increase in length of the midgut (Tandler, 1902). The second, which has been supported by animal experiments and clinical findings in patients, is that of intestinal ischaemia at some stage of intrauterine life. Tandler's theory was discredited by the findings in infants with a complete intestinal atresia that the meconium distal to the atresia contained epithelial squames, lanugo and bile, and hence the gut lumen must have been patent before the episode causing the atresia.

These findings led to the development of the vascular accident as a cause of the atresias. If the blood supply to the fetal bowel is impaired and the bowel is empty, the bowel becomes gangrenous and is absorbed. If the bowel has intestinal content this will be freed into the peritoneal cavity and then produce an inflammatory reaction, i.e. meconium peritonitis. The differing components respond to ischaemia in different ways, i.e. the highly specialized cells of the intestinal mucosa are more sensitive to anoxia and will therefore die before the smooth muscle and fibroblasts in the intestinal wall. Such differing responses to anoxia could account in part for the different types of intestinal atresia found in clinical practice (Fig. 22.8).

Experimental proof of the vascular accident theory has been shown in studies in pregnant bitches (Louw and Barnard, 1955; Louw, 1959). The uterus was opened between the 45th and 55th day of pregnancy, the abdomen of the fetal puppy opened and the blood supply to a segment of intestine interrupted. The fetal abdomen, maternal uterus and abdomen were then closed and the bitch was allowed to go to term. In 38 bitches whose puppies were born 12–14 days after intrauterine operation, intestinal atresias of a similar type to that found in the human were found. Thus the vascular accident theory has replaced the earlier Tandler theory as the causation of intestinal atresias. Furthermore, it is supported by the low incidence of other congenital anomalies in patients with jejunoileal atresia, which contrasts with the high incidence found in patients with duodenal and rectal atresias. The different types of intestinal atresia found include a stenosis, a complete septum (type I), a fibrosis cord (type II) and a gap with separation of the proximal and distal limbs of the intestine (type III). The atresias may be either single or multiple. The possible sequence of events which may occur and result in a complete atresia is illustrated in Fig. 22.9.

MANAGEMENT

Preoperative care

This has already been described earlier in this section, i.e. nasogastric aspiration and correction of fluid and electrolyte losses are the mainstays of preparation for definitive and corrective surgery.

Operation

The vast improvement in the mortality from jejunoileal atresias followed a better understanding of the functional propulsive activity of the bowel. In earlier years continuity was restored by end to end, or end-to-side or side-to-side anastomoses. This was followed by a prolonged period of ileus with a high mortality. Following experimental animal work it was show that if the grossly dilated bowel was excised proximal to the atresia and an end-to-back anastomosis performed there was a very significant improvement in the mortality (Nixon, 1960). Thus the end-to-back anastomosis following resection

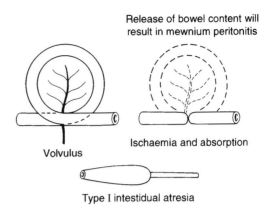

Fig. 22.9 Intrauterine volvulus leading to formation of an intestinal atresia.

of the grossly dilated intestine became the standard surgical treatment for an ileal or low jejunal atresia (Fig. 22.10).

In patients with a high jejunal atresia it was impractical to resect a significant length of intestine owing to the proximity of the bile ducts. A method of overcoming this problem was to reduce the calibre of the jejunum by tapering or refashioning the proximally dilated bowel (Fig. 22.11). Continuity was restored by an end-to-end anastomosis (Howard and Othersen, 1973).

With the improvement of parenteral nutrition in recent years another alternative method of treatment is available, i.e. to revert to the original operation of restoring continuity without resection of the dilated intestine and to rely on parenteral nutrition for a prolonged period, which would allow the dilated intestine to revert to its normal calibre.

Postoperative care

Prolonged nasogastric aspiration, replacement of fluid and electrolytes, and parenteral nutrition are required until full oral feeding is established.

COMPLICATIONS

Early

- Anastomotic leak: the standard anastomosis is a single layer with interrupted sutures. The disparity in size between the ends being anastomosed increases the technical difficulty of the anastomosis. The risk of a breakdown seems to be higher in those with high jejunal and/or multiple atresias.

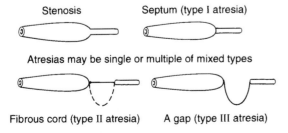

Fig. 22.8 Types of jejunoileal atresia.

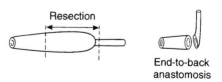

Fig. 22.10 Nixon end-to-back anastomosis.

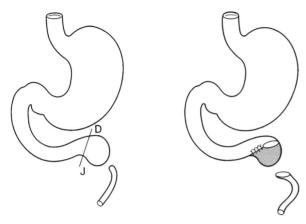

Fig. 22.11 Tapering jejunoplasty for a high jejunal atresia.

- Aspiration pneumonia: intensive-care nursing and adequate nasogastric aspiration should prevent this complication.

Late

- Metabolic complications: these include problems with hypokalaemia, hypocalcaemia and hypomagnesaemia which should be preventable but may require urgent treatment. Malabsorption and lactose intolerance may complicate the management in patients who have lost intestinal length.
- Adhesions: these may cause intestinal obstruction at a later date.
- Failure to thrive: there may be delays in growth and development, although the vast majority will have attained normal levels within 1–2 years of the original operation. This may be due to compensatory changes in the intestinal mucosa following a lengthy resection.

Meconium ileus

SURGICAL PATHOLOGY

Fibrocystic disease of the pancreas is genetically determined by an autosomal recessive gene with a recurrence risk in future pregnancies of 1 in 4. In 10–15% of patients with fibrocystic disease abnormal viscid meconium and deficient pancreatic enzymes cause a bolus type of intestinal obstruction in the newborn. The usual level of the obstruction is in the ileum, hence the term meconium ileus. The obstruction may, however, be at a higher level, i.e. jejunal, or lower in the colon. The bowel becomes grossly distended and thick walled owing to hypertrophy of the smooth muscle. Distally, the bowel is of small calibre and collapsed to produce a 'microcolon' effect. The dilated and thickened bowel is prone to undergo a volvulus. If this occurs before birth the bowel becomes gangrenous, liberating meconium into the peritoneal cavity to produce a meconium peritonitis. Atresia of the bowel may be associated with this

sequence of events, with an incidence of about 20%. If the volvulus occurs after birth then gangrene, perforation and a bacterial peritonitis may complicate the clinical picture (Fig. 22.12).

MANAGEMENT

Preoperative care

Nasogastric aspiration, replacement of fluid and electrolyte losses are the mainstay of the early management prior to a laparotomy.

Operation

The mortality from meconium ileus was originally of the order of 75%, but then the Bishop–Koop ileostomy was introduced (Bishop and Koop, 1957). This was a radical change in management and resulted in a fall in mortality to under 25%. Although the operation is not used as much today it represents an important phase in the development of neonatal surgery and is still a safe procedure. The bowel is inspected and any volvulus present is untwisted. The grossly distended bowel is excised proximal to the obstruction. The distal end of the bowel is brought out as an ileostomy and the proximal bowel is anastomosed to the side of the ileostomy. No attempt is made to empty the distal bowel of the viscid meconium (Fig. 22.13).

An alternative method of management is to correct the volvulus, resect any gangrenous bowel or associated atresia, wash out the distal bowel with acetyl cysteine and then restore continuity with an end-to-end anastomosis. In some patients this can be performed through an enterotomy in viable bowel. This procedure is associated with a considerable amount of handling of the bowel, which may result in a prolonged postoperative ileus and may indicate the need for a period of total parenteral nutrition. This is likely in patients in whom a resection is not undertaken to remove the grossly dilated bowel.

In some patients conservative treatment is possible as the obstruction may be relieved by the hygroscopic effect of a gastrografin enema (Noblett, 1969). The procedure is not without complications and it should be remembered that a volvulus is present in about 50% of patients with meconium ileus. On screening, if gastrografin is seen to enter a dilated loop of ileum a conservative regime may be tried, thus avoiding a laparotomy.

POSTOPERATIVE CARE

The continuation of nasogastric aspiration and the replacement of fluid and electrolytes is essential and, if the ileus is prolonged, parenteral nutrition is indicated (Suita *et al.*, 1984). Oral Pancrex is given (125 mg in 5 ml normal saline) every 4 hours to the stomach via the nasogastric tube even if regular aspirations are still carried out. If a Bishop–Koop ileostomy is present then Pancrex is instilled into the stoma using a short, soft

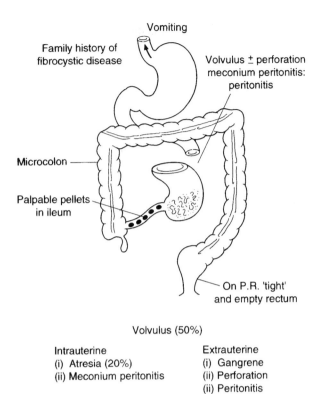

Vomiting

Family history of fibrocystic disease

Volvulus ± perforation meconium peritonitis: peritonitis

Microcolon

Palpable pellets in ileum

On P.R. 'tight' and empty rectum

Volvulus (50%)

Intrauterine	Extrauterine
(i) Atresia (20%)	(i) Gangrene
(ii) Meconium peritonitis	(ii) Perforation
	(ii) Peritonitis

Fig. 22.12 Clinical features and surgical pathology of meconium ileus.

catheter. This is started 24 hours after the operation and continued at 2-hour intervals until meconium is passed, which normally occurs within 48–72 hours. If a more conservative operation or non-operative care has been used a gastrografin enema may be repeated in order to clear the distal bowel of viscid meconium.

Intraperitoneal closure of a Bishop–Koop ileostomy is required and there is some debate relating to the timing of its closure. Originally this was delayed for a long time if the stoma was behaving as a dry mucous fistula. The author prefers to close the ileostomy as soon as the meconium distal to the obstruction is passed, i.e. with 2–4 days of the original operation.

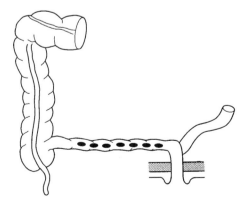

Fig. 22.13 The Bishop–Koop illeostomy.

Regrading with oral feeds is started as soon as possible, initially using 5% dextrose but then increasing to half-strength and then full-strength milk feeds. Predigested feeds such as Pregestimil play a role in the management of these patients.

Final confirmation of the diagnosis of fibrocystic disease is made by measuring the sodium content of sweat obtained by iontophoresis.

COMPLICATIONS

Early

An anastomotic leak may occur, sometimes related to the poor blood supply to the bowel.

Late

Failure to thrive is not uncommon and is related to the primary condition, postoperative adhesions and loss of intestinal length. The general complications of fibrocystic disease such as liver failure, intestinal malabsorption, portal hypertension and respiratory failure eventually lead to death. With improvements in the long-term management of these patients many are now reaching adult life.

References

Atwell, J.D. 1971: Pitfalls in the diagnosis of intestinal obstruction in the newborn. *Proceedings of the Royal Societies of Medicine* **64**, 374–377.

Bishop, H.C. and Koop, C.E. 1957: Management of meconium ileus: resection Roux-en-y anastomosis and ileostomy irrigation with pancreatic enzymes. *Annals of Surgery* **145**, 410–14.

Howard, E.R. and Othersen, H.B. 1973: Proximal jejunoplasty in the treatment of jejuno-ileal atresia. *Journal of Pediatric Surgery* **8**, 685–90.

Louw, J.H. 1959: Congenital intestinal atresia and stenosis in the newborn. Observations on its pathogenesis and treatment *Annals of the Royal College of Surgeons of England* **25**, 209–34.

Louw, J.H. and Barnard, C.N. 1955: Congenital intestinal atresia. Observations on its origin. *Lancet* **ii**, 1065–7.

Nixon, H.H. 1960: An experimental study of the propulsion in isolated small intestine, and applications to surgery in the newborn. *Annals of the Royal College of Surgeons of England* **21**, 105–24.

Noblett, H. 1969: Treatment of uncomplicated meconium ileus by gastrografin enema: a preliminary report. *Journal of Pediatric Surgery* **4**, 190–7.

Suita, S., Ikeda, K., Hayashida, Y. *et al.* 1984: Zinc and copper requirements during parenteral nutrition in the newborn. *Journal of Pediatric Surgery* **19**, 126–130.

Tandler, J. 1900: Zur Entwicklungsgeschichte des Menschlichen Duodenums im Frühen Embryonal Stadiem. *Gegenbaurs Morphologisches Jahrbuch* **29**, 187–216.

Young, D.G. 1966: Neonatal acid–base disturbances. *Archives of Diseases in Childhood* **41**, 201–3.

CHAPTER 23

Hirschsprung's disease

J.C. MOLENAAR AND C. MEIJERS

Introduction	Clinical features
Classification of Hirschsprung's disease and	Differential diagnosis
related disorders of the enteric nervous system	Management
Pathogenesis and genetics	References

Introduction

In 1886, Harald Hirschsprung (1830–1916), a Danish paediatrician, delivered a lecture in which he described two boys who presented with a characteristic clinical picture: severe difficulty with defaecation from birth, increasing abdominal distension and a deterioration in health leading to death at the age of 11 and 7 months, respectively. The autopsies revealed pronounced dilatation, bowel wall hypertrophy and mucosal ulceration of the colon (Hirschsprung, 1887).

Half a century later, the era of understanding the pathophysiology of Hirschsprung's disease dawned when Swenson and Bill (1948) detected that the dilated hypertrophied megacolon was not the cause of the disease but the late effect of dysmotility of the recto-sigmoid. They were the first to develop appropriate surgical treatment by experimentally resecting the recto-sigmoid in dogs, involving anastomosis of the residual colon to the anus with subsequent retention of continence. This anal pull-through technique was then applied successfully to children with Hirschsprung's disease. The therapeutic success obtained in this way indicated that the underlying dysmotility of the recto-sigmoid was indeed the cause of the diseased colon. The removal of this dysfunctional part of the rectocolon has remained the principle of the surgical treatment of Hirschsprung's disease, although a variety of surgical procedures has been used.

The underlying pathology of Hirschsprung's disease was discovered when Whitehouse and Kernohan (1948) and Zuelzer and Wilson (1948) showed that the wall of the distal colon lacked enteric neurons. After the demonstration that the level of aganglionosis of the submucous plexus corresponds to that of the myenteric plexus, the safer suction mucosal biopsies supplanted full-thickness biopsies (Gherardi, 1960; Aldridge and Campbell, 1968). The immature ganglion cells of the submucous plexus in the infant are less distinctive than the ganglion cells in older patients or those of the myenteric plexus, and can be mimicked by macrophages, fibroblasts, smooth muscle cells, Schwann cells and even lymphocytes (Ariel et al., 1983; Campbell and Noblett, 1969; Yunis et al., 1976). Thus it was often necessary to examine serial sections before arriving at a diagnosis.

Classification of Hirschsprung's disease and related disorders of the enteric nervous system

Hirschsprung's disease is defined as the absence of enteric neurons and the presence of hypertrophic nerve trunks in the distal bowel beginning with and including the internal anal sphincter. The aganglionsis extends over varying distances proximally but always includes the anus and at least part of the rectum. The incidence of Hirschsprung's disease is approximately 1 in every 5000 newborns (Madsen, 1964; Passarge, 1967; Goldberg, 1984; Spouge and Baird, 1985).

Several classifications of Hirschsprung's disease have been proposed. Ravitch (1958) perceived, from clinical and pathological observations, that aganglionosis was not the underlying disease in a number of patients with congenital megacolon. He therefore proposed a division between Hirschsprung's disease and pseudo-Hirschsprung's disease.

Another classification of Hirschsprung's disease is based on the distance from the internal anal sphincter encompassed by the aganglionosis, and distinguishes four classes (Boley *et al.*, 1978; Kleinhaus *et al.*, 1979). The first is an ultrashort segment, which involves only the anus and distal rectum below the peritoneal reflexion. The second is the short-segment or classic type, involving the anus, rectum and a part of the sigmoid colon. The third class, the long-segment aganglionosis, involves the colon proximal to the sigmoid colon, whereas the fourth class involves the entire colon; the latter type is also called Zuelzer–Wilson disease (Zuelzer and Wilson, 1948).

Apart from total colonic aganglionosis, total intestinal aganglionosis has been described. This is a rare congenital malformation, characterized by the absence of enteric neurons in the entire intestinal tract. Histochemical studies show normal acetyl cholinesterase (AChE) activity in the lamina propria of the small bowel and colon (Caniano *et al.*, 1985).

Apart from aganglionosis, hyperganglionosis presenting at different distances from the anus and upwards has been described, mimicking the same symptoms as in Hirschsprung's disease. Intestinal hyperglanglionosis, or neuronal intestinal dysplasia, is characterized by an above-average number of neurons in the submucous and myenteric plexuses and the presence of hyperplastic parasympathetic nerve trunks (Meier-Ruge, 1971; Howard and Garret, 1984). The abnormalities were initially thought to be confined to the colon, but later it was found that they can occur in the entire bowel.

There are two types of neuronal intestinal dysplasia: type A (15%) is characterized by hypoplasia or aplasia of the sympathetic innervation. The early clinical presentation is characterized by acute onset of severe constipation, diarrhoea and enterocolitis. Type B (70%) is characterized by normal sympathetic innervation and presents late with chronic constipation. In 15% of the cases a combination of both types is found. Neuronal intestinal dysplasia has been recognized with increasing frequency in recent years.

In patients with the clinical symptoms characteristic for Hirschsprung's disease and ganglion cells on rectal biopsy, neuronal intestinal dysplasia should be suspected as the underlying cause of the symptoms.

Pathogenesis and genetics

It is generally accepted that the development of the enteric nervous system starts in the rhombencephalic part of the neural crest (Le Douarin, 1982). Neural crest cells develop in the dorsal part of the embryonic neural tube and migrate extensively. From studies in our laboratory it was concluded that the embryonic enteric microenvironment harbours signals, recognized by the migrating neural crest cells, which enable them to migrate further through the gut to specific sites and differentiate into enteric neurons. The formation of the enteric nervous plexus is only part of the function of neural crest cells. As well as differentiating into other peripheral nerve cells and ganglia elsewhere in the body, the rhombencephalic neural crest cells are involved in the formation of different structures of ectomesenchymal origin, such as the craniofacial skeleton, the outflow tract of the heart, the adrenal medulla, the thymus and melanocytes.

Careful examination of patients with Hirschsprung's disease and their families for associated anomalies therefore could provide a better understanding of the underlying defects. A clinical geneticist is indispensable in this respect.

A positive family history exists in 3.6% of all cases (females 7.2%, males 2.6%). If Zuelzer–Wilson disease is included, the incidence of familial occurrence rises to 21% (Swenson *et al.*, 1973; Kleinhaus *et al.*, 1979). Two-generation transmission (from parent to child) is well recorded in the literature (Madsen, 1964), and even three-generation transmission has been reported (Lipson and Harvey, 1987). A nine-generation family with presumptive Hirschsprung's disease had associated Waardenburg syndrome, congenital deafness and Down's syndrome (Cohen and Gadd, 1982).

As a generation of treated and surviving patients grows to maturity and reproductive age, genetic counselling is indicated, if only to provide early and prompt surgical care and treatment of the disease (Carter *et al.*, 1981). The actual mode of inheritance will also become clearer. Genetic counselling should also take into account the Mendelian inheritance of some syndromes associated with Hirschsprung's disease. Non-syndromic cases of Hirschsprung's disease are thought to be inherited in a gender-modified multifactorial mode (Passarge, 1983). This term implies that the threshold of genes needed for expression of the trait in one gender is lower than in the other.

The importance of associated anomalies is obvious to some physicians, but this is not properly reflected in the literature. The incidence of anomalies associated with Hirschsprung's disease varies from 3.6 to 35%. The wide range is due to the diligence with which they are sought and the manner in which they are reported. Some reports show an increase in additional malformations, while others show only an increase in Down's syndrome and anomalies of the genitourinary tract

(Warkany, 1967; Boley *et al.*, 1978; Passarge, 1983). The number of reports on anomalies associated with Hirschsprung's disease has increased in recent years.

At present, genetic mutations have been identified in three genes in patients with Hirschsprung's disease. Mutations in the *RET* gene, encoding for a transmembrane tyrosine kinase receptor protein, are causative in cases of dominant forms of Hirschsprung's disease. Mutations in the *RET* gene are detected in about half of the familial cases and in 10–15% of the sporadic cases. The mutations are scattered all over the gene. The penetrance of the mutations also varies within families. Mutations in the *RET* gene also occur in familial cancer syndromes such as MEN2A and MEN2B (multiple endocrine neoplasia). It is recommended to screen for mutations in the *RET* gene, since in a few cases MEN2A mutations have been detected in patients with Hirschsprung's disease. This could mean that these patients are at risk for MEN2 type of cancer as adults.

In few familial and some sporadic cases mutations have been detected in the endothelin-B receptor gene (*EDNRB*). Patients with homozygous mutations have not only Hirschsprung's disease but also Waardenburg syndrome type 2. Patients heterozygous for *EDNRB* mutations suffer from Hirschsprung's disease only. The penetrance is variable in the case of *EDNRB* gene mutations.

The third gene that predisposes to Hirschsprung's disease is the gene that encodes the ligand for the ENDRB protein: endothelin 3 (*EDN-3*). Homozygous mutations in the *EDN-3* gene are associated with a Waardenburg type 2 phenotype.

The detection of mutations in the above-mentioned genes is time-consuming and depends on the screening methods that are used, i.e. single strand conformation polymorphism (SSCP) or denaturing gradient gel electrophoresis (DGGE). Until now mutations have been detected in only a few patients. Other genes have to be screened and the possibility cannot be excluded that Hirschsprung's disease is a polygenic disease, in which interactions of various gene products play an important role. Calculating the risks of recurrence is difficult and should be determined in each individual case. The exclusion of MEN2 mutations in the *RET* gene is important for follow-up.

Clinical features

In the neonatal period delay of the passage of the first meconium beyond 24 hours after birth in an otherwise healthy newborn is an important sign of Hirschsprung's disease. In Swenson's series, 94% patients with Hirschsprung's disease failed to pass meconium during the first 24 hours of life (Swenson *et al.*, 1973). Vomiting occurs in most newborns with Hirschsprung's disease and is usually stained with bile.

Physical examination of the baby often shows a full-term healthy baby with a distended abdomen. When the little finger is gently introduced into the anus the rectal wall always feels tight and resists further probing. Abdominal distension was the second frequent sign of Hirschsprung's disease in neonates, in 87% in Swenson's series, and constipation was found in 93% in the first month of life (Swenson *et al.*, 1973).

The appearance of diarrhoea predicts a worsening of the child's condition and is an early sign of the presence of enterocolitis. If enterocolitis is present, the baby is sick with a poor circulation and is dehydrated. The abdomen is distended, tense and painful. In the case of enterocolitis withdrawal of the examining finger from the anus leads to an explosive passage of flatus and foul-smelling liquid faeces. If the baby is otherwise in good condition additional investigations are required. In a sick baby with enterocolitis further investigations are limited to a plain X-ray of the abdomen, urgent medical treatment and decompression of the bowel.

Differential diagnosis

Although meconium plugs occur in about 1% of all newborns, only one in every 500 show symptoms (Falls and Jaffe, 1931). The low water content (Zachary, 1957) and low trypsin content (Mikity *et al.*, 1967) of meconium plugs mimic both meconium ileus and Hirschsprung's disease. Both diseases have to be ruled out before the plug can be regarded as a harmless event.

Colonic atresia also causes a low intestinal obstruction, but here a barium enema will prove its real nature.

Functional intestinal obstruction in premature babies may cause symptoms mimicking Hirschsprung's disease. Gentle dilation of the anus and small enemas of saline or diluted gastrografin usually lead to sufficient bowel movements and passage of meconium. Invasive diagnostic procedures such as suction biopsies and barium enemas should be avoided, especially in very tiny premature babies, because of the risk of bowel perforation.

Management

INVESTIGATIONS

(i) *Barium enema* studies have been regarded as not specific enough to diagnose infantile Hirschsprung's disease (Taxman *et al.*, 1986). The demonstration of a transitional zone is regarded as the most useful and reliable sign for Hirschsprung's disease, but false-positive results may be obtained. The delayed emptying of the colon 24–48 hours after the barium enema study can also be misleading. The appearance of irregular peristaltic contractions in the aganglionic rectosigmoid, however, should lead to strong suspicions for the existence of Hirschsprung's disease.

(ii) *Anorectal manometry* can be a reliable screening test for the exclusion of neonatal Hirschsprung's disease (Loening-Baucke *et al.*, 1985). However, a normal inhibitory reflex does not exclude Hirschsprung's disease.

(iii) *Suction biopsy* of the rectal wall is a painless and simple procedure. The technique of suction biopsy was well described by Noblett (1969). Rectal suction biopsies can be performed at the bedside without anaesthesia or sedation in the neonatal patient (Dobbins and Bill, 1965). The biopsy tube is introduced into the anus and positioned against the posterior bowel wall. By generating a negative pressure with the aid of a large syringe, biopsies of sufficient thickness can be obtained (mucosa, muscularis mucosae and if possible submucous tissue), without the risk of perforation. To determine the length of the aganglionic segment biopsies are taken at various distances from the dentate line (e.g. at 2, 3 and 5 cm).

The suction biopsy specimen is carefully placed on a small piece of filtration paper with saline and quick-frozen in liquid nitrogen ($-196°C$). In order to prevent freezing artefacts the specimen is first placed in cooled isopentane. Staining of the enzyme AChE can be performed according to Karnovski and Roots (1964). This staining method, described by Meier-Ruge and co-workers (1972), demonstrated that an increase in AChE activity in the lamina propria and muscularis mucosae in suction biopsies of the rectal mucosa is pathognomonic for Hirschsprung's disease. The demonstration of AChE activity in cryostat sections may be difficult to interpret as there may be excessive mucosal haemorrhage with increased red blood cell AChE activity (Lake *et al.*, 1978; Meier-Ruge, 1982). The identification of enteric neurons remains important in the diagnostic process.

Normal low AChE activity in the lamina propria mucosae in the first 8 weeks of life does not exclude the diagnosis of Hirschsprung's disease (Novak and Pfeiffer, 1989). Negative mucosal biopsies within 8 weeks after birth in combination with a strong clinical suspicion of Hirschsprung's disease are an indication for repeated mucosal or full-thickness biopsies.

Full-thickness and/or partial-thickness biopsy is necessary if the result of suction biopsy does not provide a definite diagnosis of Hirschsprung's disease, especially with persistent clinical symptoms. Such rectal wall biopsies require a general anaesthesia. The anus is slightly dilated and one stitch is placed in the midline of the posterior rectal wall 1 cm above the pectinate line. A second stitch is placed 1 cm proximally, and another again 1 cm more proximal. Gentle pulling will cause the floppy mucosa to come forward easily. The second stitch will serve as a stay suture for the mucosa to take a full-thickness biopsy horizontally from the posterior rectal wall. The other two sutures are used to hold the two edges of the created rectal wound and to serve the proper suturing of this wound with a few through-and-through haemostatic sutures.

The full-thickness biopsy specimen is fixed in formalin and routinely stained with haematoxylin and azophloxin. Ganglion cells and/or abnormal nerve fibres are then looked for. Part of the biopsy specimen may be quick-frozen and treated as described above.

TREATMENT OF HIRSCHSPRUNG'S DISEASE IN THE NEWBORN PERIOD

Ulcerative enterocolitis is the main threat for newborns suffering from Hirschsprung's disease (Teitelbaum *et al.*, 1988). All measures should be aimed at prevention or treatment of this complication. Decompression of the stomach using a proper-sized nasogastric tube should prevent further vomiting and remove the risk of aspiration.

Reliable intravenous access is necessary to correct previous losses of water and electrolytes. Monitoring the urine production and analysing its content for electrolytes are extremely important to maintain homoeostasis.

As *Clostridium difficile* in the faeces is often associated with the presence of enterocolitis, antibiotic treatment (vancomycin) should be directed against this organism (Thomas *et al.*, 1982).

Rectal washouts and anorectal cannulation are important and often therapeutic in decompressing the lower intestines. If the child's condition is deteriorating, operative decompression should be considered as an emergency. This surgical approach should enable the surgeon to examine the entire colon. In severe cases of pseudomembranous enterocolitis in which the colon is purulent and gangrenous, total colectomy can be a life-saving procedure. In less serious cases a colostomy is usually sufficient. Most surgeons prefer a routine right-sided transverse colostomy. When good pathology service is available an end colostomy just proximal to the transitional zone is preferable. In patients with long-segment aganglionosis an end colostomy as a colon-saving procedure is the treatment of choice.

Corrective surgery is carried out later under protection by the earlier transverse colostomy, or without in the case of a previously made end colostomy.

When the patient is well and does not show symptoms of enterocolitis, several methods of treatment are available.

Primary corrective surgery was advocated by Carcassonne and co-workers in 1982, and by others (So *et al.*, 1980; Chin-Che and Yen-Hsia, 1983). All accepted surgical procedures can be used with comparable good results (Duhamel, 1956; Swenson, 1959; Rehbein and Nicolai, 1963; Soave, 1963). There is a slight preference for Duhamel's technique but a primary Swenson's resection and pull-through has also been used (Shanbhogue and Bianchi, 1990). An interesting new stapling technique for the Duhamel–Martin procedure has recently been introduced using the EndoGIA stapling device instead of the original GIA instrument (Zee *et al.*, 1993). This technique allows for the Duhamel procedure to be carried out safely without using a protective colostomy, even in neonates.

Special attention is required for the operative treatment of patients with total aganglionic colon. Here a varying part of the distal ileum is often involved in the aganglionosis. An ileostomy is often unavoidable. This should be placed in ganglionic ileum only. The appearance of the ileum during the operation may be misleading, therefore correct peroperative histology is necessary. End ileostomy in definitive ganglionic tissue for a short period, used to improve the infant's condition, is preferable, followed by definitive corrective surgery as soon as possible.

All the reported cases of total intestinal aganglionosis share a fatal outcome; however, in one patient with multiple myotomies, Ziegler and co-workers (1987, 1993) achieved a survival of over 18 months.

Treatment of neuronal intestinal dysplasia can be very frustrating. A rapid clinical deterioration may require an urgent enterostomy although regular daily enemas are a more preferable method of treatment.

RESULTS

The overall outcome of the treatment of neonates suffering from Hirschsprung's disease and related disorders is difficult to define because there are no large series limited to patients in the newborn period only. In most series operative treatment in this period is limited to enterostomies followed by definitive corrective surgery just before or after 1 year of age.

One large series of 1628 patients, compiled by Ikeda and Goto (1984), shows an increasing mortality rate in the preoperative period related to the length of the aganglionic segment, the main cause of death being sepsis due to enterocolitis. In this series the diagnosis of Hirschsprung's disease could be confirmed in 48.7% within 1 month after birth, in 23.4% between 1 and 3 months and in the remaining 27.9% the diagnosis was confirmed later, in 5.7% even after the age of 5 years.

The introduction of a new operative treatment of Hirschsprung's disease by Swenson and Bill (1948), followed by proposals for other operative techniques, introduced by Duhamel (1956), Rehbein (1963) and

Soave (1963), strongly emphasized the importance of surgical correction of this disease. Over the years persistent constipation was reported in 10% of patients in the large series, irrespective of the type of operation (Joppich, 1982), and other studies reported a higher incidence of constipation (20%) (Klück *et al.*, 1986). Incontinence of variable degree was reported in 50% of patients (Misahalany and Woolley, 1987).

From the few long-term studies it appears that no operative technique can claim definitive cure of Hirschsprung's disease. Long-term follow-up is necessary and from our experience with patient organizations it has become clear that patients require long-term supervision and help, and free access to clinics with expertise in defaccation disorders should be available.

References

Aldridge, R.T. and Campbell, P.E. 1968: Ganglion cell distribution in the normal rectum and anal canal. A basis for the diagnosis of Hirschsprung's disease by anorectal biopsy. *Journal of Pediatric Surgery* **3**, 475–90.

Ariel, I., Vinograd, I., Lernau, O.Z. *et al.* 1983: Rectal mucosal biopsy in aganglionosis and allied conditions. *Human Pathology* **14**, 991–5.

Boley, S.J., Dinari, G. and Cohen, M. 1978: Hirschsprung's disease in the newborn. *Clinical Perinatology* **5**, 45–60.

Campbell, P.E. and Noblett, H.R. 1969: Experience with rectal suction biopsy in the diagnosis of Hirschsprung's disease. *Journal of Pediatric Surgery* 1969: **4**, 410–15.

Caniano, D., Ormsbee III, H.S., Polito, W. *et al.* 1985: Total intestinal aganlionosis. *Journal of Pediatric Surgery* **20**, 456–60.

Carcassonne, M., Morrisson-Lacombe, G. and Letourneau, J.N. 1982: Primary corrective operation without decompression in infants less than three months of age with Hirschsprung's disease. *Journal of Pediatric Surgery* **17**, 241–3.

Carter, C.O., Evans, K. and Hickman, V. 1981: Children of those treated for Hirschsprung's disease. *Journal of Medical Genetics* **18**, 87–90.

Chin-Che, C. and Yen-Hsia, W. 1983: Ring-clamps crushing anastomosis in retrorectal pull-through operation for Hirschsprung's disease. *Journal of Pediatric Surgery* **18**, 296–8.

Cohen, I.T. and Gadd, M.A. 1982: Hirschsprung's disease in a kindred: a possible clue to the genetics of the disease. *Journal of Pediatric Surgery* **17**, 632–4.

Dobbins, W.O. and Bill, A.H. 1965: Diagnosis of Hirschsprung's disease excluded by rectal suction biopsy. *New England Journal of Medicine* **272**, 990–3.

Duhamel, B. 1956: Une nouvelle opération pour le mégacolon congénital: l'abaissement rétro-rectal et transnasal du côlon et son application possible au traitement de quelques autres malformations. *Presse Medicale* **64**, 2249.

Falls, F.H. and Jaffe, R.H. 1931: Intestinal obstruction in the newborn due to mucous plug. *American Journal of Obstetrics and Gynecology* **22**, 409–15.

Gherardi, G.J. 1960: Pathology of the ganglionic–aganglionic junction in congenital megacolon. *Archives of Pathology* **69**, 520–3.

Goldberg, E. 1984: An epidemiological study of Hirschsprung's disease. *International Journal of Epidemiology* **13**, 479–85.

Hirschsprung, H. 1887: Stuhlträgheit Neugeborener in Folge von Dilatation und Hypertrophie des Colons. *Jahrb Kinderh* **27**, 1–7.

Howard, E.R. and Garrett, J.R. 1984: Hirschsprung's disease and other neuronal disorders of the hindgut. In Tanner, M.S. and Stocks, R.J. (eds), *Neonatal gastroenterology – contemporary issues*. Newcastle upon Tyne: Intercept, 121–37.

Ikeda, K. and Goto, S. 1984: Diagnosis and treatment of Hirschsprung's disease in Japan; an analysis of 1628 patients. *Annals of Surgery* **199**, 400–5.

Joppich, I. 1982: Late complications of Hirschsprung's disease. In Holschneider, A.M. (ed.), *Hirschsprung's disease*. Stuttgart: Hippokrates, 251–61.

Karnovski, M.J. and Roots, L. 1964: A direct-coloring thiocholine method for cholinesterases. *Journal of Histochemistry and Cytochemistry* **12**, 219–21.

Kleinhaus, S., Boley, S.J., Sheran, M. *et al.* 1979: Hirschsprung's disease. A survey of the members of the surgical section of American academy of pediatrics. *Journal of Pediatric Surgery* **14**, 588–97.

Klück, P., Tibboel, D., Leendertse-Verloop, K. *et al.* 1986: Diagnosis of congenital neurogenic abnormalities of the bowel with monoclonal anti-neurofilament antibodies. *Journal of Pediatric Surgery* **21**, 132–5.

Lake, B.D., Puri, P., Nixon, H.H. *et al.* 1978: Hirschsprung's disease. An appraisal of histochemically demonstrated acetylcholinesterase activity in suction rectal biopsy specimens as an aid to diagnosis. *Archives of Pathology and Laboratory Medicine* **102**, 244–7.

Le Douarin, N.M. 1982: *The neural crest*. Cambridge: Cambridge University Press.

Lipson, A.H. and Harvey, J. 1987: Three-generation transmission of Hirschsprung's disease. *Clinical Genetics* **32**, 175–8.

Loening-Baucke, V., Pringle, K.C. and Ekwo, E.E. 1985: Anorectal manometry for the exclusion of Hirschsprung's disease in neonates. *Journal of Pediatric Gastroenterology and Nutrition* **4**, 596–603.

Madsen, C.M. 1964: *Hirschsprung's disease*. Copenhagen: Munksgaard.

Meier-Ruge, W. 1971: Uber ein Erkrankungsbild des Colon mit Hirschsprung-Symptomatik. *Verhandlungen der Deutschen Gesellschaft für Pathologie* **55**, 506–10.

Meier-Ruge, W. 1982: Morphological diagnosis. In Holschneider, A.M. (ed.), *Hirschsprung's disease*. Stuttgart: Hippokrates.

Meier-Ruge, W., Lütterbeck, P.M., Herzog, B. *et al.* 1972: Acetylcholinesterase activity in suction biopsies of the rectum in the diagnosis of Hirschsprung's disease. *Journal of Pediatric Surgery* **7**, 11–17.

Mikity, V. G., Hodgman, J.E. and Paciulli, J. 1967: Meconium blockage syndrome. *Radiology* **88**, 740–4.

Mishalany, H.G. and Woolley, M.M. 1987: Postoperative functional and manometric evaluation of patients with Hirschsprung's disease. *Journal of Pediatric Surgery* **22**, 443–6.

Noblett, H.R. 1969: A rectal suction biopsy tube for use in the diagnosis of Hirschsprung's disease. *Journal of Pediatric Surgery* **4**, 406–9.

Novak, N. and Pfeiffer, J. 1989: Acetylcholinesterase-Negativität der lamina propria spricht in der ersten acht lebenswochen nicht gegen Morbus Hirschsprung. *Zeitschrift für Kinderchirurgie* 1988: **44**, 33–6.

Passarge, E. 1967: The genetics of Hirschsprung's disease. Evidence for heterogeneous etiology and a study of sixty-three families. *New England Journal of Medicine* **276**, 138–43.

Passarge, E. 1983: Hirschsprung's disease and other developmental defects of the gastrointestinal tract. In Emergy, A.F.H. and Rimoin, D.L. (eds), *Principles and practice of medical genetics*. Edinburgh: Churchill Livingstone.

Ravitch, M. 1958: Pseudo-Hirschsprung's disease. *Annals of Surgery* **147**, 781–95.

Rehbein, F. and Nicolai, I. 1963: Operation der Hirschsprungschen Krankheit. *Deutsche Medizinische Wochenschrift* **88**, 1595.

Shanbhogue, L.K.R. and Bianchi, A. 1990: Experience with primary Swenson resection and pull-through for neonatal Hirschsprung's disease. *Pediatric Surgery International* **5**, 446–8.

So, H.B., Schwartz, D.L., Becker, J.M. *et al.* 1980: Endorectal pull-through without preliminary colostomy in neonates with Hirschsprung's disease. *Journal of Pediatric Surgery* **15**, 470–1.

Soave, F. 1963: Une nouvelle technique chirurgicale pour le traitement de la maladie de Hirschsprung. *Journal de Chirurgie* **86**, 451.

Spouge, D. and Baird, P.A. 1985: Hirschsprung's disease in a large birth cohort. *Teratology* **32**, 171–7.

Swenson, O. 1959: Hirschsprung's disease (aganglionic megacolon) *New England Journal of Medicine* **260**, 972–6.

Swenson, O. and Bill, A.H. 1948: Resection of rectum and rectosigmoid with preservation of sphincter for benign spastic lesions producing megacolon. *Surgery* **24**, 212–20.

Swenson, O., Sherman, J.O. and Fisher, J.H. 1973: Diagnosis of congenital megacolon: an analysis of 501 patients. *Journal of Pediatric Surgery* **8**, 581–93.

Taxman, T.L., Yulish, B.S. and Rothstein, F.C. 1986: How useful is the barium enema in the diagnosis of infantile Hirschsprung's disease? *American Journal of Diseases of Children* **140**, 881–4.

Teitelbaum, D.H., Gaulman, S.J. and Caniano, D.A. 1988: Hirschsprung's disease indications of risk factors for enterocolitis. *Annals of Surgery* **207**, 240–4.

Thomas, D.F.M., Malone, M., Fernie, D.S. *et al.* 1982: Association between clostridium difficile and enterocolitis in Hirschsprung's disease. *Lancet* **i**, 78–9.

Warkany, J. 1967: *Congenital malformations*. Chicago, IL: Year Book Medical Publishers, 704–9.

Whitehouse, F.R. and Kernohan, J.W. 1948: Myenteric plexus in congenital megacolon. Study of eleven cases. *Archives of Internal Medicine* **82**, 75–111.

Yunis, E.J., Dibbins, A.W. and Sherman, F.E. 1976: Rectal suction biopsy in the diagnosis of Hirschsprung's disease. *Zeitschrift für Kinderchirurgie* **34**, 36–42.

Zachary, R.B. 1957: Meconium and faecal plugs in the newborn. *Archives of Disease in Childhood* **32**, 881–4.

Zee, D.C. van der, Bax, N.M.A., Pull ter Gunne, A.J. and Rovekamp, M.H. 1993: Use of EndoGIA stapling device in Duhamel–Martin procedure for Hirschsprung's disease. *Pediatric Surgery International* **8**, 447–8.

Ziegler, M.M., Ross, A.J. and Bishop, H.C. 1987: Total intestinal aganglionosis: a technique for prolonged survival. *Journal of Pediatric Surgery* **22**, 82–3.

Ziegler, M.M., Royal, R.E., Brandt, J., Drasnin, J. and Martin, L.W. 1993: Extended myectomy–myotomy. A therapeutic alternative for total intestinal aganglionosis. *Annals of Surgery* **218**, 504–11.

Zuelzer, W.W. and Wilson, J.L. 1948: Functional intestinal obstruction on a congenital neurogenic basis in infancy. *American Journal of Disease in Children* **75**, 40–64.

CHAPTER 24

Congenital anorectal anomalies

N.V. FREEMAN

Anorectal anomalies
Embryology
Clinical features
Assessment of other visceral anomalies
Spine and sacrum
Management
Colostomy

General surgical principles
Postoperative management
Optimal age for the definitive operation
Management of cloacal anomalies
Surgical techniques for anorectal anomalies
Results
References

Anorectal anomalies

It may come as a surprise to the reader to know that a baby, born without an anus, an internal sphincter or rectum, can with skilled surgery achieve virtually normal faecal continence, possess what appears to be an anus on the perineum and lead a normal social life.

INCIDENCE OF ANORECTAL ANOMALIES

The incidence of anorectal anomalies is approximately 1:5000 live births. In a survey of a collective series of 5454 cases from the literature, the male-to-female ratio was 55:44. In an accumulated series of 2376 cases of anorectal anomalies, 52% were 'rectal' or 'high' and 48% 'anal' or 'low' in males, and 65% 'rectal' or 'high' and 35% 'anal' or 'low' in females (Smith, 1988).

CLASSIFICATION OF ANORECTAL ANOMALIES

There are many varied and complicated classifications in use. None of which, unfortunately, has been accepted internationally. For practical purposes the question to answer is: 'does the bowel end above the pelvic diaphragm', i.e. a 'high' anomaly, or 'has the bowel almost completed its normal development', and is the problem one of stenosis or ectopia of the anal orifice, i.e. a 'low' anomaly? An 'intermediate' group is also identified in some classifications. Most anomalies are named on an anatomical basis (Fig. 24.1).

Abnormal embryonic development of the hind gut, the urogenital sinus and the Mullerian duct system may result in anomalous connections (fistulae) between the urinary and intestinal tract. The Müllerian duct system (the future vagina, uterus and Fallopian tubes) develops between the urinary tract and hind gut. Aberrant development in females may result in a fistula between the bowel and the vagina, but the never bowel and the urinary tract as in males (Fig. 24.2).

AETIOLOGY

Anorectal anomalies may be isolated, syndromic or associated with various chromosome anomalies. It is more likely, however, that some form of arrest or maldevelopment during early embryonic life (for no known cause) is responsible.

FAMILY HISTORY

Several reports have shown an incidence of more than one sibling being affected, or a parent and child being affected, but this is rare. Following studies of all the families reported in the literature, it has been concluded that heredity plays only a minor or an insignificant role in the aetiology (Smith, 1988).

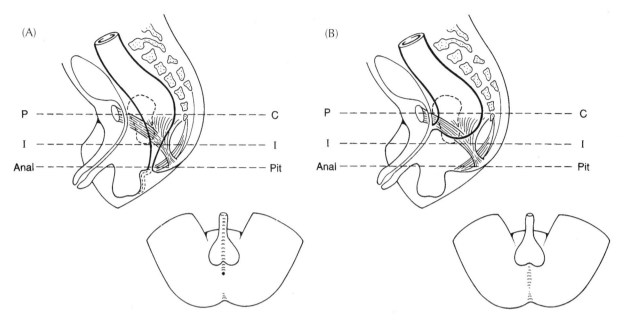

Fig. 24.1 (A) Diagram based on the saggital view of X-ray anatomical landmarks, showing the relationship of the misplaced anorectum to the pelvic muscles (levator ani complex) in a 'low' anomaly in a male patient. The view of the perineum shows the possible tract of an anocutaneous fistula. (B) Shows the relationships in a 'high' anomaly. The perineum is flat with no orifice. Meconium will be found in the urine in the majority of cases.

Embryology

The exact mechanism of the formation of the anorectum in early embryonic life has remained controversial and hypothetical. Until recently, two main events were identified which were thought to be responsible for the differentiation of the cloaca. First, the cloaca is septated by a downwards growing urorectal septum, which divides the cloaca into a urogenital and urorectal part. The prime disagreement was whether the division took place by a downward frontal septum (Torneux fold), a median fusion of two lateral ridges (lateral fold of Rathke), or a combination of both, the cloacal membrane then being divided into a separate anal and urogenital membrane. In the male a second fusion follows and the anogenital folds fuse to form the perineal and scrotal raphe and the penis. Van der Putte (1986) and colleagues from The Netherlands, working on pig embryos, have shown that the previous theories are not tenable. The course of events is as follows (Fig. 24.3A). In young embryos (9–13 mm) the cloaca presents itself in the most characteristic form. The future urinary passages, the destined anorectum and the tailgut open into the cloaca. The cloaca is separated from the amniotic cavity by the cloacal plate, which consists of a multi-layered solid epithelium. The cloacal plate extends dorsally to the tailgroove and ventrally to the tip of the genital tubercle. The 'urorectal septum' is not a true septum but a large mesenchymal mass with two tubular structures, the unfolding urinary and anorectal passages, which open into the cloaca. The 'uroenteric region' would be a more appropriate term for the 'urorectal septum'. Three major processes now take place: (a) a distinct enlargement and ventral growth of the genital tubercle, (b) degeneration of the tailgut and adjacent dorsal cloaca, and (c) lateral stretching and thinning of the dorsal part of the cloacal plate. There is no downwards growth or lateral infolding of the urorectal septum or uroenteric region to divide the cloaca. In the older embryo (15–18 mm) the urorectal septum was observed never to fuse with the cloacal plate. The previously described apparent downwards growth of the urorectal septum is brought about by the changes which occur in the dorsal part of the cloacal membrane. When the thin dorsal part of the cloacal membrane breaks, the future urinary and anorectal tracts are exposed simultaneously. The urorectal septum broadens and the distance between the anorectal and urogenital openings increases. The urogenital opening maintains its position with the tip of the tubercle. In the female this results in a narrow raphe, whereas in the male the raphe is broad. Fusion of the urogenital folds is not seen. A so-called proctodeum does not exist. In this period dense mesenchyme around the intestines indicates the development of a smooth muscle layer. The primordia of the external sphincter and levator ani can just be recognized at the end of this period. From now on the relationships exist and further maturation occurs. In embryos with an abnormal anorectum the striking difference is found in the cloacal plate, which does not reach the tailgroove

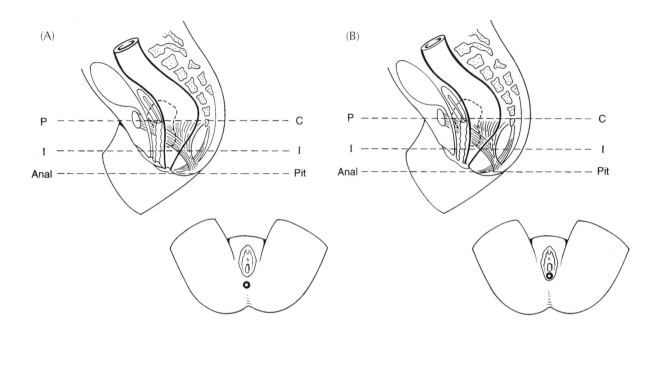

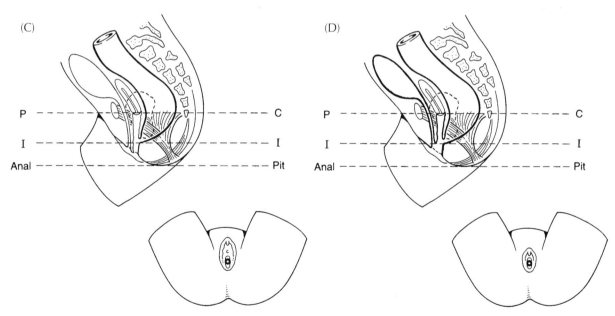

Fig. 24.2 (A) Diagrams based on the saggital view of X-ray anatomical landmarks, showing the relationship of the misplaced anorectum to the pelvic muscles (levator ani complex) in a 'low' anomaly in a female patient. The view of the perineum shows the anal orifice completely surrounded by squamous epithelium. (B) Shows the relationship in a 'low' anomaly with an anovestibular fistula. The perineum shows the 'anal' opening between the forchette and the hymen. Beware that a 'high' anomaly can have exactly the same external appearance! (C) The relationships in a 'high' anomaly with a recto-vaginal fistula. The 'anal' opening is within the vagina. (D) The appearance of a cloacal deformity. Only a single opening is noted on the perineum. The vulva is often small and the clitoris trunk like. The length of the cloacal channel can vary in length.

(Fig. 24.3B). Between the dorsal part of the cloacal plate and tailgroove a mass of mesenchyme is detected instead of epithelium. Because the dorsal part of the cloacal membrane regulates the site of the future anorectum, an abnormal ventral position of the anal opening results. The size of the mesenchymal mass in the dorsal cloaca plate will determine whether the anorectal anomaly is 'low' or 'high'. The pathogenesis of other anorectal anomalies is shown in Fig. 24.3(C).

Clinical features

It is the legal responsibility of every midwife, attending doctor or paediatrician to inspect the perineum of all new-born infants to ascertain that all the orifices are present and normal.

MALES

A careful search should be made for any communication of the bowel with the skin. When found, this track may be seen to be filled with air, white epithelial pearls or black meconium, and may be situated anywhere from the normal anal site to the tip of the penis. The presence of a 'bucket-handle' always indicates a 'low' anomaly. The urethral opening is inspected and urine collected, to establish whether or not meconium is present in the urine. Meconium may be visible either macroscopically or, on microscopic examination, as squamous or epithelial cells in the urine. Meconium in the urine establishes the existence of a fistula between the bowel and urinary tract. The configuration of the perineum may be either 'flat', with bulging on crying, or more normal looking, with a deep intragluteal groove and anal dimple. The

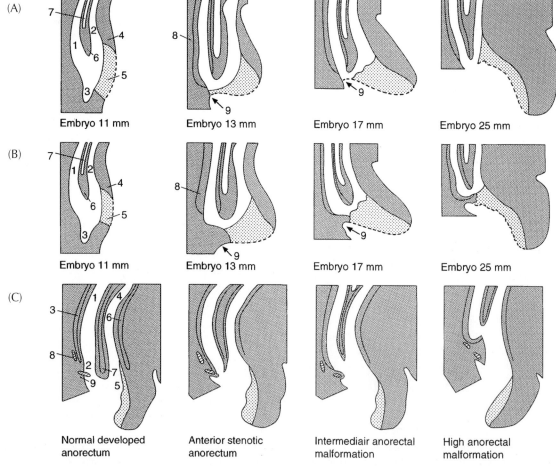

Fig. 24.3 (A) Normal development of the anorectum in the pig from 11 to 25 mm stage. (B) Pathogenesis of congenital malformations in the pig from 11 to 25 mm stage. 1, Future rectum, 2, future urinary passages; 3, tailgut; 4, genital tubercle; 5, cloacal plate; 6, uroenteric region; 7, celomic cavity; 8, smooth muscle of rectum; 9, tail groove. (C) Different types of anorectal malformations in pig embryos of 25 mm. 1, Future rectum; 2, anus; 3, smooth muscle of rectum; 4, future urinary passages; 5, orificium urethra externum; 6, smooth muscle of bladder; 7, uroenteric region; 8, levator ani muscle; 9, sphincter eternus muscle.

shape may help in determining whether the lesion is 'high' or 'low', but is more useful as a clue to the underlying development of the muscle complex.

FEMALES

The perineum is inspected so that it can be established whether the anus is in the normal site or 'ectopic' in position. An ectopic anus is situated less than one-third of the distance between the fourchette and coccyx. It is determined whether there are one, two or three orifices present which, in the newborn, is not always as easy as it sounds. If the anus is not in the normal site, is the opening within the vagina above the hymen, between the fourchette and hymen, or ectopically placed and surrounded completely by dry perineal skin? The infant's back is examined to exclude a spina bifida or a vertebral anomaly. The tip of the coccyx is palpated and a note is made of whether the buttocks are flat with little or no natal cleft, suggestive of sacral agenesis. These bony anomalies will be visible on the plain X-ray. Perineal sensation and the presence of a functioning sphincter are assessed by pinprick or nerve stimulation of the perineum.

Assessment of other visceral anomalies

The acronym VATER, or the expanded VACTERL, is a useful reminder of the other systems that are most likely to be involved in anorectal anomalies, and which need careful examination. The acronym is made up from the first letter of the system involved: vertebral, anal, cardiac, tracheo-oesophageal, renal and limb anomalies. If three or more of the anomalies are present, the child is said to suffer from the VATER or VACTERL syndrome. Since 10% of anorectal anomalies have concomitant oesophageal atresia, a 10 FG nasogastric tube should always be passed if there is any doubt, or if the baby has symptoms suggestive of oesophageal atresia. All children should, at the earliest convenient time, have an ultrasound or intravenous pyelogram (IVP) assessment of the urinary tract to exclude an anomaly, as the incidence is very high, varying from approximately 20% in 'low' (anal) lesions to 50% in 'high' (rectal) lesions.

Spine and sacrum

As many as 30% of anorectal anomalies will have an abnormal spine or sacrum. The vertebral deformities are in the form of butterfly, dysplastic or hemivertebrae, anywhere along the length of the spine. The sacral abnormality may be symmetrical or asymmetrical. The agenesis or hemisacrum may be total or subtotal. A minimum of three sacral segments is required for normal faecal and urinary continence. Intraspinal lesions

are common and may cause progressive deterioration. These lesions are best demonstrated by computerized tomography or magnetic nuclear resonance.

Management

INSPECTION

Careful inspection of the perineum in a good light supplemented by a malleable silver probe will help in the examination of the various fistulae and orifices.

RADIOLOGY (NON-CONTRAST)

The most commonly used X-ray remains the classical 'invertogram' described by Wangenstein and Rice (1930). More recently, a lateral X-ray with the buttocks raised has proved to be equally diagnostic, and does not require the baby to be held upside down for 3 min (Fig. 24.4) (Narashimha *et al.*, 1986). The purpose of the X-ray is to determine the distance of the blind pouch or the fistula from the perineum, and also to judge the relationship of the blind ending pouch to the pelvic diaphragm and the striated muscle complex. The X-ray must be a true lateral centred over the greater trochanter, and the film should include the pubis, sacrum, coccyx and perineum. The anal site should be marked with a smear of thick barium paste. Various parameters or landmarks can be drawn on the X-ray as guides (Figs 24.1 and 24.2). Gas may be seen in the bladder, urethra or in a subcutaneous tract, indicating a connection with the bowel.

RADIOPAQUE DYE STUDIES

To delineate accurately the anatomy of the fistula radiopaque dye can be injected into the orifice. If a colostomy is present, a distal loopogram should be performed prior to any definitive surgery. A Foley balloon catheter is inserted into the distal loop of the colostomy and inflated. The dye must be injected by syringe, in order to raise the hydrostatic pressure in the distal segment. Not using hydrostatic pressure may fail to outline the level of the lesion accurately or demonstrate a fistula.

In the minority of cases (approximately 15%) there is no fistula and the lesion is thought to be 'low' or 'intermediate' on plain X-ray. In these patients needle aspiration of the perineum, in the midline, is a worthwhile procedure. If meconium or gas is encountered, contrast can be injected (Muragasu, 1970). The fistula may be demonstrated by micturition cystography, either via a catheter into the bladder or by injection of contrast retrograde from the tip of the urethra.

PITFALLS

For correct interpretation, the terminal gas shadow of the atretic bowel must be smooth and rounded. This

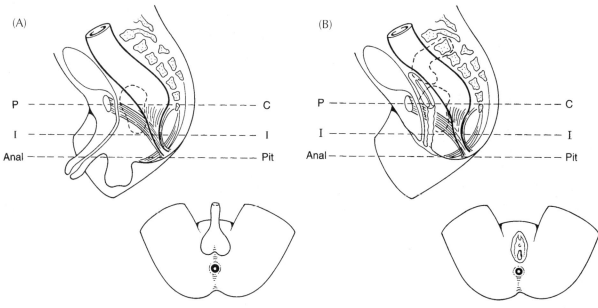

Fig. 24.4 Diagrams based on the lateral X-ray landmarks of the male (A) and female (B) infant pelvis, showing the relationship of the bowel to the pelvic muscle complex and the bony structures. The Pubo-coccygeal line (PC) is drawn from the centre of the pubis to the sacrococcygeal articulation. The line passes through the upper and middle thirds of the ischium. The ischial line is parallel to the PC line at the lowest point of the ischial bone. The anal pit line is parallel and one to two centimetre below the 'L' line. Soft tissues in the male: PC line – verumontanum, peritoneal reflection; 'I' line – bulb of the urethra. In the female: bladder neck, cervix; perineal body, triangular lig. Also note that the pelvic diaphragm (levator ani, pubo rectalis, striated muscle complex) are funnel shaped, mainly above the 'I' point.

indicates complete filling and displacement of all the distal meconium. The X-ray should be taken preferably more than 24 hours after birth, as gas does not reach the rectum much before this time.

Sticky meconium occupying the distal bowel may lead to errors in interpretation as to the level of the lesion.

A strong contraction of the levator complex at the moment of X-ray causes occlusion of the anal canal and may give a totally wrong impression of the length of a fistula or the presence of an anal canal (Fig. 24.5).

Gas may escape through a fistula to the skin, urethra or vagina, thereby preventing full distension and outline of the rectum.

Misleading levels of the gas shadow are seen when the baby cries, as the distended rectal gas shadow may be pushed beyond the 'I' point by the raised intra-abdominal pressure.

OTHER INVESTIGATIVE METHODS

Ultrasound scanning of the pelvis via the perineum may demonstrate the type and level of anomaly (Willital, 1971). This technique has not received wide application and needs an experienced operator for interpretation.

Computerized axial tomography and magnetic resonance (Mezzacappa *et al.*, 1987) are now being used more often to demonstrate the anorectal anatomy and striated muscle complex. The baby is small enough to be placed sagittally in the opening of the scanner to obtain a midline, rather than a transverse scan (Tam *et al.*, 1987).

Electromyography of the external sphincter by bipolar needle electrodes inserted into the perineum is also being used to determine the presence of the striated muscle complex (Yokoyama *et al.*, 1985).

Endoscopy of the urethra or vagina provides further information on the size and site of the fistula, and is best carried out at the start of the definitive operative procedure.

Colostomy

As there is a definite morbidity and mortality associated with colostomy, the operation should never be performed, unless strictly necessary. A colostomy is needed for all 'high' lesions, with an occasional exception. Controversy exists regarding the use of colostomy in the 'intermediate' lesions. A colostomy should never be required in 'low' lesions. Several important precautions are needed in the establishment of a colostomy. It should be defunctioning. A simple sigmoid loop colostomy,

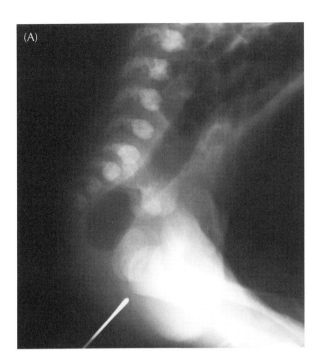
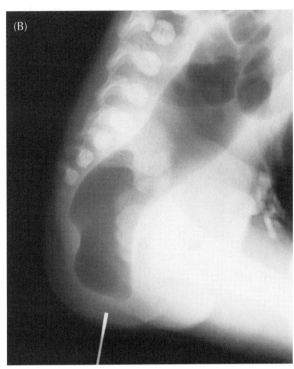

Fig. 24.5 Invertogram X-rays taken at (A) 12 and (B) 24 hours. Clinically the anomaly was suspected as being 'low', but the 12-hour film could easily have been misinterpreted as a 'high' anomaly. The appearance is due either to sticky meconium or or contraction of the levator ani muscle.

sited in the left iliac fossa, leaving enough distal sigmoid colon for the subsequent definitive pull-through operation, is satisfactory. Some authors insist on complete division of the colon with separation of the loops by a skin bridge. In most cases this is not necessary, especially if the definitive surgery is performed early in the neonatal period and the colostomy closed within a few months. When creating a colostomy the marginal blood supply must be carefully inspected and preserved, so as not to compromise the distal bowel on subsequent closure of the colostomy. At the time of colostomy the distal loop must be washed out until completely emptied of meconium. Normal saline or 1% aqueous betadine can be used for the washout. In a loop colostomy the distal segment can refill because of overspill and must be kept empty, by further washouts, if necessary.

There is seldom any real urgency to operate immediately on a baby with an anorectal anomaly. For the inexperienced surgeon the primary decision is whether to perform a colostomy or whether a simple 'anoplasty' or dilatation is all that is needed. The surgeon should not operate until he or she is certain as to the exact anatomy of malformation present.

The algorithms shown in Figs 24.6 and 24.7 outline the management in the male and female infant with an anorectal anomaly.

General surgical principles

The following general surgical principles apply to all anorectal operations. Skilled anaesthesia is necessary with full facilities for intensive monitoring, as many of these operations are very prolonged. The monitoring should include two temperature probes to measure the core–skin temperature gradient, pulse oxymetry, blood loss measurement and blood gas analysis. Venous access by means of a peripheral or a central vein is usual. In most instances the blood loss should be minimal, as the paediatric surgeon tries to operate in virtually a bloodless field. The use of diathermy throughout, even for cutting the skin, is helpful in this respect. The theatre should be designed to keep the baby warm, and should include the ability to increase the ambient air temperature individually in a theatre suite. As the baby is exposed to the surrounding temperature during induction and the insertion of intravenous lines, an overhead radiant heater in the induction room and theatre, together with a circulating water mattress on the operating table, helps to prevent further heat loss. The baby's arms, legs and head should be wrapped in cotton wool or Gamgee prior to skin preparation.

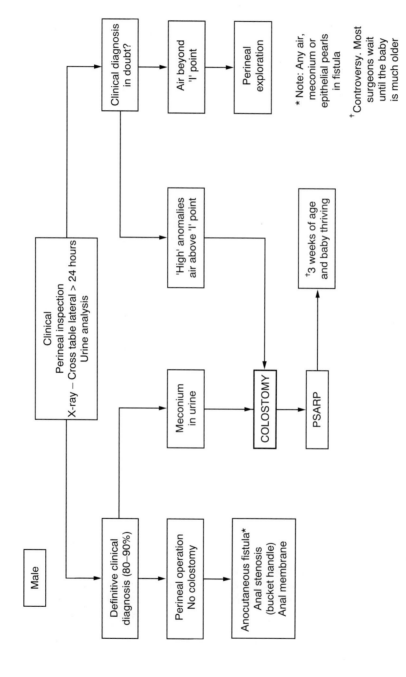

Fig. 24.6 Algorithm of the management plan in a newborn male infant with an imperforate anus.

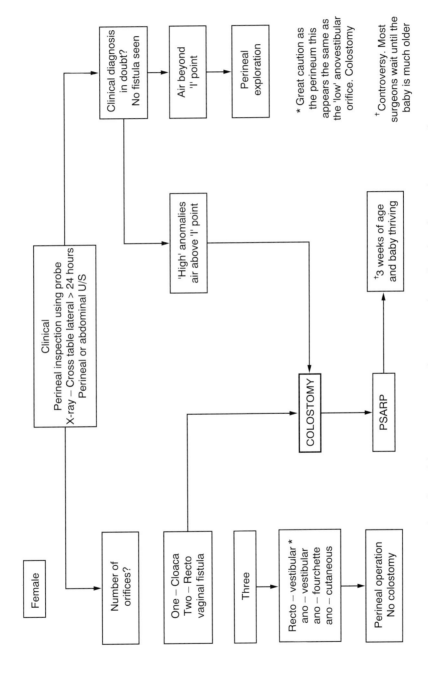

Fig. 24.7 Algorithm of the management plan in a newborn female infant with an imperforate anus.

Antiseptic fluids for skin cleansing should be warm. During surgery a large plastic drape covers the whole baby, and if the baby is well positioned on the water mattress the heat from the mattress is entrapped by the drape.

POSITION OF THE PATIENT ON THE OPERATING TABLE

The following three main positions can be used,

(a) The 'jack-knife' position: the baby is placed prone with the buttocks raised by a sandbag under the pelvis. Two small pads are placed under the shoulders to prevent hyperextension of the neck. The sandbag is best placed under the circulating water mattress.
(b) The lithotomy position: even with the use of small stirrups only the older children can be positioned comfortably in the lithotomy position.
(c) A modified lithotomy position: if the baby is a neonate or too small, then this position can be used by strapping the feet and legs together across the lower abdomen.

POSITION OF THE SURGEON

Ideal placement of the surgeon, assistant and scrub nurse around a small baby, with each having a reasonable view and access, can be difficult. The surgeon can sit at the foot of the table with the baby directly in front of him or her, in either the jack-knife or lithotomy position. Standing on the right side of the operating table is also suitable, but involves a lot of bending. A Mayo table should be fixed to the upper part of the operating table, with the lower edge at about the level of the patient's xiphisternum and raised about 6 inches from the baby's face.

BOWEL WASHOUT ON THE TABLE

The bowel should be mechanically cleansed and sterilized with 1 to 2% aqueous povodine iodine just before surgery. Warm solutions should be used at all times to prevent further heat loss from the baby.

ANTIBIOTICS

Preoperative gut sterilization using antibiotics is not necessary. Metronidazole and cloxacillin, or a similar combination, started with the induction of anaesthesia and continued for 3–5 days, usually suffices as a 'prophylaxis'. Operating with magnification, using a loupe or a dissecting microscope, is to be recommended.

Electrostimulation during the operation is essential to identify functioning bands of muscle. The anaesthetist's peripheral nerve stimulator is capable of delivering 60 mA. In older children or those with a lot of scar tissue, especially during secondary operations, a stimulator capable of delivering up to 240 mA may be necessary.

Postoperative management

The success of most anorectal operations depends on a very careful, personal, meticulous and prolonged follow-up by the surgeon. Primary healing without any breakdown of wounds, leaks or sepsis is the ideal aim. If sepsis occurs, a fibrotic stricture at the mucocutaneous junction or behind the anal canal is likely to develop.

Faecal contamination of the area may be prevented by a diverting colostomy. As stated previously, a colostomy is not always necessary and careful bowel preparation together with a low-residue diet preoperatively may be equally effective. When the bowel starts to function postoperatively and faecal soiling occurs, the area should immediately be irrigated with normal saline. It is preferable to use a hand-shower, if the patient can be transported to the appropriate bathroom. Sitting on the perineum exerts a tremendous lateral force on the midline suture lines and should be avoided for the first week to 10 days postoperatively. This may be difficult in practice but, if possible, the patient should only be permitted to stand or lie on his or her back or side. Nylon skin sutures rather than subcutaneous absorbable sutures are recommended, and should be left *in situ* for at least 10 days.

Catheterization of the patient for 3–4 days postoperatively lessens the overall movement of the patient and helps to protect the suture line from excess force, thereby allowing primary healing. When healing has occurred, at approximately 10 days, dilatations are started. With the possible exception of the first dilatation, local anaesthetic cream or no anaesthetic is better and safer than a traumatic forceful dilatation under general anaesthesia. The dilatations must be gentle and graduated. Increasing the size too rapidly and causing bleeding and tearing is to be avoided, as in the long term more scarring and fibrosis will occur. Dilatations must continue for several months until the anus is soft and supple. A regime of daily or twice-daily dilatations for 1–2 months then decreasing to once a week for 3–6 months is suitable. The author prefers the mother using her finger for dilatation, but this may not be practical at times because of the large size of the mother's finger. As Hegar dilators are expensive, simple dilators for use at home can be made from candies, disposable plastic pen tops, etc. The ideal size of the anus at which to aim can be determined from the formula: 1.3 + (weight in kg × 3), roughly 3–4 mm diameter (No. 11–12 Hegar size) in the newborn (el-Haddad and Corkery, 1985).

Optimal age for the definitive operation

In 'low' anomalies in both male and female infants simple dilatation or an anoplasty to widen the orifice can be performed in the immediate neonatal period. In 'high' anomalies, due to intestinal obstruction, a colostomy is necessary, usually within the first 24–48 hours.

Once the obstruction has been relieved the timing of the definitive pull-through operation is optional and remains controversial. At present most surgeons believe that the operation is safer, and the anatomical structures better defined, if the surgery is deferred until about 9–12 months of age. There is physiological evidence that early surgery within the first 3 months of life may have definite advantages, as the brain is immature at birth and the synaptic cortical connections, measured by evoked anal potentials, are made in the early weeks or months of postnatal life. If the bowel is placed in the correct site before 3 months of age appropriate cortical connections may develop and the outcome may improve (Freeman *et al.*, 1980, 1986).

After performing a colostomy in 'intermediate' anomalies, the definitive surgery can be delayed to suit the surgeon's preference. Otherwise, an operation in the neonate is needed to relieve the obstruction.

Management of cloacal anomalies

A colostomy is always necessary. Relief of the urinary and vaginal obstruction may require vesicostomy and drainage of the mucocolpos. The repair is best delayed until the child is about 6 months old. Even in the very experienced hands of a surgeon such as Pena, a total reconstruction may take 4–12 hours to complete.

Surgical techniques for anorectal anomalies

In low anomalies a simple 'cut-back', i.e. one blade of the scissors placed in the tract and a cut made in the midline, or a more elaborate Y–V plasty will widen the anal opening. If repositioning of the anus is required some form of transplant of the anal canal, using a limited PSAP, is needed.

In 'high' anomalies the abdominoperineal pull-through was used in the 1960s (Rhoades *et al.*, 1948). This was superseded by the sacroperineal pull-through (Stephens, 1953) in the 1970s. In 1982 Pena and de Vries described the posterior sagittal anorectoplasty which was based on Bodenhamer's (1860) operation. This procedure is the most widely practised at present and can also be employed for the more complicated cloacal deformities.

Results

It is impossible to evaluate results from the various publications, as the following important facts are not always mentioned:

(a) whether a 'high', 'intermediate' or 'low' anomaly was originally treated
(b) whether the anomaly was approached via a purely perineal, sacroperineal or abdominoperineal route
(c) the decade in which the report appeared
(d) the age of the patient at operation
(e) the actual technical details of the operation, e.g. whether the tip of the 'anus/fistula' was excised
(f) the length of follow-up.

The decade in which the publication appeared is significant. From the turn of the century the approach was a midline perineal approach (Kieswetter and Turner, 1963). This changed to an abdominoperineal approach in the 1950s following the paper by Rhoades *et al.* (1948) paper. Stephens (1953) introduced the sacroperineal operation which, together with its modifications, held sway for the next decade. The decade of the 1980s saw the return of Bodenhamer's (1860) perineal operation, now described as posterior sagittal anorectoplasty (Pena and de Vries, 1982).

AGE AT INITIAL OPERATION

The age at operation needs to be considered. Until recently it was accepted world-wide that it was unsafe and unsatisfactory to perform the definitive operation before the age of 1 year, because of possible damage to the delicate sphincteric complex. With the advances in anatomical knowledge, magnification and the use of a muscle stimulator at operation, this is no longer true. Several authors (Nixon and Puri, 1977; Freeman *et al.*, 1986) have shown superior results in those children treated early. The reason for this may lie in the postnatal development of synapses within the brain (Freeman *et al.*, 1980).

OPERATIVE DETAILS

Embryological studies on pigs (Van der Putte, 1986) have shown that the anal region is developed morphologically and contains the rudimentary sphincters. Patients in which this portion of the bowel was excised are therefore likely to suffer some loss of control (Templeton and Dietsheim, 1985). Several criteria have been used to determine and define adequate faecal continence but these have not been applied uniformly in publications.

CLINICAL CRITERIA OF FAECAL CONTINENCE

It is doubtful whether any child with a 'high' anomaly ever achieves perfect faecal continence. By 'perfect' or 'excellent' control, one implies that there are no accidents or faecal soiling, with either solid or liquid stools, controlled passage of flatus, no constipation and no use of laxatives or enemas. The manner in which 'faecal control' or 'continence' has been expressed varies in different publications. Clinical criteria can be used and classifications such as 'good', 'fair' or 'poor' or 'excellent', 'good', 'fair' or 'poor', have been used to describe the author's range of near normal control to total incontinence (Kieswetter and Turner, 1963; Senson and Donnellan, 1967; Stephens and Smith, 1967).

RADIOLOGICAL ASSESSMENT OF CONTINENCE

The clinical assessment may be supplemented by a scoring system based on certain X-ray findings on contrast examination. During the contrast examination the amount of leak around a 24 FG catheter, rectal sensation on filling and degree of puborectalis contraction are evaluated (Kelly, 1969).

MANOMETRIC ASSESSMENT

Several authors regard the data obtained by detailed physiological electromanometry studies as the most accurate way of measuring and expressing the degree of continence. The parameters which are recorded include the rectosphincteric relaxation reflex, 'the rectosphincteric contraction reflex' of the external anal sphincter, 'the anorectal resting profile', 'the anorectal squeezing pressure profile', and 'the rectal adaption reaction' (Holschneider, 1988).

DURATION OF FOLLOW-UP

There is definite evidence of improvement in continence with the passage of time. Patients should preferably be more than 10 years old before a final assessment of their faecal continence is made. The author's personal results indicate 70% 'good', 18% 'fair' and 12% 'poor' for 'high' lesions (Freeman and Bulut, 1986). Sieber, reporting from Pittsburg compared the results of the sacroperineal and abdominosacroperineal (1986) approach in 63 patients. He showed approximately a 40% 'good', 30% 'fair' and 30% 'poor' outcome. Holschneider (1988) reported the results in 174 patients, of whom 71 had 'high' lesions, and of these 59 were available for detailed follow-up assessment. There was an overall mortality of 16.6%. The deaths occurred in the 'high' (58%), 'intermediate' (27%) and 'low' (3%) groups. Overall, 50% of 'high' and 14% of 'low' anomalies remained incontinent 5 years after surgery. Only 15% of the 'high' anomalies became continent, in spite of secondary surgery.

More attention needs to be directed to the outcome of 'low' anomalies, where 100% 'good' results should be anticipated, but between 15 and 20% of children still have problems with defaecation.

Rintala *et al.* (1991) studied 83 adults, 53 females and 30 males, with low anorectal anomalies at a mean age of 35 years. Only 60% had 'good' continence and 15% had 'normal' continence. Social problems were found in 39%, and 15% had sexual problems. No

fertility has been observed over 30 years in any of the 'high' anorectal anomalies, in males, treated at Great Ormond Street Hospital, London (Kiely, 1991).

Langemeijer and Molenaar (1991) reviewed patients between 1 and 7 years after surgery for 'high' anorectal anomalies. They concluded that no patient achieves continence, although 20 of 23 patients achieved 'pseudo-continence' with the use of daily enemas. On testing with anal manometry and electrostimulation, there was no functional difference between the PSAP and the earlier type of pull-through operations. Only one patient showed evidence of an inhibitory reflex. These patients suffer from a life-long handicap and need support and follow-up. These findings are echoed by Pena's group from New York, who studied 30 patients 5–9 years after surgery: 21 showed no internal sphincter, 19 were constipated and 16 soiled (Hedlund *et al.*, 1991). Pena's (1992) results indicate that 60% of male patients, with a normal sacrum and a rectourethral fistula, have 'good' results.

References

Bodenhamer, W. 1860: *Aetiology, pathology and treatment of congenital malformations of the rectum and anus.* New York: Samuel S. & William Wood.

el-Haddad, M. and Corkery, J.J. 1985: The anus in the new born. *Paediatrics* **76**, 927–8.

Freeman, N.V. and Bulut, M. 1986: 'High' anorectal anomalies treated by early 'neonatal' operation. *Journal of Paediatric Surgery* **21**, 218–20.

Freeman, N.V., Burge, D.M., Sedgewick, E.M. and Soar, G. 1980: Anal evoked potentials. *Zeitschrift für Kinderchirugie* **31**, 22–9.

Hedlund, H., Pena, A., Rodriquez, G. and Maza J. 1991: Long term anorectal function in imperforate anus treated by posterior sagittal anorectoplasty (PSARP). Presented at the XXXVIII Meeting of British Paediatric Surgeons, Budapest, July 1991.

Holschneider, A.M. 1988: Function of the sphincters in anorectal malformations and post-operative evaluation. In Stephens, F.D. and Smith, E.D. (eds), *Anorectal malformations in children: update* 1988, **24**, March of Dimes, Birth Defects Foundation. New York: Alan R. Liss, 425–45.

Kelly, J.H. 1969: The radiographic anatomy of the normal and abnormal neonatal pelvis. *Journal of Pediatric Surgery* **4**, 432–44.

Kiely, E. 1991: Remark at BAPS, Budapest, July 1991.

Kieswetter, W.B. and Turner, C.R. After surgery for imperforate anus. A critical analysis and preliminary experience of the sacroperineal pull-through. *Annals of Surgery* **158**, 498–506.

Langemeijer, R.A.T. and Molenaar, J.C. 1991: Continence after posterior sagittal anorectoplasty. *Journal of Pediatric Surgery* **26**, 587–690.

Mezzacappa, P.M., Price, A.P., Haller, J.O., Kassner, E.G. and Hansbrough, F. 1987: MR and CT demonstration of levator sling in congenital anorectal anomalies. *Journal of Computer Assisted Tomography* **11**, 273–5.

Muragasu, J.J. 1970: a new method of roentgenological demonstration of anorectal anomalies. *Surgery* **68**, 706–12.

Narashimha, R.L.L., Prasad, G.R., Kotariya, S., Mitra, S. and Pathak, I.C. 1986: Prone cross table lateral view: an alternative to the invertogram in imperforate anus. *American Journal of Roentgenology* **140**, 227–9.

Nixon, H.H. and Puri, P. 1977: The results of treatment of anorectal anomalies: a thirteen to twenty year follow-up. *Journal of Pediatric Surgery* **12**, 27–31.

Pena, A. 1992: Current management of anorectal anomalies. *Surgical Clinics of North America* **6**, 1393–416.

Pena, A. and de Vries, P.A. 1982: Posterior sagittal anorectoplasty: important technical considerations and new applications. *Journal of Pediatric Surgery* **17**, 796–811.

Rhoades, J.E., Piper, R.L. and Randall, J.P. 1948: A simultaneous abdominal and perineal approach in operations for imperforate anus with atresia of the rectum and rectosigmoid. *Annals of Surgery* **127**, 552–6.

Rintala, R., Mildh, L. and Lindahl, H. 1991: Fecal continence and quality of life in adult patients with an operated low anorectal malformation. Presented at BAPS, Budapest, July 1991.

Sieber, W.K. 1986: Anorectal anomalies. The Pittsburg experience. Presented at the Douglas Stephens Symposium on anorectal and genito-urinary anomalies, Chicago, IL, 16–18 October 1986.

Smith, D. 1988: Incidence, frequency of types, and etiology of anorectal malformations. In Stephens, F.D. and Smith, D. (eds), *Anorectal malformations in children*: *update 1988*. March of Dimes, Birth Defects Foundation. New York: Alan R. Liss, 231–43.

Stephens, F.D. 1953: Imperforate rectum: a new surgical technique. *Medical Journal of Australia and New Zealand* 202–3.

Stephens, F.D. and Smith, E.D. 1967: Results and complications and assessment of continence. In: Stephens, F.D. and Smith, E.D. (eds), *Anorectal malformations in children*. Chicago, IL: Year Book Publishers, 339–37.

Swenson, O. and Donnellan, W.L. 1967: Preservation of the pubo rectalis sling in imperforate anus repair. *Surgical Clinics North of America* **47**, 173–7.

Tam, P.K., Chan, F.L. and Saing, H. 1987: Direct sagittal T scan: a new diagnostic approach for surgical neonates. *Journal of Pediatric Surgery* **22**, 397–400.

Templeton, J.M. and Dietsheim, J.A. 1985: High imperforate anus – quantitative results of longterm fecal continence. *Journal of Pediatric Surgery* **20**, 645–52.

Van der Putte, S.C.J. 1986: Normal and abnormal development of the anorectum. *Journal of Pediatric Surgery* **21**, 434–40.

Wangenstein, O.H. and Rice, C. 1930: Imperforate anus: a method of determining surgical approach. *Annals of Surgery* **92**, 77–9.

Willital, G.H. 1971: Advances in the diagnosis of anal and rectal atresia by ultrasonic-echo scan. *Journal of Paediatric Surgery* **6**, 454–7.

Yokoyama, J., Ikawa, H. and Katsumata, K. 1985: Abdominoextended sacroperineal approach in high type anorectal malformation – and a new operative method. *Zeitschrift für Kinderchirugie* **40**, 151–7.

CHAPTER 25

Necrotizing enterocolitis

V.E. BOSTON

Introduction
Incidence
Pathology
Risk factors
Aetiology

Management
Summary
References
Further reading

Introduction

The first description of necrotizing enterocolitis (NEC) was probably made by Generisch in 1891, when a full-term infant was reported to have had an ileal perforation of unknown cause and without distal intestinal obstruction. Since then, the characteristics of the disease have become established, together with some understanding of the aetiology.

Incidence

The incidence of NEC is reported to be approximately 0.3 per 1000 live births (Kliegman and Fanaroff, 1981; Walsh and Kliegman, 1986; Kosloske and Musemeche, 1989). Eighty per cent of all affected children are either of less than 34 weeks' gestation or weigh less than 2000 g at birth. However, up to 20% will be full-term infants (Blin et al., 1976; Wiswell et al., 1988). There is a 2:1 male-to-female ratio (Kliegman and Fanaroff, 1981; Walsh and Kliegman, 1986; Cheromcha and Hyman, 1988; Walsh et al., 1988; Amspacher, 1989) and 95% will have been fed orally before presentation (Kliegman and Fanaroff, 1981; Cikrit et al., 1984; Thilo et al., 1984; Milner et al., 1986; Kishan et al., 1988; Walther et al., 1989; Covert et al., 1989; Kosloske and Musemeche, 1989). Most commonly, the signs of NEC develop on the third day of life (Kliegman and Fanaroff,

1986; Amspacher, 1989) but approximately 15% of cases will occur on the day of birth (Thilo et al., 1984) and the disease has been recognized up to 3 months of age or older (Ramenofsky, 1977; Moss and Adler, 1982). It occurs almost exclusively in neonatal intensive care units (NICU) where its frequency is approximately 12% (Walsh and Kliegman, 1986; Gregory et al., 1987; Cheromcha and Hyman, 1988; Walsh et al., 1988; Palmer et al., 1989; Holmn et al., 1989). While NEC is uncommon, it is an important cause of morbidity and mortality. Approximately 6% of all neonatal deaths (Brans et al., 1982) and 15% of those dying after the first week of life (Wilson et al., 1981) are caused by NEC. In all affected children, mortality is reported to be between 10 and 40%, increasing to greater than 50% in high-risk babies (Cikrit et al., 1984).

Pathology

NEC is primarily a mucosal disease which extends well beyond the margins of apparently normal intestine on the serosal surface. The most frequently affected parts are the terminal ileum, ascending and transverse colon. The descending colon and, rarely, the greater part of the small intestine and stomach are also affected.

The affected intestinal mucosa is oedematous and haemorrhagic, with ulceration in more severe cases. The capillary bed of the submucosal vascular plexus demonstrates plugging with platelet aggregates which is associated with engorgement of more proximal vessels and distal venous thrombosis (Santulli *et al.*, 1975; Joshi, 1977; Kosloske and Musemeche, 1989). This process is primarily a microvascular as opposed to a macrovascular disease and the main mesenteric vessels are usually patent (Kosloske and Musemeche, 1989).

There is a notable absence of infiltration of the bowel wall with inflammatory cells early in the disease. However, bacteria can usually be identified at this stage in the mucosa and deeper layers. The serosa will usually be oedematous but may be haemorrhagic or show signs of transmural infarction in severe cases.

In the majority of cases, blebs of gas (pneumatosis intestinalis) are visible under the visceral peritoneum and these often extend into the mesentery. Gas is often visible in the interstitial tissue and possibly also in the lymphatics of the bowel wall. This is usually associated with transmural infarction.

Where perforation has occurred there are usually signs of generalized peritonitis. Loops of small intestine will often be matted together and associated with local abscess formation at the site of infarction (Santulli *et al.*, 1975; Joshi, 1977; Kosloske and Musemeche, 1989).

After a few days an inflammatory cell infiltration becomes apparent in the affected segment of intestine. In most instances this will resolve without trace but where there has been significant tissue loss caused by necrosis, repair often results in fibrosis, which may cause a stenosis of the lumen. This process may take at least 3–4 months to become established and has implications for the medium- to long-term management of these cases (Joshi, 1977; Kosloske and Musemeche, 1989).

Risk factors

There are many prenatal and postnatal risk factors which have been reported to be associated with NEC. However, using methods of multivariance analysis the only significant risk indicators appear to be low birth weight, prematurity and oral feeding prior to the onset of disease (Kliegman *et al.*, 1982; Cheromcha and Hyman, 1988; Walther *et al.*, 1989). Congenital heart disease appears to increase the incidence of NEC in affected children, particularly after corrective surgery, but this group is small and the relative risk is difficult to assess (Leung *et al.*, 1988).

Aetiology

No single mechanism can be demonstrated to account for the pathogenesis of NEC in all cases. The timing of events suggests that the common feature is a process initiated by mucosal injury which may progress to either mild or fulminant NEC depending on local circumstances. This initiating mucosal injury probably has many different causes and in some children there may be more than one mechanism at work.

FREE RADICALS

In animal models of NEC it is known that toxic free radicals of oxygen are released in the intestine in response to many different challenges, including reduced intraluminal pH, hypoxia, hypovolaemia, occlusion/reperfusion injury and cold stress (Miller *et al.*, 1988; Clark *et al.*, 1988; Miller and Clark, 1989; Cassatto *et al.*, 1989; Caplan and Hsueh, 1990). These free radicals are known to cause lipid peroxidation and thus damage cell membranes and increase vascular permeability. In NEC, there is good clinical and laboratory evidence that local production of free radicals then causes the release of the cytokines [e.g. as tumour necrosis factor (TNF), interleukin-1 (IL-1) and interleukin-6 (IL-6)] and vasoactive factors [e.g. platelet aggregation factor (PAF) and eicosanoids] (Sharon and Stenson, 1985; Llausa-Magan *et al.*, 1988; Cueva and Hsueh, 1988; Hsueh and Gonzalez-Crussi, 1988; Cheromcha and Hyman, 988; Miller and Clark, 1989; Hsueh *et al.*, 1990; Caplan and MacKendrick, 1993; Tan *et al.*, 1993. Complex feedback mechanisms between these factors causes a cascade of events which eventually results in bacterial translocation from the lumen, thrombosis of intramural vessels and transmural infarction typical of NEC.

The source of these free radicals is thought to be intestinal macrophages. In normal circumstances there is 'in-house protection' against these toxic metabolites in the form of 'scavengers' such as superoxide dismutase/catalase. Superoxide dismutase will prevent the development of NEC in an experimental model (Miller *et al.*, 1988; Caplan and Hsueh, 1990).

Local production of mucosal free radicals probably occurs through several different mechanisms which may include direct physical damage to the mucosa by infection or the products of infection, hypoxaemia, decreased perfusion and perhaps immune complex formation.

INFECTIVE AGENTS AND TOXINS

The neonatal intestine is sterile at birth and becomes colonized with increasing age. The rate and type of colonization will depend on various factors which include the environment in which the child is being nursed, whether antibiotics are being administered, the timing of the introduction of feeds and type and volume of feeds which have been employed (Long and Swenson, 1977; Goldman *et al.*, 1978; Yoshioka *et al.*, 1983; Stevenson, 1989). Premature and full-term infants colonize in different ways. This is probably related to differences in immunological status and feeding practices (Yoshioka *et al.*, 1983).

Epidemiologically, two different types of NEC are recognized. Eighty per cent are of the sporadic type, as compared to the rarer epidemic form, which clusters in both time and space (Moomjian *et al.*, 1978; Kliegman and Fanaroff, 1981; Wilson *et al.*, 1981; Brans *et al.*, 1982; Chany *et al.*, 1982; Rotbart and Levin, 1983; Anderson *et al.*, 1984; Walsh and Kliegman, 1986; Zabielski *et al.*, 1989). In microbiological terms, the epidemic form typifies an infective illness where the organism responsible for the disease, is common to all cases and where there has been nosocomial spread from child to child within the unit (Chany *et al.*, 1982; Rotbart and Levin, 1983; Mogilner *et al.*, 1983; Mollitt *et al.*, 1988; Rotbart *et al.*, 1988). This hypothesis has been further strengthened by the observation that strict infection control measures, such as hand washing, isolation and single cohort nursing, appear to reduce the incidence of the disease once cases have occurred in a NICU (Rotbart and Levin, 1983). However, in the vast majority of sporadic or epidemic cases no specific pathogen has been identified (Virnig and Reynolds, 1974; Anderson *et al.*, 1984).

Ninety per cent of affected children will have pneumatosis intestinalis (Kliegman and Fanaroff, 1982). This intramural gas has been analysed and in particular has been shown to contain hydrogen (Engel *et al.*, 1973). Biologically, this gas can only have been derived from the fermentation of carbohydrate and this implies the presence of anaerobic bacteria (Engel *et al.*, 1973; Yale *et al.*, 1974; Bousseboua *et al.*, 1989). What is not clear however, is whether the bacteria which caused the pneumatosis were the primary cause of the NEC.

Many species such as *Clostridia* produce exotoxins which are capable of inflicting mucosal damage (Lyerly *et al.*, 1988; Bousseboua *et al.*, 1989). Epidemic NEC has been documented to be associated with *Clostridium butyricum* and production of exotoxin may have been partly responsible for the development of the disease in these cases (Bousseboua *et al.*, 1989). Other less well-known species have been implicated, such as *Staphylococcus albus*, which are capable of toxin production (Scheifele *et al.*, 1987; Mollitt *et al.*, 1988). Exotoxin- or endotoxin-induced NEC is unlikely to be the main cause of mucosal damage because the vast majority of all cases are not associated with faecal culture of toxin-producing species (Virnig and Reynolds, 1974). Consequently, some other mechanism of pathogenicity must be involved in the majority.

SHORT-CHAIN FATTY ACIDS

Carbohydrate malabsorption occurs in all newborn infants. It is known that normal colonic commensals can ferment malabsorbed carbohydrate with the production

of gas and the short-chain fatty acids (SCFA) acetic, lactic, butyric and proprionic acids. Normally, these are cleared from the intestinal lumen by one or more mechanisms (Kripke *et al.*, 1989; Jenkins, 1989). When this process is occurring efficiently the intraluminal pH rarely drops below 5 and fermentation and absorption can continue to occur. However, the stools of babies who have developed NEC usually contain fatty acids and have a pH < 5, implying that the mechanism for absorption of SCFA has been overwhelmed by either excessive production or decreased absorption (Clark *et al.*, 1985). There is experimental evidence which suggests that a intraluminal pH < 5 is associated with mucosal damage (Garstin *et al.*, 1987; Miller and Clark, 1989). Thus if absorption of SCFAs is impaired, a cycle of events can occur which will eventually lead to bacterial translocation through the normally impenetrable mucosal barrier.

Excessive production, as compared to decreased absorption of SCFA, appears to account for the majority of cases (Garcia *et al.*, 1984; Anderson *et al.*, 1985; Garstin and Boston, 1987b; Cheu *et al.*, 1989; Stevenson, 1989). Increased amounts of carbohydrate reaching the terminal small bowel (which is then available for fermentation) will depend not only on the total amount of ingested feed but also on the degree to which it is malabsorbed. It is well known that neonates and in particular premature infants are prone to small intestinal lactase deficiency.

Decreased clearance can be either primary due to deficiency of mucosal systems for clearance of SCFA caused by immaturity, or secondary due to damage of the intestinal mucosa by hypoxia, decreased perfusion, contact with bacterial toxins or decreased intraluminal pH (Garcia *et al.*, 1984; Anderson *et al.*, 1985; Garstin and Boston, 1987b; Cheu *et al.*, 1989; Stevenson, 1989).

ENTERAL FEEDS

Fresh breast milk contains immunoglobulins (Ig) and white cells which are thought to confer protection to the breastfed infant (Barlow *et al.*, 1974; Kliegman *et al.*, 1979; Caplan and MacKendrick, 1993). It is an observed fact that these babies are less likely to develop NEC than their formula-fed equivalents (*Nutrition Review*, 1989; Caplan and MacKendrick, 1993). The protective effect of fresh breast milk probably has two components. Firstly, breast milk induces colonization of the neonatal intestine with bifidobacteria, which reduces the risk of subsequent colonization by pathogens (Yoshioka *et al.*, 1983). Secondly, inappropriate colonization with these pathogens is inhibited by the immunoglobulin and white cell content of fresh breast milk (Barlow *et al.*, 1974; Caplan and MacKendrick, 1993). A similar protection may be conferred by enteral IgA and IgG (*Nutrition Review*, 1989; Caplan and Mackendrick,

1993). Refrigeration kills or impairs the function of the important white cells in fresh breast milk and this could explain the reduction in the protective effect when breast milk is cold stored (Moriaritey *et al.*, 1979). By contrast, there is evidence to suggest that immune complexes to cow's milk casein can be formed in premature infants who are fed formula (Van Epps *et al.*, 1977; Miller *et al.*, 1988; Clark *et al.*, 1988). This is thought to occur because the permeability to macromolecules is increased in the immature gut and these immune complexes can then lead to direct damage to the mucosa. This may be prevented by the prenatal treatment of the fetus using steroids given to the mother (Bauer *et al.*, 1984; Halac *et al.*, 1990; Caplan and MacKendrick, 1993).

It is recognized that many premature infants physically cannot tolerate the volumes necessary to sustain an adequate calorie intake for growth, owing to disordered function of the intestine. Hyperosmolar feeds, have therefore been employed to provide increased calories for a reduced volume load. Clinical and laboratory evidence suggests that these induce mucosal damage and may be responsible for causing NEC in some cases (Sweeny *et al.*, 1974; Book *et al.*, 1975). Where possible, these should therefore be avoided in at-risk infants.

MUCOSAL BLOOD FLOW

The act of feeding has been shown to increase both the oxygen consumption of the intestine and its blood flow. This is normally controlled to ensure adequate mucosal perfusion during and after feeding. In premature infants it is known that the normal reflex vasodilatation of mucosal blood vessels which accompanies feeding does not occur as readily as in more mature babies (Crissinger and Burney, 1991, 1992). In this situation free radical release could occur, with subsequent damage.

Hypovolaemia and hypoxaemia cause shunting of blood from the intestine and have been shown to induce experimental NEC (Touloukian *et al.*, 1972; Topalian and Ziegler, 1984). This could occur with congenital heart disease, exchange transfusion, hyperviscosity, umbilical catheterization, respiratory distress and low Apgar score at birth, all of which have been suggested as risk factors for NEC (Nowicki *et al.*, 1983; LeBlanc *et al.*, 1984; Dunn *et al.*, 1985; Kliegman *et al.*, 1985; Sibbons *et al.*, 1988; Kosloske and Musemeche, 1989; Hebra *et al.*, 1993).

RAISED INTRALUMINAL PRESSURE

There is experimental evidence that mucosal ischaemia occurs with raised intraluminal pressure (Boley *et al.*, 1969). This may be caused by either intestinal obstruction or increased gas production. Premature infants often develop delay in gastrointestinal transit and this

may be related to immaturity of intramural nerve plexus function (Garstin and Boston, 1987a). There is evidence that there is increased hydrogen production in the intestine just before the onset of NEC (Garstin and Boston, 1987b; Cheu *et al.*, 1989). If this is sufficiently rapid, the evolved gas cannot be cleared and the intraluminal pressure must therefore increase.

Management

DIAGNOSIS

Clinical features

Typically the patient is a premature baby who has already been established on formula feeds and has been making good progress. The child then develops abdominal distension and becomes clinically unwell. There is an increase in the volume of gastric residue, which may be bile stained and the child who has been defaecating normally now becomes constipated and passes a blood-stained stool.

There may be a wide range of clinical manifestations, from a mild benign disturbance of intestinal function to a rapidly fulminant course characterized by signs of peritonitis, septicaemia and shock.

Bell suggested a classification of NEC, which has proven valuable not only for diagnoses but also for treatment (Bell *et al.*, 1978; Walsh and Kliegman, 1986).

Stage I

These infants will develop a mild systemic illness, associated with temperature instability, apnoea, bradycardia and general lethargy. There may be a minor degree of abdominal distension associated with vomiting and/or increased prefeed gastric residues. Some of these children will demonstrate positive occult blood on stool testing, although it must be borne in mind that while approximately 40% of NEC patients will have blood in the stools the majority of stool haematest positive neonates will not have NEC (Abramo *et al.*, 1988; Amspacher, 1989). Stage I has been called suspected NEC and many children who demonstrate these clinical signs will be suffering from the much more common feeding intolerance associated with prematurity or low birth weight. However, those who demonstrate these clinical characteristics should be regarded as at risk of developing more fulminant disease and treated accordingly.

Stage II

These babies will have a more profound systemic illness, with a mild metabolic acidosis and thrombocytopenia. Abdominal distension is apparent and bowel sounds cannot be heard. Many will demonstrate abdominal tenderness and some will have oedema and cellulitis of the abdominal wall, particularly around the umbilicus. There will be definite X-ray findings of NEC with pneumatosis intestinalis with or without free gas in the peritoneal cavity or gas in the portal vein.

Stage III

This is associated with severe life-threatening generalized sepsis. In addition to the features of stage II disease, the baby will demonstrate hypotension, metabolic acidosis, hyponatraemia, jaundice and decimated intravascular coagulation. There will be signs of generalized peritonitis, with marked abdominal tenderness and distension, and these will usually be associated with radiological signs of perforation and ascites. Stage II and III disease therefore represent unequivocal NEC.

X-ray findings

Specific X-ray findings are best demonstrated by sequential examination of at-risk children. In stage I disease the only finding on abdominal X-ray may be generalized gaseous distension of the intestine (Walsh and Kliegman, 1986). A double-contrast enema may be of help in identifying those with early disease who will demonstrate mucosal oedema and perhaps ulceration (Uken *et al.*, 1988; Kao *et al.*, 1992) (Fig. 25.1).

Pneumatosis intestinalis can sometimes be present in stage I disease. However, this X-ray finding, which is generally regarded as pathognomonic of NEC, is usually seen in the more severe stages II and III of the condition (Koloske *et al.*, 1980; Kliegman and Fanaroff, 1986). In fewer than 10% of confirmed cases this sign will not be present (Kliegman and Fanaroff, 1982). It appears as crescents or halos around the gas shadow of the lumen (when viewed in cross-section at right angles to the lumenal axis of the intestine) or a more diffuse ground-glass appearance (Fig. 25.2).

When peritonitis and oedema of the intestinal wall become established, the interface between loops of bowel increase in thickness. Fixed distension of loops, apparent on sequential abdominal X-rays, usually indicates necrosis of the affected intestine. Perforation, when it occurs, is often associated with a decrease in intraluminal gas as this escapes into the peritoneal cavity. A lateral decubitus X-ray will often demonstrate this free gas, which is particularly evident between the abdominal wall (Kolsoke *et al.*, 1988) and the liver. Free gas can occasionally be seen in the pouch of Morrison in erect pictures (Brill *et al.*, 1990). Gas may also be apparent in the region of the liver in the portal vein (Cikrit *et al.*, 1985) (Fig. 25.3). Ascites is usually associated with faecal contamination of the peritoneal cavity (Kosloske *et al.*, 1988). Both ascites and portal vein gas are usually associated with stage III disease and are generally regarded as indications for surgical intervention (Kosloske *et al.*, 1980, 1988; Cikrit *et al.*, 1985).

Abdominal ultrasound scan

Localization of oedema of affected intestine, fluid in the abdominal cavity and Morrison's pouch and gas in the liver, are similar to the conventional X-ray findings.

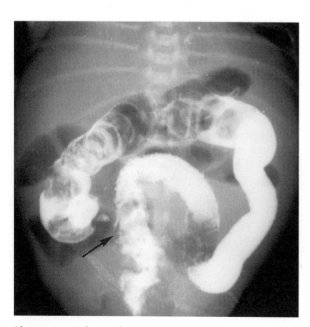

Fig. 25.1 Early involvement of the rectum with mucosal oedema and ulceration (arrow) on contrast enema.

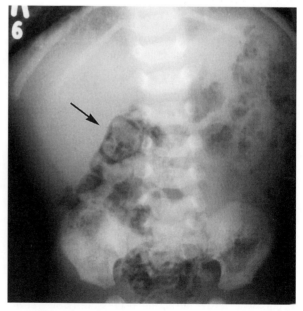

Fig. 25.2 Pneumatosis intestinalis (arrow) in the transverse colon. More diffuse involvement can also be seen in the region of the splenic flexure.

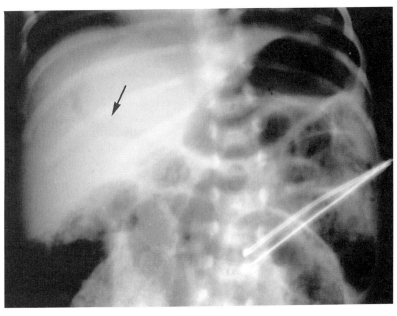

Fig. 25.3 Gas in the portal vein (arrow) in stage II and III NEC.

However, ultrasound, in addition, offers specific dynamic imaging facilities. Doppler flow techniques, which may be related to the altered dynamics of septicaemic shock, can demonstrate opening of the ductus arteriosus and loss of end diastolic flow or reversal of flow in the superior mesenteric artery (SMA) (Coombs *et al.*, 1990; Kempley *et al.*, 1991; Kempley and Gamsu, 1992).

Stool-reducing substances

While malabsorption of carbohydrate is a common occurrence, particularly in premature neonates, sequential measurement of stool carbohydrate has been shown to increase significantly prior to the onset of NEC. This simple test using 'Clinitest' tablets, appears to have a positive predicative value of approximately 70% for the development of the condition (Book *et al.*, 1976).

Breath hydrogen

Hydrogen, a product of bacterial fermentation of malabsorbed carbohydrate, is absorbed and can be measured in the expired gas. It is significantly elevated in the 24–36-hour period prior to the onset of disease (Garstin and Boston, 1987b; Cheu *et al.*, 1989). This test is easily and non-invasively performed by sampling air from the oropharynx during the expiratory phase of respiration.

Urinary D-lactate

Colonic bacterial flora can produce large quantities of D-lactate by fermentation of malabsorbed carbohydrate. This is absorbed and excreted in the urine. Urinary D-lactate excretion has been shown to be significantly elevated in children who develop NEC. Unlike the measurement of breath hydrogen, urinary D-lactate excretion does not provide an early warning of the development of the condition in at-risk infants but may be a useful indicator in those affected children who have stage I disease (Garcia *et al.*, 1984).

Urinary immunoreactive thromboxane

Thromboxane B$_2$ is a major metabolite of arachidonic acid. It has a short half-life and its more stable metabolite thromboxane B$_2$ is excreted and can be measured in the urine. Elevated levels of urinary thromboxane have been documented to occur in NEC (Hyman *et al.*, 1987).

TREATMENT

Prophylaxis before the onset of NEC

Prenatal use of dexamethasone has been shown to improve the fetal intestinal mucosal barrier and reduce the risk of NEC developing (Bauer *et al.*, 1984; Halac *et al.*, 1990). Postnatally, avoidance of stress situations induced by hypothermia, hypoxaemic or hypercarbia, metabolic acidosis, hypovolaemia and pain will reduce the risk of shunting of blood away from the newborn intestine. Drugs such as methylxanthines or prostaglandin antagonists, which are known to have an adverse effect on intestinal blood flow, should be used with caution (Nowicki and Oh, 1989; Canarelli *et al.*, 1993).

Strict infection control measures within the NICU will reduce the risk of nosocomial colonization with pathogens (Rotbart and Levin, 1983).

Mothers should be encouraged to provide fresh breast milk. This contains protective white cells and IgA (Barlow *et al.*, 1974; Kliegman *et al.*, 1979; Caplan and MacKendrick, 1993). In addition, it promotes more appropriate gut colonization with bifidobacteria and reduces the risk of colonization with pathogens (Yoshioka *et al.*, 1983). Early introduction high-volume feeds, particularly with hyperosmolar solutions, should be avoided (Sweeny *et al.*, 1974; Book *et al.*, 1975). If necessary, total or supplemental parental nutrition should be employed to maintain adequate calorie intake.

There is evidence which suggests that oral IgA given to at-risk neonates may improve the mucosal barrier to bacterial translocation.

After the onset of NEC

Stage I disease

Continuance of oral feeding is likely to cause progression of the disease in children who have NEC (Walsh and Kligman, 1986; Kosloske and Musemeche, 1959), but there are many babies who have clinical features of stage I NEC who are better treated by continuing with oral feeds.

Therefore, it is important to distinguish those babies who are suffering from NEC from those who are not. Apart from routine radiological, haematological, biochemical and bacteriological screening, all at-risk infants where possible should have sequential measurement of expired breath hydrogen, urinary D-lactate and thromboxane B_2 and stool carbohydrate.

When a firm diagnosis of NEC is established oral feeds should be discontinued and parenteral antibiotics should be commenced. The exact combination will be determined by the antibiotic policy of the unit but should include a combination active against both aerobic and anaerobic organisms. Total parenteral nutrition will be necessary to maintain the acute metabolic demands of the individual.

Stage II disease

Treatment is as with stage I disease but in addition, the systemic affects of sepsis such as endotoxic shock and disseminated intravascular coagulation need to be corrected aggressively, if necessary delaying surgical intervention even if this is indicated (Walsh and Kliegman, 1986).

The main priorities of this resuscitation are as follows:

- Endotracheal intubation and mechanical ventilation to normalize PO_2, and PCO_2.
- Maintenance of an adequate circulating blood volume, usually with a colloid. The exact volume administered will be determined by the response of the

central venous pressure, which should be maintained between 0 and 0.5 kPa.
- Cardiac output should be maintained, if necessary by the use of inotropic agents.
- The effects of total body fluid overload caused by the syndrome of inappropriate antidiuretic hormone secretion (SIADH) should be treated by the use of diuretics such as frusemide. Maintenance intravenous fluid therapy should be used with caution in these circumstances as fluid overload with cerebral oedema is a real risk.

Perforation is an absolute indication for operation. Most children will demonstrate peritonism with erythema or oedema of the anterior abdominal wall. A lateral decubitus radiograph of the abdomen will demonstrate free intraperitoneal gas in most cases. Gas in the portal vein (Fig. 25.3) is usually associated with fulminant disease associated with perforation. In the absence of signs of perforation or gas in the portal vein affected children can be treated conservatively as in stage I (Kosloske *et al.*, 1980; 1988; Cikrit *et al.*, 1985; Walsh and Kliegman, 1986; Kosloske and Musemeche, 1989).

Stage III disease

These children are profoundly unwell and usually have extensive transmural infarction and perforation which is usually associated with a high mortality. The same general principles apply as with stage II disease. Intensive cardiopulmonary resuscitation will be required before operative intervention, although in this case the child may be too unwell to tolerate open laparotomy.

Operation

Approximately half of the recognized cases of NEC will come to surgery (Walther *et al.*, 1989). However, there has been much debate as to the appropriate surgical approach in these circumstances.

Peritoneal drainage

Many children are verging on death and it has been argued that the operative trauma of an open laparotomy may carry a greater risk than simple drainage of the abdominal cavity. The objective is to reduce peritoneal soiling and decompress the abdomen. This reduces the source of continuing sepsis, reduces diaphragmatic splinting and improves ventilation.

Simple drainage should not be regarded as an alternative to open surgery, which will be required in most cases after the child's general condition improves. It has been suggested that simple peritoneal drainage is appropriate for children with congenital cyanotic heart disease or where the birth weight is less than 1500 g (Ricketts, 1986; Cheu *et al.*, 1988; Ein *et al.*, 1990). Whereas, those over 1500-g birth weight who have no evidence of congenital heart disease and who are systemically relatively well may be better managed by immediate laparotomy with or without resection (Ein *et al.*, 1990).

Access to the peritoneal cavity will facilitate lavage removal of contaminants, which are a source of absorbable endotoxin and cytokines. The procedure is usually performed under local anaesthetic. Through an incision performed in one or other of the iliac fossae, a soft latex French gauge 10 or 12 tube drain is inserted into the peritoneal cavity under direct vision. This is connected to a closed drainage system. Following removal of fluid and debris from the peritoneal cavity (which should be sent for culture, white cell count and biochemistry), an intravenous cannula can be inserted into the opposite iliac fossa for the purpose of lavage. In infants who are *in extremis*, inserting an intravenous cannula into the peritoneal cavity may be all that will be tolerated and this compromise may assist in improving the baby in the first instance before alternative strategies are contemplated.

Laparotomy

The consequences of operative trauma and the release of endotoxin caused by handling diseased intestine must be taken into account when planning a laparotomy. While ideally the surgeon will wish to solve the problem without recourse to further surgery this is frequently not possible. Expediency in the interests of safety for the child usually mean some form of limited primary operation with reconstruction at a later stage (Ein *et al.*, 1990; Anagnostopoulos *et al.*, 1991).

There has been a vogue for primary resection and direct end-to-end anastomosis of healthy bowel. It must be remembered that the affection of the intestine in NEC is greater on the mucosal than on the serosal surface. Therefore, in order to obtain a safe primary anastomosis, an extensive resection of potentially viable gut will be necessary (Kiesewetter *et al.*, 1979; Kosloske *et al.*, 1988; Griffiths *et al.*, 1989). As a general rule, resection and primary end-to-end anastomosis should only be performed if this can be done safely and without risking intestinal failure due to short gut.

In most circumstances, the child is unwell and the duration of surgery should not be prolonged. If a resection is required the proximal and distal limbs should be exteriorized at the limits of viability (as judged on the serosal surface), rather than performing an anastomosis (Cikrit *et al.*, 1984; Sen *et al.*, 1988; Dykes *et al.*, 1989). It is an advantage when subsequently closing this enterostomy, if the two stomata are placed together, thus avoiding two separate abdominal incisions.

Alternatively, a proximally based defunctioning enterostomy (usually the terminal ileum) can be performed without resection, even in the presence of perforation. This approach has the advantages of avoiding extensive mobilization of tissue and reduces the necessity for excision of potentially viable intestine. The potential risk of continuing sepsis from the site of perforation is usually prevented. Peritoneal lavage will be necessary in all cases to remove intestinal contents and reduce bacterial contamination of the peritoneal cavity. However, it is probably unnecessary in most cases to place a drain to the site of the perforation.

Generally speaking, a resection will be necessary if there is extensive serosal necrosis, whereas a proximal defunctioning enterostomy alone will be appropriate if only a single localized perforation has occurred without obvious transmural infarction.

Reintroduction of feed

As the general condition of the baby improves, intestinal function will return to normal. Gastric residue and abdominal distension will decrease and there will be passage of stool, indicating that oral feeds can be reintroduced. If this is started prematurely there is about a 5% risk of recurrence of NEC.

Malabsorption can be anticipated in most cases owing to the villous damage caused by the mucosal disease affecting the small intestine. This takes some time to improve and is usually present for many weeks after the intestine demonstrates normal peristalsis. A formula containing short-chain carbohydrates, peptones or amino acids and medium-chain triglycerides may be more readily absorbed in these circumstances and this should be used when feeding is reintroduced.

Hyperosmolar feeds which may predispose to the development of NEC should be avoided. Some weeks may pass before adequate growth and normalized intestinal absorption returns, indicating that a more normal feed can be employed.

Closure of the enterostomy

Fluid losses from the stoma may be large and difficult to control (Walsh *et al.*, 1988) and thus there is a need to restore intestinal continuity as soon as possible. This should be delayed if circumstances permit, for at least 3–4 months, during which time most secondary strictures (which occur in up to 30% of cases) will have developed (Walsh *et al.*, 1988; Sen *et al.*, 1988). Reconstruction should only be undertaken after patency of the distal intestine has been determined by a contrast enema (Fig. 25.4) (Radhakrishnan *et al.*, 1991).

Long-term management

Extensive gut resections may result in calorie or protein malabsorption which may necessitate long-term total or supplemental parental nutrition (Walsh *et al.*, 1988; Anagnostopoulos *et al.*, 1991). However, it is unusual for this to result in a failure to thrive and most survivors will attain normal growth on normal enteral feeds. It must be said, however, that children so affected have a high mortality and the numbers which survive are

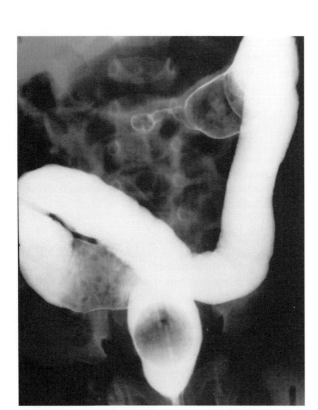

Fig. 25.4 Barium enema taken about 3 months after the acute phase of NEC showing a stricture in the transverse colon.

small. With loss of the terminal ileum selective malabsorption of vitamin B_{12} and iron can be managed using replacement therapy, which is usually unnecessary in the long term. Similarly, bile acid malabsorption in the terminal small intestine, which causes diarrhoea, is usually self-limiting, but can be treated in the short term by the use of cholestyramine (Walsh *et al.*, 1988; Skidmore *et al.*, 1989).

It is now increasingly recognized that children who have suffered stage II or III disease are at risk of developing psychomotor retardation (Simon *et al.*, 1993). This has long-term implications for education and family support (Kliegman and Fanaroff, 1986; Walsh *et al.*, 1988; Kosloske and Musemeche, 1989).

Summary

NEC is a serious disease which occurs almost exclusively in neonatal intensive care units. It is of obscure aetiology primarily affecting premature or small-for-date babies who have been fed orally. Preventive measures may reduce the incidence in at-risk children, but the greatest impact on prognosis will be early diagnosis followed by appropriate treatment. Many children can be managed conservatively, whereas others with extensive or progressive disease will require operative intervention. Most babies will survive but in a minority there are significant long-term complications, including short gut syndrome and neurological sequelae.

References

Abramo, T.J., Evans, J.S., Kokomoor, F.W. and Kantak, A.D. 1988: Occult blood in stools and necrotizing enterocolitis. *American Journal of Disease in Children* **142**, 451–2.

Amspacher, K.A. 1989: Necrotising enterocolitis: the never-ending challenge. *Journal of Perinatal Neonatal Nursing* **3**, 58–68.

Anagnostopoulos, D., Valioulis, J., Sfougaris, D., Maliaropoulos, N. and Spyridakis, J. 1991: Morbidity and mortality of short bowel syndrome in infancy and childhood. *European Journal of Pediatric Surgery* **1**, 273–6.

Anderson, C.L., Collin, M.F., O'Keefe, J.P. *et al.* 1984: A widespread epidemic of mild necrotizing enterocolitis of unknown cause. *American Journal of Disease in Children* **138**, 979.

Anderson, D.M., Rome, E.S., Kliegman, R.M. 1985: Relationship of endemic necrotizing enterocolitis (NEC) to alimentation. *Pediatric Research* **19**, 331A.

Barlow, B., Santulli, T.V., Heird, W.C., Pitt, J., Blanc, W.A. and Schullinger, J.N. 1974: An experimental study of acute neonatal enterocolitis: the importance of breast milk. *Journal of Pediatric Surgery* **9**, 587–95.

Bauer, C.R., Morrison, J.C., Poole, W.K. *et al.* 1984: A decreased incidence of necrotizing enterocolitis after prenatal glucocorticoid therapy. *Pediatrics* **73**, 682–7.

Bell, M.J., Ternberg, J.L., Feigin, R.D. *et al.* 1978: Neonatal necrotizing enterocolitis: therapeutic decisions based upon clinical staging. *Annals of Surgery* **187**, 1–6.

Boley, S.J., Agrawal, G.P. Warren, A.R. *et al.* 1969: Pathophysiologic effects of bowel distention on intestinal blood flow. *American Journal of Surgery* **117**, 228–34.

Book, L.S., Herbst, J.J. and Jung, A.L. 1976: Carbohydrate malabsorption in necrotizing enterocolitis. *Pediatrics* **57**, 201–4.

Book, L.S., Herbst, J.J., Atherton, S.O. and Jung, A.L. 1975: Necrotizing enterocolitis in low-birth-weight infants fed an elemental formula. *Journal of Pediatrics* **87**, 602–5.

Bousseboua, H., Coz, Y.L., Dabard, J. *et al.* 1989: Experimental cecitis in gnotobiotic quails monoassociated with *Clostridium butyricum* strains isolated from patients with neonatal necrotizing enterocolitis and from healthy newborns. *Infection and Immunity* **57**, 932–6.

Brans, Y.W., Escobedo, M.B., Hayashi, R.H., Huff, R.W., Kagan-Hallet, K.S. and Ramamurthy, R.S. 1982: Perinatal mortality in a large perinatal center: five-year review of 31,000 births. *American Journal of Obstetrics and Gynecology* **148**, 284–9.

Brill, P.W., Olson, S.R. and Winchester, P. 1990: Neonatal necrotizing enterocolitis air in Morison pouch. *Radiology* **174**, 469–71.

Canarelli, J.P., Poulain, H., Clamadieu, C., Ricard, J., Maingourd, Y. and Quintard, J.M. 1993: Ligation of the patent ductus arteriosus in premature infants – indications and procedures. *European Journal of Pediatric Surgery* **3**, 3–5.

Caplan, M.S. and Hsueh, W. 1990: Necrotizing enterocolitis: role of platelet activating factor, endotoxin, and tumor necrosis factor [Review]. *Journal of Pediatrics* **117**, S47–51.

Caplan, M.S., MacKendrick, W. 1993: Necrotizing enterocolitis: a review of pathogenetic mechanisms and implications for prevention [Review]. *Pediatric Pathology* **13**, 357–69.

Cassutto, B.H., Misra, H.P., Pfeiffer, C.J. 1989: Intestinal post-ischemic reperfusion injury: studies with neonatal necrotizing enterocolitis. *Acta Physiologica Hungarica* **73**, 363–9.

Chany, C, Moscovici, O., Lebon, P. and Rousset, S. 1982: Association of coronavirus infection with neonatal necrotizing enterocolitis. *Pediatrics* **69**, 209–18.

Cheromcha, D.P. and Hyman, P.E. Neonatal necrotizing enterocolitis inflammatory bowel disease of the newborn. *Digestive Diseases and Sciences* **33**, 78S–84S.

Cheu, H.W., Brown, D.R. and Rowe, M.I. 1989: Breath hydrogen excretion as a screening test for the early diagnosis of necrotizing enterocolitis. *American Journal of Disease in Children* **143**, 156–9.

Cheu, H.W., Sukarochana, K. and Lloyd, D.A. 1988: Peritoneal drainage for necrotizing enterocolitis. *Journal of Pediatric Surgery* **23**, 557–61.

Cikrit, D., Castandrea, J., West, K.W., Schreiner, R.L. and Grosfeld, J.L. 1984: Necrotizing enterocolitis: factors affecting mortality in 101 surgical cases. *Surgery* **96**, 648–55.

Cikrit, D., Mastandrea, J., Grosfeld, J.L., West, K.W. and Schreiner, R.L. 1985: 1985: Significance of portal vein air in necrotizing enterocolitis: analysis of 53 cases. *Journal of Pediatric Surgery* **20**, 425–30.

Clark, D.A., Fornabaio, D.M., McNeill, H., Mullane, K.M., Caravelia, S.J. and Miller, M.J.S. 1988: Contribution of oxygen-derived free radicals to experimental necrotizing enterocolitis. *American Journal of Pathology* **130**, 537–42.

Clark, D.A., Thompson, J.A., Weiner, L.B., McMillan, J.A., Schneider, A.J. and Rokahr, J.E. Necrotizing enterocolitis: intraluminal biochemistry in human neonates and a rabbit model. *Pediatrics* **19**, 919–21.

Coombs, R.C., Morgan, M.E., Durbin, G.M., Booth, I.W. and McNeish, A.S. 1990: Gut blood flow velocities in the newborn: effects of patent ductus arteriosus and parenteral indomethacin. *Archives of Disease in Childhood* **65**, 1067–71.

Covert, R.F., Neu, J., Elliott, M.J., Rea, J.L. and Gimotty, P.A. 1989: Factors associated with age of onset of necrotizing enterocolitis. *American Journal of Perinatology* **6**, 455–60.

Crissinger, K.D. and Burney, D.L. 1992: Influence of luminal nutrient composition on hemodynamics and oxygenation in developing intestine. *American Journal of Physiology* **263**, G254–60.

Crissinger, K.D. and Burney, D.L. 1991: Postprandial hemodynamics and oxygenation in developing piglet intestine. *American Journal of Physiology* **260**, G951–7.

Cueva, J.P. and Hsueh, W. Role of oxygen derived free radicals in platelet activating factor induced bowel necrosis. *Gut* **29**, 1207–12.

Dunn, S.P., Gross, K.R., Shcerer, L.R., Koenning, S., Desanto, A. and Grosfeld, J.L. 1985: The effect of polycythemia and hyperviscosity on bowel ischemia. *Journal of Pediatric Surgery* **20**, 324–7.

Dykes, E.H., Fitzgerald, R.J. and O'Donnell, B. 1989: Surgery for neonatal necrotising enterocolitis in Ireland 1980–1985. *Intensive Care Medicine* **15**, S24–6.

Ein, S.H., Shandling, B., Wesson, D. and Filler, R.M. 1990: A 13-year experience with peritoneal drainage under local anesthesia for necrotizing enterocolitis perforation. *Journal of Pediatric Surgery* **25**, 1034–6; discussion 1036–7.

Engel, R.R., Virnig, N.L., Hunt, C.E. and Levitt, M.D. 1973: Origin of mural gas in necrotizing enterocolitis. *Pediatric Research* **7**, 292.

Garcia, J., Smith, F.R., Cucinell, S.A. 1984: Urinary D-lactate excretion in infants with necrotizing enterocolitis. *Journal of Pediatrics* **104**, 268–70.

Garstin, W.H.I. and Boston, V.E. 1987: Sequential assay of expired breath hydrogen as a means of predicting necrotising enterocolitis in susceptible infants. *Journal of Pediatric Surgery* **22**, 208–10.

Garstin, W.H.I., Boston, V.E. 1987: Assessment of hindgut function in premature infants. *Journal of Pediatric Surgery* **22**, 353–5.

Garstin, W.H.I., Kenny, B.D., McAneaney, D. and Boston, V.E. 1987: The role of intraluminal tension and pH in the development of necrotising enterocolitis: an animal model. *Journal of Pediatric Surgery* **22**, 205–7.

Genersich, A. 1891: Bauchfellentzundung Beim Neugebornen in Folge von Perforation des Ileums. *Virchows Archives* **126**, 485–94.

Goldman, D.A., Leclair, J. and Macone, A. 1978: Bacterial colonisation of neonates admitted to an intensive care environment. *Journal of Pediatrics*; **93**, 288–93.

Gregory, J.R., Campbell, J.R., Harrison, M.W. and Campbell, T.J. 1987: Neonatal necrotizing enterocolitis: a 10 year experience. *American Journal Surgery* **141**, 562–7.

Griffiths, D.M., Forbes, D.A. Pemberton, P.J. and Penn, I.A., 1989: Primary anastomosis for necrotizing enterocolitis: a 12 year experience. *Journal of Pediatric Surgery* **24**, 515–18.

Halac, E., Halac, J., Begue, E.F. *et al.* 1990: Prenatal and postnatal corticosteroid therapy to prevent neonatal necrotizing enterocolitis: a controlled trial. *Journal of Pediatrics* **117**, 132–8.

Hebra, A., Brown, M.F., Hirschl, R.B. *et al.* 1993: Mesenteric ischemia in hypoplastic left heart syndrome. *Journal of Pediatric Surgery* **28**, 606–11.

Holman, R.C., Stehr-Green, K. and Zelasky, M.T. 1989: Necrotizing enterocolitis mortality in the United States 1979–85. *American Journal of Public Health* **79**, 987–9.

Hsueh, W., Gonzalez-Crussi, F. 1988: Ischemic bowel necrosis induced by platelet activating factor: an experimental model. *Archives of Experimental Pathology* **13**, 208–39.

Hsueh, W., Sun, X., Rioja, L.N. and Gonzalez-Crussi, F. 1990: The role of the complement system in shock and tissue injury induced by tumour necrosis factor and endotoxin. *Immunology* **70**, 309–14.

Hyman, P.E., Abrams, C.E. and Zipser, R.D. 1987: Enhanced urinary immunoreactive thromboxane in neonatal necrotizing enterocolitis: a diagnostic indicator of thrombotic activity. *American Journal of Disease in Children* **141**, 686–9.

Jenkins, D.J.A. 1989: The link between colon fermentation and systemic disease [Editorial]. *American Journal of Gastroenterology* **84**, 1362–4.

Joshi, V.V. 1977: Implications of pathologic findings in the treatment of neonatal necrotising enterocolitis. *Pediatrics* **59**, 954–5.

Kao, S.C., Smith, W.L., Franken, E.A. Jr, Sato, Y., Sullivan, J.H. and McGee J.A. 1992: Contrast enema diagnosis of necrotizing enterocolitis. *Pediatric Radiology* **22**, 115–17.

Kempley, S.T. and Gamsu, H.R. 1992: Superior mesenteric artery blood flow velocity in necrotising enterocolitis. *Archives of Disease in Childhood* **67**, 793–6.

Kempley, S.T., Gamsu, H.R., Vyas, S. and Nicolaides, K. 1991: Effects of intrauterine growth retardation on postnatal visceral and cerebral blood flow velocity. *Archives of Disease in Childhood* **66**, 1115–18.

Kiesewetter, W.B., Taghizadeh, F., Bower, R.J. 1979: Necrotizing enterocolitis: is there a place for resection and primary anastomosis? *Journal of Pediatric Surgery* **14**, 360–3.

Kishan, J., El-Mauhoub, M. and Kumar, A. Risk factors for necrotizing enterocolitis in premature infants. *American Journal of Disease in Children* **142**, 701.

Kliegman, R., Pittard, W.B. and Fanaroff, A.A., 1979: Necrotizing enterocolitis in neonates fed human milk. *Journal of Pediatrics* **95**, 450–3.

Kliegman, R., Stork, E. and Fanaroff, A. 1985: Lack of relationship between umbilical arterial catheter complications and necrotizing enterocolitis. *Pediatric Research* **19**, 349A.

Kliegman, R.M. and Fanaroff, A.A. 1981: Neonatal necrotizing enterocolitis: a nine year experience: epidemiology and uncommon observations. *American Journal of Disease in Children* **135**, 603–7.

Kliegman, R.M. and Fanaroff, A.A. 1986: Necrotizing enterocolitis. *New England Journal of Medicine* **310**, 1093–103.

Kliegman, R.M. and Fanaroff, A.A. 1982: Neonatal necrotizing enterocolitis in the absence of pneumatosis intestinalis. *American Journal of Disease in Children* **136**, 618–20.

Kliegman, R.M., Hack, M., Jones, P. and Fanaroff, A.A. 1982: Epidemiologic study of necrotizing enterocolitis among low-birth-weight infants. *Journal of Pediatrics* **100**, 440–4.

Kosloske, A., Musemeche, C.A., Ball, W.S. Jr, Ablin, D.S. and Bhattacharyya, N. 1988: Necrotizing enterocolitis: value of radiographic findings to predict outcome. *American Journal of Roentgenology* **151**, 771–4.

Kosloske, A.M. and Musemeche, A. 1989: Necrotizing enterocolitis of the neonate. *Clinical Perinatology* **16**, 97–111.

Kosloske, A.M., Papile, L.A., Burstein, J. 1980: Indications for operation in acute necrotizing enterocolitis of the neonate. *Surgery* **87**, 502–8.

Kripke, S.A., Fox, A.D., Berman, J.M., Settle, R.G. and Rombeau, J.L. 1989: Stimulation of intestinal mucosal growth with intracolonic infusion of short-chain fatty acids. *Journal of Parenteral and Enteral Nutrition* **13**, 109.

LeBlanc, M.H., D'Cruz, C. and Pate, K. 1984: Necrotizing enterocolitis can be caused by polycythemic hyperviscosity in the newborn dog. *Journal of Pediatrics* **105**, 804–8.

Leung, M.P., Chau, K., Tam, A.Y.C., Chan, F.M., Lai, C., Yeung, C. 1988: Necrotizing enterocolitis in neonates with symptomatic congenital heart disease. *Journal of Pediatrics* **113**, 1044–6.

Llausas-Magana, E., Hsueh, W., Arroyave, C.M., Arroyave, J.L., Torre-Amione, G. and Gonzalez-Crussi, F. 1988: Cobra venom factor, an activator of the complement system, enhances the bowel necrosis induced by platelet-activating factor. *Immunopharmacology* **15**, 31–8.

Long, S.S., Swenson, R.M. 1977: Development of anaerobic fecal flora in healthy newborn infants. *Journal of Pediatrics* **91**, 298–301.

Lyerly, D.M., Krivan, H.C. and Wilkins, T.D. 1988: *Clostridium difficile*: its disease and toxins. *Clinical Microbiology Reviews* **1**, 1–18.

Miller, M.J.S. and Clark, D.A. 1989: Profile and sites of eicosanoid release in experimental necrotizing enterocolitis. *Advances in Prostaglandin, Thromboxane and Leukotriene Research* **19**: 556–9.

Miller, M.J.S., McNeill, H., Mullane, K.M., Salvatore, J., Clark, C. and Clark, D.A. 1988: SOD prevents damage and attenuates eicosanoid release in a rabbit model of necrotizing enterocolitis. *American Journal of Physiology* **255**, G556–65.

Milner, M.E., de la Monte, S.M., Moore, G.W. and Hutchins, G.M. 1986: Risk factors for developing and dying from necrotizing enterocolitis. *Journal of Pediatric Gastroenterology and Nutrition* **5**, 359–64.

Mogilner, B.M., Bar-Yochai, A., Miskin, A., Shif, I. and Aboudi, Y. 1983: Necrotizing enterocolitis associated with rotavirus infection. *Journal of Medical Science* **19**, 894–6.

Mollitt, D.L., Tepas, J.J. and Talbert, J.L. 1988: The role of coagulase-negative staphylococcus in neonatal necrotising enterocolitis. *Journal of Pediatric Surgery* **231**, 60–3.

Moomjian, A.S., Peckham, G.J., Fox, W.W., Pereira, G.R. and Schaberg, D.A. 1978: Necrotizing enterocolitis endemic VS epidemic form. *Pediatric Research* **12**, 530.

Moriaritey, R.R., Finer, N.N. and Cox, S.F. *et al.* 1979: Necrotising enterocolitis and human milk. *Journal of Pediatrics* **94**, 295–6.

Moss, T.J. and Adler, R., Necrotizing enterocolitis in older infants, children, and adolescents. *Journal of Pediatrics* **100**, 764–6.

Nowicki, P.T. and Oh, W. 1989: Methylxanthines and necrotising enterocolitis revisited. *Journal of Pediatrics Gastroenterology and Nutrition* **9**, 137–8.

Nowicki, P.T., Stonestreet, B.S., Hansen, N.B., Yao, A.C. and Oh, W. 1983: Gastrointestinal blood flow and oxygen consumption in awake newborn piglets: effect of feeding. *American Journal of Physiology* **245**, G697–702.

Nutrition Review 1989: Immunoglobulin feeding prevents necrotizing enterocolitis in formula-fed very-low-birthweight infants. *Nutrition Review* **47**, 186–8.

Palmer, S.R., Biffin, A. and Gamsu, H.R. 1989: Outcome of neonatal necrotising enterocolitis: results of the BAPM/CDSC surveillance study, 1981–84. *Archives of Disease in Childhood* **64**, 388–94.

Polin, R.A., Pollack, P.F., Barlow, B. *et al.* Necrotizing enterocolitis in term infants. *Journal of Pediatrics* **89**, 460–2.

Radhakrishnan, J., Blechman, G., Shrader, C., Patel, M.K., Mangurten, H.H. and McFadden, J.C. 1991: Colonic strictures following successful medical management of necrotizing enterocolitis: a prospective study evaluating early gastrointestinal contrast studies. *Journal of Pediatric Surgery* **26**, 1043–6.

Ramenofsky, M.I. 1977: Necrotizing enterocolitis occurring in an infant three months of age. *Journal of Pediatric Surgery* **12**, 597–9.

Ricketts, R.R. 1986: The role of paracentesis in the management of infants with necrotizing enterocolitis. *American Surgery* **52**, 61–5.

Rombeau, J.L. and Kripke, S.A. 1990: Metabolic and intestinal effects of short-chain fatty acids. *Journal of Parenteral and Enteral Nutrition* **14**, 181S–5S.

Rotbart, H.A. and Levin, M.J. 1983: How contagious is necrotizing enterocolitis? *Pediatric Infectious Disease* **2**, 406–13.

Rotbart, H.A., Nelson, W.L., Glade, M.P. *et al.* 1988: Neonatal rotavirus-associated necrotizing enterocolitis: case control study and prospective surveillance during an outbreak. *Journal of Pediatrics* **112**, 87–93.

Santulli, T.V., Schullinger, J.N., Heird, W.C. *et al.* 1975: Acute necrotizing enterocolitis in infancy: a review of 64 cases. *Pediatrics* **55**, 376–87.

Scheifele, D.W., Bjornson, G.L., Dyer, R.A. and Dimmick, J.E. 1987: Delta-like toxin produced by coagulase-negative staphylococci is associated with neonatal necrotizing enterocolitis. *Infection and Immunity* **55**, 2268–73.

Sen, S., Rajadurai, V.S. and Ford, W.D.A. 1988: Late onset bowel stenosis after neonatal necrotizing enterocolitis. *Pediatrics Journal* **24**, 366–8.

Sharon, P., Stenson, W.F. 1985: Metabolism of archidonic acid in acetic acid colitis in rats: similarity to human inflammatory bowel disease. *Gastroenterology* **88**, 55–63.

Sibbons, P., Spitz, L., van Velzen, D. and Bullock, G.R. 1988: Relationship of birth weight to the pathogenesis of necrotizing enterocolitis in the neonatal piglet. *Pediatric Pathology* **8**, 151–62.

Simon, N.P., Brady, N.R., Stafford, R.L. and Powell, R.W. 1993: The effect of abdominal incisions on early motor development of infants with necrotizing enterocolitis. *Developmental Medicine and Child Neurology* **35**, 49–53.

Skidmore, M.D., Shenker, N., Kliegman, R.M., Shurin, S. and Allen, R.H. 1989: Biochemical evidence of asymptomatic vitamin B_{12} deficiency in children after ileal resection for necrotizing enterocolitis. *Journal of Pediatrics* **115**, 102–5.

Stevenson, D.K. Breath hydrogen in preterm infants. *American Journal of Disease in Children* **143**, 1262–3.

Sweeny, M.J., deLemos, R.A., Rogers, J.H., Jr and McLaughlin, G.W. 1974: Experimental production of necrotizing enterocolitis in new-born goats. *Pediatric Research* **8**, 380.

Tan, X., Hsueh, W. and Gonzalez-Crussi, F. Cellular localization of tumor necrosis factor (TNF)-alpha transcripts in normal bowel and in necrotizing enterocolitis. TNF gene expression by Paneth cells, intestinal eosinophils, and macrophages. *American Journal of Pathology* **142**, 1858–65.

Thilo, E.H., Lazarte, R.A. and Hernandez, J.A. Necrotizing enterocolitis in the first 24 hours of life. *Pediatrics* **73**, 476–80.

Topalian, S.L. and Ziegler, M.M. 1984: Necrotizing enterocolitis: a review of animal models. *Journal of Surgery Research* **37**, 320–36.

Touloukian, R.J., Posch, J.N. and Spencer, R. 1972: The pathogenesis of ischemic gastroenterocolitis of the neonate: selective gut mucosal ischemia in asphyxiated neonatal piglets. *Journal of Pediatric Surgery* **7**, 194–205.

Uken, P., Smith, W., Franken, E.A., Frey, E., Sato, Y. and Ellerbroek, C. 1988: Use of barium enema in the diagnosis of necrotizing enterocolitis. *Pediatric Radiology* **22**, 24–7.

Van Epps, D.E., Bankhurst, A.D. and Williams, R.C., Jr 1977: Casein-mediated neutrophil chemotaxis a parallel between surface binding and chemotaxis. *Inflammation* **2**, 115–23.

Virnig, N.L. and Reynolds, J.W. 1974: Epidemiological aspects of neonatal necrotizing enterocolitis. *American Journal of Disease in Children* **128**, 186–90.

Walsh, M.C. and Kliegman, R.M. 1986: Necrotising enterocolitis: treatment based on staging criteria. *Pediatric Clinics of North America* **33**, 179–8.

Walsh, M.C., Kliegman, R.M. and Fanaroff, A.A. 1988: Necrotizing enterocolitis: a practitioner's perspective. *Pediatrics in Review* **9**, 219–26.

Walther, F.J., Verloove-Vanhorick, S.P., Brand, R. and Ruys, J.H. 1989: A prospective survey of necrotising enterocolitis in very low birthweight infants. *Paediatric Perinatal Epidemiology* **3**, 53–61.

Wilson, R., Kanto, W., McCarthy, B. *et al.* 1981: Epidemiologic characteristics of necrotizing enterocolitis: a population-based study. *American Journal of Epidemiology* **114**, 880–7.

Wiswell, T.E., Robertson, C.F., Jones, T.A. and Tuttle, D.J. 1988: Necrotizing enterocolitis in full-term infants. *American Journal of Disease in Children* **142**, 532–5.

Yale, C.E., Balish, E.P.J. and Wis, M. 1974: The bacterial etiology of pneumatosis cystoides intestinalis. *Archives of Surgery* **109**, 89–94.

Yoshioka, H., Iseki, K., Fujita, K. Development and differences of intestinal flora in the neonatal period in breast-fed and bottle-fed infants. *Pediatrics* **72**, 317–21.

Zabielski, P.B., Groh-Wargo, S.L. and Moore, J.J. 1989: Necrotizing enterocolitis: feeding in endemic and epidemic periods. *Journal of Parental and Enteral Nutrition* **13**, 520–4.

Further reading

Caplan, M.S. and MacKendrick, W. 1993: Necrotizing enterocolitis: a review of pathogenetic mechanisms and implications for prevention [Review]. *Pediatric Pathology* **13**, 357–69.

Grosfeld, J.L., Cheu, H., Schlatter, M., West, K.W. and Rescorla, F.J. 1991: Changing trends in necrotizing enterocolitis. Experience with 302 cases in two decades. *Annals of Surgery* **214**, 300–6; discussion 306–7.

CHAPTER 26

The vitellointestinal duct

J.D. ATWELL

Surgical embryology
Pathology
Clinical features

Management
References

Surgical embryology

The vitellointestinal duct is an embryological remnant representing the original communication between the primitive intestinal tract and the yolk sac (Fig. 26.1). The vitellointestinal duct arises from the midgut region of the primitive alimentary tract, and the yolk sac atrophies when it has finished its purpose of being a site of blood production from the islands of Pander. Under normal circumstances the duct then disappears completely. The structure of the vitellointestinal duct is the

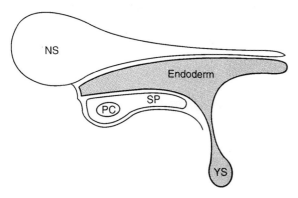

Figure 26.1 Longitudinal section of an embryo showing the primitive gut (endoderm), the vitellointestinal duct (VID) and the yolk sac (YS). NS, nervous system; PC, pericardial coelom; SP, septum transversum.

same as the normal distal small bowel, although there may be areas of ectopic pancreatic tissue and gastric mucosa. The blood supply and venous drainage of the duct are via the vitelline artery and vein, respectively.

Pathology

Anomalies of the vitellointestinal duct occur when part of the duct remains and the pattern of defects found is variable (Fig. 26.2). The duct may persist in its entirety, i.e. a complete vitellointestinal duct, or there may be partial remnants of the duct, i.e. incomplete vitellointestinal duct anomalies, which include a Meckel's diverticulum, a vitelline band, a Meckel's diverticulum with a band, an umbilical sinus and an enterocystoma with or without attachment to the umbilicus or the intestine.

The changes that occur are probably due to changes in the blood supply to the duct by the vitelline artery. The complete disappearance or partial disappearance leaving a Meckel's diverticulum resembles type III intestinal atresia found in the small intestine and the persistent band with or without a Meckel's diverticulum resembles the type II intestinal atresia.

Ectopic gastric mucosa is often found within a Meckel's diverticulum, which then may be subject to all the complications of peptic ulceration with either acute or chronic haemorrhage, abdominal pain or perforation leading to a local or generalized peritonitis.

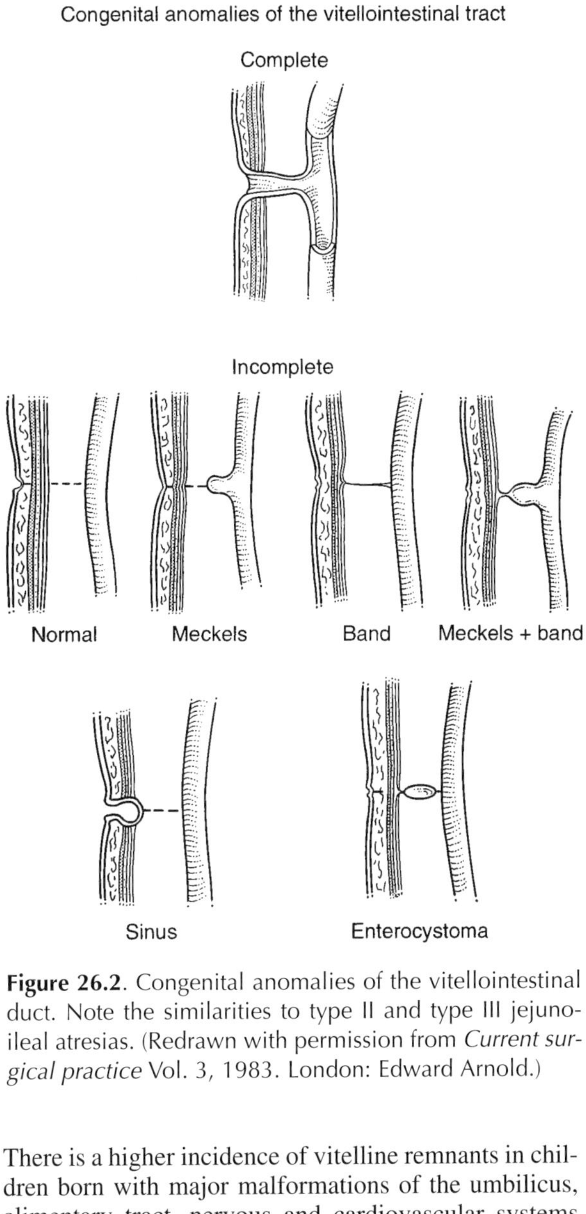

Congenital anomalies of the vitellointestinal tract

Complete

Incomplete

Normal   Meckels   Band   Meckels + band

Sinus   Enterocystoma

Figure 26.2. Congenital anomalies of the vitellointestinal duct. Note the similarities to type II and type III jejuno-ileal atresias. (Redrawn with permission from *Current surgical practice* Vol. 3, 1983. London: Edward Arnold.)

There is a higher incidence of vitelline remnants in children born with major malformations of the umbilicus, alimentary tract, nervous and cardiovascular systems (Simms and Corkery, 1980).

Clinical features

COMPLETE VITELLOINTESTINAL DUCT

With a persistent complete vitellointestinal duct there is often no visible lesion at birth. However, within 1–3 weeks following delivery the umbilical cord separates and an area of intestinal mucosa appears at the umbilicus. This has the appearance of a perfectly fashioned ileostomy and milk or flatus may be passed from the lumen, thus establishing the diagnosis. This may be confirmed by outlining the tract with the introduction of some contrast material. The duct may

occasionally prolapse outwards as an intussusception, and therefore there is no reason to delay surgical treatment.

INCOMPLETE VITELLOINTESTINAL DUCT

The most common of these lesions is the Meckel's diverticulum, with a stated incidence in the population of 2%. The diverticulum may be asymptomatic. If symptomatic this is invariably due to the development of complications such as abdominal pain (due to peptic ulceration or diverticulitis), bleeding (either acute or chronic from peptic ulceration or diverticulitis), perforation (either due to peptic ulceration or diverticulitis) or intestinal obstruction (due to associated bands, adhesions or from the length of the diverticulum). Unusual presentations include intussusception which may be either in an antegrade or retrograde direction. Occasionally a patient may present with a simultaneous acute haemorrhage and perforation, such patients, often under 3 years of age, will be found to have haemoglobin levels as low as 5.0 g/dl or less.

Management

COMPLETE VITELLOINTESTINAL DUCT

The diagnosis is not usually a problem although the condition is rare. The surgical treatment is to explore the abdomen and excise the duct with restoration of continuity of the small bowel. As this situation occurs in the neonatal period it is easy to resect the diverticulum with a wedge of distal ileum which is left intact on the mesenteric border (Fig. 26.3).

INCOMPLETE VITELLOINTESTINAL DUCT

The majority of these patients present either as an emergency with an acute abdomen or for investigation of rectal bleeding or recurrent abdominal pain.

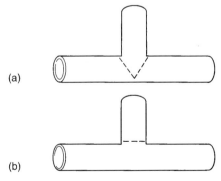

(a)

(b)

Figure 26.3. Lines of resection for a Meckel's diverticulum in (a) the neonate and (b) the older child.

ACUTE ABDOMEN WITH A MECKEL'S DIVERTICULUM

The acute abdomen may be due to perforation or severe haemorrhage or a combination of both. Initial resuscitation with replacement of blood followed by an urgent laparotomy under antibiotic cover is required. Excision of the diverticulum is the treatment of choice with either a transverse or the preferable V-shaped incision (Fig. 26.3) across the base of the diverticulum. Ectopic gastric mucosa if present is often in the junctional region between the ileum and the diverticulum thus the mucosa must be inspected to ensure that any gastric mucosa is excised.

Meckel's with or without a band present with the signs and symptoms of intestinal obstruction, i.e. vomiting, abdominal distension and absolute constipation. Diagnosis of a small bowel obstruction is confirmed by erect and supine plain radiographs of the abdomen which will reveal distended loops of bowel with fluid levels. After correction of any biochemical and haematological deficiency an urgent laparotomy is required to divide any adhesions, resect gangrenous bowel if present with the diverticulum and restore continuity.

Recurrent abdominal pain, anaemia and rectal bleeding

The patient presenting with recurrent abdominal pain, rectal bleeding and/or anaemia presents difficulties in both diagnosis and management. In such patients considerable judgement is required in distinguishing those patients who require full investigation from those in whom it is safe to observe.

Haematological investigations are required to exclude a bleeding diathesis and to quantify the degree of anaemia. Local causes of rectal bleeding, such as anal fissures and polyps, must be excluded. Barium meals and follow-through examinations in order to demonstrate a Meckel's diverticulum are usually non-contributable. The sodium pertechnate scan is useful in demonstrating ectopic gastric mucosa in either a Meckel's diverticulum or a duplication cyst (Garvie *et al.*, 1978) (Fig. 26.4).

In patients with symptoms suggestive of a Meckel's diverticulum it is usual to monitor the haemoglobin levels at regular intervals. A falling haemoglobin level and exclusion of other causes of bleeding will lead to the need for an exploratory laparotomy.

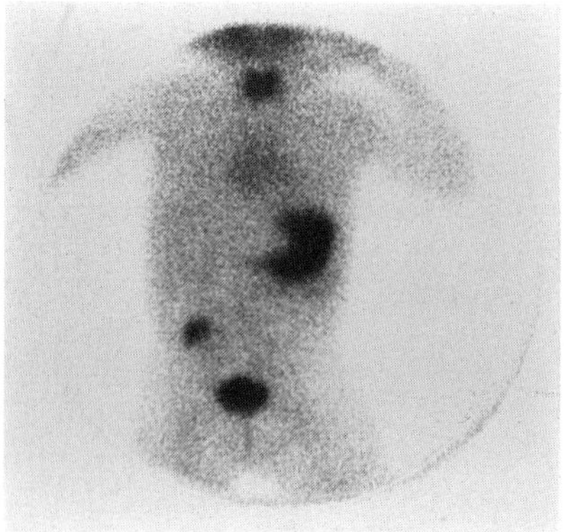

References

Garvie, N.W., Harrison, G.S.M. and Ackery, D.M. 1978: Diagnosis of an ileal duplication with sodium pertechnate 99 Tc^m. *British Journal of Radiology* **51**, 825–6.

Simms, M.M. and Corkery, J.J. 1980: Meckel's diverticulum: its association with congenital malformation and significance of atypical morphology. *British Journal of Surgery* **67**, 216–19.

Figure 26.4. Sodium pertechnate ^{99m}Tc scan used to demonstrate ectopic gastric mucosa.

CHAPTER 27

Biliary atresia and choledochal cyst

E.R. HOWARD AND M. DAVENPORT

Biliary atresia
Choledochal cyst

References

Biliary atresia

Biliary atresia is an obliterative, inflammatory process affecting both the intrahepatic and extrahepatic parts of the biliary tree which presents as persisting, cholestatic jaundice. The incidence of biliary atresia is similar throughout the world (Psacharopoulos *et al.*, 1980; Shim *et al.*, 1980; Houwen *et al.*, 1988), ranging from 0.8 to 1.0 per 10 000 live births.

HISTORICAL FEATURES

Isolated cases of biliary atresia were reported during the nineteenth century and in 1892 a review of 49 cases was published by John Thomson of Edinburgh. Holmes in 1916, was the first to discuss possible surgical treatment for this condition and he suggested that biliary atresia could be divided into 'correctable' and 'non-correctable' depending on the presence or absence of any residual segment of bile duct in the proximal biliary tree. William Ladd of Boston recorded the first successful operations for biliary atresia in 1928 but the results of surgical intervention remained poor and Bill (1978) could only collect 52 surgical successes from the world literature between 1927 and 1970.

The current management of extrahepatic biliary atresia follows the observations of Kasai and Suzuki (1959) that bile drainage may be established from residual microscopic channels in the residual bile duct tissue of the porta hepatis. Kasai *et al.* (1968) showed that these channels often communicate with residual intrahepatic ducts and he devised the operation of portoenterostomy in which a Roux-en-Y loop of jejunum is anastomosed to the edges of resected bile duct tissue at the level of the liver capsule in the porta hepatis. A large number of patients with effective bile drainage after this procedure has now been reported and the oldest survivor is now more than 33 years old (Kasai *et al.*, 1989).

AETIOLOGY

The true aetiology of biliary atresia is still unknown but the current view is that it is probably heterogeneous (Silveira *et al.*, 1991a) (see Table 27.1). The original theory of biliary atresia as a failure of recanalization of the biliary tract held sway for the greater part of this century and has usually been linked to Ylppö (1913). This hypothesis was challenged during the 1960s and 1970s by Landing (1974) and Brent (1962) when they originated the concept of an 'infantile cholangiopathy'. They suggested that the normally formed biliary tract was subject to an insult such as a viral infection in the late prenatal or perinatal period. Neonatal hepatitis and choledochal cyst were linked into this hypothesis as variants because of similar 'inflammatory' histological features. An important argument against such a linkage is the lone association of biliary atresia with other extrahepatic anomalies such as polysplenia, situs inversus

Table 27.1 Aetiological hypotheses in biliary atresia

Hypothesis	Comments	References
Developmental	Early gestational insult: explains association with extrahepatic anomalies	Smith *et al.* (1991), Davenport *et al.* (1993)
Viral	Animal models especially reovirus type 3	Morecki *et al.* (1982), Hart *et al.* (1991), Parashar *et al.* (1992)
Metabolic	Animal models L-Proline, monohydroxy bile acid	Jenner and Howard (1975), Vacanti and Folkman (1979)
Genetic	Occasional familial cases	Strickland *et al.* (1985)
Abnormal pancreatobiliary ductal union	Higher incidence of common channel	Miyano *et al.* (1979), Chiba *et al.* (1990)

and abnormalities of the portal vein (Karrer *et al.*, 1991; Davenport *et al.*, 1993). We are not aware of such an association in cases of neonatal hepatitis or choledochal cyst. The well-recognized occurrence of extrahepatic anomalies with biliary atresia suggests a disturbance of organogenesis in the embryo at around 30–40 days postfertilization because of the timing in the critical developmental stage for each organ.

Some authors believe that perinatal viral infections, such as rubella (Strauss and Bernstein, 1968) and the hepatotropic reovirus type 3 (Parashar *et al.*, 1992), are important in the aetiology of biliary atresia. However, ultrastructural examination of tissue resected at surgery in humans (Jenner 1978; Nmazaki *et al.*, 1980) has failed, so far, to identify either the infective agent or any evidence of viral particles. Experimental inoculation of mice with reovirus type III causes hepatitis, biliary tract inflammation and fibrosis of extrahepatic ducts with proximal duct dilatation (Banjura *et al.*, 1980; Parashar *et al.*, 1992). However, the histological changes in this murine model are not entirely characteristic of changes found in the portal tracts of patients with biliary atresia and progression to biliary cirrhosis has never been demonstrated. Morecki *et al.* (1982) showed antibodies to type III reovirus in 68% of a group of infants with biliary atresia compared to 8% of age-matched controls but a similar study from France failed to show any differences between subjects and controls (Dussaix *et al.*, 1984). Time-space clustering, suggesting an environmental factor, has been shown in some series (Strickland and Shannon, 1982), but not in others (Houwen *et al.*, 1988).

A possible genetic relationship has been suggested by some authors in isolated cases (Strickland *et al.*, 1985; Davenport *et al.*, 1993). Discordant and even concordant twins have been described with biliary atre-

sia (Silveira *et al.* 1991b) and one report (Hart *et al.*, 1991) has described intrauterine cytomegalovirus associated with neonatal hepatitis in one of a pair of twins whilst the other developed biliary atresia. Familial cases have also been described, although only in particular ethnic groups (e.g. North American Indians; Smith *et al.*, 1991). Isolated cases of biliary atresia have also been described with the trisomy syndromes 17–18 (Alpert *et al.*, 1969; Strauss *et al.*, 1972) and 21 (Danks, 1965), congenital listerosis (Bercroft, 1972) and following maternal amphetamine misuse (Levin, 1971).

Experimental studies have usually failed to implicate ischaemia as a cause of progressive duct injury (Klippel, 1972). Devascularization or ligation of the fetal extrahepatic bile duct has been attempted in some animal models *in utero*. Lesions similar to the less common 'correctable' variants of biliary atresia have been produced in some studies (Pickett and Briggs, 1969; Spitz, 1980), whilst in others the results have been less conclusive (Holder and Ashcroft, 1967).

Several reports have suggested possible metabolic abnormalities. Intraperitoneal infusion of L-proline in mice is associated with enlargement of proximal bile ducts and epithelial proliferation similar to clinical biliary atresia, although, as in the viral studies, there are no associated intrahepatic changes (Vacanti and Folkman, 1979). Four infants with biliary atresia were shown to have low levels of L-proline and high levels of the precursor L-glutamic acid, perhaps suggesting an enzyme deficiency associated with disturbed growth of the biliary tree. Jenner and Howard (1975) studied the possible toxic effects of monohydroxy bile acids on bile ducts in a rabbit model of bile duct obliteration, and postulated that some cases of biliary atresia could result from high levels of monohydroxy bile acids, which are synthesized by the developing liver. The toxic effects of these bile acids could be potentiated by a relative deficiency of sulphation in the early fetus.

Anatomical variants in the junction of bile and pancreatic ducts (Miyano *et al.,* 1979; Chiba *et al.,* 1990) have also been considered as possible aetiological factors in biliary atresia. Chiba *et al.* (1990) studied the distal cholangiographic appearance of 28 cases of biliary atresia and found an increased frequency of a long common channel compared with cases of biliary hypoplasia and neonatal hepatitis. This hypothesis has also been used to explain a rare occurrence of two siblings, one with biliary atresia and one with a choledochal cyst (Ando *et al.,* 1991).

PATHOLOGY

The morphology of the extrahepatic ducts in atresia varies from case to case. The currently accepted classification is based on that proposed by the Japanese Society of Pediatric Surgeons, which divides cases into three principal types (Chiba *et al.,* 1987; Ohi and Ibrahim, 1992): atresia of the common bile duct (type 1), atresia of the common hepatic duct (type 2), and atresia of the right and left hepatic ducts (type 3). There are further subdivisions to include the morphology of the gallbladder and the distal common bile duct. Histological features of the tissue at the porta hepatitis may also be classified. The gross appearance of the remnant biliary tree is not thought to be of prognostic importance, although we have recently observed that a particular morphological appearance of the biliary remnant (absence of the common bile duct) was associated with those cases of biliary atresia associated with splenic malformation.

There is a wide variation in the histological appearance of the proximal duct at the level of the porta hepatis and in most cases microscopic biliary ductules can be found. Correlation between the histology of residual tissue and postoperative bile flow has varied from series to series but it seems that satisfactory bile flow may be anticipated when the maximum size of residual ducts exceeds 150 μm (Kasai *et al.,* 1975). However, bile flow may be achieved regardless of duct size and even in cases in which ducts have not been identified in the tissue resected at surgery (Lawrence *et al.,* 1981). The size of biliary ductular remnants is the only histological feature known to have prognostic importance (Hitch *et al.,* 1979; Gauthier and Eliot, 1981).

Absence of the proximal biliary tree has been termed biliary agenesis by some authors (Schwartz *et al.,* 1990), although in three of the five cases reported the gallbladder and common bile duct were still present. Features of the splenic malformation syndrome were seen in the two infants treated at King's College Hospital with no biliary remnants whatsoever (Davenport *et al.,* 1993).

Studies of extrahepatic duct remnants excised at surgery (Fig. 27.1) have shown a wide variety of histological appearances which have been classified into three main types (Gauthier and Eliot, 1981). Type 1 shows no residual duct tissue and the connective tissue contains few inflammatory cells, type 2 shows lumina lined by cuboidal epithelium with diameters usually less than 50 μm, and type 3 cases show evidence of residual bile ducts with residual epithelium of the columnar type. Bile, mostly within macrophages, was found in 68% of type 3 cases. Histological studies of the liver have shown that intrahepatic bile ducts are patent from the intralobular portion of the liver to the porta hepatis during the first 2 or 3 months after birth in nearly all patients. The nature of involvement of the intrahepatic biliary ducts in cases of biliary atresia is controversial, with some authors suggesting that the ductular damage is panductular from the outset and others believing that intrahepatic involvement is a secondary phenomenom (Sherlock, 1987). Takahiro *et al.* (1983) showed with repeated cholangiography and electron microscopy that intrahepatic ducts tended to remain obstructed in children who underwent surgery after 80 days of life, suggesting an irreversible process.

Liver histology in biliary atresia, if sampled early, shows the classical features of biliary obstruction: fibrosis and oedema expand the portal tracts with large numbers of peripheral proliferating bile duct ductules in association with interlobular bile ducts. Bile is seen within dilated canaliculi and hepatocytes. Multinucleate giant hepatocytes may also be present, although these cells are more commonly seen in neonatal hepatitis. The most likely source of histopathological confusion is with alpha-1-antitrypsin deficiency, where a pattern of intrahepatic biliary atresia can be mimicked.

ASSOCIATED ANOMALIES

A range of extrahepatic anomalies has been observed in up to 20% of infants with biliary atresia. The most common association is known as the polysplenia syndrome, which consists of polysplenia, portal vein anomalies, malrotation and situs inversus (Karrer *et al.,* 1991). Other anomalies are described in Table 27.2. In our series of 308 cases treated since 1975, 23 infants (7.5%) had polysplenia, two had a double spleen and two had asplenia. All 27 showed anomalies which may occur in the polysplenia syndrome and we now use the term biliary atresia splenic malformation syndrome to describe all such infants (Davenport *et al.,* 1993). In our series they had a lower birth weight and a higher incidence of maternal problems (e.g. diabetes) compared with the non-syndromic cases. The extrahepatic appearance of the biliary tree was also different, with a much higher incidence of absence of parts of the bile duct. Both features suggest that the aetiology of this subgroup may differ from the more usual case.

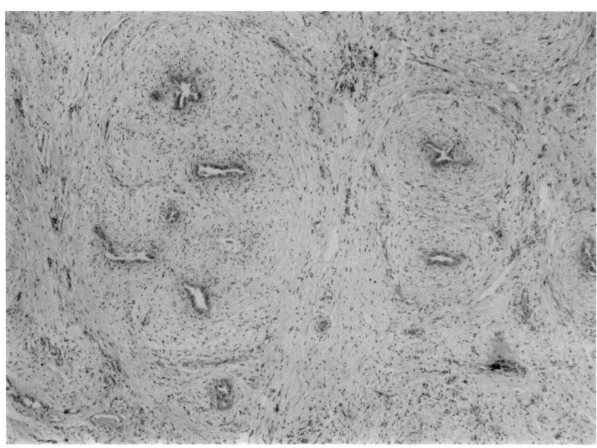

Fig. 27.1 Histological section from the porta hepatis of a case of biliary atresia. The small residual bile ductules, surrounded by concentric rings of fibrous tissue, are clearly seen.

Table 27.2 Extrahepatic anomalies reported in biliary atresia

Feature	Variations
Splenic anomalies	Polysplenia
	Double spleen
	Asplenia
Portal vein anomalies	Preduodenal
	Absence
	Cavernomatous transformation
Situs inversus	
Malrotation	
Cardiac anomalies	
Annular pancreas	
Immotile cilia syndrome (Kartagener's syndrome)	
Duodenal atresia	
Oesophageal atresia	
Polycystic kidney	
Cleft palate	
Jejunal atresia	

Based upon over 350 cases treated at King's College Hospital (1975–92) (Davenport *et al.*, 1993).

CLINICAL FEATURES

The majority of cases of biliary atresia present with jaundice, pale stools and dark urine due to the conjugated nature of the hyperbilirubinaemia. There is a slight female predominance in most series (Lilly *et al.*, 1989; Karrer *et al.*, 1990; Howard *et al.*, 1991). Antenatal diagnosis of a rare cystic lesion has been made on one occasion (Greenholz *et al.*, 1986) but most cases present outside the neonatal period because of persistent jaundice. Infants have usually been born at term of normal birth weight and are usually feeding and gaining weight appropriately but they may present occasionally with a coagulopathy and abnormal bleeding due to vitamin K deficiency. Examination of these infants may reveal hepatomegaly and splenomegaly. Ascites and wasting may be seen as a late presentation when hepatic fibrosis or biliary cirrhosis has supervened.

A preoperative diagnosis of biliary atresia in an infant with conjugated hyperbilirubinaemia can be made from a combination of clinical features, ultrasonography, radioisotope studies and liver biopsy. The differential diagnosis of conjugated jaundice in infancy is wide ranging (Table 27.3) and medical conditions such as alpha-1-antitrypsin deficiency, cystic fibrosis and maternal intrauterine infection (e.g. hepatitis and cytomegalovirus) must be excluded. The most common diagnostic difficulty concerns the separation of biliary atresia from neonatal hepatitis and although liver biopsy and interpretation by an experienced histopathologist is usually adequate for discrimination other tests may be required in 15–20% of cases. Newer, more specific hepatobiliary radioisotopes such as the technetium-labelled iminodiacetic acid compounds, e.g. ^{99m}Tc di-isopropyliminodiacetic acid (DISIDA) (Spivak *et al.*, 1987) have replaced the older ^{131}I-Rose Bengal faecal

excretion test and are easier to interpret and more reliable. Duodenal intubation for bilirubin and direct cholangiography via an (ERCP) (Wilkinson *et al.*, 1991; Guelrud *et al.*, 1991) or via direct percutaneous intrahepatic puncture (Howard and Nunnerly, 1979) may help, although neither method is absolutely reliable because of the high false-negative rate. Direct visualization of the liver and gallbladder and cholangiography via gallbladder puncture can be performed using laparoscopic techniques. Whichever diagnostic tests are used the emphasis must be on rapid diagnosis because the cholangiopathic process and liver damage is progressive (Hussein *et al.*, 1991). The diagnosis of atresia versus hepatitis may occasionally remain in doubt until laparotomy, and operative cholangiography performed through the fundus of the gallbladder is then crucial. Ten per cent of atresia cases have patent distal common bile ducts communicating with the gallbladder (Lilly *et al.*, 1989) and it is therefore essential to demonstrate continuity with the intrahepatic ducts if atresia is to be excluded. Aspiration of bile from the gallbladder and cholangiography are particularly useful in confirming the presence of a type 1 lesion with patency of the proximal common bile duct and in the rare cases of true biliary hypoplasia. This latter diagnosis is found in cases of Alagille's syndrome (Alagille *et al.*, 1975) (arteriohepatic dysplasia) and other features should be sought such as an 'elfin' face, the murmur of pulmonary stenosis and a 'butterfly' appearance of the vertebrae on X-ray. Preoperative diagnosis followed by definitive surgery should be possible in most cases.

SURGICAL MANAGEMENT

The key to successful surgery in biliary atresia is adequate exposure of the porta hepatis (Fig. 27.2). This is

Table 27.3 Differential diagnosis of conjugated hyperbilirubinaemia

Medical (after Mowat, 1987)	Surgical	
Metabolic e.g. galactosaemia, fructosaemia, tyrosinaemia, cystic fibrosis, alpha-1-antitrypsin deficency, hypothyroidism, hypothyroidism, parenteral nutrition	**Choledochal cyst** spontaneous perforation of the bile duct (Davenport *et al.*, 1991a), inspissated bile syndrome (Heaton *et al.*, 1991)	**Bile duct lesions** e.g. choledochal cyst, spontaneous perforation, inspissated bile syndrome
Biliary hypoplasia e.g. Alagille's syndrome	**External pressure** e.g. duplication cyst	
Intrauterine infection e.g. syphilis, hepatitis B, toxoplasma, malaria, cytomegalovirus, rubella		

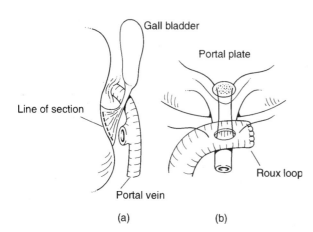

Gall bladder

Portal plate

Line of section

Roux loop

Portal vein

(a)   (b)

Fig. 27.2 Schematic representation of a portoenterostomy procedure and reconstruction using a 40 cm Roux jejunal loop. (a) Elevation of obliterated biliary tree before its division at the level of the portal plate. (b) Placement of stay sutures between portal plate and Roux loop.

achieved by complete mobilization of the liver itself by division of the falciform, left and right triangular ligaments. This manoeuvre allows the liver to be everted fully into the wound (Fig. 27.3).

Correctable lesions (Fig. 27.4), either cystic dilatations or residual segments of duct to which conventional biliary enteric anastomoses can be performed in the porta hepatis, are rarely found. It is often difficult to decide from macroscopic appearances whether cystic structures in the porta hepatis communicate with intrahepatic ducts and, unless there is clear evidence of a large lumen containing definite bile, portoenterostomy is recommended as the operation of choice. The long-term results in this group of infants treated with conventional surgical techniques have been poor (Lilly

et al., 1987). None the less hepaticojejunostomy, if thought suitable, may be performed with an end-to-side anastomosis between a large duct remnant and a 45 cm Roux-en-Y loop of jejunum.

The technique of portoenterostomy for the usual, more severe form of atresia was developed by Kasai and Suzuki (1959) following the observation that bile ductules are usually present in the fibrous tissue remnants at the porta hepatis. The operation consists of an initial mobilization of gallbladder and cystic duct which allows identification of the remnants of the common bile duct. These are dissected free from the hepatic artery and portal vein. After transection of the distal common bile duct the fibrous remnants of gallbladder and bile ducts are elevated and dissected proximally to the porta hepatis. The bifurcation of the portal vein must be clearly exposed. The cone of the proximal biliary remnant is transected flush with, but not within, the liver capsule (Fig. 27.5) and angulated scissors have been designed for this purpose (Davenport and Howard, 1992). Anastomosis of the fibrous edges of the transected tissue to a 45 cm Roux-en-Y loop of jejunum with interrupted sutures completes the operation. Polydioxanone (PDS) is the authors' preferred suture material for all biliary anastomoses.

The level of tissue transection in the porta hepatis is critical and attempts to deepen the dissection into liver substance have resulted in rapid obliteration of the small residual bile channels. We do not depend on frozen section examination of tissue transected at the porta hepatis as is sometimes recommended (Altman, 1976) because the primary operation should be so radical that little more in the way of resection is possible whatever is revealed on histological examination.

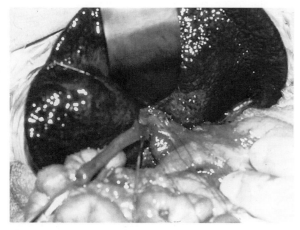

Fig. 27.3 Complete mobilization of the liver in a portoenterostomy operation. Note the accessibility of the porta hepatis.

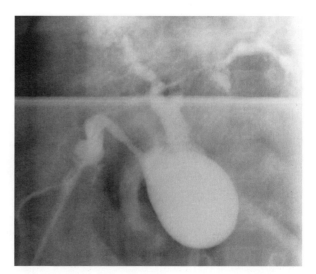

Fig. 27.4 Percutaneous cholangiogram in a jaundiced infant showing a type 1 cystic variety of biliary atresia. At operation the cyst contained bile and was treated by hepaticojejunostomy.

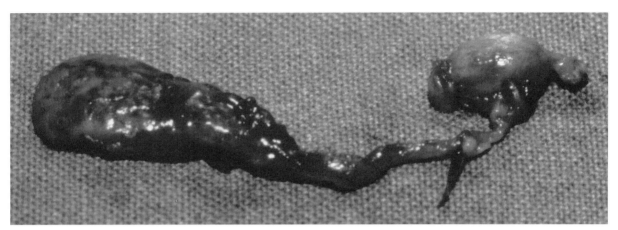

Fig. 27.5 Resected specimen of gallbladder and residual, atretic, bile duct tissue from a 7-week-old infant with biliary atresia.

Most of the modifications of the original porto-enterostomy procedure (e.g. Suruga I, II; Sawaguchi; see Ohi (1991b) for discussion) were designed to prevent cholangitis, which is one of the more frequent complications of portoenterostomy, on the assumption that reflux of intestinal content to the hilar anastomosis was the most important precipitating cause. Most variations included an exteriorization of the Roux loop and total or partial external diversion of bile. The dissection in the porta hepatis remains unmodified in all of these variations. Any bile which drains from these stomas may be re-fed to the patient to reduce fluid and electrolyte loss. However, a reduction in the incidence of cholangitis has never been proven with these exteriorization techniques and the stoma itself causes morbidity due to either dehydration and salt loss or the formation of mucocutaneous varices. Stomas also make any subsequent hepatic transplant procedure more difficult.

Other surgical procedures have been designed to prevent reflux of intestinal contents up the Roux loop. A valve effect may be created in the Roux loop by removing the seromuscular layer of a segment of bowel and intussuscepting the denuded mucosa distally as a nipple valve (Tanaka *et al.*, 1987; Saeki *et al.*, 1991). Anastomosis of the gallbladder to the transected tissue of the porta hepatis (portocholecystostomy; Lilly, 1979a) has also been used in the 15% of patients who are proven to have a patent distal common bile duct. However, a reduction in the incidence of cholangitis must be compared with an increase in technical complications, including obstruction of the mobilized gallbladder and small common bile duct and prolonged leaks of bile.

Repeat operation after a failed portoenterostomy has been advocated, particularly for those children whose jaundice increases again after a period of satisfactory bile flow (Ohi *et al.*, 1985; Lilly *et al.*, 1989). In general, however, the results of reoperation are disappointing. Reoperation consists either of further excision of bile duct remnants still present in the porta hepatis or of curettage of fibrous tissue at the site of previous anastomosis. Seven out of 33 cases subjected to reoperation in one series became jaundice free, three after a repeat portoenterostomy and four after curettage (Ohi *et al.*, 1985).

The postoperative management of these infants varies from centre to centre and has seldom been subject to controlled trial. Cholestyramine, phenobarbitone, ursodeoxycholic acid (Ullrith *et al.*, 1987) and steroids (Karrer and Lilly, 1985) have all been used with varying efficacy, usually in an attempt to improve postsurgical biliary excretion.

Bile flow after portoenterostomy has been reported in up to 90% of cases undergoing operation before 10 weeks of age (Miele-Vergani *et al.*, 1989), but maximal bile flow may not be seen for up to 1 year after operation. Bile salts tend to be excreted preferentially to cholesterol and phospholipid and serum concentrations of these substances may take many months to fall to within normal range (Lilly and Javitt, 1976). Lack of bile may lead to reduced serum levels of fat-soluble vitamins A and E, but these do not often seem to cause clinical symptoms. Long-term survivors frequently show evidence of osteomalacia and osteoporosis, the latter being independent of vitamin D (Kobayashi *et al.*, 1974). Intestinal malabsorption rather than reduced hepatic metabolism of vitamin D appears to be responsible for rickets and the condition responds rapidly to additional vitamin D supplements (Kooh *et al.*, 1979). Low plasma zinc levels and high plasma copper levels have been noted in children treated for biliary atresia although the clinical relevance is obscure (Endo *et al.*, 1991). Developmental delay may be seen in infants and children with end-stage liver failure and has been related to lack of growth and vitamin E levels in infants and the degree of liver dysfunction in older children (Stewart *et al.*, 1987).

Table 27.4   Complications after surgery

Cholangitis	
Portal hypertension	Oesophageal varices
	Stomal varices
	Anorectal varices
Ascites	
Poor nutrition	Malabsorption
	Vitamin D, A, K and E deficiency
Splenomegaly	Hypersplenism
Intrahepatic cyst formation	

COMPLICATIONS AFTER SURGERY

Ascending bacterial cholangitis

Most series show an incidence of cholangitis from 25 to 50% (Lilly *et al.*, 1989; Karrer *et al.*, 1990; Howard *et al.*, 1991) (Table 27.4). Diagnosis is made from the triad of pyrexia, elevated serum bilirubin and acholic stools. The causative organism is usually a Gram-negative bacillus which may be cultured from blood, bile or a liver biopsy. Prompt treatment with broad-spectrum antibiotics is essential as liver function deteriorates with each attack. Whilst the aetiology is believed to be an ascending infection along the Roux loop, other routes of entry such as the portal venous system (Danks *et al.*, 1974) and hepatic lymphatics (Hirzig *et al.*, 1978) have also been suggested. Suspected infection should be treated early and with vigour but there is no evidence that prophylactic antibiotics confer any further benefit.

Cholangitis occurs most frequently during the year following surgery and episodes after this time should suggest the possibility of mechanical obstruction within the Roux loop. Late-onset cholangitis should be investigated urgently with an hepatic radionuclide excretion scan and with percutaneous transhepatic cholangiography (Fig. 27.6).

Portal hypertension

Measurements of portal pressure during initial operations for biliary atresia have shown elevated values in a majority of infants (Kasai *et al.*, 1981) and portal hypertension remains a significant problem in many long-term survivors. Biliary atresia is the second most common cause of portal hypertension in children after portal vein thrombosis (Howard *et al.*, 1988). Kasai *et al.* (1981) suggested that the cause is a presinusoidal block due to obliteration of portal venous radicals. It is not possible to predict the development or severity of portal hypertension. The degree of fibrosis in the diagnostic liver biopsies, the age at which the portoenterostomy is performed and any subsequent attacks of

cholangitis have no clear relationship with the development of varices (Kang *et al.*, 1993). Satisfactory bile flow and clearance of jaundice does not exclude the development of portal hypertension, although our series of cases did show that the more severe grades of varices were seen in children with unremitting jaundice and a derangement of liver biochemistry (Davenport *et al.*, 1991b).

Bleeding from oesophageal varices should be treated by resuscitation, correction of any coagulopathy and early endoscopy. Control should be obtainable by injection sclerotherapy in most cases although a Sengstaken tube may be needed occasionally (Stringer *et al.*, 1989). Further injections may be needed over a longer period to achieve variceal regression and obliteration. Surgical treatment of portal hypertension with mesocaval

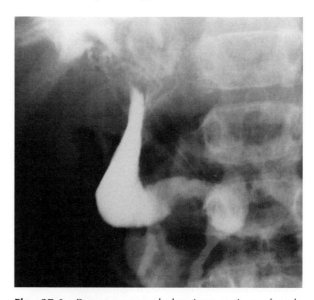

Fig. 27.6   Percutaneous cholangiogram in a female 7-year-old child. She had undergone portoenterostomy in infancy and had remained well, with a normal serum bilirubin, until a single attack of jaundice. The cholangiogram confirmed an obstruction in the lower end of the Roux-en-Y loop from adhesions.

and splenorenal shunts (Alpert, 1976) has been used in the past but is probably best avoided in view of the compromised liver function of most of these patients. Deteriorating liver function and recurrent variceal bleeds should be an indication for liver transplantation.

Although oesophageal varices are the commonest manifestation of portal hypertension, varices can also develop in other sites of portosystemic communication and although overt rectal bleeding due to anorectal varices and haemorrhoids is uncommon we have seen this in four cases of biliary atresia (Heaton *et al.*, 1992).

A degree of hypersplenism causing anaemia, neutropenia and thrombocytopaenia is commonly seen but should be treatable by conservative measures including dietary iron supplementation. Some authors advocate partial splenic embolization (Brandt *et al.*, 1989) using angiographic techniques to ameliorate the haematological consequences of this complication.

RESULTS

The unexpectedly poor long-term results for type 1 cases treated by conventional anastomotic techniques have been mentioned previously and confirmed in a number of centres in Europe (Howard *et al.*, 1991) and Japan (Kasai *et al.*, 1989). The effectiveness of portoenterostomy has gradually improved since its introduction in 1957 when a 10% success rate was reported (Kasai and Suzuki, 1959; Kasai *et al.*, 1968). Kasai's report (Kasai *et al.*, 1989) of some 245 cases of biliary atresia showed that 81% were able to achieve postoperative bile excretion whilst clearance of jaundice occurred in 46%. Seventy-six per cent of the most recent cohort (1982–7) achieved clearance of jaundice following surgery. Such results have now been reported from a number of centres throughout the world. We have analysed a cohort of 185 infants with biliary atresia treated during the 1980s at King's College Hospital (Howard *et al.*, 1990) and shown that the probability of medium-term survival (to 5 years) was 60% following portoenterostomy (Fig. 27.7). Other centres have reported similar recent results, e.g. 57% of 131 infants (1973–88) from Denver, USA, with sustained relief from jaundice of over 1 year (Lilly *et al.*, 1989).

The single most important determinant of a good outcome following portoenterostomy is the age at operation, thus 86% of infants operated before 8 weeks became jaundice free whilst only 41% of infants operated on from 8 to 12 weeks became jaundice free (Karrer and Lilly, 1985). The relationship of age to long-term outcome, however, is far from clear. For instance, in a large Japanese series (Kasai *et al.*, 1989) 10 year survival of 74% was seen in infants undergoing surgery at less than 60 days of age compared to 26% survival in infants operated on from 61 to 90 days, with no long-term survivors if the infant was older than 120

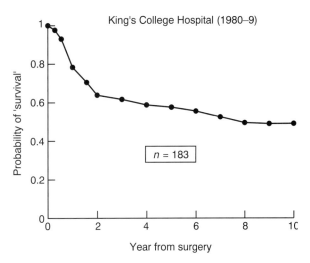

Fig. 27.7 Actuarial survival after surgical treatment of 185 infants at King's College Hospital, London (1980–1989). The endpoints in this analysis were death or transplantation. Note that two further infants with biliary agenesis diagnosed during this period were not amenable to surgery.

days at surgery. In contrast, neither Suruga *et al.* (1985) nor Tagge *et al.* (1991) found any relationship between age at surgery and the establishment of long-term bile flow or survival. In our own much larger series of 185 infants treated in the 1980s (Howard *et al.*, 1991) there appeared to be a plateau in survival expectation with age at surgery. Although there was a survival advantage if the operation was performed within 60 days a progressive disadvantage after that time could not be demonstrated. Even infants operated on after 100 days had a probability of survival to 5 years of about 50%. Survival figures from the Biliary Atresia Registry suggest a similar plateau effect, although they indicate that this occurred rather later, at 100 days (Karrer *et al.*, 1990). There may be a range of severity in the disease, particularly in the intrahepatic pathology, which is independent of age.

Other factors which have a significant effect on surgical outcome include the experience of the surgeon. Better results are obtained in those centres treating five or more new cases per year (McClement *et al.*, 1985). This observation provides an argument for centralization of the treatment for these children. The incidence of postoperative cholangitis may also influence outcome (Suruga *et al.*, 1985).

Although long-term survival is unquestionable in biliary atresia, biochemical liver function is seldom normal (Laurent *et al.*, 1990; Ohi *et al.*, 1991a). In a survey of long-term survivors, 85 patients over 5 years of age were analysed (Laurent *et al.*, 1990). Although 95% were apparently asymptomatic, the majority showed obvious abnormalities of liver histology and liver function tests, especially liver enzymes which were persistently elevated. A histological diagnosis of cirrhosis, however, does appear to be compatible with long-term survival.

Since the late 1980s liver transplantation has become an option for children who either fail to respond to porto-enterostomy or develop features of chronic liver failure later despite apparent bile drainage, and these children now form the most frequent single indication for paedi-atric liver transplantation (Otte *et al.*, 1988). In the largest series from the USA, 217 (54%) of 400 paedi-atric transplants had a diagnosis of biliary atresia (Starz *et al.*, 1989). Similarly, 43 (83%) of 52 children trans-planted in Belgium had biliary atresia (Otte *et al.*, 1988). The frequency of postoperative technical prob-lems is higher in a paediatric population than in an equivalent adult population and vascular anastomoses (especially the hepatic arterial anastomosis; Tan *et al.*, 1988) are prone to thrombosis because of the inherent small size of the vessels. However, the success of the procedure over the last decade has been attributed to the use of more efective and safer immunosuppressive agents such as cyclosporin A and FK 506 and increas-ing experience in transplantation in smaller children and infants. The use of smaller organ grafts and split livers has contributed to the increase in paediatric transplantation.

The role of the portoenterostomy procedure in the management of biliary atresia has been questioned and transplantation has been suggested as the primary modality of treatment for these children. This argument ignores the good results that can be obtained with porto-enterostomy and the risks associated with transplanta-tion. The best centres report a 1-year patient survival of 80% at 2 years for children (not infants) (Otte *et al.*, 1988), but the long-term side-effects of current immunosuppressive regimens are unknown. Primary transplantation would be an option if the outcome of portoenterostomy could be reliably predicted before initial surgery. However, the only published predictor of long-term survival is the age at the time of porto-enterostomy and even that is unreliable in individual cases. Current opinion (Lilly *et al.*, 1989; Wood *et al.*, 1990; Vacanti *et al.*, 1990) suggests that the two proce-dures should therefore be regarded as complementary rather than competitive.

The decision for hepatic transplantation should be made before the hazards of ascites, gastrointestinal bleeding, failure to thrive and repeated episodes of cholangitis reduce the chances of successful grafting. Bilirubin excretion after portoenterostomy has been suggested as a guide to outcome (Vazquez-Estevez *et al.*, 1989) but this can only be determined accurately in the presence of a small bowel stoma.

Most infants born with biliary atresia should be treat-ed with a standard portoenterostomy and liver trans-plantation is now a practical option for those children who fail to respond.

Choledochal cyst

The term choledochal cyst refers to a congenital lesion of the biliary tree (either intrahepatic or extrahepatic) characterized by dilatation, which may be cystic or, less commonly, fusiform in appearance.

Douglas provided one of the earliest and best clinical descriptions of a choledochal cyst of the common bile duct in 1852. A jaundiced, pyrexial, 17-year-old girl presented with a painful swelling in the right hypochon-drium after a 3-year history of intermittent pain and 3 months of jaundice. Although percutaneous drainage of 900 ml of bile reduced the symptoms she died 1 month later. Post-mortem examination revealed a huge chole-dochal cyst, an undilated gallbladder and fibrotic changes in the wall of the cyst.

INCIDENCE

Although the true incidence of choledochal cyst is unknown it is clear that there is a marked racial varia-tion. The highest rates are seen in Chinese and Japanese (Yamaguchi, 1980) populations. Although about 60% of cases are diagnosed in the first 10 years of life an ini-tial presentation in adult life is well known. There is a marked female predominance of about 4:1 in most series, whatever the racial origin.

AETIOLOGY

Numerous hypotheses have been put forward to explain the aetiology of choledochal cysts. These can be classi-fied into three categories: obstruction of the distal com-mon bile duct causing dilatation (Ito *et al.*, 1984), congenital weakness of the walls of the bile ducts, and bile duct damage from the reflux of pancreatic juices into the biliary tree via an abnormal pancreaticobiliary junction (Babbit, 1969). Choledochal cysts have been produced experimentally by removing epithelium and ligating the distal portion of bile ducts in puppies, and also by anastomosising the pancreatic duct directly to the biliary tract (Ohkawa *et al.*, 1982).

ANOMALOUS PANCREATICOBILIARY JUNCTION AND CHOLEDOCHAL CYSTS

Abnormally high levels of amylase are frequently found in bile taken from choledochal cysts (Tan and Howard, 1988) and this is believed to occur because of reflux through an abnormal junction of the biliary and pancreatic ducts proximal to the ampulla of Vater. This abnormality produces a common biliary–pancreatic channel which is at least 2 cm in length (Jona *et al.*, 1979). In fetal life the pancreaticobiliary junction lies outside the duodenum and migrates into the wall to lie within the sphincter complex before birth (Wong and Lister, 1981). Arrest of this process may be the cause of the common channel anomaly. Common channels, although seen occasionally as a normal variant, are also associated with other pathological conditions such as gallbladder cancer. In one series a common channel was identified in 1.5% of ERCP, of which 18 of 24 (75%) were in patients with choledochal cysts and four of 24 (16.6%) had gallbladder carcinoma (Yamauchi *et al.,* 1987). Approximately 60–70% of choledochal cysts can be shown to have a common channel and Komi *et al.* (1992) have recently devised a complex classification of anomalous pancreaticobiliary junctions based on the radiographic appearances of 51 cases of choledochal cyst (Fig. 27.8). They also suggested that certain subtypes may lead to chronic pancreatitis even following appropriate surgery for cystic disease.

PATHOLOGICAL FEATURES

The most widely accepted classification of choledochal cysts was first described by Alonso-Lej *et al.* (1959) and modified by Todani *et al.* (1977). The five types are illustrated in Fig. 27.9.

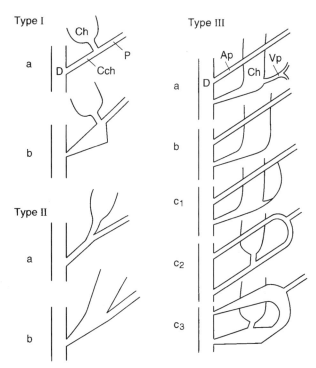

The new Komi classification of APBD. Ch, choledochus; P, pancreatic duct, Cch, common channel; duodenum; Ap, accessory pancreatic duct; Vp, ventral pancreatic duct.

Fig. 27.8 Illustration of the Komi *et al.* (1992) classification of anomalous pancreaticobiliary junctions. This classification was based on the radiographic appearances of 51 cases of choledochal cyst. (Reproduced with permission.)

The most common variant is the type I cyst, which describes a dilatation of the common bile duct proximal to a narrow segment of distal common bile duct. Type I cysts are subdivided into cystic (50%) (Fig. 27.10a) and fusiform (10%) (Fig. 27.10b) variants based on external morphology. Intrahepatic ducts may or may not be involved in the dilatation.

A type II cyst is a congenital diverticulum of the common bile duct. It is very rare and only five genuine examples have been reported (Alonso-Lei *et al.,* 1959; Iuchtman *et al.,* 1971). Type III cysts are also known as choledochoceles and are dilatations of the intraduodenal portion of the common bile duct (Venu *et al.,* 1984). They may be associated with recurrent jaundice and are best diagnosed by ERCP. Type IV cysts involve both the intrahepatic and extrahepatic biliary tree, whereas type V cysts are confined to within the liver substance itself (Fig. 27.10c). The latter two variants may be complicated by portal hypertension and cirrhosis (Tan and Howard, 1988).

Caroli's disease (Caroli, 1968) refers to a condition in which there are multiple, often bilateral, irregular segmental dilatations of the intrahepatic bile ducts. Unlike other types of choledochal cyst, Caroli's disease may be associated with hepatic fibrosis and cystic disease of the kidneys. This condition is not, however, related to polycystic disease of the liver, in which the cysts do not communicate with the biliary tract and contain mucus rather than bile. Caroli defined two types of intrahepatic dilatation: a rarer form which is not associated with cirrhosis and portal hypertension, and a more common type associated with congenital hepatic fibrosis and usually presenting in childhood. Medullary sponge kidneys and, occasionally, the Lawrence–Moon–Biedl syndrome may be found in association with the latter type of Caroli's disease.

Histologically, the wall of a choledochal cyst is partially replaced by chronic inflammation and fibrous tissue, and the epithelial lining may be wholly or partially absent. In a study of the age-related effects on 40 choledochal cysts, Komi *et al.* (1986) stated that under 2 years of age there is epithelial desquamation and fibrosis but minimal inflammation, by the age of 15 years an epithelial lining could not be identified in the majority of cysts, and in those excised from adults there were pronounced metaplastic changes. Adenocarcinoma was found in five of the 23 excised cysts. Shimada *et al.* (1991) recently suggested a biochemical mechanism for these changes when they observed high levels of phospholipid A_2 in bile from cases with a common channel. This mediator produces a cytotoxic phospholipid which may cause direct damage to biliary mucosa.

The histological appearance of the liver varies from a mild inflammatory infiltration to frank biliary cirrhosis. Portal hypertension and oesophageal varices may occur and this uncommon complication has even been seen in a 3-month-old infant.

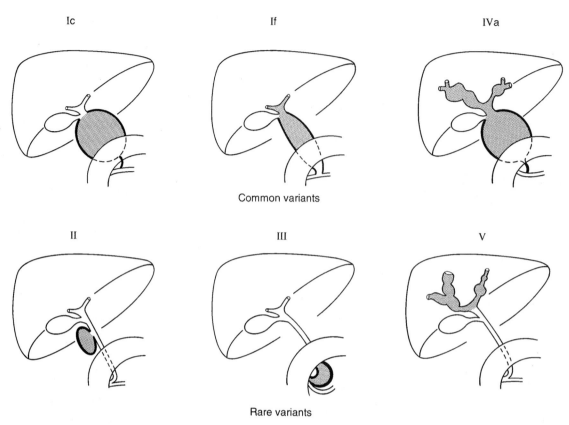

Fig. 27.9 Classification of choledochal cysts.

CLINICAL FEATURES

The classic presentation of pain, mass and jaundice (Fig. 27.11) varies in incidence from series to series. It is not, however, a universal presentation and was present in only 38% of the 740 cases collected by Flanigan (1975) and in only 25% of the series reported from King's College Hospital (Tan and Howard, 1988; Howard, 1991). Infants with choledochal cysts commonly present with jaundice alone and the condition must be distinguished from biliary atresia in this age group.

Choledochal cyst should always be considered in an older child who presents with recurrent abdominal pain and raised serum amylase (Karjoo *et al.,* 1973; Gauthier *et al.,* 1986), as pancreatitis is a well-recognized complication of the common channel anomaly. The refluxing amylase may be absorbed through areas in the cyst wall denuded of epithelium and this may cause an hyperamylasaemia. Recurrent abdominal pain may be associated with high levels of serum amylase and pancreatitis, although macroscopic pancreatic changes may not be very obvious at laparotomy. Stringel and Filler (1982) described this lack of pancreatic change at operation as 'fictitious pancreatitis'.

Uncommon presentations of choledochal cyst have included spontaneous and traumatic rupture (Tagart, 1956; Valayer and Alagille, 1975; Yamashiro *et al.,* 1982), dysfibrinogenaemia (Levy *et al.,* 1987), liver abscess (Karjoo *et al.,* 1973) and oesophageal varices due to cirrhosis (Kim, 1981; Tan and Howard, 1988).

MANAGEMENT

Diagnosis

Non-invasive investigations with ultrasound or computed tomography are commonly used to confirm the clinical diagnosis and in most cases these are the definitive tests. Plain X-rays of the abdomen (Fig. 27.12) and barium studies of the upper gastrointestinal tract may show duodenal displacement and excretion radionuclide scans may also be useful (Fig. 27.13). However, delayed scans are often needed to demonstrate isotope accumulation in the cysts of jaundiced patients.

Accurate preoperative anatomical definition of the biliary tree may be obtained by percutaneous transhepatic cholangiography or ERCP, although these methods may be associated with complications of bile leakage and pancreatitis and are not recommended for routine diagnosis. Prenatal diagnosis with ultrasonography was first reported in 1983 (Howell *et al.,* 1983) and two of our own cases were diagnosed as early as at 17 weeks' gestation (Howard, 1991).

Surgery

Internal drainage and radical excision have been the two main approaches used in the surgical management of choledochal cyst. Most authors have now concluded that internal drainage procedures, whilst technically easier, have an unacceptably high complication rate in the long term (O'Neil and Clatworthy, 1971; Lilly, 1979b; Joseph, 1990). It is now recommended that, except in the unusual situations of acute cholangitis or severe portal hypertension, the treatment in the majority of cases should be complete cyst excision.

Surgery is usually performed through an upper abdominal transverse incision (Howard, 1985, 1991). Cholangiography may be performed initially via the gallbladder to confirm the extent of both biliary dilatation and intrahepatic involvement in smaller cysts. In larger cysts it is unhelpful as the large volume of contrast required to fill the cyst obscures the detailed anatomy of the distal common bile duct. In very young

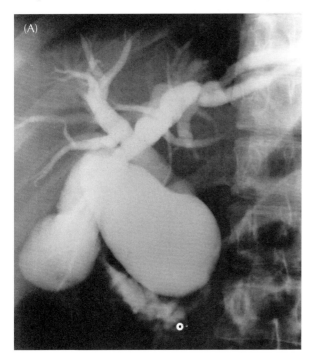

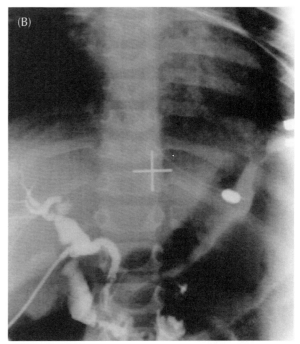

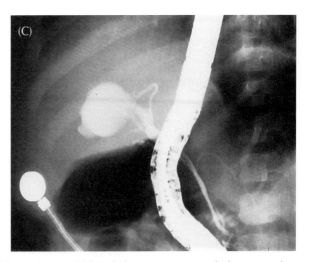

Fig. 27.10   (A) Large type Ic choledochal cyst demonstrated in a 16-year-old female by percutaneous cholangiography; (B) type If choledochal cyst demonstrated by operative cholangiography in a 5-month-old infant; (C) type V choledochal cyst within the right lobe of the liver of a 4-month-old infant. The cyst was first detected on prenatal ultrasound examination. The lesion remains asymptomatic.

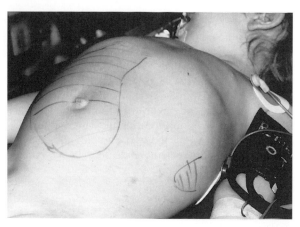

Fig. 27.11 Female 2-year-old infant who presented with jaundice and a large mass in the right side of the abdomen caused by a choledochal cyst. The spleen was also enlarged.

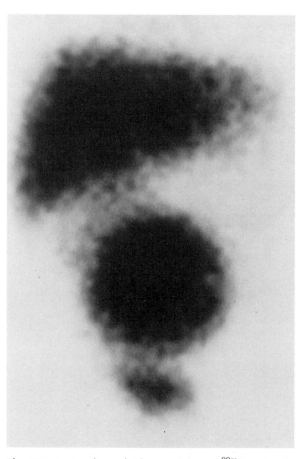

Fig. 27.13 A radionucleide scan (using a ^{99m}Tc iminodi-acetic acid derivative) in an 8-month-old infant who had been jaundiced for 1 month showing a large choledochal cyst. A type Ic choledochal cyst was excised.

infants it is necessary to exclude biliary atresia which may be associated with cystic dilatation in either the proximal or distal regions of the atretic bile duct. These cystic segments must not be confused with true choledochal cysts. Bile is aspirated at the start of the operation and analysed immediately for amylase content. A high amylase level would indicate the presence of a common pancreaticobiliary channel.

The choledochal cyst and the gallbladder are dissected free of the hepatic artery and the portal vein. The proximal end of the cyst, usually at the level of the bifurcation of the common hepatic bile duct, is encircled and then divided. This mobilization assists the distal dissection which proceeds to the level of the pancreas. The narrowed segment of the common bile duct is then divided and the lower end sutured or ligated. An hepticojejunostomy using a 40 cm Roux loop of jejunum is used for bile drainage. It is occasionally prudent to leave a portion of the distal cyst wall because of inflammation and scarring, but the mucosa in the distal portion of the cyst can be removed by submucosal dissection (Lilly, 1978).

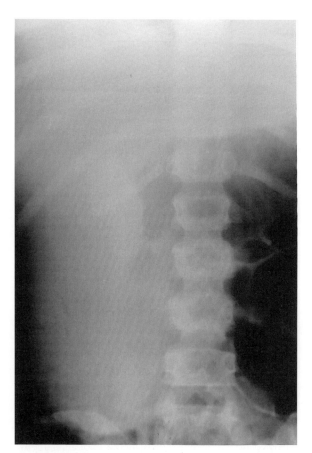

Fig. 27.12 Plain X-ray of a jaundiced child showing a large mass in the right side of the abdomen, which was a choledochal cyst.

Endoscopic or operative sphincterotomy has been used in some cases of fusiform choledochal cyst. Ng *et al.* (1992) reported good results in five of six children subjected to endoscopic sphincterotomy, but with a mean follow-up of only 4 years. They suggest that endoscopic sphincterotomy should be restricted to children with mild fusiform dilatation and a demonstrable distal stenosis. Despite theoretical objections because of the long-term risk of malignancy, Todani *et al.* (1985) suggested that carcinoma seldom, if ever, develops in this fusiform type. We are not in favour of the sphincterotomy approach to treatment in patients who possess a common channel as the risk of future attacks of pancreatitis and cholangitis remains. We have personal experience of a child with fusiform dilatation of the common bile duct who underwent a sphincteroplasty in infancy and required cyst resection after 10 years for these complications.

Other rarer variants of these choledochal anomalies may require more individualized surgery. Type II choledochal cysts can be treated by excision of the diverticulum and reconstruction of the bile duct (Iuchtman *et al.,* 1971). Type III cysts (choledochoceles) can be either removed via a transduodenal approach (Powell *et al.,* 1981) or ablated by endoscopic sphincterotomy (Venu *et al.,* 1984). The management of intrahepatic cystic disease is more complex. If the cystic disease is localized to one lobe then this can be excised completely as a formal hepatic lobectomy (Watts *et al.,* 1974). If the intrahepatic biliary tree dilatation is combined with extrahepatic dilatation then radical excision of the extrahepatic biliary tree and Roux loop reconstruction should improve biliary drainage. Long-term follow-up is mandatory as intrahepatic cysts may develop complications including stone formation and malignant change.

COMPLICATIONS

Many of the reported complications including recurrent cholangitis and pancreatitis have followed internal cyst drainage procedures, such as choledochocyst enterostomy, despite the construction of a wide anastomosis (Tan and Howard, 1988). These complications may be caused by the mixing of bile or pancreatic juice in the common channel with enterokinase from the duodenum or jejunum. Cyst resection and conversion to a hepticojejunostomy should be curative.

A few patients who have undergone cyst excision and hepaticojejunostomy may present with a late recurrence of pancreatitis. This may be secondary to proximal pancreatic duct or sphincter stenosis, pancreatic duct calculi or congenital anatomical anomalies of the pancreatic ducts. Examination with ERCP is imperative in these cases and sphincterotomy may relieve the symptoms.

Carcinomatous change may occur in choledochal cysts, particularly in adults. The increased risk has been calculated at between five and 35 times more than cholangiocarcinoma in undilated ducts (Todani *et al.,* 1977; Reveille *et al.,* 1990). However, malignancy may occur in children and Iwai *et al.* (1990) recently reported a 12-year-old girl with adenocarcinoma of the distal cyst wall. Flanigan (1975) reviewed 24 cases of malignant change and suggested an overall incidence of 2.5%. Histologically, these tumours may be either adenocarcinoma or squamous carcinoma. The prognosis is poor following the development of carcinoma and Kagawa *et al.* (1978) described 47 cases where the average survival after diagnosis was only 8.5 months. The cause of metaplastic and neoplastic change is still not understood but stasis and bacterial overgrowth generate secondary bile acids which may be mutagenic (Reveille *et al.,* 1990). All biliary mucosa is at risk of neoplastic change and this is not reduced by simple internal drainage operations.

References

Alagille, D., Odievre, M., Gautier, M. and Domegues, J.P. 1975: Hepatic ductular hypoplasia associated with characteristic facies, vertebral malformations, retarded physical, mental and skeletal development and cardiac murmer. *Journal of Pediatrics* **86**, 63–71.

Alonso-Lej, F., Rever, W.B. and Pessagno, D.J. Congenital choledochal cyst with a report of 2, and an analysis of 94 cases. *Surgery, Gynecology and Obstetrics: International Abstracts of Surgery* **108**, 1–30.

Alpert, L.I., Strauss, L. and Hirschhom, K. 1969: Neonatal hepatitis and biliary atresia. *New England Journal of Medicine* **280**, 16–20.

Alpert, R.P. 1976: Portal decompression by interposition mesocaval shunt in patients with biliary atresia. *Journal of Pediatric Surgery* **11**, 809–13.

Altman, R.P. 1976: The portoenterostomy procedure for biliary atresia. *Annals of Surgery* **188**, 357–61.

Ando, K., Miyano, T., Kimura, K., Shinomura, H. and Ohya, T. 1991: Congenital biliary atresia and congenital biliary dilatation in siblings. *Journal of Pediatric Surgery* **26**, 1399–400.

Babbitt, D.P. 1969: Congenital choledochal cysts: new etiological concept based on anomalous relationships of the common bile duct and pancreatic bulb. *Annals of Radiology* **12**, 231–5.

Banjura, B., Moreki, R. and Glaser, H. 1980: Comparative studies of biliary atresia in the human newborn and REO virus-induced cholangitis in weanling mice. *Laboratory Investigations* **43**, 456–62.

Becroft, D.M.O. 1972: Biliary atresia associated with prenatal infection by *Listeria monocytogenes*. *Archives of Disease in Childhood* **47**, 656.

Bill, A.H. 1978: Biliary atresia. *World Journal of Surgery* **2**, 557–9.

Brandt, C.T., Rothbarth, L.J., Kumpe, D.A., Karrer, F.M. and Lilly, J.R. 1989: Splenic embolisation in children. *Journal of Pediatric Surgery* **24**, 642–5.

Brent, R.L. 1962: Persistent jaundice in infancy. *Journal of Pediatrics* **61**, 111–44.

Caroli, J. 1968: Diseases of intrahepatic bile ducts. *Israel Journal of Medical Science* **4**, 21–35.

Chiba, T., Kasai, M. and Suzuki, T. Variation in the course of vessels in the vicinity of the hepatic port in biliary atresia. *Journal of Pediatric Surgery* **22**, 963–6.

Chiba, T., Ohi, R. and Mochizuki, I. 1990: Cholangiographic study of the pancreatobiliary ductal junction in biliary atresia. *Journal of Pediatric Surgery* **25**, 609–12.

Danks, D.M. 1965: Prolonged neonatal obstructive jaundice. A survey of modern concepts. *Clinical Pediatrics* **4**, 499–510.

Danks, D.M., Campbell, P.E., Clarke, A.M., Jones, P.G. and Solomon, J.R. 1974: Extrahepatic biliary atresia. *American Journal of Diseases in Childhood* **128**, 684–6.

Davenport, M. and Howard, E.R. 1992: Portoenterostomy scissors: a new instrument for surgery in the porta hepatis. *Annals of the Royal College of Surgeons of England* **74**, 68–9.

Davenport, M., Heaton, N.D. and Howard, E.R. 1991a: Spontaneous perforation of the bile duct in infants. *British Journal of Surgery* **78**, 1068–70.

Davenport, M., Kang, N., Driver, M. and Howard, E.R. 1991b: The development of oesophageal varices in extrahepatic biliary atresia. In Ohi, R. (ed.), *Biliary atresia: Proceedings of the 5th International Sendai Symposium*. Tokyo: ICOM Associates, 233–7.

Davenport, M., Savage, M., Mowat, A.P. and Howard, E.R. 1993: Biliary atresia splenic malformation syndrome. *Surgery* **113**, 662–8.

Douglas, A.H. 1852: Case of dilatation of the common bile duct. *Monthly Journal of Medical Science (London)* **14**, 97.

Dussaix, E., Hadchouel, M., Tardieu, M. and Alagille, D. 1984: Biliary atresia and the reovirus type 3 infection. *New England Journal of Medicine* **310**, 658.

Endo, M., Fuchimoto, Y., Ukiyama, E. *et al.* 1991: Evaluation of post-operative zinc and copper dynamics in infants and children with special reference to progression of liver cirrhosis. In Ohi, R. (ed.), *Biliary atresia: Proceedings of the 5th International Sendai Symposium*. Tokyo: ICOM Associates, 1991: 210–14.

Flanigan, D.P. 1975: Biliary cysts. *Annals of Surgery* **182**, 635–43.

Gauthier, F., Brunelle, F. and Valayer, J. 1986: Common channel for bile and pancreatic ducts. Presentation of 12 cases and discussion. *Chirugie Pediatrique* **27**, 148–52.

Gauthier, M. and Eliot, N. 1981: Extrahepatic biliary atresia: morphological study of 98 biliary remnants. *Archives of Pathology and Laboratory Medicine* **105**, 397–402.

Greenholz, S.K., Lilly, J.R., Shikes, R.H. and Hall, R.J. 1986: Biliary atresia in the newborn. *Journal of Pediatric Surgery* **21**, 1147–8.

Guelrud, M., Jaen, D., Mendoza, S., Plaz, J. and Torres, P. 1991: ERCP in the diagnosis of extrahepatic biliary atresia. *Gastrointestinal Endoscopy* **37**, 522–6.

Hart, M.H., Kaufman, S.S., Vanderhoof, J.A., Kaufman, J.A., Erdman, S., Linder, J. *et al.* 1991: Neonatal hepatitis and extrahepatic biliary atresia associated with cytomegalovirus in twins. *American Journal of Disease in Childhood* **145**, 302–4.

Heaton, N., Davenport, M. and Howard, E.R. 1991: Intraluminal biliary obstruction. *Archives of Disease in Childhood* **66**, 1395–8.

Heaton, N.D., Davenport, M. and Howard, E.R. 1992: Symptomatic hemorrhoids and anorectal varices in children with portal hypertension. *Journal of Pediatric Surgery* **27**, 833–5.

Hirsig, J., Kara, O. and Rickham, P.P. 1978: Experimental investigations into the etiology of cholangitis following operation for biliary atresia. *Journal of Pediatric Surgery* **13**, 55–7.

Hitch, D.C., Shikes, R.H. and Lilly, J.R. 1979: Determinants of survival after Kasai's operation for biliary atresia using actuarial analysis. *Journal of Pediatric Surgery* **14**, 310–14.

Holder, T. and Ashcraft, K.W. 1967: The effects of bile duct ligation and inflammation in the fetus. *Journal of Pediatric Surgery* **2**, 35–40.

Holmes, J.B. 1916: Congenital obliteration of the bile duct: diagnosis and suggestions for treatment. *American Journal of Disease in Childhood* **11**, 405–31.

Houwen, R.H.J., Kerremans, I.I., van-Steensel-Mol, H.A., Van Romunde, L.K., Bijleveld, C.M. and Schweizer, P. 1988: Time-space distribution of extrahepatic biliary atresia in the Netherlands and West Germany. *Zeitschrift für Kinderchirugie* **43**, 68–71

Howard, E.R. 1985: Choledochal, cysts. In Schawartz, S.I. and Ellis, H. (eds), *Maingot's abdominal operations*, 8th ed. Norwalk, CA: Appleton-Century-Crofts.

Howard, E.R. 1991: Choledochal cysts. In Howard, E.R. (ed.), *Surgery of liver disease in childhood*. London: Butterworths, 78–90.

Howard, E.R. and Nunnerly, H.B. 1979: Percutaneous cholangiography in prolonged jaundice of childhood. *Journal of the Royal Society of Medicine* **72**, 495–502.

Howard, E.R. Stringer, M.D. and Mowat, A.P. 1988: Assessment of injection sclerotherapy in the management of 152 children with oesophageal varices. *British Journal of Surgery* **75**, 404–8.

Howard, E.R., Davenport, M. and Mowat, A.P. 1991: Portoenterostomy in the eighties: the King's College Hospital experience. In Ohi, R. (ed.), *Biliary atresia: Proceedings of the 5th International Sendai Symposium*. Tokyo: ICOM Associates, 111–15.

Howell, C.G., Templeton, J.M., Weiner, S., Glassman, M., Betts, J.M. and Witzleben, C.L. 1983: Antenatal diagnosis and early surgery for choledochal cyst. *Journal of Pediatric Surgery* **18**, 387–93.

Hussein, M., Howard, E.R., Mieli-Vergani, G. and Mowat, A.P. 1991: Jaundice at 14 days of age: exclude biliary atresia. *Archives of Disease in Childhood* **66**, 1177–9.

Ito, T., Ando, H., Nagaya, M. and Sugito, T. 1984: Congenital dilatation of the common bile duct in children – the etiological significance of the narrow segment distal to the dilated common bile duct. *Zeitschrift für Kinderchirugie* **39**, 40–4.

Iuchtman, M., Martins, M.S. and Scheidemantel, R.E. 1971: Congenital diverticulum of the choledochus; report of a case. *International Surgery* **55**, 280–22.

Iwai, N., Deguchi, E., Yanagihara, J. *et al.* 1990: Cancer arising in a choledochal cyst in a 12 year old girl. *Journal of Pediatric Surgery* **25**, 1261–3.

Jenner, R.E. 1978: New perspectives on biliary atresia. *Annals of the Royal College of Surgeons of England* **60**, 367–74.

Jenner, R.E. and Howard, E.R. 1975: Unsaturated mono-hydroxy bile acids as a cause of idiopathic obstructive cholangiopathy. *Lancet* **ii**, 1073–4.

Jona, J.Z., Babbitt, D.P., Starshak, R.J., LaPorta, A.J., Glicklich, M. and Cohen,R.D. 1979: Anatomic observations and etiologic and surgical considerations in choledochal cyst. *Journal of Pediatric Surgery* **14**, 315–20.

Joseph, V.T. 1990: Surgical techniques and long-term results in the treatment of choledochal cyst. *Journal of Pediatric Surgery* **25**, 782–7.

Kagawa, Y., Kashihara, S., Kuramoto, S. and Maetani, S. 1978: Carcinoma arising in a congenitally dilated biliary tract. *Gastroenterology* **74**, 1286–94.

Kang, N., Davenport, M., Driver, M. and Howard, E.R. 1993: Hepatic histology and the development of esophageal varices in biliary atresia. *Journal of Pediatric Surgery* **28**, 63–6.

Karjoo, M., Bishop, H.C., Borns, P. and Hotzapple, P.G. 1973: Choledochal cyst presenting as recurrent pancreatitis. *Pediatrics* **51**, 289–91.

Karrer, F.M. and Lilly, J.R. 1985: Corticosteroid therapy in biliary atresia. *Journal of Pediatric Surgery* **20**, 683–95.

Karrer, F.M., Hall, R.J. and Lilly, J.R. 1991: Biliary atresia and the polysplenia syndrome. *Journal of Pediatric Surgery* **26**, 524-7.

Karrer, F.M., Lilly, J.R., Stewart, B.A. and Hall, R.J. 1990: Biliary Atresia Registry, 1976–1989. *Journal of Pediatric Surgery* **25**, 1076–81.

Kasai, M. and Suzuki, S. 1959: A new operation for 'non-correctable' biliary atresia. *Shujitsu* **13**, 733–9.

Kasai, M., Kiura, K., Asakura, Y., Suzuki, H., Taira, Y. and Ohashi E. 1968: Surgical treatment of biliary atresia. *Journal of Pediatric Surgery* **3**, 665–75.

Kasai, M., Mochizuki, I., Ohkohchi, N., Chiba, T. and Ohi, R. 1989: Surgical limitations for biliary atresia: indications for liver transplantation. *Journal of Pediatric Surgery* **24**, 851–4.

Kasai, M., Okamoto, A., Ohi, R., Yabe, K. and Matsumura, Y. 1981: Changes of portal vein pressure and intrahepatic blood vessels after surgery for biliary atresia. *Journal of Pediatric Surgery* **16**, 152–9.

Kasai, M., Watenabe, I. and Ohi, R. 1975: Follow-up studies of long-term survivors after hepatic portoenterostomy for 'non-correctable' biliary atresia. *Journal of Pediatric Surgery* **10**, 173–82.

Kim, S.H. 1981: Choledochal cyst. Survey by the surgical section of the American Academy of Pediatrics. *Journal of Pediatric Surgery* **16**, 27–32.

Klippel, C.H. 1972: A new theory of biliary atresia. *Journal of Pediatric Surgery* **7**, 651–4.

Kobayashi, A., Kawai, S., Utsunomiya, T. and Ohbe, Y. 1974: Bone disease in infants and children with hepatobiliary disease. *Archives of Disease in Childhood* **49**, 641–6.

Komi, N., Takehara, H., Kunimoto, K., Miyoshi, Y. and Yagi, T. 1992: Does the type of anomalous arrangement of pancreaticobiliary ducts influence the surgery and prognosis of choledochal cyst? *Journal of Pediatric Surgery* **27**, 728–31.

Komi, N., Tamura, T., Tsuge, S., Miyoshi, Y., Udaka, H. and Takehara, H. 1986: Relation of patient age to premalignant alterations in choledochal cyst epithelium: histo-chemical and immunohistochemical studies. *Journal of Pediatric Surgery* **21**, 430–3.

Kooh, S.W., Jones, G., Reilly, B.J. and Fraser, D. 1979: Pathogenesis of rickets in chronic hepatobiliary disease in children. *Journal of Pediatrics* **74**, 870–4.

Ladd, W.E. 1928: Congenital atresia and stenosis of the bile duct. *Journal of the American Medical Association* **91**, 1082–4.

Landing, B.H. 1974: Considerations of the pathogenesis of neonatal hepatitis, biliary atresia and choledochal cyst: the concept of infantile obstructive cholangiopathy. *Progress in Pediatric Surgery* **6**, 113–39.

Laurent, J., Gauthier, F., Bernard, O., Hadchouel, M., Odievre, M., Valayer, J. and Alagille, D. 1990: Long-term outcome after surgery for biliary atresia. *Gastroenterology* **99**, 1793–7.

Lawrence, D., Howard, E.R., Tzannatos, C. and Mowat, A.P. 1981: Hepatic portoenterostomy for biliary atresia. *Archives of Disease in Childhood* **56**, 460–3.

Levin, J.N. 1971: Amphetamine with biliary atresia. *Journal of Pediatrics* **79**, 130.

Levy, J., Pettei, M.J. and Weitz, J.I. 1987: Dysfibrinogenaemia in obstructive liver disease. *Journal of Pediatric Gastroenterology and Nutrition* **6**, 967–70.

Lilly, J.R. 1978: Total excision of choledochal cyst. *Surgery, Gynecology and Obstetrics* **146**, 254–6.

Lilly, J.R. 1979a: Hepatic portocholecystostomy for biliary atresia. *Journal of Pediatric Surgery* **14**, 301–4.

Lilly, J.R. 1979b: The surgical treatment of choledochal cysts. *Surgery, Gynecology and Obstetrics* **149**, 36–42.

Lilly, J.R. and Javitt, N.B. 1976: Biliary lipid excretion after hepatic portoenterostomy. *Annals of Surgery* **184**, 369–75.

Lilly, J.R., Hall, R.J., Vasquez-Estvez, J., Karrer, F. and Shikes, R.H. 1987: The surgery of 'correctable' biliary atresia. *Journal of Pediatric Surgery* **22**, 522–5.

Lilly, J.R., Karrer, F.M., Hall, R.J. *et al.* 1989: The surgery of biliary atresia. *Annals of Surgery* **210**, 289–96.

McClement, J.W., Howard, E.R. and Mowat, A.P. 1985: Results of surgical treatment for extrahepatic biliary atresia in United Kingdom 1980–82. *British Medical Journal* **290**, 345–7.

Miele-Vergani, G., Howard, E.R., Portmann, B. and Mowat, A.P. 1989: Later referral for biliary atresia – missed opportunities for effective surgery. *Lancet* **i**, 421–3.

Miyano, T., Suruga, K. and Suda, K. 1979: Abnormal choledochopancreatico–ductal junction related to the etiology of infantile obstructive jaundice diseases. *Journal of Pediatric Surgery* **14**, 16–26.

Moreki, R., Glaser, J.H., Cho, S., Balistreri, W.F. and Horwitz, M.S. 1982: Biliary atresia and reovirus type 3 infection. *New England Journal of Medicine* **307**, 481–4.

Mowat, A.P. 1987: Hepatitis and cholestasis in infancy: intrahepatic disorders. In *Liver disorders in childhood*. London: Butterworths, 37–71.

Ng, W.D., Liu, K., Wong, M.K. *et al.* 1992: Endoscopic sphincterotomy in young patients with choledochal dilatation and a long common channel: a preliminary report. *British Journal of Surgery* **79**, 550–2.

Nmazaki, Y., Oshima, T., Tanaka, A. *et al.* 1980: Neonatal liver disease and cytomegalovirus infection. In Kasai, M. and Shiraki, K. (eds), *Cholestasis in infancy.* Tokyo: University of Tokyo Press, 61–66.

O'Neil, J.A. and Clatworthy, H.W. 1971: Management of choledochal cyst: a 14 year follow-up. *American Surgeon* **37**, 230–7.

Ohi, R. 1991a: Biliary atresia: long-term results of hepatic portoenterostomy. In Howard, E.R. (ed.), *Surgery of liver disease in children.* London: Butterworth-Heinemann, 60–71.

Ohi, R. 1991b: Biliary atresia: modification to the original portoenterostomy operation. In Howard, E.R. (ed.), *Surgery of liver disease in childhood.* London: Butterworth-Heinemann, 72–7.

Ohi, R. and Ibrahim, M. 1992: Biliary atresia. *Seminars in Liver Disease* **1**, 115–24.

Ohi, R., Hanamatsu, M., Mochizuki, I., Ohkohchi, N. and Kasai, M. 1985: Reoperation in patients with biliary atresia. *Journal of Pediatric Surgery* **20**, 256–9.

Ohkawa, H., Sawaguchu, S., Yamazaki, Y., Ishikawa, A. and Kikuchi, M. 1982: Experimental analysis of the ill-effect of anomalous pancreaticobiliary ductal union. *Journal of Pediatric Surgery* **17**, 7–13.

Otte, J.B., Yandza, T., de Ville de Goyet, J., Tan, K.C., Salizzoni, M. and de Hemptinne, B. 1988: Pediatric liver transplantation: report on 52 patients with a 2 year survival of 86%. *Journal of Pediatric Surgery* **23**, 250–3.

Parashar, K., Tarlow, M.J. and McCrea, M.A. 1992: Experimental reovirus type 3-induced murine biliary tract disease. *Journal of Pediatric Surgery* **27**, 843–847.

Pickett, L.K. and Briggs, H.C. 1969: Biliary obstruction secondary to hepatic vascular ligation in the fetal sheep. *Journal of Pediatric Surgery* **4**, 95–101.

Powell, C.S., Sawyers, J.L. and Reynolds, V.H. 1981: Management of adult choledochal cysts. *Annals of Surgery* **193**, 666–76.

Psacharopoulos, H.T., Mowat, A.P. and Williams, R. 1980: Epidemiological study of hepatitis syndrome in infancy in south-east England: incidence and early course. In Kasai, M. and Shiraki, K. (eds), *Cholestasis in infancy.* Tokyo: University of Tokyo Press, 11–17.

Reveille, R.M., Van Stiegmann, G. and Everson, G.T. 1990: Increased secondary bile acids in a choledochal cyst. *Journal of Pediatric Surgery* **99**, 525–7.

Saeki, M., Nakano, M., Hagane, K. *et al.* 1991: Effectiveness of an intussusceptive anti-reflux valve to prevent ascending cholangitis after hepatic portoenterostomy in biliary atresia. *Journal of Pediatric Surgery* **26**, 800–3.

Schwartz, M.Z., Hall, R.J., Reubner, B., Lilly, J.R., Broge, T. and Toyama, W.M. 1990: Agenesis of the extrahepatic bile ducts: report of five cases. *Journal of Pediatric Surgery* **25**, 805–7.

Sherlock, S. 1987: The syndrome of disappearing intrahepatic bile ducts. *Lancet* **ii**, 493–6.

Shim, K.T., Kasai, M. and Spence, M.A. 1980: Race and biliary atresia. In Kasai, M. and Shiraki, K. (eds), *Cholestasis in infancy.* Tokyo: University of Tokyo Press, 67–74.

Shimada, K., Yanagisawa, J. and Nakayama, F. 1991: Increased lysophosphatidylcholine and pancreatic enzyme content in bile of patients with anomalous pancreaticobiliary junction. *Hepatology* **13**, 438–44.

Silveira, T.R., Salzano, F.M., Howard, E.R. and Mowat, A.P. 1991a: Congenital structural abnormalities in biliary atresia: evidence for aetiopathogenic heterogeneity and therapeutic implications. *Acta Paediatrica Scandinavica* **80**, 1192–9.

Silveira, T.R., Salzano, F.M., Howard, E.R. and Mowat, A.P. 1991b: Extrahepatic biliary atresia and twinning. *Brazilian Journal of Medical and Biological Research* **24**, 67–71.

Smith, B.M., Laberge. J.-M., Schreiber, R., Weber, A.M. and Blanchard, H. 1991: Familial biliary atresia in three siblings including twins. *Journal of Pediatric Surgery* **26**, 1331–3.

Spitz, L. 1980: Ligation of the common bile duct in the fetal lamb: an experimental model for the study of biliary atresia. *Pediatric Research* **14**, 740–8.

Spivak, W., Sarker, S., Winter, D., Glassman, M., Donion, E. and Tucker, K.J. 1987: Diagnostic utility of hepatobiliary scintigraphy with ^{99m}Tc-DISIDA in neonatal cholestasis. *Journal of Pediatrics* **110**, 855–61.

Starzl, T.E., Demetris, A.J. and Van Theil, D. 1989: Liver transplantation – Part I. *New England Journal of Medicine* **321**, 1014–22.

Stewart, S.M., Uauy, R., Waller, D.A. *et al.* 1987: Mental and motor correlates in patients with end-stage biliary atresia. *Pediatrics* **79**, 882–8.

Strauss, L. and Bernstein, J. 1968: Neonatal hepatitis in congenital rubella: a histopathological study. *Archives of Pathology* **86**, 317–27.

Strauss, L., Valderrama, E. and Alpert, L.I. 1972: Biliary tract anomalies: the relationship of biliary atresia to neonatal hepatitis. *Birth Defects* **8**, 135–48.

Strickland, A.D. and Shannon, K. 1982: Studies in the etiology of extrahepatic biliary atresia: time–space clustering. *Journal of Pediatrics* **100**, 749–53.

Strickland, A.D., Shannon, K. and Coln, C.D. 1985: Biliary atresia in two sets of twins. *Journal of Pediatrics* **107**, 418–19.

Stringer, G. and Filler, R.M. 1982: Fictitious pancreatitis in choledochal cyst. *Journal of Pediatric Surgery* **17**, 359–61.

Stringer, M., Howard, E.R. and Mowat, A.P. 1989: Endoscopic sclerotherapy in the management of esophageal varices in 61 children with biliary atresia. *Journal of Pediatric Surgery* **24**, 438–42.

Suruga, K., Miyano, T., Ogawa, T., Sasaki, K. and Deguchi, E. 1985: A study of patients with long-term bile flow after hepatic portoenterostomy for biliary atresia. *Journal of Pediatric Surgery* **20**, 252–5.

Tagart, R.E.B. 1956: Perforation of a congenital cyst of the common bile duct. *British Journal of Surgery* **44**, 18–21.

Tagge, D.U., Tagge, E.P., Drongowski, R.A., Oldham, K.T. and Coran, A.G. 1991: A long-term experience with biliary atresia. *Annals of Surgery* **214**, 590–8.

Takahiro, I., Horisawa, M. and Ando, H. 1983: Intrahepatic bile ducts in biliary atresia – a possible factor determining prognosis. *Journal of Pediatric Surgery* **18**, 124–30.

Tan, K.C. and Howard, E.R. 1988: Choledochal cyst: a 14 year surgical experience with 36 patients. *British Journal of Surgery* **75**, 892–5.

Tan, K.C., Yandza, T., de Hemptinne, B., Clapuyt, P., Claus, D. and Otte, J.B. 1988: Hepatic artery thrombosis in pediatric liver transplants. *Journal of Pediatric Surgery* **23**, 927–30.

Tanaka, K., Inomata, Y., Matsuoka, S. *et al.* 1987: A valved hepatic portoduodenal intestinal conduit for biliary atresia. In Ohi, R. (ed.), *Biliary atresia.* Tokyo: Professional Postgraduate Services, 169–72

Thomson, J. 1892: *Congenital obliteration of the bile ducts.* Edinburgh: Oliver & Boyd.

Todani, I., Watanabe, Y., Narusue, M., Tobuchi, K. and Okajima, K. 1977: Congenital bile duct cysts. Classification, operative procedure and review of 37 cases including cancer arising from a choledochal cyst. *American Journal of Surgery* **134**, 263–9.

Todani, T., Watanabe, Y., Fijii, T., Toki, A., Uemura, S. and Koike, Y. 1985: Cylindrical dilatation of the choledochus: a special type of congenital bile duct dilatation. *Surgery* **98**, 964–8.

Ullrich, D., Rating, D., Schroter, W., Hanefield, F. and Bircher, J. 1987: Treatment with ursodeoxycholic acid renders children with biliary atresia suitable for liver transplantation. *Lancet* **ii**, 1324.

Vacanti, J.P. and Folkman, J. 1979: Bile duct enlargement by infusion of L-proline: potential significance in biliary atresia. *Journal of Pediatric Surgery* **14**, 814–18.

Vacanti, J.P., Shamberger, R.C., Eraklis, A. and Lillehei, C.W. 1990: The therapy of biliary atresia combining the Kasai portoenterostomy with liver transplantation: a single centre experience. *Journal of Pediatric Surgery* **25**, 149–52.

Valayer, J. and Alagille, D. 1975: Experience with choledochal cyst. *Journal of Pediatric Surgery* **10**, 65–8.

Vazquez-Estevez, J., Stewart, B., Shikes, R.H., Hall, R.J. and Lilly, J.R. 1989: Biliary atresia: early determination of prognosis. *Journal of Pediatric Surgery* **24**, 48–51.

Venu, R.P., Geenan, J.E., Hogan, W.J. *et al.* 1984: Role of ERCP in the diagnosis and treatment of choledochocele. *Gastroenterology* **87**, 1144–9.

Watts, D.R., Lorenzo, G.A. and Beal, J.M. 1974: Congenital dilatation of the intrahepatic ducts. *Archives of Surgery* **108**, 592.

Wilkinson, M.L., Mieli-Vergani, G., Ball, C., Portmann, B. and Mowat, A.P. 1991: Endoscopic retrograde cholangiopancreatography in infantile cholestasis. *Archives of Disease in Childhood* **66**, 121–3.

Wong, K.C. and Lister, J. 1981: Human fetal development of the hepato-pancreatic duct junction – a possible explanation of congenital dilation of the biliary tract. *Journal of Pediatric Surgery* **16**, 139–45.

Wood, R.P., Mangnas, A.N., Stratta, R.J. *et al.* 1990: Optimal therapy for patients with biliary atresia: portoenterostomy ('Kasai' procedures) versus primary transplantation. *Journal of Pediatric Surgery* **25**, 153–62.

Yamaguchi, M. 1980: Congenital choledochal cyst. Analysis of 1,433 patients in the Japanese literature. *American Journal of Surgery* **140**, 653–60.

Yamashiro, Y., Sato, M. and Hoshino, A. 1982: Spontaneous perforation of a choledochal cyst. *European Journal of Pediatrics* **138**, 193–5.

Yamauchi, S., Koga, A., Matsumoto, S., Tanaka, M. and Nakayama, F. 1987: Anomalous junction of pancreaticobiliary duct without congenital choledochal cyst: a possible risk factor for gallbladder cancer. *American Journal of Surgery* **82**, 20–4.

Ylppö A. 1913: Zwei Falle von kongenitalem Gallengangsverschluss: Fett- und Bilirubin Stoffwechselversuche bei einem derselben. *Zeitschrift für Kinderheilk* **9**, 319.

CHAPTER 28

Hydrocephalus

E.P. GUAZZO AND J.D. PICKARD

Historical
Cerebrospinal fluid circulation and function
Definitions and terminology
Pathophysiology
Clinical features and investigation
Management

Indications for a shunt
Operative techniques
Shunt complications
Shunts and the paediatric general surgeon
Results
References

Historical

'Water on the brain' and enlarged heads in infancy and childhood were readily recognized by the ancients. Effective lifelong care of hydrocephalus continues to present many challenges. The presence of fluid within the cavities of the brain was first recorded in the Edwin Smith surgical papyrus written around the seventeenth century BC. Hippocrates (260–377 BC) also noted the presence of fluid within the cavities of the brain and is credited with the first tapping of the ventricles in hydrocephalus, though this was probably done after the patient's death. He also recognized that accumulation of this fluid within the cavities of the brain resulted in an abnormal head enlargement. Prior to this, the ventricles were considered to be filled with a vital spirit. In the second century AD Galen provided the first description of the ventricular cavities but it was not until 1764 that Contugno gave the first satisfactory account of cerebrospinal fluid (CSF). Magendie began the first systematic studies of CSF in 1825 and gave the fluid its name. Using gelatine and dyes, the Swedish anatomists Axel Key and Magnus Retzius (1875) undertook detailed studies of the subarachnoid space and in 1935 Lewis Weed demonstrated the circulation of the CSF as we know it today (Fishman, 1992) (Fig. 28.1).

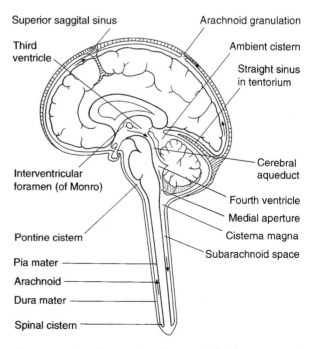

Fig. 28.1 Circulation of cerebrospinal fluid.

Cerebrospinal fluid circulation and function

CSF is predominantly produced by the choroid plexus of the ventricular system, with the brain parenchyma and the ventricular ependyma being significant extrachoroidal sites of production. CSF is normally crystal clear, colourless and predominantly composed of water (Table 28.1). Pathological processes affecting the central nervous system result in characteristic changes in the composition of CSF which are helpful in diagnosis. The choroidal production of CSF is relatively constant, at 20 ml/hour. It is an energy-dependent process that is not affected significantly by changes in intracranial pressure (ICP). It is reduced in the short term by carbonic anhydrase inhibitors. Extreme dehydration and hypotension will lower the production rate. CSF flows through the ventricular system to emerge from the fourth ventricle. It traverses the subarachnoid space and drains through the unidirectional open channels of the arachnoid villi as a result of the hydrostatic pressure difference between CSF pressure and venous sinus pressure. Hence, the rate of CSF absorption increases with increasing ICP. Some CSF may be absorbed by diffusion into the brain substance or drained by lymphatics accompanying brain capillaries. Absorption via the arachnoid villi associated with spinal nerve arachnoid sleeves also occurs. At any time there is approximately 150 ml of CSF: 50 ml within the ventricular system and 100 ml in the subarachnoid space. In total, 450 ml of CSF is produced per day, and therefore the total volume of CSF is exchanged approximately three times per day (Rekate and Oliver, 1990).

The primary function of CSF is to provide buoyancy and allow the brain to float, protecting it from repetitive trauma on each occasion the head moves. Moment-to-moment movement of CSF through the foremen magnum compensates for the changes in cerebral blood volume with each heartbeat. CSF contains little protein, with bicarbonate being its only buffer. It also serves as a transport medium allowing the circulation of various neurotransmitters and local hormones and as a modified lymphatic system for the brain and spinal cord. It has been referred to as the third circulation (Millhorat, 1975).

Table 28.1 Composition of cerebrospinal fluid

Parameter	Content
Osmolarity	295 mosm/l
Water content	99%
Sodium	138 mmol/l
Potassium	2.8 mmol/l
Glucose	60 mg/dl
Total protein	35.0 mg/dl

Definitions and terminology

Donald Matson (1969) described hydrocephalus not as a single entity, but as the end result of a diverse group of conditions that result in accumulation of CSF within the head which is usually under increased pressure and associated with ventricular enlargement. The term 'active hydrocephalus' is used when the intraventricular pressure is elevated. Active hydrocephalus may be either progressive or compensated. It is progressive when the elevation in intraventricular pressure is sufficient to cause progressive ventricular enlargement and a progressively worsening clinical syndrome of uncontrolled hydrocephalus. The term 'compensated active hydrocephalus' is used when the ventricles are enlarged but no longer progressively dilating despite moderate elevation of ICP and the absence of clinical signs. If the process 'arrests', the ventricular pressure returns to normal and is no longer a stimulus for ventricular enlargement. The ventricles may or may not decrease in size and there is an absence of signs of raised intracranial pressure. The processes leading to hydrocephalus rarely arrest and the majority of individuals who are thought to be 'arrested' do not have normal ICP and exhibit pathological pressure waves when monitored.

Dandy and Blackfan (1914) used dye studies to differentiate between 'communicating' and 'non-communicating' hydrocephalus, that is, to differentiate whether there was communication between the ventricular system and the subarachnoid pathways. This functional classification is useful in helping to determine treatment and the site of shunt placement.

Pathophysiology

Hydrocephalus can occur at any stage of life and the presentation varies according to age. It is a dynamic disorder of CSF circulation and rarely an all-or-none phenomenon. There is either a congenital or acquired imbalance between the production and absorption of CSF, resulting in accumulation of CSF and secondary ventricular enlargement. Obstruction to CSF flow is the hallmark of hydrocephalus (McCullough, 1989). Very rarely, if ever, hydrocephalus is the result of overproduction of CSF due to a rare tumour of the choroid plexus. These tumours occur within the ventricular system and are usually associated with a degree of obstruction to flow which contributes to the hydrocephalus. The CSF produced has a high protein content and this may impair absorption. Furthermore with the successful removal of choroid plexus papilloma, more than 50% of these children will require shunting to achieve good control of their hydrocephalus.

Obstruction to flow may occur at any point in the CSF pathway. Conditions that predispose to hydrocephalus can be classified into three basic disease processes (Table 28.2). Congenital hydrocephalus typically presents during the neonatal period or in early infancy (Fig. 28.2). Common congenital anomalies of the CSF pathways include stenosis, occlusion or forking of the aqueduct of Sylvius, fourth ventricular outlet obstruction or more complex anomalies such as the Dandy–Walker syndrome. Some 80% of children with spina bifida cystica require treatment for progressive hydrocephalus which usually results from a combination of the Arnold–Chiari malformation and basal cistern arachnoid fibrosis.

Tumours that obstruct CSF flow typically occur in or adjacent to the ventricular system or in the posterior fossa, where space is limited and the propensity for obstruction is greater. Primary neoplasms of the central nervous system are the most common solid malignancy of childhood. More than 50% of these tumours occur in the posterior fossa and typically these children present with symptoms of raised intracranial pressure from hydrocephalus. Metastatic tumours to the brain are rare in the paediatric population. Third ventricular colloid

Table 28.2 Classification of hydrocephalus in children

Obstruction to CSF flow or absorption

Congenital causes:	Aqueduct stenosis, forking or atresia
	Dandy–Walker syndrome
	Spina bifida
	Hindbrain abnormalities
Space-occupying lesions	Congenital cysts
	Posterior tumours of childhood (medulloblastoma, astrocytoma)
Inflammatory	Postinfective (TB, fungal meningitis)
	Ventricular haemorrhage of prematurity
	Post-traumatic hydrocephalus

Overproduction of CSF (rare if ever)
Choroid plexus papilloma

cysts or arachnoid cysts within the ventricular system can also obstruct CSF flow (Fig. 28.3).

Inflammatory conditions, be they of infective origin such as following meningitis, or the result of irritation from substances such as blood, lead to impairment of CSF absorption at the arachnoid villi or a fibrosis of the subarachnoid pathways. Management of bacterial meningitis has improved substantially in recent decades and the incidence of postbacterial meningitic hydrocephalus has declined. Hydrocephalus may still occur following infection with more resistant organisms such as tuberculosis or fungi. The incidence of intraventricular haemorrhage of prematurity is declining but it still remains a common cause of hydrocephalus in this group. Traumatic intracranial haemorrhage may also lead to hydrocephalus and should not be forgotten as a reason for late deterioration in children with head injuries.

The pathogenesis of the ventricular dilatation remains poorly understood. Ventricular enlargement is not a uniform process. It occurs mainly at the expense of the periventricular white matter. The grey matter is relatively spared until the process is well advanced. There is a disproportionate reduction in blood flow in the periventricular white matter in the presence of hydrocephalus, which is reversed once successful treatment of hydrocephalus has been instituted (Pickard, 1984). Animal models have shown that the first event in the presence of hydrocephalus is the transependymal movement of ventricular fluid into the periventricular white matter. This increase in hydrostatic pressure in the periventricular white matter may cause the preferential reduction in blood flow and hence reduction in myelin lipid and subsequent white matter thinning. As further ventricular enlargement occurs, the periventricular white matter becomes gliotic, with an increase in astroglial scar tissue reflecting the brain tissue damage around the ventricles. As the process advances the changes become

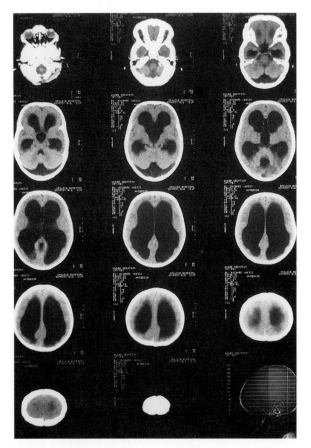

Fig. 28.2 CT scan of an infant with congenital hydrocephalus due to obstruction of CSF flow at the level of the basal cisterns. All of the ventricles are markedly enlarged, as is the cisterna magna, indicating that the level of obstruction is distal to this point in the CSF circulation.

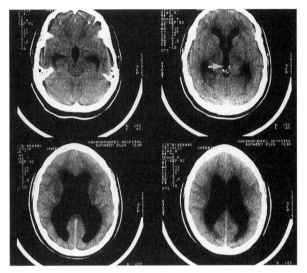

Fig. 28.3 CT scan of a child with acquired hydrocephalus secondary to a pineal region cyst (arrowed) obstructing the outlet of the third ventricle. The third and lateral ventricles are very dilated.

irreversible. Early treatment will result in complete reversal of the periventricular oedema but delays or multiple shunt revisions, particularly if complicated by infection, will result in chronic gliosis and long-term damage to the periventricular white matter.

Clinical features and investigation

In the neonate, rapid head enlargement crossing percentile lines is the usual clinical finding. The presence of hydrocephalus *in utero* is rare. Most neonates develop hydrocephalus after birth. Most infants with congenital hydrocephalus are asymptomatic and it is only late in the process that they develop signs of irritability, decreased appetite, vomiting and poor head control. For this reason regular and accurate head circumference measurements are important in all infants and will detect hydrocephalus before the onset of clinical symptoms (Fig. 28.4).

The usual clinical findings are of a full fontanelle, dilated veins and separated sutures. MacEwan's sign (a tympanitic sound obtained on percussing the vault of a hydrocephalic skull) or the brilliant transillumination that occurs in hydrocephalus should be rare findings as they indicate advanced hydrocephalus. The setting sun sign (paralysis of upward gaze and the prominence of the upper part of the sclera) again is a late sign although initially it may occur intermittently.

Papilloedema is rare in infants. In older children once the sutures begin to fuse, the clinical symptoms and signs of raised ICP are more common. Morning headache associated with vomiting and subsequent drowsiness are typical. Sixth nerve palsies due to their

stretching as the brainstem descends may occur. A history of trauma, infection or interventricular haemorrhage should be sought. Cerebellar signs are common when the hydrocephalus is due to a posterior fossa tumour.

Transfontanelle ultrasound, computed tomography (CT) and magnetic resonance imaging (MRI) have displaced plain X-rays, used to display diastasis of the sutures, and ventriculography as the methods of choice to investigate children suspected of having hydrocephalus. Ultrasound has the benefit of being a non-invasive bedside test which can be repeated regularly while the fontanelle remains open. It has suffered from its lack of sensitivity but skilled ultrasonographists with modern equipment can provide very detailed information on the intracranial compartment. CT has revolutionized neurosurgery and, in particular, the management of hydrocephalus, with its ability to reveal the aetiology of hydrocephalus and possibly the reason for shunt mal-

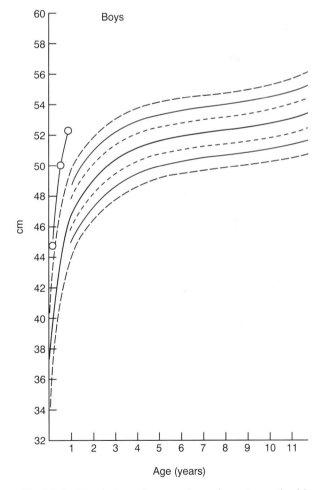

Fig. 28.4 Head circumference chart of an 11-month-old male infant with progressive macrocephaly due to congenital hydrocephalus. The reason for his late referral was that he was asymptomatic and the head circumference had not been serially plotted and its large size not noticed.

function. The size of the ventricles can be measured and compared to previous scans. Elevation of intracranial pressure secondary to active hydrocephalus is suggested by periventricular lucency. MRI is very helpful in more complex cases with multiple congenital lesions and in definition of the anatomy at the foramen magnum.

Intracranial pressure measurements and CSF infusion studies may be helpful in difficult diagnostic cases. Neuropsychological assessment and developmental progress may also be used as adjuncts to decisions over whether or not a shunt is required (Guazzo, 1993).

Management

Various non-operative therapies have been tried to control hydrocephalus, including wrapping of the head. Medications to reduce CSF production such as carbonic anhydrase inhibitors, steroids or diuretics play a small role, primarily in the premature infant population and may serve in helping to control the hydrocephalus until the child is well enough to undergo surgery (Scott, 1990).

Surgical therapies have been the prime management of hydrocephalus for hundreds of years and many surgical techniques have been used in attempts to control progressive hydrocephalus (Pudenz, 1981). Most have been efforts to divert CSF from the obstructed intracranial compartment to another part of the body, including the distal ureter, fallopian tube, pleural cavity, gallbladder, stomach, sagittal sinus, internal jugular vein and cisterna magna. In most cases, they were inefficient, dangerous, overdrained and rapidly blocked, and frequently became infected. With the development of valve-regulated shunt mechanisms and improved materials the incidence of complications has fallen. Most children are now treated with a ventriculoperitoneal (VP) shunt which is made of three components. A ventricular catheter is sited in the ventricle, inserted via either a frontal or parieto-occipital approach, usually on the right side of the head (Fig. 28.5). This, in turn, is connected to a valve plus reservoir mechanism, of which there are many types. The peritoneal catheter is tunnelled and then inserted into the peritoneum in the right upper quadrant with spare tubing to allow the child to grow. This is a significant advantage of the peritoneal cavity over the atrium for the siting of the distal end of the shunt (Ruge and McClone, 1993). Repeat or chronic peritoneal sepsis or multiple previous abdominal procedures with subsequent adhesions may indicate that a ventriculoatrial (VA) shunt is the better option.

Lumboperitoneal shunts, draining fluid from the lumbar subarachnoid space to the peritoneal cavity, are rarely used and only in communicating hydrocephalus where they may be followed by secondary descent of the cerebellar tonsils. They are dangerous in other circumstances. Devices that allow regular tapping of

the ventricles are frequently used in the premature neonatal population to control hydrocephalus until the child is large enough to undergo a VP shunt.

Lespinasse, using a rigid cystoscope, was the first to fulgurate the choroid plexus in two infants with hydrocephalus. One child died immediately and the other died 5 years later. Coagulating or removing the choroid plexus is difficult to do because of its location in all ventricles. Furthermore, extrachoroidal production of CSF rapidly increases in many children and hence this procedure is of limited value. However, endoscopic third ventriculostomy to treat hydrocephalus secondary to aqueductal stenosis has met with success in skilled hands. Endoscopic management of intraventricular cysts or large arachnoid cysts to establish their communication with normal CSF pathways may overcome the need for any shunting procedure (Mainwaring *et al.*, 1989).

Indications for a shunt

Insertion of a shunt implies a lifelong commitment for the patient, the family and the neurosurgeon, and is not a decision to be taken lightly. In the main, the decision is clear where there is active, progressive hydrocephalus supported by radiological evidence of ventriculomegaly. However, the presence of ventriculomegaly on

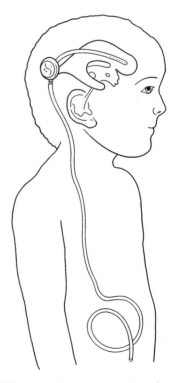

Fig. 28.5 Diagrammatic representation of a typical right-sided ventriculoperitoneal shunt in a child. A ventricular catheter was inserted via the right parieto-occipital route.

radiological investigation, in the absence of any supporting features, does not necessarily mean there is active hydrocephalus and in these children a shunt may be incorrect. Other more elaborate investigations including CSF pressure studies may be appropriate before a decision is made. The goals of treatment are to control the ICP and head growth, to protect the cerebral mantle from progression compression and to use a treatment that has a low risk of complications.

Wherever possible a shunt should be avoided. With improved neurosurgical operative techniques, obstructing lesions such as tumours are more readily and safely removed and the need for a shunt avoided. Benign cystic structures such as intraventricular colloid cysts or congenital archnoid cysts may be successfully managed microsurgically or via endoscopy and a shunt is avoided.

Operative techniques

The authors' technique for shunt insertion is described and references are given for alternative methods (Epstein, 1989; Rekate, 1989; Millhorat, 1989). As with all surgical procedures, a scrupulous technique is the best way to achieve a satisfactory result and prevent complications. With meticulous surgical technique and attention to preoperative, intraoperative and postoperative detail, it is possible to reduce the incidence of complications.

The child is given a general anaesthetic with an endotracheal tube and is positioned on the operating table with the head turned to the left and a sandbag under the right shoulder to straighten the angle between the neck and clavicle. The necessary amount of hair is shaved immediately prior to surgery, the intended incisions are marked, the skin is prepared with antiseptic Betadine and allowed to dry, and the child draped with an adhesive plastic drape and towels. An appropriate dose of flucloxicillin is given during this period. Particularly for neonates and infants, heat loss must be minimized by avoiding prolonged exposure, using heat lamps and warming the theatre. The intended incisions are infiltrated with local anaesthetic and adrenaline mixture, with care taken to ensure the appropriate dose for body weight. The peritoneal cavity is identified and opened via a right upper quadrant 2 cm transverse skin crease incision and muscle splitting approach. The authors' preference is for a burr hole valve, which is positioned immediately above the lambdoidal suture, 3–4 cm from the midline in a burr hole of sufficient size to allow the valve to sit well down avoiding pressure on the overlying skin. The incision is 4–5 cm in length, curved and positioned to ensure that when the valve is in place it does not underlie the skin incision.

The shunt components are kept in their sterile packets until immediately before use and not handled unnecessarily. A long shunt passer is tunnelled in the subcutaneous plain from the scalp incision to the abdominal incision, avoiding interposing incisions. The proximal end of the peritoneal catheter is then withdrawn to the scalp wound and the valve connected. The previously measured ventricular catheter with stylet in place is introduced into the brain via a small dural opening to prevent CSF leakage, and aimed towards the midline of the forehead halfway between the nasion and the hairline. The intention is to place the tip of the catheter 2 cm distal to the foramen of Munro. A minimum of CSF is allowed to escape to prevent rapid ventricular decompression during the procedure. The valve is connected to the ventricular catheter and then anchored with sutures to the pericranium. The shunt should be spontaneously functioning prior to the insertion of the full length of peritoneal catheter into the peritoneal cavity. The wounds are closed in layers with careful attention to skin apposition.

Many commercial varieties of shunt are available and, as yet, one particular shunt has not been proven to be significantly better than others (Post, 1985). Therefore the chosen device should be familiar and simple to use.

Shunt complications

Underdrainage (malfunction), infection and overdrainage account for the majority of shunt complications. The incidence of epilepsy attributable to shunt insertion is small, although epilepsy complicating the condition that resulted in hydrocephalus may occur. Trauma to the brain at shunt insertion should be rare, provided the appropriate technique is used. There are particular risks associated with shunt revision which will be discussed later.

UNDERDRAINAGE: MALFUNCTION

Shunt malfunction implies underdrainage and the actuarial probability of shunt failure is 80% in 12 years, with the highest risk being in the first year after shunt insertion (30%) (Saint-Rose et al., 1989). The most common cause of shunt malfunction is related to choroid plexus occlusion of the ventricular catheter. Many methods attempting to avoid this have been tried, including altering the ventricular catheter type and varying its position. The choroid plexus progressively occludes the holes in the distal end of the ventricular catheter causing it to obstruct (Fig. 28.6a–c). If the ventricular catheter tip is inserted away from the choroid plexus, the child's head grows and changes shape so that the catheter position alters, allowing it to come into contact with the choroid plexus. The optimal position may well be in the frontal horn region away from the choroid plexus. Connective tissue, brain tissue, meninges, ependyma or foreign bodies may also cause obstruction. Valve failure, tube fracture or disconnec-

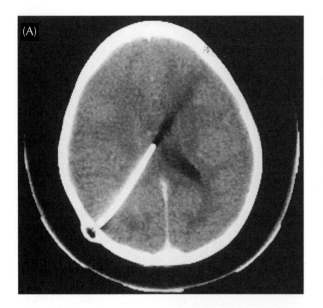
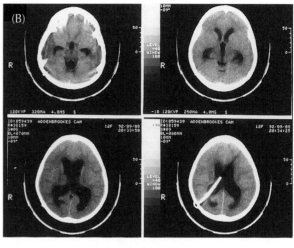

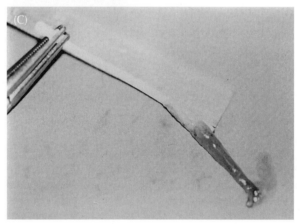

Fig. 28.6 CT scan of a 12-year-old female, who has a right VP shunt, taken (A) when she was well, and (B) CT scan of the same child when she was symptomatic of shunt malfunction: the ventricles are now enlarged, confirming the diagnosis of shunt malfunction. (C) The ventricular catheter removed at the time of shunt revision – choroid plexus is seen occluding the catheter tip.

tion, migration and other material failures are less common. The use of connectors encourages disconnections and fracture as these form points of fixation preventing the silicone tube from moving freely.

Most ventricular catheters are inserted blind and malposition of the ventricular catheter may occur, leading to early shunt failure (Fig. 28.7). Intraoperative ultrasound or endoscopic placement may be used to reduce such malpositioning. Lower end malposition or intestinal trauma or perforation should occur rarely.

In the majority of children the symptoms of malfunction are clear (Table 28.3) but in others the symptoms may be intermittent and insidious. A high index of suspicion must be maintained and a detailed history should be taken. The child's parents may recognize the symptoms of malfunction from a previous episode and they should

be listened to carefully. Clinical evidence of malfunction, such as abnormal head enlargement, full fontanelle, separation of sutures or signs of raised ICP are sought but their absence does not exclude shunt malfunction.

Table 28.3 Symptoms of shunt malfunctions

Infants	Toddlers	Children
Head enlargement	Head enlargement	Headache
Full tense fontanelle	Headache	Vomiting
Split sutures	Vomiting	Drowsiness
Setting sun sign	Irritability	Decline in academic performance

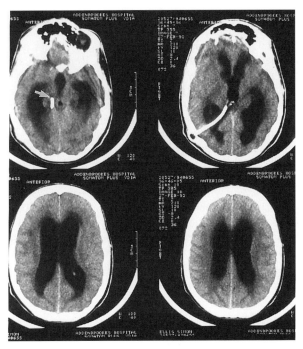

Fig. 28.7 CT scan illustrating continuing hydrocephalus following shunt insertion due to malpositioning of the ventricular catheter (arrowed). The tip of the catheter is outside the lateral ventricle. Periventricular lucency remains indicative of active hydrocephalus.

Assessment of the valve reservoir chamber can be notoriously difficult, particularly if it has been in place for a long period. Thick scar tissue or calcification may make it difficult to palpate. The valve reservoir chamber should pump easily. If it is empty or does not fill quickly after emptying a proximal ventricular catheter block is suggested. If the valve reservoir does not empty a distal occlusion is probable. Examination and palpation of the complete shunt system is mandatory. Collection of CSF at points of fracture or disconnection may be evident. Plain X-rays can demonstrate disconnections (Fig. 28.8). The principal investigation is a CT scan, which can be of great value when compared with a CT scan taken when the child was well is very useful (Fig. 28.6A and B).

Shunt revision is not without morbidity or mortality. The surgeon should prepare the patient in theatre so as to allow access to the complete shunt. Prior to revision, clinical examination and subsequent investigation should have determined the site of malfunction and often only this part of the shunt needs revision. Ventricular catheters firmly adherent to the choroid plexus present a very difficult problem as major haemorrhage can occur if the choroid vessels are torn. The safest option may be to leave the ventricular catheter in place.

INFECTION

Infection remains a serious complication of shunt implantation with a patient morbidity/mortality rate of 30–40% and those who survive risking intellectual, cognitive and neurological deficit. Altogether, 90% of shunt infections occur within 6 months of insertion and 70% within 1 month. Hence, in the majority of patients, shunt infection is a complication of shunt surgery and attention to surgical details such as technique, appropriate skin preparation and asepsis are considered the most important in reducing their incidence (Choux *et al.*,

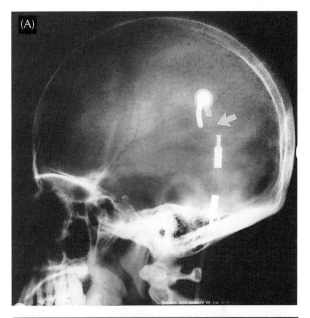

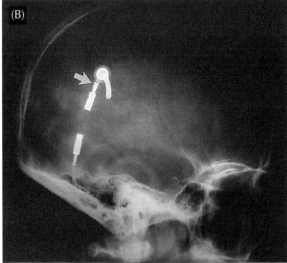

Fig. 28.8 Plain lateral skull X-ray (A) when the shunt was connected and the child asymptomatic, and (B) demonstrating disconnection (arrowed). The child was now suffering symptoms suggestive of shunt malfunction.

1992). The use of prophylactic antibiotics is less clear. *Staphylococcus epidermidis* and *Staphylococcus aureus* are the predominant infecting organisms. Flucloxacillin is an appropriate prophylactic antibiotic because of its narrow-spectrum bacteriocidal properties and high affinity for plasma proteins which facilitate antibacterial activity throughout the operation. Only a single pre-operative dose is given.

Often, when shunts become infected, the process is insidious and not obvious. There may be evidence of shunt malfunction with no clinical evidence of infection. In other cases, there may be evidence of a meningitic process, cellulitis along the shunt tract or wound infection. The presence of abdominal symptoms indicate a lower end infection. The white cell count may not be raised, though the C-reactive protein is often elevated. Using an aseptic technique under neurosurgical guidance, the shunt reservoir may be tapped to confirm the presence of colonization or infection.

Infection of ventriculoatrial shunts may precipitate the serious cardiac features of endocarditis, recurrent infected emboli or signs of right heart failure. Immune complex nephritis is a rare but recognized complication of VA shunt infection.

Removal of the shunt, a period of temporary external ventricular drainage and the administering of appropriate antibiotics that penetrate the CSF are required to eradicate shunt infection. Regular examinations of the CSF are taken to ensure that the infection has been completely eradicated and the white cell count has fallen to normal in the CSF prior to reinsertion of the shunt.

OVERDRAINAGE

The gravity effect due to the hydrostatic column of CSF between the inlet and outlet of a shunt causes most shunts to overdrain as they are differential pressure valves only. This 'siphon' effect may produce slit ventricle syndrome, subdural haematomas, encysted fourth ventricles or postshunt craniosynostosis. Flow-regulated valves have been developed in an attempt to reduce the incidence of these complications (Saint-Rose *et al.*, 1987).

Shunts and the paediatric general surgeon

Abdominal symptoms and complaints are common in childhood. The presence of a ventriculoperitoneal shunt lengthens the differential diagnosis. Abdominal symptoms of peritonitis related to the peritoneal catheter tip or more commonly formation of a pseudocyst as the omentum walls off the infection are indicative of peritoneal catheter infection. An abdominal ultrasound will demonstrate the pseudocyst.

Appendicitis is common in childhood and should not be managed differently when a VP shunt is present. Only when there is frank abdominal sepsis will the peritoneal catheter require externalization. Reinsertion into the peritoneal cavity is usual once the abdominal sepsis has resolved. Rarely, a peritoneal catheter may perforate the intestine. A temporary period of externalization is required until the catheter can be reinserted into the peritoneal cavity.

Endoscopic surgery is increasingly being used to treat abdominal conditions that previously required laparotomy. This requires the insufflation of the peritoneal cavity with carbon dioxide to pressures of 30 cm H_2O, often combined with the Trendelberg position. The ability of various VP shunts to prevent the retrograde flow of carbon dioxide into the cranial cavity has not been tested. Temporary occlusion of the peritoneal catheter while the procedure is undertaken may be the safest option.

Results

Significant advances have been made in understanding the pathophysiology of hydrocephalus and the exact indications for intervention. The majority of children will require a ventriculoperitoneal shunt, though wherever possible this is avoided by removing the obstructive lesion or increasingly by using endoscopic techniques. The insertion of a shunt implies a lifelong commitment to ensuring that it functions appropriately. In most cases, complications of shunts present acutely, but regular periodic review is important to look for evidence of the child failing to progress, a subtle, slow decline in intellectual performance or other insidious signs which may be the only markers of shunt dysfunction.

References

Choux, M., Genitori, L., Lang, D. and Gabriel, L. 1992: Shunt implantation: reducing the incidence of shunt infection. *Journal of Neurosurgery* **77**, 875–80.

Dandy, W.E. and Blackfan, K.D. 1914: Internal hydrocephalus. An experimental, clinical and pathological study. *American Journal of Disease in Children* **8**, 406–82.

Epstein, M.H. 1983: Surgical management of hydrocephalus. In Schmidek, H.H. and Sweet, W.H. (eds.), *Operative neurosurgical technique*, 2nd ed., vol. 1. Philadelphia, PA: W.B. Saunders.

Fishman, R.A. (ed.) 1992: *Cerebrospinal fluid in diseases of the nervous system*, 2nd ed. Philadelphia, PA: W.B. Saunders.

Guazzo, E.P. 1993: Recent advances in paediatric neurosurgery. *Archives of Disease in Childhood* **69**, 335–8.

Mainwaring, K.H., Rekate, H. and Kaplan, A. 1989: Hydrocephalus management by endoscopy. *Annals of Neurology* **26**, 488.

Matson, D.D. 1969: *Neurosurgery of infancy and childhood*. Springfield, IL: Charles C. Thomas, 199.

McCullough, D.C. 1989: Hydrocephalus: aetiology, pathological effects, diagnosis and natural history. In *Paediatric neurosurgery*, 2nd ed. Philadelphia, PA: W.B. Saunders, 180–99.

Millhorat, T.H. 1975: The third circulation revisited. *Journal of Neurosurgery* **45**, 628.

Millhorat, T.H. 1989: Treatment of hydrocephalus. In Symon, L. (ed.) *Rob and Smith's operative surgery – neurosurgery*, 4th edn. London: Butterworths, 1989: 123–34.

Pickard, J.D. 1984: Adult communicating hydrocephalus. In Harrison M.J.G. (ed.), *Contemporary neurology*. London: Butterworths, 543–54.

Post, E.M. 1985: Currently available shunt systems – a review. *Neurosurgery* **16**, 257–60.

Pudenz, R.H. 1981: The surgical treatment of hydrocephalus – an historical review. *Surgery and Neurology* **15**, 15–26.

Rekate, H. and Oliver, W. 1990: Current concepts of CSF production and absorption in hydrocephalus. In Scott, M.R. (ed.), *Concepts of neurosurgery,* vol. 3. Baltimore, MD: Williams & Wilkins, 11–12.

Rekate, H.L. 1989: Treatment of hydrocephalus. In *Paediatric neurosurgery*, 2nd ed. Philadelphia, PA: W.B. Saunders, 200–18.

Ruge, J.R. and McLone, D.G. 1993: Cerebrospinal fluid diversion procedures. In Apuzzo, M.J. (ed.), *Brain surgery*, vol. 2. New York: Churchill Livingstone.

Saint-Rose, C., Hoffman, H.J. and Hirsch, J.F. 1989: Shunt failure. In Marlin, A.E. (ed.) *Concepts in paediatric neurosurgery*, vol. 9. Basel: Karger, 7–20.

Saint-Rose, C., Hooven, M.D. and Hirsch, J.F. 1987: A new approach to the treatment of hydrocephalus. *Journal of Neurosurgery* **66**, 213–26.

Scott, M.R. (ed.) 1990: Hydrocephalus. In *Concepts in neurosurgery*, vol 3. Baltimore, MD: William & Wilkins.

CHAPTER 29

Spinal dysraphism

J. GARFIELD

Classification of spinal dysraphism
Clinical features
Developmental anatomy and mechanism
of production of neurological deficit

Associated anomalies
Management
Results
Further reading

Classification of spinal dysraphism

As in other spinal disorders, lesions may be classified as extradural, intradural or intramedullary. In spinal dysraphism there may be a combination of two or all three of these features.

Clinical features

The traditional classification of the manifestations of dysraphism is cutaneous, orthopaedic, urological or neurological. This order reflects the frequency of occurrence, but any combination of the different types of manifestation is to some extent capricious, although it may be related to the severity of disorganization of the spinal skeletal and neurological anatomy. The degree, but not the type, of cutaneous manifestation, is often related to the severity of anatomical disorganization, but sometimes a relatively severe urological disorder may be accompanied by trivial or even negligible cutaneous abnormality.

There are many problems in determining the extent to which an orthopaedic or urological disorder can be ascribed to the spinal disorganization of dysraphism. Thus a primarily orthopaedic lower limb structural abnormality may be ascribed erroneously to a neuroanatomical disorganization; for example, talipes demonstrated by ultrasound *in utero*, and present at birth, is a relatively common disorder, but it is rare for this to be accompanied by any of the accepted manifestations of dysraphism, and for investigations, including magnetic resonance imaging (MRI) to reveal any spinal abnormality. To what extent defects of lower limb bone growth requiring leg equalizing procedures can be ascribed to lumbar dysraphism remains unproven, unless there are overt neurological manifestations accompanied by observed muscle wasting (atrophy) and disuse. The possible relationship with congenital dislocation of the hip is even less clear.

Urological disorders, both structural and functional, are relatively common in children. Therefore it may be very difficult to differentiate those which can be ascribed either fully (i.e. a true neurogenic bladder disturbance) or in part to dysraphism from those which are due entirely to structural or non-neurological functional disorders of the urinary tract. A combination of structural abnormalities and a neurogenic element presents particular difficulties of diagnosis and management.

These examples should make the paediatric specialist cautious before concluding that the evidence is sufficient to embark on spinal surgery, with the object of halting or improving established orthopaedic or urological disorders. The indications for prophylactic spinal surgery in the absence of orthopaedic, urological or neurological abnormalities may be contentious but raise somewhat different questions (see below).

Developmental anatomy and mechanism of production of neurological deficit

The basic development of the neuraxis, the process and order of its normal closure and the defects in the process which lead to the grosser abnormalities is described in Chapter 30. There is a wide variety of skeletal and neuroanatomical anomalies in lumbar dysraphism. The anomalies of dysraphism, which are relatively minor compared to those of spina bifida, are more suggestive of infolding or inclusion of tissues that can be regarded as vestigial remnants of germ layers which, in normal development, would have disappeared. Examples are fat within the theca merging into the lower end of the spinal cord, and striated muscle in association with the filum terminale. The intrathecal dermoid cyst, which may be partly intramedullary, with its connection to the skin by a patent or occluded tract lined by squamous epithelium, is more readily explained by a premature infolding of the non-neural element of primitive ectoderm. It is debatable whether the so-called 'low conus' (see below) represents the failure of 'ascent' of the lower end of the spinal cord from its fetal to its normal skeletal level due to tethering of the cord to the dura and extradural tissues. Thus a low conus may or may not be associated with 'tethering' as seen at operation, or with other anomalies such as an intrathecal lipoma.

The precise mechanism of a neurological deficit, or of a neurogenic bladder dysfunction, or a neurologically induced orthopaedic lower limb deformity, may be difficult to define, whatever intraspinal anomaly is present. Possible mechanisms include congenital absence of neural elements (e.g. anterior horn cells or dorsal root ganglia), traction on relatively normal neural elements and compression by masses such as lipomas or dermoid cysts, are all possible mechanisms. It may be difficult in an individual child to decide which is the major or sole factor and for that reason the indications for surgery are often empirical, and are based upon the radiological demonstration of what are relatively gross anatomical abnormalities.

Associated anomalies

INTRASPINAL ANOMALIES: CLASSIFICATION

(1) Skeletal:
   laminar arch and spinous process defects
   vertebral body anomalies; absent: fused; hemivertebrae
   bony spurs of diastematomyelia
(2) Extradural:
   fibrous bands
   squamous epithelial tubes
   lipomata
   blind dural prolongation
(3) Intradural extramedullary
   tethering of conus to dura with or without specific tethering fibrous bands (Fig. 29.1)
   thickened and/or tight filum terminale (Fig. 29.2)
   lipomata
   dermoid tube and cysts within the cauda equina
   tethering of roots to dura at intervertebral foramena (Fig. 29.3)
(4) Intradural intramedullary:
   bifid spinal cord symmetrical or asymmetrical
   low conus medullaris
   lipomata (Figs 29.4–29.6)
   dermoid
   diastematomyelia
   mixed tissue masses.

With the exceptions of diastematomyelia and dermoid cysts, many of these malformations occur in combination, which may make it difficult to assess the part played by each anomaly in producing the clinical manifestations of the disorder, and to plan surgical strategy.

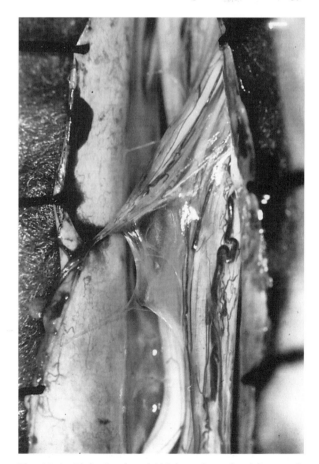

Fig. 29.1 Tethering band (thickened arachnoid) extending from the gathered roots of the cauda equina to the dura.

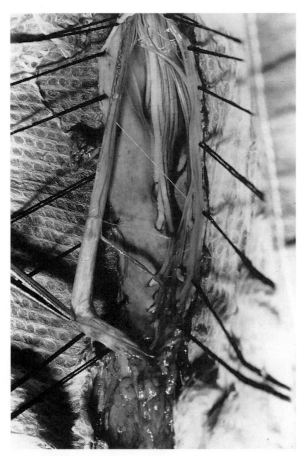

Fig. 29.2 Thickened filum terminale (pulled aside) extending into the extradural lipoma in the sacral canal.

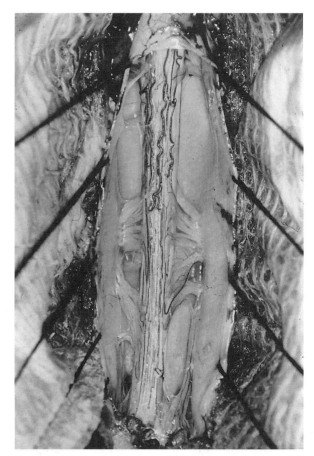

Fig. 29.3 Spinal cord extending down to the lower limit of theca, with nerve roots ascending or running horizontally to reach the exit foramina.

Apart from the bony spurs associated with diastematomyelia, purely skeletal abnormalities are the least significant. Conversely, the more florid the intradural and especially the intramedullary disorganization, the greater the neurological deficit.

LAMINAR ARCH AND SPINOUS PROCESS DEFECTS

The term radiological spina bifida occulta is often used to imply that the child is perfectly normal, there are no cutaneous abnormalities and the radiological abnormality is a chance or irrelevant finding. The simplicity of this definition may be misleading, however, if the reason for taking an X-ray of the spine has any basis in lower limb or urological symptoms, and any confirmation of the normality of the intraspinal anatomy by special investigations (e.g. myelography or MRI) must raise the question of the indications for that investigation. In view of these reservations, figures for the true incidence of radiological spina bifida occulta are difficult to obtain, and it may well be that with the tendency towards greater use of non-invasive investigations (MRI) the true

incidence will fall, as more intraspinal abnormalities are shown. Although bifid spinous processes or laminar arch defects are easily visible radiologically in adults, this is not so with children, especially for the lowest lumbar and sacral segments. Wide laminar arch defects from L2 downwards are commonly associated with intraspinal abnormalities, especially lipomata and intradural masses of mixed tissue. There is no evidence that laminar arch defects are associated with later spinal instability, but they do add to the difficulties of surgical access in the absence of definable tissue planes.

VERTEBRAL BODY ANOMALIES

In the child without any surface stigmata these are not usually associated with intraspinal neural abnormalities, with the lower limb orthopaedic manifestations of dysraphism, or with urological or neurological disorders. However, if they result in scoliosis and the development of a pelvic tilt they may produce disorders of gait and stance without any neurological basis. Vertebral body anomalies such as hemivertebrae or

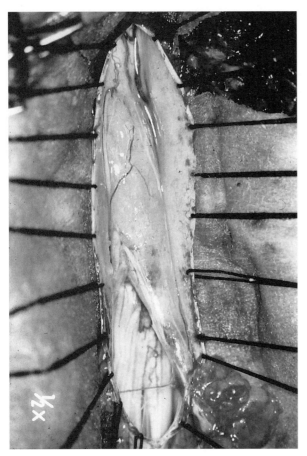

Fig. 29.4 Intradural lipoma arising above within spinal cord, extending downwards to the dura, continuous with the extradural lipoma.

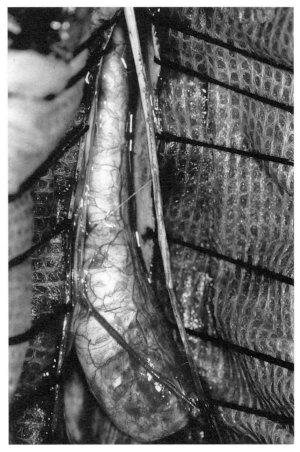

Fig. 29.5 Intradural dermoid cyst extending downwards from the lower end of the spinal cord.

severe scalloping may not be true manifestations of dysraphism, but rather skeletal evidence of neurofibromatosis, or the trait of that syndrome.

Rarely, an anterior meningocele may produce erosion or excavation of the posterior aspect of lumbar vertebrae, as can also be produced by intradural or extradural lipoma. This is similar to the situation seen in adults in the sacrum in association with arachnoid (Tarlov) cysts.

BONY SPURS WITH DIASTEMATOMYELIA

Characteristically, these are bony spurs which are based anteriorly in the midline on the posterior aspects of one or more vertebral bodies, and which project backwards for a variable distance. They most commonly occur in the region of the thoracolumbar junction, rather more so from the lower thoracic than the upper lumbar vertebrae, which is an important distinction from the other skeletal manifestations of dysraphism which are most common at the lower lumbar and sacral levels. The associated abnormalities (see Intradural intramedullary) are usually related to the height (i.e. posterior projec-

tion) of the spur, and the degree to which the spur has 'divided' or 'transfixed' the dural sac and the spinal cord. Spurs may or may not be visible on plain radiographs, especially in anteroposterior projections.

EXTRADURAL FIBROUS BANDS

These are relatively common abnormalities but do not, in themselves, have any neurological or urological significance. They are thin, often multiple, and run from the dura posteriorly, usually in the midline, to the laminar or underlying ligamentum flava, which are not well developed in children. Their diameter (less than 1 mm), and their position are sufficient indications of their nature to permit removal with impunity. There usually is not any underlying intradural anomaly in continuity with these bands. They are most common at the lumbosacral level.

EXTRADURAL SQUAMOUS EPITHELIAL TUBES

These are similar in position to the extradural fibrous

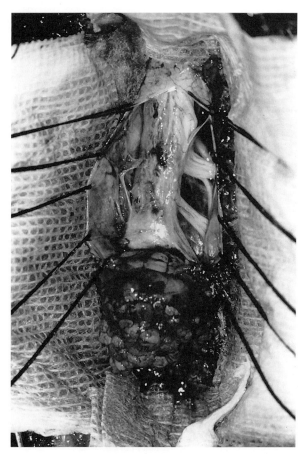

Fig. 29.6 Spinal cord extending down to, and attached to, the lower end of theca, with extradural lipoma.

bands, but are thicker and many have extensions into the subcutaneous tissues having passed between the laminae or fibrous tissue, found in place of the laminae. Their developmental origin may be similar to the true dermoid cysts, the more superficial extensions are the less well-developed squamous cell inclusion. In the majority of cases these blind tubes do not extend within the dura, and their midline position and obvious termination posteriorly either within or just outside the spinal canal in the subcutaneous tissues, indicate that it is safe to remove them. Occasionally parts of these tubes can be more obviously akin to dermoid cysts, and contain sebaceous material, reaching a small cutaneous punctum (see section on Cutaneous stigmata), but these more dilated parts of the tube usually end well short of the dura.

EXTRADURAL LIPOMATA

These are relatively common in lumbar dysraphism and may be associated and in continuity with extensive subcutaneous lipomata (lipomatous meningomyelocele) and/or with intradural lipomata, which may in turn be in continuity with the spinal cord, there forming a

true intramedullary lipoma (see below). The extradural lipomata are usually associated with extensive laminar arch defects. Fortunately, functioning neural elements are rarely present within the extradural lipomata, particularly when the lipomata are in the midline posteriorly. If they are more extensive, and extend round the sides of the theca or occupy the sacral canal below the termination of the sacral sac, functioning nerve roots may run through the fatty tissue, posing problems during surgical removal. Without thorough radiological examination, it should always be assumed that an extradural lipoma is associated with a significant intradural extension which may also extend intramedullary. It is doubtful whether the presence of excess fat in the extradural space acts as a lesion which is responsible for neurological deficit simply by compression of the theca. Deficit is more likely to be associated with intradural anomalies.

TETHERING OF CONUS

This term has been used widely and somewhat indiscriminately to describe any situation in which the conus, be it low or in the normal position, appears radiologically to be tethered or held to the dura. Apparent lack of movement of the conus, shown radiologically, may or may not mean that the conus is truly tethered to the dura and that an element of traction is responsible for the neurological deficit. Proof of the adverse effects of traction or tightness of the conus and/or filum terminale is often lacking. At operation the conus may be firmly and directly adherent to the dura, or there may be tethering bands which are no more than discrete fibrous thickenings of the arachnoid and clearly do not contain any neural elements. Less commonly one or more roots of the cauda equine may be tethered or stuck to the dura in the region of an intravertebral foremen through which the roots do not pass, but continue down within the theca to the appropriate exit foramena.

Anomalies of the filum terminale may take several forms. With a conus that extends as low as a lumbosacral junction the filum terminale may not be within the theca, and it is represented by a vestigial extradural band. The filum may be abnormally thick, and contain neural, glial or fatty tissue and even striated muscle. It is not easy to judge the tension or tightness of the filum terminale at operation unless it clearly retracts when divided at its lower end. The beneficial effects of this manoeuvre are generally accepted but difficult to prove.

DERMOID CYSTS

Of all the intradural abnormalities these are potentially the most dangerous due to recurrent infection, enlargement and progressive entanglement with the roots of the cauda equina, and progressive expansion of any intramedullary portion. Infection enters through a skin punctum and a vestigial squamous-lined tube which leads to the dura. The effects caused by dermoids are due to a combination of these complications, and therefore once the diagnosis has been made surgery is indicated, after any overt episode of infection has been treated. Antibiotics can do no more than control, albeit temporarily, meningeal infection, but are not likely to eradicate chronic infection within the dermoid cyst.

The intramedullary extension of dermoid cysts is variable. Only a minority of these lesions are clearly separate from the conus with which they are closely associated and which form part of a thickened filum terminale. Many appear to reach the conus, and the line of demarcation from cord tissue is rarely distinct, as becomes obvious when viewed through the operating microscope. This creates major problems when attempting excision, prudence usually dictating partial removal, especially if the sphincters are still functioning normally. Unfortunately the intramedullary lesions may be very extensive, sometimes reaching to a midthoracic level, in which case more than partial evacuation of their contents (sebaceum, hair and squamous epithelium) is precluded.

LOW CONUS MEDULLARIS

This has been described in the context of tethering. When the conus is very low, e.g. sacral, the emerging nerve roots will ascend to reach their respective exit foramena. Quite apart from diastematomyelia, the cord may be asymmetrical in configuration, with usually a partial or rarely a complete separation into two longitudinal structures with nerve roots emerging from each structure.

DIASTEMATOMYELIA

Although a well-described entity, diastematomyelia is a relatively rare form of dysraphism compared with the other anomalies. It occurs most commonly in the low thoracic or thoracolumbar region. In its full form there is a bony spur (see above) projecting backwards, usually in the midline between completely separated halves of the spinal cord, each contained within its own dural sac over the length of one or less commonly two skeletal vertebral segments. The greater longitudinal growth of the vertebral column compared with that of the spinal cord may cause tractional pressure by the bony spur, which is believed to account for any progression of the neurological deficit.

INTRADURAL LIPOMA

This is often associated with extradural lipoma. Its extent and relationship are similar to those occurring with dermoid cysts without the element of recurrent infection. The degree of delineation from the conus varies, but is usually more favourable surgically compared with that of dermoid cysts.

A MIXED TISSUE MASS

This is one of the anomalies least amenable to treatment, seen characteristically at the sacral level, where it is inseparable from the low conus. Macroscopically, the mass is composed of a mixture of dense hard fibrous tissue, portions of which appear cartilagenous or even bony, there are emerging nerve roots, and the whole structure is often firmly attached to or projecting through the dura. Microscopy confirms an assortment of appearances representing origins in the ectoderm, mesoderm and sometimes endoderm.

Management

The advent of accurate non-invasive methods of investigation and especially MRI, has been of very great benefit in the management of children with lumbar dysraphism, or suspected dysraphism. But is also creates problems in that radiological demonstration of an abnormality may sway the surgeon towards an aggressive approach, when in fact a conservative approach is more appropriate. Therefore the urological and orthopaedic assessments are generally of greater importance than the neurological, when it comes to making final decisions about management, and equating the clinical problem with the radiological appearances.

The stages of management can be classified as follows:

1. Observation and confirmation of: (a) abnormalities observed at or soon after birth including cutaneous stigmata; (b) failure or delay in development of normal bladder function and/or recurrent urinary infection and later deterioration in bladder function; (c) skeletal/orthopaedic abnormalities affecting the lower limbs, including defects of growth; (d) neurological deficits.
2. Spinal radiology.
3. Surgery, 'therapeutic' or 'prophylactic'.
4. Further review and repeated investigations.

(1a) ABNORMALITIES OBSERVED AT OR SHORTLY AFTER BIRTH

The overt manifestations of spina bifida are covered in Chapter 30. In the neonatal period one cutaneous abnormality that requires early investigation which may lead to prophylactic surgery is the tell-tale pit of the dermoid cyst. Other cutaneous stigmata such as hair (the faun's tail), transverse or vertical cutaneous angiomata, scars or subcutaneous lipomata, require later urological and orthopaedic assessment, but this is not urgent. Although there is some dispute, the early recognition of congenital dislocation of the hip does not in itself require spinal investigation to exclude lumbar dysraphism, neither do severe degrees of bilateral talipes equinovarus at birth in the absence of cutaneous stigmata. Subcutaneous lumbar lipomata without other cutaneous stigmata and without lower limb skeletal abnormalities require full urological assessment.

(1b) BLADDER FUNCTION

Defects of bladder function with sequelae such as recurrent urinary infection, are the most important manifestations of dysraphism which demands very thorough urological and spinal investigation, and which most commonly leads to spinal surgery. The relevant types of presentation, and the appropriate investigations are described in Chapter 30. Much can be learned from the description of the infant's urinary stream, including constant wetting of nappies, which is an early sign of incontinence. Neurosurgical referral usually follows assessment by paediatricians and urologists, but it is important that orthopaedic and neurological surgeons to whom infants may be referred directly by general practitioners are aware of the early signs of bladder dysfunction. Day incontinence persisting beyond the age at which control is usually achieved is one of the more obvious signs of neurogenic bladder dysfunction. Enuresis which may have a similar origin, is more difficult to assess but should certainly prompt the neurosurgeon to refer a child with cutaneous stigmata of dysraphism for full urological assessment. The urologist may sometimes have difficulty in distinguishing a non-neurogenic structural functional cause of bladder dysfunction from a purely neurogenic cause, and diagnosis is even more difficult when they coexist. In such circumstances, if all urological procedures have not improved significantly bladder function, the neurogenic element may be a sufficient basis for spinal surgery, provided that a spinal anomaly has been clearly demonstrated.

Overt and detectable abnormal neurological signs with a urologically proven neurogenic bladder dysfunction may or may not be present. The most likely abnormal signs are absence of ankle jerks, and some reduction of appreciation of pinprick in the perineal and perianal regions, and/or on the outer side of the feet. The detection of such deficits is difficult in young children and must rely on the apparent response to a painful stimulus. With an anomalous low spinal cord, the neurological picture may be confused by the addition of signs of an upper motor neurone lesion (e.g. brisk tendon reflexes) emanating from a disturbed conus medullaris. In the majority of cases some relevant detectable neurological deficit is present, but its absence alone cannot be accepted as certain evidence that a bladder disturbance is not neurogenic.

The importance of the urological aspects of dysraphism cannot be emphasized too strongly because, although in any individual case it is difficult to predict the urological benefit of spinal surgery, in this author's experience overall it has been the urological rather than the orthopaedic or neurological deficits that have responded most favourably to spinal surgery.

(1c) SKELETAL AND LOWER LIMB ABNORMALITIES

These are the most common overt manifestations of lumbar dysraphism. Talipes equinovarus deformity may be unilateral or asymmetrical and is very rarely as severe as in so-called idiopathic talipes. Other features are equinus with short tendo Achilles, wasting of the peroneal compartment, valgus deformity and a small foot with loss of the normal plantar arch. Inequality of leg length and thinning of the whole limb from birth may become more apparent as time passes. These orthopaedic abnormalities may be associated with only minor neurological deficits such as absence of the ankle jerk. The direct correlation between these orthopaedic deformities and remediable intraspinal pathology is often uncertain (see above) but orthopaedic assessment should always lead to neurological and urological review, especially when cutaneous stigmata are present. Abnormalities of gait noticed by parents may be due to a mixture of defects of growth, foot deformities and neurological deficit, congenital dislocation of the hip having been excluded. If there are indications for orthopaedic procedures such as elongation of the tendo Achilles, tendon transfers and midtarsal stabilization, neurosurgical assessment and operations should usually precede the orthopaedic procedure because any lessening of muscle imbalance will improve the prospects of orthopaedic correction. Rarely, sensory loss is severe enough to produce chronic perforating ulcers, osteomyelitis of phalanges and even metatarsal heads. Spinal surgery is unlikely to improve even the milder degrees of sensory loss.

(1d) NEUROLOGICAL DEFICITS

As already indicated, detectable neurological deficits, especially in infants, are not common, and as a primary presenting feature are rare. Therefore, although deficits must be sought with care in children whose referral has been for urological or orthopaedic reasons, it is most unlikely that the referral will have been prompted by parents' awareness of weakness, and even less so of sensory loss, in their child's lower limbs. Even in a lower limb which is thin, with obvious wasting of calf and peroneal muscles, motor power may appear normal with the usual objective tests. The most readily detected and most significant deficits are impaired appreciation of pain in the peroneal region and over the outer borders of the feet, and absence of the ankle jerks. With diastematomyelia and a bony spur projecting through the spinal cord in the thoracolumbar region, abnormal neurological signs may be entirely of an upper motor neurone lesion; and there may be an upper motor neurone element in disorders of a conus medullaris which is low and associated with some of the anomalies already described.

(2) SPINAL RADIOLOGY

Confirmation of a diagnosis of occult dysraphism and demonstration of the level of termination of the conus are done radiologically. The clinical features are usually associated with a cluster of plain film anomalies affecting the vertebral bodies and neural arches. These include disc hypoplasia or vertebral fusion, a defect in the development of the laminae usually comprising underdevelopment or fenestration and, characteristically, an increase in the interpedicular measurement which may either involve the whole of the lumbar canal or be confined to a single vertebral segment. The plain film demonstration of a diastematomyelia is often difficult on plain films, as the cartilaginous element is not visible and a bony diastem is often obscured by superimposition of the spinous process.

Demonstration of the lower cord and conus has traditionally been through myelography using a variety of contrast media – oil-based, gas or water-soluble – introduced via the cisternal, suboccipital, lateral C1–2 or lumbar route. Computed tomography (CT) confirms the bony features and may demonstrate a diastem. It gives no other detail of structures within the spinal canal or theca but latterly has been a valuable supplement to myelography in, for example, defining a split cord, although still giving no intramedullary detail. Success in the demonstration of the anatomy of the lower cord and cauda equine by ultrasound has been variable owing to bone artefact. Like myelography, it may still have a role to play if MRI is not possible or is contraindicated due, for example, to the patient's claustrophobia or the presence of a cardiac pacemaker.

The diagnosis is otherwise confirmed and the anatomy is best demonstrated by MRI. This has the advantage over CT scanning and myelography of being non-invasive, eliminating the use of ionizing radiation and providing multiplanar images. Splits in the cord and involvement of the conus or cauda in a fibro-fatty lipoma or dermoid are clearly shown, particularly when there are both intra-dural and extra-dural components.

(3) SURGERY: THERAPEUTIC OR PROPHYLACTIC

Strictly speaking, the term therapeutic surgery should be reserved for cases in which there is good evidence that urological, orthopaedic or neurological disorders are related to potentially remediable intraspinal anatomy that has been demonstrated radiologically. Prophylactic surgery may be applied to cases where there is no detectable disorder beyond external cutaneous stigmata or a subcutaneous lipoma, but where an intraspinal anomaly has been demonstrated which might technically be amenable to some surgical manoeuvre. The objective in therapeutic surgery is to improve the disorder or to prevent further deterioration: whereas in prophylactic surgery it is to prevent the development of a disorder at some later date.

The place of prophylactic surgery, as defined, is still a matter of some debate, although some neurosurgeons hold more positive views than do others. To operate on a child who is urologically, orthopaedically and neurologically intact is in some ways a weightier undertaking than to operate on a child who already has a sphincter or orthopaedic disorder, because of the risk, however small, of disturbing bladder function. Therefore, for prophylactic surgery there should be a high probability of an anatomically favourable anomaly being present, such as tethering bands, a conus locally adherent to the dura, a thickened filum terminale and an intradural extramedullary lipoma. The dermoid cyst is in a special category. Unfortunately, in neither prophylactic nor therapeutic surgery can the objective be achieved with certainty, however, apparently favourable the findings seem at operation.

Principles of surgery for spinal dysraphism

1. Children with subcutaneous lumbosacral lipomata should not be operated on without first excluding an intradural lesion by imaging.
2. Exposure must be of sufficient length to allow the dura to be approached through normal anatomy (e.g. laminae) before exposing the dura beneath the laminar arch defects or fibrous tissue.
3. Extradural tubes or bands should not be divided or removed except when strictly in the midline posteriorly, without first establishing by opening the dura that they do not contain neural structures.
4. Provided there has been preoperative imaging, it is reasonable to remove extradural dermoid cysts or tubes, stopping excision at the dura, without formally opening the dura.
5. If nerve roots are seen ascending to their exit foramena, the structure from which they arise (e.g. low conus or complex intradural anomaly) must not be jeopardized, whatever its histological structure may prove to be.
6. When lesions such as intradural lipomata or intradural dermoid cysts are closely applied to the conus, it is probable that there is an intramedullary element, which may vary greatly in its extent. The use of the operating microscope is essential in trying to define any line of demarcation between the cord and the lesion. Even the decision on how far to pursue the lesion may be very difficult. As a rule, it is wiser to be less rather than more aggressive if serious and irreversible postoperative bladder dysfunction is to be avoided.
7. Closure of the dura should always be attempted, but may not be possible, especially when it has been involved in the anomaly. Therefore in all cases care should be taken in the exposure to preserve the muscle layers and the fibrous tissue

present in place of laminar arches, because these can provide an effective layer for closure.

8. Division of a thickened or tight filum terminale should be done as low down as possible, close to its dural attachment at the lower limit of the dural sac.

9. In diastematomyelia the dura on each side of the bony spur must be carefully exposed throughout its depth before removing the spur with nibblers. Thereafter the dural opening should ensure that there is no residual tethering or fixation by the central section of the dura.

10. When the spinal cord appears to have been replaced by two asymmetrical longitudinal structures, it may be difficult to identify the true conus and filum terminale. In those circumstances the division of the filum terminale should be avoided, unless there is very obvious tension.

(4) REVIEW

After consideration, it may well be felt that operation is not indicated, at least after the first round of clinical assessments and investigations. In some cases there may be good evidence that any orthopaedic or urological disorders are not related to lumbar dysraphism, and these children will remain under orthopaedic or urological care. Those who may be considered for prophylactic surgery by some surgeons, but not by others, should ideally be kept under long-term paediatric review. Children in whom the initial conservative decision was a result of some debate, should be kept under joint review by the relevant specialists, including the neurosurgeons. It may be necessary to repeat urological investigations so that any adverse change in bladder function is recognized as early as possible.

Results

For a number of reasons it is very difficult to assess the direct effects and benefits of spinal surgery, not least because the prognosis of the natural history in any individual case is difficult to foresee. This is particularly so in children who show no more clinical signs than the external stigmata. Establishing the nature of the natural history requires careful follow-up for an indefinite period, and certainly well into adult life.

It is rare for orthopaedic abnormalities to be corrected by spinal surgery alone and the majority will require orthopaedic lower limb procedures. Whether these have been made more effective by spinal surgery in a particular case is usually very difficult to judge.

At present, the neurogenic bladder dysfunction, especially of recent onset, appears to respond most clearly to spinal surgery, such as division of tethering bands, release of a spinal cord which is attached to the dura, division of a tight filum terminale, and removal of intradural dermoid cysts.

In conclusion, current practice may be summarized as follows: infants born with external stigmata should be reviewed regularly, with particular attention being paid to the development of bladder control and recurrent urinary infections. Before the normal age of bladder control, simple urological assessment is necessary.

The use of imaging (MRI) in a child with external stigmata but who is otherwise normal is justified if the clinician would favour prophylactic surgery for what appears radiologically to be a remediable spinal lesion. The alternative approach is careful long-term review with repeat urological investigation.

The external sign of a dermoid cyst is a clear indication for spinal imaging and prophylactic surgery. Before ascribing any orthopaedic or urological disorders to dysraphism, it is essential to exclude with great care the presence of any primary urological or orthopaedic abnormality.

If the above criteria apply and spinal imaging shows a potentially correctable abnormality, then spinal surgery is indicated, accepting that a neurogenic cause may be superimposed on a structural orthopaedic or urinary disorder.

It is very difficult to predict what can be achieved technically at operation and to what extent this will improve any urological or orthopaedic disorder. However, on the basis of the assessments described, there are often strong grounds for surgery by those who have experience of the great variety of operative findings, which are often difficult to interpret and to unravel.

ACKNOWLEDGEMENT

With thanks to Peter Cook for his contribution to the Radiology section of this chapter.

Further reading

Hoffman, H., Taecholarn, C., Hendrick, E. and Humphreys, R. 1985: Management of lipomyelomeningoceles. *Journal of Neurosurgery* **62**, 1–8.

O'Neil, P. and Singh, J. 1991: Occult spinal dysraphism in children. The need for early neurological referral. *Child's nervous system* **7**, 309–11.

Pierre-Kahn, A., Lacombe, J., Pichon, J. *et al.* 1986: Intraspinal lipomas with spina bifida. Prognosis and treatment in 73 cases. *Journal of Neurosurgery* **65**, 756–61.

Regal, D. and Clone, D 1994: Tethered spinal cord. In Cheek, W.R. (ed.), *Paediatric neurosurgery,* 3rd ed. Philadelphia, PA: W.B. Saunders, 77–95 (this chapter contains 128 references to the majority of significant publications).

Till, K. 1974: The value of prophylactic surgical treatment. In *Recent progress in neurological surgery*. Amsterdam: Excerpta Medical, No. 320, 60–6.

CHAPTER 30

Spina bifida

J.D. ATWELL

Historical	**Associated anomalies**
Surgical embryology	**Management**
Incidence	**Results**
Aetiology	**A handicapped child in the family**
Classification	**References**

Historical

The earliest record of a sacral spina bifida was found in the adult skeleton of a central European of the Neolithic period (fifth millennium BC). Sacral defects were not necessarily associated with a severe neurological deficit. Prehistoric remains with defects above the sacrum are rare, possibly owing to early deaths in infancy with poorly mineralized skeletons. The precise origin of the term spina bifida is difficult to determine but in the sixteenth century Morgagni reviewed the condition and its pathophysiology. He described the association of spina bifida with hydrocephalus and anencephaly and considered them to be of a similar nature. He also suggested that the abnormalities of the lower limbs, bladder and rectum were secondary to nerve damage within the spinal cord (Van Gool and Van Gool, 1986).

The ninteenth century was marked by the development of anatomy and pathology and their associated museums. Detailed descriptions and preparations of myelomeningoceles were reported (Cleland, 1883). Even early experimental work with the chick embryo suggested that myelomeningoceles and anencephaly were two extremes of the same developmental disturbance (Lebedeff, 1881). This was the first report to suggest that the defect was due to a failure of closure of the neural tube and the surrounding mesoderm and that this may have been secondary to a kyphosis.

The first classification of the types of spina bifida and indications and techniques for surgical closure of the defect was by Von Recklinghausen in 1886. Shortly after this, Arnold (1884) described the prolongation of the tonsils and vermis of the cerebellum through the foramen magnum and Chiari (1895) described the prolongation of the medulla into the foramen magnum. The combination of these defects (the Arnold–Chiari malformation) caused hydrocephalus due to a partial obstruction of the flow of cerebrospinal fluid (CSF) from the exit foramina at the base of the brain.

As there was no satisfactory treatment for the control of hydrocephalus no advances were made in the management of spina bifida until well into the twentieth century. In 1939 Torkildsen described a method of shunting CSF from the lateral ventricles to the cisterna magna using a rubber tube. In 1951 the neurosurgeon Eugene Spitz inserted a ventriculoatrial shunt into a boy with hydrocephalus (Nulsen and Spitz, 1951). The shunt had been designed by Holter. Thus by the end of the 1950s well-tried methods of controlling hydrocephalus by either ventriculoatrial or ventriculoperitoneal shunts were well established (Pudenz and Russell, 1957). This radical method of being able to control hydrocephalus led to a reappraisal of the methods of treating myelomeningoceles in the newborn period (Sharrard et al., 1963; Rickham and Mawdsley, 1966).

Surgical embryology

The nervous system is derived from the embryonic ectoderm. An elongated area known as the neural plate gives rise to the brain and spinal cord. The neural plate first appears in the presomite stage and overlies the notochord. It then thickens and becomes depressed to form the neural groove. Elongation of the neural plate occurs with the development of the somites and segmentation of the embryo. The primitive neural plate then folds in to form the neural tube. At the same time there is a condensation of the para axial mesoderm to form the coverings of the cord, the vertebral column and its associated muscles (Fig. 30.1). This is a very simplified account of the embryology of the spinal cord and its coverings but it allows an understanding and appreciation of the various types of central nervous system defects found in clinical practice.

Incidence

The incidence of spina bifida and associated central nervous system (CNS) malformations varies in different parts of the UK (Fig. 30.2). On average it is 2.5 per 1000 live births, with a range of 1.1–4.2 (Harper, 1916; Coffey and Jessop, 1955) per 1000 live births. One example is the high incidence in south Wales (1 in 250 births) compared with that found in East Anglia (1 in 500 births) (Laurence, 1964). There is no doubt that environmental factors are important as in Boston between 1890 and 1920 the average incidence was 2 per 1000 live births but between 1920 and 1949 there were peaks with a threefold increase to 6 per 1000 live births (MacMahon and Yen, 1971). This is similar to the increased incidence in UK between 1950 and 1970. Since then the incidence has fallen (Fig. 30.3) and this has not been due to improvements in antenatal diagnosis and the use of therapeutic abortions (Northern Region Fetal Abnormality Survey, 1988). Although that is a factor, the main alteration appears to be due to some change in the environment.

Aetiology

The factors which alter the development of the spinal cord and column occur early in pregnancy as the neural plate is differentiating at the presomite stage (18 days) and is complete by the fourth week when segmentation of the embryo is fully established. The aetiology of spina bifida is unknown. However, since many factors are known to have an effect during early development and its causation is probably multifactorial. This is supported by the variations of spina bifida found in clinical practice: for instance, some defects appear to be due to an arrest of development whereas in others there is evidence of disordered development such as myelodysplasia (see under Classification of defects).

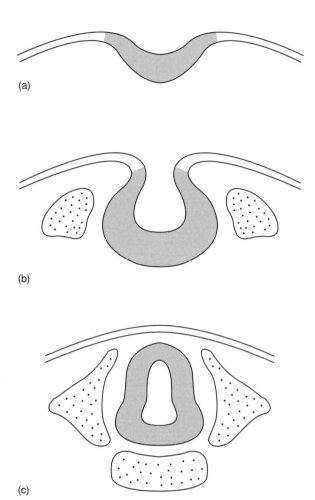

(a)

(b)

(c)

Fig. 30.1 Embryological development of the spinal cord.

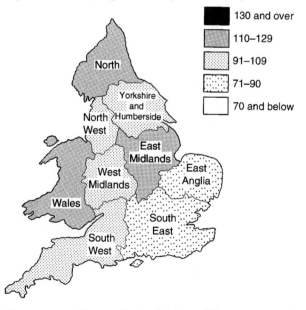

■	130 and over
▨	110–129
▥	91–109
⣿	71–90
☐	70 and below

Fig. 30.2 Incidence of spina bifida in different regions of England and Wales. (From the Northern Region Fetal Abnormality Survey, 1988.)

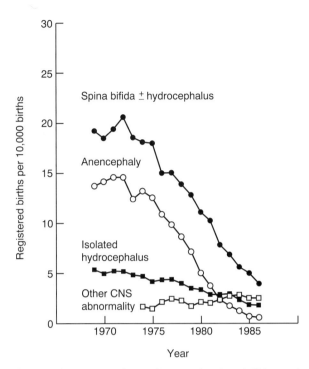

Fig. 30.3 Decreased incidence of spina bifida and hydrocephalus from 1970 to 1985. (From the Northern Region Fetal Abnormality Survey, 1988.)

Genetic and familial factors are important. The risk of a first born being affected is about 1 in 250 (range 1 in 250 to 1 in 500) (Coffey and Jessop, 1955; Laurence, 1964; Durham Smith, 1965) but this increases to about 1 in 20 or 1 in 25 risk in the next pregnancy (Williamson, 1965). If two children in the same family have been affected the risk increases to 1 in 10 (Carter and Fraser Roberts, 1967). There is also an increased risk of spina bifida and associated malformations when a male or female individual with spina bifida has their own family, to 3 in 100 (Carter and Evans, 1973). Maternal age may be relevant as there appeared to be a significant excess of children with spina bifida in young mothers ($p > 0.01$ to $p > 0.001$) (Smithells and Chinn, 1965). There was a similar finding in the ages of mothers of anencephalic infants.

Viral infections are alleged to be associated with a high incidence of spina bifida, although this has not been confirmed (Coffey and Jessop, 1959). There is a seasonal variation which would support this hypothesis (Guthkelch, 1962), with a higher incidence of spina bifida in births during December to May than in those born in June to November. In another series there was an excess of winter births but no seasonal variation in conceptions (Smithells and Chinn, 1965). An epidemic of spina bifida occurred in Boston in 1929–32 and was attributed to the influenza epidemic of 1918–19 having an effect on young females which affected their future

pregnancies (Janerich, 1971). Similar findings have been made on the effects of starvation in childhood on future pregnancies. Birth order is important, as the incidence of spina bifida is higher in first- and second-born children. This is difficult to substantiate as there are more first-born children than third-, fourth- and fifth-born, therefore statistical evaluation is fraught with difficulties. Geographical variations have already been discussed under the section on incidence. Vitamin deficiencies in experimental animals have been implicated (vitamin A deficiency) in the aetiology and more recently the prevention of neural tube defects has been advocated by giving folic acid supplements during a pregnancy (Laurence *et al.*, 1981; Smithells *et al.*, 1983; MRC Vitamin Study Group, 1991; Folic Acid Report, 1991). Noxious chemicals have been implicated, such as trypan blue in the experimental animal and solanine found in the skin of potatoes subjected to late blight (Renwick, 1972). Later clinical trials disproved the latter hypothesis, as withholding potatoes from the diet before conception and during pregnancy did not prevent the birth of a second spina bifida or anencephalic infant (Lorber, 1973). Chromosomal defects and syndromes are associated with spina bifida but these are rare (see Chapters 5 and 52). In a series of mothers with hydramnios, 45% of the infants had CNS malformations but hydramnios is not a common finding in mothers with a spina bifida infant. The incidence of threatened abortion and hydramnios was higher in spina bifida pregnancies than in controls (Smithells *et al.*, 1983).

Classification

CNS malformations are classified into different groups depending on the severity of the lesion (Table 30.1). It is also important to define the level of the defect, i.e. cervical, thoracic, thoracolumbar, lumbar, lumbosacral or sacral.

Table 30.1 Types of spina bifida

Spinal dysraphism

Spina bifida occulta
(i) radiological
(ii) clinical
Extradural
Intradural with or without surface stigma
Intramedullary (see Chapter 29)

Meningocele

Meningomyelocele or myelomeningocele

Myelocele

Hydromyelia

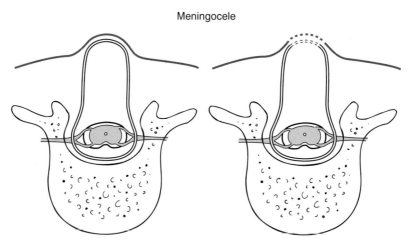

Meningocele

Fig. 30.4 Transverse section through a meningocele. Note that there is no abnormality of the spinal cord.

MENINGOCELE

In a meningocele (Fig. 30.4) there is a herniation of the coverings of the cord (dura and pia mater, and the pia arachnoid) through the bifid neural arch. The swelling is usually covered by skin and dura but sometimes this is very attenuated and the fluid contents of the sac are visible. The neural tube is fully developed and by definition there is no neurological deficit.

MENINGOMYELOCELE OR MYELOMENINGOCELE

The terms are synonymous. The dura mater and skin are deficient over the posterior aspect of the defect but the cord is still protected by the pia arachnoid (Fig. 30.5).

There may be evidence of myelodysplasia and diastematomyelia and usually there is evidence of a neurological deficit. The extent of the deficit depends on the level of the defects. They are usually lumbar or lumbosacral in position.

MYELOCELE

This is an open lesion with the neural plate exposed (Fig. 30.6). The central canal opens on to the surface at the upper end of the neural groove. The dura mater is deficient and stops at the margin of the defect. Myelodysplasia and diastematomyelia are common associated anomalies. The defects are usually thoracolumbar or lumbar and the neurological defect is often

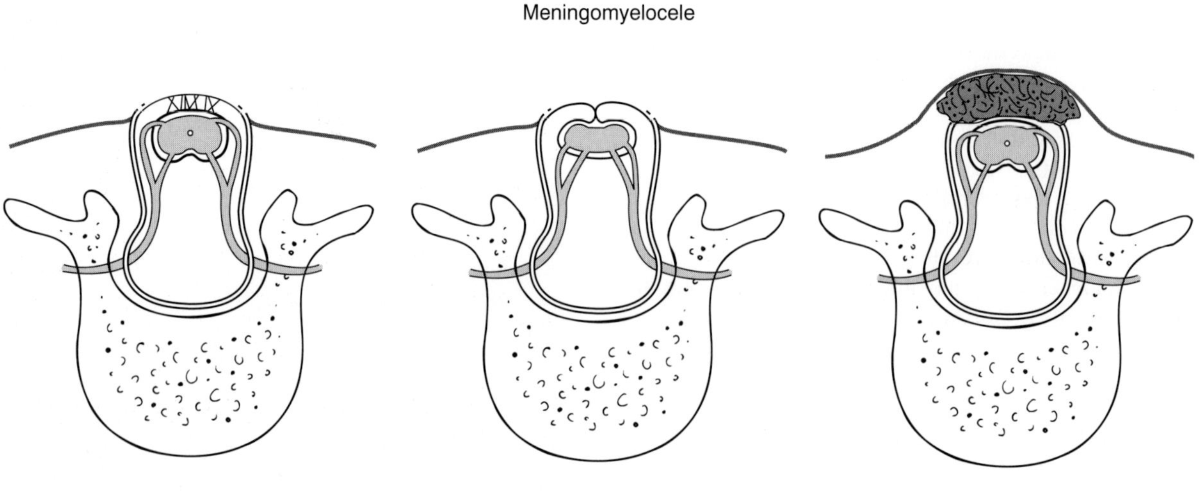

Meningomyelocele

Lipomatous meningomyelocele

Fig. 30.5 Transverse section through a meningomyelocele or myelomeningocele. Note that the nervous tissue is still protected by the pia arachnoid but that the dura mater is deficient.

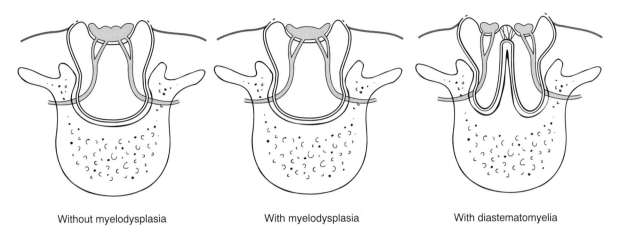

Without myelodysplasia   With myelodysplasia   With diastematomyelia

Fig. 30.6 Transverse section through a myelocele. Note that the neural plaque is exposed and the central canal opens on to the surface at the proximal end of the plaque.

severe with evidence of intrauterine paralysis of muscle groups leading to dislocation of the hips, talipes and arthrogryposis. In many series of spina bifida cystica the thoracolumbar myelocele is the most common lesion.

In reported series of spina bifida cystica the terms myelomeningocele, meningomyelocele and myelocele have been interchangeable, thus comparisons between the severity of the different types has been difficult. Lesions with an exposed neural plate with or without myelodysplasia are usually associated with severe neurological dysfunction.

SURFACE STIGMA

These are important in assessing patients with spinal dysraphism as they are closed lesions whereas in the above open lesions the pathology is visible. Areas of angiomatous tissue are commonly seen at the margins of myeloceles and meningomyeloceles and in others there may be an excess of pigmentation, lack of pigmentation and excessive hair (faun's tail).

Associated anomalies

These can be subdivided into two main groups: primary associated anomalies and problems associated with neurological dysfunction.

PRIMARY ANOMALIES

These include vertebral anomalies such absent vertebrae, hemivertebrae, bifid vertebrae and butterfly vertebrae. In some patients there is gross disorganization and precise definition of the anomalies is impractical (Fig. 30.7). These congenital defects of the spine result in the deformities of kyphosis and kyphoscoliosis

(Fig. 30.8). As the ribs develop from the vertebrae it is not unusual to find absent or fused ribs.

Probably the next highest group of anomalies comprises those associated with the renal tract. The incidence found in three separate reported series is shown in Table 30.2. Problems such as dilated ureters and vesicoureteric reflux have been excluded because in this group of patients they are more likely to be the result of neurological dysfunction affecting the bladder.

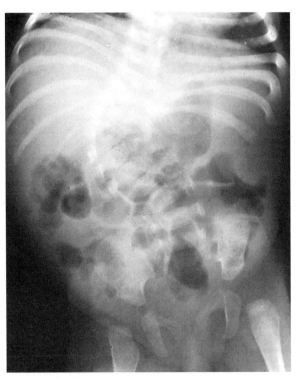

Fig. 30.7 Severe vertebral anomalies associated with spina bifida cystica.

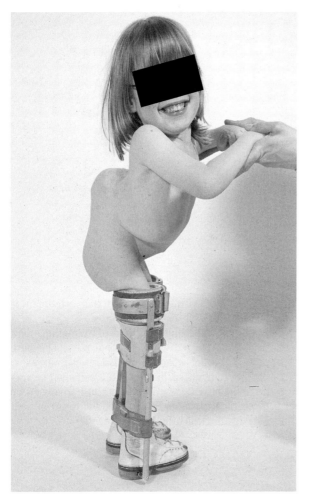

Fig. 30.8 Severe kyphosis in a patient with a thoracolumbar myelocele.

Congenital heart disease and other serious defects are relatively rare in patients with spina bifida but the incidence is greater than expected in normal controls (Table 30.2).

The Arnold–Chiari malformation, resulting in hydrocephalus, is almost a universal finding. In some patients aqueduct stenosis causes severe hydrocephalus and in these patients initial skull circumference is likely to be above the 90th percentile, whereas in the Arnold–Chiari malformation the circumference is often at or below the 50th percentile.

SECONDARY ANOMALIES DUE TO NEUROLOGICAL DYSFUNCTION

These can be subdivided into motor (paralysis), sensory (loss of touch, temperature and proprioception) and autonomic (sphincter paralysis of the bladder and bowel).

In some patients the paralysis has occurred *in utero* and is associated with an abnormal fetal position. Thus the hips may be dislocated, talipes, either equino varus or calcaneo valgus, is present and sometimes there is arthrogryposis affecting the knee. Sensory impairment may result in secondary pressure sores, burns and the development of Charcot's joints.

The neurological deficit may be related to the surgical treatment, i.e. closure of the spinal defect causing spinal shock which may be temporary or permanent. In others the neurological dysfunction may be primary or secondary.

Involvement with the autonomic system results in sphincter paralysis with problems associated with a neurogenic bladder and bowel. Associated paresis of the pelvic floor muscles may increase the severity of sphincter incontinence with rectal prolapse and occasionally complete procidentia in a newborn female.

A REGIONAL SERVICE FOR THE TREATMENT OF SPINA BIFIDA CYCTICA

The early and intensive treatment of the back lesion led to the development of other methods of treatment for the associated defects such as the control of hydrocephalus (Chapter 28), the management of urinary and faecal incontinence (Chapter 65) and the early treatment of orthopaedic problems such as congenital dislocation of the hip (CDH) and talipes (Chapter 82). Thus there was a need to develop a multidisciplinary team with a co-ordinator who was responsible for the overall management of the patient (Fig. 30.9). In this way the patient benefited by being able to see several consultants on the same day with the resultant reduction in time spent at multiple outpatient sessions. Unfortunately, when these patients reached adult life this ideal was not possible and as a result attendance for follow-up appointments decreased.

EARLY DETECTION AND PREVENTION OF SPINA BIFIDA CYSTICA

Measures to reduce the incidence of spina bifida or to make the diagnosis early in pregnancy to allow a termination are of vital interest to the family and the community. The development of screening programmes therefore became an urgent clinical need and a UK collaborative study (1977) on maternal serum α-fetoprotein levels was undertaken. It showed that in 301 pregnancies affected by neural tube defects it was possible to diagnose 88% of patients with anencephaly and 79% of patients with open spina bifida by screening the pregnant population between 16 and 18 weeks of gestation. These findings were confirmed by further studies (Ferguson Smith *et al.*, 1978) when 36 or 6122 pregnancies were tested between 15 and 20 weeks' gestation. The test was positive in 87.5% of anencephalics and 71.4% of open spina bifida.

Table 30.2 Primary congenital anomalies associated with spina bifida cystica

Defect	Series		
	Durham Smith **(101 patients)**	**Smithells** **(258 patients)**	**Atwell** **(96 patients)**
Renal tract anomalies	9	7	16 in 10 patients
Hypospadias	2	–	1
Horseshoe kidney	1		3
Renal agenesis	–		3
Double ureters	3		3
Renal ectopia	–		5
Renal hypoplasia	–		1
Urethral diverticulum	1		–
Bladder exstrophy	1		–
Posterior urethral valves	1		–
Congenital heart disease	3	10	2
Other serious defects			
Diaphragmatic hernia	–	2	–
Oesophageal atresia and tracheo-oesophageal fistula	1	–	1
Anorectal anomalies	5	–	–
Exomphalos	2	–	–

The finding of a raised serum α-fetoprotein led to the need to perform an amniocentesis to confirm the raised level of α-fetoprotein in the amniotic fluid. The risk of an amniocentesis causing an abortion is between 1.0 and 1.5% and this is the main disadvantage of the technique.

The development of maternal ultrasonography has been important in the safe antenatal detection of neural tube defects. It is particularly useful for:

- establishing the precise duration of pregnancy
- excluding fetal death
- excluding multiple pregnancy
- reducing the risk of amniocentesis
- direct demonstration or exclusion of the neural tube defect.

In addition, ultrasonography has led to the development of intrauterine therapeutic procedures (see Chapter 4).

Prevention of the first and subsequent neural tube defects is better than the early detection of such defects (Smithells *et al.*, 1983; MRC Vitamin Study Group, 1991; Folic Acid Report, 1991). This has been studied by an expert advisory group of the Department of Health, Scottish Office Home and Health Department, Welsh Office and Department of Health and Social Services, Northern Ireland (Folic Acid Report, 1991). They reviewed the effect of folic acid on the prevention of neural tube defects. Their recommendation to prevent a first occurrence of a neural tube defect was 'extra folate/folic acid is recommended for all women prior to conception and during the first 12 weeks of pregnancy'.

In order to prevent a recurrence of a neural tube defect their recommendations were: adequate counselling about the risks in any future pregnancy, and folic acid supplement at a daily dose of 5 mg for those women who wish to become pregnant and that this should continue until the 12th week of pregnancy.

Management

INITIAL ASSESSMENT

A detailed family history is obtained especially for a previous history of CNS anomalies, the number of pregnancies and or abortions, age of the parents, and history of any drugs or viral infections during the pregnancy especially in the first month.

A detailed examination is then made of the back defect. The level is noted and the size of the neural plate (zona granulosa), the size of the membranes covering the defect (zona membranosa) and the overall size of the defect are measured. On occasions there is evidence of a rupture of the sac with leakage of CSF. There may be a diastematomyelia but this is usually an operative finding.

The hydrocephalus is assessed clinically by charting the occipitofrontal circumference on the appropriate

Management of Spina Bifida

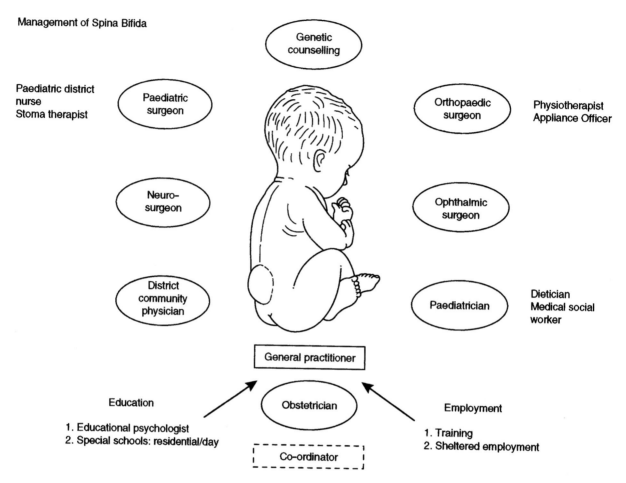

Fig. 30.9 Regional service for the care of infants born with spina bifida cystica. Note the need for a multidisciplinary team.

charts. The degree of hydrocephalus is also assessed by noting the amount of separation of the skull sutures, the prominence of the scalp veins, size and tension of the anterior fontanelle and eye signs of either evidence of a nerve palsy (usually the sixth cranial nerve) or 'sunsetting' of the eyes.

The extent of skeletal deformity is then assessed. The degree of kyphosis is important as in severe cases this means that a wheelchair existence is not feasible without extensive spinal surgery. The presence of congenitally dislocated hips (paralytic type) is noted together with talipes equinovarus or calcaneovalgus. The knee joint is sometimes abnormal, with arthrogryposis affecting all the joints of the lower limbs. Wasting of muscle groups noted on the initial examination is evidence of intrauterine paralysis and thus a poor prognosis for functional recovery.

The sphincters are examined, and it is determined whether the anus is patulous or rectal prolapse is present. It is established whether the bladder is palpable or expressible, and whether urine dribbles out or there is evidence of intermittent micturition. In many patients with paralysis of the pelvic floor there is a 'flush bottom' appearance, i.e. loss of the natal cleft.

Investigations are also essential in the initial evaluation of the patient and include radiographs of the spine to assess vertebral anomalies, and ultrasound imaging to confirm the degree of hydrocephalus and the thickness of the cerebral mantle and also to determine whether there are any primary associated renal anomalies such as renal agenesis or horseshoe kidney (see Table 30.2).

Following the examination and investigations a decision must be made concerning the future management of the infant. This decision must be made after a full discussion with one or both of the parents and the medical advice is fundamentally important as the parents must understand the full implications of looking after a physically handicapped child who may also have some mental impairment from the associated hydrocephalus. Thus one has to attempt a prognosis: will the child walk unaided or with calipers or be in a wheelchair? Will he or she be incontinent of urine and faeces? Will he or she have a normal intelligence quotient or have impairment of the mental faculties?

PLAN OF TREATMENT

The three possible plans of treatment are early closure of the back (Sharrard *et al.*, 1963; Rickham and Mawdsley, 1966), late closure of the back (Keys Smith and Durham Smith, 1973) and selective treatment (Lorber, 1973).

Early closure

This method of treatment followed the development of the Spitz–Holter valve to control the associated hydrocephalus. The promising early results (Sharrard *et al.*, 1963) led to the abandonment of a controlled trial which, in hindsight, may have been unfortunate. The plan was to close the back lesion within 24 hours of delivery, with some evidence accumulating that those closed within 4 hours had a better end result than those closed within 24 hours (personal observation). This policy was completely non-selective and attempts were made to treat all patients irrespective of the severity of the lesion.

Late closure

This was a variation of the original treatment of spina bifida when the defect was allowed to epithelialize, i.e. skin cover was obtained by the ingrowth of epithelium from the periphery of the defect. In an account of the natural history of spina bifida cystica this occurred with survival of approximately 30% of patients. Later repair of the cystic lesion of the back could then be undertaken, especially as it was felt that the risk of an exacerbation of the hydrocephalus was reduced. The risks of death from an ascending ventriculitis or from hydrocephalus are increased in this method of management.

Selective treatment policy

The early closure method was in widespread use between the late 1950s and the early 1970s, but then it was realized that the overall results of treatment were disappointing in the severe cases, i.e. patients with an extensive thoracolumbar myelocele. This led to the development of selection which required established criteria for its use:

- severe hydrocephalus
- severe kyphosis
- size, level and type of defect, with or without myelodysplasia
- associated malformations
- personal and social factors.

One problem in assessment was the number of factors necessary for selection. Fortunately several factors were usually positive. Severe hydrocephalus without other positive criteria was not sufficient to adopt a selective policy. Serious associated malformations have a relatively low incidence in spina bifida but the problems of paralytic CDH, talipes and arthrogryposis were included as they are associated with intrauterine paralysis. Similarly, the degree of sphincter paralysis could be used in the assessment of the individual patient, as double incontinence is a severe handicap even without other physical and mental deficits.

Results

There are difficulties in assessing the results of the intensive treatment of spina bifida. Firstly, there is the question of terminology, as stated earlier in this chapter, i.e. the presence of a neural plaque is associated with a greater degree of handicap (Hunt *et al.*, 1973). Secondly, the incidence of defects at different levels varies from centre to centre, e.g. in a series (Durham Smith, 1965) of 295 patients only 18 were thoracolumbar whereas in a personal series of 96 patients, 46 were thoracolumbar and 75 had an open neural plaque, i.e. were myeloceles.

MORTALITY

The most common earliest cause of death was either from infection due to an ascending ventriculitis or from a failure to control severe hydrocephalus. With intensive early closure of the back lesion the mortality is between 20 and 30% (Fig. 30.10). Using selective criteria for the treatment of spina bifida the mortality increases and in one series of 37 patients 25 received no treatment and died by 9 months of age, i.e. a 67% mortality (Lorber, 1973). This change is seen in Fig. 30.10, which covers a series of patients with spina bifida treated between 1969 and 1977.

MOBILITY AND FUNCTIONAL RESULTS

Mobility was assessed in one series of 113 patients of whom 80 survived (Hunt *et al.*, 1973). Five patients had minimal disability, i.e. walking without appliances and with a normal range of intelligence. Only one of these patients was incontinent. Seventy-one patients had moderate to severe disability. In the severe group of 39 only one was continent and none could walk 20 yards. In the moderate disability group none could run, some could walk a few steps and nearly all had calipers. In 12 patients with very severe handicap ten could not walk at all and all but one was severely retarded and all were incontinent. These authors also showed that a skull circumference at birth above the 90th percentile was associated with a greater degree of disability. These and similar findings led to the use of 'adverse' criteria used in making decisions about the suitability of surgical treatment (Lorber, 1973). These include gross paralysis, thoracolumbosacral lesions, kyphosis, multiple congenital defects and severe hydrocephalus. In one series of 25 untreated patients 21 had two or more adverse criteria.

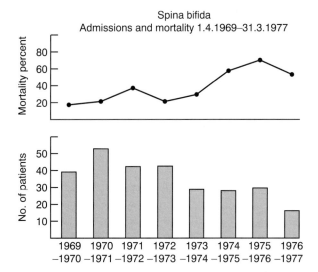

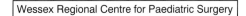

Fig. 30.10 Mortality of the early treatment of spina bifida cystica, showing the increasing mortality with selective treatment. The graph shows the decreasing incidence of spina bifida starting in the early 1970s.

A handicapped child in the family

The arrival of a newborn with a serious congenital malformation causes extreme emotional stress to both the mother and the whole family. It is important that someone with experience in the degree of handicap of the affected newborn fully discusses the situation with the family and outlines in detail as far as possible the degree of handicap expected, i.e. will the child walk? Will he or she be doubly incontinent? Will the hydrocephalus be associated with mental retardation? All of these are important questions to be answered and will help the parents in coming to an understanding of the clinical situation and any conclusions about the treatment given.

In one review of family stress associated with spina bifida cystica (Hare *et al.*, 1966) the reactions of relatives and neighbours, effect on marital harmony, effect of multiple visits to hospital and risks of any future pregnancy are discussed. It is not unusual to find that separation of the parents or divorce follows, some mothers become depressed and overweight, and some may even become thyrotoxic. Families with a severely handicapped child need support in order to sustain adequate care of the child. This requirement led to the development of societies such as the Association for Spina Bifida and Hydrocephalus in the UK and the Association for the Aid of Crippled Children in the USA. Both societies have prepared suitable literature to provide information to the parents (Swinyard, 1966;

Association for Spina Bifida and Hydrocephalus, 1966) Similar publications have been published by the Department of Health and Social Security (1973). In some instances the arrival of a malformed newborn draws the members of the family into a close unit group and they cope amazingly well (Hunt, 1973).

The education of the physically handicapped child who may also have some mental disability is another source of worry to the parents. Similarly, as the child grows and the parents get older management is more difficult and anxiety about sheltered employment and the long-term future of their child come to the fore. Finally, the future lies in prevention (Bower and Stanley, 1996).

References

Arnold, J. 1894: Myelocyste, Transposition von Gewebskeimen und Symbodie. *Beitrag Pathologie Anatomie* **16**, 1–28.

Association for Spina Bifida and Hydrocephalus 1968: *Your child with spina bifida. A practical guide to parents.* London: Association for Spina Bifida and Hydrocephalus.

Bower, C.M. and Stanley, F.J. 1996: Issues in prevention of spina bifida. *Journal of the Royal Society of Medicine* 436–42.

Carter, C.O. and Evans, K. 1973: Children of adult survivors with spina bifida cystica. *Lancet* **ii**, 924–6.

Carter, C.O. and Fraser Roberts, J.A. 1967: The risk of recurrence after two children with central-nervous-system malformations. *Lancet* **i**, 306–8.

Chiari, H. 1895: Über Veranderungen des Kleinhirns des Pons und der Medulla Oblongata in folge von congenitaler Hydrocephalie des Grosshirns. In *Clinical neurosurgery*. Baltimore, MD, Williams & Wilkins, 1958, Vol. 5.

Cleland, J. 1883: Contribution to the study of spina bifida, encephalocele and anencephalus. *Journal of Anatomy and Physiology* **17**, 257.

Coffey, V.P. and Jessop, W.J.E. 1955: Congenital anomalies. *Irish Journal of Medical Science* **349**, 30–48.

Coffey, V.P. and Jessop, W.J.E. 1959: Maternal influenza and congenital deformities: a prospective study. *Lancet* **ii**, 935–8.

DHSS 1973: *Care of the child with spina bifida.* London: DHSS.

Durham Smith, E. 1965: Spina bifida and the total care of spina myelomeningocele. In Ravitch, M.M. (ed.), *Pediatric surgical monographs*. Springfield, IL: Charles C. Thomas.

Ferguson Smith, M.A., Mayh, M., Vince, J.D. *et al.* 1978: Avoidance of anencephalic and spina bifida births by maternal serum alpha-fetoprotein screening. *Lancet* **i**, 1330–3.

Folic Acid and the Prevention of Neural Tube Defects, Report from an Expert Advisory Group 1991: Department of Health, Scottish Office Home and Health Department, Welsh Office and Department of Health and Social Services, Northern Ireland.

Guthkeleh, A.N. 1962: Studies in spina bifida cystica III. Seasonal variations in frequency of spina bifida births. *British Journal of Preventive and Social Medicine* **16**, 159–62.

Hare, E.H., Laurence, K.M., Payne, H. and Rawnsley, K. 1966: Spina bifida cystica and family stress. *British Medical Journal* **2**, 757–60.

Harper, J.A. 1916: *Bulletin Lying in Hospital*, **10**, 143.

Hunt, G.M. 1973: Implications of the treatment of myelomeningocele for the child and his family. *Lancet ii*, 1308–10.

Hunt, G., Lewin, W., Gleave, J. and Gardner, D. 1973: Predictive factors in open myelomeningocele with special reference to sensory level. *British Medical Journal* **4**, 197–201.

Janerich, D.T. 1971: Relationship between the influenza pandemic and the epidemic of neurological malformations. *Lancet* **i**, 1165.

Laurence, K.M., James, N., Miller, M.H., Tennant, G.B. and Campbell, H. 1981: Double blind randomised controlled trial of folate treatment before conception to prevent recurrence of neural tube defects. *British Medical Journal* **282**, 1509–11.

Laurence, K.M. 1964: The natural history of spina bifida. *Archives of Disease in Childhood* **39**, 41–57.

Lebedeff, A. 1881: Über die Enstehung der Anencephalie und Spina Bifida bei Vogeln und Menschen. *Virchows Archives of Pathology, Anatomy and Physiology* **86**, 263.

Lorber, J. 1973: Early results of selective treatment of spina bifida cystica. *British Medical Journal* **ii**, 201–4.

Lorber, J. 1968: *Your child with spina bifida*. London: Association for Spina Bifida and Hydrocephalus.

MacMahon, B. and Yen, S. 1971: Unrecognised epidemic of anencephaly and spina bifida. *Lancet* **i**, 31–3.

MRC Vitamin Study Group 1991: Prevention of neural tube defects. Results of the Medical Research Council Vitamin Study. *Lance* **238**, 131–7.

Northern Regional Fetal Abnormality Survey 1988: *First progress report*.

Nulsen, F.E. and Spitz, E.B. 1951: Treatment of hydrocephalus by direct shunt from ventricle to jugular vein. *Surgical Forum* **2**, 399–403.

Pudenz, R.H. and Russell, F.E., Hurd, A.H. *et al.* 1957: Ventriculo-auriculostomy. A technique for shunting cerebrospinal fluid into the right auricle. *Journal of Neurosurgery* **14**, 171–9.

Recklinghausen, F. Von 1886: Untersuchungen über die Spina Bifida. *Archives fur Pathologie und Anatomie* **105**, 243–373.

Renwick, J.H. 1972: Hypothesis: anencephaly and spina bifida are usually preventable by avoidance of a specific but unidentified substance present in certain potato tubers. *British Journal of Preventive and Social Medicine* **26**, 67–88.

Rickham P.P. and Mawdsley, T. 1966: The effect of early operation on the survival of spina bifida cystica. *Developmental Medicine and Child Neurology Suppl.* **2**, 20–6.

Sharrard, W.J.W., Zachary, R.B., Lobber, J. and Bruce A.M. 1963: A controlled trial of immediate and delayed closure in spina bifida cystica. *Archives of Disease in Childhood* **38**, 18–22.

Smith, G. Keys and Durham Smith, E. 1973: Selection for treatment in spina bifida cystica. *British Medical Journal* **ii**, 189–97.

Smithells, R.W. and Chinn, E.R. 1965: Spina bifida in Liverpool. *Developmental Medicine and Child Neurology* **7**, 258–68.

Smithells, R.W., Nevin, N.C., Sheppard, S. *et al.* 1983: Further experience of vitamin supplementation for prevention of neural tube defect recurrences. *Lancet* **i**, 1027–31.

Swinyard, C.A. 1966: *The child with spina bifida*. New York: Association for the Aid of Crippled Children.

Torkildsen, A. 1939: New palliative operation in cases of inoperable occlusion of the sylvian aqueduct. *Acta Chirurgica Scandinavica* **82**, 117–23.

UK Collaborative Study on Alpha-fetoprotein in Relation to Neural Tube Defects 1977: *Lancet* **i**, 1323–32.

Van Gool, J.D. and Van Gool, A.B. 1986: *A short history of spina bifida*. London: Society for Research into Hydrocephalus and Spina Bifida.

Williamson, E.M. 1965: Incidence and family aggregation of major congenital malformation of central nervous system. *Journal of Medical Genetics* **2**, 161–72.

CHAPTER 31

Ambiguous genitalia and intersex

I.A. HUGHES AND P. MALONE

Introduction
Embryology of sex development
Genetics of sex determination
Genetics and endocrinology of sex
differentiation
Causes of ambiguous genitalia

Causes of virilized females
Investigations
Gender assignment
Management
Long-term results
References

Introduction

Sex determination followed by sex differentiation (together known as sex development) is normally a staged sequence of events programmed at fertilization depending on whether the zygote is heterogametic (46XY) or homogametic (46XX). A simple format for this process is illustrated in Fig. 31.1, which depicts a pathway referred to as the Jost paradigm (Jost, 1970). This is derived from fetal castration experiments performed in rabbits followed by either testosterone replacement or testis regrafting. In the absence of a gonad (testis or ovary) and whatever the karyotype, a female phenotype differentiates. Testosterone replacement ensures normal male internal genital development on the ipsilateral side but also maintenance of female genital ducts. Only whole testis grafting produces ipsilaterally the presence of male and the absence of female internal genitalia. The pivotal role of the testis as an organ producing androgens for fetal virilization and another non-steroidal product (anti-Müllerian hormone, AMH) to cause regression of female development underpins the explanation in most instances of how ambiguous genitalia and intersex can arise.

Hermaphroditos, according to Greek mythology, was the son of Hermes and Aphrodite and achieved an inter-

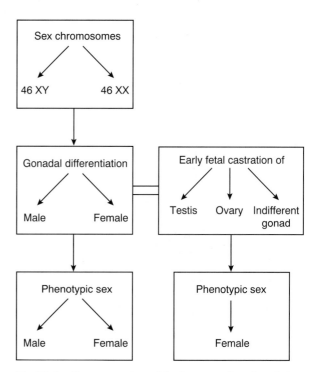

Fig. 31.1   Representation of the Jost paradigm in relation to sex development.

sex state on death by becoming joined in one body with the nymph Salmacis. Thus has the term hermaphrodite been coined to define an individual who possesses the germ cell elements (not just the stroma) of both a testis and an ovary. The prefices true and pseudo have traditionally been used to classify disorders of intersex, with male pseudohermaphroditism and female pseudo-hermaphroditism a confusing terminological outcome. Rather, this chapter adopts a functional classification of intersex based on causes of the virilized female and the undervirilized male. Hermaphroditism is retained for its true purpose.

The embryology, molecular genetics and endocrine control of normal sex development (Grumbach and Conte, 1992; Wachtel, 1993) are reviewed briefly in order to illustrate how, in the majority of instances, the causes of intersex can be readily explained. It is also noteworthy that the identification of a number of genes involved in sex development occurred as a result of careful investigation of patients with intersex disorders.

Embryology of sex development

The pathway of germ cell migration, the dual genital duct system and the common external genital anlagen are shown in Figs 31.2–4. The indifferent or primitive developing gonad is identical in early male and female embryos and develops as a thickened ridge of coelomic epithelium on the medial aspect of the mesonephros between 5 and 6 weeks of gestation.

This region is known as the genital ridge where a number of genes involved in testis determination are expressed at this stage in embryogenesis. Primordial germ cells originate in the extra-embryonic mesoderm at the base of the allantoic diverticulum near the caudal end of the primitive streak. They need to migrate from the yolk sac through the mesentery of the hind gut to the genital ridge. What signals the start and finish of this complex migratory route largely still remains unknown but growth factors and transcription factors appear to play a role. Some germ cells also migrate to the mesonephros or the developing fetal adrenal glands. Incorporation of

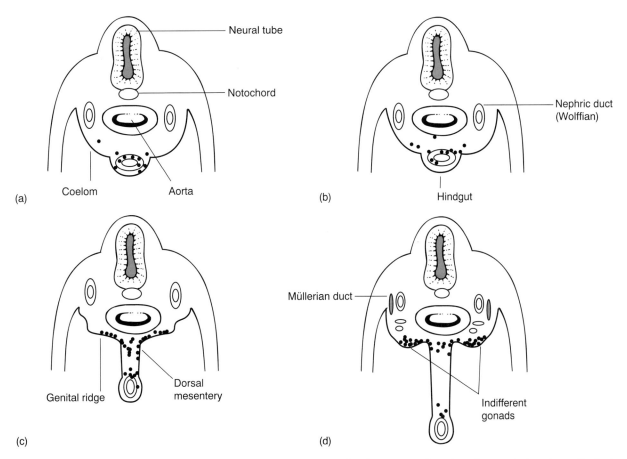

Fig. 31.2 Migration of germ cells from hindgut to the genital ridge. (Reproduced with permission from *Topical Endocrinology*, Issue 3.)

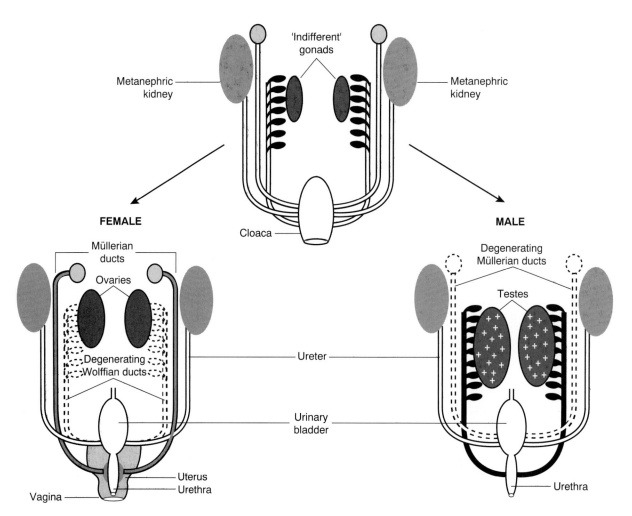

Fig. 31.3 Differentiation of the internal genital ducts. (Reproduced with permission from *Topical Endocrinology*, Issue 3.)

clumps of germ cells within surrounding somatic cells (precursors of Sertoli, Leydig and interstitial cells) of the genital ridge heralds the initial formation of the gonad. Expression of a number of testis-determining genes leads to formation of a testis from the indifferent gonad. The appearance of Sertoli cells and the formation of seminiferous cords form the first histological evidence of fetal testicular development. Interstitial cells outside the seminiferous cords develop later into Leydig cells which are responsible for synthesizing critical amounts of androgen necessary for the differentiation of male internal and external genitalia. The indifferent gonad appears to develop as an ovary in the absence of the influence of testis-determining genes (see later).

Histological evidence of development occurs later in the ovary and is characterized by primordial germ cells surrounded by supporting granulosa cells and thecal cells originating from the interstitial mesenchyme. Together, these cells form ovarian follicles which surround the oocytes. Primary oocytes are arrested in development during prophase of the first meiotic division and peak in number to 7 million at midgestation. The first meiotic division is not completed until ovulation (approximately 14 years later) and the second meiotic division occurs when the ovum is fertilized. The number of oocytes is reduced to 2 million by birth and to only 5% of the peak fetal numbers when puberty is reached. The process of oocyte atresia is considerably accelerated in Turner's syndrome.

The internal genitalia are represented initially as a dual duct system comprising the Wolffian and Müllerian ducts. Subsequent sex-specific differentiation of the ducts is dependent on the presence or absence of a testis. The Wolffian duct derives from the mesonephric tubules of the primitive kidney and under the influence of a high local concentration of testosterone develops into the vas deferens, epididymis and seminal vesicle. Metanephric tubules differentiate as the definitive kidney. The Müllerian ducts develop in parallel with the Wolffian ducts and give rise in the female to the

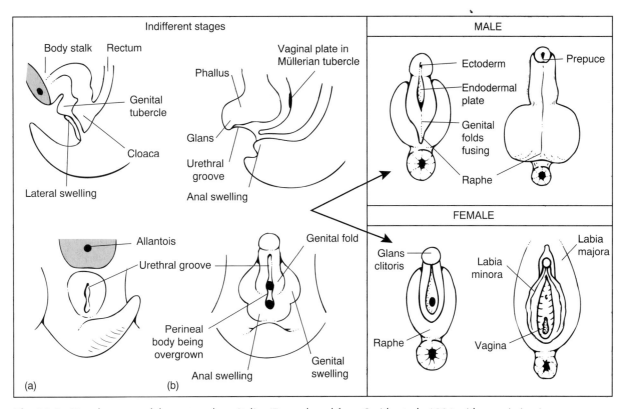

Fig. 31.4 Development of the external genitalia. (Reproduced from Smith *et al.*, 1984 with permission.)

Fallopian tubes, uterus and upper one-third of the vagina. Associated congenital malformations of the renal and genital tracts are not uncommon. Regression of Müllerian duct development in the male is mediated via AMH secreted by the Sertoli cells of the fetal testis and acting on its target receptor. The process starts at 8 weeks and is completed by 10 weeks of gestation.

The external genitalia develop from an anlage common to both sexes comprising the urogenital sinus, genital tubercle and swellings and urethral folds. The genital tubercle elongates in the male under the influence of androgens to form the penis and the urethral folds fuse ventrally to develop the penile urethra. The urogenital orifice migrates forwards to the tip of the developing penis. The scrotum is formed by posterior fusion of the labioscrotal folds. External genital differentiation in the male starts at 10 weeks and is completed by 16 weeks of gestation. At this stage the penis and clitoris are approximately a similar size but thereafter, penile length increases about ten-fold until term. Testicular descent occurs later in gestation and is described in Chapter 34. The genital tubercle bends caudally in the female and undergoes limited growth to form the clitoris. The genital swellings enlarge to form the labia majora which remain unfused except for posteriorly, where the fourchette is formed. The urethral folds form the labia minora. The urogenital sinus gives rise at the site of the Müllerian tubercle to the prostate gland in the male, while in the female it forms

the vestibule of the vagina. Development of the vagina by later canalization of the uterovaginal plate appears to be independent of hormones.

Genetics of sex determination

The study of 46XX males with testis formation in the absence of a Y chromosome was critical to the identification of the principal testis-determining gene. The explanation lies with translocation of Y chromosomal material adjacent to the pseudoautosomal region to the terminal part of the X chromosome during paternal meiosis (Affara *et al.*, 1986; Sinclair *et al.*, 1990). This Y chromosomal gene termed SRY (sex-determining region of the Y) encodes a protein which functions as a transcription factor and therefore influences other genes probably involved in gonadal determination. The majority of 46XX males are SRY positive. Other evidence for the role of SRY in testis determination is found in the study of 46XY females with pure gonadal dysgenesis in whom 10–15% of patients have mutations of the SRY gene. However, the molecular genetic explanation for the remaining majority of these patients remains unexplained. Further proof of the role of SRY came when sex reversal was induced in the mouse when the SRY mouse homologue was introduced into a female mouse embryo (Koopman *et al.*, 1991).

Table 31.1 Sex reversal and genes involved in testis determination

Syndrome	Gene	Chromosome
XX male, XY female	SRY	Y
Denys–Drash	WT-1	11
Campolmelic dysplasia	SOX9	17
Xp duplication	DSS locus	X

Table 31.1 details other syndromes associated with sex reversal (either complete or partial) and the genes which are now implicated in testis determination as a result of their study. How these gene products interrelate to one another when expressed in the genital ridge remains unclear. The Wilms' tumour protein (WT-1) gene is expressed in the fetal kidney, genital ridge and fetal gonad and is expressed earlier than SRY in the genital ridge. The WT-1 protein contains zinc finger structures which bind to DNA in order to manifest its function as a transcription factor. Mutations of the WT-1 gene give rise to the Denys–Drash syndrome, which is characterized by a glomerulosclerotic nephropathy, Wilm's tumour and genital anomalies (Pelletier *et al.*, 1991). In an affected XY male, there may be complete sex reversal or an intersex phenotype.

Sex reversal is a feature of the rare skeletal disorder, camptomelic dysplasia (Houston *et al.*, 1983). The study of one such 46XY patient with a translocation involving the long arm of chromosome 17 led to the isolation of a gene which has homology to the SRY gene. The gene is part of the SOX family of genes, so-called because the protein contains an HMG box (conserved amino acid motif of a high mobility group) which is also shared by SRY (hence SRY-like HMG-box). A large family of SOX genes has been identified as being involved in developmental regulation and SOX9 is attributed a role in testis determination. Mutations in SOX9 have been reported in camptomelic dysplasia (Wagner *et al.*, 1994; Kwok *et al.*, 1995). Complete XY sex reversal or isolated hypospadias can be the clinical outcome of the same SOX9 mutation. Such diversity in phenotype expression is not unusual in single gene disorders of sex development.

The steroidogenic factor-1 (SF-1) gene encodes a nuclear transcription factor which is involved in the regulation of adrenal and gonadal steroidogenesis but in addition, has a developmental role in the hypothalamus (Ingraham *et al.*, 1994). Targeted disruption of this gene in the mouse results in absent adrenals and gonads but preservation of Müllerian structures in either sex. Formation of the ventromedial nucleus of the hypothalamus is impaired and pituitary gonadotrophins are deficient. No human homologue of this phenotype has been identified yet but these studies illustrate an important role for SF-1 in sex development. As in the case of

WT-1, the SF-1 gene is expressed before SRY in the genital ridge and both genes may interplay with SRY in repressing ovarian development.

It has been assumed that the panoply of sex-determining genes is involved in testis determination only and ovarian development is just the result of a default pathway. This is clearly not the case, as exemplified by XO individuals. Furthermore, complete sex reversal can occur in 46XY individuals who have duplications of part of the short arm of the X chromosome (Bardorni *et al.*, 1994). In the presence of an intact SRY gene, this suggests that two active copies of an X-linked gene can override the effect of SRY and other known testis-determining genes. The dosage-sensitive sex reversal (DSS) locus on Xp21 spans a region containing a number of genes which when deleted in males gives rise to a contiguous gene deletion syndrome characterized by congenital adrenal hypoplasia, hypogonadotrophic hypogonadism, mental retardation, glycerol kinase deficiency and Duchenne muscular dystrophy. The combination of adrenal hypoplasia and gonadotrophin deficiency is a syndrome caused by mutations in a gene contained within the Xp21 locus. This gene is labelled DAX-1, standing for DSS, AHC (adrenal hypoplasia congenita) on the X chromosome, gene 1. It is likely that DAX-1 is the candidate DSS gene and when duplicated in males is able to inhibit the male pathway of sex development.

Another genetic control mechanism essential for early male sex development is the regression of Müllerian structures. A Sertoli cell peptide, AMH, mediates this process via mesenchymal cells surrounding the epithelium of the Müllerian duct during a short period of AMH sensitivity lasting up to 8 weeks of gestation. AMH is a member of the transforming growth factor-β family and binds to a specific serine/threonine kinase receptor. Serum levels of AMH are high in male fetuses during the second trimester, rise again during early infancy and fall gradually towards puberty. Measurement of serum AMH can be a useful marker of the presence of testicular tissue. Surgeons are long familiar with the persistence of Müllerian structures found rarely in some males explored for undescended testes. This syndrome is now explained in most cases by the presence of mutations which are identified either in the AMH gene or (when serum AMH levels are normal or elevated) in the AMH receptor gene (Josse *et al.*, 1997).

Genetics and endocrinology of sex differentiation

In the male, sex differentiation is dependent on a high local concentration of fetal testosterone in early gestation for Wolffian duct development and the conversion of testosterone to dihydrotestosterone (DHT) in the genital anlage to amplify the androgen signal for external male genital differentiation. Leydig cells become differentiated in early gestation, possibly autonomously at first, but primarily under the influence of placental human chorionic gonadotrophin (HCG) as a trophic factor. Later in gestation, fetal pituitary luteinizing hormone (LH) secretion maintains testosterone production to promote growth of the phallus and a further high local concentration of testosterone to enable the testes to descend into the scrotum by term.

The pathways of androgen biosynthesis and metabolism are illustrated in Fig. 31.5, which also indicates the enzymes and their cognate genes. The critical steps required to generate androgen production sufficient for adequate masculinization include signal transduction via the LH receptor, provision of cholesterol substrate for initiating steroidogenesis, conversion of Δ^5 to Δ^4 steroids by 3β-hydroxysteroid dehydrogenase, 17α-hydroxylation of precursor steroids and their conversion by lyase activity to weak androgens, and finally the conversion to testosterone by one of the isoenzymes of 17α-hydroxysteroid dehydrogenase. Type III isoenzyme is preferentially expressed in the testis but some peripheral conversion of androstenedione to testosterone takes place through action of the type II isoenzyme. The placenta and ovary are the preferential sites of expression of the type I isoenzyme.

Testosterone is a prohormone for both an androgen of greater biological activity (DHT) and an oestrogen through the action of the aromatase enzyme complex. In both instances, the conversions are irreversible. Type II isoenzyme of 5α-reductase is expressed early in androgen-dependent tissues and is critical in the male for external genital development and formation of the prostate. In adult life, DHT appears to be the principal androgen which causes androgenetic alopecia in genetically prone males. Oestrogens are formed by aromatization of androgen substrate in the ovary, placenta, skin and adipose tissue. Their role in morphological fetal sex development is unclear, although the fetus is exposed to large amounts of oestrogen throughout pregnancy.

The action of testosterone, as well as DHT and other androgens, is mediated via binding of the steroid to an intracellular protein which forms part of a large superfamily of ligand-activated nuclear transcription factors (Tsai and O'Malley, 1994). Thus all steroid receptors, thyroid hormone and retinoic acid receptors belong to this class of transcription factors. They share a protein structure which comprises an amino-terminal domain involved in transcriptional activation, a carboxy-terminal domain primarily involved in ligand binding and a central domain which mediates binding of the hormone–receptor complex to DNA. The central domain is conserved throughout the nuclear receptor family and is characterized by two zinc finger motifs which are involved in linking with helix grooves in DNA. The protein structure is similar to the WT-1 and DAX-1

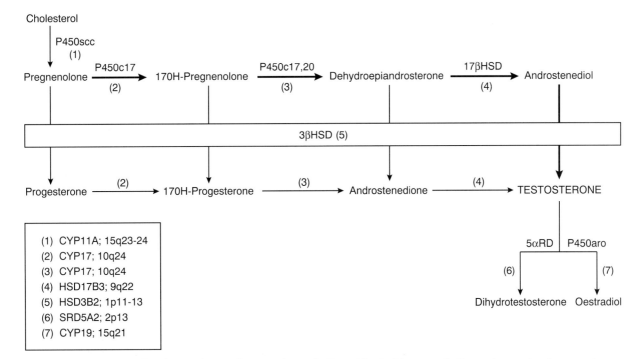

Fig. 31.5 Pathways of androgen biosynthesis and metabolism. The bold arrows indicate the predominant pathway, using Δ^5-steroids as substrates. The inset details the relevant genes and their chromosomal locations.

proteins, previously described as transcription factors relevant for testis determination. The androgen receptor is thus a vital final link in the chain of events leading to normal sex development. Since the receptor acts as a transcription factor, all the known biological events of androgen action (sex differentiation, skeletal and muscle growth, erythropoiesis, growth of sexual hair, voice breaking and male pattern baldness) must be mediated by the products of androgen responsive genes. Nowhere is this more vividly illustrated than by the complete androgen insensitivity syndrome, a paradigm of hormone resistance, when an affected XY individual with testes and normal androgen production and metabolism is completely sex reversed and has a normal female phenotype apart from absent or scanty pubic and axillary hair. The pathway of male sex development detailing the important genetic control points is summarized in Fig. 31.6.

Causes of ambiguous genitalia

THE UNDERVIRILIZED MALE

Reference to Figs 31.5 and 31.6 indicates a multitude of potential causes which may give rise to undervirilization. This can either be complete so that the phenotype is female and there is no intersex problem *per se*, or of

Table 31.2   Causes of the undervirilized male

Testicular dysgenesisidysplasia
  True hermaphroditism
  Mixed gonadal dysgenesis
  Klinefelter's syndrome
  Pure and partial XY gonadal dysgenesis

Defects in androgen production and metabolism
  Leydig cell aplasia or hypoplasia
  Steroidogenic enzyme defects
  5α-Reductase deficiency

Defects in androgen action
  Complete androgen insensitivity syndrome
  Partial androgen insensitivity syndrome

Miscellaneous
  Syndromal complex (e.g. Smith–Lemli–Optiz, Beckwith–Weidemann, Denys–Drash)
  Isolated hypospadias
  Possible environmental toxins (e.g. xenobiotics, anti-androgens)

partial degree, resulting in a wide variety of phenotype from either isolated hypospadias or isolated micropenis to a clitoral-like phallus with perineal hypospadias and minimal labial fusion. A similar appearance of the external genitalia can be produced by many different causes. Table 31.2 classifies the causes into three main broad categories. Each group is subdivided into examples of causes for which the list is not exhaustive.

TESTICULAR DYSGENESIS OR DYSPLASIA

This is often used as an all-embracing term to represent an abnormality in testis development and consequently in function. Insufficient fetal androgen production manifests as failure of Wolffian duct and particularly, external genital development. Incomplete Müllerian duct regression is the consequence of insufficient AMH production at the critical period in embryogenesis. The third component of the testis, germ cell function, is invariably absent. Assessing testicular function in postnatal life provides only indirect evidence of the cause but an HCG stimulation test to assess Leydig cell reserve and histological examination of a testicular biopsy are the minimum requirements to classify an intersex case into the broad category of testicular dysgenesis.

Since a panoply of testis-determining genes is now being identified, it is not surprising that testicular dysgenesis may arise as a result of defects of genes involved in developmental regulation. A prime example is a deleterious mutation in the SRY gene which results in pure XY gonadal dysgenesis. Nevertheless, only a minority of such patients have an SRY gene mutation so that other testis-determining genetic abnormalities

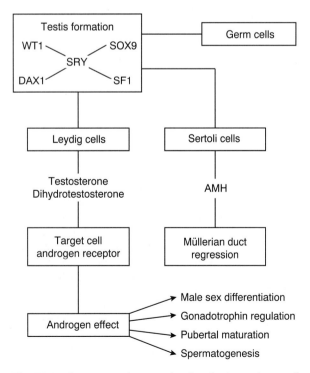

Fig. 31.6   Some genetic control points in the pathway of male sex development.

remain to be identified to explain both the pure and partial forms of XY gonadal dysgenesis. Sex chromosome abnormalities must also be considered within this group. These include mixed gonadal dysgenesis (45XO/46XY), true hermaphroditism (46XX/XY mosaicism as well as 46XX and 46XY karyotypes) and Klinefelter's syndrome (47XXY). The degree of undervirilization can vary considerably among these syndromes. In mixed gonadal dysgenesis, for example, penile growth is often normal but a severe hypospadias requires correcting. Short stature is also an accompanying feature in later life. Klinefelter's syndrome is seldom associated with hypospadias, small testes being the characteristic feature in later life owing to seminiferous tubule dysgenesis. In most gonadal dysgenesis cases associated with Y chromosomal genetic material, there is the risk of gonadal neoplasia in adult life which should be considered when planning surgical management (Savage and Lowe, 1990).

DEFECTS IN ANDROGEN PRODUCTION AND METABOLISM

Reference to Fig. 31.5 indicates which enzymatic steps are critical for adequate androgen production. Complete 46XY sex reversal is the phenotypic expression of the failure to transport cholesterol across the inner mitochondrial membrane and also when the defect is associated with failure to 17α-hydroxylate precursor steroids. The former disorder has been recognized indirectly for many years because of the accumulation of lipid, particularly in the adrenal glands, and is known as congenital lipoid adrenal hyperplasia (Bonette *et al.*, 1964). A P450 enzyme, required for side-chain cleavage in order to convert cholesterol to pregnenolone, is encoded by the CYP11A gene on chromosome 15q and was initially thought to be deficient in this disorder. All studies to date have shown no mutation in the CYP11A gene (Fukami *et al.*, 1995). However, a protein required for cholesterol transport (steroidogenic acute regulatory protein, StAR) is non-functional in lipoid adrenal hyperplasia (Lin *et al.*, 1995). The defect is shared by the adrenals and gonads but not by the placenta. A complete female phenotype also occurs in a 46XY male with 17α-hydroxylation deficiency. The enzymatic reaction is also required in adrenal steroidogenesis except for mineralocorticoid synthesis. Hypertension thus occurs in later life through excess production of deoxycorticosterone, a potent mineralocorticoid.

The remaining defects in androgen biosynthesis and metabolism give rise phenotypically to varying degrees of undervirilization of the external genitalia. 17α-Hydroxylation of precursors is followed by a lyase reaction which cleaves the C17–20 carbon bond to form androgen substrates. The same enzyme, encoded by a CYP17 gene on chromosome 10, catalyses both reactions. When only 17,20-lyase deficiency occurs, an affected male has a micropenis and severe hypospadias. Similar phenotypes occur with deficiencies of each of the 3β-hydroxysteroid dehydrogenase (Simard *et al.*, 1993), 17α-hydroxysteroid dehydrogenase (Geissler *et al.*, 1994) and 5α-reductase enzyme reactions (Wilson *et al.*, 1993). Only 3β-hydroxysteroid dehydrogenase deficiency also affects the adrenals so that signs of cortisol and aldosterone deficiency are accompanying features. Sometimes, the undervirilization in all three enzyme defects is so severe at birth that an apparent normal female is raised as a girl only to develop signs of virilization (enlarged clitoris, deepening of voice, hirsutism, muscular build) at puberty. This phenomenon is attributed to a combination of residual enzyme activity stimulated by pubertal LH concentrations and substrate use of isoenzymes unaffected by deleterious mutations. For example, the 5α-reductase enzyme which converts testosterone to the more active androgen DHT is expressed in two isoforms: type I isoenzyme, encoded by a gene on chromosome 2, is present in liver and skin but is not fully expressed until puberty, whereas the type II isoenzyme is expressed during fetal life in androgen-dependent tissues and is encoded by a gene on chromosome 5. The syndrome of 5α-reductase deficiency, as reported in a large inbred population in the Dominican Republic, is due to mutations only affecting the type II isoenzyme (Peterson *et al.*, 1977). Affected individuals are typically raised female but have profound virilization at puberty so that in this culture gender change is undertaken. Inbred populations affected by 5α-reductase deficiency are also reported in Pakistan and New Guinea as well as isolated cases. Expression of type I isoenzyme activity at puberty as well as some residual type II isoenzyme activity is a plausible explanation for virilization at puberty. Those electing to remain male generally do not have breast development (in contrast to partial androgen insensitivity), the prostate remains small and spermatogenesis is seldom normal.

The production of androgens by the testis is dependent initially on trophic stimulation by LH acting via a transmembrane receptor coupled to G proteins to initiate signal transduction via adenylyl cyclase. Leydig cell hypoplasia has long been recognized as a histological entity associated with complete or incomplete virilization in an affected male (Bertezène *et al.*, 1976). Indirect evidence suggested an abnormality in the LH receptor based on cell membrane binding studies. The precise defect is now recognized to be inactivating mutations affecting the LH receptor gene (Kremer *et al.*, 1995). Affected 46XY cases are usually phenotypic females but partial virilization and even isolated micropenis are described. Intriguingly, mutations affecting other parts of the LH receptor molecule can be activating in nature and result in a syndrome of familial male-limited precocious puberty (Kremer *et al.*, 1993).

DEFECTS IN ANDROGEN ACTION

A state of hormone resistance is defined by the absence of a biological response despite the production and transport to target tissues of normal or increased concentrations of the trophic hormone. The resistance may be absolute and complete or some partial responsiveness may occur. The latter biological response with respect to androgens results in a relatively large number of 46XY intersex cases in whom a diagnosis of partial androgen insensitivity is considered a possibility. The disorder is expressed in the hemizygous state (XY individuals affected), there is no shortening of the lifespan in affected individuals and several natural animal models of the disorder exist (Batch *et al.*, 1992).

The complete form of androgen insensitivity syndrome (CAIS) in humans also referred to as testicular feminization, typically presents as primary amenorrhoea in an adolescent female. Breast development is normal, whereas pubic and axillary hair growth is absent or scanty. The external genitalia are female but the vagina is usually shorter than normal and blind-ending. There are no female internal genitalia because of normal AMH action from the fetal testis. The testes are usually intra-abdominal but may present as swellings within inguinal herniae. The karyotype is 46XY and adult patients are taller than normal females. The differential diagnosis in the completely sex-reversed XY female is limited to pure gonadal dysgenesis, 17α-hydroxylase deficiency and Leydig cell hypoplasia. Concentrations of LH and testosterone are increased while follicle-stimulating hormone (FSH) levels are usually normal. A HCG stimulation test may be required to exclude Leydig cell hypoplasia. CAIS is generally only recognized before puberty if the testes herniate as inguinal swellings, usually in early infancy. Bilateral inguinal herniae are unusual in girls so the karyotype should always be checked in such cases. Because of the X-linked inheritance, a history of surgery for bilateral herniae in an older sister hitherto unrecognized as having CAIS is relatively common. A biopsy should be performed when in doubt about the macroscopic nature of a gonad-containing hernia.

The partial form of androgen insensitivity syndrome (PAIS) usually presents with intersex in the newborn. The appearance of the external genitalia typically shows perineoscrotal hypospadias, a bifid scrotum, micropenis with chordee and testes which may be cryptorchid. Such a phenotype may also be identified in a 46XY infant with any one of the numerous disorders which lead to undervirilization (Table 31.2). The plasma testosterone and DHT, and urinary androgen metabolize response to HCG stimulation will usually exclude a defect in androgen biosynthesis or metabolism. Testicular dysgenesis is ultimately a histological diagnosis, although the presence of Müllerian duct remnants suggests that category of causes. The spectrum of genital abnormalities in PAIS can be wide, ranging from almost a CAIS phenotype with just isolated clitoromegaly to an otherwise normal male with an isolated hypospadias (Batch *et al.*, 1993b).

The androgen receptor is encoded by a gene on the long arm of the X chromosome and is expressed in many tissues including skin fibroblasts. Androgens bind with higher affinity to fibroblasts grown from genital as compared with non-genital skin (Evans *et al.*, 1984). Saturation analysis of androgen receptor binding using radiolabelled androgen provides a measure of binding affinity and the receptor concentration. Androgen binding to genital skin fibroblasts is usually undetectable or extremely low in CAIS. In the case of PAIS, androgen binding is usually detectable but the binding affinity is abnormal. Occasionally, androgen binding is normal in fibroblasts from a CAIS patient, and quite often in a patient with PAIS. The results of androgen binding assays in genital skin fibroblasts provide a useful pointer as to which functional domain of the androgen receptor is likely to be affected by a mutation (Fig. 31.7).

In common with other members of the large superfamily of nuclear receptor transcription factors, the androgen receptor is subdivided into three functional domains encoded by eight exons labelled A to H, as in Fig. 31.7. Absent androgen binding or altered binding affinity is associated with mutations which affect the C-terminal hormone binding domain of the receptor (Patterson *et al.*, 1994b). Most are point mutations resulting in amino acid substitutions. A number of mutations in the first exon which encodes the N-terminal domain has been described which produce frame-shift and premature stop codons resulting in the synthesis of a truncated receptor. Such mutations are usually characterized by decreased or absent androgen binding in patients with the CAIS phenotype. Mutations causing androgen insensitivity are distributed throughout the gene and now number more than 150 novel examples (Patterson *et al.*, 1994a). Several interesting mutations have been described involving exons B and C which encode the zinc finger binding motifs of the DNA binding domain. Since the hormone binding domain is unaffected, androgen binding in genital skin fibroblasts is normal.

The functional consequences of mutations are important to assess in order to determine whether it is possible to predict responsiveness to androgens, particularly at puberty. A mutant receptor can be re-created *in vitro*, linked to a reporter gene, the expression of which in this case can be controlled by increasing concentrations of androgen. In such a study of mutations identified in patients with PAIS (Bevan *et al.*, 1996), some mutant receptors were able to respond to high doses of androgen *in vitro* and this correlated with the clinical response *in vivo*. One PAIS patient with a mutation in the hormone binding domain virilized spontaneously at

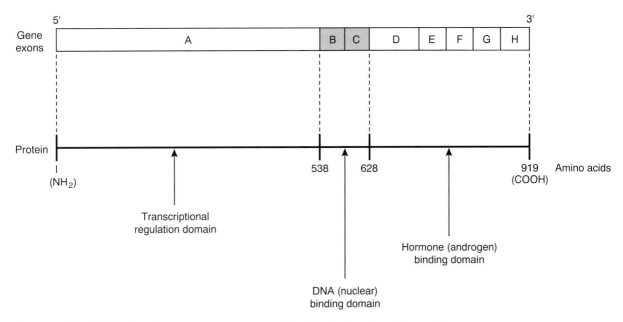

Fig. 31.7 The X-linked androgen receptor gene and functional domains of the protein.

puberty. The mutant and normal receptors responded almost identically to androgen stimulation *in vitro*. In contrast, other mutant receptors showed no response even when stimulated by supraphysiological concentrations of androgens. Patients harbouring such mutations tended to be more undervirilized and were raised as females. Such complex *in vitro* tests do not yet offer an early predictive test of androgen responsiveness for the neonate with a PAIS phenotype but further analysis of long-term outcome in patients raised as males should provide useful information concerning the biological consequences of different mutant receptors. Some promise has been shown with the use of sex hormone-binding globulin measurements (Sinnecker and Köhler, 1989). Exogenous androgens induce a fall in concentrations in normal males, while no change is observed in patients with CAIS. However, the response to androgens is variable in patients with PAIS, which is the subgroup in whom a clearcut difference from normals could be of practical benefit. However, this could be combined with the more pragmatic approach of a 2–3-month course of androgen currently used by many clinicians before taking a final decision on the sex of rearing. Since androgen insensitivity syndrome is an X-linked recessive disorder, knowledge of the mutation in an index case may be used for subsequent prenatal diagnosis and carrier detection (Hughes and Patterson, 1994). It is important to realize that phenotypic variability in the expression of a particular mutation in PAIS, both intra- and inter-familial, can pose difficulties in predicting outcome (Batch *et al.*, 1993). Furthermore, it should be noted that approximately 30% of mutations arise *de novo*.

MISCELLANEOUS CAUSES

A number of syndromes associated with genital anomalies has already been mentioned in relation to the identification of testis-determining genes. Other syndromes which can pose problems of intersex as well as other system disorders include Smith–Lemli–Opitz, Beckwith–Weidemann and unclassified malformation syndromes. There remains a large group of 46XY infants with ambiguous genitalia where the phenotype is compatible with PAIS and in whom all relevant investigations appear to have excluded an underlying cause. These are usually isolated cases but when a first-born child is affected this poses added problems of counselling in relation to future pregnancies. A comprehensive mutation screen of all known genes involved in sex development is desirable but not entirely practical in such cases. Selective mutation screening can only be undertaken when clinical, biochemical and histological investigation has been undertaken appropriately.

Minor genital anomalies such as simple hypospadias, isolated small penis or undescended testes are not generally classified as intersex problems. However, their study may provide useful information concerning the increasing incidence of male urogenital abnormalities, including testicular cancer and declining sperm counts (Sharpe and Skakkebaek, 1993). Consequently, the increasing evidence for oestrogenic and anti-androgenic biological effects from environmental toxins perhaps having some adjunctive role in the aetiology of genital anomalies should not be ignored (de Kretser, 1996).

Causes of virilized females

Sex differentiation is normal in 46XX females who have virilization confined only to the external genitalia. Wolffian duct development does not occur (presumably because androgen excess occurs later in embryogenesis) and Müllerian ducts differentiate normally in the absence of fetal testicular AMH secretion. The presence of normal female internal genitalia, even when the virilized external genitalia have a male appearance, is an observation of fundamental importance for sex of rearing and predicting the outlook for fertility in adult life. Table 31.3 lists causes of virilization in female infants; the congenital adrenal hyperplasias comprise by far the most common group of disorders causing intersex in general (Walker and Hughes, 1994).

Congenital adrenal hyperplasia (CAH) is a family of autosomal recessive disorders and characterized by adrenocorticotropic hormone (ACTH)-induced hyperplasia of the adrenal cortex during fetal life as a result of primary cortisol deficiency. The pathways of adrenal steroid biosynthesis, the key enzymes involved and their cognate genes are illustrated in Figs 31.8 and 31.9.

A deficiency of 21-hydroxylase enzyme activity accounts for more than 90% of the causes of CAH. The

Table 31.3   Causes of virilization in female infants

Increased fetal androgens
  Congenital adrenal hyperplasias
  Persistent fetal adrenal steroidogenesis
  Placental aromatase deficiency

Increased maternal androgens
  Ovarian androgen-secreting tumours
  Adrenal androgen-secreting tumours
  Ingestion of progestational agents

Miscellaneous
  Isolated idiopathic clitoromegaly
  Clitoromegaly in neurofibromatosis
  Isolated labial fusion

clinical hallmark is virilization of the external genitalia in an affected female infant due to increased adrenal androgen production. The severity may range from mild isolated clitoromegaly or isolated labial fusion to marked clitoromegaly resembling a penis, scrotalization of the labia and the formation of a penile urethra. In this situation, the newborn infant may be mistaken for a 'male' with undescended testes. The affected male

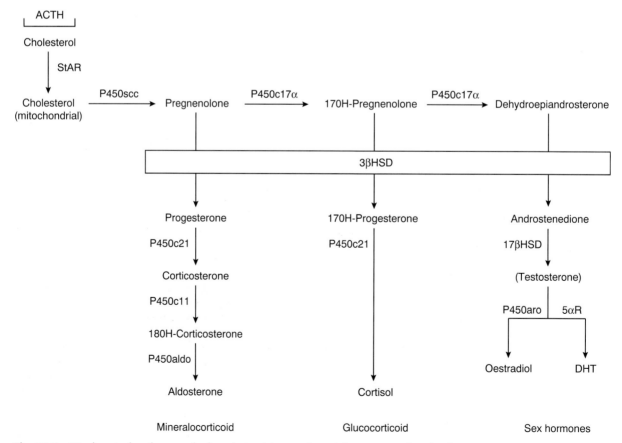

Fig. 31.8   Biochemical pathways of adrenal steroidogenesis and the enzymes involved.

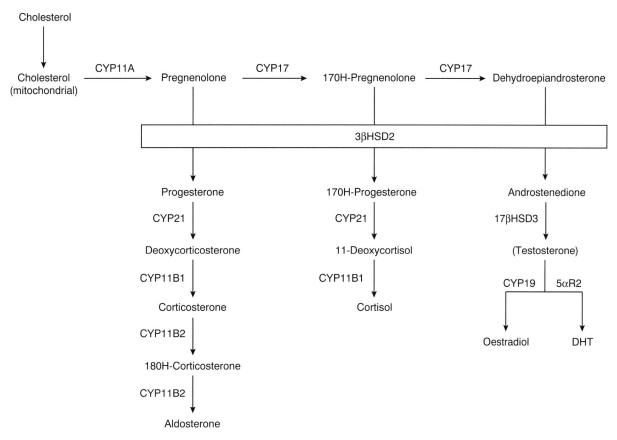

Fig. 31.9 Pathways of adrenal steroidogenesis indicating genetic control.

has normal genitalia at birth apart from the occasional increase in scrotal skin pigmentation. At least 75% of all 21-hydroxylase deficient infants have an associated defect in aldosterone synthesis. This manifests clinically in its most severe form as an acute salt-wasting state during the second or third week of life. Early biochemical features are hypokalaemia and increased urinary sodium excretion before the plasma sodium concentration starts to fall. The most sensitive index of mineralocorticoid insufficiency is an elevated plasma renin activity, and hypoglycaemia may also occur with an adrenal salt-wasting crisis. The affected male salt loser may be mistaken for having pyloric stenosis. The latter disorder, when associated with prolonged vomiting, is characterized biochemically by a hypokalaemic alkalosis rather than the hyperkalaemic acidosis, hyponatraemia and azotaemia characteristic of the CAH infant in severe salt-losing crisis.

Approximately 5% of CAH cases result from a deficiency of the 11β-hydroxylase enzyme. Virilization tends to be more severe than in the 21-hydroxylase defect. Salt wasting does not occur since increased production of deoxycorticosterone, the potent mineralocorticoid, compensates for aldosterone deficiency.

Hypertension eventually occurs in the untreated state. A mild degree of virilization occurs in a female infant with 3β-hydroxysteroid dehydrogenase deficiency due to increased production of dehydroepiandrosterone, which is a weak androgen. The infant with severe enzyme deficiency will also be a salt loser. Males with CAH due to either 21-hydroxylase or 11β-hydroxylase enzyme deficiencies are not virilized at birth, despite plasma concentrations of testosterone which may fall within the normal adult male range. There is no ready explanation for this apparent paradox.

Virilized external genitalia in an infant with 46XX karyotype are invariably due to CAH. The diagnosis is clinched by documenting elevated concentrations of 17OH-progesterone, which can be determined in plasma, filter paper blood spot or saliva specimens. Caution should be exercised with the interpretation of results in sick preterm infants without adrenal disease who may have elevated levels of 17OH-progesterone as a result of an adrenal response to stress. In the case of 11β-hydroxylase deficiency, the specific marker is an elevated plasma 11-deoxycortisol concentration (see Fig. 31.8). A number of precursor steroid levels are elevated in 3β-hydroxysteroid dehydrogenase deficiency, but the most specific marker is 17OH-pregnenolone. A change from the fetal to an adult pattern of adrenal steroid secretion can be delayed in some preterm infants so that Δ^5 steroids are persistently elevated. These produce weak androgens which may cause isolated and transient clitoromegaly in a preterm female infant.

Other causes of a virilized female infant, as listed in Table 31.3, are extremely uncommon. Placental aromatase deficiency is an interesting rare disorder which highlights the normal function of the maternal–fetoplacental steroid unit in providing a system for oestrogen production and a mechanism to protect against the effect of androgens produced by the fetal adrenals which, although of weak potency, are produced in large amounts.

Androgens are prohormones for oestrogen production utilizing the cytochrome P450 aromatase enzyme complex. A single enzyme is widely expressed in the ovary, testis, placenta, adipose tissue, skin and brain, with the specificity of tissue expression controlled by tissue-specific gene promoters. The most abundant source of aromatase is the placental syncytiotrophoblast. With placental aromatase deficiency, both the mother and a female fetus can be virilized as a result of the excess fetal adrenal androgens not being aromatized to oestrogens. Adequate oestrogen synthesis during embryogenesis is clearly required neither for sex differentiation nor for fetal survival.

Investigations

The problem of intersex at birth is a matter for urgent investigation. There is no place for guesswork in deciding the sex of the infant and registration of the birth must be delayed until a decision has been made on the sex of rearing. A multidisciplinary team is required to manage these infants and their families adequately and should consist of experts in neonatology, endocrinology, surgery, genetics, biochemistry and ideally a nurse specialist who can counsel and support the families through the difficult and upsetting times that lie ahead.

The aims of investigation are to establish a precise diagnosis (but it must be understood that this is not always possible) and to establish criteria for deciding on the most appropriate sex of rearing. The most important initial investigation is the peripheral karyotype and a provisional result is generally available within 48–72 hours.

Investigation of the virilized female is far more straightforward than for the undervirilized male and the results are available sooner. Measurement of a plasma 17OH-progesterone concentration is now routinely available and is the investigation of first choice in view of the frequency of 21-hydroxylase deficiency. Samples should also be saved for measurement of other steroids such as 11-deoxycortisol and 17OH-pregnenolone if that

becomes necessary. Chromatographic analysis of urinary steroid metabolites is a useful adjunct to plasma steroid measurements, particularly in the rarer enzyme defects. Occasionally, the cause of virilization (especially in isolated clitoromegaly) is not established but investigations in that case should also include examining the mother for a maternal source of androgens.

Once the karyotype has been established in the undervirilized male, the investigations listed in Table 31.4 should be followed. The HCG stimulation test is of paramount importance and preferably should be undertaken in early infancy when Leydig cells are active. Numerous protocols for the test are in existence but a useful option is described in Table 31.4. Collection of appropriate samples and distribution to relevant laboratories can assure the success or otherwise of establishing a precise diagnosis. In the undervirilized male it is vital to identify the internal genital structures and locate the gonads. Ultrasound is useful in this respect and can also identify any associated renal tract anomalies. Laparoscopy is increasingly used and provides an opportunity to obtain samples for histological examination. When genital reconstructive surgery is undertaken, this is an opportunity to obtain a genital skin biopsy to establish a fibroblast cell line for androgen binding studies. The cells are also a source for DNA and RNA for molecular studies which can complement results obtained by extracting DNA from blood samples.

In both the undervirilized male and the virilized female it is important to delineate the lower genitourinary anatomy prior to reconstructive surgery. For these purposes a sinogram and cystoscopy are helpful particularly with reference to the relationship of the external sphincter mechanism and the junction of the vagina with the urethra.

Table 31.4 Investigations in the undervirilized male

Biochemical	LHRH stimulation test
	Testosterone, LH, FSH
	HCG stimulation test[a]
	17OH-progesterone
	Androstenedione
	Testosterone
	Dehydroepiandrosterone
	Urinary androgen metabolites
Radiological	Pelvic ultrasound
	Sinogram (vaginogram)
Genetic	Peripheral karyotype
	Genital skin biopsy for RNA source
	Blood for DNA analysis

[a]1500 units daily for 3 days; samples collected on days 1 and 4.

Gender assignment

The decision regarding the sex of rearing in a virilized female investigated in infancy should never be in doubt, even in the most severely virilized infants (Whitaker, 1991). As the internal genitalia and ovaries are normal, the outlook for fertility, given adequate steroid replacement and surgical correction, is potentially normal. These patients should be reared as girls. There are still recorded examples of severely virilized female infants with CAH who have been raised male and the diagnosis not established until late childhood or adolescence. In these circumstances, sex reversal may not be appropriate and surgery is planned for removal of the ovaries and Müllerian structures.

Gender assignment in the undervirilized male is more complicated. The decision is linked closely to the functional anatomy of the external genitalia, the nature of the surgical procedures required, the underlying cause (if established) and whether useful information has been obtained from a trial of androgen treatment. The latter may be given in the form of a course of 25–50 mg Sustanon as monthly injections over 3 months. The surgeon is best able to judge whether the technical problems in correcting a severe defect in growth and differentiation of the penis and scrotum can be overcome. An assessment of the penile body and glans size is an important factor. Nomograms of penile size are available and measurements are made of the stretched penis from the pubic symphysis to the tip of the glans (Lee *et al.*, 1980). At term, the normal penile length is 3.5 ± 0.4 cm. If severe chordee is present a measurement of the diameter is helpful with the normal at term being 1.0–1.5 cm. If the length $\times$ diameter of the penis is less than 2.0×0.9 cm it is in a grey area and a trial of androgen treatment will be helpful. If the length $\times$ diameter is less than 1.5×0.7 cm there is little hope of producing a sexually functional penis and a gender reassignment is generally advised (Savage, 1982). Even in these circumstances a trial of androgen therapy may be useful to help convince parents of the need for sex reversal. It is important that the parents are actively involved in the decision making of gender assignment and they should be comfortable with the ultimate decision that is reached.

Management

The management of all patients with ambiguous genitalia requires the co-ordinated efforts of a paediatric endocrinologist and an experienced surgeon.

As CAH is an autosomal recessive disorder there is a 25% chance of subsequent children being affected. Prenatal diagnosis is possible using a number of methods, including DNA analysis, HLA haplotyping and measurement of steroid concentrations in amniotic fluid (Hughes *et al.*, 1987; Strachan, 1990). Virilization of an affected female fetus can be prevented by giving dexamethasone to the mother. Treatment needs to start as early as 6–7 weeks' gestation and hence before the diagnosis can be made. The appropriate diagnostic tests can be performed at 10–12 weeks' gestation by chorion villus biopsy or at 16 weeks by amniocentesis when treatment can be discontinued in an unaffected female or an affected male fetus. The prevention of virilization is not always total but subsequent surgery is always less than in the untreated case. There is no evidence that such prenatal treatment has any harmful effects on the fetus (Levine and Pang, 1994; Wudy *et al.*, 1994).

All patients require lifelong hydrocortisone replacement and as the majority are salt losers mineralocorticoids are also needed. Treatment needs to be closely monitored by a paediatric endocrinologist. Increased dosages are required when patients undergo surgery. It is important to recognize that mineralocorticoids cannot be administered parenterally and if enteral feeding is disrupted fluid and electrolyte balance needs to be carefully managed.

It is not the purpose of this book to provide a detailed description of the operative procedures used, but the general principles will be discussed. Excellent descriptions of these procedures are provided elsewhere (Passerini-Glazel, 1989; Gustafson and Donahoe, 1995).

The principles of surgical correction in the virilized female are as follows:

- Clitoral reduction: the glans clitoris is mobilized off the corpora cavernose, preserving the two neurovascular bundles. The corpora are then resected back to the bifurcation and the glans are reattached to the corpora and recessed in a skin hood. This should preserve normal sensation and some erectile function in adult life.
- Feminizing genitoplasty: this involves reduction of the labioscrotal folds and using the redundant clitoral shaft skin to form labia minora.
- Vaginoplasty: when there is a low confluence of the vagina and urethra a posterior-based U-skin flap vaginoplasty is sufficient to produce a good result. For patients with a high confluence a more complex procedure is required. A new approach was developed in 1989 by Passerini-Glazel and this has now become the accepted standard. It uses the clitoral shaft skin and the distal detubularized segment of the urogenital sinus to reconstruct the distal vagina after it is separated from the urethra.

There is little doubt that these procedures produce excellent cosmetic results. The functional results of nerve-preserving clitoral reduction are encouraging. In one study, eight out of nine patients old enough to be sexually active experienced normal sensation and achieved orgasm (Newman *et al.*, 1992). However, the functional results following early vaginoplasty remain in doubt. In one study satisfactory vaginal function was reported in only 21% of patients following vaginoplasty at a mean age of 21 months. With revision surgery at puberty over 80% achieved satisfactory function but in the majority of cases the revisional surgery was minor (Bailez *et al.*, 1992). Long-term results of the Passerini procedure are not yet available. These findings have led to debate on the ideal timing of vaginoplasty, with some centres recommending delaying surgery until late adolescence or young adulthood (Oesterling *et al.*, 1987). However, the consensus remains in favour of early surgery during the first year of life. The clitoral reduction, feminizing genitoplasty and vaginoplasty are performed as a single-stage procedure (Passerini-Glazel, 1989; Donahoe and Gustafson, 1994; de Jong and Boemers, 1995). It is hoped that early surgery will minimize the emotional disturbance suffered by both the child and parents.

In the undervirilized male who is to be reared female there is similar controversy regarding the timing of surgery. In general most accept the need for early phallic reduction and feminizing genitoplasty and the authors also believe in early vaginoplasty, for the reasons listed above. The principles of reconstruction are:

- clitoral reduction
- feminizing genitoplasty
- gonadectomy: all testicular tissue must be removed at an early stage to remove the focus of testosterone production and because of the high risk of malignant degeneration in later life (Woodhouse, 1992)
- vaginoplasty: in these patients a neovagina needs to be constructed. In the past vaginoplasty has been performed in adolescence utilizing skin flap or free graft techniques (McIndoe and Bannister, 1938; Johnson *et al.*, 1991; Martinez-Mora *et al.*, 1992). However, present evidence favours the use of sigmoid colon colovaginoplasty and this has the added advantage that it can be performed in early infancy (Martinez-Mora *et al.*, 1992; Freundt *et al.*, 1992; Hitchcock and Malone, 1994). In the authors' experience of older patients with colovaginoplasty, normal sexual function is achievable.

Many undervirilized males with mixed gonadal dysgenesis and true hermaphroditism will be reared as males. The principles of surgical reconstruction are:

- removal of all inappropriate gonadal tissue: this will require a laparotomy in most cases
- remove inappropriate ductal structures: the rudimentary vagina needs only be resected as far as can conveniently be reached as problems with the retained vaginal stump rarely arise (Aaronson, 1985)
- correction of hypospadias: preoperative androgen therapy is often recommended to increase the size of the genitalia. The surgical techniques and timing will be dealt with in detail in Chapter 61.

Debate continues to surround the management of the dysgenetic 'testes' in patients reared as males. The 'testis' has a 30% incidence of gonadoblastoma, of which 30% will progress to malignancy. Neoplasms may occur before puberty but the risk is said to rise rapidly after puberty. It would be wrong to remove all gonads, and those that can be placed in the scrotum and produce adequate amounts of testosterone may be preserved until the patient has undergone spontaneous puberty. At this stage gonadectomy is probably best advised. For patients with intra-abdominal testes that cannot be brought to the scrotum early removal is best as they have a higher risk of malignant change and endocrine function is usually impaired. The combined skills of the paediatric endocrinologist and surgeon are needed to ensure that the onset of puberty is normal.

Long-term results

For patients with CAH it seems likely that a combination of immediate diagnosis, correct medical and surgical treatment and proper counselling of parents will lead to near-normal psychosexual development (Woodhouse, 1991). There is little long-term information on karyotypic males reared as females or on the success of those reared as males.

ACKNOWLEDGEMENT

The secretarial assistance of Mrs Nina Hardman is gratefully appreciated.

References

Aaronson, I. 1985: True hermaphroditism: a review of 41 cases with observations on testicular histology and function. *British Journal of Urology* **57**, 775–9.

Affara, N.A., Ferguson-Smith, M.A., Tolmie, J. *et al.* 1986: Variable transfer of Y specific sequences in XX males. *Nucleic Acids Research* **14**, 5375–87.

Bailez, M.M., Gearhart, J.P., Migeon, C. and Rock, J. 1992: Vaginal reconstruction after initial construction of the external genitalia in girls with salt-wasting adrenal hyperplasia. *Journal of Urology* **148**, 680–2.

Bardoni, B., Zanaria, E., Guioli, S. *et al.* 1994: A dosage sensitive locus at chromosome Xp21 is involved in male to female sex reversal. *Nature Genetics* **7**, 497–501.

Batch, J.A., Davies, H.R., Evans, B.A.J. *et al.* 1993a: Phenotypic variation and detection of carrier status in the partial androgen insensitivity syndrome. *Archives of Disease in Childhood* **68**, 453–7.

Batch, J.A., Evans, B.A.J., Hughes, I.A. *et al.* 1993b: Mutations of the androgen receptor gene identified in perineal hypospadias. *Journal of Medical Genetics* **30**, 198–201.

Batch, J.A., Patterson, M.N. and Hughes, I.A. 1992: Androgen insensitivity syndrome. *Reproductive Medicine Review* **1**, 131–50.

Berthezène, F., Forest, M.G., Grimand, J.A. *et al.* 1976: Leydig cell agenesis: a cause of male pseudohermaphroditism. *New England Journal of Medicine* **295**, 969–72.

Bevan, C.L., Brown, B.B., Davies, H.R. *et al.* 1996: Functional analysis of six androgen receptor mutations identified in patients with partial androgen insensitivity syndrome. *Human Molecular Genetics* **5**, 265–73.

Bonette, J., Roidot, M., Manuel, M.C. *et al.* 1964: Sur un cas d'hyperplasia lipoïdique congenitale des surrénales (syndrome de Prader). Étude anatomoclinique. *Archives Francaise Pédiatrie* **21**, 851–9.

Donahoe, P.K. and Gustafson, M.L. 1994: Early one-stage surgical reconstruction of the extremely high vagina in patients with congenital adrenal hyperplasia. *Journal of Pediatric Surgery* **29**, 352–8.

Evans, B.A.J., Jones, T.R. and Hughes, I.A. 1984: Studies of the androgen receptor in dispersed fibroblasts: investigation of patients with androgen insensitivity. *Clinical Endocrinology* **20**, 93–105.

Freundt, I., Toolenaar, T.A.M., Huikeshoven, F.J.M. *et al.* 1992: A modified technique to create a neovagina with an isolated segment of sigmoid colon. *Surgery, Gynaecology and Obstetrics* **174**, 11–16.

Fukami, M., Sato, S., Ogata, T. *et al.* 1995: Lack of mutations in P450scc gene (CYP11A) in six Japanese patients with congenital lipoid adrenal hyperplasia. *Clinical Paediatric Endocrinology* **4**, 39–46.

Geissler, W.M., Davis, D.L., Wu, L. *et al.* 1994: Male pseudohermaphroditism caused by mutations of testicular 17β-hydroxysteroid dehydrogenase 3. *Nature Genetics* **7**, 34–9.

Grumbach, M.M. and Conte, F.A. 1992: Abnormalities of sex differentiation. In Wilson, J.D. and Foster, D.W. (eds), *Williams textbook of endocrinology*, 8th ed. Philadelphia, PA: W.B. Saunders, 853–951.

Gustafson, M.L. and Donahoe, P.K. 1995: Surgical reconstruction of intersex abnormalities. In Spitz, L., Coran, G. (eds), *Rob and Smith's operative surgery, paediatric surgery*, 5th ed. London: Chapman & Hall, 773–86.

Hitchcock, R.J.I. and Malone, P.S. 1994: Colovaginoplasty in infants and children. *British Journal of Urology* **73**, 196–9.

Houston, C.S., Optiz, J.M., Spranger, J.W. *et al.* 1983: The campomelic syndrome: review, report of 17 cases, and follow-up on the currently 17 year old boy first reported by Maroteaux *et al.* in 1971. *American Journal of Medical Genetics* **15**, 2–28.

Hughes, I.A., Dyas, J., Riad-Fahmy, D. *et al.* 1987: Prenatal diagnosis of congenital adrenal hyperplasia: reliability of amniotic fluid steroid analysis. *Journal of Medical Genetics* **24**, 344–7.

Hughes, I.A. and Patterson, M.N. 1994: Prenatal diagnosis of androgen insensitivity. *Clinical Endocrinology* **40**, 295–6.

Ingraham, H.A., Lala, D.S., Ikada, Y. *et al.* 1994: The nuclear receptor steroidogenic factor I acts at multiple levels of the reproductive axis. *Genes and Development* **8**, 2302–12.

Johnson, N., Batchelor, A. and Lilford, R.J. 1991: Experience with tissue expansion vaginoplasty. *British Journal of Obstetrics and Gynaecology* **98**, 564–8.

Jong, T.P. de and Boemers, T.M. 1995: Neonatal management of female intersex by clitorovaginoplasty. *Journal of Urology* **154**, 830–2.

Josse, N., Picard, J.-Y., Imbeaud, S. *et al.* 1997: Molecular genetics of the persistent Müllerian duct syndrome. *Clinical Endocrinology* (in press).

Jost, A. 1970: Hormonal factors in sex differentiation of the mammalian foetus. *Philosophical Transactions of the Royal Society, London: Biology* **259**, 119–30.

Koopman, P., Gubbay, J., Vivian, N. *et al.* 1991: Male development of chromosomally female mice transgenic for SRY. *Nature* **351**, 117–21.

Kremer, H., Kraaij, R., Toledo, S.P.A. *et al.* 1995: Male pseudohermaphroditism due to a homozygous missense mutation of the luteinizing hormone receptor gene. *Nature Genetics* **9**, 160–4.

Kremer, H., Mariman, E., Otten, B.J. *et al.* 1993: Cosegregation of missense mutations of the luteinizing hormone receptor gene with familial male-limited precocious puberty. *Human Molecular Genetics* **2**, 1779–83.

Kretser, D.M. de 1996: Declining sperm counts. Environmental chemicals may be to blame. *British Medical Journal* **312**, 457–8.

Kwok, C., Weller, P.A., Guidi, S. *et al.* 1995: Mutations in SOX9, the gene responsible for campomelic dysplasia and autosomal sex reversal. *American Journal of Human Genetics* **57**, 1028–36.

Lee, P.E., Mazur, T., Danish, R. *et al.* 1980: Micropenis 1. Criteria, etiologies and classification. *Johns Hopkins Medical Journal* **146**, 156–63.

Levine, L.S. and Pang, S. 1994: Prenatal diagnosis and treatment of congenital adrenal hyperplasia. *Journal of Paediatric Endocrinology* **7**, 193–200.

Lin, D., Sugawara, T., Strauss, J.F. *et al.* 1995: Role of steroidogenic acute regulatory protein in adrenal and gonadal steroidogenesis. *Science* **267**, 1828–31.

McIndoe, A.H. and Bannister, J.B. 1938: An operation for the cure of congenital absence of the vagina. *Journal of Obstetrics and Gynaecology of the Empire* **45**, 490–4.

Martinez-Mora, J., Isnard, R., Castellvi, A. and Lopez Ortiz, P. 1992: Neovagina in vaginal agenesis: surgical methods and long-term results. *Journal of Pediatric Surgery* **27**, 10–14.

Newman, K., Randolph, J. and Parson, S. 1992: Functional results in young women having clitoral reconstruction as infants. *Journal of Pediatric Surgery* **27**, 180–4.

Oesterling, J.E., Gearhart, J.P. and Jeffs, R.D. 1987: A unified approach to early reconstructive surgery in the child with ambiguous genitalia. *Journal of Urology* **138**, 1079–82.

Passerini-Glazel, G. 1989: A new 1 stage procedure for clitorovaginoplasty in severely masculinized female pseudohermaphrodites. *Journal of Urology* **142**, 565–8.

Patterson, M.N., Hughes, I.A., Gottlieb, B. *et al.* 1994a: The androgen receptor gene mutations database. *Nucleic Acids Research* **22**, 3560–62.

Patterson, M.N., McPhaul, M.J. and Hughes, I.A. 1994b: Androgen insensitivity syndrome. In Sheppard, M.C. and Stewart, P.M. (eds), Hormones, enzymes and receptors. *Clinical Endocrinology and Metabolism* **8**, 379–404.

Pelletier, J., Bruering, W., Kashton, C.E. *et al.* 1991: Germline mutations in the Wilms tumour suppressor gene are associated with abnormal urogenital development in Denys–Drash syndrome. *Cell* **67**, 437–47.

Peterson, R.E., Imperato-McGinley, J., Gautier, T. *et al.* 1977: Male pseudohermaphroditism due to steroid 5α-reductase deficiency. *American Journal of Medicine* **62**, 170–91.

Savage, M.O. 1982: Ambiguous genitalia, small genitalia and undescended testes. *Clinics in Endocrinology and Metabolism* **11**, 127–58.

Savage, M.O. and Lowe, D.G. 1990: Gonadal neoplasia and abnormal sexual differentiation. *Clinical Endocrinology* **32**, 519–33.

Sharpe, R.M. and Skakkebaek, N.E. 1993: Are oestrogens involved in falling sperm counts and disorders of the male reproductive tract? *Lancet* **341**, 1392–5.

Simard, J., Rhéaume, E., Sanchez, R. *et al.* 1993: Molecular basis of congenital adrenal hyperplasia due to 3β-hydroxysteroid dehydrogenase deficiency. *Molecular Endocrinology*. **7**, 716–28.

Sinclair, A.H., Berta, P., Palmer, M.S. *et al.* 1990: A gene from the human sex determining region encodes a protein with homology to a conserved DNA-binding motif. *Nature* **346**, 240–4.

Sinnecker, G. and Köhler, S. 1989: Sex hormone binding globulin response to the anabolic steroid stanozolol: evidence for its suitability in biological androgen sensitivity test. *Journal of Clinical Endocrinology and Metabolism* **68**, 1195–200.

Smith, C.P.W., Williams, O.L. and Treadgold, S. 1984: *Basic human embryology*, 3rd ed. London: Pitman.

Strachan, T. 1990: Molecular pathology of congenital adrenal hyperplasia. *Clinical Endocrinology* **32**, 373–93.

Tsai, M.-J. and O'Malley, B.W. 1994: Molecular mechanisms of action of steroid/thyroid receptor superfamily members. *Annual Reviews in Biochemistry* **63**, 451–86.

Wachtel, S.S. 1993: *Molecular genetics of sex determination*. London: Academic Press.

Wagner, T., Wirth, J., Meyer, J. *et al.* 1994: Autosomal sex reversal and campomelic dysplasia are caused by mutations in and around the SRY-related gene SOX9. *Cell* **79**, 111–12.

Walker, J. and Hughes, I.A. 1994: Ambiguous genitalia. *Current Paediatrics* **4**, 161–7.

Whitaker, R.H. 1991: Surgical management of the virilised female. In Gonzales, E.T., and Roth, D. (eds), *Common problems in pediatric urology*. St Louis, MO: Mosby Year Book, 394–401.

Wilson, J.D., Griffin, J.E. and Russell, D.W. 1993: Steroid 5α-reductase 2 deficiency. *Endocrine Reviews* **14**, 577–93.

Woodhouse, C.R.J. 1991: Problems of intersex, gender identity and micropenis. In *Long term paediatric urology*. London: Blackwell Scientific, 176–91.

Woodhouse, C.R.J. 1992: Late malignancy in urology. *British Journal of Urology* **70**, 345–51.

Wudy, S.A., Homoki, J. and Teller, W.M. 1994: Successful prenatal treatment of congenital adrenal hyperplasia due to 21-hydroxylase deficiency. *European Journal of Pediatrics* **153**, 556–9.

PART III

General surgery of infancy and childhood

CHAPTER 32

Herniae and hydroceles

A.E. MACKINNON

Introduction	Umbilical herniae
Inguinal herniae	Other herniae
Hydroceles	References
Femoral herniae	Further reading

Introduction

This group of pathological conditions represents the most common indications for surgery in children. Even so, particularly with inguinal herniae in infancy, the technical aspects can be amongst the most demanding in paediatric surgery. Conversely surgery is often recommended for umbilical herniae in spite of the fact that resolution may well occur throughout childhood.

Inguinal herniae

Evidence of a surgical approach to the management of inguinal herniae dates back nearly 2000 years. Skinner and Grosfeld (1993) outline the historical development of hernia surgery with herniotomy being described at the turn of the century.

EMBRYOLOGY AND ANATOMY

The gonad begins to develop at the fifth week of intrauterine life (Lemeh, 1960). Elongation of the body stalk results in a relative caudal migration but the first phase of the testicular descent is under the influence of Müllerian inhibiting hormone (Hutson and Beasley, 1992). At the lower pole of the gonad a strand of mesenchymal cells develops into a band-like structure which becomes the gubernaculum in the male and the round ligament in the female. At about the eighth week

of development a peritoneal prolongation appears, passing through the layers of developing abdominal wall muscle along the course of the developing gubernaculum or round ligament and into the labioscrotal fold. The testis then migrates down the peritoneal canal or processus vaginalis, which is still patent at birth in about 90% of children. Failure of this process leads to the potential of an inguinal hernia or hydrocele.

Figure 32.1 illustrates the possible variations that arise when the processus vaginalis fails to close in part or in whole. Theoretically, if a wide canal persists then a hernia may develop, and if narrow a hydrocele. However, a wide processus may be associated with no clinical abnormality, a hydrocele or both hernia and hydrocele, particularly if the neck is partly obturated by omentum or a Richter's type of hernia. Incomplete hernia sacs, or bubonoceles (Fig. 32.1d), are said to account for 95% of inguinal herniae (Herzfeld, 1938).

Once the abdominal muscles have developed the processus vaginalis emerges through the deep inguinal ring lying anterolateral to the cord structures, or round ligament in the female. It then passes along the inguinal canal lying anterior to these structures and emerges through the superficial ring to pass into the scrotum in boys, or labium major in girls. The inguinal canal has virtually no length at birth, the deep and superficial rings lying one upon the other. The canal has achieved a significant length at about 4 years of age, allowing an alternative operative approach.

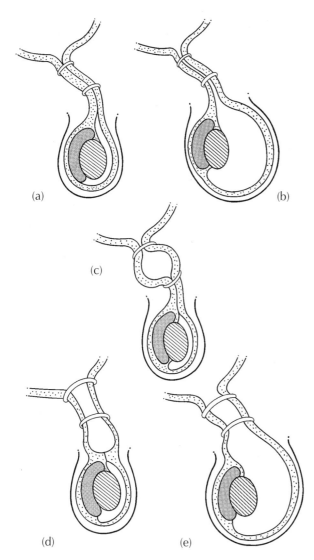

Fig. 32.1 Outcome of processus vaginalis: (a) normal obliteration; (b) communicating hydrocele; (c) hydrocele of cord; (d) inguinal hernia: bubonocele; (e) inguinal hernia: complete.

The medial boundary of the deep inguinal ring comprises the deep inferior epigastric vessels. The surface marking of the deep ring therefore is a point just above and medial to the point where the femoral artery passes under the inguinal ligament. This is the key to placing the incision during surgery. The sac wall in the majority of inguinal herniae comprises solely the processus vaginalis. However, on occasions significant variations occur, the most common in boys being the presence of an undescended testis (Brown and MacKinnon, 1976). In girls the ovary may prolapse on a mesovarium and this may be accompanied by a sliding element involving the fallopian tube (Atwell, 1962b). Less commonly the wall of large intestine or bladder (Shaw and

Santulli, 1967) may be involved. The presence of a Meckel's diverticulum (Littré's hernia) has also been recorded in infancy (Baillie, 1958). Inguinal herniae may also be associated with specific syndromes including Ehlers–Danlos, Hurler Hunter (Grosfeld, 1989) and testicular feminization (Atwell, 1962a; Nielsen and Bulow, 1976). The latter is important in girls, particularly when there are bilateral herniae, as this may be the initial presentation. This has led to some authors recommending karyotyping all such cases.

Direct inguinal herniae are extremely rare in children, although it has been suggested there may be a direct element in 1%. However, it is possible that this is an iatrogenic finding.

CLINICAL FEATURES

The most common presentation is of an intermittent swelling in the groin at the point of the deep inguinal ring, possibly extending to the scrotum or labium. If, on examination, this is not present it may be demonstrated by raising the intra-abdominal pressure if the child cries or can be made to laugh or cough. If there is still no visible evidence then supportive signs include thickening of the cord structures, or if there is a very wide sac, then rolling the cord between finger and pubic tubercle may give a feeling of rubbing two layers of silk together.

Some boys around the age of 8 years present with a testis that lies high in the scrotum for which orchidopexy is not justified but then they represent later with a clear inguinal hernia. These may represent 'incomplete' examples of the ascending testis (Atwell, 1962b).

Confusion over the diagnosis is uncommon. However, in male infants, it can be difficult to differentiate herniae from hydroceles. It may not be easy to decide whether one can 'get above' the hernia, the classic distinguishing feature in adults. Herniae in this age group may transilluminate as brightly as a hydrocele.

It is commonly taught that, unless incarcerated, herniae do not cause symptoms. In older children this is largely true, but in perhaps 80% of infants discomfort is present, as can be judged by the parents noticing a clear improvement following surgery.

INCIDENCE

At birth, approximately 95% of infants are said to have a patent processus vaginalis. This figure falls to 40% at 1 year and 20% at 2 years (Devlin, 1988). Based on large series of patients the overall incidence of herniae is 1–2%, with a preponderance of male to female of 4:1. Clinically evident bilateral herniae occur in 10% but if the contralateral groin is explored nearly 50% are found to have a patent processus vaginalis (Roe *et al.*, 1951). Not surprisingly the younger the child the higher the incidence of finding a contralateral patency. In boys, right-sided herniae account for 60–70% of cases,

20–25% are left sided and 5–15% may be bilateral (Atwell, 1962b; Scorer and Farrington, 1971). Contralateral herniae are found twice as often when the index side is left. Laterality is equal in girls.

The question has to be addressed whether or not to perform bilateral exploration in every case as suggested by some authors (Duckett, 1952; McGregor *et al.*, 1980). If a positive finding is present in half the cases but 30% of adult post mortems reveal the presence of an open processus vaginalis, then a policy of bilateral exploration will lead to unnecessary surgery in about 80%. Careful clinical examination will reveal some cases of bilaterality in which case both groins should be explored particularly if the index side is left. The younger the patient the greater this chance, so that for most preterm infants bilateral exploration is advisable to avoid a double exposure to the risks of surgery.

Methods to detect bilateral patency have included contrast radiography (Guttman *et al.*, 1972), trans-peritoneal probing (Kiesewetter and Oh, 1980) and laparoscopy. The former has been shown to reveal a contralateral patent processus in about 30% of cases, which approximates to the natural incidence of clinically non-significant patency.

MANAGEMENT

As soon as a child's hernia is detected he or she should be referred for surgery. Any infant under one year of age and certainly those below 6 months should be seen urgently for fear of incarceration developing. Examination should confirm the diagnosis whenever possible although clear evidence from parents or health workers can be accepted. Particular attention must be paid to the opposite side, noting associated pathology such as cryptorchidism.

The vast majority of children are best operated on as a day case (Davies *et al.*, 1990). Preoperative haemo-globin estimation is necessary below the age of 3 years to ensure that it is at least 10 g/dl. Concomitant medical conditions may necessitate inpatient surgery. This also applies to infants up to 12 months of age who had significant respiratory problems as a neonate, particularly if preterm, because of their impaired respiratory function in the first year of life (Atwell *et al.*, 1973). Infants less than 44 weeks postconceptional age (PCA) are at risk of postoperative apnoea (Bryan *et al.*, 1973): consideration should be given to postponing surgery until after this age and monitoring for 12–24 hours after surgery should be performed even up to 60 weeks PCA. These risks are greater for preterm infant (Liu *et al.*, 1983) and remain critically so up to 52 weeks PCA (Steward, 1982; Welborn *et al.*, 1990). Special consideration has to be given to the timing of surgery in infants who develop a hernia while in special care units. The risks of anaesthesia have to be set against the risk of incarceration. However it should be possible to manage the latter problem without complications developing while the infant remains in hospital. The safest policy is to arrange for surgery to be undertaken immediately prior to discharge from the baby unit.

INCARCERATED HERNIAE

Although incarceration of inguinal herniae may occur at any age in childhood this complication occurs more often in the first 6 months of life particularly in babies born preterm. At this age it is estimated that up to 50% of herniae may present with an episode of incarceration (Palmer, 1978). Regrettably, nearly half of such cases could have been prevented by expeditious surgery (Davies *et al.*, 1990).

The clinical features are often insidious in onset, with the baby being non-specifically disturbed. A tender red swelling in the groin later becomes obvious, with features of intestinal obstruction. It is an absolute rule that any baby appearing miserable in a non-specific way must be examined with the nappy off. The differential diagnosis includes testicular torsion and suppurative inguinal lymphadenopathy.

In girls the ovary may enter the hernia sac and be irreducible without being strangulated. This is a situation requiring expeditious though not emergency surgery as incarceration may supervene (Boley *et al.*, 1991). The management of an infant with an incarcerated hernia is by resuscitation, reduction and repair. Considerable fluid loss may occur within a few hours, in which case intravenous fluids need to be given before any attempt at reduction. To reduce the hernia the fingers of one hand are placed at the neck of the sac to support it and prevent the hernia simply being pushed

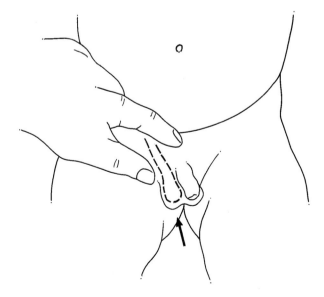

Fig. 32.2 Method for reducing an inguinal hernia.

around under the skin (Fig. 32.2). Gentle pressure by these fingers may help to reduce some of the oedema. At the same time the fingers of the opposite hand exert pressure on the lower end of the hernia. If there is any difficulty in performing this reduction then the patient should be sedated with morphine after ensuring intravenous access. The historical manoeuvre of placing the lower limbs in gallows traction is of dubious use and places the patient at risk of inhalation if he or she vomits.

The organ most at risk of ischaemia is the gonad. Even so it is less likely to undergo atrophy if reduction can be achieved non-operatively (Puri *et al.*, 1984). Once reduced the hernia should be repaired within a few days for fear of recurrence. The best approach to these herniae is by the preperitoneal route. This avoids having to dissect a very friable sac and allows dissection at the very upper end of its neck. Moreover, the cord structures are more easily separated at this level and full inspection of incarcerated bowel to ensure its viability is possible even if it reduces back within the peritoneal cavity. In children it is extremely rare to have to resect bowel but failure to make adequate inspection has led to deaths. Surgery for incarcerated herniae must be performed by a paediatric surgeon (Puri *et al.*, 1984).

OPERATIVE TREATMENT

Inguinal herniotomy is one of the most satisfying procedures in surgery. The correct procedure is based on a knowledge of anatomy, may be technically challenging but seems simple in the hands of the expert surgeon, and is highly effective with rare recurrence. The various procedures described here are planned in the belief that the shutter mechanism of the inguinal canal should not be laid open unless necessary as, for example, with an orchidopexy. The chosen procedure depends mainly on the patient's age. The operation is performed under general anaesthesia with local or regional infiltration with bupivacaine.

Low approach

This is the classical procedure for children below about 3–4 years of age since the inguinal canal has no significant length before then. The cord is exposed outside the superficial ring and the processus vaginalis dissected after opening the cord coverings. A transverse incision is made in the lower abdominal skin crease (Fig. 32.3a) approximately 2 cm long just cephalad of where the cord structures can be palpated as they cross the pubic bone. The fat and Scarpa's fascia are divided carefully to minimize bleeding and avoid the use of diathermy in the operation, thus removing risk to the vas. The wound is then retracted caudally so that the dissection is continued perpendicular to the skin surface to explore the anterior aspect of the cord as it emerges from the superficial ring. It can be recognized by a shiny bluish colour. The superficial layer is picked up and divided with scissors (Fig. 32.3b) and the opening spread to allow the cremaster to be picked up. It is recognized by its interweaving pinkish fibres (Fig. 32.3c). This layer draws with it the internal spermatic fascia and processus vaginalis, and therefore division again with scissors has to be careful. Experience alone facilitates recognition of these tissue planes. The cremaster is split open to allow the processus vaginalis to be grasped with a mosquito forcep (Fig. 32.3d) and be drawn up on

(a)

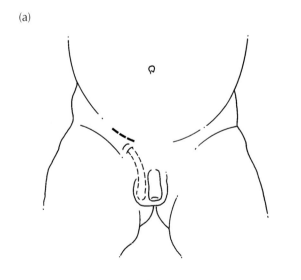

(b)

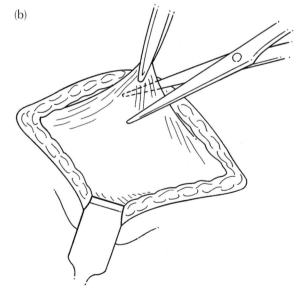

Fig. 32.3 (a) and (b).

(c)

(d)

(e)

(f)

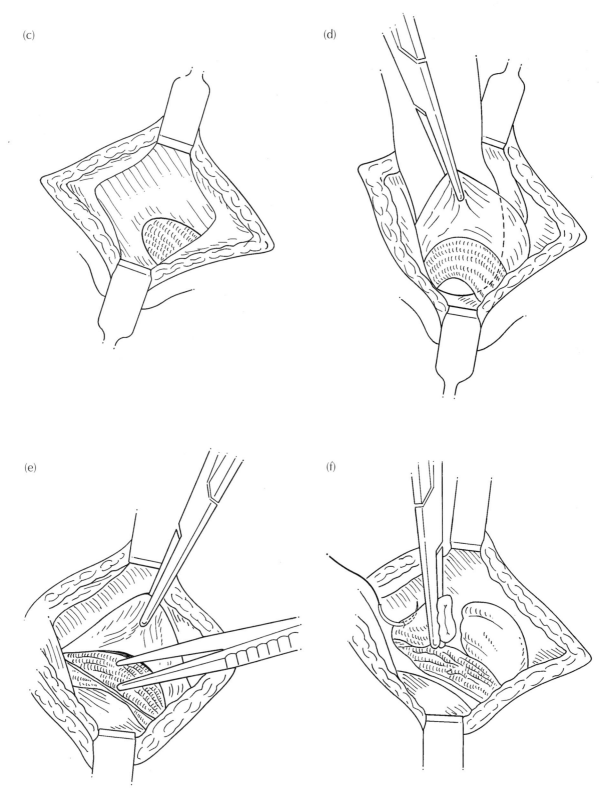

Fig. 32.3 Low approach to inguinal herniotomy: (a) skin incision; (b) division of superficial cord coverings; (c) cremaster muscle seen over cord emerging from superficial inguinal ring; (d) processus vaginalis being lifted forward with index finger supporting behind; (e) processus vaginalis being dissected free from cord; (f) processus vaginalis transfixed and divided.

to the index finger of the left hand for a right-sided hernia and vice versa. The cord structures may then be teased off the sac using the edge of blunt dissecting forceps while the sac is pulled up on to the supporting finger, using it like an anvil, by the thumb. Dissection is carried around the sac, never grasping the vas, until a clear plane is seen between cord and sac (Fig. 32.3e). A mosquito forcep is then placed across the sac which is divided distally. The sac is dissected to its neck, transfixed with 3-0 polyglactin and divided (Fig. 32.3f). There is no need to excise the distal end of the sac which in a complete hernia is the tunica vaginalis. Any oozing from the pampiniform plexus is best controlled by firm pressure. In most cases the sac wall is thin enough for simple inspection to reveal that there is no sliding element or abdominal structure such as the fallopian tube. The wound is then closed with 4-0 catgut or polyglactin sutures to the fat and subcuticular layer. Finally, in boys the correct scrotal placement of the testis is ensured. A similar procedure may be performed using a periscrotal incision, which is thought to be cosmetically superior by some surgeons (Fig. 32.4).

The most common difficulties in this operation are caused by inability to recognize the structures involved due to inexperience, or failing to keep the dissection perpendicular to the skin over the cord, thus wandering off line in the prepubic fat. Once the external cremaster layer has been opened a well-formed condensation of connective tissue may mimic the sac. Finally, the dissection around the sac may seem to be never ending. This usually is due to the surgeon dissecting around the end of a bubonocele and once this is recognized the sac can be cleared easily.

Sliding herniae present special difficulties. Firstly, the anatomy has to be realized. Quite often an ovary or a fallopian tube may be freed from the wall sufficiently to permit simple transfixion of the sac. In other instances and where bowel or bladder is involved the simplest and almost always effective procedure is to place a purse-string suture around the external aspect of the neck of the sac and thus invert the sliding viscus at the same time as closing the processus.

High approach

Once there is a significant length to the canal at about 4 years of age the above procedure necessitates pulling the sac down the inguinal canal, which is feasible. An alternative is to expose the neck of the sac at the deep inguinal ring through a short opening in the external oblique but without opening the canal along its full length. This requires accurate placement of the incision and line of dissection. A skin crease incision 2 cm long

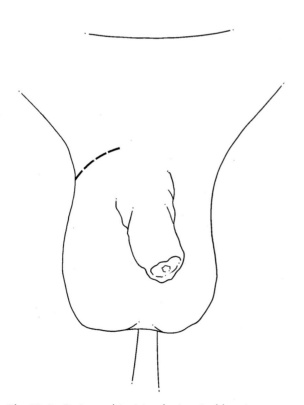

Fig. 32.4 Periscrotal incision for inguinal herniotomy.

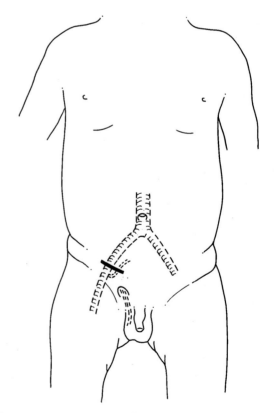

Fig. 32.5 Incision over deep inguinal ring for 'high approach'.

is made over the deep ring (Fig. 32.5) (see Embryology and anatomy). The external oblique is then incised for 1.5 cm perpendicularly below the skin. The inguinal nerve can often be seen through the aponeurosis and this confirms the correctness of the dissection site. The internal oblique muscle is split with mosquito forceps as it becomes the cremaster muscle, the edges being held open by blunt dissecting forceps. The cremaster must be fully split and likewise the internal spermatic fascia (or transversalis fascia), thus revealing the cord or round ligament with the hernia sac in front. If it is difficult to lift the sac forwards there may be one of three problems: the hernia may not be fully reduced, the dissection may not have been bold enough to split the transversalis fascia or, finally, parietal peritoneum has been grasped in error. From this point on the dissection is similar to the low approach, the wound requiring one suture of 3-0 polyglactin to the external oblique aponeurosis.

Preperitoneal approach

This was first described by Cheatle in 1921 and is advocated in particular for incarcerated herniae (Jones and Towns, 1983). However, it is also probably the optimum procedure in infancy and for recurrent herniae. This technique is slightly more difficult to learn than the two previous procedures but with experience the dissection of cord structures from the sac is easier and because the merging of the neck of the sac and parietal peritoneum is in view there should be no possibility for recurrence. The approach also allows inspection of the posterior wall of the canal looking for a direct element and the femoral canal.

The incision is made in the skin fold, as with the low approach, but is twice as long (Fig. 32.6a). The subcutaneous fat and Scarpa's fascia are divided and then separated cephalad from the external oblique aponeurosis for 2–3 cm. A transverse muscle splitting incision is then made in the external and internal oblique and transversus abdominis muscles, often splitting the lateral margin of the rectus sheath (Fig. 32.6a). The transversalis fascia may then be split (Jones and Towns, 1983) and the plane between it and the peritoneum opened caudally, but this leaves the peritoneum unsupported and at risk of being torn. Alternatively, the lower margin of the anterior abdominal wall is elevated and the upper margin, peritoneum and transversalis fascia are retracted cephalad with a deeper retractor. The neck of the processus vaginalis then is defined by blunt dissection medially and laterally. It often lies more medial than one at first might expect and recognition of its appearance requires experience and is the key to the operation. The transversalis fascia is then opened in front of the sac and careful dissection continued on either side working posteriorly until eventually a mosquito forcep can be placed behind the sac and clipped to the edge of the external oblique for support. The contents of the hernia must be reduced before this step, or dissection will be almost impossible. If there is any question of viability of contained bowel the sac is opened at its neck and the bowel inspected. Very rarely is resection necessary but it can easily be accomplished from this exposure. It is occasionally necessary to pass an instrument extremely carefully through the deep ring to stretch the inguinal orifices and permit reduction. The sac is then separated from the vas and vessels (Fig. 32.6b), rather surprisingly by dissecting around the lateral side. The anterior wall is grasped and drawn medially, then the lateral wall is drawn medially until the cord structures are seen and freed. The supporting mosquito may then be replaced in the plane between cord and sac before the sac is cross-clamped (Fig. 32.6c), divided and transfixed at its neck with 3-0 polyglactin. If the peritoneum has been damaged it can be closed as if at a laparotomy, but even after an episode of incarceration the sac is much easier to handle than through a lower approach. The muscles are closed with 3-0 polyglactin and the fat and skin with 4-0 catgut. Finally, as always, the testes must be seen to be fully descended. This operation is ideal for orchidopexy for a concomitant cryptorchid testis.

(a)   (b)   (c)

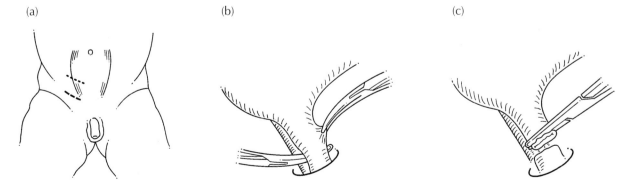

Fig. 32.6 (a) Incision on skin (long bars) for preperitoneal approach, and in muscle fascia (short bars); (b) dissection behind sac separating it from cord structures; (c) sac clamped and divided.

POSTOPERATIVE CARE

Most patients can be discharged on the same day and are likely to require a mild analgesic for less than 48 hours. Early activity should not be detrimental to the surgery but common sense dictates avoidance of possible contact sports for 10 days. In some patients there may be thickening and bruising of the scrotum which resolves in 1–2 weeks. This can be mistaken for an early recurrence which seems to be incarcerated but this is rare. Many units arrange for a visit by the district nurse on the following day but the need for this is doubtful. Children should be able to return to school after 2–3 days, or even sooner.

COMPLICATIONS

Large series indicate a low incidence of postoperative problems (Ingimarsson and Spak, 1983; Harvey *et al.*, 1985). Recurrence of inguinal herniae should be rare (Atwell, 1962b). At re-exploration the cause is not usually evident. Tearing of the sac at its neck is suggested as a cause and almost certainly some recurrences are caused by picking up the side of the hernia sac and treating it as a bubonocele but not reaching the true neck. Hydrocele fluid may collect in the distal end of an incompletely excised sac but this resolves spontaneously in almost every instance.

Infection may occur in the superficial layers in sporadic cases but if clusters occur then theatre management should be reviewed. Deep infection is an occasional complication of using non-absorbable sutures to transfix the sac. Iatrogenic cryptorchidism may occur even when care is taken to ensure that the testis lies in the lower pole of the scrotum at the end of surgery. More serious is the small incidence of testicular atrophy which is made more likely if unnecessary testicular mobilization is performed. Risk of injury to the vas can be minimized by not using diathermy during the operation. One study suggested an injury rate of 1.6% (Weiner, 1962).

Hydroceles

The embryology of hydroceles is the same as for indirect inguinal herniae. In girls they present as a swelling along the line of the round ligament and are often called hydroceles of the canal of Nuck. In males the majority are confined to the tunica vaginalis (Fig. 32.1b) but they may be associated with a hernia which is not clinically evident. Commonly they first arise following a systemic viral illness or after the creation of a peritoneal cerebrospinal fluid (CSF) shunt or peritoneal dialysis, as can a hernia. Hydroceles of the cord (Fig. 32.1c) are clinically obvious but could be confused with a rare crossed ectopic testis. The serious differential diagnosis of a hydrocele in the scrotum is a testicular teratoma which can be partly cystic and therefore transilluminate.

Teratomas have been described as feeling like a hydrocele (MacKinnon and Cohen, 1978). It is therefore imperative that a normal testis can be felt on the posterior wall of a hydrocele sac or if it is too tense to feel then transillumination will reveal its position. It must be remembered that herniae also transilluminate in young children.

MANAGEMENT

In the first year of life hydroceles resolve spontaneously in over 90% of cases. If very gross, parents often press for surgery and if their request is acceded to recurrence is frequent. Under such circumstances the best action is to wait for resolution. Hydroceles seldom present in the second year of life and at this age could be left alone but thereafter surgery is advisable as resolution is unlikely.

The operative procedure is the same as for herniae but often the processus vaginalis in the inguinal canal is very narrow and easily missed. It must be traced cephalad until it is seen to widen out at the peritoneum. The best route to identify the processus is the high approach in the majority of children, which ensures transfixion of the sac at its neck. Equally important is to ensure thorough drainage of hydrocele either by passing an instrument such as a mosquito forcep down the distal limb or by pushing the testis into the prepubic fat and widely draining it. This is performed as spontaneous reabsorption of the fluid is slow. Recurrence is rare and may require re-exploration and in these cases the preperitoneal route allows certainty of displaying the relevant anatomy.

Femoral herniae

Much less common than inguinal herniae (Tan and Lister, 1984), femoral herniae have an equal sex incidence in children. They are occasionally secondary to disruption of pelvic anatomy by orthopaedic surgery (Salter, 1961). The sac may contain any pelvic organ, small bowel or omentum. Incarceration is very infrequent. They have to be distinguished clinically from inguinal herniae by their inferior and more medial position, and from enlarged lymph nodes.

OPERATION

These herniae may be tackled from below at the lower end of the femoral canal. However, it is not always easy to separate the sac from the fat surrounding it and by far the easiest procedure is to use the preperitoneal approach as described for inguinal herniae, suturing the medial end of the inguinal ligament to the pectinate ligament with a 3-0 polyglactin suture. A compound curved needle facilitates this manoeuvre.

Umbilical herniae

These are the most common herniae in children. The umbilicus is a scar so it is not surprising that it cicatrizes, leading to resolution in most cases. This occurs in the first year of life but a significant chance remains of spontaneous closure of the defect at the age of 5 years (Hall *et al.*, 1981). Parents often needlessly fear that the thin sac will rupture but strangulation is rare (Vyas and MacKinnon, 1983). The other parental fear is that the child will be teased, but this depends more often on family attitudes than on peer opinions.

Indications for surgery are rather vague but some children do seem to get discomfort and social pressures are sometimes sufficiently strong. In the first 3 months of life strapping the abdominal wall so as to obturate the hernia can be performed but is probably of no real benefit.

Operative repair is quite simple, performed under general anaesthesia with local anaesthetic infiltration for postoperative comfort. The loose skin is grasped with an Allis forcep and a curved incision made around 50% of the circumference of the defect (Figs 32.7a and b), and must lie within the umbilicus.

By a combination of blunt and sharp dissection the plane around the base of the hernia sac is developed (Fig. 32.7c). The skin is then dissected off the sac but if some peritoneum remains attached this causes no problem. The lateral ends of the sac are grasped with haemostats and the sac is excised (Figs 32.7d and e). There are no significant vessels to ligate. Any contained omentum must be reduced prior to closure, which can be performed by a double row of 3-0 polyglactin mounted on a cutting needle (Fig. 32.7f). A formal Mayo procedure is not necessary. The skin margin may need to be trimmed before closing if there is gross redundancy and the deep aspect has to be sutured to the line of closure of the hernia sac. To prevent a haematoma forming the wound is dressed with a pledglet in the umbilicus held in place with a folded dressing swab and 3-inch-wide sticking plaster.

PARAUMBILICAL HERNIAE

These are not rare in children and lie just above or occasionally below the umbilicus. They can be distinguished from a true umbilical hernia because the latter has a circular orifice whereas the paraumbilical hernia has a transverse elliptical orifice. They differ in their outcome since these seldom if ever resolve spontaneously so are more likely to require repair.

EPIGASTRIC HERNIAE

These comprise a small herniation of extraperitoneal fat, single or multiple, in the midline through the linea alba. They lie one-third to one-half the distance from the umbilicus to the xiphisternum. Rarely, they cause pinpoint discomfort related to the lesion but often parents attribute non-specific abdominal pain to them. Only if necessary should they be operated on, in which case the protruding fat may be excised or reduced and the hole closed with a single suture.

DIVARICATION OF THE RECTI

This occurs frequently in infants. It is important to know that no action is required, although it can be difficult to reassure parents.

Other herniae

Rare herniae of the abdominal wall may also occur in children. These include Spigelian herniae and lateral abdominal wall herniae. The latter may arise through the potential defects where latissimus dorsi and external oblique muscles overlap at the iliac crest below or costal margin above. Such herniae may also be associated with neurogenic lesions (Placzek and MacKinnon, 1980). The method of repair depends on the local anatomy but often there is no true sac.

(a)

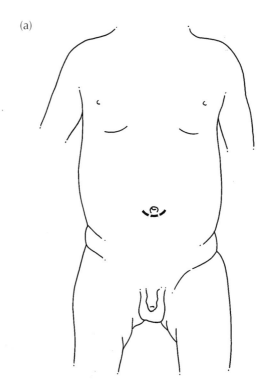

Fig. 32.7   Umbilical herniorrhaphy; (a) incision.

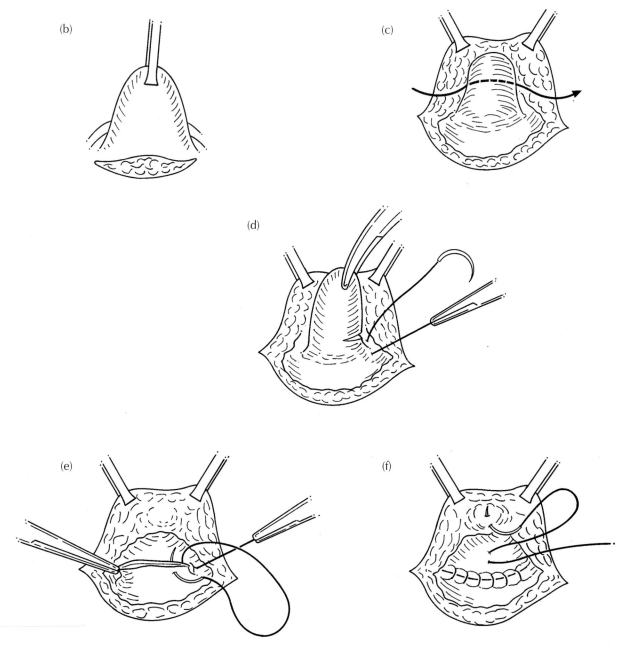

Fig. 32.7 Umbilical herniorrhaphy; (b) umbilicus pulled forwards for dissection; (c) dissection behind sac; (d) preparation to excise sac; (e) sac excised and repair started; (f) repair complete.

References

Atwell, J.D. 1962a: Inguinal hernia and the testicular feminisation syndrome in infancy and childhood. *British Journal of Surgery* **49**, 367–71.

Atwell, J.D. 1962b: Inguinal herniae in female infants and children. *British Journal of Surgery* **50**, 294–7.

Atwell, J.D., Burns, J.M.S., Dewar, A.K. and Freeman, N.V. 1973: Paediatric day case surgery. *Lancet* **ii**, 895–7.

Baillie, R.C. 1958: Incarceration of a Meckel's inguinal hernia in an infant. *British Journal of Surgery* **45**, 562–4.

Boley, S.J., Cahn, D., Lauer, T., Weinberg, G. and Kleinhaus, S. 1991: The irreducible ovary: a true emergency. *Journal of Pediatric Surgery* **26**, 1035–8.

Brown, S. and MacKinnon, A.E. 1976: The scrotal pouch operation for undescended testis. *Annals of the Royal College of Surgeons of England* **61**, 377–80.

Bryan, M.H., Hardie, M.G., Reilly, B.J. and Swyer, P.R. 1973: Pulmonary function studies during the first year of life in infants recovering from the respiratory distress syndrome. *Pediatrics* **52**, 169–78.

Cheatle, G.L. 1921: An operation for inguinal hernia. *British Medical Journal* **2**, 1025–6.

Davies, N., Najmaldin, A. and Burge, D.M. 1990: Irreducible inguinal hernia in children below two years of age. *British Journal of Surgery* **77**, 1291–2.

Devlin, H.B. 1988: *Management of abdominal hernias.* London: Butterworths, 75.

Duckett, J.W. 1952: Treatment of congenital inguinal hernia. *Annals of Surgery* **135**, 879–85.

Grosfeld, J.L. 1989: Current concepts in inguinal hernia in infants and children. *World Journal of Surgery* **13**, 506–15.

Guttman, F.M., Bertrand, R. and Ducharme, J.C. 1972: Herniography and the paediatric contralateral hernia. *Surgery, Gynaecology and Obstetrics* **135**, 551–5.

Hall, D.E., Roberts, K.B. and Charney, E. 1981: Umbilical hernia: what happens after age 5 years? *Journal of Pediatrics* **98**, 415–17.

Harvey, M.H., Johnstone, M.J.S. and Fossard, D.P. 1985: Inguinal herniotomy in children: a five year survey. *British Journal of Surgery* **72**, 485–7.

Herzfeld, G. 1938: Hernia in infancy. *American Journal of Surgery* **39**, 422–8.

Hutson J.M. and Beasley, S.W. 1992: *Descent of the testis.* London: Edward Arnold.

Ingimarsson, O. and Spak, I. 1983: Inguinal and femoral hernias: long-term results in a community hospital. *Acta Chirurgica Scandinavica* **149**, 291–7.

Jones, P.F. and Towns, F.M. 1983: An abdominal extraperitoneal approach for the incarcerated inguinal hernia of infancy. *British Journal of Surgery* **70**, 719–20.

Kiesewetter, W.B. and Oh, K.S. 1980: Unilateral inguinal hernias in children. *Archives of Surgery* **115**, 1443–5.

Lemeh, C.H. 1960: A study of the development and structural relationships of the testis and gubernaculum. *Surgery, Gynecology and Obstetrics* **110**, 164–72.

Liu, L.M.P., Cote, C.J., Goudsouzian, N.G. *et al.* 1983: Life threatening apnoea in infants recovering from anaesthesia. *Anaesthesiology* **59**, 506–10.

McGregor, D.B., Halverson, K. and McKay, C.B. 1980: The unilateral paediatric inguinal hernia: should the contralateral side be explored? *Journal of Paediatric Surgery* **15**, 313–17.

MacKinnon, A.E. and Cohen, S.J. 1978: Archenteronoma (yolk sac tumours). *Journal of Pediatric Surgery* **13**, 21–3.

Nielsen, D.F. and Bulow, S. 1976: The incidence of male hermaphroditism in girls with inguinal hernia. *Surgery, Gynecology and Obstetrics* **142**, 875–6.

Palmer, B.V. 1978: Incarcerated inguinal hernia in children. *Annals of the Royal College of Surgeons of England* **60**, 121–4.

Placzek, M.M. and MacKinnon, A.E. 1980: Lateral meningocele and defect of abdominal wall. *Postgraduate Medical Journal* **56**, 142–4.

Puri, P., Guiney, E.J. and O'Donnell, B. 1984: Inguinal hernia in infants; the fate of the testis following incarceration. *Journal of Pediatric Surgery* **19**, 44–6.

Roe, M.I., Copelson, L.W. and Clatworthy, H.W. 1951: The patent processus vaginalis and the inguinal hernia. *Surgical Clinics of North America* **71**, 1371–6.

Salter, R.B. 1961: Innominate osteotomy in the treatment of dislocation and subluxation of the hip. *Journal of Bone and Joint Surgery* **43B**, 518–39.

Scorer, C.G. and Farrington, G.H. 1971: *Congenital deformities of the testis and epididymis.* London: Butterworths.

Shaw, A. and Santulli, T.V. 1967: Management of sliding hernias of the urinary bladder in infants. *Surgery, Gynecology and Obstetrics* **124**, 1315–16.

Skinner, C.G. and Grosfeld, J.L. 1993: Inguinal and umbilical hernia repair in infants and children. *Surgical Clinics of North America* **73**, 439–49.

Steward, D.J. 1982: Preterm infants are more prone to complications following minor surgery than are term infants. *Anaesthesiology* **56**, 304–6.

Tan, P.K.H. and Lister, J. 1984: Femoral hernia in children. *Archives of Surgery* **119**, 1161–4.

Vyas, I.D. and MacKinnon, A.E. 1983: Strangulated umbilical hernia in a child. *Postgraduate Medical Journal* 1983; **59**, 794–5.

Weiner, D.O. 1962: Bilateral exploration in inguinal hernia in juvenile patients. *Surgery* **51**, 393–406.

Welborn, L.G., Rice, L.J., Hannallah, R.S., Broadman, L.M., Ruttimann, U.E. and Fink, R. 1990: Postoperative apnoea in former preterm infants: prospective comparison of spinal and general anaesthesia. *Anaesthesiology* **72**, 838–42.

Further reading

Devlin, H.B. 1992: *Management of abdominal hernias.* London: Butterworths.

Hutson, J.M. and Beasley, S.W. 1992: *Descent of the testis.* London: Edward Arnold.

Scorer, C.G. and Farrington, G.H. 1971: *Congenital deformities of the testis and epididymis.* London: Butterworths.

Skinner, M.A. and Grosfeld, J.L. 1993: Inguinal and umbilical hernia repair in infants and children, in hernia surgery. *Surgical Clinics of North America* **73**, 439–49.

CHAPTER 33

The prepuce and circumcision

J.I. CURRY AND D.M. GRIFFITHS

Introduction
Development and natural history
of the foreskin

Surgical treatment
Conclusions
References

Introduction

The foreskin, or prepuce, forms a substantial part of the workload of the paediatric surgeon both in the operating theatre and in the outpatients' department. Some 127 paediatric operations were performed in the year 1994 in Southampton General Hospital, and at present some 21 000 circumcisions are performed annually in the UK by both general and paediatric surgeons, with some 7% of boys having the operation on the National Health Service (NHS) by the age of 15 years (Rickwood and Walker, 1989). This chapter aims to document the natural history of the foreskin and so outline the approach to diagnosis and surgical management.

Development and natural history of the foreskin

At 8 weeks' gestation the prepuce develops as a circumferential epidermal thickening which extends over the base of the glans penis. Growth at this stage is more rapid on the dorsum and by 12 weeks' gestation the urethra still opens on the ventral surface of the penis and the prepuce is deficient here, hence the hooded type of foreskin seen in hypospadias. The ventral aspect of the prepuce and the terminal urethra are formed by outgrowths from the inferior aspect of the glans, carrying the adherent dorsal prepuce. The glans and prepuce then fuse in the midline ventrally to form the terminal urethra and the ventral aspect of the prepuce.

By 16 weeks, growth of the prepuce has reached the tip of the penis and there is a common squamous epithelium between the undersurface of the prepuce and the glans. The now potential space is formed by a process of desquamation until an actual space exists.

The smegma produced by the glands around the corona of the glans collects under the pseudomucosa as white lumps, so-called preputial pearls. These can become sufficiently prominent to convince the mother that her son has cancer. As the adhesions lyse, the cheesy material is discharged. If it becomes infected it liquifies and resembles pus, often stimulating the use of antibiotics when simple lavage may be more appropriate. At birth, separation of the prepuce from the underlying glans is incomplete and the term 'adhesions' in this context is somewhat of a misnomer as they are not pathological. Figure 33.1 charts the increasing incidence of retractility of the prepuce from birth to 5 years. Thus it can be seen that the foreskin is not usually fully retractile in the first 3 years of life. Oster (1968) has shown that even up until the age of 15 years a few residual adhesions between the foreskin and the glans are present in over 10% of boys. Functionally the prepuce serves to protect the delicate, underlying glans from ammoniacal dermatitis while the child is in nappies and it is presumably no coincidence that achieving

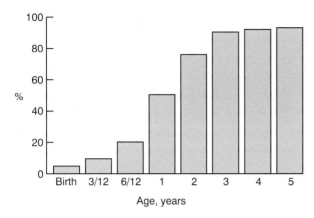

Fig. 33.1 Percentage of boys with a retractile prepuce. (After Gairdner, 1949.)

continence coincides with approximately 95% of boys having a retractile foreskin. The advice given to parents and other health care workers should be dependent on the child's age. In the newborn period and the first year or 2 of life they should just wash the penis gently. When 3–4 years of age, the child, with the parents, should be encouraged to gently retract and wash the prepuce and underlying glans to encourage lysis of the adhesions. When the foreskin becomes fully retractile he should practice routine penile hygiene.

Surgical treatment

INDICATION

Operating on the prepuce is only advocated for medical reasons (Editorial, 1979).

Phimosis (Greek: 'muzzled')

This is a condition which affects the terminal part of the foreskin and causes a tight ring. This ring prevents retraction of a foreskin which is no longer adherent to the glans.

Phimosis is either primary, in which the foreskin has never been retractile but ballooning on micturition indicates that the preputial adhesions are broken down, or secondary when the phimosis develops after the prepuce has been retractile. Conditions causing such phimosis include balanitis xerotica obliterans (BXO) and trauma.

BXO is a condition which affects the prepuce and glans and has a peak incidence around the age of 8 years. The presentation is typically with a phimosis in a child who may have previously been able to retract the foreskin. The presentation can also include dysuria, obstructive symptoms ranging from a poor stream with ballooning to severe obstruction and retention, haema-

turia and paraphimosis. The clinical findings are characteristic, with a scarred whitish foreskin which does not retract. Similar plaques can be found on the glans and if involving the meatus can cause meatal stenosis. Histologically, the prepuce shows a superficial dermal thick hyaline zone with a dense band of lymphocytes at the deep border (Bale and Martin, 1987). This condition is argued by some to be the only true condition which requires circumcision both for the symptoms it causes and the potential predisposition to malignant change. Spontaneous regression has been reported (Rickwood *et al.*, 1980) but must be regarded as an exception to the rule. With regards to the meatus, at the time of surgery a decision will need to be made regarding its patency and whether a meatotomy needs to be performed. If on removal of the plaque from the meatus there is an area of raw glans then a mild topical steroid can be used in the postoperative period to settle this inflammation. Meatal stenosis is the major long-term complication from this condition (up to 28% according to Griffiths *et al.*, 1985) and the parents should be informed of this when the child is first seen in the clinic.

The foreskin should be sent for histological analysis to confirm the diagnosis but an experienced paediatric surgeon will have little difficulty in recognizing this condition clinically.

Trauma may occur if a physiologically non-retractile foreskin is withdrawn over the glans, causing a tear in the foreskin with subsequent healing by scarring. This scarring may narrow the potential diameter of the prepuce and prevent further retraction when the foreskin is mobile.

It can be seen that the major dilemma is differentiating the child with a non-retractile foreskin who has a true phimosis, in whom surgery would be needed, from the child who has normal preputial adhesions in whom surgery would be unwarranted. To this end, if the child is less than 5 years old, has on inspection a soft, non-scarred, non-retractile prepuce and has a good urinary stream then it is likely that he has a normally adherent foreskin and not a phimosis (Rickwood and Walker, 1989).

Paraphimosis (Greek: 'almost muzzled')

If a tight prepuce is retracted over the glans and not replaced then this constricting band inhibits venous return and the glans swells. This swelling in turn prevents return of the prepuce and a vicious circle ensues. Return of the prepuce can sometimes be achieved using EMLA cream and gentle compression on the ward but usually necessitates general anaesthetic and even a dorsal slit. Circumcision is usually deferred to allow the oedema to settle.

There may be a tendency to paraphimosis. By definition, there will be some boys whose foreskin is neither non-retractile due to a phimosis, nor normally retractile as they have an intermediate preputial tightness. The foreskin retracts fully, but there is an obvious constriction band round the shaft and if left they would develop a true paraphimosis. Many of these bands will improve with regular retraction in the bath and at micturition, but the boy must be reminded to replace the foreskin every time. If the constriction band fails to improve after 6–12 months of regular retraction, or the boy refuses to co-operate, then an elective circumcision as a child is less traumatic than an emergency admission as an adolescent with a girlfriend and a paraphimosis!

Balanitis and posthitis (inflammation of the glans and prepuce, respectively)

In Rickwood's paper of 1989, 34% of 420 referrals to the outpatients' department were for balanitis and this figure was similar in the Griffiths cohort of 1985 (40%). Inflammation of the glans and prepuce affects less than 4% of boys, who are usually under the age of 4 years (Rickwood and Walker, 1989). The episodes themselves are usually self-limiting and are probably due to bacteria infecting the smegma which collects behind the 'adhesions'. They probably have no long-term sequelae.

Symptomatic treatment is employed to bathe the penis in a mild antiseptic and antibiotics are usually prescribed although no infecting organism is identified. In view of this, surgery should be restricted to those children who have recurrent episodes (more than three) causing distress to the child and scarring in an otherwise morphologically normal prepuce.

Trauma

Trauma to the prepuce, such as occurs with a zip fastener, may produce enough damage to necessitate circumcision, or if the skin of the shaft is amputated then the prepuce can be used to provide skin cover.

Urinary tract infections (UTI)

In an American series (Wiswell *et al.*, 1993), infants who were uncircumcised had a tenfold increase in the incidence of UTI compared those who were circumcised and in their meta-analysis of nine previous studies they found between a fivefold and 89-fold increase in UTI in those who were uncircumcised. The exact place of circumcision in recurrent UTI is not clear but it is becoming a procedure being performed increasingly as the first operative procedure in a boy not responding to prophylaxis before any other procedure is performed to correct a structural abnormality (e.g. reimplantation for vesicoureteric reflux). There is as yet no prospective evidence to suggest that routine neonatal circumcision would reduce the incidence of complicated UTI, especially those that lead to renal scarring.

Social, religious and pleasure

The most common indication in this category would be circumcision as part of the parent's religious beliefs. Such circumcisions have been occurring as far back as 2300 BC (noticed on Egyptian mummies) and probably further back, as evidenced by hieroglyphics. Muslims and Jews circumcise their male children but in the Jewish community this rite is performed by the Rabbi. NHS purchasers now vary in their attitude to religious circumcisions and many do not now offer this service. This may lead to an increase in the rate of serious complications especially if the procedure is performed by a person who is not medically trained (Madden and Boddy, 1991).

It will be the case that some mothers will request circumcision because they are certain from their own experience that circumcised men are sexually more satisfying and more satisfied. These mothers may not be dissuaded from circumcision and if you refuse then they will persevere until they find a less qualified surgeon and anaesthetist.

Malignancy

Proponents of circumcision have advocated it as a means of reducing the incidence of penile carcinoma but no conclusive evidence exists to support this. The same is also the case for their partners with reference to carcinoma of the cervix (Poland, 1990). Lack of proper hygiene has been suggested as a causative factor in carcinoma of the penis and it would seem good advice to recommend the regular cleaning of the glans (which is impossible with a phimosis) (Frisch *et al.*, 1995).

CONTRAINDICATIONS TO CIRCUMCISION

- Hypospadias: the prepuce may be used in the repair of a hypospadias; for example, in the operation described by Duckett the inner lining of the foreskin is separated on a vascular pedicle from the outer lining, then brought round to the front of the shaft of the penis, tubularized on a stent and interposed between the distal urethral orifice and the terminal glans. A similar procedure can also be performed by directly laying the prepuce on to the urethral plate.
- Buried penis: the foreskin is used as a donor of skin to elevate and surround the penile shaft.
- Correction of chordee without hypospadias: the prepuce is used to create penile shaft coverage when the chordee has been corrected at surgery.
- Correction of urethral stenosis following trauma: although not a contraindication to circumcision as such the prepuce has been found to be useful in bridging a gap in the urethra created by resection of a stricture secondary to trauma.

SURGERY OF THE FORESKIN

Circumcision is the main surgical procedure advocated but some foreskins are suitable for an alternative procedure, preputial plasty (Cuckow *et al.*, 1994). Firstly, the technique of reduction of paraphimosis is described, followed by circumcision and preputial plasty.

Reduction of paraphimosis

Boys with a paraphimosis will usually need a general anaesthetic to replace the foreskin. Most will have enough discomfort from the swollen glans to make any effort to manipulate it, at best, unkind.

Once the child is anaesthetized pressure should be exerted on the region of the glans to reduce the swelling. This may take 10–15 min of pressure. If the foreskin is still unable to be reduced then consideration should be given to performing a dorsal split at the point of the constriction band on the foreskin. The technique is identical to that performed in a preputial plasty (see later). It is advisable not to perform a circumcision at this stage because it can be very difficult to assess the amount of skin that needs to be excised as the tissues are very oedematous and the wound healing is less good. Regular retraction and prompt replacement of the foreskin may result in avoiding a circumcision.

Circumcision

An artery forcep is used to dilate the phimosis (if necessary) so that the foreskin can be retracted and cleaned with aqueous povidone iodine (Seton Health Care, UK). Any residual adhesions present between the glans and foreskin are gently broken down at this stage. Care should be taken not to introduce the forcep into the urethral meatus (Fig. 33.2A). Clips are placed on the dorsal and ventral surface of the foreskin and elevated. A sinus forceps or standard small bone cutter is placed around the corona of the glans with the jaws open, the instrument being held in the right hand (Fig. 33.2B). The operator's left thumb then pushes against the glans to displace it below the jaws which are then opposed on the foreskin with the glans safely below. A knife or scissors are then used to produce a straight cut (Fig. 33.2C). Any excess pseudomucosa is trimmed with scissors to leave a rim of approximately 5 mm (Fig. 33.2D). Haemostasis is vital at this stage prior to closure. The wound can be closed with interrupted or subcuticular absorbable suture (e.g. 5/0 chromic cat gut) (Fig. 33.2E).

No postoperative dressing is needed but some form of cream on the glans is useful to prevent sticking to the underclothes (e.g. chloromycetin eye ointment).

Preputial plasty

Following the technique as above, the foreskin is retracted over the glans (Cuckow *et al.*, 1994). An incision is made at the constriction ring from A to B as indicated (Fig. 33.3A and B). The incision is then sutured transversely using absorbable sutures (Fig. 33.3C and D). This is in effect a dorsal slit. Functionally, the results can be excellent but occasionally the cosmetic result is less so, with the foreskin having a dog-eared appearance. Within 7 days the boy is encouraged to retract his foreskin regularly to permit cleaning.

COMPLICATIONS

The series from Southampton reported by Griffiths *et al.* (1985) quoted an overall rate of morbidity of 6.4% but the incidence of 'minor' postoperative problems noticed only by the community paediatric nurse was much higher in terms of oozing, vomiting (related to the use of opiates as part of the anaesthetic) and the length of time before the children were back to wearing normal clothes. Complication rates vary depending on the series, with a range from 0.06% (Speert, 1953) to 55% (Patel, 1966), but a realistic figure would be between 2 and 10% (Fraser *et al.*, 1981; Kaplan, 1983; Griffiths *et al.*, 1985). Williams and Kapila (1993) reviewed the complications in detail. The most common problems include the following.

Haemorrhage

The quoted incidence of haemorrhage is in the region of 1–2%. Most commonly it occurs in the first 24 hours postoperatively and can occasionally be managed by local pressure. Topical vasoconstrictors have been used but give troublesome side-effects from systemic absorption. Meticulous haemostasis is required prior to closure of the wound to avoid this, and agitation of the raw area with a swab can reveal vessels needing attention which might otherwise have been missed. It is recommended that the child is taken back to theatre for exploration if haemorrhage occurs. Major haemorrhage has been reported, but never requiring transfusion.

Sepsis

This is seen on the glans and if it occurs is usually mild with only local inflammatory changes. In very young children, however, especially those still in nappies, the infection can be quite severe, causing ulceration and necrosis with the long-term consequences of meatal or urethral stenosis. Septicaemia and death have been reported.

Meatal stenosis

As already mentioned this can be a consequence of BXO but can also occur following circumcision for other reasons if meatal ulceration occurs. In its most severe form it can be a cause of recurrent pyelonephritis and obstructive uropathy.

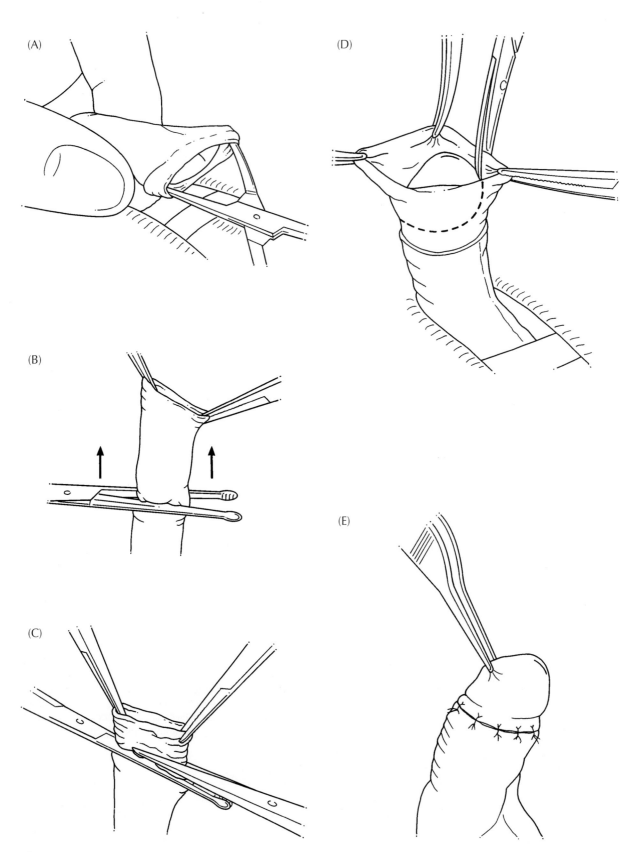

Figs 33.2 Circumcision.

(A)

(C)

(B)

(D)

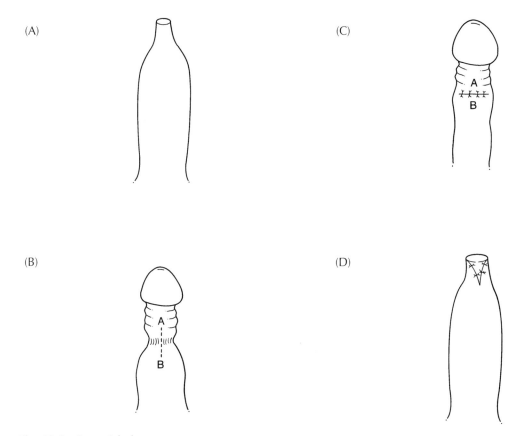

Figs 33.3 Preputial plasty.

Iatrogenic trauma

Inadvertent injury and even amputation of the glans have been reported following circumcision (often in an out-of-hospital setting) and will usually require specialist expertise to reconstruct. The terminal urethra lies in close proximity to the frenulum and stitches placed too deeply can penetrate the urethra and cause fistulae. In common with most surgical procedures the experience or inexperience of the operator will have a direct effect on the outcome and the common practice of leaving circumcisions to unsupervised junior surgeons with little exposure in the above techniques is certainly one to be discouraged.

Psychological problems

The literature and even the media show evidence of not only the physical but the emotional scarring this 'mutilating' operation has had on some men and to this end there is now advice available to help men return to the uncircumcised state (Bigelow, 1994a, b). Even in the neonatal period marked behavioural changes have been noted in association with this procedure.

Conclusions

Rickwood and Walker (1989) stated that in the Mersey region up to two-thirds of all circumcisions were performed inappropriately owing to the misdiagnosis of preputial pathology, especially phimosis, in very young boys.

With a better understanding of the natural history of the prepuce it is likely that the number of operations performed will reduce and that there will be a change in the ratio of prepuce-sparing procedures performed, compared to standard circumcisions. If the outpatient workload is to be reduced then there needs to be a programme of education aimed at general practitioner trainees to teach what is and what is not normal so as to reduce the number of unnecessary referrals.

References

Bale, P.M. and Martin, H.C.O. 1987: Balanitis xerotica obliterans in children. *Paediatric Pathology* **7**, 617–27.

Bigelow, J. 1994a: The joy of uncircumcising. Personal view. *British Medical Journal* **309**, 676–7.

Bigelow, J. 1994b: *The joy of uncircumcising! Restore your birthright and maximise sexual pleasure.* Folkestone: Hour Glass Press.

Cuckow, P.M., Rix, G. and Mouriquand, P.D.E. 1994: Preputial Plasty: A good alternative to circumcision. *Journal of Paediatric Surgery* **29**, 561–3.

Editorial 1979: *British Medical Journal* **i**, 1163.

Frank, J.D. 1995: Circumcision, meatotomy and meatoplasty. In *Rob and Smith's operative surgery: paediatric surgery.* London: Chapman & Hall Medical.

Fraser, I.A., Allen, M.J., Bagshaw, P.F. and Johnstone, M. 1981: A randomised trial to assess childhood circumcision with the plastibell device compared to a conventional dissection technique. *British Journal of Surgery* **68**, 593–5.

Frisch, M., Friis, S., Kjaer, S.K. and Melbye, M. 1995: Falling incidence of penis cancer in an uncircumcised population (Denmark 1943–90). *British Medical Journal* **311**, 1471.

Gairdner, D. 1949: The fate of the foreskin. *British Medical Journal* **2**, 1433–9.

Griffiths, D.M., Atwell, J.D. and Freeman, N.V.A. 1985: Prospective survey of the indications and morbidity of circumcision in children. *European Urology* **11**, 184–7.

Kaplan, G.W. 1983: Complications of circumcision. *Urological Clinics of North America* **10**, 543–9.

Madden, P. and Boddy, S.-A. 1991: Should religious circumcisions be performed on the NHS? *British Medical Journal* **302**, 47.

Oster, J. 1968: Further fate of the foreskin. *Archives of Disease in Childhood* **43**, 200–3.

Patel, H. 1966: The problem of routine circumcision. *Canadian Medical Association Journal* **95**, 576.

Poland, R.L. 1990: The question of routine neonatal circumcision. *New England Journal of Medicine* **322**, 1312–15.

Rickwood, A.M.K., Hemalatha, V., Batcup, G. and Spitz, L. 1980: Phimosis in boys. *British Journal of Urology* **52**, 147–50.

Rickwood, A.M.K. and Walker, J. 1989: Is phimosis over-diagnosed in boys and are too many circumcisions performed as a consequence? *Annals of the Royal College of Surgeons, England* **71**, 275–7.

Speert, H. 1953: Circumcision of the newborn; an appraisal of the present status. *Obstetrics and Gynaecology* **2**, 164–72.

Williams, N. and Kapila, L. 1993: Complications of circumcision. *British Journal of Surgery* **80**, 1231–6.

Wiswell, T.E. and Hachey, W.E. 1993: Urinary tract infection and the uncircumcised state; an update. *Clinical Paediatrics* **32**, 130–4.

CHAPTER 34

The undescended testis

A. BIANCHI

Introduction
Embryology
Normal testicular descent
Histology of the cryptorchid testis
The hypothalamo-pituitary–gonadal axis
Incidence of testicular undescent
The cause of testicular undescent
Normal testicular position: the retractile testis
Classification of testicular undescent
Unusual forms of testicular undescent

Associated pathology
Testicular transfer to the scrotum (orchidopexy)
Treatment
Complications associated with orchidopexy
for the palpable testis
The impalpable testis
Summary of surgical approach
Conclusion
References
Further reading

Introduction

Several issues surrounding the mechanisms of normal descent, the aetiology of undescent and the normality of the undescended testis remain as controversial today as in John Hunter's time (Hunter, 1786). Questions relating to management, both medical and surgical, remain the subject of interesting debate. The role of hormone or drug therapy, largely discredited as a treatment for undescent, is being assessed in relation to improved fertility. Surgical techniques have changed, with new variations on the operation of orchidopexy. The management of the impalpable testis continues to provoke marked controversy. In essence therefore, even today the field of normal and abnormal testicular descent remains a subject for fruitful research.

Embryology

Early gonadal differentiation from the urogenital ridge is sexually indifferent in mammals. Gonadal induction to form a testis is regulated by genes on the short arm of the Y chromosome. At least two genes, ZFY and SRY

(sex-determining region of Y) are known to be involved. The more specific SRY encodes for a DNA binding protein, is testis specific and is expressed at an appropriate stage of embryonic gonadal development (Editorial, 1990). Gonadal differentiation towards a testis and the subsequent onset of testicular hormone production appear to 'switch on' cellular genetic programmes controlling a cascade of secondary changes leading to virilization of the basic female (Warne, 1992). It is these same hormones, testosterone and Müllerian inhibiting substance (MIS), that influence the descent of the testis to the scrotum (Fig. 34.1).

Normal testicular descent

Hutson and Beasley (1992) suggested that testicular descent occurs in two separate phases, each controlled by different hormones.

PHASE 1: TRANSABDOMINAL DESCENT

Transabdominal migration of the testis from the urogenital ridge to the internal inguinal ring does not depend on androgens. The migratory process is associated with

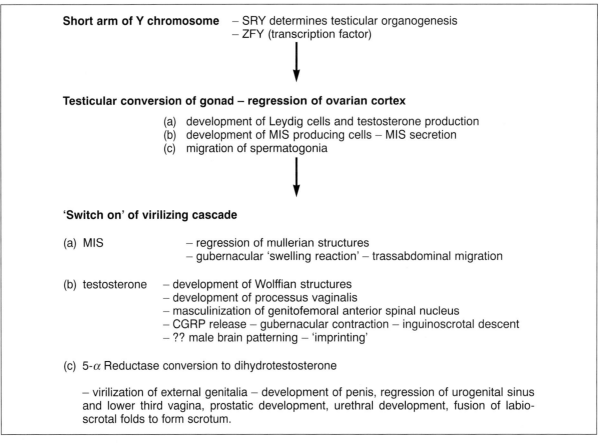

Fig. 34.1 Male sex development.

thickening and shortening of the gubernaculum, the 'gubernacular swelling reaction', which anchors the testis to the lateral abdominal wall. Such 'swelling reaction' occurs only in the male but is also found in patients with complete androgen insensitivity, thus confirming its androgen independence. Observations of the persistent Müllerian duct syndrome, male pseudohermaphrodites with dysplastic gonads and oestrogen-treated fetal male mice indicate MIS as the controlling factor in transabdominal testicular migration.

PHASE 2: INGUINOSCROTAL TESTICULAR DESCENT

Just prior to this phase of descent the short thickened male gubernaculum anchors the testis at the internal inguinal ring. Within it lies the developing peritoneal sac, the processus vaginalis, surrounded by the developing cremaster muscle which is innervated by the genitofemoral nerve. Experimental and clinical studies have ascertained the major role of androgens in the inguinoscrotal phase of testicular descent. It has been suggested that androgens produced by the fetal testis act

to masculinize irreversibly the anterior spinal nucleus of the genitofemoral nerve (sexual dimorphism) (Hutson and Beasley, 1992). In response to androgens the nerve releases the neurotransmitter calcitonin gene-related peptide (CGRP) which stimulates strong rhythmic contractions in the CGRP-receptor rich gubernaculum, thus inducing inguinoscrotal testicular migration.

NORMAL POSTNATAL TESTICULAR HISTOLOGY AND DEVELOPMENT

At term the seminiferous tubules are filled with gonocytes, spermatogonia and Sertoli cells. Leydig cells are easily identifiable in the interstitial tissues. These demonstrate accentuated growth during the second to sixth month after birth and subsequently regress, becoming more difficult to identify until the ninth year when they again become prominent. During the first years of life spermatogonia are quantifiable as the 'tubular fertility index' (TFI) which represents the percentage of tubules seen to contain spermatogonia. After 6 years of age the TFI rises and by the eighth year primary spermatocytes appear. Development of a tubular lumen and Sertoli cell maturation is followed by the onset of spermatogenesis.

Histology of the cryptorchid testis

In 1929 Cooper noted that the younger the child and the further the level of testicular descent the closer was the histology of the cryptorchid testis to normal. The prepubertal cryptorchid testis has a typical appearance, with a broad empty interstitium surrounding small or degenerate tubules containing few or no germ cells. The appearances are different, however, during the early years of life. At least up to 2 years of age the cryptorchid testis contains normal numbers of germ cells and the tubule diameter is maintained, after which there is a progressive reduction in germ cell numbers and a failure of maturation of the spermatogonia to form spermatocytes. From the outset the number of Leydig cells is markedly reduced and their development is impaired, coinciding with the absence of the normal surge in testosterone output during the first 6 postnatal months. The reduced Leydig cell mass may reflect a failure of gonadotrophin stimulation during fetal life and highlights the relevance of the hypothalamo-pituitary–gonadal axis to testicular development and descent.

The hypothalamo-pituitary–gonadal axis

Testicular function and male reproduction is controlled by the hypothalamo-pituitary–gonadal axis. Its function commences as early as 4–6 weeks after conception when luteinizing hormone-releasing hormone (LHRH) is detectable in the hypothalamus, and undergoes continuing development until puberty. This 'hypothalamic oscillator' in the arcuate nucleus releases LHRH which stimulates secretion of luteinizing hormone (LH) and follicle-stimulating hormone (FSH) from the anterior pituitary, which in turn influence the development of the fetal testis. The whole is regulated by a negative feedback mechanism. It is noteworthy that anencephalic and apituitary fetuses have very low LH and FSH levels and demonstrate markedly hypotrophic genitalia with small intra-abdominal testes containing severely reduced germ cell and Leydig cell numbers. Pituitary LH influences Leydig cell function and hence androgen secretion. FSH appears to be instrumental in the transformation of primordial germ cells into spermatogonia and in the differentiation of Sertoli cells.

Human chorionic gonadotrophin (HCG) is a glycoprotein produced by the placenta. It is of similar structure to LH and FSH and has similar androgen stimulatory effects. As placental HCG levels decline, their function is taken up by the fetal pituitary, which induces sufficient testosterone release from the fetal testis for development of the genital tubercle and for testicular growth (Grumbach and Kaplan, 1974). Immediately postnatally, the cryptorchid child, with his markedly diminished Leydig cell mass, fails to produce a testosterone surge and generates a lower peak LH level on LHRH stimulation, reflecting the possible failure of the hypothalamo-pituitary–gonadal axis during fetal and subsequent gonadal development.

Incidence of testicular undescent

Recent studies reported a real increase in testicular undescent from 2.7% (Scorer, 1964) for the term child to 4.3% (Jackson et al., 1986a, b). The incidence of undescent is higher with increasing prematurity. It is accepted that testicular descent continues during the first 3–6 months postnatally, such that the true incidence of undescent reduces to 1.58% (Jackson et al., 1986a, b) and remains unchanged thereafter (Campbell, 1959). The right testis is undescended slightly more often (53–58%) than the left (42–47%). Bilateral undescent is less common and occurs in 10–25% of cases. Approximately 14% of cryptorchid boys have a family history of testicular undescent. Undescent is a common association with hypospadias and other forms of undervirilization. It occurs with endocrine disorders, with anomalies of the abdominal wall, e.g. prune belly syndrome, ectopic bladder, gastroschisis and with numerous chromosomal and polymalformation syndromes which can be referenced in appropriate specialized texts.

The cause of testicular undescent

The reason for testicular undescent remains unclear but 'may lie with the testis itself' (Hunter, 1786). It may possibly relate to a failure of the hypothalamo-pituitary–gonadal axis or to an abnormal or failed development or migration of the gubernaculum. Thus aberrant gubernacular migration may account for testicular ectopia whereas failure of hormonal induction or of gonadal response may lead to retention along the normal pathway of descent.

Normal testicular position: the retractile testis

Testicular retractility is a normal feature during the prepubertal years, and is caused by a brisk cremasteric contraction in response to minor stimuli in the area of distribution of the genitofemoral nerve. The reflex is weakest after birth and becomes progressively stronger after the first year of life. The normal retractile testis may thus lie at any site between the external inguinal ring and the scrotum. It should be able to descend spontaneously into the lowermost scrotum when the child is warm and relaxed. On clinical examination the normal testis can be brought to low scrotum on a demonstrably long spermatic cord, without pain or even the slightest discomfort to the child. Normal testicular volume is less than 2 ml up to 11 years of age rising to 5 ml by 12 years and 12–14 ml by 15 years. Any variation on these criteria should be regarded as abnormal, the testicle falling within the 'spectrum of testicular undescent'.

Classification of testicular undescent

The undescended testis may be palpable or impalpable. The palpable testes may be imperfectly descended, lying along the normal pathway of descent. Within this group are testes which lie in high scrotum and do not descend spontaneously beyond this point. Such testes, called 'gliding or mobile' testes, should be regarded as undescended since they are often smaller and show the histological features of cryptorchidism (Cucchi *et al.*, 1993). Alternatively, the palpable testes may lie in an aberrant or ectopic position. The various common positions are outlined in Fig. 34.2.

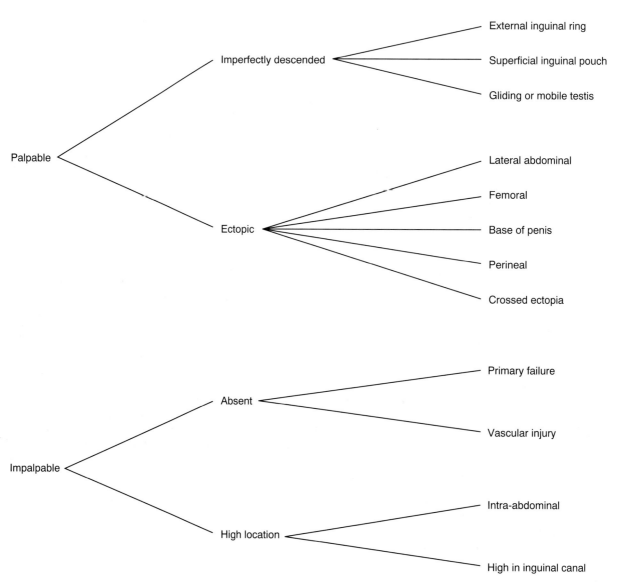

Fig. 34.2   Classification of the undescended testis.

The impalpable testis may be absent (anorchia) because of a primary failure of development or more commonly because of loss from a vascular accident, e.g. torsion. It is much more likely however to be found lying high in the inguinal canal or intra-abdominally. Recent studies (Hadziseimovic, 1983) have reported these testes to contain normal numbers of germ cells during the first 6 months postnatally. The impalpable testis constitutes some 15–20% of all undescended testes, with anorchia occurring in only 6–10% of these. It is therefore always important to attempt to locate an impalpable testis.

Unusual forms of testicular undescent

ASCENDING TESTIS

There have been several reports (Atwell, 1985; Fenton *et al.*, 1990) of testes which have ascended from a confirmed scrotal position at birth to a position consistent with undescent. It is suggested that the reason is a failure of proportional elongation of the spermatic cord in line with body growth such that the testis is progressively retracted out of the scrotum.

IATROGENIC UNDESCENT

This complication follows surgery (division of processus vaginalis, orchidopexy) in the inguinal area. It is due to fibrous tethering of the spermatic cord to the operative scar such that the testis is retracted out of the scrotum with increasing body growth. Iatrogenic undescent is different from 'recurrence of undescent' which is most commonly due to inadequate testicular mobilization or choice of an inappropriate surgical technique for a testis on a short vascular pedicle.

Associated pathology

PATENT PROCESSUS VAGINALIS: TORSION

Failure of the testis to reach the lowermost scrotum is associated with persistent patency of the processus vaginalis which presents as a hydrocele or an indirect inguinal hernia. The factors responsible for fusion of the processus vaginalis remain unclear. It is interesting that the imperfectly descended testis is always associated with processal patency, whereas fusion of the processus occurs with testicular ectopia even though the testis has never been near the scrotum. Incomplete testicular descent results in an abnormally mobile testis which is liable to torsion. It may happen at any age and is not uncommon during intrauterine life. Torsion is usually of the extravaginal variety, occurring on the spermatic cord and resulting in loss of the testis and blind-ending testicular vessels and vas.

EPIDIDYMAL AND VASAL ANOMALIES

Epididymo-testicular dissociation and anomalies of the epididymis and vas deferens are found in 17% of unilateral undescent and 26% of bilateral undescent cases. The higher the gonad is retained the greater the incidence. It is evident that such anomalies also have a definite bearing on infertility related to testicular undescent.

SPERMATOGENESIS

The hallmark of cryptorchidism is a 'failure of maturation of seminiferous tubules with a consequent inability to produce sperm'. The problem may relate to a failure of the hypothalamo-pituitary–gonadal axis, to an intrinsically abnormal gonad, to the deleterious effect of a higher temperature on the undescended testis or to a combination of these factors. The relatively normal tubular architecture and number of germ cells in undescended testes at birth, and the subsequent failure of maturation and progressive loss of spermatogonia particularly after the second year of life has been reported (Mengel *et al.*, 1974; Hadziselimovic *et al.*, 1975). It has been suggested that cryptorchidism be regarded as a 'progressive disease process' which, by implication, it should be possible to halt or reverse (Hadziselimovic *et al.*, 1975). Studies in animals and humans have repeatedly confirmed the deleterious effect of a higher temperature on spermatogenesis. It is logical therefore to attempt to transfer the testis to a normal, lower temperature scrotal environment as soon as possible and before spermatogenic injury has occurred.

NEOPLASIA

It seems likely that the higher content of dysgenetic tissue within the undescended testis relates to the increased incidence of neoplasia (Sohval, 1956). The incidence reduces with a greater degree of testicular descent. The contralateral scrotal testis also contains a larger than normal content of dysgenetic material, such that one in five testicular tumours associated with undescent occurs in the scrotal testis. In recent studies the risk of tumour in an undescended testis has been placed at five to ten times that of the normal population (Woodhouse, 1991; Stone *et al.*, 1991), previous figures of 35–50 times being excessively high. Sixty per cent of tumours are seminomas and present at the usual age for testicular tumours of 20–40 years. The incidence of 'carcinoma *in situ*' is 1.7–2% and is considered to arise from abnormal gonocytes within the undescended testis. Following such a diagnosis there is a 5% risk of a similar lesion for the contralateral scrotal testis. Long-term follow-up is therefore always relevant.

PSYCHOLOGICAL DISTURBANCE IN THE CHILD AND THE PARENTS

The particular relevance of normal genitalia to the

development of body image, gender acceptance and personality in the adolescent is beyond question (Gross and Replogle, 1963; Hazebroek, 1986). The issue is of equal importance to the parents, for whom fears relating to their child's future virility and fertility generate much anxiety and distress. Preservation of the testes and placement in a normal scrotal position providing a normal genital appearance from an early age is therefore a serious consideration.

HORMONE SECRETION AND SEXUAL ORIENTATION AND FUNCTION

Leydig cell function and hence testosterone secretion does not appear to be noticeably affected after the first 6 months of life and neither is it altered by testicular position. Unless there is bilateral gonadal atrophy, patients with undescended testes do not show failure of virilization and develop normal libido and potency. It would appear that sufficient hormone was present during fetal life for 'male' brain imprinting.

URINARY TRACT ANOMALIES

Some 3–9% of patients admitted for orchidopexy have major renal anomalies, commonly pelviureteric junction obstruction or absent ipsilateral kidney. This incidence is not considered sufficient to warrant routine investigation for all patients with testicular undescent.

Testicular transfer to the scrotum (orchidopexy)

TIMING

Since the incidence of undescent remains stable after 6 months of life and since deleterious effects of excessive temperature become increasingly evident after the second year, it seems logical to suggest that the undescended testis be transferred to a normal scrotal environment within six months and the second year of life. All children should therefore be reviewed on their first birthday. Persistent undescent is pathological and is an indication for testicular transfer to the scrotum.

INDICATIONS FOR ORCHIDOPEXY

Perhaps the most relevant indication for testicular transfer to the scrotum, i.e. orchidopexy is to provide 'normal' genitalia as early as possible. The lower temperature scrotal position enhances spermatogenesis and may even be associated with a reduction in neoplasia (Martin and Menck, 1975). In a scrotal situation the testis is easier to self-examine and monitor. Coincidental operative division of the processus and fixation of the testis eliminates the risk of torsion and inguinal hernia.

INDICATIONS FOR ORCHIDECTOMY

Orchidectomy is only indicated for proven *in situ* or florid malignancy. Otherwise it should only be considered for testes which have no psychological, spermatogenic or hormonal value. It is rarely indicated before puberty and should only be performed after careful consultation with a fully informed consenting patient mature enough to realize the possible implications for sexual function.

CLINICAL EXAMINATION AND DIAGNOSIS

At the first postnatal examination the presence, size (volume), consistency and the most caudal position to which the testis will descend are recorded. The presence of a hydrocele and the degree of scrotal hypoplasia are noted. Persistent undescent, at review on the child's first birthday, is an indication for treatment. Knowledgeable detailed correct examination and record keeping is crucial to correct therapy and eventual audit. It should be possible for the testis to reach and retain the lowermost scrotal position without any discomfort to the child.

INVESTIGATIONS

The most relevant, and for the palpable testis often the only investigation, is a thorough clinical examination. In view of the low incidence of anorchia and the increased risk of neoplasia, it is always important to attempt to locate an impalpable gonad. The investigation of a child with impalpable testes is best approached as a team which includes the endocrinologist and the geneticist. Serum LH and FSH levels may give an indication of hypothalamo-pituitary function and feedback. Alone they are insufficient for exclusion of an intra-abdominal testis. Assessment of gonadal testosterone response to HCG stimulation (1500 IU HCG i.m. for 3 days or 4500 IU as a single i.m. dose) will determine the presence of hormonally functional testicular tissue. However, a low or absent response does not exclude a dysplastic or hormonally non-functional primordial gonad. Laparoscopy constitutes the only definitive investigation, as all other modalities carry a degree of morbidity and are not definitive in the event of a negative result. At laparoscopy the location and status of the testis, the epididymis, the testicular vessels and the vas can be determined bilaterally. The presence of residual Müllerian structures can be ascertained. An atretic vas alone does not exclude a high testis. It is therefore always necessary to visualize blind-ending testicular vessels. A testicular biopsy may be taken.

SURGICAL EXPLORATION OF THE INGUINAL AREA

Surgical exploration of the inguinal canal is disruptive and inappropriate solely as a form of investigation, and is only acceptable as part of a definitive operative intervention. All information can be better obtained at laparoscopy. Passage of the vas and testicular vessels through the internal inguinal ring is evidence of previous testicular presence. If the testis is not palpable in the groin, it will have atrophied. Surgical exploration is not necessary since it is exceptional to find any residual dysgenetic tissue. The situation however is different should the testis not be palpable after previous orchidopexy for a testis on a short vascular pedicle. Total testicular atrophy cannot be assumed and postpubertal groin exploration is appropriate, with a view to orchidectomy or testicular placement (subcutaneously or scrotally) for easy self-monitoring.

MANAGEMENT OF THE CHILD WITH IMPALPABLE TESTES

Management is similar for unilateral and bilateral undescent, as well as for the child with a single residual testis after natural or iatrogenic loss. It involves an assessment of:

- the presence, location and quality of the testis, epididymis and vas

- the nature of the testicular vascular pedicle
- the age of the child in relation to spermatogenesis
- the risk of neoplasia.

These various relationships are delineated in Fig. 34.3.

Treatment

MEDICAL THERAPY

The intricate hormonal interactions involved in testicular descent prompted the use of hormonal therapy for testicular undescent. LHRH and HCG have had only limited success, for those testes which already lay in the high scrotum. These hormones seem to act by reducing cremasteric contractility. It is likely that responding testes would have descended spontaneously at puberty anyway. It is now accepted that LHRH and HCG therapy was based on an erroneous concept (Hutson and Beasley, 1992) and has no role in the management of undescent. There may, however, be a possible new role for hormonal manipulation for the induction of maturation of spermatogonia and hence improved fertility.

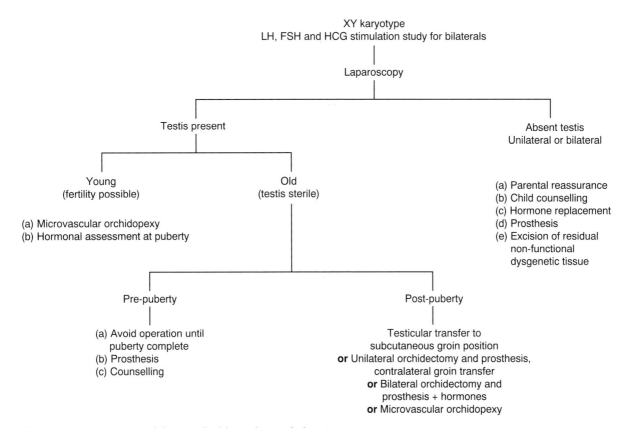

Fig. 34.3   Management of the impalpable undescended testis.

SURGICAL MANAGEMENT

Surgery remains the mainstay of treatment for testicular undescent. Orchidopexy for the palpable testis is relatively straightforward.

CONVENTIONAL ORCHIDOPEXY

The technique of conventional orchidopexy mobilizes the testis through an inguinal approach as described by Schuller in 1889 and Bevan in 1899 and 1903. Placement of the testis in a dartos pouch constructed through a separate scrotal incision was recommended by Schoemaker in 1932. These authors made the point that the palpable testis was held up by a shorter than normal processus vaginalis, the testicular vessels and vas having sufficient length for tension-free transfer to the scrotum. These features have been reiterated more recently (Hazebroek *et al.*, 1987; Bianchi and Squire, 1989) and form the basis for the transscrotal orchidopexy (Bianchi and Squire, 1989; Iyer *et al.*, 1995).

TRANSSCROTAL ORCHIDOPEXY

This procedure is performed through a skin crease incision in the neck of the scrotum. Dissection of the spermatic cord under direct vision allows safe separation of the short processus vaginalis from the vessels and the vas. High ligation and division of the processus allows the testis to be placed, without any tension, in an ipsilateral subdartos pouch, constructed through the same incision. No other fixation is necessary. This approach has the advantage of minimal dissection through a single incision, and of avoiding disruption of the inguinal canal. It is comfortable for the child, aesthetically pleasing and particularly suitable for day case surgery. Complication rates are presently similar for both the conventional and the transscrotal approach.

Complications associated with orchidopexy for the palpable testis

FAILED ORCHIDOPEXY

This is usually due to insufficient testicular vessel and vasal mobilisation at the first procedure. Following full mobilization the testis will usually reach the scrotum without tension.

RECURRENCE OF UNDESCENT

Recurrence is largely due to an inappropriate choice of surgical technique for a testis on a short vascular pedicle, which therefore will only reach the scrotum under tension. These testes, though palpable, originally lay high in the inguinal canal and could not be manipulated much below the external inguinal ring. Conventional orchidopexy is insufficient.

TESTICULAR REASCENT

Testes which become tethered to the operative scar after previous appropriate orchidopexy at a young age may be retracted out of the scrotum with increasing body growth. Release of fibrous adhesions will allow the testis to be returned to the scrotum without tension.

TESTICULAR ATROPHY

Postoperative atrophy is largely iatrogenic and is due to division of, or major injury to the main testicular vessels by rough handling or excessive tension. It is rarely due to spontaneous regression for primary intrinsic reasons.

VAS AND VASAL VESSEL INJURY

This is always iatrogenic and relates to inappropriate dissection technique. Vasal injury may well be partly responsible for the infertility associated with testicular undescent. Investigation is relevant since an injured or divided vas is amenable to microsurgical reconstruction.

COMPLICATIONS COMMON TO ANY OPERATION

Bruising, scrotal haematoma, wound disruption, testicular extrusion and infection are uncommon and become less likely with increasing experience and expertise.

The impalpable testis

HIGH INGUINAL AND INTRA-ABDOMINAL TESTIS

Some 20% of undescended testes lie high in the inguinal canal or intra-abdominally (Bianchi, 1995a). These testes have a short vascular pedicle and will not reach the scrotum. Several surgical options have been proposed, as follows.

MULTISTAGE ORCHIDOPEXY

This procedure, either with (Corkery, 1975) or without a silastic wrap (Levitt *et al.*, 1978) is carried out in at least two stages. The risk of injury to the testis, testicular vessels and vas increases with the increasing fibrosis and hence increasing difficulty on each subsequent occasion. It is possible that the reported successes may relate to insufficient mobilization at the first procedure.

FOWLER–STEPHENS TECHNIQUE

This procedure, which divides the main testicular vessels and relies on the delicate vasal and cremasteric collaterals for testicular survival and growth (Fowler and Stephens, 1959), is associated with a 50–100% atrophy rate. Variations proposed towards increasing testicular survival include mobilization of the vas in the centre of a wide peritoneal band in order to avoid injury to the flimsy vasal vessels (Snyder and Duckett, 1984), and the delayed or staged Fowler–Stephens approach which initially interrupts the main testicular vessels either at open operation (Ransley *et al.*, 1984) or laparoscopically (Bloom, 1991), and at a second procedure transfers a surviving testis to the scrotum. Paternity studies in a rat model by Tsang *et al.* (1993) have highlighted the severe spermatogenic injury to surviving testes following such sudden and chronic interruption of the dominant circulation.

MICROVASCULAR ORCHIDOPEXY

This implies the immediate return of a full circulation to the transferred testis (Bianchi, 1995b). The procedure involves high mobilization of the testicular vascular pedicle but also carefully safeguards the vas and vasal collaterals. Following high division of the dominant blood supply the testis is transferred to the scrotum and immediately revascularized by one arterial and one or two venous anastomoses to the inferior epigastric vessels. The procedure is technically demanding, but is often successful and is associated with 92% testicular survival and growth at puberty (Bianchi, 1990). The limited warm hypoxia of some 45–90 min duration had little effect on paternity in the rat (Tsang *et al.*, 1993).

REFLUO TECHNIQUE

This technique stems from the observation of Domini and Lima (1989; Lima *et al.*, 1989) that testicular loss following the Fowler–Stephens procedure was due to venous infarction because of inadequate venous return through the vasal collaterals. Their technique provides full venous drainage by microvascular anastomosis of the testicular vein to the inferior epigastric vein, but relies on the arterial input from the vasal collaterals. In the rat model the Refluo technique was associated with only minimal spermatogenic injury (Tsang *et al.*, 1993). The authors accept full microvascular revascularization (both arterial and venous anastomoses) whenever feasible, and recommend the Refluo approach (venous anastomosis only) as an acceptable 'fallback' position.

LAPAROSCOPIC ORCHIDOPEXY

This has been suggested as a one-stage alternative for the non-palpable testis (Hadziselimovic *et al.*, 1987; Al-Shareef *et al.*, 1996). The intra-abdominal testis is mobilized laparoscopically on intact vessels and vas and is then transferred by traction with a haemostat passed up from the scrotum. A considerable number of intra-abdominal testes were brought, on intact vessels and vas, to a low scrotal position, which was subsequently maintained. This striking feature is contrary to the usually finding of insufficient vessel length on full testicular mobilization at open operation. Furthermore, 28.6% of testes were excised, having been classed as 'atrophic' or 'high with vessels too short'. It is precisely the 'high' testes on 'short vessels' that require a microvascular approach rather than excision. The definition of the term 'atrophic' was not given.

Summary of surgical approach

Microvascular orchidopexy, in rapidly returning a full normal blood supply, is now the treatment of choice and the gold standard for the high inguinal and intra-abdominal testis on a short vascular pedicle. The procedure is applicable to children under 2 years of age, when the testicular vessels are still comparatively well developed. The Refluo concept provides an acceptable 'fallback' position, with the Fowler–Stephens procedure as the final poor compromise in view of the high incidence of spermatogenic injury and testicular atrophy. Laparoscopic orchidopexy as a one-stage procedure for the non-palpable testis is an interesting suggestion. The indications for this technique require careful evaluation.

THE 'LONG LOOP' VAS

The term describes a vas and accompanying vessels which pass down the inguinal canal for a variable distance and then loop back to link up with a high testis on a short vascular pedicle. This anatomical variant is said to be associated with a well-developed collateral circulation and thus to be ideal for the Fowler–Stephens approach. Assessment of this circulation at the time of surgery has made it abundantly clear that the collateral circulation from the vasal vessels is insufficient. Immediate full revascularization is the treatment of choice with any additional benefit from a better collateral circulation being regarded as a bonus.

PRUNE BELLY SYNDROME

Bilateral intra-abdominal testes form one element of the triad required for diagnosis of the prune belly syndrome. The cause of testicular undescent is unclear but may relate to interference with gubernacular attachment by the large distended bladder or to inadequacy of the abdominal musculature to raise intra-abdominal pressure to assist the passage of the testis out of the abdomen. It is interesting that these testes are often found to have a long vascular pedicle, particularly during the first months of life. The condition is associated with a high incidence of epididymo-vasal anomalies which, together with poor prostatic function and weak ejaculatory ability may account for the high incidence of infertility.

Conclusion

Over 60% of cryptorchid testes are easily palpable distal to the external inguinal ring. If untreated, 90% of bilateral cryptorchids are sterile. Even the untreated unilateral cryptorchid is infertile in 50.6% of cases and subfertile in 28.8%. It is well accepted that testes exposed to a higher body temperature sustain a reduction in spermatogenesis. Indeed, even the relatively low-lying gliding or mobile testis shows progressive deleterious changes typical of cryptorchidism. Such changes become more marked after the second year of life, such that all undescended testes should be transferred to the scrotum before this time. The role of hormones (LHRH, HCG, testosterone) for induction of testicular descent has been discredited (Hutson and Beasley, 1992). In future, new mediators such as CGRP may play a role in the medical and surgical management of undescent. For the present, conventional or transscrotal orchidopexy remains the appropriate treatment for the palpable testis below the external inguinal ring. The high inguinal and intra-abdominal testis also deserves early transfer to the scrotum at a time when the number of germ cells is said to be normal. The operation of microvascular orchidopexy is the treatment of choice. Indeed, it is illogical and unacceptable to transfer the testis on a less than adequate circulation.

The hallmark of the cryptorchid testis is the failure of maturation of the seminiferous tubules and spermatogonia, with consequent inability to produce sperm. This may reflect a failure of the hypothalamo-pituitary–gonadal Axis commencing during fetal life. The place for hormones such as LHRH, HCG, testosterone and the LHRH analogue buserelin (Nasser, 1995) in enhancing maturation of spermatogonia is presently being assessed. The ultimate goal of achieving a fertile testis on a full and adequate blood supply, in the scrotum from an early age, for the child born with testicular undescent, is now excitingly close.

References

Al-Shareef, Z.H., Al-Shlash, S., Koneru, S.R., Town, E., Al-Dhohayan, A. and Al-Brekett, K. 1996: Laparoscopic orchidopexy: one stage alternative for non palpable testes. *Annals of the Royal College of Surgeons of England* **78**, 115–18.

Atwell, J.D. 1985: Ascent of the testis. Fact or fiction? *British Journal of Urology* **57**, 474–7.

Belloli, G., D'Agostino, S. and Campobasso, P. 1994: Epididymal and vasal abnormalities in undescended testes and azoospermia. *Pediatric Surgery International* **9**, 95–8.

Bevan, A.D. 1899: Operation for undescended testicle and congenital inguinal hernia. *Journal of American Medical Association* **33**, 773–7.

Bevan, A.D. 1903: The surgical treatment of undescended testicle. *Journal of American Medical Association* **41**, 718–24.

Bianchi, A. 1990: Management of the impalpable testis: the role of microvascular orchidopexy. *Pediatric Surgery International* **5**, 48–53.

Bianchi, A. 1995a: The impalpable testis. *Annals of the Royal College of Surgeons of England* **77**, 3–6.

Bianchi, A. 1995b: Microvascular transfer (testis). In *Rob and Smith's operative surgery*, 5th ed. London: Chapman & Hall, 726–33.

Bianchi, A. and Squire, B.R. 1989: Transscrotal orchidopexy: orchidopexy revised. *Pediatric Surgery International* **4**, 189–92.

Bloom, D.A. 1991: Two-step orchidopexy with pelviscopic clip ligation of the spermatic vessels. *Journal of Urology* **145**, 1030–3.

Campbell, H.E. 1959: The incidence of malignant growth of the undescended testicle: a reply and re-evaluation. *Journal of Urology* **81**, 663–8.

Cooper, E.R.A. 1929: The histology of the retained testis in the human subject at different ages and its comparison with the scrotal testis. *Journal of Anatomy* **64**, 5–27.

Corkery, J.J. 1975: Staged orchidopexy – a new technique. *Journal of Pediatric Surgery*, **10**, 515–18.

Cucchi, L., Serao, A., Schiaffino, E., Caccia, F. and Canova, G. 1993: Il testicolo mobile: una condizione sottovalutata. *Medico e Bambino* **4**, 27–32.

Domini, R. and Lima, M. 1989: L'autotrapianto microvascolare 'refluo' del testicolo: una nuova soluzione tecnica. *Rassegna Italiana di Chirurgia Pediatrica* **31**, 213–23.

Editorial 1990: The secret of sex? *Lancet* **336**, 348–9.

Fenton, E.J.M., Woodward, A.A., Hudson, I.L. and Marschner, I. 1990: The ascending testis. *Pediatric Surgery International* **5**, 6–9.

Fowler, R. and Stephens, F.D. 1959: The role of testicular vascular anatomy in the salvage of high undescended testes. *Australian and New Zealand Journal of Surgery* **29**, 92–106.

Gross, R.E. and Replogle, R.L. 1963: Treatment of the undescended testis. *Postgraduate Medicine* **34**, 266–70.

Grumbach, M.M. and Kaplan, S.L. 1974: Fetal pituitary hormones and the maturation of central nervous system regulation of anterior pituitary function. In Gluck, L. (ed.), *Modern perinatal medicine*. Chicago, IL: Year Book Medical Publishers, 247.

Hadziseimovic, F. (ed.) 1983: Histology and ultrastructure of normal and cryptorchid testes. In *Cryptorchidism*. Berlin: Springer, 35–58.

Hadziselimovic, F., Herzog, B. and Seguchi, H. 1975: Surgical correction of cryptorchidism at 2 years: electron-microscopic and morphometric investigations. *Journal of Pediatric Surgery* **10**, 19–26.

Hadziselimovic, F., Huff, D., Duckett, J. *et al.* 1987: Long term effect of luteinizing-hormone-releasing-hormone analogue (buserelin) on cryptorchid testes. *Journal of Urology* **138**, 1043–5.

Hazebroek, F.W.J. 1986: Psychosexual aspects of cryptorchidism. In de Muinck Keizer-Schrama S.M.P.F. and Hazebroek, F.W.J. (eds), *The treatment of cryptorchidism: why, how, when. Clinical studies in prepubertal boys* **5.3.3**, 219–21.

Hazebroek, F.W.J., de Muinck Keizer-Schrama S.M.P.F., Van Maarschalkerweerd, M., Visser, H.K.A. and Molenaar, J.C. 1987: Why leuteinizing-hormone-releasing-hormone nasal spray will not replace orchidopexy in the treatment of boys with undescended testes. *Journal of Pediatric Surgery* **22**, 1177–82.

Hunter, J. 1786: Observations on certain parts of the animal economy. In Palmer, R. (ed.). *Observations on certain parts of the animal economy*. London: Longmans, Green & Co.

Hutson, J.M. and Beasley, S.W. 1992: Hormonal treatment. *Descent of the testis*. London: Edward Arnold, 154.

Iyer, K.R., Kumar, V., Huddart, S. and Bianchi, A. 1995: The scrotal approach. *Pediatric Surgery International* **10**, 58–60.

Jackson, M.B., Chilvers, C., Pike, M.C., Ansell, P. and Bull, D. and the John Radcliffe Hospital Cryptorchidism Study Group 1986a: Boys with late descending testes: the source of patients with 'retractile' testes undergoing orchidopexy. *British Medical Journal* **293**, 789–90.

Jackson, M.B., Chilvers, C., Pike, M.C., Ansell, P. and Bull, D. and the John Radcliffe Hospital Cryptorchidism Study Group 1986b: Cryptorchidism: an apparent substantial increase since 1960. *British Medical Journal* **293**, 1401–4.

Levitt, S.B., Kogan, S.J., Engel, M., Weiss, R.M., Martin, D.C. and Ehrlich, R.M. 1978: The impalpable testis: a rational approach to management. *Journal of Urology* **120**, 515–20.

Lima, M., Gentile, C., Ruggieri, G. *et al.* 1989: Autotrapianto testicolare sperimentale: premessa all' autotrapianto testicolare 'refluo' in eta pediatrica. *Rassegna Italiana di Chirurgia Pediarica* **31**, 243–6.

Martin, D.C. and Menck, H.R. 1975: The undescended testis: management after puberty. *Journal of Urology* **114**, 77–9.

Mengel, W., Hienz, H.A., Sippe, W.G. and Hecker, W.C. 1974: Studies on cryptorchidism: a comparison of histological findings in the germinative epithelium before and after the second year of life. *Journal of Pediatric Surgery* **9**, 445–50.

Nasser, A.H.M. 1995: Laparoscopic-assisted orchidopexy. A new approach to the impalpable testes. *Journal of Paediatric Surgery* **30**, 39–41.

Ransley, P.G., Vordermark, J.S., Caldamone, A.A. and Bellinger, M.F. 1984: Preliminary ligation of the gonadal vessels prior to orchidopexy for the intra abdominal testicle: a staged Fowler–Stephens procedure. *World Journal of Urology* **2**, 266–8.

Schoemaker, J. 1932: Uber Kryptorchismus und seine Behandlung. *Chirurgie* **4**, 1–3.

Schuller, M. 1889: On inguinal testicle and its operative treatment by transplantation into the scrotum. *Annals of Anatomy and Surgery* **4**, 89–102.

Scorer, C.G. 1964: The descent of the testis. *Archives of Disease in Childhood* **39**, 605–9.

Snyder, H.McC. and Duckett, J.W. 1984: Orchidopexy with division of spermatic vessels: a review of 10 years experience [Abstract]. *Journal of Urology* **131**, 126A.

Sohval, A.R. 1956: Testicular dysgenesis in relation to neoplasm of the testicle. *Journal of Urology* **75**, 285–91.

Stone, J.M., Cruickshank, D.G., Sandeman, T.F. and Matthews, J.P. 1991: Laterality, maldescent, trauma and other clinical factors in the epidemiology of testis cancer in Victoria, Australia. *British Journal of Cancer* **64**, 132–8.

Tsang, T.M., Bianchi, A., Carneiro, P.M.R., Chan, Y.F. and McLean, J. 1993: A study of warm testicular ischaemia and paternity in rats. *Pediatric Surgery International* **8**, 41–4.

Warne, G.L. 1992: The baby of uncertain sex. *Pediatric Surgery International* **7**, 244–8.

Woodhouse, C.R.J. 1991: Undescended testes. *Long-term paediatric urology*. Oxford: Blackwell Scientific.

Further reading

Bianchi, A. 1990: Microvascular orchidopexy for high undescended testes. In Frank, J.D. and Johnston, J.H. (eds) *Operative paediatric urology 12*. Edinburgh: Churchill Livingstone, 113–22.

de Muinck Keizer-Schrama, S.M.P.F. and Hazebroek, F.W.J. 1986: *The treatment of cryptorchidism: why, how, when. clinical studies in prepubertal boys*.

Fonkalsrud, E.W. 1986: Undescended testes. In Welch, K.J., Randolph, J.G., Ravitch, M.M., O'Neill, J.A., Jr and Rowe, M.I. (eds), *Pediatric surgery*, 24th ed. Chicago, IL: Year Book Medical Publishers, 793–807.

Hadziselimovic, F. 1983: *Cryptorchidism: management and implications*. Berlin: Springer.

Hadziselimovic, F., Herzog, B. and Girard, J. 1987: Cryptorchidism. In *International Symposium on Pediatric and Surgical Andrology*. Springer International European Journal of Pediatrics **146**, S1–68.

Hutson, J.M. and Beasley, S.W. 1992: *Descent of the testis*. London: Edward Arnold.

CHAPTER 35

Torsion of the testis and appendages: varicocele

N. ADE-AJAYI AND R.A. WHEELER

Introduction
Embryology
Clinical features and management
Surgical treatment

Differential diagnosis
Varicoceles in children
References

Introduction

Torsion of the spermatic cord as a result of abnormal rotation of the testis in relation to its surrounding structures, or rotation of testicular appendages leading to their infarction comprise the most common causes of acute scrotal inflammation in children. The natural history of the illness and the treatment and prognosis depend on the anatomical relations of the testis.

Embryology

The descent of the testis behind the processus vaginalis to its final site in the scrotum and the subsequent investment of the medial, anterior and lateral surfaces with tunica vaginalis confers stability on the testis, preventing abnormal rotation along the axis of the spermatic cord. During this process of descent, lack of fixation to the posterior wall of the processus may allow testicular rotation to occur with consequent torsion of the cord and testicular loss, presenting as perinatal (extravaginal) torsion. If testicular invagination into the posterior wall of the scrotal processus is continued to the point where the posterior epididymal surface is invested with a visceral coat of tunica, and the reflection from visceral to parietal coats occurs at the level of the spermatic cord, the testis is afforded no protection against axial rotation and torsion of the cord may result, this time within the confines of the parietal tunica vaginalis.

Clinical features and management

The scene is thus set for two distinct varieties of spermatic cord torsion. Extravaginal torsion is perhaps 100 times less common than intravaginal torsion. Torsion involving the testis or its appendages is reported as occurring in 1 in 160 men by the age of 25 years. Both spermatic cord and appendage torsion occur primarily in adolescence, whereas in the prepubertal group the incidence of both conditions is equal (Williamson, 1976).

The cause of torsion has not been found. Speculation has surrounded the significance of trauma, an ambient temperature $< 2°C$, a nocturnal elevation in testosterone levels and a positive correlation with spermatic cord length.

With cord torsion comes venous congestion, reduced arterial inflow and ultimately arterial thrombosis. The speed with which irreversible damage occurs is positively correlated with the number of twists in the cord, as are the chances of atrophy correlated with the duration of ischaemia time and testicular necrosis has been reported after a history of only 2 hours.

Perinatal torsion was first described by Taylor in 1897 and is considered as prenatal in 75% and postnatal (within the neonatal period) in 25%. It presents as an apparently painless, erythematous unilateral scrotal swelling (although reported to be bilateral in 12%). There is rarely systemic disturbance and both sides are equally affected. In most cases the testis is in an extravaginal location. In a review of 98 testes only 8% were intravaginal and bilateral torsion occurred in 15 patients, 12 synchronously (Das and Singer, 1990).

Intravaginal torsion, described in 1840 by Delasiauve, is associated with the near-complete investment of the testis and epididymis with tunica vaginalis. This results in a 'bell clapper' deformity and torsion usually presents with all the features of acute scrotal inflammation. The testis itself is exquisitely tender and traditionally lies, together with the contralateral side, horizontally (Angell, 1963). Torsion is more common on the left side, perhaps because of the longer left spermatic cord. The testis may be imperfectly descended, with an increased risk of torsion of the spermatic cord, and this risk increases further in paraplegics with an undescended testis (Phillips and Holmes, 1972). One-third of patients have had previous transient episodes of testicular pain (Cass, 1982), systemic symptoms of nausea, vomiting and fever are common and right lower quadrant pain and dysuria are not unusual.

The differential diagnosis in the perinatal group includes pathology related to a patent processus or its contents, inflammation, infarction, infection or neoplasm of the gonad or its appendages and ectopic tissues. Physical examination rather than technological investigation is therefore used to determine whether an early operation is required. Whether the torsion was of an extravaginal or intravaginal testis, the obvious fear is that the underlying predisposition to abnormal rotation will apply bilaterally, thus there is a need to explore and fix the contralateral side. Additionally, because the diagnosis of intrascrotal neoplasm cannot be confidently excluded, with teratomas, granulosa cell and yolk sac tumours being reported in the newborn, many surgeons perform an elective scrotal exploration (Das and Singer, 1990). As so few testes in the prenatal group will be viable, this exploration is not done as an emergency. In the baby who was born with normal scrotal testes and who develops perinatal torsion, immediate operation is indicated, in the hope of preserving both testes. Nevertheless, many UK surgeons believe that any surgical intervention is valueless, the incidence of neoplasm and of metachronous extravaginal torsion being low. The exploration of neonatal torsion is still, therefore, controversial.

The management of intravaginal torsion is more clear cut. The differential diagnosis includes torsion of the testicular appendages, epididymo-orchitis, trauma, hernia or hydrocoele, Henoch–Schönlein purpura (HSP) and idiopathic scrotal oedema. Physical examination continues to play the major role in resolving the diagnosis, and scrotal exploration can be viewed as a safe, rapid and reliable diagnostic as well as therapeutic procedure. Attempts at visualizing a twisted spermatic cord with real-time ultrasonography are frustrated by the non-specific findings. Doppler studies of vessel patency have been found to be promising (Kass *et al.*,

1993) but are not sufficiently reliable to make a confident negative diagnosis (Steinhardt *et al.*, 1993), while radionuclide studies are only of use to demonstrate the vascular pattern of testicular infarction, at a late stage in the natural history. Imaging also causes a significant time delay which is unacceptable in these circumstances. Physical examination may allow confident diagnosis of hernia and hydrocele, torted appendage, idiopathic scrotal oedema and HSP. Infection, the results of trauma and epididymitis due to sterile urine reflux may all produce such non-specific signs that a confident diagnosis is impossible and exploration in these circumstances is indicated. Some authors propose that closed reduction of the torsion either with or without locally infiltrated anaesthetic (Davidson, 1984) followed by an elective testicular fixation, is an acceptable alternative to immediate open exploration; however, this view has not met with support amongst British paediatric surgeons.

Surgical treatment

The scrotum may be explored through various incisions. The posterior raphe approach allows access to both scrotal compartments with a good cosmetic result, whilst paired transverse incisions have the advantage that if there is infection on one side, it can be isolated from the contralateral side. With the diagnosis confirmed, the testis is derotated until the torsion of the cord is resolved. The torsion is usually in the direction of external rotation and sometimes of 720°. The testis is then wrapped in a moist swab and contralateral testicular fixation performed using a three-point fixation technique with a non-absorbable suture (the use of absorbables having been shown to be associated with recurrent torsion (May and Thomas, 1980). The damaged side is then reinspected. It is common practice to incise the tunica albuginea to reduce the intratesticular pressure and reduce reperfusion injury. If the testis is viable, it is returned to the scrotum and fixed either as above, or using a scrotal pouch, thought by some to offer better protection against recurrent torsion (Mishriki *et al.*, 1992).

The prognosis for testicular survival after torsion of the spermatic cord in the perinatal group is uniformly gloomy, with few palpable testes surviving. Superficially, in the intravaginal group the outlook is better, with salvage rates of up to 80% reported, but this reflects the subjective perioperative assessment rather than objective long-term data. In a series of torted testes examined for 2 or more years postoperatively up to 66% were found to have atrophied (Bartsch *et al.*, 1980), with the duration of torsion correlating with the degree of atrophy. Furthermore, there is evidence of both ipsilateral and contralateral testicular damage resulting in reduced production of sperm and reduced sperm quality. It was originally feared that this might represent a process of autoimmune orchiopathia, the retained damaged testis giving rise to auto-antibodies which then damaged the contralateral side (Williamson and Thomas, 1984). However, these studies could not be confirmed and the undoubted observation of post torsion subfertility has been variously ascribed (Anderson and Williamson, 1990) to damage to the contralateral testis during fixation, damage to the blood–testis immune barrier and subsequent development of seminal plasma antibodies (Wardle *et al.*, 1989), recurrent transient bilateral torsions or a bilateral congenital defect in spermatogenesis associated with the anomaly of tunical investment.

A viable post-torsion testis should be preserved (Anderson and Williamson, 1990), although it is noted that there is a three-fold increase in the risk of testicular cancer associated with spermatic cord torsion (Chilvers *et al.*, 1987). Testicular prostheses are available in various sizes but it seems reasonable to advise against repeated changes of prosthesis as the child advances through puberty and suggest that an appropriate prosthesis is inserted once puberty is passed.

Differential diagnosis

Torsion of the appendages (Fig. 35.1) may be difficult to differentiate from a twisted spermatic cord. First reported by Colt in 1922, of the four common appendages it is the appendix testis which is most constant (92%) and most often torted (90%) (Skoglund *et al.*, 1970). Usually unilateral, appendage torsion may be bilateral and has been reported as simultaneous with an ipsilateral spermatic cord torsion (Redman and O'Donnell, 1977). If a blue–black tender spot can be seen at the upper pole of an otherwise normal testis and a confident diagnosis made then it is permissible to offer the child and his parents the option of non-operative treatment. With analgesia, the symptoms can be controlled and the infarcted appendage will involute. Alternatively, excision of the infarcted tissue will shorten the convalescent period and reduce the overall need for pain relief, as well as having has the advantage of confirming the diagnosis. Oedema of the scrotal skin may well preclude a confident diagnosis, in which case exploration is essential.

Varicoceles in children

Varicoceles in children are common but are rarely symptomatic and do not appear to cause irreversible pathology during childhood. The problems with fertility ascribed to them are still a matter of discussion but develop during adult life so that the management of this condition during childhood is viewed as largely prophylactic.

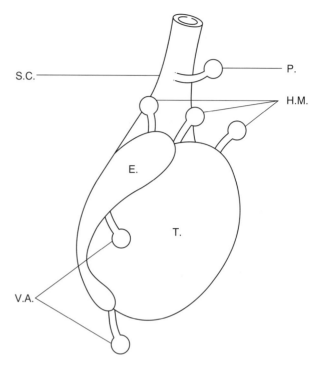

Fig. 35.1 Types of gonadal appendage found in clinical reports of torsion (after Campbell, 1951). SC, spermatic cord; E, epididymis; T, testis; p, paradidymis, organ of Giraldes, mesonephric tubular remnant; HM, hydatid of Morgagni, appendix testis, paramesonephric duct remnant; when sited on the head of the epididymis (appendix of epididymis) this is usually considered a mesonephric vestige; VA, vas aberrans, organ of Haller, mesonephric vestige.

Varicocele, first noted in the first century AD by Celsus, describes an abnormal dilatation of the testicular (spermatic) veins, extending from the pampiniform plexus proximally into the reducing number of testicular veins in the inguinal canal. It rarely extends to involve the distal retroperitoneal testicular vein (Hanley and Harrison, 1962).

Unusual before the age of 10 (Steeno *et al.*, 1976), varicoceles are often detected in adolescence and 15% of males will ultimately develop this condition. Active case-finding does not seem to change the incidence of the condition, although it may reduce the age of presentation (Nagar and Levran, 1993). Most commonly unilateral and left sided (78–93%), bilateral varicoceles are less common (2–20%) and unilateral right varicoceles rare (1–7%) (Saypol, 1981). There is no difference in the incidence in the Black population. The diagnosis is made on finding a mass of veins in an enlarged scrotum, sometimes associated with an ache in the groin or sensation of heaviness in the scrotum. The testis tends to lie horizontally (Wheeler and Atwell, 1991). The diagnosis is qualified by size, using a grading system: grade 1, <1 cm diameter; grade 2, 1–2 cm; grade 3, >2 cm. In a series of 78 10–17-year-olds, the distribution by grade was 1:32%, 2:4% and 3:64% (Nagar and Levran, 1993). Whether the grading is of anything more than descriptive interest is debatable. The originators of the system suggested that the degree of varicocele bore no relation to associated *infertility* (Dubin and Amelar, 1970) although a low sperm count has been positively correlated with varicocele grade (Fariss *et al.*, 1981) and the effect on testicular volume (Kass and Reitelman, 1995).

Investigation of the varicocele has been directed more towards the underlying and contralateral testis than the varix itself. Doppler ultrasonography is effective at confirming the diagnosis of varicosity and demonstrating impalpable varices, relying on the observation that only patients with a varicocele will have reflux of venous blood down the testicular vein during quiet respiration and allowing classification of the grade of varix according to the waveform produced (Hirsh *et al.*, 1980). However, these authors advise caution in the interpretation of Doppler assessments because they observed that valsalva-induced reflux could be elicited in otherwise normal subjects and could lead to a high false-positive rate. Formal investigation of testicular volume by calipers (Lipschultz and Corriere, 1977) orchidometry (Takihara *et al.*, 1983) and ultrasound (Constabile *et al.*, 1992) allows accurate comparison of affected and contralateral sides. This has revealed that in a child with a unilateral varix, there may be bilateral reduction in size when compared with an age-matched cohort (Lipschultz and Corriere, 1977) and ipsilateral testicular volume loss correlates positively with the grade of the varix (Steeno *et al.*, 1976). The significance of these observations is unknown.

Testicular biopsy has also revealed conflicting evidence, but in summary there appears to be an initial mild and reversible injury associated with the presence of a varicocele to both the tubular and interstitial structures in the ipsilateral testis. These changes progress with time and the contralateral testis can then undergo similar changes. Once Leydig cell hyperplasia can be demonstrated, the damage to the testis may be irreversible.

Another aspect of investigation is the hypothalamo-pituitary–gonadal axis. Abnormal hormone synthesis and spermatogenesis have been demonstrated in patients with a varicocele, these abnormalities being reversible by treatment of the varix (Hudson *et al.*, 1986). One aspect of the endocrine abnormality is that there is an excessive production of luteinizing hormone (LH) in response to the administration of gonadotropin-releasing hormone (Gn-RH). This response is now used routinely to identify individuals with testicular dysfunction (Kass and Reitelman, 1995).

Seminal analysis in adolescents can be problematic because it is not always possible to obtain samples and because normal age-dependent ranges are poorly defined. A progressive deterioration of sperm density and motility has been observed in the adults managed without operation (Gorelick and Goldstein, 1993) and it seems likely that the adolescent with a varicocele is undergoing the early stages of this deterioration.

The objective of treatment is to interrupt the column of venous blood distal to the varix, leaving no potential channels for recurrence whilst maintaining an adequate blood supply and drainage to the testis and epididymis.

This is usually achieved surgically, although transvenous embolization or sclerotherapy under radiological control has its advocates (Porst *et al.*, 1984). The surgical debate initially centred on whether the approach should be scrotal, inguinal or retroperitoneal. Advocates of the lower approaches took support from the view that varicoceles involve only cremasteric veins and that testicular veins are normal (Murley, 1994), whilst those supporting the high approach point to the hypothesis that testicular, cremasteric and vasal vessels may all contribute to the varix formation (Ivanissevich, 1966). Whilst recognizing the potential contributory channels, some authors suggest that despite the numerous potential collateral channels, it is only the minute collateral branches of the testicular veins which are closely applied to the surface of the testicular artery that have potential for allowing recurrence after testicular vessel ligation (Kass and Reitelman, 1995). It is for this reason that they and others (Matsuda *et al.*, 1992) propose the ligation of the whole spermatic cord, above the entry of the vas deferens. This leaves the testis and epididymis reliant on the artery of the vas and the anastomosis with the cremasteric artery (Palomo, 1949). Providing the child has not had previous groin surgery and the testis is scrotal, no ill-effects from this ligation have been noted and catch-up growth is comparable to the artery-sparing procedures (Okuyama *et al.*, 1988). Although applicable to left-sided varicoceles, the division and ligation of the testicular vessels above the level of vas may not solve the problem of all right-sided varicoceles, some of which may fill as a result of scrotal venous cross-over (Matsuda *et al.*, 1992). This rare group may benefit from preliminary venography to differentiate abnormalities of distal testicular vein drainage (such as drainage into the right renal vein or renal capsule) from abnormalities confined to the pampiniform plexus, the latter group then undergoing simple inguinoscrotal varicocelectomy.

The debate has now extended to whether the ligation of the testicular vessels should be performed laparoscopically (Lynch *et al.*, 1993); with protagonists (Sandison and Jones, 1991; Al-Shareef *et al.*, 1993) balancing incision lengths, operating time, analgesic requirements, benefits of laparoscopic magnification and early ambulation and discharge to suit their preferred practice. This debate will require more finesse if it is to be meaningful in the context of paediatric surgery. Prolonged follow-up will be required to solve the dispute, particularly in this case of surgery for prophylaxis.

CHAPTER 36

Infantile hypertrophic pyloric stenosis

P.K.H. TAM

Introduction
Historical aspects
Epidemiology
Pathology and pathogenesis
Clinical features

Diagnosis
Treatment
Results
References

Introduction

Infantile hypertrophic pyloric stenosis is a common cause of vomiting in infancy. Once an invariably lethal condition, it is now associated with an almost negligible mortality rate. The main reason for this remarkable success was undoubtedly Ramstedt's introduction of pyloromyotomy as a simple, effective surgical cure. Results of treatment have further been enhanced by earlier diagnosis, improved preoperative management and safer neonatal anaesthesia. Nevertheless, morbidity has not been completely eliminated. More importantly, despite much research, the cause remains unknown.

Historical aspects

The earliest description of the condition is attributed to Hildanus who in 1627 reported the occurrence of 'spastic vomiting' in an infant (von Hilden, 1646). There was no pathological confirmation as the child survived. In 1717, Blair, a botanist and surgeon from Dundee, described the autopsy findings of a 5-month-old boy who had 'violent vomiting' since the age of 1 month (Blair, 1717). The pylorus was 'cartilaginous' and obstructing; the only incongruous finding was that the stomach, despite being thick-walled, had a small cavity. In 1788, Beardsley gave a clear account of a male child with non-bilious ejectile vomiting which began in the first

week of life and continued until his death at 5 years of age (Beardsley, 1788). A scirrhous pylorus had been felt months before the child's death and the postmortem findings were typical of pyloric stenosis. There were other reports in the literature (e.g. Williamson, 1841; see Ravitch, 1960) but the medical world remained generally unaware of the disorder. The condition became recognized as a distinct clinical entity in 1887 when Hirschsprung presented the clinical and pathological findings of two unequivocal cases of infantile hypertrophic pyloric stenosis (Hirschsprung, 1888). He made no suggestions for therapy.

In 1893, the first surgical attempt to treat the condition by means of a jejunostomy was made but the patient died (Cordua, 1893). Schwyzer (1896), a pathologist, commenting on this condition in 1894, already predicted that 'surgical interference alone will be of any avail or benefit to the patient – either ... dilating the stenosed pylorus, or else simple gastroenterostomy'. In 1900, Lobker reported the first successful operation for this condition by performing a gastroenterostomy. By 1910, a total of 49 gastroenterostomies had been reported, with a 61% mortality (Weber, 1910). Divulsion of the pylorus with instruments and digitally via a gastrotomy was reported in three young adults with pyloric stenosis probably resulting from chronic duodenal ulcers (Loreta, 1887). In 1900, Nicholl successfully treated a baby with hypertrophic pyloric stenosis by this method. By 1908, 44 operations of this type had been reported, with a 53% mortality (Ibrahim, 1908).

Pyloroplasty was first performed successfully for hypertrophic pyloric stenosis by Dent in 1902 (Cautley and Dent, 1904) using the Heineke–Mikulicz method. Within 15 years, Dent had 10 successes out of 12 attempts but the technical difficulties of suturing the thickened pylorus prevented the approach from becoming popular. In 1907, Fredet, a French surgeon came closest to finding the final solution by performing successfully a Heineke–Mikulicz pyloroplasty on the divided muscles without incising the mucosa and submucosa (Fredet and Guillemot, 1910). Weber independently adopted a similar approach in 1908 (Weber, 1910). In 1911, Ramstedt (1912) attempted to follow Weber's example and found that he was unable to achieve complete transverse closure of the longitudinal myotomy wound as the sutures cut through. The baby vomited for 8 days. Ramstedt attributed this to an incomplete relief of the obstruction and decided that in the next case he would not suture the split muscle. In 1912, he successfully performed the operation which now bears his name and the procedure rapidly became accepted as the standard procedure for the condition.

Epidemiology

The incidence of pyloric stenosis among Caucasians is generally quoted as 2–3 per 1000 live births and a range of 1.4–8.8 had been reported in different years from different institutions (Webb *et al.*, 1983; Kerr, 1980). An increasing incidence has been described in the UK since 1956 when McLean reported a change of incidence for Aberdeen from 2.4 during 1938–41 to 4.5 during 1950–3. Subsequent reports from other parts of the UK (Knox *et al.*, 1983; Kerr, 1980; Webb *et al.*, 1983; Tam and Chan, 1991) and in the USA (Jedd *et al.*, 1988) appeared to confirm the rising trend in the 1970s and 1980s, although similar observations have not been made elsewhere (Hitch *et al.*, 1987). The incidence is less than 1 per 1000 births in Negroes and Asians irrespective of whether they are brought up in their countries of origin or the western world (Tam, 1994). A seasonal variation in incidence is well described, peaks having been observed in winter in Belfast (Dodge, 1975) and in spring and autumn in Washington (Kwok and Avery, 1967). These findings could be at least partly attributable to the seasonal variation in birth rates.

There is a male preponderence, with an average male-to-female ratio of 4:1. In some series, the gender discrepancy is increasing (Jedd *et al.*, 1988; Tam and Chan, 1991). Firstborns are more often affected and comprise 40–60% of all cases. It had been suggested that this finding was a statistical artefact (Huguenard and Sharples, 1972) but in several series where comparison was made against the firstborn preponderence in the normal population, a true difference could be detected. The firstborn preponderence in pyloric steno-

sis appears to affect male infants but no female infants (Jedd *et al.*, 1988). Infants with blood group A appear to have a lower risk of developing pyloric stenosis (Dodge, 1967).

Infants with pyloric stenosis were twice as likely to have been breastfed than normal infants (Dodge, 1975). This observation was confirmed by Jedd *et al.* (1988) but did not support the previously stated association with young maternal age, maternal stress and use of doxylamine succinate pyridoxide hydrochloride during pregnancy. A recent population-based case–control study, however, showed that infants with pyloric stenosis were significantly less likely to have been exclusively breastfed during the first week of life, suggesting a protective effect of breastfeeding in pyloric stenosis (Pisacane, 1996).

The average age of onset of symptoms is 3–4 weeks but up to 20% of infants may be symptomatic from birth (Andrassy *et al.*, 1977). A longitudinal population study with ultrasonography showed that muscle hypertrophy was not present in the early newborn period of infants who later developed pyloric stenosis (Rollins *et al.*, 1989). This suggests that pyloric stenosis is an acquired condition and not a congenital disorder. The average duration for the pylorus to develop the classical finding of hypertrophy has not been defined. Prenatal demonstration of gastric dilatation followed by eventual occurrence of pyloric hypertrophy has been described (Katz *et al.*, 1988). Repeated imaging studies in some symptomatic infants have shown that the transition from pyloric spasm to hypertrophy can occur within a few days (Tam and Chan, 1991), an observation which is not easily explained. Rarely, fully developed hypertrophic pyloric stenosis has been described in neonates (Zenn and Redo, 1993).

Associated anomalies have been described in 6–33%. (Scharli *et al.*, 1969; Al-Salem *et al.*, 1990) but the true incidence is unknown. In one series, upper urinary tract anomalies were found retrospectively in 2.7%, inguinal hernia in 3.4%, undescended testes in 3.0% and hypospadias in 0.9% but the incidence of urinary tract anomalies increased to 20.6% on prospective evaluation with intravenous urography (Atwell and Levick, 1981). A recent review identified a 1.4% incidence of urinary tract anomalies, representing a seven-fold increase over the incidence in the general population (Bridair *et al.*, 1993). Other associated anomalies include oesophageal atresia (Glasgow *et al.,* 1973), hiatus hernia (Irjima *et al.*, 1996), malrotation, (Croitoru *et al.*, 1991), Hirschsprung's disease (Whalen and Asche, 1985) and congenital diaphragmatic hernia (Al-Salem *et al.*, 1990).

Although the aetiology of pyloric stenosis is unknown, there is no doubt that genetic factors play an important role. The condition has been described in association with Smith–Lemli–Opitz syndrome, ovarian dysgenesis, dominantly inherited polycystic kidneys, and various chromosomal disorders including trisomy 18, trisomy 21, Turner's syndrome, X/XX mosaicism and chromosome 9 duplication (Chung *et al.*, 1993).

Twin studies show a concordance rate of 7–14% in dizygotic twins and 27–80% in monozygotic twins (Mitchell and Risch, 1993). Three-generation occurrence of pyloric stenosis has been described (Keizer, 1952). Overall, there is an 18-fold increase of incidence in first-degree relatives compared to the general population (Mitchell and Risch, 1993). With an affected mother, there is a 20% risk for the son and a 7% risk for the daughters to develop pyloric stenosis. With an affected father, the respective risks are 5% and 2.5%.

Analyses of pooled family data suggest that the inheritance of pyloric stenosis is explained by either multifactorial threshold or multiple interacting loci, with no single locus accounting for more than a five-fold increase in the risk to first-degree relatives (Mitchell and Bisch, 1933). Modern molecular genetic techniques may hold the key to unravelling this mystery (Chung *et al.*, 1993). Family linkage analysis suggests that the neuronal nitric oxide synthase (NOS1) gene is a susceptibility locus for pyloric stenosis (Chung *et al.*, 1996).

Pathology and pathogenesis

The pylorus is enlarged to become an olive-shaped mass, giving rise to a clinically palpable 'tumour'. There is a two- to four-fold increase in the thickness of the circular muscle and to a lesser extent of the longitudinal muscle which causes an encroachment on the submucosa and pyloric lumen. Earlier studies suggest a mixture of hypertrophy and hyperplasia (Belding and Kernohan, 1953) but modern investigations have proven that the muscle pathology is a pure hypertrophy (Tam, 1985). The muscle fibres run in all directions and result in an irregular pattern reminiscent of a leiomyoma. The muscle hypertrophy is accompanied by an increase in connective stroma and deposits of extracellular matrix proteins, particularly chondroitin sulphate which may contribute to the cartilaginous texture of the 'tumour' (Cass and Zhang, 1991).

While some of the longitudinal muscle is continuous between the pylorus and the duodenum, a block of fibrous tissue separates the circular muscles of the two segments. The pyloric vein demarcates the pyloroduodenal junction externally. There is, however, an infolding of the duodenal mucosa here and the thickened pyloric muscle protrudes into the duodenum similar to the vaginal cervix. Mucosal perforations during pyloromyotomy occur most frequently at the site of the duodenal 'fornix'. This risk is said to be accentuated on the lesser curvature as a result of muscle asymmetry (Cass and Bond, 1990). The gastropyloric junction is frequently indistinct, with the 'tumour' gradually tapering into the thickened antrum. With long-standing pyloric obstruction, which is rare nowadays, the stomach muscles undergo secondary hypertrophy.

From being regarded as a primary muscular abnormality in the days of Hirschsprung, pyloric stenosis is now increasingly recognized as a neuromuscular disorder. Early histological studies suggest a reduction in the number of ganglion cells as well as ganglion cell abnormalities, variously interpreted as representing immaturity (Friesen *et al.*, 1956), severe degeneration or mild degeneration from overstimulation (Spitz and Kaufman, 1975). These findings were not substantiated by semi-quantification (Tam, 1985) ultrastructural (Challa *et al.*, 1977) and immunohistochemical (Tam, 1986) studies. Modern studies have, however, identified a number of neuromuscular abnormalities, some of which have been speculated to have pathogenetic implications.

Cholinergic activity is much reduced in the nerve fibres in the hypertrophied muscles but is relatively normal in the myenteric plexus (Kobayash *et al.*, 1994a). Several neuropeptides are affected. There is a reduction of substance P in both the myenteric plexus and muscles which is interpreted to be a result of overstimulation of substance P-containing nerves which are responsible for muscle contraction (Tam, 1986). Vasoactive intestinal peptide (pyloric relaxation), enkephalin (pyloric contraction) and neuropeptide Y are reduced in the nerve fibres of the muscle and unaffected in the myenteric plexus (Wattchow *et al.*, 1987; Malmfors and Sundler, 1986; Shen *et al.*, 1990). The peptidergic nerve fibres are often swollen, suggesting degeneration. Defective intramuscular innervation of the muscle layer is further suggested by reduced immunoreactivity of a synaptic vesicle-specific protein in the muscle but not the myenteric plexus (Okazaki *et al.*, 1994). The nerve-supporting cells (Kobayashi *et al.*, 1994b), the interstitial cells of Cajal (Langer *et al.*, 1995) intestinal pacemaker cells (Vanderwinden *et al.*, 1996a; Yamakata *et al.*, 1996), nerve growth factor (Kobayashi *et al.*, 1995), are all deficient in pyloric stenosis and may play a part in its pathogenesis. The possible involvement of nitric oxide innervation i.e. discussed below.

The aetiology of pyloric stenosis remains unknown and while a neurogenic origin has often been postulated on the basis of the neurological abnormalities described above, it has been impossible to determine whether the findings are the cause, result or an association. Similarly, gastrointestinal hormones and other biologically active substances have been implicated but not proven to cause pyloric stenosis. The aetiological role of gastrin was suggested by Dodge (1970) who induced pyloric stenosis in puppies by prolonged perinatal pentagastrin administration. A raised serum gastrin level was reported in infants with pyloric stenosis (Spitz and Zail, 1976; Gasasa *et al.*, 1977) but the results were not reproduced by others (Rogers *et al.*, 1975, Christofides *et al.*, 1983). In any case it has been observed that hypergastrinaemia can result from antral distension secondary to pyloric obstruction. Decreased plasma concentrations of enteroglucagon, neurotensin, motilin and gastric inhibitory polypeptides are present in pyloric stenosis (Christofides *et al.*, 1983). In contrast, levels of prostaglandin E_2 and F_2 are increased in the gastric juice of infants with pyloric stenosis (La Ferla *et al.*, 1986). The significance of these findings is unclear.

Among the many theories of pathogenesis, the most favoured one is that of a pyloric spasm followed by hypertrophy, although how spasm is initiated has been poorly understood. The most promising explanation has come from the recent finding that nitric oxide synthase activity is absent in the nerve fibres in the hypertrophied circular muscle in pyloric stenosis (Vanderwinden *et al.*, 1992; Kobayashi *et al.*, 1995). Nitric oxide synthase catalyses the formation of nitric oxide, which is involved in the non-adrenergic, non-cholinergic inhibitory neurotransmission mediating relaxation of the pylorus, and its deficiency results in pyloric spasm. In 'knock-out' mice with nitric oxide synthase gene deletion, there is hypertrophy of the circular muscle of the pylorus and stomach, showing that lack of nitric oxide can lead to pyloric stenosis (Huang *et al.*, 1993). Genetic mapping of families with at least three affected individuals suggests that the nitric oxide synthase gene is a susceptibility locus for pyloric stenosis (Chung *et al.*, 1996). Nevertheless, the exact aetiological role of nitric oxide in the general population of pyloric stenosis awaits further study.

Clinical features

The classical presentation is non-bilious vomiting which usually begins at 3–4 weeks of age. The vomiting may not be forcefully projectile at the start but soon becomes so. It is effortless and not preceded by discomfort. The child appears to be hungry all the time and feeds voraciously. There is an average delay of a week before the infant is admitted to hospital. Occasionally symptoms start as early as the first week of life and rarely as late as 14 months. Haematemesis occurs in 15–20% of cases and is usually mild and resolves spontaneously on relief of obstruction. Rarely infants are encountered with significant blood loss requiring transfusion preoperatively. The cause of haemetemesis is usually oeophagitis (Takeuch *et al.*, 1993) and only very rarely gastric erosion.

Preterm infants account for 9–20% of modern series of pyloric stenosis (Muayed *et al.*, 1984, Evans, 1982). Their average onset of symptoms is in the fifth week of life and vomiting is often not projectile. Recognition of the condition is often delayed in those having transpyloric feeding (Latchaw *et al.*, 1989; Cosman *et al.*, 1992). Similar difficulties in diagnosis may arise in patients with associated anomalies such as oesophageal atresia, malrotation, incarcerated hernia, intracranial pathology, cleft lip and palate (Scharli *et al.*, 1969).

Because of increased awareness and earlier diagnosis, other symptoms described in the past are now much less frequently observed. Starvation may result in constipation, passage of greenish 'hungry stool, starvation diarrhoea', failure to thrive, weight loss and lethargy. Jaundice occurs in 2% of patients as a result of unconjugated hyperbilirubinaemia due to hepatic glucuronyl transferase deficiency. Surgery results in spontaneous resolution.

Wasting and severe dehydration are seldom seen today. There is often a worried look when the infant is about to vomit. Gastric contractions passing from left to right across the epigastrium can be seen in 75–95% of cases and are suggestive but not pathognomonic of pyloric stenosis. The definitive sign of pyloric stenosis is a palpable olive-shaped mass ('tumour') in the right upper quadrant. The infant's stomach could be emptied before the examination. A small feed with dextrose water helps to relax the abdominal muscles during the examination. The hypertrophied pylorus contracts and hardens during feeding and can often be rolled under the fingers. The demonstration of a palpable mass requires skill, experience and patience, and repeated examinations may sometimes be necessary. Over-reliance on imaging studies in recent years has resulted in a decline in the incidence of detection of a palpable mass in some institutions from 90% in the 1970s to 60% in the 1980 (Tam and Chan, 1991).

Differential diagnosis for non-bilious vomiting in early infancy includes overfeeding, gastro-oesophageal reflux and medical conditions. A careful history should distinguish these causes. Gastro-oesophageal reflux is the condition most likely to confuse but vomiting usually starts earlier, in the first week of life. Pyloric stenosis and gastro-oesophageal reflux can also co-exist. On rare occasions, anomalies causing gastric outlet obstruction such as webs and duplications can mimic pyloric stenosis. The caudate lobe of the liver, aberrant pancreatic tissue and the upper pole of the kidney may sometimes be mistaken for a hypertrophied pylorus but are unlikely to result in errors of diagnosis in symptomatic infants.

Diagnosis

Imaging studies for diagnosis are only required in patients without a palpable mass. There is a worrying trend that increased reliance on imaging studies since the 1970s has resulted in a decreased rate of clinical diagnosis but has not led to earlier diagnosis (Tam and Chan, 1991). In places where the ultrasonographic expertise is available, ultrasonography has replaced barium meal examination as the investigation of choice for the diagnosis of pyloric stenosis. Since its introduction in 1977 (Teele and Smith, 1977), there have been many refinements in the use of ultrasonography for this purpose and sensitivity, specificity and accuracy rates approaching 100% are achievable (Hernanz-Schulman *et al.*, 1994). The main advantage of ultrasonography is that it is non-ionizing and can be safely repeated in cases of evolving pyloric stenosis. However, despite the introduction of quantifiable diagnostic criteria, the accuracy of ultrasonography remains operator dependent. The most commonly accepted measurements for the diagnosis of pyloric stenosis include a muscle thickness of 4 mm or above, an anteroposterior diameter of 15 mm or above and a muscle length of 19 mm or above. There are many ancillary signs such as double-track, shoulder and nipple signs similar to those in barium studies. Real-time imaging allows continuous dynamic assessment and demonstration of vigorous unproductive gastric peristalsis and non-passage of fluid through a consistently linear pyloric canal.

Contrast studies of the upper gastrointestinal tract for the diagnosis of pyloric stenosis have been in use since 1932. The typical findings are a distended stomach with delayed passage of contrast through an elongated, narrowed pyloric canal – the 'string sign'. Other ancillary signs include the 'beak sign' representing the beginning of the elongated pyloric canal and often associated with the 'string sign', the 'mucosal nipple sign' from the protrusion of the redundant pyloric mucosa into the antrum, the 'shoulder sign' produced by the impression of the hypertrophied pyloric muscle on the distal antrum and the 'double-track sign' caused by barium encircling the thickened pyloric mucosa. Gastric retention of contrast alone without accompanying radiological changes in the pyloric canal does not provide sufficient evidence to distinguish pyloric stenosis from pyloric spasm and other causes of delayed gastric emptying. Occasionally, contrast examinations are indicated to evaluate the possibilities of gastro-oesophageal reflux and malrotation as alternative causes of infantile vomiting.

A new alternative method of diagnosis is upper gastrointestinal endoscopy. In one series (De Backer *et al.*, 1994), a diagnostic rate of 97% was achieved. The procedure can be performed without general anaesthesia and other conditions such as reflux oesophagitis can also be evaluated. The expertise, however, is not widely available and it is unlikely to replace ultrasonography as the popular choice of investigation for pyloric stenosis.

The characteristic biochemical change in pyloric stenosis is hypochloraemic alkalosis. This is mainly a result of excessive loss of gastric fluids rich in hydrogen and chloride (130–150 mmol/l), along with smaller sodium (60–100 mmol/l) and potassium (10–15 mmol/l) losses. In established pyloric stenosis, the patient is dehydrated, and serum pH and bicarbonate levels are elevated, and the serum chloride and to lesser extents potassium and sodium levels are lowered.

The mechanism of the biochemical abnormalities is complex. The initial response to metabolic alkalosis from hydrogen and chloride loss is excretion of an alkaline urine to restore normal blood pH. As dehydration worsens, maintenance of extracellular volume through sodium conservation becomes a more important priority. There is increased sodium resorption by the renal tubules in exchange for potassium through an aldosterone-mediated mechanism. Some of the potassium loss is replaced by hydrogen excretion, resulting in paradoxical aciduria. In the absence of available chloride, bicarbonate accompanies sodium resorption and alkalosis is worsened. Hypokalaemia aggravates alkalosis and vice versa, and a vicious circle is thus completed.

The development of biochemical abnormalities is correlated to the duration of vomiting (Breaux *et al.*, 1989). Although severe changes are less frequent nowadays, some degree of alkalosis (serum bicarbonate ⩾ 26 mmol/l) still exists in two-thirds of patients in modern series (Shanbhogue *et al.*, 1992). Serum chloride levels, especially following rehydration, correlate well with acid–base status: a chloride level ⩾ 106 mmol/l accurately predicts an absence of alkalosis (Goh *et al.*, 1990; Shanbhogue *et al.*, 1992).

Treatment

The standard treatment for pyloric stenosis is surgery. It is possible to treat pyloric stenosis medically but this involves prolonged antispasmodic therapy and hospitalization. In one series (Rasmussen *et al.*, 1987), the median length of hospital stay was 40.5 days with a mortality of 5.3% and a morbidity of 17% which included respiratory complications and atropine poisoning. Slightly better results can be obtained if only patients with milder symptoms are selected for conservative treatment (Jacoby, 1962; Swift and Prossor, 1991). The suggested protocol involves reduced volumes of feeds (180–270 ml in the first 24 h), 0.1 ml 0.7% alcoholic solution of atropine methylnitrate before four feeds on the first day and before three feeds in subsequent days. Alternatively, pipenzolate bromide may be used as an antispasmodic. The modern results of surgical treatment are so vastly superior that it is difficult to justify conservative treatment except under extreme circumstances.

Surgical management of pyloric stenosis begins with the correction of dehydration and biochemical abnormalities. There is no place for emergency operation until this has been achieved. A nasogastric tube is passed to decompress the stomach and allow gastric loss to be measured. The stomach should initially be irrigated with normal saline until it is cleared of milk curds and mucus as this will aid postoperative recovery. Intravenous fluid and electrolytes are administered according to the patient's clinical and biochemical status. The major electrolyte deficits are chloride and sodium. Potassium will also become depleted in advanced cases. These should be replaced accordingly.

A useful regimen is as follows.

1. No dehydration/alkalosis:
   100 ml 0.18% saline–5% dextrose/kg per day + replacement of gastric loss with an equal volume of normal saline. Add 20 mmol KCl to each litre of infused fluid.
2. Mild dehydration/alkalosis:
   130 ml 0.45% saline–5% dextrose/kg per day + replacement of gastric loss with an equal volume of normal saline. Add 40 mmol KCl to each litre of infused fluid. Check serum electrolytes and acid–base after 12–24 hours. Revert to regimen 1 when appropriate.
3. Moderate dehydration/alkalosis:
   150 ml 0.45% saline–5% dextrose/kg/per day + replacement of gastric loss with an equal volume of normal saline. Add 40 mmol KCl to each litre of infused fluid. Check serum electrolytes and acid–base after 12 hours. Revert to regimens 2 and 1 in succession when appropriate.
4. Severe dehydration/biochemical changes:
   similar to regimen 3 plus any other resuscitatory measures as necessary.

Transfusion is given if haematemesis has resulted in severe anaemia. The emphasis is on regular clinical (including urine output) and biochemical assessment and surgery is arranged only when normality in fluid and electrolyte balance has been achieved.

Ramstedt's pyloromyotomy is the standard operation for pyloric stenosis and is generally performed under general anaesthesia. The claim that local anaesthesia is associated with fewer postoperative complications and less vomiting (Bristol and Bolton, 1981) has not been substantiated (Gray *et al.*, 1984). There is no doubt that the operation is facilitated by muscle relaxation with general anaesthesia. If the expertise of safe paediatric anaesthesia and surgery is not available, the infant should be transferred to a hospital with such facilities.

The most commonly used incision is a transverse incision in the right upper quadrant midway between the xiphisternum and the umbilicus extending from the lateral border of the rectus towards the coastal margin. After the external oblique aponeurosis is incised transversely, the abdominal muscles may be split vertically with a pair of straight Mayo's scissors or cut transversely. The author's preference is the muscle-splitting approach but muscle cutting provides greater access and is particularly recommended for the inexperienced

surgeon. The liver edge underlies part of his incision and is supposed to provide some splintage for postoperative wound healing, thus minimizing dehiscence.

Upper midline and right paramedian incisions are now seldom used by paediatric surgeons for this procedure. Tan and Bianchi (1986) described a circumumbilical incision which gives excellent cosmetic results. Because of a high rate of wound sepsis, meticulous care is taken to clean the umbilicus and the skin folds before incision. The umbilical skin is incised above the umbilicus for 50–75% of its circumference. The peritoneum is entered via a similar curved incision in the linea alba. For greater access, the incision can be extended laterally into the rectus sheath to allow separation of the recti.

On entering the peritoneal cavity, the firm pyloric 'olive' is readily identified by palpation and can be grasped by a pair of atraumatic tissue-holding forceps (Russian or Denis–Browne) for delivery out of the wound. Alternatively, part of a wet gauze is inserted into the peritoneal cavity. On withdrawal, it will carry with it the omentum to allow identification of the body of stomach and retrieval of the pylorus. It is possible (Grogono, 1993) but not generally recommended to carry out pyloromyotomy within the peritoneal cavity. Once it is delivered out of the wound, the pyloric mass is held between the surgeon's left thumb on the duodenal side and the left index finger on the antral side (Fig. 36.1).

An incision is made along the length of the pyloric mass on its relatively avascular antero-superior aspect to include the serosa and superficial part of the hypertrophied muscle. The risk of perforation is greatest at

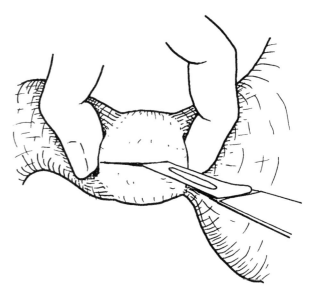

Fig. 36.1 The incision is made along the length of the pyloric tumour on the relatively avascular anteriosuperior aspect.

the site where the duodenal mucosal fold projects into the pylorus. The external landmark of the distal limit of the incision is the white line just proximal to the pre-pyloric vein and the position is confirmed by invaginating the duodenal lumen against the gritty pyloric mass with the surgeon's left thumb. Proximally, the incision should extend well into the antrum. The blunt end of an empty scalpel holder is inserted into the hypertrophied muscle with its flat surface along the length of the incision until it comes against the mucosa. It is then turned 90°, splitting the muscle and allowing the mucosa to bulge out (Fig. 36.2). Alternatively, the muscle is split with a pyloric spreader or a pair of artery forceps with the tips pointing upwards away from the mucosa. The mucosa is examined for possible perforations. Testing for leakage by injection of air via the nasogastric tube is advisable for the inexperienced surgeon.

Various technical modifications have been described, most of which are unnecessary. A V-shaped extension at the distal end of the myotomy incision has been used to reduce the risk of duodenal mucosal injury (Rowe *et al.*, 1995) and a double V-shaped extensions at both ends of the myotomy incision has also been employed to widen the pyloric canal (Ohri *et al.*, 1991). A myotomy incision with its distal part curving down on the anterior surface has been suggested to reduce mucosal perforations (Cass and Zhang, 1990).

When a mucosal perforation is recognized, it can usually be repaired safely with simple absorbable sutures

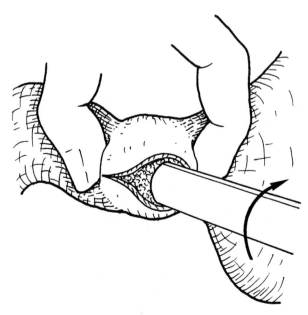

Fig. 36.2 The blunt end of an empty scalpel holder is inserted into the hypertrophied muscle along the length of the incision until it comes against the mucosa. It is then turned through 90° allowing the mucosa to bulge out and thus relieving the obstruction.

with or without an omental patch (Royal *et al.*, 1995). Alternatively, a duodenal perforation may be imbricated beneath the seromuscular layer of the duodenum by a horizontal mattress suture (Hight *et al.*, 1981). It may occasionally be necessary to close the original incision, rotate the pylorus and perform a new pyloromyotomy on the antero-inferior surface instead.

Minor oozing from venous engorgement at the myotomy site will usually stop when the pylorus is returned to the peritoneal cavity. For more severe bleeding, cautery or sutures may be required for haemostasis.

The wound should be closed with strong, slow-absorbing sutures. Pyloromyotomy has an unjustified reputation for burst abdomen which is related to improper techniques rather than to the condition itself. Local infiltration of 0.25% bupivacaine reduces post-operative wound pain.

Laparoscopic pyloromyotomy has recently been introduced (Alain *et al.*, 1996). There are some theoretical advantages of a minimally invasive approach but whether the excellent results of the open method can be surpassed remains debatable. The basic requirements include expertise in laparoscopic techniques, special attention to anaesthesia and the availability of special miniaturized instruments. In brief, a pneumoperitonium of less than 10 cm water is created and three 4 mm ports consisting of an endoscope in the umbilicus and an instrumentation canula in each upper quadrant are used. Some authors (Lobe, 1995) apply retraction sutures through the abdominal wall proximal and distal to the pyloric mass for fixation. Grasping forceps are introduced through the right part to secure the pylorus while an endotome and spreading forceps are applied successively through the left port for pyloromyotomy.

Endoscopic balloon dilatation for hypertrophic pyloric stenosis has been tried with limited success (Tam and Carty, 1989, 1991; Ogawa *et al.*, 1996). An experienced endoscopist is required for the procedure which involves the passage of a 15 mm diameter balloon catheter with built-in guide wire through the narrowed pyloric canal. This is followed by insufflation of the balloon for 5–10 min. The clinical outcome is variable and therefore the procedure in its present form cannot be considered for primary use until further developments take place.

There are several postoperative feeding regimens, which differ in the time of introduction of feeds and the speed with which full feeds are established. The reason for withholding feeds in the early postoperative period is based on the manometric findings that gastric peristalsis is absent in the initial 4–6 hours and is depressed for an additional 16–24 hours (Scharli and Leditschke, 1968). Another study (Nour *et al.*, 1993) suggested that gastric emptying returns to normal by the seventh day after operation. However, a prospective, randomized study (Wheeler *et al.*, 1990) comparing three regimens involving gradual regrading of feeds over 48 hours, rapid regrading of feeds over 16 hours and starvation for the initial 24 hours followed by full feeds revealed no difference in the incidence of vomiting and duration of hospital stay between the treatment groups. In another study (Georgeson *et al.*, 1993), early feeding even resulted in a shorter postoperative stay despite being associated with increased incidence and frequency of minor vomiting. Prolonged fasting of a hungry baby in the postoperative period results in distress and is unnecessary.

Results

The excellent results of modern surgical treatment of pyloric stenosis can be attributed to improved diagnosis, correct fluid and electrolyte therapy, safe paediatric anaesthesia and, above all, an effective and simple operation. Mortality should approach zero, except in the rare occurrence of associated life-threatening medical anomalies. Complications are usually minor (Tam, 1994) and most patients can be discharged from hospital within 2 days postoperatively. There is continuing debate as to whether the high standards can be achieved in specialist centres only (Atwell, 1993) or in non-specialist hospitals as well (Eriksen and Anders, 1991; Curley *et al.*, 1997). A series comparing the results before and after the appointment of a specialist paediatric surgeon in the same hospital showed a significant reduction in morbidity in the specialist era: rates of wound infection decreased from 15.5% to 2.8%, wound dehiscence from 6.7% to 0 and duodenal perforation from 12.8% to 0 (Brain and Roberts, 1996). In a recent survey of 17 specialist centres in the UK (British Association of Paediatric Surgeons, personal communication), over a quarter of patients were deemed to have inadequate or inappropriate management before transfer to the specialists. The overall complication rate was 6%: normal pylorus 0, mucosal perforation 1%, incomplete myotomy 1%, wound dehiscence 0.7%, wound infection 2.6%, incisional hernia 0.3% and others 0.3%. These results are superior to those reported from non-specialist hospitals and argue strongly for the concentration of care for this condition in specialist centres.

Minor degrees of postoperative vomiting are not uncommon and can be ignored. Persistent vomiting is a different matter and can be due to gastritis, reflux oesophagitis, medical causes or more seriously, mucosal perforation and incomplete myotomy. Gastritis is usually self-limiting. Unrecognized mucosal perforation will result in peritonitis and sepsis in the early postoperative period in addition to vomiting. Prompt reoperation to repair the defect is required. Incomplete myotomy is not always easy to recognize. In this instance, postoperative vomiting is not only persistent but also forceful and is often described by the mother or the nurse as being 'the same as that before the operation'. Imaging studies are difficult to interpret. Normal gastric emptying can help to exclude the complication but incomplete myotomy cannot be positively diagnosed by imaging studies as the sonographic and radiological appearances of hypertrophic pyloric stenosis persist for weeks and months after adequate myotomy. The need to reoperate is often decided on clinical grounds. Preparation for surgery includes attention to fluid and nutritional requirements. Incomplete myotomy is said to occur frequently on the gastric side. The remedy consists of either completion of the myotomy or making a new incision antero-inferiorly or posteriorly. Alternatively, residual stenosis can be eradicated endoscopically by balloon dilatation if the expertise is available (Tam and Carty, 1991).

Wound infection remains the most common complication. The umbilicus is an important source of infection and extra efforts to sterilize this area preoperatively are well rewarded (Fitzgerald, 1984). The main disadvantage of the circumumbilical approach, putting aside the question of access, is its higher wound infection rate: 16% compared to 5.5% in the conventional approach despite more frequent use of antibiotic prophylaxis (Huddart *et al.*, 1993). The occurrence of mucosal perforation and inexperience of the surgeon are other factors associated with an increased risk of wound infection. The occurrence of wound dehiscence and incisional hernia are related to surgical techniques and are avoidable. The finding of a normal pylorus occurs in up to 2% in some series but should become much rarer with improved diagnosis.

Results of laparoscopic pyloromyotomy are only beginning to appear. The largest reported series (Alain *et al.*, 1996) consisted of 70 patients with two complications, both being gastric mucosal perforation. In another series (Najmaldin and Tan, 1995), 37 patients were treated laparoscopically and one developed subcutaneous emphysema which resolved spontaneously. The possible benefits of the laparoscopic approach, such as reduction of postoperative pain, are difficult to measure. Against the background of the consistent success of the conventional Ramstedt's operation, it is likely that laparoscopic pyloromyotomy will remain an alternative approach practised by enthusiasts in selected centres. More data will be necessary before a proper appraisal of the different approaches can be made.

The fate of the pyloric 'tumour' appears to differ depending on the method of treatment (Armitage and Rhind, 1951). After the medical treatment, the tumour persists for months or years and then disappears. After gastroenterostomy it persists indefinitely into adult life. After pyloromyotomy the incision heals by fibrosis after 9–13 days, becoming a narrow scar after 25 days and disappearing after 18–24 months (Wollstein, 1922). The pathological abnormalities in the circular muscle layer and enteric nervous system in pyloric stenosis have been observed to resolve within four months after pyloromyotomy (Vanderwind *et al.*, 1996b). Sonographically, pyloric muscle hypertrophy resolves in 2–12 weeks (Okorie *et al.*, 1988). There is conflicting evidence as to whether functional sequalae exist in the long term after treatment of pyloric stenosis. Reported abnormalities include increased gastric acid secretion (Wanscher and Jensen, 1971), raised fasting somatostatin (which inhibits acid and gastrin release) content with increased gastric somatostatin binding sites (Martinez-Urrutia *et al.*, 1995), increased duodenogastric reflux and rapid (Tam, 1985) or delayed (Wanscher and Jensen, 1971) gastric emptying. These data provide an explanation for the reported increased prevalence of ulcer dyspepsia in adults treated for pyloric stenosis in their childhood (Wanscher and Jensen, 1971). Other workers (Rasmussen *et al.*, 1988; Ludtke *et al.*, 1994), however, have shown that treated patients have a normal frequency of ulcer dyspepsia and gastric emptying rate on a long-term follow-up.

References

Alain, J.L., Grousseau, D., Congis, B., Ugazzi, M. and Ferrier, G. 1996: Extramucosal pyloromyotomy by laparoscopy. *Journal of Pediatric Surgery* **6**, 10–12.

Al-Salem, A.H., Grant, C. and Khwaja, S. 1990: Infantile hypertrophic pyloric stenosis and congenital diaphragmatic hernia. *Journal of Pediatric Surgery* **25**, 607–8.

Andrassy, R.J., Hoff, R.C. and Larsen, G.L. 1977: Infantile hypertrophic pyloric stenosis during the first week of life. *Clinical Pediatrics* **16**, 475–6.

Armitage, G. and Rhind, J.A. 1951: The fate of the tumour in infantile hypertrophic pyloric stenosis. *British Journal of Surgery* **39**, 39–43.

Atwell, J.D. 1993: Comment on infantile pyloric stenosis: where should it be treated? *Annals of the Royal College of Surgeons* **75**, 34–7.

Atwell, J.D. and Levick, P. 1981: Congenital hypertrophic pyloric stenosis and associated anomalies in the genitourinary tract. *Journal of Pediatric Surgery* **16**, 1029–35.

Beardsley, H. 1788: Congenital hypertrophic stenosis of the pylorus. In *Cases and observations by the Medical Society of New Haven*, New Haven, CT: F. Meigs, 81.

Belding, H.H. and Kernohan, J.W. 1953: A morphologic study of the myenteric plexus and musculature of the pylorus with special references to changes in hypertrophic pyloric stenosis. *Surgery, Gynaecology and Obstetrics* **97**, 322–4.

Blair, P. 1717: An account of dissection of a child, communicated in a letter to Dr Brook Taylor, R.S. Sear. *Philosophical Transactions*, **30**, 63.

Brain, A.J.L. and Roberts, D.S. 1996: Who should treat congenital hypertrophic pyloric stenosis: the general or specialist paediatric surgeon? *Journal of Pediatric Surgery* **31**, 1535–7.

Breaux, C.W., Hood, J.S. and Georgeson, K.Z. 1989: The significance of alkalosis and hypochloremia in hypertrophic pyloric stenosis. *Journal of Pediatric Surgery* **24**, 1250–2.

Bridair, M., Kalota, S.J. and Kaplan, G.W. 1993: Infantile hypertrophic pyloric stenosis and hydronephrosis: is there an association? *Journal of Urology* **150**, 153–5.

Bristol, J.B. and Bolton, P.A. 1981: The results of Ramstedt's operation in a district general hospital. *British Journal of Surgery* **68**, 590–2.

Casara, J.M., Lafuente, J.M., Boix-Ochoa, J. *et al.* 1977: Gastrin and gastric acidity in hypertrophic pyloric stenosis. *Annales de Chirurgic Infantile* **18**, 363–9.

Cass, D.T. and Bond, G. 1990: Asymmetrical nature of the muscular anatomy of the infantile pylorus; a possible consideration in pyloromyotomy. *British Journal of Surgery* **77**, 919–21.

Cass, D.T. and Zhang, A.L. 1991: Extracellular matrix changes in congenital hypertrophic pyloric stenosis. *Pediatric Surgery International* **6**, 190–214.

Cautley, E. and Dent, C. 1904: Congenital hypertrophic stenosis of the pylorus. *British Journal of Children's Diseases* **1**, 10.

Challa, V.R., Jona, J.Z. and Markesbery, W.R. 1977: Ultrastructural observations of the myenteric plexus of the pylorus in infantile hypertrophic pyloric stenosis. *American Journal of Pathology* **88**, 309–22.

Christofides, N.D., Mallett, E., Ghatei, M.A. *et al.* 1983: Plasma enteroglucagon and neurotensin in infantile pyloric stenosis. *Archives of Disease in Childhood* **58**, 52–5.

Chung, E., Coffey, R., Parker, K., Tam, P. *et al.* 1993: Linkage analysis of infantile pyloric stenosis and markers from chromosome 9 11–33: no evidence for a major gene in this candidate region. *Journal of Medical Genetics* **30**, 393–5.

Chung, E., Curtis, D., Chen, G., Marsden, P.A. *et al.* 1996: Genetic evidence for the neuronal nitric oxide synthase gene NOS1 as a susceptibility for infantile pyloric stenosis. *American Journal of Human Genetics* **58**, 363–70.

Cordua, E. 1893: Referred to by Grisson, 1904. *Deutsche Zeitschrift für Chirurgie* **75**, 111.

Cosman, B.C., Sudekum, A.G., Oakes, D.D. and de Vries, P.A. 1992: Pyloric stenosis in premature infants. *Journal of Pediatric Surgery* **27**, 1534–6.

Croitoru, D., Neilson, I. and Guttman, T.M. 1991: Pyloric stenosis associated with malrotation. *Journal of Pediatric Surgery* **26**, 1276–8.

Curley, P.J., McGregor, B., Ingoldby, C.J.H. and MacFaul, R. 1997: The management of pyloric stenosis in a district hospital. *Journal of Royal College of Surgeons* **42**, 265–8.

De Backer, A., Bove, T., Vandenplas, Y., Peeters, S. and Deconinck, P. 1994: Contribution of endoscopy to early diagnosis of hypertrophic pyloric stenosis. *Journal of Pediatric Gastroenterology and Nutrition* **18**, 78–81.

Dodge, J.A. 1967: Blood groups and congenital hypertrophic pyloric stenosis. *British Medical Journal* **4**, 781–2.

Dodge, J.A. 1970: Production of duodenal ulcers and hypertrophic pyloric stenosis by administration of pentagastrin to pregnant and newborn dogs. *Nature* **225**, 284–5.

Dodge, J.A. 1975: Infantile hypertrophic pyloric stenosis in Belfast. *Archives of Disease in Childhood* **50**, 171–8.

Erikson, C.A. and Anders, C.J. 1991: Audit of results of operation for infantile pyloric stenosis in a district general hospital. *Archives of Disease in Childhood* **66**, 130–3.

Evans, N.J. 1982: Pyloric stenosis in premature infants after transpyloric feeding [Letter]. *Lancet* **ii**, 665.

Fitzgerald, R.J. 1984: Letter commenting on paper. 'The results of Ramstedt's operation; room for complacency?' *Annals of the Royal College of Surgeons* **66**, 449.

Fredet, P. and Guillemot, L. 1910: Le stenose du pylore par hypertrophie musculaire chez des nourrissons. *Annales de Gynecologie et d'Obstetrique* **67**, 604.

Friesen, S.R., Boley, J.O. and Miller, D.R. 1956: The myenteric plexus of the pylorus: its early normal development and its changes in hypertrophic pyloric stenosis *Surgery* **39**, 21–9.

Georgeson, K.G., Corbin, T.V., Griffen, J.W., Breaux, C.W., Jr 1993: An analysis of feeding regimens after pyloromyotomy for hypertrophic pyloric stenosis. *Journal of Pediatric Surgery* **28**, 1478–80.

Glasgow, M.J., Bandrevico, V. and Cohen, D.H. 1973: Hypertrophic pyloric stenosis complicating oesophageal atresia. *Surgery* **74**, 530.

Goh, D.W., Hall, S.K., Gornall, P., Buick, R.G., Green, A. and Cockery, J.J. 1990: Plasma chloride and alkalaemia in pyloric stenosis. *British Journal of Surgery* **77**, 922–3.

Gray, D.W., Gear, M.W. and Stevens, D.W. 1984: The results of Ramstedt's operation: room for complacency? *Annals of the Royal College of Surgeons of Edinburgh* **66**, 280–2.

Grogono, J.L. 1993: Laparoscopic operations in paediatric surgery [Letter]. *British Journal of Surgery* **80**, 264.

Hernanz-Schulman, M., Sells, L.L., Ambrosino, M.M., Heller, R.M. *et al.* 1994: Hypertrophic pyloric stenosis in the infant without a palpable olive: accuracy of sonographic diagnosis: *Radiology* **193**, 771–6.

Hight, D.W., Benson, C.D., Philippant, A.I. and Hertzler, J.H. 1981: Management of mucosal perforation during pyloromyotomy for infantile pyloric stenosis. *Surgery* **77**, 85–6.

Hirschsprung, H. 1888: Falle von angeborener Pylorusstenose beobachtet bei Sauglingen. *Jahrbuch für Kinderheilkunde* **27**, 61.

Hitchcock, N.E., Gilmour, A.I., Gracey, M. and Burke, V. 1987: Pyloric stenosis in W. Australia. *Archives of Disease in Childhood* **62**, 512–3.

Huang, P.L., Dawson, T.M., Bredt, D.S., Sugden, S.H. and Fishanan, M.L. 1993: Targeted disruption of the neuronal nitric oxide synthase gene. *Cell* **75**, 1273–86.

Huddart, S.N., Bianchi, A., Kumar, V. and Gough, D.C.S. 1993: Ramstedt's pyloromyotomy: circumumbilical versus transverse approach. *Pediatric Surgery International* **8**, 395–6.

Huguenard, J.R. and Sharples, G.E. 1972: Incidence of congenital pyloric stenosis within sibships. *Journal of Pediatrics* **81**, 45–9.

Ibrahim, J. 1908: Die Pylorus stenose der Sauglinge. *Ergebnissee der Inneren Medizin und Kinderheilkunde* **1**, 208.

Irjima, T., Okamatou, T., Matsumura, M. and Yatsuzuka, M. 1996: Hypertrophic pyloric stenosis associated with hernia. *Journal of Pediatric Surgery* **31**, 277–9.

Jacoby, N.M. 1962: Pyloric stenosis; selective medical and surgical treatment. *Lancet* **i**, 119–21.

Jedd, M.D., Melton, J., Griffin, M.R. *et al.* 1988: Factors associated with infantile hypertrophic pyloric stenosis. *American Journal of Diseases of Children* **142**, 334–7.

Katz, S., Basel, D. and Brauski, D. 1988: Prenatal gastric dilatations and infantile hypertrophic pyloric stenosis. *Journal of Pediatric Surgery* **23**, 1021–2.

Keizer, D.P.R. 1952: Third generation pyloric stenosis. *Pediatrics* **7**, 1.

Kerr, A.M. 1980: Unprecedented rise in incidence of infantile hypertrophic pyloric stenosis. *British Medical Journal* **281**, 714–5.

Knox, E.G., Armstrong, E. and Haynes, R. 1983: Changing incidence of infantile hypertrophic pyloric stenosis. *Archives of Disease in Childhood* **58**, 582–5.

Kobayashi, H., O'Briain, D.S. and Puri, P. 1994a: A defective cholinergic innervation in pyloric muscle of patients with hypertrophic pyloric stenosis. *Pediatric Surgery International* **9**, 338–41.

Kobayashi, H., O'Briain, D.S. and Puri, P. 1994b: Selective reduction in intramuscular nerve supporting cells in infantile hypertrophic pyloric stenosis. *Journal of Pediatric Surgery* **29**, 651–4.

Kobayashi, H., O'Briain, D.S. and Puri, P. 1995: Immunohistochemical characterization neural cell adhesion molecule (NCAM), nitric oxide synthase and neurofilament protein expression in pyloric muscle of patients with pyloric stenosis. *Journal of Pediatric Gastroenterology and Nutrition* **20**, 319–25.

Kwok, R.H. and Avery, G. 1967: Seasonal variation of congenital hypertrophic pyloric stenosis. *Journal of Pediatrics* **70**, 963.

La Ferla, G., Watson, J., Fyfe, A.H.B. and Drainer, I.K. 1986: The role of prostaglandins E_2 and F_2 in infantile pyloric stenosis. *Journal of Pediatric Surgery* **21**, 410–2.

Langer, J.C., Berezin, I. and Daniel, G.G. 1995: Hypertrophic pyloric stenosis: ultrastructural abnormalities of enteric nerves and the interstitial cells of Cajal. *Journal of Pediatric Surgery* **30**, 1535–43.

Latchaw, L.A., Jacio, N.N. and Harris, B.H. 1989: The development of pyloric stenosis during transpyloric feedings. *Journal of Pediatric Surgery* **24**, 823–4.

Lobe, T.G. 1995: *Pyloromyotomy in pediatric surgery*, Spitz, L. and Coran, A.G. (eds), 5th edn. London: Chapman & Hall, 320–7.

Lobker, H. 1900: Protokolle, Discussionen, Kleinere Mittheilungen, *Verhandlungen der Deutschen Gessellschaft fur Chirurgie*, 128.

Loreta, P. 1887: Divulsioni del piloro e del cardias. *Gazz. d. osp.* Milano **8**, 803.

Ludtke, F.E., Bertus, M., Voth E., Michelski, S. and Lapsien, G. 1994: Gastric emptying 16 to 26 years after treatment of hypertrophic pyloric stenosis. *Journal of Pediatric Surgery* **29**, 523–6.

Macdessi, J. and Oates, R.K. 1993: Clinical diagnosis of pyloric stenosis: a declining art. *British Medical Journal* **306**, 553–5.

McLean, M.M. 1956: The incidence of infantile pyloric stenosis in the North East of Scotland. *Archives of Diseases in Childhood* **31**, 481–2.

Malmfors, G. and Sundler, F. 1986: Peptidergic innveration in infantile hypertrophic pyloric stenosis. *Journal of Pediatric Surgery* **21**, 303–6.

Martinez-Urrutia, M.J., Lassalette, L., Lama, R., Barrios, V. and Tovar, J.A. 1995: Gastric somatostatin content and binding in children with hypertrophic pyloric stenosis: a long term follow up study. *Journal of Pediatric Surgery* **30**, 1443–6.

Mitchell, L.E. and Risch, N. 1993: The genetics of infantile hypertrophic pyloric stenosis, a reanalysis. *American Journal of Diseases in Childhood* **147**, 1203–11.

Muayed, R., Jabar, K., Young, D.G. and Raine, P.A.M. 1984: Pyloric stenosis in sick premature babies. *Lancet* **ii**, 344–5.

Najmaldin, A. and Tan, H.L. 1995: Early experience with laparoscopic pyloromyotomy for infantile hypertrophic pyloric stenosis. *Journal of Pediatric Surgery* **6**, 10–12.

Nicholl J.H. 1906: Congenital hypertrophic stenosis of the pylorus. *British Medical Journal* **2**, 571.

Nour, S., Mangnall, Y., Dickson, J.A.S., Pearse, R. and Johnson, A.G. 1993: Measurement of gastric emptying in infants with pyloric stenosis using applied potential tomography. *Archives of Disease in Childhood* **68**, 484–6.

Ogawa, Y., Higashimoto, Y., Nishijima, E., Muraji, T. *et al.* 1996: Successful endoscopic balloon dilatation for hypertrophic pyloric stenosis. *Journal of Pediatric Surgery* **31**, 1712–14.

Ohri, S., Sackier, J. and Singh, P. 1991: Modified Ramstedt's pyloromyotomy for treatment of infantile hypertrophic pyloric stenosis. *Journal of the Royal College of Surgeons Edinburgh* **36**, 94–6.

Okazaki, T., Yamakata, A., Fujiwara, T., Nishiye, H. *et al.* 1994: Abnormal distribution of nerve terminals in infantile hypertrophic pyloric stenosis. *Journal of Pediatric Surgery* **29**, 655–8.

Okorie, N.M., Dickson, J.A.S., Carver, R.A. and Steiner, G.M. 1988: What happens to the pylorus after pyloromyotomy. *Archives of Disease in Childhood* **63**, 1339–40

Pisacane, A., de Luca, U., Crisuolo, L. *et al.* 1996: Breast feeding and hypertrophic pyloric stenosis: population based case on control study. *British Medical Journal* **312**, 745–6.

Ramstedt, C. 1912: Zur operation der angeborenen Pylorusstenose *Medizinische Klinik* **8**, 1702.

Rasmussen, L., Hansen, L.P. and Pedersen, S.A. 1987: Infantile hypertrophic pyloric stenosis: the changing trend in treatment in a Danish country. *Journal of Pediatric Surgery* **22**, 953–5.

Rasmussen, L., Hansen, L.P., Qvist, N. and Pedersen, S.A. 1988: Infantile hypertrophic pyloric stenosis and subsequent ulcer dyspepsia. *Acta Chirurgica Scandinavica* **154**, 657–8.

Ravitch, M.M. 1960: The story of pyloric stenosis. *Surgery* **48**, 1117–43.

Rogers, I.M., Drainer, I.K., Moore, M.R. *et al.* 1975: Plasma gastrin in congenital hypertrophic pyloric stenosis. *Archives of Disease in Childhood* **50**, 467–71.

Rollins, M.D., Shields, M.D., Quinn, R.J.M. and Wooldridge, M.A.W. 1989: Pyloric stenosis: congenital or acquired? *Archives of Disease in Childhood* **64**, 138–47.

Rowe, M.I., O'Neill, J.A. Jr, Grosfeld, J.L., Foukelsrud, G.W. and Coran, A.G. 1995: Hypertrophic pyloric stenosis. In Rowe, M.I. *et al.* (eds), *Essentials of pediatric surgery*. St Louis, MO: Mosby, 481–5.

Royal, R.E., Ling, D.N., Gruffo, D.L. and Ziegler, M.M. 1995: Repair of mucosal perforation during pyloromyotomy; surgeon's choice. *Journal of Pediatric Surgery* **30**, 1430–2.

Scharli, A.F. and Leditschke, J.F. 1968: Gastric motility after pyloromyotomy in infants: a reappraisal of post-operative feeding. *Surgery* **64**, 1133–7.

Scharli, A.F., Sieber, W.K. *et al.* 1969: Hypertrophic pyloric stenosis at the Children's Hospital of Pittsburgh from 1912–1967. *Journal of Pediatric Surgery* **4**, 108–14.

Schwyzer, F. 1896: A case of congenital hypertrophy and stenosis of the pylorus. *New York Medical Journal* **64**, 674.

Shanbhogue, L.K.R., Sikdaar, T., Jackson, M. and Lloyd, D.A. 1992: Serum electrolytes and capillary blood gases in the management of hypertrophic pyloric stenosis. *British Journal of Surgery* **79**, 251–3.

Shen, X., She, Y., Wang, W. and Wong, L. 1990: Immunohistochemical study of peptidergic nerves in infantile hypertrophic pyloric stenosis. *Pediatric Surgery International* **5**, 110–3.

Spitz, L. and Kaufman, J.C.G. 1975: The neuropathological changes in congenital hypertrophic pyloric stenosis. *South African Journal of Surgery* **13**, 234–42.

Spitz, L. and Zail, S.S. 1976: Serum gastrin levels in congenital hypertrophic pyloric stenosis. *Journal of Pediatric Surgery* **11**, 33–35

Swift, P.G.F. and Prossor, J.G. 1991: Modern management of pyloric stenosis – must it always be surgical? [Letter]. *Archives of Disease in Childhood* **66**, 667.

Takeuchi, S., Tamate, S., Nakahira, M. and Kadowaki, H. 1993: Esophagitis in infants with hypertrophic pyloric stenosis: a source of hematemesis. *Journal of Pediatric Surgery* **28**, 59–62.

Tam, P.K.H. 1985: Observations and perspectives of the pathology and possible aetiology of infantile hypertrophic pyloric stenosis – a histological, biochemical, histochemical study and immunocytochemical study. *Annals of the Academy of Medicine, Singapore* **14**, 525–9.

Tam, P.K.H. 1986: An immunohistochemical study with neuron-specific enolase and substance P of human enteric innervation – the normal developmental pattern and abnormal deviations in Hirschsprung's disease and pyloric stenosis. *Journal of Pediatric Surgery* **21**, 227–32.

Tam, P.K.H. and Carty, H. 1989: Non-surgical treatment for pyloric stenosis. *Lancet* **ii**, 393.

Tam, P.K.H. and Chan, J. 1991: Increasing incidence of hypertrophic pyloric stenosis. *Archives of Disease in Childhood* **66**, 530–1.

Tam, P.K.H. and Carty, H. 1991: Endoscopy-guided balloon dilatation for infantile hypertrophic pyloric stenosis. *Pediatric Surgery International* **6**, 306–8.

Tam, P.K.H. 1994: Stomach and gastric outlet. In Freeman, N.V. *et al.* (eds), *Surgery of the newborn*. Edinburgh: Churchill Livingstone, 89–106.

Tan, K.C. and Bianchi, A. 1986: Circumumbilical incision for pyloromyotomy. *British Journal of Surgery* **73**, 399.

Teele, R.L. and Smith, E.A. 1977: Ultrasound in the diagnosis of idiopathic hypertrophic pyloric stenosis. *New England Journal of Medicine* **296**, 1149–50.

Vanderwinden, J.M., Mailleux, P., Schiffmann, S.N., Vanderhaeghen, J.J. and DeLaet, M.H. 1992: Nitric oxide synthase activity in infantile hypertrophic pyloric stenosis. *New England Journal of Medicine* **327**, 511–5.

Vanderwinden, J.M., Lin, H., Delaet, M.H. and Vanderwinden, J.J. 1996a: Study of interstial cells of Cajal in infantile hypertrophic pyloric stenosis. *Gastroenterology* **111**, 279–88.

Vanderwinden, J.M., Lin, H., Menu, R., Conreur, J.L. *et al.* 1996b: The pathology of infantile hypertrophic pyloric stenosis after healing. *Journal of Pediatric Surgery* **31**, 1530–4.

Von Hilden, F. 1646: *(Hildanus) Opera Quae Extant Monia.* Frankfurt: Bejerus, 541.

Wanscher, B. and Jensen, H.E. 1971: Late follow up studies after operation for congenital pyloric stenosis. *Scandinavian Journal of Gastroenterology* **6**, 597–9.

Wattchow, D.A., Cass, D.T., Furness, J.B. *et al.* 1987: Abnormalities of peptide-containing nerve fibres in infantile hypertrophic pyloric stenosis. *Gastroenterology* **92**, 443–8.

Webb, A.R., Lari, J. and Dodge, J.A. 1983: Infantile hypertrophic pyloric stenosis in S. Glamorgan 1970–1979. *Archives of Disease in Childhood* **58**, 582–5.

Weber, W. 1910: Ueber einen Technische neuering bei der Operation der Pylorus Stenose des Sangling. *Berliner Klinik Wochenschrift* **47**, 673.

Whalen, T. and Asch, W.J. 1985: Report of two patients with hypertrophic pyloric stenosis and Hirschsprung's disease. *American Surgeon* **51**, 480–1.

Wheeler, R.A., Najmaldin, A.J. and Stoodley, N. *et al.* 1990: Feeding regimes after pyloromyotomy. *British Journal of Surgery* **77**, 1018–9.

Williamson, T. 1841: A case of scirrhus of the stomach, probably congenital. *Edinburgh Monthly Journal of Medical Science* **1**, 23.

Wollstein, M. 1922: Healing of hypertrophic pyloric stenosis after the Fredet–Ramstedt operation *American Journal of Diseases of Children* **23**, 511.

Yamakata, A., Fujiwara, T., Kato, Y., Okazaki, T. *et al.* 1996: Lack of intestinal pacemaker (C-KIT-positive) cells in infantile hypertrophic pyloric stenosis. *Journal of Pediatric Surgery* **31**, 96–9.

Zenn, M.R. and Redo, S.F. 1993: Hypertrophic pyloric stenosis in the newborn. *Journal of Pediatric Surgery*, **28**, 1577–8.

CHAPTER 37

Intussusception

D.G. YOUNG

Introduction
Clinical features
Pathology
Diagnosis

Treatment
Results
References

Introduction

Intussusception, i.e. the invagination of the bowel within itself (Fig. 37.1) causing intestinal obstruction, was described in detail by John Hunter in the eighteenth century (Hunter, 1793). In the nineteenth century, many unsuccessful attempts at treatment were made but in 1871, Hutchinson, who had been opposed to surgery in young children for relief of intestinal obstruction, operated successfully on a 2-year-old child. He reduced the intussusception and achieved the recovery of the child instead of the usual rapidly fatal outcome (Hutchinson, 1878). Another successful operation on a 7-month-old infant after initial attempts at reduction of the intussusception by hydrostatic or air insufflation methods had failed was reported by Marsh (1876). In the same period, Hirschsprung in Copenhagen was rationalizing and standardizing the non-operative treatment by hydrostatic reduction in a young patient (Hirschsprung, 1876). With this method, he achieved very successful results, reporting a mortality of only 35% in 107 cases (Hirschsprung, 1905). Hutchinson subsequently enunciated the following propositions over a century ago (Clark, 1900), and it is interesting to see these in the light of the management of intussusception today:

I.   It is absurd to institute any comparison between treatment by insufflation or injection and that by laparotomy. The rule of practice ought to be invariably to try the former measures in the early

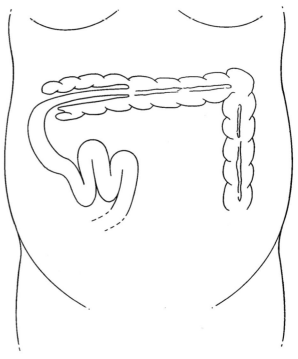

Fig. 37.1 Diagrammatic representation of intussusception showing the ileum prolapsing through the ileocaecal valve and drawing the caecum up into intussusceptum, having reached the mid-transverse colon.

stages. It is only when they have failed that laparotomy ought to be thought of. The two measures are not competitive, but the one is supplementary to the other. Statistical tables instituting a contrast as regards the relative success of the two measures are mere waste of labour.

II. Whilst fully admitting that insufflation and injection treatment ought to be tried first, it is to be borne in mind that these measures are not without risk. They are to be practised with judgement and caution and not persevered in too long. In not a few instances when done too boldly, rupture of the bowel has resulted.

III. It is probable that there is not much reason for preference for insufflation, or injection of air, over injection of water. If the latter is done, the patient's body should be in the inverted position, at any rate during part of the time. As regards the details of the process, I prefer to do it by hydrostatic pressure rather than by a syringe, believing that it is more easy to estimate the amount of distensile force which is used.

IV. If the patient be an infant, say under two years of age, it will be well to be content with repeated attempts by injection. The results by laparotomy in infants have been so almost invariably fatal, that it is safer to trust to the other measures.

V. If the patient be more than two years of age, and a patient attempt at treatment by injection have failed, a prompt resort to laparotomy is to be recommended. It is desirable that this should be done early, before the serous surfaces have become adherent, or the reduction of the incarcerated portion has been made difficult by swelling.

VI. In the performance of the operation the difficult part is the withdrawal of the incarcerated portion of bowel. It is very important to remember that this is often most easily accomplished not by traction of the upper end, but by pressure on the lower, or by the two at the same time.

VII. The older the patient, the slower in all probability will be the progress of symptoms in intussusception, and the longer the period during which it is practicable to effect relief by operation. Thus in adults an intussusception case may be protracted over weeks and even over months. The conditions present even after a very long interval may still be such as to permit of a successful operation.

At the end of the nineteenth century, Clark emphasized the necessity of two conditions for successful operation – early diagnosis and early operation – in intussusception, and in acute abdominal obstructions generally (Clark, 1900). Abdominal section gave by far the better results. The most successful laparotomies were in children under 2 years of age. Manipulation might be tentatively employed in the very earliest stages. Inflation had not been found a successful method of treatment.

Series of patients with intussusception have been reported from most countries. In England and Wales, the reported incidence varies from 1.5 to 4.3 per 1000 live births (Stringer *et al.*, 1992a). In Scotland, the incidence has been 1.4 per 1000 live births since the mid-1980s and there has been little change in incidence since the 1970s, although before that there had been a decline (Pollet and Helms, 1972). While in England and Wales the incidence is currently just over 1 per 1000 live births the incidence in China appears to be higher, as Shanghai Children's Hospital report 500 cases annually, but there is a lack of detailed information (Guo *et al.*, 1986). The peak incidence occurs between 4 and 10 months of life, and two-thirds of patients presenting under 1 year of age.

There has been much discussion on the seasonal incidence of intussusception. In an initial Glasgow series (Strang, 1959) of 400 cases two peaks of incidence were found. This pattern has not been confirmed in later series (Dennison and Shaker, 1970; Hutchinson *et al.*, 1980). Intussusception occurs throughout the year, although overall there is a slight increase during the summer period in reported series.

Most of the series report a preponderance of males, with the male-to-female ratio ranging from 3:2 to 2:1. In 1199 cases in Glasgow (1946–88) there were 786 male patients.

Clinical features

Classical presentation of intussusception is of an otherwise fit and well-nourished infant with sudden onset of signs and symptoms (Table 37.1).

The classical presentation is of vomiting, intermittent abdominal pain, passage of blood per rectum and a mass palpable in the abdomen between the spasms of pain. The infant becomes lethargic. A less common sign at presentation is diarrhoea and prolapse of the intussusception (often mistaken for rectal prolapse). The incidence of prolapse has been reported as 3% (Ravitch, 1959) but in Glasgow this has only been documented in 1% of patients.

The vomiting is initially of gastric contents. If there is delay in the diagnosis, intestinal obstruction becomes superimposed. The vomitus may become stained with bile. Other signs of intestinal obstruction also supervene. In a collection of over 2000 cases the incidence of vomiting was 85% (Stringer *et al.*, 1992a).

Abdominal pain is marked and with each spasm of pain the infant draws up his legs and becomes pale. This pallor is often striking. After these spasms of intestinal colic, the infant becomes more lethargic between the recurrent bouts. Pain, which is a variable feature of intussusception, was absent in 13% of a Toronto series (Ein, 1976).

The characteristic stool of the infant admitted with intussusception is described as being like redcurrant jelly. This is due to the excess mucus secreted from the intussuscepted bowel due to early venous congestion.

Table 37.1 Signs and symptoms of 1199 patients admitted to RHSC Glasgow (1946–88)

Symptom	Percentage of patients
Vomiting	80
Pain	78
Mass	65
Bleeding	61
Diarrhoea	16
Palpable mass per rectum[a]	4

[a]Mass on rectal examination was only documented in 799 patients.

Blood then passes into the lumen of the colon and may mix with some mucus, hence the production of this reddish jelly. The infant's bowels usually move after the initial spasm of pain. There may be no blood in this stool and the blood may appear only on subsequent motions. Some infants do not have a bowel action and blood may be found on the examiner's glove following rectal examination. This sign is less frequent than that of vomiting or pain, and occurs in just over half of patients. The triad of abdominal pain, vomiting and blood per rectum was documented in from 20–50% of patients (Stringer *et al.*, 1992a). It is important to realize that not all signs and symptoms are present in many patients, and vigilance is necessary to prevent delay before the diagnosis is established. The presence of diarrhoea can be particularly misleading. This was present in 16% in the Glasgow series and had on occasion been mistakenly interpreted as a sign of gastroenteritis, thus delaying the correct diagnosis.

Pathology

There has been much discussion on the aetiology of intussusception. In a few patients, a specific lead point is found, such as a Meckel's diverticulum, heterotopic pancreatic tissue, intestinal polyp, enterogenous cyst, adenoma, neurofibroma, Henoch–Schönlein purpura, coagulation disorders and hypertrophy of the lymphoid tissue. This latter condition may be a common cause of intussusception. The distal small bowel, being the site of large collections of lymphoid tissue, is also the usual site of initiation of an intussusception. It may be that hypertrophied Peyer's patches protrude into the lumen of the bowel during waves of peristalsis, initiating the intussusception, and once the intussusception has commenced in the lower ileum, recurrent activity of the bowel feeds the intussusception through the ileocaecal valve and for a variable distance along the colon. Viral infections have been widely incriminated as causative of the lymphoid hyperplasia, but proof of this

is lacking. The relationship of intussusception to upper respiratory infections suggested that viruses were aetiological agents (Dennison, 1948). Subsequent studies which did isolate viruses were negated by the fact that control patients had a similar positive yield of viruses.

The intussuscepted bowel undergoes impairment of its blood supply as the mesentery of the enfolded bowel is compressed within the tunnel thus created. If allowed to persist, this may proceed to venous obstruction, followed by arterial obstruction. As a consequence, gangrene of the intussusceptum may occur. A few case reports record sloughing of the intussusceptum with the bowel wall continuity maintained by autoanastomosis (Robb and Souter, 1962). Gangrene has also occurred in intrauterine intussusception with ileal atresia occurring as a consequence of the intussusception (Parkkulainen, 1958; Laird and Kerr, 1968).

Diagnosis

Diagnosis is made primarily on the basis of the history followed by careful clinical examination. The typical signs are a lethargic baby in whom a sausage-shaped mass is felt across the mid-abdomen when one palpates the abdomen between spasms. It is not always easy to palpate the mass and often each time pressure is applied through the abdominal wall on the mass, the infant tightens the rectus muscles and the clinician can only appreciate that there is an area of tenderness in the ascending or transverse colon. Rectal examination may reveal the mass (4%) where the intussusceptum has advanced into the rectum.

Investigations which are helpful in establishing a diagnosis are abdominal X-ray (Stephenson *et al.*, 1989; Lee *et al.*, 1994; Lazar *et al.*, 1995), ultrasound examination (Holt and Samuel, 1978; Barr, 1994) and contrast enema. Computerized tomography (Parienty *et al.*, 1981) has not been of significant benefit over these investigations. The abdominal X-ray may show the soft tissue mass in the colon with dilated loops of small bowel in the right lower quadrant (Fig. 37.2). The diagnosis should be made before the plain films show marked changes of low intestinal obstruction (Fig. 37.3). Ultrasound examination has been very useful in confirming the diagnosis of intussusception (Fig. 37.4) and the addition of colour Doppler to the ultrasonic examination can assist in defining the viability of the bowel (Lagalla *et al.*, 1994).

Contrast enema (Fig. 37.5) for diagnosis, largely with barium studies until the 1990s, has been replaced by the use of air insufflation. Either hydrostatic (Ravitch, 1954) or air (Kirsk, 1995; Miller *et al.*, 1995) techniques are used for diagnosis and then continued as a therapeutic procedure to reduce the intussusception in the majority of patients.

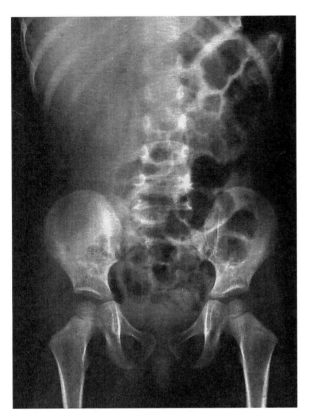

Fig. 37.2 X-ray of the abdomen showing dilated small bowel loops in the lower abdomen and soft tissue mass in the ascending and transverse colon.

Treatment

Not all infants or children who develop an intussusception require active intervention. Spontaneous reduction of intussusception has been described and has been visualized using ultrasound examination. Intussusception occurs in patients with cystic fibrosis (Holsclaw *et al.*, 1971) and they seem to have a high rate of spontaneous reduction. In the vast majority of infants, intussusception does not reduce and requires active therapeutic intervention.

Essential initial treatment of intussusception is to ensure that the infant has an adequate circulating volume. Development of the intussusception causes a significant early loss of fluid from the circulation into the bowel and the baby seldom shows the classical signs of dehydration. However, simple measurement of peripheral skin temperature will reveal a difference of more than 3°C between peripheral and core temperatures, indicating hypovolaemia. Rapid intervention should be undertaken to replace the intravenous fluids by crystalloid, colloid or plasma, until the core peripheral temperature difference is less than 3°C. If the baby has been vomiting a nasogastric tube is

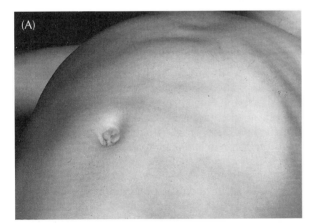

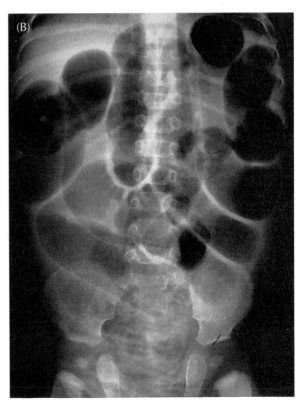

Fig. 37.3 (A) Visible loops of bowel in an obstructed infant with intussusception. (B) X-ray of the abdomen of an infant with intussusception and superimposed intestinal obstruction. The soft tissue mass is almost obscured by the dilated small bowel.

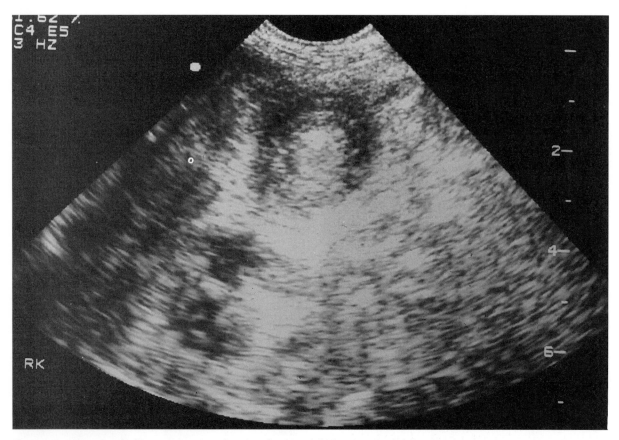

Fig. 37.4 Ultrasound of intussusception showing the pseudokidney or sign of the intussusception.

passed and the stomach emptied. Once stabilized, further confirmatory tests for the clinical diagnosis of intussusception are performed and continued to definitive treatment.

NON-OPERATIVE MANAGEMENT

Barium or air enema is carried out under screening and following confirmation of the diagnosis is continued as a therapeutic procedure. With barium, the reservoir is kept at 30 cm above the patient's buttocks and the pressure of the column of barium into the bowel pushes the intussusception back (Fig. 37.5).

For the intussusception to be completely reduced the colon must be filled out normally and there should be reflux along the ileum for some distance. Air currently has many protagonists advising that air enema is a safer and more successful therapeutic method of treatment (Fig. 37.6). Again, the important point is to ensure that excess pressures are not induced within the lumen of bowel as perforation may occur. Gradual and steady pressure not exceeding 120 cm of water is successful in reducing the intussusception in the majority of patients. Pressures above this are more likely to

induce perforation. These non-operative methods in the reducible intussusception obviate a laparotomy, but they do have a higher recurrence rate than those treated by operative reduction. The highest success rates recorded are from China and at the end of their series a 95% success rate was achieved (Guo *et al.*, 1986).

OPERATIVE MANAGEMENT

Infants and children in whom there has been failure of the conservative approach of management of their intussusception require surgery. A second group requiring operation comprises those who have peritonism at presentation. This group should not undergo a therapeutic enema reduction attempt as the infant may have gangrenous or potentially gangrenous bowel in which perforation would be predicted.

With the stabilized infant under general anaesthesia, laparotomy is performed through a right transverse incision just above the umbilical level. The intussusception may be reduced by gentle finger pressure on the apex of the intussuscepted bowel in the descending or transverse colon, often without needing to bring the bowel

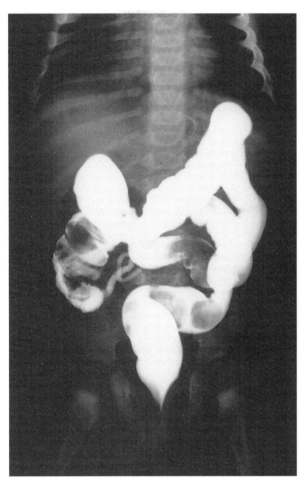

Fig. 37.5 Barium enema showing intussusception in the ascending colon.

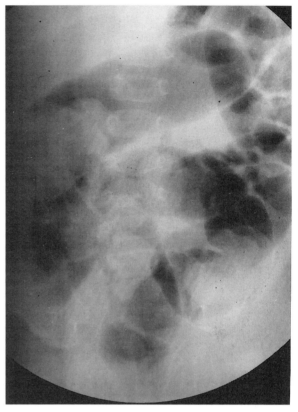

Fig. 37.6 Pneumatic reduction (air enema) showing intussusception in transverse colon.

out of the abdominal cavity. The intussusception should be pushed back from the distal end (Fig. 37.7), and not pulled at the proximal entrance. Reduction is often easily achieved as far as the ascending colon but further reduction may then be difficult. The intussuscepted bowel can then be brought on to the surface and by pressure of the bowel reduction is usually possible. If during this process there is splitting of the serosa, these areas are best oversewn before returning the bowel to the abdominal cavity. If there is a pathological lead point, resection is performed. If the bowel cannot be reduced, the intussuscepted segment is resected and the bowel reconstituted with end-to-end anastomosis. If the bowel is reduced but appears of doubtful viability, it is best to return it to the abdominal cavity and wait for 15 min before inspecting it again. Reinspection may reveal a substantial improvement in the discoloured bowel and a decision to leave it or to resect needs to be made at this time. It should be noted that it is common for the bowel to be very

bruised and it may be quite discoloured from haemorrhage into the wall. Bowel which in an adult one would consider must be resected is often quite viable in the infant, who has greater powers of recovery. Careful postoperative surveillance is necessary in this latter situation if resection is not performed, as delayed perforation of the bowel may occur within the next week.

With the current expertise in fluid, electrolyte and nutritional management, there is rarely inclination for staged operative procedures such as the Mikulicz procedure (Gross and Ware, 1948) or for a side-to-side anastomosis (White and Dennison, 1952). The decision to remove the appendix at the time of laparotomy is an arbitrary one on which surgeons hold various views, but for which there is little evidence to justify either removing it or leaving it *in situ*.

Results

The results of treatment of intussusception have been reviewed (Stringer *et al.*, 1992a) and a summary of the findings from collected series shows the higher rate of

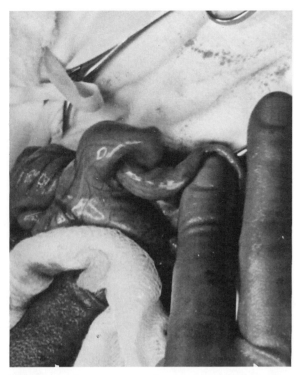

Fig. 37.7 Operative photograph of ileocolic intussusception which has been reduced until the intussusceptum is in the terminal ileum.

successful non-operative management by air enema than by barium enema (Table 37.2). The former are based on the large Chinese series in which, as well as the very high incidence, there is a very high success rate reported with pneumatic reduction. In series from other centres this better success rate with air is also noted, although no other series reaches the near 95% success rate reported from China (Guo *et al.*, 1986). Reduction by operation is usually successful but resection rates have increased to 17% in Glasgow as a consequence of the limited number of patients submitted to operation (Hutchison *et al.*, 1980). Recurrence rates have been highest following hydrostatic reduction and lowest

Table 37.2 Cumulative results of series of patients reported by Stringer *et al.* (1992) with hydrostatic and pneumatic attempted reduction of intussusception

	Hydrostatic	**Pneumatic**
Patients (*n*)	1781	9750
Attempted reduction (%)	67	99 (92)
Successful reduction (%)	40	92 (81)
Perforation (%)	0.3	(0.3)
Recurrence (%)	6	(4)

following surgery, with pneumatic reduction intermediate (6%, 3% and 4%, respectively). An additional complication of operative reduction is subsequent intestinal obstruction due to adhesions. Adhesion obstruction can occur years after operation and our most recent experience was with a child 4 years after operative reduction who presented with one-third of his small bowel gangrenous from an internal hernia secondary to a small adhesion band.

MORTALITY

Mortality overall is under 1% and should decrease further. There were 33 reported deaths from intussusception in England and Wales between 1984 and 1989 (Stringer *et al.*, 1992b). The authors concluded that 20 of these patients had avoidable factors which if successfully addressed could result in further reduction in the mortality. These factors were delay in diagnosis, inadequate intravenous fluid administration, inadequate antibiotic therapy, delay in recognizing recurrent or residual intussusception, particularly in patients with non-operative reduction, and surgical complications.

References

Barr, L.L. 1994: Sonography in the infant with acute abdominal symptoms. *Seminars in Ultrasound CT and MRI* **15**, 275–9.

Clark, H.E. 1900: Case report of a child who made a successful recovery from acute intussusception. *Glasgow Medical Journal* **53**, 209–10.

Dennison, W.M. 1948: Acute intussusception in infancy and childhood. *Glasgow Medical Journal* **29**, 71–80.

Dennison, W.M. and Shaker, M. 1970: Intussusception in infancy and childhood. *British Journal of Surgery* **57**, 679–84.

Ein, S. 1976: *Journal of Pediatric Surgery* **11**, 563–4.

Gross, R.E. and Ware, P.F. 1948: Intussusception in children. *New England Journal of Medicine* **239**, 645–52.

Guo, J.Z., Ma, X.-Y. and Zhou, Q.-H. 1986: Results of air pressure enema reduction of intussusception: 6396 cases in 13 years. *Journal of Pediatric Surgery* **21**, 1201–3.

Hirschsprung, H. 1876: Tilfaelde af Subakut Tarhinvagination. *Hospitals-Stidende* **3**, 321–7.

Hirschsprung, H. 1905: Falle von Darminvagination bei Kindern, Behandelt im Konigin. Louisen Kinderhospital in Kopenhagen Wahrend der Jahre 1871–1904. *Mitt Grenzgeb Medico-Chirurgi* **14**, 555–74.

Holsclaw, D.S., Rocmans, C. and Schwachman, H. 1971: Intussusception in patients with cystic fibrosis. *Pediatrics* **48**, 51.

Holt, S. and Samuel, E. 1978: Multiple concentric ring sign in the ultrasonographic diagnosis of intussusception. *Gastrointestinal Radiology* **3**, 307.

Hunter, J. 1793. On intussusception. *Transactions of a Society for the Improvement of Medical and Chirurgical Knowledge* **7**, 103–15.

Hutchinson, J. 1874: A successful case of abdominal section for intussusception. *Medico-Chirurgical Transactions* **57**, 31–76.

Hutchison, I.F., Olayinola, B. and Young, D.G. 1980: Intussusception in infancy and childhood. *British Journal of Surgery* **67**, 209–12.

Kirks, D.R. 1995: Air intussusception reduction: 'winds of change'. *Pediatric Radiology* **25**, 89–91.

Lagalla, R., Caruso, G., Novarra, V., Derchi, L.E. and Cardinale, A.E. 1994: Colour Doppler ultrasonography in paediatric intussusception. *Journal of Ultrasound Medicine* **13**, 17–4.

Laird, A.P. and Kerr, M.M. 1968: Antenatal jejunal intussusception. *Kinderchirurgie Supplement zu Band* 5.

Lazar, L., Rathaus, V., Ferez, I. and Katz, S. 1995: Interrupted air column in the large bowel on plain abdominal film: a new radiological sign of intussusception. *Journal of Pediatric Surgery* **30**, 1551–3.

Lee, J.M., Kim, H., Byon, J.Y., Lee, H.G., Kim, C.Y., Shin, K.S. and Bahk, Y.W. 1994: Intussusception: characteristic radiolucencies in plain abdominal radiograph. *Pediatric Radiolog* ' **25**, 293–5.

Marsh, 1876: A case in which abdominal section was successfully performed for intussusception in an infant seven months old. *Medico Chirurgical Transactions* **59**, 79–84.

Miller, S.F., Landes, A.B., Dautenhahn, L.W., Pereira, J.K., Connolly, B.L., Babyn, P.S., Abton, D.J. and Danemann, A. 1995: Ability of fluoroscopic images obtained during air enemas to depict bad points and other abnormalities. *Radiology* **197**, 493–6.

Parienty, R.A., Lepreux, J.F. and Cruson, B. 1981: Sonographie and CT features of ileocolic intussusception. *American Journal of Radiology* **136**, 608.

Parkkulainen, K.V. 1958: Intrauterine intussusception as a cause of intestinal atresia. *Surgery* **44**, 1106.

Pollet, J.E. and Helms, G. 1980: The decline in incidence of intussusception in childhood in north east Scotland. *Journal of Epidemiology and Community Health* **34**, 42.

Ravitch, M.M. 1954: Reduction of intussusception by barium enema. *Surgery, Gynaecology and Obstetrics* **99**, 431–5.

Ravitch, M.M. 1959: *Intussusception in Infants and Children.* Springfield, IL: Charles C. Thomas.

Robb, W.A.T. and Souter, W. 1962: Spontaneous sloughing and healing of intussusception: historical review and report of a case. *British Journal of Surgery* **49**, 542–6.

Stephenson, C.A., Seibert, J.J. and Strain, J.D. 1989: Intussusception: clinical and radiographic factors influencing reducibility. *Pediatric Radiology* **20**, 57–60.

Strang, R. 1959: Intussusception in infancy and childhood. A review of 400 cases. *British Journal of Surgery* **46**, 484–95.

Stringer, M.D., Pablot, S.M. and Brereton, R.J. 1992a: Pediatric intussusception. *British Journal of Surgery* **46**, 484–95.

Stringer, M.D., Pledger, G. and Drake, D.P. 1992b: Childhood deaths from intussusception in England and Wales 1984–1989. *British Medical Journal* **3304**, 737–9.

White, M. and Dennison, W.M. 1952: Irreducible intussusception in infants. *British Journal of Surgery* **40**, 137–40.

CHAPTER 38

Gastro-oesophageal reflux in childhood

E.W. FONKALSRUD

Introduction
Physiological basis for gastro-oesophageal reflux
Complications of gastro-oesophageal reflux
Associated disorders
Delayed gastric emptying

Diagnosis evaluation
Medical treatment
Surgical treatment
References

Introduction

Although transient reflux of gastric fluid into the oesophagus with rapid clearing is a normal physiological event, when acid reflux occurs frequently and with more than usual volume, or is not tolerated by the person, a variety of gastrointestinal and respiratory symptoms may result. Gastro-oesophageal reflux (GOR) is one of the most frequent symptomatic clinical disorders affecting the gastrointestinal tract in persons of all ages. Extensive surveys of healthy adults in the USA have shown that 7–10% have heartburn on a daily basis and that 25–40% have it at least monthly (Richter, 1992). Since the late 1970s, GOR has been recognized more frequently in infants and children owing to an increased awareness of the condition, and also to the more sophisticated diagnostic techniques for identifying the disorder. It is currently estimated that approximately one in every 350 children will experience sufficiently severe symptomatic GOR that surgical treatment will be necessary.

Physiological basis for gastro-oesophageal reflux

The concept of GOR disease has gradually evolved since the mid-1930s when it was first demonstrated that symptoms could be produced by the action of gastric acid on oesophageal mucosa (Winkelstein, 1935). In the 1940s and 1950s, the cause of pathological reflux was generally believed to be mechanical, most often associated with a hiatus hernia. It is now apparent that although many patients with reflux disease have a hiatus hernia, many with severe symptomatic GOR have no demonstrable hiatus hernia. In the 1960s it was recognized that a weak or atonic lower oesophageal sphincter (LOS) was the major factor permitting reflux (Skinner and Booth, 1970).

The anti-reflux mechanism in humans can be considered as a mechanical model in which the body of the oesophagus functions as a propulsive pump, the stomach as a reservoir and the LOS as a valve. The LOS is a physiological valve-like mechanism with three major components: the oesophageal hiatus which is a sling formed by the crura of the diaphragm, the angle of His, which is the acute angle formed by the greater curvature of the gastric fundus and the lower oesophagus, and the high-pressure zone of the distal oesophagus which extends from within the abdomen into the low mediastinum. The lower oesophagus comprises of an internal layer of circular muscle fibres and an external layer with longitudinal fibres. The circular muscles extend on to the gastric fundus, with the thickest portion being directly above the gastro-oesophageal junction, corresponding to the high-pressure zone and correlating with the LOS. When the internal muscle contracts, the oesophageal lumen is narrowed and the angle of His is tightened. Thus, there is no clear anatomical sphincter, but rather a combination of factors which creates the conditions necessary for the dynamic function of the LOS. Oesophageal manometry has made it possible to localize the LOS and to determine when the pressure is sufficiently low that it no longer functions as a major barrier to GOR.

A combination of factors appears to influence the development of symptomatic GOR, including a weak LOS, the presence of a hiatus hernia, the motility and clearance capacity of the oesophagus, the resistance of the oesophageal epithelium to injury, and the amount, frequency and duration of fluid of low pH refluxing into the oesophagus. Furthermore, the function of the stomach with respect to the volume of gastric fluid produced, the degree of distention and the intragastric pressure, as well as the effectiveness of motility and the ability to empty at a normal rate, greatly influence the severity of acid reflux. Normal gastro-oesophageal function, therefore, is a complex mechanism that depends on effective oesophageal motility, timely relation and contractility of the LOS, the mean intraluminal pressure in the stomach, the effectiveness of contractility and emptying of the stomach and the resistance to gastric outflow. More than one of these mechanisms may be abnormal in the same child with symptomatic reflux. In GOR disease, particularly in those children with neurological disorders, there appears to be a high prevalence of autonomic neuropathy in which oesophageal transit and gastric emptying are frequently delayed, producing a foregut motility disorder (Cunningham *et al.*, 1990).

The resistance to GOR is provided by the barrier of the LOS and depends on the sphincter pressure, its overall length and the length of the lower oesophagus exposed to the positive-pressure environment of the abdomen. The greater the length of intra-abdominal oesophagus, the more competent this valve-like mechanism becomes. For infants and young children, the intra-abdominal oesophagus is believed to range from 1.5 to 2.5 cm in length. Competence is not maintained if the intragastric pressure due to gastric muscular contraction, and/or elevated intra-abdominal pressure from any cause, exceeds oesophageal muscle tone. Normally, intragastric pressure resulting from stomach contractions rarely exceeds that of the lower oesophagus, unless other factors, e.g. delayed gastric emptying, hypermotility or vomiting, occur. A mean intra-abdominal pressure of less than 10 cm H_2O is necessary for the LOS to function with competence.

Certain drugs may increase the LOS, including cholinergic agents, gastrin, urecholine, metoclopramide and peptones. A large number of other drugs and some hormones may decrease the LOS, including secretin, cholecystokinin, nicotine, alcohol glucagon, prostaglandins, progesterone, oestrogens, theophylline, isoproterenol, vasopressin, atropine, morphine, diazepam, meperidine and calcium channel blockers.

The damage to the oesophageal mucosa caused by gastric acid depends on the duration of contact as well as the volume of reflux. Symptomatic GOR is not commonly related to gastric acid hypersecretion, although the symptoms can often be improved by giving the patient H_2-blocking agents. If alkaline duodenogastric reflux is also present, the virulence of GOR is increased (Pellegrini *et al.*, 1978). The combination of gastric acid, bile salts, pancreatic secretions and pepsin may be devastating to the oesophagus.

Complications of gastro-oesophageal reflux

The LOS mechanism allows the passage of food into the stomach but simultaneously prevents its regurgitation, thereby keeping acid within the stomach. Incompetence of the LOS may cause various of clinical symptoms which are broadly categorized into nutritional, respiratory, those from oesophageal inflammation and miscellaneous. Pathological reflux often produces more than one type of symptom in the same patient. The most common symptom of reflux disease in infants is recurrent vomiting; characteristically it occurs with or shortly after feeding and usually does not contain bile. It is often effortless, but may occasionally be projectile and thus confused with pyloric or duodenal obstruction. Repeated vomiting with failure to thrive secondary to calorie deprivation is the most common symptom complex during the first 2 years of life. When acid reflux repeatedly extends to the oral cavity in young children, severe dental decay may occur and may be one of the initial manifestations of the condition.

Repeated vomiting with periodic aspiration of gastric contents in children can produce recurrent bronchitis or pneumonia, particularly during sleep when swallowing and oesophageal clearance of acid are least efficient. The insidious aspiration of gastric contents can often be demonstrated on pulmonary scintiscan studies. Typically, pneumonia is frequent with repeated attacks and involving different pulmonary lobes. Furthermore, several studies suggest that the reflux of small amounts of acid into the mid or upper oesophagus may produce reflux laryngospasm and/or bronchospasm frequently accentuating the symptoms of asthma. Moreover, various bronchodilator medications used for the treatment of asthmatic children decrease the LOS pressure which has the untoward effect of increasing the likelihood of reflux and aspiration. Reflux-induced laryngospasm is also believed to be a cause of obstructive apnea in infants and possibly a cause of recurrent stridor, acute hypoxia and sudden infant death syndromes (SIDS). There is no conclusive study, however, that proves that GOR causes apnea or SIDS in infants, although the marked improvement in elimination of respiratory symptoms following surgical treatment strongly suggests the existence of a causal relationship. It is rare that a documented death in infancy has been attributed to aspiration of gastric contents. GOR has occasionally been implicated as a possible cause of recurrent laryngitis and otitis media.

Repeated acid reflux into the lower oesophagus frequently causes oesophagitis with chronic inflammation of all layers. For infants with reflux oesophagitis, crying is a common complaint, whereas for older children heartburn is the most frequent symptom. Untreated persistent oesophagitis may progress to stricture of varying lengths of the lower oesophagus and cause dysphagia. Chronic oesophagitis is believed to be a major cause of shortening of the oesophagus. In older children, chronic oesophagitis from repeated gastric reflux is considered to be a major factor leading to the development of columnar epithelium in the lower oesophagus (Barrett's oesophagus), which is generally recognized as a premalignant condition.

Less common symptoms in young children include gastrointestinal bleeding and anaemia from oesophagitis. When GOR is associated with posturing with flexion of the extremities and extension of the neck and torso, it is termed the Sandifer syndrome. In older children, the presentation is similar to that in adults with heartburn, retrosternal discomfort and a bitter taste in the mouth being the most common symptoms. They may also experience easily induced episodes of regurgitation or vomiting while bending over, during Valsalva manoeuvres or even following gastric distention with a large meal.

GOR has a different course and prognosis depending on the age of onset. The majority of newborn infants have an incompetent LOS mechanism as well as a high intra-abdominal pressure when they cry or strain. They often vomit or spit up during the first few months of life, a condition described by Neuheuser and Berenberg (1947) and referred to as chalasia. Boix-Ochoa and Canals (1976) demonstrated by manometry that the normal infant's LOS does not mature to become an effective antireflux mechanism until 5–7 weeks postnatally, following which there is a considerable decrease in the frequency of vomiting. Virtually all infants have some degree of GOR but most are asymptomatic with a marked decrease in the frequency of vomiting by the time solid food is introduced into the diet, usually by 4 months of age. Those with persistent and severe symptomatic reflux are believed to have delayed maturation or incomplete development of the antireflux mechanism. Fewer than 10% of infants and children with symptomatic GOR have an anatomical hiatus hernia.

The function of the LOS in infants is related to the position in which they are placed to sleep. Reflux is increased while in the supine position, whereas prone positioning of a baby decreases reflux which improves the quality of sleep and reduces crying time. The incidence of SIDS, however, is increased in infants sleeping in the prone position.

Associated disorders

Symptomatic GOR is a frequent occurrence in infants who have undergone repair of oesophageal atresia malformations (Ashcraft *et al.*, 1977). Furthermore, it is likely that recurrent oesophageal anastomotic strictures following repair of this anomaly may be caused by the repeated reflux of acid into the oesophagus. The prevalence of oesophageal reflux in these patients may be due in part to the short oesophagus associated with the original malformation, compounded by the repair, in which the lower oesophagus is elevated with sufficient tension in order to complete the anastomosis. Lower oesophageal motility in these patients is invariably abnormal and increases the adverse effects of reflux by delaying oesophageal clearance of acid.

It is generally recognized that the majority of children who undergo extended oesophagomyotomy for achalasia will develop GOR following the procedure. A fundoplication is recommended at the time of the myotomy in most of these patients.

Symptomatic GOR is more prevalent in infants with malformations that cause an increase in intra-abdominal pressure, e.g. omphalocele, gastroschisis, diaphragmatic hernia, ascites and any cause of chronic abdominal distention. Table 38.1 lists several malformations in which symptomatic GOR is commonly present and adds appreciably to the overall morbidity.

Neurologically impaired children often do not achieve their potential development because of malnutrition. The incidence of GOR is considerably increased in these children who commonly require tube feedings because of uncoordinated swallowing and who frequently experience aspiration. Vomiting and the lack of a reliable route for administration of medications make seizure control difficult. When gastrostomy alone is performed in these patients GOR is often produced or made worse. Many surgeons therefore routinely perform a fundoplication for all neurologically impaired children who require a feeding gastrostomy (Stringel *et al.*, 1989).

Delayed gastric emptying

In recent years, delayed gastric emptying (DGE) has been documented with increasing frequency in infants and children who experience symptoms of GOR (Fonkalsrud *et al.*, 1987; Papaila *et al.*, 1989). The use of scintiscans with incorporation of radioisotope (technetium-99m sulphur colloid) in a normal diet for the age group studied has made it possible to quantitate reliably the magnitude of gastric retention at various time-intervals after eating. Retention of more than 50% of the isotope meal after 90 min is generally considered to be abnormal. Pyloroplasty is usually not performed unless more than 60% of the isotope is retained in the

Table 38.1   Major malformations associated with gastro-oesophageal reflux

Neurological
Mental retardation from any cause
Brain injury from any cause
Cerebral palsy
Down's syndrome
Microcephaly
Seizure disorders
Mobius syndrome
Cornelia–de Lange syndrome
Hydrocephalus

Gastrointestinal
Gastric outlet obstruction from any cause
Oesophageal atresia
Pharyngeal swallowing uncoordination
Congenital duodenal obstruction (Ladd's bands, diaphragm)
Congenital abdominal wall defects (omphalocele, gastroschisis)
Short bowel syndrome
Hirschsprung's disease
Portal hypertension
Ascites

Cardiac
More frequent in anomalies causing left heart failure

Respiratory
Congenital diaphragmatic hernia
Tracheal or subglottic stenosis
Cleft palate
Pierre Robin syndrome
Phrenic nerve palsy
Bronchopulmonary dysplasia

Prematurity

Multiple anomalies

stomach at 90 min. It is estimated that approximately half of the children with symptomatic GOR have some delay in gastric emptying without demonstrable mechanical obstruction.

Refluxing children at high risk for DGE include those with serious neurological disorders, including brain damage from any cause, retardation, cerebral palsy, Down's syndrome and microcephaly. Both an acute and chronic decrease in LOS pressure, as well as altered gastric motility have been produced experimentally in a feline model by a global brain injury with increase in intracranial pressure (Vane *et al.*, 1982). Although occasional children with DGE have been observed to have slight thickening of the antral muscle and thus may be considered to have the antral dysmotility syndrome, the majority of patients have a grossly normal appearing gastric antrum.

Diagnostic evaluation

When the clinical history is compatible with symptomatic GOR, a variety of diagnostic studies is available to evaluate the extent of the reflux and the potential causes or contributing factors, and to determine the severity of pathological sequelae (Table 38.2).

Radiographs of the chest may identify and indicate the severity of recurrent pulmonary infections due to aspirations, but they are not helpful in specifically diagnosing reflux. The barium cine oesophagram can provide helpful information regarding the presence and magnitude of a hiatus hernia, as well as evidence of oesophageal inflammation. If a stricture is present, the severity and length can be determined. Furthermore, this study is helpful in identifying oesophageal motility

Table 38.2 Diagnostic studies to evaluate gastro-oesophageal reflux

Chest X-ray
Barium oesophagram
Twenty-four hour oesophageal pH monitoring
Gastric isotope emptying study
Oesophagoscopy with biopsy
Pulmonary scintiscan
Oesophagogastric manometry
Oesophageal motility study

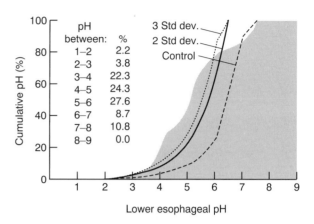

Fig. 38.1 Computerized 24-hour oesophageal pH monitoring study from a 14-month-old boy with symptomatic GOR and DGE showing cumulative pH recordings at each pH level and indicated as a percentage of the total time monitored. The shaded area to the right of the dashed line (control) indicates the normal range, with a pH of 4 less than 5% of the monitored time. The straight line indicates 2 and the dotted line 3 standard deviations from normal. The shaded area which extends to the left of the dotted line shows the values for the patient, which are also shown in numeric form on the left.

disorders and is necessary to rule out mechanical obstruction in the pylorus or duodenum which might cause repeated vomiting. The cine oesophagram often demonstrates GOR; however, the study may be positive in 20–30% of children who have no reflux complications.

OESOPHAGEAL pH MONITORING

The most sensitive and specific test for diagnosing GOR and identifying its temporal relationships to feeding and other physiological events is intraoesophageal pH monitoring (Boix-Ochoa *et al.*, 1980). Various probes are available which are small enough to be used easily in the newborn infant. The oesophageal pH probe is passed into the oesophagus, transnasally, positioned in the distal esophagus 1–4 cm above the LOS and attached to a pH meter. Monitoring continuously over a 24-hour period allows measurement of the effect of various physiological activities on the reflux of gastric juice into the oesophagus over a complete circadian cycle (De Meester *et al.*, 1980). Monitoring is carried out without analgesia and with the patient participating in normal daily activities, limited only by the presence of the pH probe and the recording unit. Ambulatory monitoring with a four-channel telemetry recorder is a cost-effective and accurate way of assessing reflux. Normal oesophageal pH is between 5.5 and 7.0, whereas an episode of reflux is considered to be a fall in pH to below 4.0. Oesophageal exposure to gastric acid is assessed by (1) cumulative time during which the oesophageal pH is below 4.0, expressed as the percentage of the total, upright and supine monitored time; (2) frequency of reflux episodes recorded as number of episodes per 24 hours; (3) duration of the episodes expressed as the number of episodes longer than 5 min per 24 hours; and (4) time in minutes of the longest episode recorded. Data compiled from these recordings determine a child's refluxing profile and are analysed by a computer program. The variance from normal is determined by standard deviations (Fig. 38.1).

In our experience, 24-hour oesophageal pH monitoring is 100% accurate in diagnosing reflux when the

recorded pH is below 4.0 for more than 5% of the total time monitored. When the oesophageal pH monitoring studies are greater than 2 standard deviations from normal, fundoplication is often recommended.

Tests to reproduce the symptoms of oesophagitis by placing dilute acid in the oesophagus (Bernstein test), and the Booth acid clearance test, currently have little place in the evaluation of GOR in childhood.

GASTRIC EMPTYING STUDY

The relationship between gastric dysmotility and GOR has recently been elucidated as a result of the clinical application of sophisticated radionuclide studies originally developed by Griffith *et al.* (1966). By combining technetium-99m sulphur colloid with liquid or semi-solid food as appropriate for age (e.g. formula, pureed food, egg sandwich), a more accurate assessment of gastric emptying can be quantified than when barium sulphate and radiographic studies are used. Infants and children who retain more than 50% of the isotope feeding in the stomach after 90 min, in the absence of mechanical obstruction, are considered to have DGE (Velasco *et al.*, 1982). It is unclear how long gastric dysmotility will persist in an infant or young child; however, if the patient is symptomatic and does not improve with medical therapy, it is our opinion that pyloroplasty should be performed (Fig. 38.2).

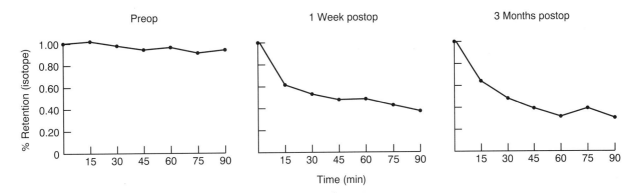

Fig. 38.2 Serial radionuclide gastric emptying studies performed in a 7-month-old girl with neurological impairment and symptomatic GOR. The preoperative study shows 90% retention at 90 min. One week following Nissen fundoplication and antroplasty there was 48% isotope retention at 90 min. Three months postoperation a repeat study showed only 29% isotope retention at 90 min.

OESOPHAGOSCOPY

Oesophagoscopy is occasionally helpful in determining the presence of oesophagitis but is unable to diagnose GOR in the absence of moderate to severe oesophagitis. In patients with mild oesophagitis the mucosal turnover rate is rapid and the typical inflamed surface may not be apparent. A biopsy is therefore necessary to determine the presence and severity of oesophagitis. This examination is particularly helpful in identifying the presence of columnar epithelium in the lower oesophagus of adolescents. Biopsy of the oesophagus can be performed with a suction capsule without need for oesophagoscopy. Direct endoscopic evaluation of the severity of oesophageal stricture and the results of dilatation are particularly helpful, both before and after antireflux surgery.

PULMONARY SCINTISCAN

Scintigraphic scanning of the lungs and upper oesophagus following ingestion of a meal containing technetium-99m sulphur colloid may demonstrate the presence of GOR and pulmonary aspiration in patients with recurrent pulmonary infection; however, the study is only confirmatory and is less sensitive than oesophageal pH monitoring in establishing the presence of GOR.

OESOPHAGOGASTRIC MANOMETRY

Manometry of the LOS is an accurate method for quantitating the resistance of the lower sphincter to reflux of gastric juice. Because of the asymmetry of the LOS, manometry in older children is performed with a catheter containing at least four pressure transducers or water-perfused side holes located around the circumference of the catheter. The catheter is passed into the stomach and slowly withdrawn, recording pressures every 0.5–1.0 cm. The study indicates the length and the resting pressure in the LOS, as well as the length of intra-abdominal oesophagus. If the LOS pressure is below 10 mmHg in young children, there is a high correlation with a continuously incompetent sphincter mechanism permitting frequent reflux. When the LOS pressure is greater than 20 mmHg, it may be intermittently incompetent depending on other factors such as DGE, intra-abdominal pressure and medications. In the past, continuous manometric recording of the LOS during an anti-reflux operation was used as a determinant of how tight to make the fundoplication; however, since anaesthesia reduces the LOS to a variable degree, this technique has largely been abandoned.

OESOPHAGEAL MOTILITY STUDY

Peristaltic contractions in the oesophageal body can be fairly accurately recorded using a continuously perfused five lumen catheter assembly attached to a multichannel recorder. The recording is evaluated for the frequency of non-peristaltic and low-amplitude contractions which interfere with normal swallowing. The recent advance of ambulatory 24-hour oesophageal motility monitoring allows assessment of oesophageal body function over an entire circadian cycle under a variety of physiological conditions (Stein *et al.*, 1990). Ineffective peristalsis of low amplitude and duration and irregular sequence may result from oesophagitis, oesophageal atresia, prolonged distention as with achalasia or a large number of neuromuscular and metabolic disorders, e.g. scleroderma. It is estimated that at least one-third of infants and children with symptomatic GOR have associated motility disorders of the oesophagus. Uncoordinated or ineffective oesophageal peristalsis contributes to prolonged stasis of acid in the oesophagus with poor clearance. It is imperative that a loose fundoplication be constructed in symptomatic children with GOR who have oesophageal dysmotility.

Medical treatment

The three pillars of the non-operative therapy for symptomatic GOR in infants and children are posture, feeds and medication. Oesophageal pH studies have shown that in patients with respiratory manifestations of GOR, most reflux occurs when the patient is flat in bed, either supine or prone. Elevation of the upper body at 60° maintained for 24 hours a day favours oesophageal clearance and effectively reduces symptoms of reflux in two-thirds of infants while awake and during sleep. Maintaining the prone position with 30° elevation has superior antireflux characteristics and greatly reduces irritability (Myers and Herbst, 1982). For children it is helpful to elevate the head of the bed 8 inches during sleep, and it is advisable to avoid eating for at least 2 hours before bedtime. Most young children who experience symptomatic improvement with positional therapy do so within 1–2 weeks after treatment is started. Positional therapy is considered to be a gravitational phenomenon and, when discontinued, the reflux may continue unchanged. Thus, in order to be effective the upright position needs to be continued indefinitely. Reducing the degree of upright positioning or shortening the period of elevation diminishes the effectiveness of this therapy.

Frequent small feeds of thickened formula or food minimize gastric distention and favour reduction of GOR. Minimizing swallowing of air by limiting the use of pacifiers and by frequent burping further relieves gastric distention and reflux. When rice cereal is used to thicken the feeding, the infant will receive a boost in caloric intake which may be particularly helpful for patients with failure to thrive. A low-fat diet is desirable because fats tend to delay gastric emptying. The combination of positional therapy and thickened small feeds may allow a young child to outgrow reflux; however, most families are unable to afford the constant time commitment required, thus making this therapy impractical for protracted periods.

Medical therapy for GOR includes the use of antacids, hydrogen ion-blocking drugs, proton pump inhibitors and a group of prokinetic medications that increase oesophageal peristalsis, increase the LOS pressure and enhance gastric emptying. Metoclopramide hydrochloride administered daily achieves all of these desired effects, but the side-effects of sedation, diarrhea, dystonia and extrapyramidal reactions limit its use to short periods in many patients. Cisapride is a noncholinergic stimulant of oesophageal peristalsis and LOS pressure which has been used extensively in Europe and on a limited basis in the USA. This drug is currently the most effective medication for treating GOR with the least number of side-effects. Bethanechol has been used clinically in previous years, but has been found to be less effective than metoclopramide or cisapride. None of these medications can be given for the many months or years which may be necessary for severe GOR to resolve, and thus they are used largely for short-term therapy for patients with mild reflux.

Antacids and hydrogen ion-blocking drugs, e.g. cimetidine and ranitidine, reduce the adverse effects of gastric acid on the oesophageal mucosa and in the lung when aspirated, and are particularly helpful during the night. The proton pump-inhibiting drug omeprazole is the most powerful agent currently available for blocking production of gastric acid and may be helpful in treating patients with oesophagitis. None has an effect on reducing GOR, however, and thus they are considered as adjuncts in the management of mild reflux, and in the preoperative and postoperative period for patients with severe GOR.

Surgical treatment

The primary indication for performing an antireflux operation on infants and children is the control of intractable and symptomatic GOR which has been clearly demonstrated by oesophageal pH monitoring and cine oesophagram. An isotope gastric emptying study is routinely performed on all children considered for operation. Although oesophageal motility studies, oesophagoscopy, biopsy and manometry are often very helpful in evaluating children with the GOR syndrome, these studies are often not performed on patients with neurological impairment. More extensive preoperative evaluation is often unnecessary since the costs of the studies may not be justified by the small amount of practical information gained. In view of the low cost and low risk of complications following fundoplication, operation is commonly performed early in symptomatic children before more severe complications of GOR develop.

The major objectives of operative repair are to increase the high-pressure zone in the lower oesophagus by accentuating the angle of His and increasing the length of the abdominal oesophagus. A properly constructed antireflux operation should allow normal swallowing, produce no troublesome alteration of oesophageal, gastric or intestinal motility, and allow burping, while eliminating the reflux of acid or gastric contents. Operative treatment is usually undertaken after an unsuccessful trial of a few weeks of medial therapy; however, for patients with severe complications of reflux, such as aspiration, growth failure or oesophagitis with stricture, antireflux surgery may be performed shortly after the diagnosis is established.

Attempts to prevent reflux by tightening the lower oesophagus with a prosthetic ring have been unsuccessful in children since the obstruction produced by the prosthesis greatly interferes with the swallowing mechanism, which is frequently abnormal in refluxing patients. Furthermore, if any acid does reflux into the oesophagus, clearance will be impeded. This procedure does not achieve any of the objectives for repair listed above.

Reflux

Fundoplication

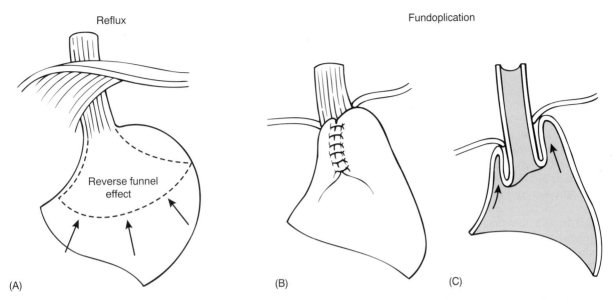

(A)   (B)   (C)

Fig. 38.3 (A) Reverse funnel effect between stomach and oesophagus when angle of His is straightened and LOS is loose; (B) Completed fundoplication; (C) Nipple valve-like mechanism created by 360° wrap which reduces reflux without increasing the LOS pressure significantly.

The most widely used antireflux procedure is that originally described by Nissen and Rosetti (1959). This technique consists of wrapping the gastric fundus 360° around the gastro-oesophageal junction, thus achieving the three objectives of repair. Furthermore, this creates a nipple-like valve mechanism which corrects the reverse funnel effect in the stomach of many children that promotes reflux (Fig. 38.3). Several modifications of the fundoplication have been made for children since the original operation was designed for adults with large hiatus hernias. The modified Nissen fundoplication can be performed transabdominally or through the left chest, but the vast majority of children are repaired through an abdominal approach. Transthoracic repair is reserved for children with severe strictures, severe oesophageal shortening or a large transverse lying liver, or for complex reoperations.

Good exposure of the oesophageal hiatus can be obtained through either an upper midline incision extending superiorly through the xiphoid or a high transverse incision extending across both rectus muscles. A nasogastric tube is used to deflate the stomach and assist in identifying the posterior wall of the oesophagus. The triangular ligament between the left lobe of the liver and the diaphragm is divided, allowing the liver to be retracted to the right. The upper third of the greater curvature of the stomach is mobilized by dividing the gastrocolic ligament, carefully cauterizing or ligating all vessels (Fig. 38.4). The short gastric vessels are divided and the spleen is reflected to the left. The peritoneum is incised on each side of the oesophagus and the crura are clearly exposed. Care is taken to avoid injury to the small vagal branch extending from the left vagus to the

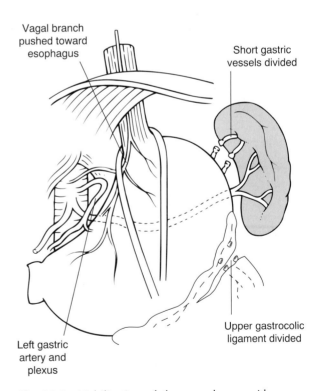

Fig. 38.4 Mobilization of the oesophagus with vagus nerves kept adjacent to the oesophagus. Short gastric and upper gastrocolic ligament vessels are divided to permit free mobilization of upper fundus.

diaphragm. The oesophagus is mobilized with a blunt right-angle clamp and elevated with umbilical tape, following which it is further exposed by blunt and sharp dissection over a distance of 2–4 cm depending on the size of the patient. Both vagus nerves are carefully preserved and are usually maintained immediately adjacent to the oesophagus. If the vagus nerves are damaged during the operation, pyloroplasty should be performed. The crura of the diaphragm are then secured together posterior to the oesophagus with silk sutures, often supported with Teflon pledgets. The right crus is often attenuated and care must be taken to avoid injury to the adjacent aorta and liver. This repair should be made loose to avoid oesophageal obstruction. The suture closest to the oesophagus incorporates a small bite of oesophageal muscularis to minimize the risk of subsequent herniation at this site.

A traction suture is then placed through the greater curvature 2–3 cm inferior to the cardio-oesophageal junction and the upper fundus is gently drawn beneath the oesophagus and elevated on the right side. The gastric fundus is then sutured together anterior to the oesophagus with interrupted silk (Fig. 38.5).

A loose or floppy fundoplication is constructed placing a large blunt clamp beneath the wrap which is opened an appropriate amount for the size of the patient. Since many refluxing children have oesophageal dysmotility, a loose fundoplication is essential to avoid making the swallowing disorder worse. Intraoesophageal bougies have been found to be less accurate in evaluating the tightness of the wrap, and also cumbersome and occa-sionally harmful to the oesophagus and pharynx. The fundoplication is made over a distance of 1.5–3 cm depending on the size of the patient. The upper edge of the wrap is sutured to the diaphragm anteriorly on each side of the diaphragm to prevent migration or slippage. A child with such a short oesophagus that a fundoplication could not be performed is rarely, if ever, encountered.

A temporary gastrostomy is placed in most patients using a No. 10 or 12 Foley catheter inserted through a small incision in the left upper abdomen. The tube is placed through a purse-string suture in the anterior stomach by the greater curvature 3–4 cm distal to the lower end of the wrap. The stomach is sutured to the abdominal wall around the tube. The nasogastric tube is removed at the end of the operation. The gastrostomy tube is left open to gravity drainage for approximately 24 hours, following which it is aspirated every 2–4 hours. Feeds are gradually advanced until a full schedule is achieved. Most patients can be discharged from the hospital by the fourth or fifth postoperative day.

The gastrostomy can be removed within 2 weeks in most patients unless it is necessary for feeding purposes, in which case a silastic catheter or gastrostomy button may be inserted. Gastrostomy may be particularly helpful for infants and young children who often swallow large volumes of air with their feeds. These patients may be unable to burp for a few weeks, placing them at risk for developing gas bloat and disruption of the fundoplication. No major complications with the use of gastrostomy have been observed in over 900 children undergoing antireflux surgery.

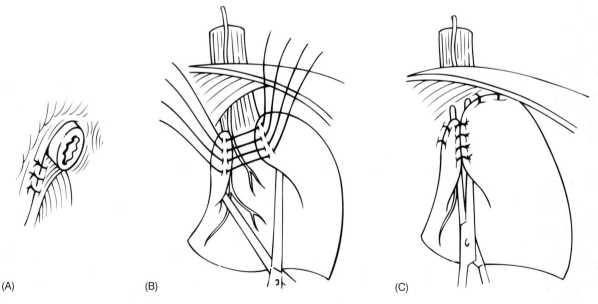

(A)   (B)   (C)

Fig. 38.5   Nissen fundoplication showing: (A) suture approximation of crura posterior to oesophagus; (B) placement of silk sutures through the stomach on each side of the oesophagus; and (C) completed fundoplication with a large clamp opened widely beneath the wrap to ensure that it is loose. The upper edge of the wrap is sutured to the diaphragm at the hiatus.

The Nissen fundoplication is an extremely effective procedure for the control of GOR in children, with more than 92% experiencing long-term resolution of their symptoms (Dedinsky *et al.*, 1987; Fonkalsrud *et al.*, 1992). Relief of reflux symptoms was achieved in almost all children and pulmonary symptoms were either relieved or cured in more than 96% of patients. Weight gain was achieved in almost all failure-to-thrive infants, and was particularly noteworthy in children with feeding disorders who required gastrostomy tube placement. Improvement in asthmatic symptoms occurred in more than 91% of involved patients, with reduced requirements for medication and a decreased frequency of nocturnal wheezing. Asthmatic symptoms, however, were not completely relieved or cured in any patient. More than 75% were able to burp after meals within 1 month after fundoplication. Occasional children, particularly those with neurological impairments, will experience repeated episodes of gagging or wretching following the operation, which can often be relieved by aspirating the gastrostomy tube frequently, and with sedation.

Postoperative complications occur in approximately 15% of patients, the most common being wrap herniation or breakdown (slipped Nissen) and gas bloat. Intestinal obstruction resulting from internal hernia or adhesions occurs in 4% of patients. Complications are more frequent in children with neurological impairment and other major disorders. Approximately 6% of patients will require at least one reoperation for complications. Pulmonary infections or atelectasis occur in approximately 7% of patients, and are most frequent in those with severe pulmonary symptoms preoperatively and those with central nervous system impairment. The postoperative mortality is less than 1% and occurs most often in neurologically impaired children. The long-term mortality is related primarily to associated diseases rather than to GOR.

For children with DGE and reflux, a gastric antroplasty or extended pyloromyotomy has been performed following fundoplication in more than 250 patients in our hospital (Fig. 38.6).

The incision extends for 2.5–3.5 cm through the antral muscularis and pylorus extending on to the duodenum less than 3 mm, but without intentional mucosal incision. The antral muscle is separated widely with a pyloromyotomy clamp and then sutured together in a transverse direction using interrupted 4-0 Maxon absorbable sutures. Reconstruction of the antrum and pylorus after the myotomy shortens the antrum and enhances long-term gastric emptying. A small opening was made in the duodenal mucosa of one-third of the patients, which was repaired with a few additional sutures prior to closure of the muscle. The antroplasty rarely added more than 15 min to the operative time when performed with a fundoplication. A standard Heineke–Mikulicz pyloroplasty with both muscularis

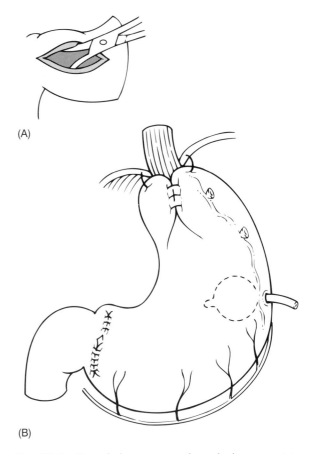

(A)

(B)

Fig. 38.6 Extended myotomy through lower gastric antrum and pylorus with transverse closure. Mucosa is not intentionally opened. Upper edge of fundoplication is sutured to diaphragm at hiatus.

and mucosal reconstruction has been used, but there was no benefit compared with the simpler mucosa-sparing antroplasty.

Transient dumping for less than 3 weeks occurred in three children with standard pyloroplasty, but in none of 215 patients with antroplasty, with a mean follow-up of 6 years. None of the patients developed a leak, obstruction or other complications from the antroplasty or pyloroplasty procedures. Repeat gastric emptying studies performed from 1 week to 2 years after operation showed that no patient had more than 51% retention at 90 min. Each of 50 children evaluated showed more rapid emptying of the stomach, particularly within the first 30 min after feeding, when compared with the preoperative study, but none had emptied all gastric contents at 90 min. None of the children have experienced any clinical evidence of alkaline reflux. Recurrent reflux, disruption of the fundoplication and para-oesophageal hernia were more than three times less frequent in patients who had a pyloroplasty with fundoplication than in those who had fundoplication

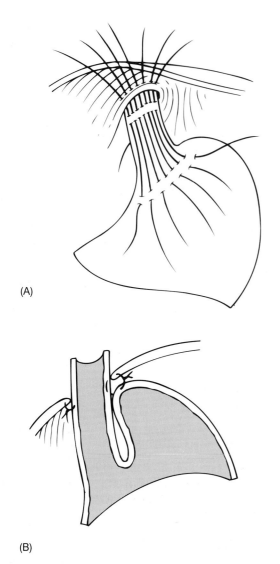

(A)

(B)

Fig. 38.7 (A) Shows the placement of interrupted non-absorbable sutures through the upper cardia of the stomach, or esophagus and diaphragm for Thal fundoplication. (B) Shows the relationship of the stomach and oesophagus in sagittal section.

alone. It is likely that a fundoplication constructed in a child with uncorrected DGE produces a closed loop obstruction which places stress on the wrap and favours slippage or disruption. An occasional patient with recurrent vomiting will have a near normal oesophageal pH monitoring study with marked delay in the isotope gastric emptying study. The author has performed extended antral myotomy without fundoplication in 12 such patients with excellent results.

For children who experience recurrent symptomatic reflux several months following a Nissen fundoplication, reoperation is often necessary. The anatomy of the gastroesophageal junction should be clearly defined by cine oesophagrams and gastric emptying should be quantitated by an isotope feeding study. The majority of patients can be safely reconstructed through a trans-abdominal approach, but in occasional patients a left thoracotomy may be preferable. Because there is often extensive scar tissue at the site of the previous wrap, placing the vagus nerves at risk, a pyloroplasty is commonly performed at the time of a redo fundoplication. Reoperation may be technically difficult if the short gastric vessels were not divided at the initial operation since the spleen may be adherent to the wrap, or even drawn posterior to the oesophagus.

An occasional patient may experience marked gastric atony with distension associated with severe neurological impairment and feeding disorder. In such patients pyloroplasty may not be sufficient to provide adequate gastric emptying. A gastrojejunostomy tube has been particularly helpful in providing enteric feeds to these patients until the stomach begins to contract adequately. Stimulants to gastric contraction such as cisapride, metoclopramide or erythromycin have been of minimal benefit in treating these patients.

For children with distal oesophageal stricture due to GOR, it is best to perform a fundoplication before beginning a course of oesophageal dilatations. In the absence of acid reflux the stricture commonly dilates more easily and is less likely to recur. In rare cases, with long-standing stricture and oesophageal shortening, it may be necessary to resect the oesophagus and perform a colonic or jejunal interposition procedure.

Although the Nissen fundoplication is preferred as the operation of choice for the treatment of GOR in infants and children by the majority of paediatric surgeons, equally good results have been reported by Ashcraft *et al.* (1984) using the modified Thal anterior fundoplication. Technically this procedure is slightly less demanding than the Nissen fundoplication inasmuch as the main goal is to reconstruct the angle of His without making a complete wrap. The primary feature of the operation is the elevation of the upper gastric cardiac and suturing it to the anterior two-thirds of the oesophagus and the diaphragm at the hiatus (Fig. 38.7).

This technique has been particularly useful for children with a large liver, short oesophagus or complex reconstruction, and for patients who undergo an extended oesophagocardiac myotomy for achalasia. Children are slightly more capable of burping during the early postoperative period following the Thal fundoplication than following the Nissen; however, the Thal procedure is slightly more likely to loosen and permit recurrent reflux than is the Nissen repair.

The Toupet partial fundoplication has been used by a few paediatric surgeons in recent years with a low incidence of complications and with good short-term results. This procedure is a posterior fundoplication in which the gastric fundus is brought behind the intra-abdominal oesophagus and sewn to each limb of the hiatal crura. The remainder of the transposed fundus is secured to each side of the lateral oesophagus with a separate suture line, resulting in a 180–200° wrap. Gas bloat and recurrent paraoesophageal hernia are believed to be less frequent following the Toupet procedure than the Nissen fundoplication. Most surgeons, however, prefer to construct a complete 360° wrap, as with the Nissen procedure, since the long-term results in the hands of surgeons who perform the operation on a frequent basis have been excellent with respect to relieving the symptoms of GOR, with a low morbidity.

The Borema gastropexy, in which the lesser curvature of the stomach is sutured to the abdominal wall, is successful in partially reducing the extent of GOR, but the results following this operation have been much less consistent than with the fundoplication procedures. Similarly, the operative procedures designed primarily to reconstruct the phreno-oesophageal ligament have found little support in the surgical treatment of GOR in childhood.

Laparoscopic Nissen fundoplication has been evaluated by a few paediatric surgeons (Lobe *et al.*, 1993); however, the operative time is considerably longer than when fundoplication is performed by the standard open technique. It is unclear at this time whether the incidence of complications, success of the operation in relieving reflux or the length of hospitalization and total costs will be improved by the laparoscopic technique. At this time laparoscopic fundoplication may be best suited for adults and children more than 4 years of age.

References

Ashcraft, K.W., Goodwin, C. *et al.* 1977: Early recognition and aggressive treatment of gastroesophageal reflux following repair of esophageal atresia. *Journal of Pediatric Surgery* **12**, 317–21.

Ashcraft, K.W., Holder, T.M., Amoury, R.A. *et al.* 1984: The Thal fundoplication for gastroesophageal reflux. *Journal of Pediatric Surgery* **19**, 480–3.

Boix-Ochoa, J. and Canals, J. 1986: Maturation of the lower esophageal sphincter. *Journal of Pediatric Surgery* **11**, 749–55.

Boix-Ochoa, J., La Fuente, J.M. and Gil-Vernet, J.M. 1980: 24-hour pH monitoring in gastroesophageal reflux. *Journal of Pediatric Surgery* **15**, 74–8.

Cunningham, K., Riddell, P., Maddern, P. *et al.* 1990: Relationships between autonomic nerve dysfunction, gastric emptying, and esophageal transport in gastroesophageal reflux. *Gastroenterology* **98**, A34–40.

De Meester, T.R., Wang, C.I., Wernly, J.A. *et al.* 1980: Technique, indications, and clinical use of 24-hour esophageal pH monitoring. *Journal of Thoracic and Cardiovascular Surgery* **79**, 656–70.

Dedinsky, G.K., Vane, D.W., Black, C.T. *et al.* 1987: Complications and reoperation after Nissen fundoplication in childhood. *American Journal of Surgery* **153**, 177–83.

Fonkalsrud, E.W., Ament, M.E. and Vargas, J. 1992: Gastric antroplasty for the treatment of delayed gastric emptying and gastroesophageal reflux in children. *American Journal of Surgery* **153**, 177–83.

Fonkalsrud, E.W., Berquist, W., Vargas, J. *et al.* 1987: Surgical treatment of the gastroesophageal reflux syndrome in infants and children. *American Journal of Surgery* **154**, 11–18.

Griffith, J.H., Owen, G.M., Kirkman, S. *et al.* 1966: Measurement of rate of gastric emptying using chromium-51. *Lancet* **i**, 1244–5.

Lobe, T.E., Schropp, K.P. and Lunsford, K. 1993: Laparoscopic Nissen fundoplication. *Journal of Pediatric Surgery* **28**, 358–61.

Myers, W.F. and Herbst, J.J. 1982: Effectiveness of positioning therapy for gastroesophageal reflux. *Pediatrics* **69**, 768–72.

Neuhauser, E.B.D. and Berenberg, W. 1947: Cardioesophageal relaxation as a cause of vomiting in infants. *Radiology* **48**, 480–6.

Nissen, R. and Rosetti, M. 1959: *Die Behandlunq von Hiatushernie und Reflux-oesophagitis mit Gastropexie und Fundoplication.* Stuttgart: Georg Thieme.

Papaila, J.G., Wilmont, D., Grosfeld, J.L. *et al.* 1989: Increased incidence of delayed gastric emptying in children with gastroesophageal reflux. *Archives of Surgery* **124**, 933–6.

Pellegrini, C.A., De Meester, T.R., Wernly, J.A. *et al.* 1978: Alkaline gastroesophageal reflux. *American Journal of Surgery* **135**, 177–84.

Richter, J.E. 1992: Surgery for reflux disease – reflections of a gastroenterologist. *New England Journal of Medicine* **326**, 825–7.

Skinner, D.B. and Booth, D.J. 1970: Assessment of distal esophageal function in patients with hiatal hernia and/or gastroesophageal reflux. *Annals of Surgery* **172**, 627–37.

Stein, H.J., Eypasch, E.P., De Meester, T.R. *et al.* 1990: Circadian esophageal motor function in patients with gastroesophageal reflux disease. *Surgery* **108**, 769–78.

Stringel, G., Delgado, M., Gertin, L. *et al.* 1989: Gastrostomy and Nissen fundoplication in neurologically impaired children. *Journal of Pediatric Surgery* **24**, 1044–8.

Vane, D.W., Shiffler, M., Grosfeld, J.L. *et al.* 1982: Reduced LES pressure after acute and chronic brain injury. *Journal of Pediatric Surgery* **17**, 960–3.

Velasco, N., Hill, L.B. and Gannan, R.M. 1982: Gastric emptying and gastroesophageal reflux: effects of surgery and correlation with esophageal motor function. *American Journal of Surgery* **144**, 58–62.

Winkelstein, A. 1935: Peptic esophagitis: a new clinical entity. *Journal of the American Medical Association* **104**, 906–10.

CHAPTER 39

Acquired conditions of the anorectum and perineum

S.W. BEASLEY

Introduction
Clinical features

Introduction

Several conditions may affect the anorectal and perineal areas in children (Table 39.1); most are unrelated and minor, but sometimes they may be a manifestation of more extensive disease, such as the perianal disease that is seen in Crohn's disease.

By far the most common condition is the anal fissure. This may present at any age with pain on defecation and small amounts of bright red blood on the surface of the stool or immediately after defecation. The fissure is found in the midline and normally heals within days. It may be a reflection of a tendency to constipation and treatment of the underlying constipation will reduce the likelihood of its recurrence.

Clinical features

RECTAL BLEEDING

A variety of conditions produces apparent rectal bleeding in children. They are best considered in relation to the way in which they present, as this will give some clues as to their likely cause (Table 39.2).

NEONATAL BLEEDING

The two important surgical causes of rectal bleeding in the neonate are necrotizing enterocolitis (see also Chapter 25), and malrotation in which volvulus of the midgut has supervened.

Neonatal necrotizing enterocolitis

Necrotizing enterocolitis is an acquired condition that most often occurs in premature infants who have undergone major perinatal stress. Predisposing factors and observed associations include prematurity, hyaline membrane disease, birth asphyxia, fetal distress during labour, prolonged rupture of membranes, multiple births, caesarian section, congenital heart disease, jaundice, catheterization of the umbilical vessels, administration of hyperosmolar oral feeds and perinatal sepsis. The infant becomes lethargic and unwell with abdominal distension and vomiting, at which stage there is often passage of loose stools containing a variable amount of blood. The observation of intramural gas on plain radiology (pneumatosis intestinalis), portal venous gas or free gas in the peritoneal cavity from perforation (pneumoperitoneum), is suggestive of the diagnosis. Initial management involves cessation of oral feeds,

Table 39.1 Acquired conditions of the anorectum and perineum in children

Anal fissure
Rectal polyp
Rectal prolapse
Perianal abscess and fistula
Inflammatory bowel disease
Straddle injuries
Labial adhesions

Table 39.2 Presentation of rectal bleeding in children

Clinical setting	Typical causes
Neonatal	Necrotizing enterocolitis Volvulus with ischaemia Haemorrhagic disease of the newborn (vitamin K deficiency) Anal fissure Swallowed maternal blood
Small amount of bright blood in a well child	Anal fissure (by far the most common) Rectal polyps Unrecognized rectal prolapse Haemorrhoids (idiopathic)
Ill child with an acute abdominal condition	Intussusception Gastroenteritis Henoch–Schönlein purpura
Major haemorrhage from gastrointestinal tract	Oesophageal varices Peptic ulcer Meckel's diverticulum Tubular duplications
Chronic illness with diarrhoea	Crohn's disease Ulcerative colitis Non-specific colitis

decompression of the bowel by nasogastric drainage, intravenous fluid resuscitation and broad-spectrum antibiotics effective against bowel organisms. Surgery is required if there is clinical or radiological evidence of full-thickness bowel necrosis, i.e. free gas or peritonitis, or when there is ongoing clinical deterioration despite intensive and appropriate supportive care.

Malrotation with volvulus

Volvulus of the midgut can occur at any age, but is most commonly seen in the neonatal period. It is a complication of malrotation and occurs because the mesentery of the midgut is very narrow (the 'universal mesentery'), predisposing it to twisting. The first sign of volvulus is bile-stained vomiting and if the significance of this is not recognized immediately, ischaemia of the midgut may ensue, leading to gross abdominal distension and signs of peritonitis. The diagnosis can be confirmed with a barium meal which shows either obstruction of the second part of the duodenum or failure of the duodenum to cross the midline and reach the level of the pylorus. Treatment involves surgery to broaden the mesentery of the small bowel. If peritonitis is already present, contrast radiology is not necessary and the child should be taken to theatre as soon as possible.

Other neonatal causes

Anal fissures may occur at any age, including in the neonatal period. If the infant has swallowed maternal blood, either during delivery or from a cracked nipple, blood may be evident in the stools. Haemorrhagic disease of the newborn also may produce blood in the stools and is prevented by routine administration of vitamin K_1.

A SMALL AMOUNT OF BLOOD IN A WELL CHILD

This is a common presentation, and the cause of the bleeding can often be determined by the history alone.

Anal fissure

An anal fissure occurs when passage of a hard stool splits the mucosa of the anus, usually in the midline posteriorly or anteriorly. The child suffers pain on defecation and a small amount of bright red blood may be seen on the surface of the stool, or immediately following it. The fissure heals rapidly, but where it has been recurrent, it may produce a small mound of oedematous skin, just external to the fissure, as a 'sentinel pile'. The diagnosis can be confirmed by gently parting the anus laterally to expose the anal mucosa anteriorly and posteriorly. Healing of the fissure is facilitated by treating the underlying constipation. Liquid paraffin oil (Parachoc® or Agarol®) is effective in softening the stools and acting as a lubricant. Sometimes an anal fissure can develop after an episode of severe diarrhoea.

Rectal polyp

A juvenile polyp is a benign hamartomatous lesion that is usually located in the rectum and should be suspected when there is intermittent rectal bleeding in the absence of constipation or pain on defecation, and where there is no fissure evident on clinical examination. The diagnosis is made on digital examination of the rectum or on proctoscopy, at which time the polyp can be removed. A rectal polyp may prolapse, in which situation it must be distinguished from rectal prolapse. If the polyp has prolapsed, its base can be ligated without anaesthesia. Otherwise, the polyp can be located through a proctoscope, withdrawn to demonstrate its stalk, and sutured. Recurrence is unusual and malignancy virtually unknown.

Rectal prolapse

Prolapse of the rectum is diagnosed from the history, as it is almost always observed by the parents. When the prolapsed rectum becomes congested or traumatized, it may ulcerate and bleed. Prolapse is common in toddlers, and although it may occur frequently over several months, it almost always resolves spontaneously without any residual sequelae. In a minority of children with rectal prolapse, there is an underlying organic cause (Table 39.3).

Predisposing factors in idiopathic rectal prolapse are believed to be excessive straining during defecation in a child with constipation, and precipitate or explosive defecation. The prolapse appears at the anus painlessly, and usually returns spontaneously, although manual replacement is sometimes required. The differential diagnosis includes prolapse of a rectal polyp and intussusception, in which the intussusceptum presents at the anus. Haemorrhoids are rare in children.

AN ILL CHILD WITH AN ACUTE ABDOMINAL CONDITION

In this clinical setting, the symptom of rectal bleeding is additional to other more obvious features suggesting significant pathology. Intussusception presents with symptoms of vomiting, colicky abdominal pain, pallor and lethargy, usually in children between 3 months and 2 years of age. In only about half the patients is there evidence of blood in the stools, the characteristic 'red-currant jelly' stool (see also Chapter 37).

Patients with severe gastroenteritis may have vomiting and colicky abdominal pain, and blood may be mixed with the loose stools. In children under 2 years of age, the initial diagnosis may be difficult to distinguish from intussusception.

In Henoch–Schönlein purpura there is arthralgia and a typical rash over the extremities, but these may not appear until after the commencement of abdominal symptoms. Submucosal haemorrhages in the bowel wall may cause abdominal pain, the passage of blood rectally and, occasionally, intussusception.

MAJOR HAEMORRHAGE PER RECTUM

In these patients the haemorrhage may be severe enough to cause anaemia or require transfusion. Causes range from oesophageal varices and peptic ulcer to bleeding Meckel's diverticulum and tubular duplications of the bowel (see also Chapters 26 and 41).

Where a Meckel's diverticulum contains ectopic gastric mucosa, the acid it produces may ulcerate the mucosa of adjacent ileum. Bleeding may be profuse and

Table 39.3 Causes of rectal prolapse

Cause	Comments
Idiopathic	By far the most common type
Neurological (paralysis of anal sphincters)	Myelomeningocele (spina bifida) Sacral agenesis
Ectopica vesicae (bladder exstrophy)	Or cloacal exstrophy
Following anorectoplasty for a congenital anorectal malformation (e.g. imperforate anus)	Note that redundant rectal mucosa may prolapse after anorectoplasty and resemble rectal prolapse
Nutritional	Marasmic undernourished hypotonic infants
Cystic fibrosis	Prolapse is seen also in children with malabsorption and chronic diarrhoea

presents as brick-red stools. Sometimes the child complains of vague abdominal pain. The bleeding usually stops spontaneously without the need for emergency surgery. The definitive investigation is surgery, but in many instances a technecium scan may demonstrate a hotspot in the region of the ectopic gastric mucosa.

PERIANAL ABSCESS

This is a common condition in infants, particularly in the first year of life, and arises from infection in one of the anal glands which opens into the crypts of the anal valves. Although there is an internal opening at the level of the anal valves, the abscess itself almost always points superficially through the skin 1–2 cm from the anal verge. Drainage of the abscess alone is inadequate as recurrence is almost certain. Appropriate treatment involves opening the entire fistulous tract from the internal opening in the anal canal to the abscess cavity under general anaesthesia.

Some children may develop a superficial subcutaneous infection in the buttock or near the anus. This tends to occur secondary to a nappy rash or poor hygiene, as a result of infection with skin organisms. Antibiotics and simple drainage are curative.

INFLAMMATORY BOWEL DISEASE

Since the late 1970s, there has been a dramatic increase in the incidence of Crohn's disease in children. The incidence of ulcerative colitis has remained unchanged. Crohn's disease can involve any part of the gastro-intestinal tract, and is characterized by a transmural inflammatory process. Perianal disease is common. Perianal abscesses and fissures tend to be chronic and indolent and, unlike the usual type of anal fissure, are often laterally placed (see also Chapter 40).

The great variability of presentation in Crohn's disease may lead to considerable delay between the onset of symptoms and diagnosis. A diagnosis of Crohn's disease should be considered in any child who has an unusual perianal abscess or fissure away from the midline. There may be a history of recurrent abdominal pain and weight loss. In the adolescent, the first manifestations of disease may be growth failure with delayed onset of puberty. In ulcerative colitis perianal disease is uncommon.

FEMALE GENITALIA

Labial adhesions

This is a common acquired condition of girls in which there is midline adherence of the labia minora which usually commences posteriorly and may extend as far anteriorly as the clitoris.

Labial adhesions (or fused labia) should not be confused with congenital absence of the vagina as such an error in diagnosis may cause parents much unnecessary anxiety. Labial adhesions have never been reported at birth.

Fused labia can be separated without anaesthesia by sweeping them apart with the blunt end of a thermometer or by exerting gentle lateral traction on the labia minora. Occasionally, particularly in older children, they may be more densely adherent, and require separation under general anaesthesia. There is a tendency for refusion following separation, so parents should be encouraged to apply Vaseline® ointment to the raw area on the medial side of the labia minora for about 2 weeks, until complete re-epithelialization has occurred.

Imperforate hymen

This condition is very much less common than labial adhesions, and often presents at birth. The vagina secretes mucus which accumulates beneath the imperforate hymen to form a mucocolpos. Sometimes an imperforate hymen is not noticed until puberty, when an adolescent presents with primary amenorrhoea and haematocolpos, or with cyclical attacks of abdominal pain. Removal of the hymen is curative.

STRADDLE INJURIES

Straddle injury is the term applied to a spectrum of injuries that may be sustained by blunt trauma to the perineum. These injuries are seen in a variety of situations such as when a child slips on a wet floor whilst getting out of a bath, falls astride a fence or bar during play, or lands heavily on the horizontal bar of a bicycle. In females, these accidents often cause significant bleeding from a tear in the region of the labia minora that extends towards the posterior fourchette. Adequate assessment may be difficult in the emergency room and the girl will require admission for examination under anaesthesia, at which time the laceration is sutured.

In boys, a straddle injury is more likely to damage the anterior urethra (see Chapter 72). If the urethra has been disrupted, there may be extravasation of urine into the scrotum and perineum. A carefully performed retrograde urethrogram will demonstrate leakage of contrast. Treatment involves either suprapubic catheter drainage of urine or primary urethral repair, depending on the level and severity of injury. Where a laceration penetrates the rectum, a colostomy for faecal diversion is warranted.

In both sexes, the possibility of sexual abuse should be considered whenever a child presents with a perineal injury. A careful history should determine whether the story provided is consistent with the nature and severity of the injuries observed. If the history and physical findings are in any way suggestive of sexual abuse, it is wise to involve the appropriate specialist sexual abuse team, or police surgeon, for further management (see Chapter 75).

CHAPTER 40

Inflammatory bowel disease

C.M. DOIG

Introduction	**General conclusions**
Crohn's disease	**References**
Ulcerative colitis	

Introduction

Despite the fact that the initial patient described by Crohn *et al.* (1932) was a 16-year-old boy, inflammatory bowel disease is still believed to occur in late teens and adult life (Smith *et al.*, 1975; Mayberry *et al.*, 1979; Lee and Costello, 1985).

INCIDENCE

The incidence of inflammatory bowel disease, especially Crohn's disease, in juveniles has shown an increase since the 1970s, in contrast to a steady incidence of ulcerative colitis, despite a fall in the young population (Barton *et al.*, 1989). This is thought to be a true increase and not due to better diagnosis and increased awareness of the problem. In the 1980s the incidence in the UK in children under the age of 15 was found to be almost 800, more than 300 of whom were suffering from ulcerative colitis and nearly 450 Crohn's disease (Table 40.1) (Ferguson *et al.*, 1986). There was a regional variation in the reporting of such cases, perhaps reflecting the local interest (or otherwise) in the disease in children, information coming from paediatricians, paediatric surgeons and adult gastroenterologists. The incidence in the London area was 7.32 per 100 000 children, 6.47 in Wessex and 9.2 in the north-west of England, in contrast to less than 1 in Northern Ireland. The reports from Scotland were only one-third of those who were admitted to hospital, as reflected by hospitals statistics (SHIPS) (Barton *et al.*, 1989).

The true incidence of childhood inflammatory bowel disease is probably higher than estimated, e.g. Crohn's disease being nearer 10 than 2.9 per 100 000 and for ulcerative colitis 6.8 rather than nearly 2 (Ferguson *et al.*, 1986). This incidence is similar to other childhood diseases such as Duchenne's muscular dystrophy, thalassaemia and haemophilia.

Although ulcerative colitis occurs in Asian children and adults, Crohn's disease is uncommon (Chong and Walker-Smith, 1986; McConnell *et al.*, 1992; Probert *et al.*, 1993a) and is virtually unknown in Asia itself. Both diseases are common in the Jewish population (Gilat *et al.*, 1986; Yang *et al.*, 1993). There is a strong familial incidence, with 30% of children having a relative with one or other disease, although the close relative may not

Table 40.1 Survey showing incidence of inflammatory bowel disease in children under the age of 15 years (Ferguson *et al.*, 1986)

Diagnosis	Male	Female	Total
Crohn's disease	261	186	447
Ulcerative colitis	157	148	305
Not stated, unclassified, other colitides	19	15	34

necessarily suffer from the same disease (four in my own series) (Mayberry, 1985; Farmer and Michener, 1986; Lashner *et al.*, 1986; Sanderson *et al.*, 1986; Monsen *et al.*, 1987). The distribution between genders is different from that in adult practice, with an equal distribution between boys and girls (Doig, 1989).

The diseases seem to be multifactorial in origin, with both environmental and genetic factors contributing to susceptibility (Satsangi *et al.*, 1994).

AGE

Although these diseases are common in adolescents they can and do occur in children below the age of 10 years. In the previously mentioned survey almost half the children were under 10 years old at the initial presentation (Fig. 40.1) (Ferguson *et al.*, 1986). However, in view of the sometimes long delay in making the diagnosis, especially of Crohn's disease (Burbidge *et al.*, 1975), partly because of the unusual presentation but also because of the diagnosis not being considered, the child may well be much older before diagnosis is made and treatment started. Awareness of these diseases occurring in children means that children are investigated and diagnosed sooner (Kirschsner, 1988a).

Crohn's disease

AETIOLOGY

The aetiology of Crohn's disease is unknown, although various theories have been put forward (Kumar and Alexander-Williams, 1993): infective (Tanaka *et al.*, 1991), dietary and autoimmune. Mycobacteria have been implicated (Chiodini *et al.*, 1984; Graham *et al.*, 1987; Sanderson and Hermon-Taylor, 1992). However, the pathological features would suggest chronic cell-mediated immune reactions which can cause mucosal ulceration (Madara and Stafford, 1989) and autoimmune reactions to bacterial antigens, as the neutrophils from patients with Crohn's disease appear to have impaired ability to deal with granuloma-forming organisms (Curran *et al.*, 1991). Evidence is appearing to implicate immunological mechanisms in damaging the tissues in Crohn's disease, with increased T cells in the lymph nodes (Ibbotson and Lowes, 1995). It would appear that there is a general activation of mucosal T cells (Ferguson *et al.*, 1987). Certain foods have been implicated (Mayberry *et al.*, 1980). Vascular injury may also be an early event (Wakefield *et al.*, 1989), with vasculitis due to multifocal infarction in the mesentry resulting in platelet dysfunction (Collins and

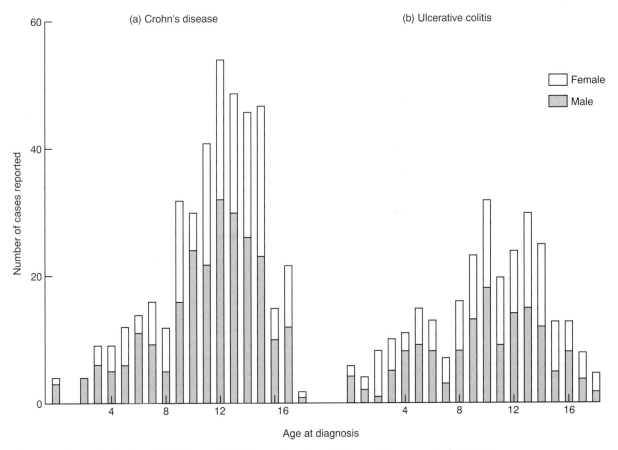

Fig. 40.1   Age distribution of children with inflammatory bowel disease (Ferguson *et al.*, 1986).

Rampton, 1995). Even the lack of breastfeeding or diarrhoeal disease has been implicated (Koletzko *et al.*, 1989) as well as tobacco smoke (Persson *et al.*, 1980).

PATHOLOGY

Crohn's disease is characterized by transmural oedema with fissures, patchy in nature, giving a cobblestone appearance to the mucosa (Fig. 40.2). Histological study shows the formation of granuloma with giant cells, but not associated with caseation (Fig. 40.3). This is a panenteric disease and skip lesions are common. It is not always possible to determine the affected area by inspection at surgery (Butterworth *et al.*, 1992), although fat encroachment on to the serosa is helpful (Sheehan *et al.*, 1992). If the ulcerative process continues unchecked, the formation of fistulae into the adjacent tissue, e.g. bowel, bladder or skin, occurs while fibrosis leads to stricture formation. Granulomatous deposits can be found in the lungs (Puntis *et al.*, 1990) as well as skin tags. Such anal disease can be devastating and painful and in more than half the cases it is associated with disease elsewhere (Elliot, 1987; Palder *et al.*, 1991).

There seems to be an increased risk of colorectal cancer developing in young-onset Crohn's disease (Gillen *et al.*, 1994; Choi and Zelig, 1994; Connell *et al.*, 1994). Dysplasia may occur, especially in rectal Crohn's disease, with the danger of the later development of carcinoma (Korelitz *et al.*, 1990).

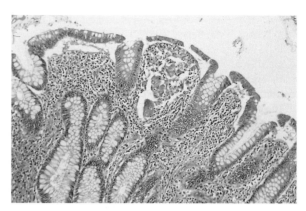

Fig. 40.3 Microscopy slide showing granuloma within the mucosa in Crohn's disease.

CLINICAL FEATURES

Vague abdominal pain, a classical presentation, occurs in only 30%, with diarrhoea in 50% and weight loss in a quarter of children (Doig, 1989). Lethargy and anorexia may predominate. Unhealing chronic perianal abscesses and fistulae are suggestive of the disease. Since abdominal pain and diarrhoea are common in children, thought must be given as to whether investigation is required (Mayberry, 1989). Unhealing chronic perianal abscesses, fistulae and anal fissures (Palder *et al.*, 1991) may need investigation. It is important that these changes should not be attributed to sexual abuse.

Extra-abdominal signs and symptoms such as skin rashes, e.g. erythema nodosum, may be the initial presentation of Crohn's disease, occurring in 10% of children, and should alert the doctor to the possible diagnosis (Elliot, 1987). Other extra-abdominal presentations include mouth ulcers in 20% (Fig. 40.4) uveitis and arthritis in 10%. These problems mean that children present to opthalmologists, orthopaedic surgeons and even dentists (Scully *et al.*, 1982) – at least four

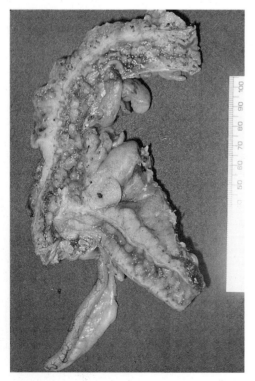

Fig. 40.2 Operative specimen of Crohn's disease showing typical mucosa.

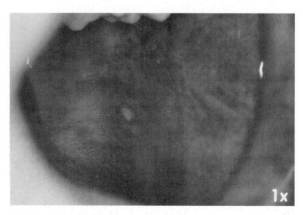

Fig. 40.4 Typical apthous ulcer in the mouth of a child with Crohn's disease.

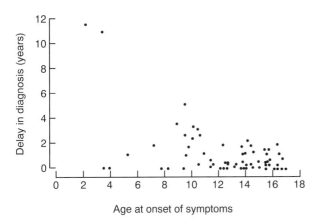

Age at onset of symptoms

Fig. 40.5 Comparison between age of presentation and time of diagnosis in Crohn's disease (Scottish figures) (Barton and Ferguson, 1990).

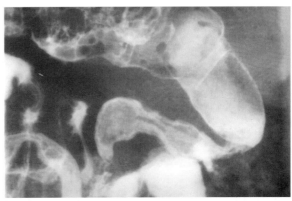

Fig. 40.7 The figure illustrates barium in the small bowel showing ileal involvment in Crohn's disease.

children of my own series were diagnosed by dentists. Such a diversity of presentation means that children do not automatically appear at gastrointestinal clinics, but can end up at growth clinics under the care of rheumatologists (MacFarlane *et al.*, 1986a) or psychiatrists (Jenkins *et al.*, 1988). Additional mental problems can lead to delay in diagnosis which may affect recovery (Andrews *et al.*, 1987). Such problems of misdiagnosis lead to delay in the diagnosis which can be up to 12 years from time of presentation to diagnosis, with a 3-year delay not being unusual (Fig. 40.5) (Barton and Ferguson, 1990).

DIAGNOSIS

An indication of an inflammatory process may be gained from blood tests, e.g. the sedimentation rate may be raised. An orosomucoid agglutination test will help to indicate whether the process is active (Macfarlane *et al.*, 1986b). However, these tests are non-specific.

A plain X-ray rarely shows obstruction (Fig. 40.6). Barium studies of the small bowel or colon, or both, will help to pinpoint the areas involved (Raine, 1984). Crohn's disease can affect the whole of the gastrointestinal tract from mouth to anus so that both studies may be necessary, although the most common site is the ileocaecal area. A small bowel enema taking the solution directly to the area in question will show on abnormal appearance of the mucosa (Fig. 40.7). Narrowing in the ileum, a classical Contor sign, leads to obstruction (Fig. 40.8), while associated stricture formation and/or fistulae suggest advanced disease with complications. As there is a field effect, the studies may show that more than one area is involved (Nolan, 1981).

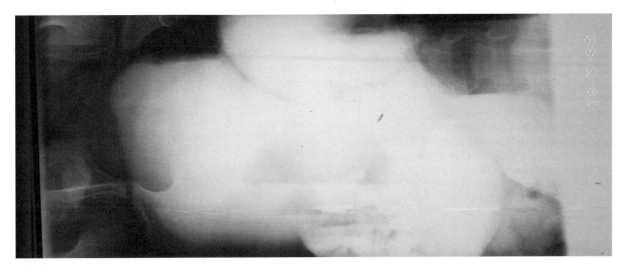

Fig. 40.6 Plain abdominal radiograph showing intestinal obstruction as an acute presentation of Crohn's disease.

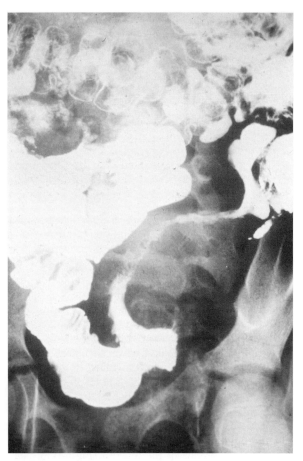

Fig. 40.8 Barium meal showing classical ileal stricture in Crohn's disease.

mucosa looks normal (Chong *et al.*, 1985). Experienced histopathologists should be available to report the specimens (Theodossi *et al.*, 1994). Tissue can also be obtained from skin lesions and perianal fistulae.

Without a tissue diagnosis the treatment can only be empirical, for instance assuming that ileal disease is likely to be Crohn's disease. Even with tissue for histology, the pathology may not be easily determined to make a definitive diagnosis. Often after diagnosis of non-specific colitis it may be some years before it becomes obvious as to which category of disease the child belongs. It is particularly important in such children to exclude infections such as *Yersinia* and *Campylobacter*. Delay in diagnosis may lead to the onset of obstructive symptoms or even external fistulae.

TREATMENT

Medical

Screening systems have been devised to determine the activity of the disease (Wright *et al.*, 1987) and hence the usefulness of medical treatment. Height and weight estimations are essential (Lloyd-Still and Green, 1979) and sexual development and bone age are significant. However, it is necessary to measure the modalities to be able to use them. Even in clinics accustomed to the care of patients with inflammatory bowel disease, such measurements are not always taken or are performed only once during the course of an individual's disease (Barton and Ferguson, 1989). This makes it difficult to

A sucrulphate scan is non-invasive means of determining ulceration (Dawson *et al.*, 1985). Since sucrulphate, which is used in the treatment of ulcers, binds to acutely ulcerated areas, the areas involved can be picked up on scanning (Fig. 40.9); however, it will not distinguish between two inflammatory diseases and is more useful in large bowel disease (George *et al.*, 1987). Using labelled white cells, a non-invasive test can determine the site and state of the disease and even though this is non-specific it can help with management (Fitzgerald *et al.*, 1992).

It is useful in Crohn's disease to perform upper endoscopy to determine the state of the upper tract, in view of the high incidence of upper gastrointestinal problems (Lenaerets *et al.*, 1989). Since colonic Crohn's disease is more common in children than would be expected (O'Donaoghue and Dawson, 1977; Grybowski and Spiro, 1978; Castile *et al.*, 1980), colonoscopy or flexible sigmoidoscopy should be performed. For a definitive diagnosis histological examination of tissue removed by endoscopy and biopsy is necessary. Multiple biopsies are necessary even if the

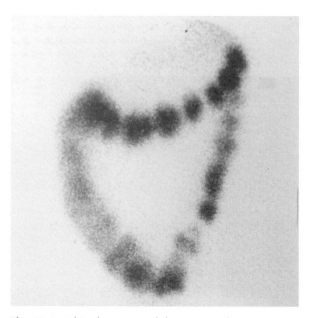

Fig. 40.9 This shows sucrulphate scans showing active colon disease in a child with Crohn's disease.

determine the course of the disease and the efficiency of the treatment. The disease can be low-grade chronic type or with an acute exacerbation.

There is a very wide range of treatments available (Table 40.2) suggesting the lack of knowledge about the cause of the disease and illustrating that there is no one ideal treatment. Failure to grow is common (Kirschsner, 1988b; Griffiths *et al.*, 1993) but may improve with correct treatment (Layden *et al.*, 1976). Effective control of the disease should mean a normal or near normal lifestyle, both educationally and socially, with normal growth and development. Complications occur if the disease is poorly controlled, e.g. abscesses, fistulae between loops of the bowel, to the skin or to the bladder, and strictures leading to obstruction. Although fistulae may heal with intravenous feeding, most of these complications require surgery.

Steroids form the mainstay of treatment, systemically and locally in anal disease. The acute problems will require intravenous feeding (Strobel *et al.*, 1979; Matuchansky, 1986; Carlson *et al.*, 1994) to rest the bowel and improve nutrition, especially prior to surgery (Payne-James and Silk, 1988). Elemental diets (e.g. Vivonex, Norwich-Eaton, Surrey, UK), given orally or by nasogastric tube, help both in the acute phase and in the more quiescent disease (Morin *et al.*, 1980; O'Morain *et al.*, 1983; Sanderson *et al.*, 1987; Gaffier *et al.*, 1990). However, this improves the nutritional state of the patient rather than the disease (Payne James and Silk, 1988) by means of improving insulin-like growth factors (Thomas *et al.*, 1993). It has been suggested that steroids can be avoided by the use of such diets (Teahon *et al.*, 1990; Raouf *et al.*, 1991; Gorad *et al.*, 1993), although relapse does occur. Remission (Lennard-Jones, 1990; Royall *et al.*, 1994) can also be achieved by dietary manipulations to reduce intestinal inflammation (Mansfield *et al.*, 1995). The treatment of chronic disease is similar, with advice regarding diet sometimes leading to improvement, but elimination diets should not be used alone (Levi, 1985; Greenberg

Table 40.2 Range of medical treatment for Crohn's disease (from Ferguson *et al.*, 1986)

Treatment	*n*	Percentage
Systemic steroids	48	71
Local steroids	15	22
Sulphasalazine	49	72
Enteral nutrition	11	16
Parental nutrition	4	6
Azathioprine	10	15
Iron	28	41
Folic acid	17	25
Hydroxycobalamin	6	9
Metronidazole	7	10

et al., 1988) since food intolerances are very variable (Pearson *et al.*, 1993). Metronidazole can help in anal disease where surgery is best avoided (Palder *et al.*, 1991; Sutherland *et al.*, 1991).

Cyclosporins (Peltekian *et al.*, 1987) and immunosuppressive drugs (Kozarek *et al.*, 1989; Baron *et al.*, 1991) have been used in both Crohn's disease (Brynskov *et al.*, 1989) and ulcerative colitis (Lichtiger and Present, 1990) but have serious side-effects (Singleton *et al.*, 1979). Salazapirine, or one of the five new amino salicylic acid derivatives, should be used in colonic Crohn's disease (Ferguson, 1992). All of these drugs attempt to modify and reduce the disease process but are not curative.

Failure to grow in these children can be due to the actual disease, malabsorption because of involvement of the small bowel, anorexia, or more specifically to the use of steroids for treatment of the disease. The nutritional state for children with Crohn's disease is almost always poor, leading to growth failure (Homer *et al.*, 1977; Booth and Harries, 1984): 75% of them will lose protein from the intestine, leading to negative nitrogen balance (Thomas *et al.*, 1992). Mucosal damage results in poor mannitol absorption and increased absorption of lactose. Steatorrhoea is common. Children's basal metabolic rate is greater than adults so that the metabolic effects of deficiencies are greater. Endocrine problems, e.g. pancreatic dysfunction (Hegnhoi *et al.*, 1990), may represent a general effect of malnutrition or the severity of the disease. Metabolic changes may have an effect on skeletal maturation (Evans and Walker-Smith, 1990). Metabolic alkalosis and electrolyte loss increase the problems of nutrition. Anaemia is common, with poor absorption of iron, vitamin B_{12} and folic acid. The deficiency of other vitamins, e.g. A and C (Doig, 1989), maintains the disease process since these are necessary for healing (Pettit *et al.*, 1988). Low amounts of other enzymes, e.g. selenium and zinc, which are also necessary for healing, account for continuing ulceration (Sandiford and Alexander, 1981; Main *et al.*, 1982).

Certain treatments may improve some biochemical abnormalities but not others. Thus steroid treatment will improve deficient enzymes and trace element absorption but not the haematological entities. In contrast, elemental diet improves factors relating to anaemia but not the trace elements (Doig, 1989). Education of the patient and family about good nutrition and dietary advice regarding supplements and specific diets is important. Prognosis is similar to that of adults (Gazzard, 1984) but although growth should occur if the child is adequately treated, this is not always the case. Treatment may also delay growth and sexual development (Kirschsner *et al.*, 1978). Therefore surgical treatment may be required despite the absence of complications in order that the child is able to grow and develop normally.

Surgical

The reasons for surgery in juvenile Crohn's disease are dominated by failure to grow and develop sexually – 70% in my own series (Table 40.3) in contrast to previous series where complications were the most common reason for surgery (Raine, 1984).

This unwillingness to operate for non-surgical reasons has meant in the past that surgery was delayed until complications presented. Surgery in the presence of very active disease and fistulae not surprisingly led to poor results, with postoperative complications and the need for still more surgery (Block *et al.*, 1977; Fonkalsrud *et al.*, 1979; Puntis *et al.*, 1984). The possibility of high recurrence rates also placed surgery low on the treatment list (Grybowski and Spiro, 1978). By the time fistulae have developed severe problems will be encountered at and after surgery. If fistulae, either entercutaneous or entervesical, do not close with adequate conservative treatment, i.e. total parentral nutrition, surgical treatment is indicated (Irving, 1983; Francois *et al.*, 1990). In most cases conservative treatment is successful. Narrowing of the small bowel seen radiologically in association with poor weight gain may be a reason for surgery, although only one child in my own series presented with an acute obstruction. Surgical treatment in the management of juvenile Crohn's disease is indicated earlier than in adult practice, mainly to achieve normal growth before puberty.

Although some children had been so acutely ill that surgery was necessary early in their disease, timing of surgery is usually about 3 years after diagnosis. Nutrition must be improved before surgery, if possible, by intravenous feeding or elemental diet for a week prior to operation (Blair *et al.*, 1986).

The operation performed depends on the site of the most severe disease. It is unnecessary to remove completely all the affected bowel. Anastomosis can be performed within microscopically diseased bowel without complications (Heuman *et al.*, 1983; Lee, 1984; Kumar and Alexander-Williams, 1993). Stricturoplasty can be used for short obstructing sections (Alexander-Williams *et al.*, 1986; Dehn *et al.*, 1989; Sayfan *et al.*, 1989). Stricturoplasty can produce reasonable results

on its own (Tjandra and Fazio, 1994) and can be used to avoid massive small bowel resection. The site of the disease does not appear to have much influence on the outcome (Davies *et al.*, 1990).

The most common operation performed for Crohn's disease is modified right hemicolectomy with an area of terminal ileum (Doig, 1989). Some children with only small bowel disease require more than one small bowel resection and others require only colonic resection for large bowel disease. Permanent stomata should preferably not be left in such children, these operations being performed only in the presence of abscesses and infection when an anastomosis would be hazardous.

Although perineal and anal disease can be devastating, faecal diversion (Orkin and Telander, 1985; Winslet *et al.*, 1994) has been enough to allow healing, but its efficacy for colonic disease is less predictable (Zelas and Jagelman, 1980; Harper *et al.*, 1985; Fasoli *et al.*, 1990). Resection of severe proximal colonic disease also can lead to improvement in the anal lesions.

Postoperative complications include wound infection and abscesses but these have not been associated with breakdown of anastomosis in my own series, nor did any of these children have postoperative fistulae. Children and parents are very carefully counselled and as much information as possible is given preoperatively to prepare for a stoma or other problems. Children should be allowed to meet others with the same problem. Postoperative psychological problems should therefore be rarely encountered.

Almost all children grow after surgery, justifying its use in such children (Fig. 40.10) (O'Donaghue and Dawson, 1977; Castile *et al.*, 1980; Coran *et al.*, 1983a; Booth and Harries, 1984; Postuma and Moroz, 1985; Hyams *et al.*, 1989; Hegnoi *et al.*, 1990; Evans and Walker-Smith, 1990; McLain *et al.*, 1990; Davies *et al.*, 1990; Thomas *et al.*, 1992). Although 40% of children may have recurrent disease, few will require further surgery and they will have normal development and become fully grown adults. Drug treatment may still be required, in particular steroids. Surgery must not be delayed so that catch-up growth is not possible (Homer *et al.*, 1977; Alpertstein *et al.*, 1985; Shivananda *et al.*, 1989; Kumar and Alexander-Williams, 1993). Earlier surgery for Crohn's disease is now also being advocated in adults (Andrews *et al.*, 1989).

Table 40.3 Reasons for surgery in Crohn's disease (own series)

Reason	*n*
Failed medical treatment	17
Failure to grow	8
Fistulae	5
Stricture formation	5
Acute abdomen	5
Bleeding	1

Ulcerative colitis

AETIOLOGY

Although Crohn's disease and ulcerative colitis are clinically separate diseases, there is some overlap since age, gender distribution, genetics and immunology are similar. What appears to be ulcerative colitis can subsequently turn out to be Crohn's disease.

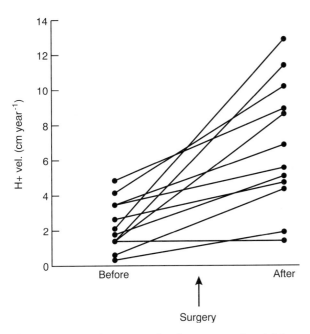

Fig. 40.10 Catch-up growth after surgery in children with Crohn's disease (Manchester).

Cigarette smoking, or rather cessation of smoking (Harries *et al.*, 1982; Gryde and Allan, 1983; Logan *et al.*, 1984; Burns, 1986; Persson *et al.*, 1990) may lead to a possible risk of colitis in adults and such an environment may have an influence on children. Diet has also been implicated in the development of ulcerative colitis (Thornton *et al.*, 1980) involving carbohydrates (Panza *et al.*, 1987) or processed fats (Guthy, 1983). Even oral contraceptives have been implicated (Lesko *et al.*, 1985). It would appear, as in Crohn's disease, that there are many reasons for the development of colitis.

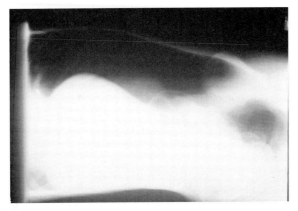

Fig. 40.11 Plain abdominal radiograph showing colon perforation after colonoscopy.

PATHOLOGY

This disease only affects the colon and rectum and in two-thirds of patients is confined to the distal colon and rectum (Allan and Hodgson, 1992).

Histologically, crypt abscesses and mucosal ulcers are found, with the formation of pseudopolyps. In about one-quarter of children proctitis alone is present, while in half the whole colon and rectum are involved (Ferguson, 1992). Damage is permanent even when the colitis is adequately treated and metaplasia leading to cancer is a real risk after 10 years of disease (Gyde *et al.*, 1980; Langholz *et al.*, 1992).

CLINICAL FEATURES

Unhealing chronic perianal abscesses and fistulae indicate anal disease (Palder *et al.*, 1991), and it is important that these changes should not be attributed to sexual abuse.

Ulcerative colitis presents, as in adult practice, with diarrhoea, often with abdominal pain, general malaise and weight loss. Proctitis alone is less common (25%) than in adults (Singleton *et al.*, 1979; Allan and Hodgson, 1992), more commonly the whole bowel being abnormal.

Extra-intestinal manifestations are rare but arthropathy, liver disease (Sachar, 1991) and skin rashes, e.g. *Pyoderma gangrenosum* (Levitt *et al.*, 1991) occur. Mouth ulcers are much less common. Complications of the disease process are rare, although bleeding may be the initial sign. Toxic megacolon with a grossly distended abdomen in a very ill patient usually arises during treatment. Perforation with associated peritonitis is a result of an acute exacerbation.

DIAGNOSIS

Diagnosis is usually made much more quickly than in Crohn's disease. Differential diagnosis includes food sensitivity and infection causes, as well as anal fissures, constipation and polyps.

Blood investigations may show an iron deficiency anaemia and hypoprotein anaemia. Erythocyte sedimentation rate may or may not be normal. High orosomucoid agglutination (MacFarlane *et al.*, 1986) or serum levels of c-reactive protein (Fagan *et al.*, 1982) are not specific to the disease. Sigmoidoscopy (and colonoscopy) with biopsy is the best means of diagnosis (Holmquist *et al.*, 1988), but there is a risk of perforation (Fig. 40.11). Again, the biopsy should be performed whether the bowel looks abnormal or not.

Ulcerative colitis only affects the large bowel so that a barium enema (Fig. 40.12) or double-contrast enema will show the lack of haustrations, and the rigidity of the bowel with crypt ulcers and mucosal abscesses. Toxic megacolon and perforation can be seen on a plain abdominal radiograph.

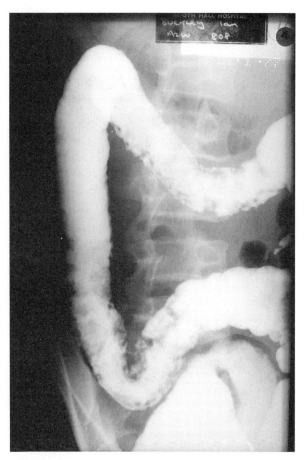

Fig. 40.12 Barium enema showing lack of haustrations indicating ulcerative colitis.

TREATMENT

Medical

The standby of the medical treatment of colitis is steroids, either systemically (during an acute exacerbation) or rectally (prednisolone) as a foam enema (Somerville *et al.*, 1985). Oral corticosteroids are used in active disease despite worries about side-effects. A low dosage on alternate days is a reasonable regime. In most children this keeps the disease under control and the child is able to carry on a normal life. However, as with Crohn's disease, steroid use in young children and adolescents causes problems, with failure to grow and develop.

Sulphasalazine (Booth, 1991) and salazopyrin (Jarnerot, 1987) can be used to induce a remission either orally or topically (Ginsberg *et al.*, 1988) and can also be used indefinitely or associated with low-dosage steroids (Bondesen, 1986). Recently, in view of a possible immune response leading to colitis, there has been an interest in cytokines. Azathoprine (of less value

in Crohn's disease) (Jewell and Truelove, 1974), 6-mercaptopurine, methotrexate (Kozarek *et al.*, 1989; Baron *et al.*, 1990) and cylosporine (Hyams and Treem, 1989) have all been suggested but have serious side-effects. Topical treatment has also been suggested with local anaesthetics (Bjorck *et al.*, 1991).

Again, such a variety of drugs (Hawkey and Hawthorne, 1988; Rachmilewitz, 1992) means that there is no single effective treatment. Effective control of the disease should result in a normal lifestyle, both educationally and socially, with normal growth and development but with an abnormal life expectancy (Probert *et al.*, 1993b). If medical treatment alone is used to control the disease the patient must be kept under long-term review by means of infrequent, but regular colonoscopy or sigmoidoscopy to check the occurrence of dysplasia (Korelitz *et al.*, 1990; Axon, 1994). A lasting remission can be achieved and most children do not need surgical treatment. Disease limited to the distal portion of the colon can progress to a more extensive disease with a poor prognosis (Mir-Midjilessi *et al.*, 1986).

Unlike Crohn's disease, surgery is performed usually because of the complications of the disease. Only after some 10 years of disease is it necessary to consider removing the colon because of the risk of cancer developing in dysplastic bowel.

SURGICAL

The reasons for surgery are inability to control the disease with drugs, to deal with complications such as toxic dilatation or postperforation, or because of complications of the treatment. A range of surgical treatment is available but only with complete removal of the colon and rectum can the child be deemed cured. Hemicolectomies or local resection are inadequate treatment for ulcerative colitis. Perforation, as a result of either colonoscopy or biopsy, abscess formation with dilatation, or ischaemic bowel, requires urgent resuscitation and ileostomy to bypass the area.

If the rectum is severely involved, panproctocolectomy is the treatment of choice. This necessitates a permanent ileostomy but does guarantee cure. Most children are so unwell, unable to attend school or lead normal lives that they accept such a permanent stoma, especially as it means no further drugs or hospital check-ups. Comparisons between children suffering from inflammatory bowel disease on medical treatment, and those who have had surgery with or without stomas show no difference in the lifestyle, body image and general well-being in the two groups who had undergone surgery. In comparison, those on medical treatment were the least happy about life in general and themselves (Lask *et al.*, 1987).

Ileoanal anastomosis have been performed to try to avoid a stoma, but these patients continue to have loose, frequent stools (Carty *et al.*, 1993) and are little better

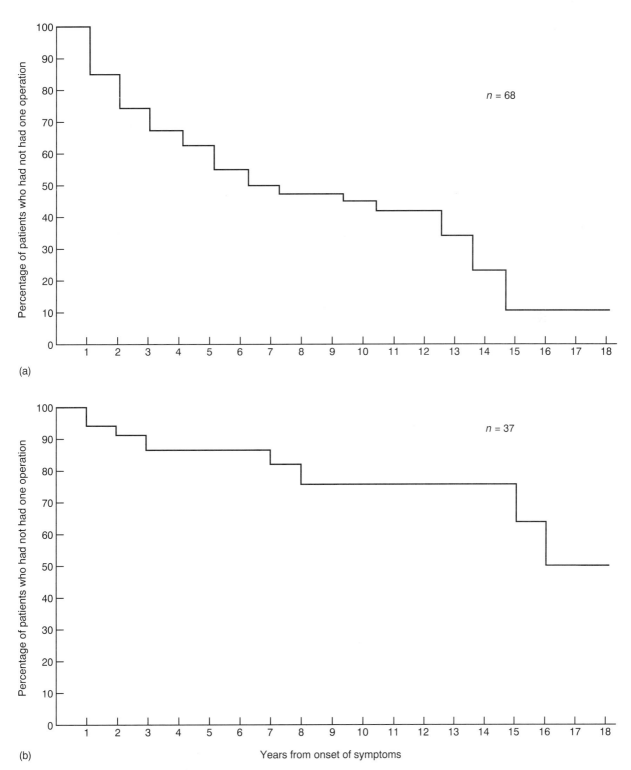

Fig. 40.13   Life charts indicating need for surgery in children with juvenile inflammatory bowel disease after 14-year period: (a) in Crohn's disease (b) in juvenile ulcerative colitis (from Sedgewick *et al.*, 1991).

than before surgery. Adaptation can occur but takes some time. Ileorectal anastomosis leaves the rectum, which then requires regular monitoring for disease and possible malignant change (Parc *et al.*, 1989). An endorectal operation (e.g. Soave operation) still has the problem that the small bowel is anastomosed to the anus (Zwiren *et al.*, 1981; Coran *et al.*, 1983b; Stryker *et al.*, 1985), but there is less pelvic dissection and therefore less chance of damage to the pelvic nerves or urinary tract.

A pouch can be created with the terminal ileum, thereby making a reservoir prior to anal anastomosis, in adults and children (Parks and Nicholls, 1978; Fonkalsrud, 1981; Canty *et al.*, 1983). In children the results have been poor, with frequent stools still a problem (Pezim and Nicholls, 1985). The pelvis is less capacious, making the operation technically more difficult, and complications are significant. Inflammation in the pouch (Nicholls *et al.*, 1989; Madden *et al.*, 1990; Keighley *et al.*, 1993) occurs in 40%, probably owing to instability of the bacterial flora in the pouch (Ruseler-van Embden *et al.*, 1994). Further surgery on the pouch may be required. In view of this pouches are best left until the child is older, e.g. late teens or early twenties. There is an uncertainty in the long-term about the occurrence of dysplasia and possible neoplasia in the pouches (Shepherd, 1990).

To allow for the possibility of a pouch being made later, a colectomy and ileostomy are routinely performed, leaving a rectal stump which can later be removed at the time of the formation of the pouch. This is only possible if the rectum is not severely involved. It may be necessary to convert to a permanent stoma and remove the rectum and anus if the disease process in the stump progresses, but this is a minor procedure. There is a risk that the defunctional stump may show changes histologically similar to Crohn's disease (Warren *et al.*, 1993).

Although complications are common in the early postoperative period, long-term problems are rare and most patients are off treatment (Michener *et al.*, 1979). There is a long definite but small increased risk of colonic carcinoma in those who have had long-term ulcerative colitis (Kvist *et al.*, 1989; Sachar, 1994). Whether the patient is medically or surgically treated, urinary calculi may occur in 4% (Bennett and Hughes, 1972).

General conclusions

It is important that the care and treatment of juvenile inflammatory bowel disease should be carried out by doctors who are interested and experienced in the problem. Combined medical and surgical involvement and clinics mean that timing of surgery, if necessary, is a mutual decision. Monitoring of the various modalities, e.g. blood tests, weight, height, sexual development and bone age, is used in the discussion to help in reaching the correct decision regarding the treatment of a particular child. The possible development of cancer when the child is older must always be kept in mind.

In the long term, within 14 years of the diagnosis of juvenile Crohn's disease, only 14% of patients will not have undergone surgery (Sedgewick *et al.*, 1991a) while, in contrast, over the same period only 25% of children with juvenile ulcerative colitis will have required surgery (Sedgewick *et al.*, 1991b) (Fig. 40.13a, b). It is important to remember that even with high recurrent rates (Coran *et al.*, 1983a), the improvement in lifestyle, and the ability to play and behave as a normal child with a sense of well-being mean that surgery should be contemplated early, so that these unfortunate children can become normal adults (Farthing, 1991). It is now also being realized in adult practice (Mitchell *et al.*, 1988) that lifestyle is important and that earlier surgery for Crohn's disease should be considered (Scott and Hughes, 1994). There may be considerable interruption of schooling and emotional difficulties, especially with interpersonal relationships (Bruce, 1986). Morbidity in young adults who have suffered juvenile onset inflammatory bowel disease leads to significant problems socially, environmentally, educationally and at work (Ferguson *et al.*, 1994). Thus correct, adequate and early treatment for these young people with either drugs or surgery is important for their long-term future.

References

Alexander-Williams, J., Allan, A., Morel, P., Hawker, P.C., Dykes, P.W. and O'Connor, H. 1986: The therapeutic dilatation of enteric strictures due to Crohn's disease. *Annals of the Royal College of Surgeons, England* **68**, 95–7.

Allan, R.N. and Hodgson, H.J.F. 1992: Inflammatory bowel disease. In Pounder, R.E. (ed.), *Recent bowel disease: frontiers in aetiology*, vol. 9. Edinburgh: Churchill Livingstone, 1–25.

Alperstein, G., Daum, F., Fisher, S.E. *et al.* 1985: Linear growth following surgery in children and adolescents with Crohn's disease: relationship with pubertal status. *Journal of Pediatric Surgery* **20**, 129–33.

Andrews, H.A., Lewis, P. and Allan, R.N. 1989: Prognosis after surgery for colonic Crohn's disease. *British Journal Surgery* **76**, 1184–90.

Andrews, Wh., Barczak, P. and Allan, R.N. 1987: Psychiatric illness in patients with inflammatory bowel disease. *Gut* **28**, 1600–4.

Axon, A.T.R. 1994: Cancer surveillance in ulcerative colitis – a time for reappraisal. *Gut* **35**, 587–9.

Baron, T.H., Truss, C.D. and Elson, C.O. 1991: Steroid sparing effect of oral methotrexate in refractory inflammatory bowel disease. *Gastroenterology* **100**, A195.

Barton, J.R. and Ferguson, A. 1989: Failure to record variables of growth and development in children with inflammatory bowel disease. *British Medical Journal* **298**, 865–6.

Barton, J.R. and Ferguson, A. 1990: Clinical features, morbidity and mortality of Scottish children with inflammatory bowel disease. *Quarterly Journal of Medicine* **75**, 423–9.

Barton, J.R., Gillon, S. and Ferguson, A. 1989: Incidence of inflammatory bowel disease in Scottish children between 1968 and 1983; marginal fall in ulcerative colitis, threefold rise in Crohn's disease. *Gut* **30**, 618–22.

Bennett, R.C. and Hughes, E.S.R. 1972: Urinary calculi and ulcerative colitis. *British Medical Journal* **i**, 494–6.

Bjorck, S., Dahlstrom, A. and Ahlman, H. 1991: Topical treatment with lignocaine in patients with ulcerative colitis. *Gastroenterology* **100**, A198–210.

Blair, G.K., Yaman, M. and Wesson, D.E. 1986: Preoperative home elemental enteral nutrition in complicated Crohn's disease. *Journal of Pediatric Surgery* **21**, 769–71.

Block, G.E., Moossa, A.R. and Simonowitz, D. 1977: The operative treatment of Crohn's disease in childhood. *Surgery, Gynaecology and Obstetrics* **144**, 713–7.

Bondesen, S. and a Danish 5-ASA Study Group 1986: Topical 5-amino-salicylic acid (5-ASA) versus prednisalone in ulcerative proctosigmoiditis (Abstract). *Scandinavian Journal of Gastroenterology* **120**, 21–6.

Booth, I. 1991: Chronic inflammatory bowel disease. *Archives of Diseases in Childhood* **66**, 742–44.

Booth, I.W. and Harries, J.T. 1984: Inflammatory bowel disease in childhood. *Gut* **25**, 188–202.

Bruce, T. 1986: Endorectal sequelae of chronic inflammatory bowel disease in children and adolescents. *Clinical Gastroenterology* **15**, 89–104.

Brynskov, S., Freund, L., Ramussen, S.N., Lauritsen, K. and de-Muckadell, O.S. 1989: A placebo controlled double blind randomized trial of cyclosporine therapy in active chronic Crohn's disease. *New England of Journal Medicine* **321**, 845–50.

Burbige, E.J., Huang, S.S. and Bayless, T.M. 1975: Clinical manifestations of Crohn's disease in children in adolescents. *Pediatrics* **55**, 866–71.

Burns, D.G. 1986: Smoking in inflammatory bowel disease and the irritable bowel syndrome. *South African Medical Journal* **69**, 232–3.

Butterworth, R.J., Williams, G.T. and Hughes, L.E. 1992: Can Crohn's disease be diagnosed at laparotomy? *Gut* **33**, 140–2.

Canty, T.G., Self, T. and Bonaldi, L. 1983: The lateral reservoir technique of ileal endorectal pull-through for ulcerative colitis and familial polyposis in children. *Journal of Pediatric Surgery* **18**, 862–71.

Carlson, G.L., Gray, P., Barber, D., Shaffer, J.L., Mughal, M. and Irving, M.H. 1994: Total parenteral nutrition modifies the acute phase response to Crohn's disease. *Journal of the Royal College of Surgeons, Edinburgh* **39**, 360–4.

Carty, N.J., Johnson, C.D. and Corder, A. 1993: Restorative procto-colectomy is a major advance in the management of ulcerative colitis. *Annals of the Royal College Surgeons, England* **75**, 275–80.

Castile, R.G., Telander, R.L., Cooney, D.R., Ilstrup, D.M. and Perrault, J. 1980: Crohn's disease in children: assessment of the regression of the disease, growth and prognosis. *Journal of Pediatric Surgery* **15**, 462–9.

Chiodini, R.J., Van Kruiningen, H.J. and Thayer, W.R. 1984: Possible role of mycobacteria in inflammatory bowel disease. *Digestive Diseases and Sciences* **29**, 1073–85.

Choi, P.M. and Zelig, M. 1994: Similarity of colorectal cancer in Crohn's disease and ulcerative colitis: implications for carcinogenesis and prevention. *Gut* **35**, 950–4.

Chong, S.K.F., Blackshaw, A.J., Boyle, S., Williams, C.B. and Walker-Smith, J.A. 1985: Histological diagnosis of chronic inflammatory bowel disease in childhood. *Gut* **26**, 55–9.

Chong, S.K.F. and Walker-Smith, J.A. 1986: Chronic inflammatory bowel disease in children from the Asian immigrant community in London. Ethnic, religious and occupational groups. *Frontiers in Gastroenterological Research* **11**, 129–34.

Collins, C.E. and Rampton, D.S. 1995: Platelet dysfunction: a new dimension in inflammatory bowel disease. *Gut* **36**, 5–8.

Connell, W.R., Sheffield, J.P., Kamm, M.A., Ritchie, J.K., Hawley, P.R. and Lennard-Jones, J.E. 1994: Lower gastrointestinal malignancy in Crohn's disease. *Gut* **35**, 347–52.

Coran, A.G., Klein, M.D. and Sarahan, T.M. 1983a: The surgical management of terminal ileal and right colon Crohn's disease in children. *Journal of Pediatric Surgery* **18**, 592–4.

Coran, A.G., Sarahan, T.M., Dent, T.L., Fiddian-Green, R., Wesley, J.R. and Jordan, F.T. 1983b: The endorectal pull-through for the management of ulcerative colitis in children and adults. *Annals of Surgery* **197**, 99–105.

Crohn, B.B., Ginzburg, L. and Oppenheimer, G.D. 1932: Regional ileitis: a pathological and clinical entity. *Journal of the American Medical Association* **99**, 1323–9.

Curran, F.T., Young, D.J., Allan, R.N. and Keighley, M.R. 1991: Candidacidal activity of Crohn's disease neutrophils. *Gut* **32**, 55–60.

Davies, G., Evans, C.M., Shand, W.S. and Walker-Smith, J.A. 1990: Surgery for Crohn's disease in childhood: influence of sites of disease and operative procedure on outcome. *British Journal of Surgery* **77**, 891–4.

Dawson, D.J., Khan, A.N., Miller, V., Radcliffe, J.F. and Shreeve, D.R. 1985: Dissection of inflammatory bowel disease in adults and children: evaluation of a new isotope technique. *British Medical Journal* **291**, 1227–30.

Dehn, T.C.B., Kettlewell, M.G.W., Mortensen, N.J.McC., Lee, E.C.G. and Jewell, D.P. 1989: Ten-year experience of stricturoplasty for obstructive Crohn's disease. *British Journal of Surgery* **76**, 339–41.

Doig, C.M. 1989: Surgery of inflammatory bowel disease in children, with reference to Crohn's disease. *Journal of the Royal College of Surgeons, Edinburgh* **34**, 189–96.

Elliot, E.J. 1987: Crohn's disease in childhood. *Gastroenterology in Practice* **3**, 52–8.

Evans, C.M. and Walker-Smith, J.A. 1990: Inflammatory bowel disease in childhood. In Allen, R.N. *et al.* (eds), *Inflammatory bowel disease*, 2nd ed. Edinburgh: Churchill Livingstone, 523–46.

Fagan, E.A., Duck, R.F., Maton, P.N. *et al.* 1982: Serum levels of c-reactive protein in Crohn's disease and ulcerative colitis. *European Journal of Clinical Investigation* **12**, 351.

Farmer, R.G. and Michener, W.M. 1986: Association of inflammatory bowel disease in families. *Frontiers in Gastroenterological Research* **11**, 17–26.

Farthing, M.J.G. 1991: Crohn's disease in childhood and adolescence. In Anagnostides, A.A., Hodgson, H.J.F. and Kirsner, J.B. (eds), *Inflammatory bowel disease*. London: Chapman & Hall Medical, 12–25.

Fasoli, R., Kettlewell, M.G.W., Mortensen, N. and Jewell, D.P. 1990: Response to faecal challenge in defunctioned colonic Crohn's disease: prediction of long-term course. *British Journal of Surgery* **77**, 616–7.

Ferguson, A. 1992: Inflammatory bowel disease in children and adolescents. *Hospital Update* **18**, 721–32.

Ferguson, A., Rifkind, E.A. and Doig, C.M. 1986: Prevalence of chronic inflammatory bowel disease in British children. *Frontiers in Gastroenterological Research* **11**, 68–72.

Ferguson, A., Sedgewick, D.M. and Drummond, J. 1994: Morbidity of juvenile onset inflammatory bowel disease: effects on education and employment in early adult life. *Gut* **35**, 665–8.

Ferguson, A., Troncone, R., Barton, J.R. and Entrican, J. 1987: Atophy, hypersensitivity and food intolerance in inflammatory bowel disease. *Inflammatory bowel disease; frontiers in aetiology*, Proceedings of the BSG International Workshop, 40–3.

Fitzgerald, P.G., Topp, T.J., Walton, J.M., Jackson, J.R. and Gillis, D.A. 1992: The use of indium 111 leukocyte scans in children with inflammatory bowel disease. *Journal of Pediatric Surgery* **27**, 1298–300.

Fonkalsrud, E.W. 1981: Endorectal ileal pull-through with lateral ileal reservoir for benign colorectal disease. *Annals of Surgery* **194**, 761–6.

Fonkalsrud, E.W., Ament, M.E., Fleisher, D. and Byrne, W. 1979: Surgical management of Crohn's disease in children. *American Journal of Surgery* **138**, 15–21.

Francois, Y., Descos, L. and Vignal, J. 1990: Conservative treatment of low recto-vaginal fistula in Crohn's disease. *International Journal of Colorectal Diseases* **5**, 12–4.

Gaffier, M.H., North, G. and Holdsworth, C.D. 1990: Controlled trial of polymeric versus elemental diet in the treatment of active Crohn's disease. *Lancet* **335**, 816–9.

Gazzard, B. 1984: Long term prognosis of Crohn's disease in childhood and adolescence. *Gut* **25**, 325–8.

George, A., Merrick, M.V. and Palmer, K.R. 1987: Tc-sulcralfate scintigraphy and colonic disease. *British Medical Journal* **295**, 578.

Gilat, T., Grossman, A., Fireman, Z. and Rosen, P. 1986: Inflammatory bowel disease in Jews. In McConnell, R., Rozen, P., Langman, M. and Gilat, T. (eds), *The genetics and epidemiology of inflammatory bowel disease*. Basel: Karger, 135–41.

Gillen, C.D., Andrews, H.A., Prior, P. and Allan, R.N. 1994: Crohn's disease and colorectal cancer. *Gut* **35**, 651–5.

Ginsberg, A.L., Beck, L.S., McIntosh, T.M. and Nochomovitz, L.E. 1988: Treatment of left-sided ulcerative colitis with 4-aminosalicylic acid enemas: a double blind placebo controlled trial. *Annals of International Medicine* **108**, 195–9.

Gorad, D.A., Hunt, J.B., Payne-James, J.J. *et al.* 1993: Initial response and subsequent course of Crohn's disease treated with elemental diet or prednisolone. *Gut* **34**, 1198–202.

Graham, D.Y., Markesich, D.C. and Yoshimura, H. 1987: Mycobacteria and inflammatory bowel disease. Results of culture. *Gastroenterology* **92**, 426–42.

Greenberg, G.R., Fleming, C.R., Jeejeebhoy, K.N., Rosenberg, I.J., Sales, D. and Tremaine, W.J. 1988: Controlled trial bowel rest and nutritional support in the management of Crohn's disease. *Gut* **29**, 1309–15.

Griffiths, A.M., Nguyen, P., Smith, C., MacMillan, J.H. and Sherman, P.M. 1993: Growth and clinical course of children with Crohn's disease. *Gut* **34**, 939–43.

Grybowski, J.D. and Spiro, H.M. 1978: Prognosis in children with Crohn's disease. *Gastroenterology* **74**, 807–17.

Guthy, E. 1983: Atiologie des Morbus Crohn: was spricht fur Fette als mogliche Urasche? *Deutsche Medizinische Wochenshrift* **108**, 1729–33.

Gyde, S.N. and Allan, R.N. 1983: Cigarette smoking and ulcerative colitis. *New England Journal of Medicine* **308**, 1476.

Gyde, S.N., Prior, P., McCartney, J.C., Thompson, H., Waterhouse, J..H. and Allan, R.N. 1980: Malignancy in Crohn's disease. *Gut* **21**, 1024–9.

Harper, P.H., Lee, E.C.G., Kettlewell, M.G.W. and Jewell, D.P. 1985: Role of the faecal stream in the maintenance of Crohn's colitis. *Gut* **26**, 279–84.

Harries, A.D., Baird, A. and Rhodes, J. 1982: Non-smoking: a feature of ulcerative colitis. *British Medical Journal* **284**, 706.

Hawkey, C.J. and Hawthorne, A.B. 1988: Medical treatment of ulcerative colitis: scoring the advances. *Gut* **29**, 1298–303.

Hegnhoi, J., Hansen, C.P., Rannem, T., Sobark, H., Anderson, L.B. and Anderson, J.R. 1990: Pancreatic function in Crohn's disease. *Gut* **31**, 1076–9.

Heuman, R., Boeryd, B., Bolin, T. and Sjodahl, R. 1983: The influcnce of disease at the margins of resection on the outcome of Crohn's disease. *British Journal of Surgery* **70**, 519–21.

Holmquist, L., Rudic, N., Ahren, C. and Fallstrom, S.P. 1988: The diagnostic value of colonoscopy compared with rectosigmoidoscopy in children and adolescents with symptoms of chronic inflammatory bowel disease of the colon. *Scandinavian Journal of Gastroenterology* **23**, 577–84.

Homer, D.R., Grand, R.J. and Colodny, A.H. 1977: Growth, course and prognosis after surgery for Crohn's disease in children and adolescents. *Pediatrics* **59**, 717–25.

Hyams, J.S., Grand, R.J., Colodny, A.H., Schuster, S.R. and Erkalis, A. 1989: Course prognosis after colectomy and ileostomy for inflammatory bowel disease in childhood and adolescence. *Journal of Pediatric Surgery* **17**, 400–5.

Hyams, J.S. and Treem, W.R. 1989: Cyclosporin treatment of fulminating colitis. *Journal of Pediatric Gastroenterology* **9**, 383–7.

Ibbotson, J.P. and Lowes, J.R. 1995: Potential role of superantigen induced activation of cell mediated immune mechanisms in the pathogenesis of Crohn's disease. *Gut* **36**, 1–4.

Irving, M. 1983: Assessment and management of external fistulas in Crohn's disease. *British Journal of Surgery* **70**, 233–6.

Jarnerot, G. 1987: New 5-aminosalicyclic acid based drugs: an evaluation of properties and possible role in the treatment of inflammatory bowel disease. In Jarnerot, G. (ed.), *Inflammatory bowel disease*. New York: Raven Press, 153–4.

Jenkins, A.P., Treasure, J. and Thompson, R.P.H. 1988: Crohn's disease presenting as anorexia nervosa. *British Medical Journal* **296**, 699–700.

Jewell, D.P. and Truelove, S.C. 1974: Azathioprine in ulcerative colitis: final report on controlled therapeutic trial. *British Medical Journal* **iv**, 627–30.

Keighley, M.R.N., Grobler, S. and Bain, I. 1993: An audit of restorative proctocolectomy. *Gut* **34**, 680–4.

Kirschsner, B.S. 1988a: Inflammatory bowel disease. *Pediatric Clinics of North America* **35**, 189–208

Kirschsner, B.S. 1988b: Nutritional consequences of inflammatory bowel disease on growth. *Journal of the American College of Nutrition* **7**, 301–8.

Kirschsner, B.S., Voinchet, O. and Rosenberg, I.H. 1978: Growth retardation in inflammatory bowel disease. *Gastroenterology* **75**, 504–11.

Koletzko, S., Sherman, P., Corey, M., Griffiths, A. and Smith, C. 1989: Role of infant feeding practices in development of Crohn's disease in childhood. *British Medical Journal* **298**, 1617–8.

Korelitz, B.I., Lauwers, G.Y. and Sommers, S.C. 1990: Rectal mucosal dysplasia in Crohn's disease. *Gut* **31**, 1382–6.

Kozarek, R.A., Patterson, D.J., Gelfand, M.D., Botoman, V.A., Ball, T.J. and Wilske, K.R. 1989: Methotrexate induces clinical and histologic remission in patients with refractory inflammatory bowel disease. *Annals of Internal Medicine* **110**, 353–6.

Kumar, D. and Alexander-Williams, J. 1993: *Crohn's disease and ulcerative colitis; surgical management* London: Springer, **15**, 38–40.

Kvist, N., Jacobsen, O., Kvist, H.K. *et al.* 1989: Malignancy in ulcerative colitis. *Scandinavian Journal of Gastroenterology* **24**, 497–506.

Langholz, E., Munkholm, P., Davidsen, M. and Binder, V. 1992: Colorectal cancer risk and mortality in patients with ulcerative colitis. *Gastroenterology* **103**, 1444–51.

Lashner, B.A., Evans, A.P., Kirsner, J.B. and Hanauer, S.B. 1986: Prevalence and incidence of inflammatory bowel disease in family members. *Gastroenterology* **91**, 1396–400.

Lask, B., Jenkins, J., Nabarro, L. and Booth, I. 1987: Psychosocial sequelae of stoma surgery for inflammatory bowel disease in childhood. *Gut* **28**, 1257–60.

Layden, T., Rosenberg, J., Nemchausky, B., Elson, C. and Rosenberg, I. 1976: Reversal of growth arrest in adolescents with Crohn's disease after parenteral alimentation. *Gastroenterology* **70**, 1017–21.

Lee, E.C.G. 1984: Aim of surgical treatment of Crohn's disease. *Gut* **25**, 217–22.

Lee, F.I. and Costello, F.T. 1985: Crohn's disease in Blackpool – incidence and prevalence 1968–80. *Gut* **26**, 274–8.

Lenaerets, C., Roy, C.C., Valliancourt, M., Weber, A.M., Morin, C.L. and Seidman, E. 1989: High incidence of upper gastrointestinal tract involvement in children with Crohn's disease. *Pediatrics* **83**, 777–81.

Lennard-Jones, J.E. 1990: Nutrition in Crohn's disease. *Annals of the Royal College Surgeons, England* **72**, 152–4.

Lesko, S.M., Kaufman, D.W., Rosenberg, L. *et al.* 1985: Evidence for an increased risk of Crohn's disease in oral contraceptive users. *Gastroenterology* **89**, 1046–9.

Levi, A.J. 1985: Diet in the management of Crohn's disease. *Gut* **26**, 985–8.

Levitt, M.D., Ritchie, J.K., Lennard-Jones, J.E. and Phillips, R.K. 1991: Pyoderma gangrenosum in inflammatory bowel disease. *British Journal of Surgery* **78**, 676–8.

Lichtiger, S. and Present, D.H. 1990: Preliminary report: cyclosporin in the treatment of severe ulcerative colitis. *Lancet* **336**, 16–9.

Lloyd-Still, J.D. and Green, O.C. 1979: A clinical scoring system for chronic inflammatory bowel disease in children. *Digestive Diseases and Sciences* **24**, 620–4.

Logan, R.F.A., Edmond, M., Somerville, K.W. and Langman, M.J.S. 1984: Smoking and ulcerative colitis. *British Medical Journal* **288**, 751–3.

McConnell, R.B. and Vadheim, C.M. 1992: Inflammatory bowel disease. In King, R.A., Rotter, J.I. and Motulsky, A.O. (eds), *The generic basis of common disease*. Oxford: Oxford University Press, 326–48.

MacFarlane, P.I., Miller, V. and Ratcliffe, J.F. 1986a: Clinical and radiological diagnosis of Crohn's disease in children. *Journal of Pediatric Gastroenterology and Nutrition* **5**, 87–92.

MacFarlane, P.I., Miller, V., Wells, F. and Richards, B. 1986b: Laboratory assessment of disease activity in childhood Crohn's disease and ulcerative colitis. *Journal of Pediatric Gastroenterology and Nutrition* **5**, 93–6.

McLain, B.I., Davidson, P.N., Stokes, K.B. and Beasley, S.W. 1990: Growth after bowel resection for Crohn's disease. *Archives of Diseases in Childhood* **65**, 760–2.

Madara, J.L. and Stafford, J. 1989: Interferon-γ directly affects barrier function of cultured intestinal epithelial monolayers. *Journal of Clinical Investigation* **83**, 724–7.

Madden, M.V., Farthing, M.J.G. and Nicholls, R.J. 1990: Inflammation in ileal reservoirs: 'pouchitis'. *Gut* **31**, 247–9.

Main, A.N.H., Hall, M.J., Russell, R.I., Fell, G.S., Mills, P.R. and Shenkin, A. 1982: Clinical experience of zinc supplementation during intravenous nutrition in Crohn's disease: value of serum and using zinc measurements. *Gut* **23**, 984–91.

Mansfield, J.C., Giaffer, M.H. and Holdsworth, C.D. 1995: Controlled trial of oligopeptide versus amino acid diet in treatment of active Crohn's disease. *Gut* **36**, 60–6.

Matuchansky, C. 1986: Parentral nutrition in inflammatory bowel disease. *Gut* **27** (Suppl), 81–4.

Mayberry, J.F. 1985: Progress report. Some aspects of the epidemiology of ulcerative colitis. *Gut* **26**, 968–74.

Mayberry, J.F. 1989: Recent epidemiology of ulcerative colitis and Crohn's disease. *International Journal of Colorectal Diseases* **4**, 59–66.

Mayberry, J., Rhodes, J. and Hughes, L.E. 1979: Incidence of Crohn's disease in Cardiff between 1934 and 1977. *Gut* **20**, 602–8.

Mayberry, J.F., Rhodes, J. and Newcombe, R.G. 1980: Increased sugar consumption in Crohn's disease. *Digestion* **20**, 323–6.

Michener, W.M., Farmer, R.G. and Mortimer, E.A. 1979: Long term prognosis of ulcerative colitis with onset in childhood or adolescence. *Journal of Clinical Gastroenterology* **1**, 301–5.

Mir-Midjilessi, D.H., Michener, W.M. and Farmer, R.G. 1986: Course and prognosis of idiopathic ulcerative proctosigmoiditis in young patients. *Journal of Pediatric Gastroenterology and Nutrition* **5**, 570–5.

Mitchell, A., Guyatt, G., Singer, J. *et al.* 1988: Quality of life in patients with inflammatory bowel disease. *Journal of Clinical Gastroenterology* **10**, 306–10.

Monsen, U., Brostrom, O., Nordenvall, B., Sorstad, J. and Hellers, G. 1987: Prevalence of inflammatory bowel disease among relatives of patients with ulerative colitis. *Scandinavian Journal of Gastroenterology* **22**, 214–8.

Morin, C.L., Roulet, M., Roy, C.C. and Weber, A. 1980: Continuous elemental enteral alimentation in children with Crohn's disease and growth failure. *American Gastroenterological Association* **79**, 1205–10.

Nicholls, R.J., Holt, S.D.H. and Lubowski, D.Z. 1989: Restorative proctocolectomy with ileal reservoir. Comparison of two stages vs three stage procedures and analysis of factors that might affect outcome. *Diseases of the Colon and Rectum* **32**, 323–6.

Nolan, D.J. 1981: Radiology of Crohn's disease of the small intestine: a review. *Journal of the Royal Society of Medicine* **74**, 294–300.

O'Donaghue, D.P. and Dawson, A.M. 1977: Crohn's disease in childhood. *Archives of Disease in Childhood* **52**, 627–32.

O'Morain, C., Segal, A.M., Levi, A.J. and Valman, H.B. 1983: Elemental diet in acute Crohn's disease. *Archives of Diseases in Childhood* **53**, 44–7.

Orkin, B.A. and Telander, R.L. 1985: The effect of intra-abdominal resection or fecal diversion on perianal disease in pediatric Crohn's disease. *Journal of Pediatric Surgery* **20**, 343–7.

Palder, S.V., Shandling, B., Bilik, R., Griffiths, A.M. and Sherman, P. 1991: Perianal complications of pediatric Crohn's disease. *Journal of Pediatric Surgery* **26**, 513–5.

Panza, E., Francheschi, S., La Vecchia, C. *et al.*, 1987: Dietary factors in the aetiology of inflammatory bowel disease. *Italian Journal of Gastroenterology* **18**, 205–9.

Parc, P., Legrand, M., Frileux, P., Tiret, E. and Ratelle, R. 1989: Comparative clinical results of ileal pouch anal anastomosis and ileorectal anastomosis in ulcerative colitis. *Hepatogastroenterology* **36**, 235–9.

Parks, A.G. and Nicholls, R.J. 1978: Proctocolectomoy without ileostomy for ulcerative colitis. *British Medical Journal* **2**, 85–8.

Payne-James, J.J. and Silk, D.B.A. 1988: Total parentral nutrition as primary treatment in Crohn's disease. *Gut* **29**, 1304–8.

Pearson, M., Teahon, K., Levi, A.J. and Bjornason, I. 1993: Food intolerance and Crohn's disease. *Gut* **34**, 783–7.

Peltekian, K.M., Williams, C.N., MacDonald, A.S., Roy, P. and Czolponska, E. 1987: Open study of cyclosporin in Crohn's disease. *Gastroenterology* **92**, A1571.

Persson, P.-G., Ahlbom, A. and Hellers, G. 1990: Inflammatory bowel disease and tobacco smoke – a case–control study. *Gut* **31**, 1377–81.

Pettit, S., Shaffer, J., Johns, W., Bennet, R. and Irving, M. 1988: Does local intestinal ascorbate deficiency predispose to fisula formation in Crohn's disease? *Journal of the Royal College of Surgeons, Edinburgh* **33**, 41–2.

Pezim, M.E. and Nicholls, R.J. 1985: Quality of life after restorative proctocolectomy with pelvic ileal reservoir. *British Journal of Surgery* **72**, 31–3.

Postuma, R. and Moroz, S.P. 1985: Pediatric Crohn's disease. *Journal of Pediatric Surgery* **20**, 478–82.

Probert, C.S.J., Jayanthi, V., Hughes, A.O., Thompson, J.R., Wicks, A.C.B. and Mayberry, J.F. 1993a: Prevalence and family risk of ulcerative colitis and Crohn's disease: an epidemiological study among Europeans and South Asians in Leicestershire. *Gut* **34**, 1547–51.

Probert, C.J.S., Jayanthi, V. and Mayberry, J.F. 1993b: British gastroenterologists' care profile for patients with inflammatory bowel disease: the need for a patient's charter. *Journal of the Royal Society of Medicine* **86**, 271–2.

Puntis, J., McNeish, A.S. and Allan, R.N. 1984: Longterm prognosis of Crohn's disease with onset in adolescence and childhood. *Gut* **25**, 329–336.

Puntis, J.W.L., Tarlow, M.J., Raafat, F. and Booth, I.W. 1990: Crohn's disease of the lung. *Archives of Disease in Childhood* **65**, 1270–7.

Rachmilewitz, D. 1992: New forms of treatment for inflammatory bowel disease. *Gut* **33**, 1301–2.

Raine, P.A.M. 1984: BAPS collective review – chronic inflammatory bowel disease. *Journal of Pediatric Surgery* **19**, 18–22.

Raouf, A.H., Hildrey, V., Daniel, J. *et al.* 1991: Enteral feeding as sole treatment for Crohn's disease: controlled trial of whole protein *v* amino acid based feed and a case study of dietary challenge. *Gut* **32**, 702–7.

Royall, D., Jeejeebhoy, K.N., Baker, J.P. *et al.* 1994: Comparisons of amino acid *v* peptide based enteral diets in active Crohn's disease: clinical and nutritional outcome. *Gut* **35**, 783–7.

Ruseler-van Embden, J.G.H., Schouten, W.R. and van Lieshout, L.M.C. 1994: Pouchitis: result of microbial imbalance? *Gut* **35**, 658–64.

Sachar, D.B. 1991: Ulcerative colitis and sclerosing cholangitis. *Gastroenterology* **100**, 1469–70.

Sachar, D.B. 1994: Cancer in inflammatory bowel disease. *Current opinions in Gastroenterology* **6**, 543–6.

Sanderson, I.R., Chong, S.K.F. and Walker-Smith, J.A. 1986: Familial incidence of chronic inflammatory bowel disease. *Frontiers in Gastroenterological Research* **11**, 12–6.

Sanderson, I.R., Udeen, S., Davies, P.S.W., Savage, M.O. and Walker-Smith, J.A. 1987: Remission induced by an elemental diet in small bowel Crohn's disease. *Archives of Diseases in Childhood* **62**, 123–7.

Sanderson, J.D. and Hermon-Taylor, J. 1992: Mycobacterial diseases of the gut: some impact from molecular biology. *Gut* **33**, 145–7.

Sandiford, J.A. and Alexander, R. 1981: Zinc deficiency in Crohn's disease. *Journal of the Royal College of Surgeons, Edinburgh* **26**, 357–9.

Satsangi, J., Jewell, D.P., Rosenberg, W.M.C. and Bell, J.I. 1994: Genetics of inflammatory bowel disease. *Gut* **35**, 696–700.

Sayfan, J., Wilson, D.A.L., Allan, A., Andrews, H. and Alexander-Williams, J. 1989: Recurrence after stricturoplasty or resection for Crohn's disease. *British Journal of Surgery* **76**, 335–8.

Scott, N.A. and Hughes, L.E. 1994: Timing of ileocolonic resection for symptomatic Crohn's disease – the patient's view. *Gut* **35**, 656–7.

Scully, C., Cochran, K.M., Russell, R.I. and Ferguson, M.M. 1982: Crohn's diseases of the mouth: an indicator of intestinal involvement. *Gut* **23**, 198–201.

Sedgewick, D.M., Barton, J.R., Hamer-Hodges, D.W., Nixon, S.J. and Ferguson, A. 1991a: Population based study of surgery in juvenile onset Crohn's disease. *British Journal of Surgery* **78**, 171–5.

Sedgewick, D.M., Barton, J.R., Hamer-Hodges, D.W., Nixon, S.J. and Ferguson, A. 1991b: Population based study of surgery in juvenile onset ulcerative colitis. *British Journal of Surgery* **78**, 176–8.

Sheehan, A.L., Warren, B.F., Gear, M.W.F. and Shepherd, N.A. 1992: Fat wrapping in Crohn's disease: pathological basis and relevance to surgical practice. *British Journal of Surgery* **79**, 955–8.

Shepherd, N.A. 1990: The pelvic reservoir: apocalypse later? *British Medical Journal* **301**, 886–7.

Shivananda, S., Hordijk, M.L., Pena, A.S. and Mayberry, J.F. 1989: Crohn's disease: risk of recurrence and re-operation in a defined population. *Gut* **30**, 990–5.

Singleton, J.W., Law, D.H., Kelley, J.R.M.L., Mekhijan, H.S. and Stardevant, R.A.L. 1979: NCCDS: adverse reaction to study drugs. *Gastroenterology* **77**, 870–83.

Smith, I.S., Young, S., Gillespie, G., O'Connor, J.O. and Bell, J.R. 1975: Epidemiological aspects of Crohn's disease in Clydesdale 1961–70. *Gut* **16**, 62–7.

Somerville, K.W., Langman, M.J.S., Kane, S.P., MacGilchrist. A.J., Watkinson, G. and Salmon, P. 1985: Effect of treatment of symptoms and quality of life in patients with ulcerative colitis: a comparative trial of hydrocortisone acetate foam and prednisalone 21-phosphate enema. *British Medical Journal* **291**, 866–7.

Strobel, C.T., Byrne, W.J. and Ament, M.E. 1979: Home parentral nutrition in children with Crohn's disease. An effective management alternative. *Gastroenterology* **76**, 272–9.

Stryker, S.J., Telander, R.L. and Perrault, J. 1985: Anorectal evaluation after colectomy and endorectal ileoanal anastomosis in children and young adults. *Journal of Pediatric Surgery* **20**, 656–60.

Sutherland, L., Singleton, J., Sessions, J. *et al.* 1991: Double blind, placebo controlled trial of metronizadole in Crohn's disease. *Gut* **32**, 1071–5.

Tanaka, K., Wilks, M., Coates, P.J., Farthing, M.J.G., Walker-Smith, J.A. and Tabaqchatis, S. 1991: Mycobacterium paratuberculosis and Crohn's disease. *Gut* **32**, 43–5.

Teahon, K., Bjarnason, I., Pearson, M. and Levi, A.J. 1990: Ten years' experience with an elemental diet in the management of Crohn's disease. *Gut* **31**, 1113–7.

Theodossi, A., Spiegelhalter, D.J., Jass, J. *et al.* 1994: Observer variation and discriminatory value of biopsy features in inflammatory bowel disease. *Gut* **35**, 961–84.

Thomas, A.G., Holly, J.M.P., Taylor, F. and Miller, V. 1993: Insulin like growth factor-I, insulin like growth factor binding protein-1, and insulin in childhood Crohn's disease. *Gut* **34**, 944–7.

Thomas, A.G., Miller, V., Taylor, F., Maycock, P., Scrimgeour, C.M. and Rennie, M.J. 1992: Whole body protein turnover in childhood Crohn's disease. *Gut* **33**, 675–7.

Thornton, J.R., Emmett, P.M. and Heaton, K.W. 1980: Diet and ulcerative colitis. *British Medical Journal* **1**, 293–4.

Tjandra, J.J. and Fazio, V.W. 1994: Stricturoplasty without concomitant resection for small bowel obstruction in Crohn's disease. *British Journal of Surgery* **81**, 561–3.

Wakefield, A.J., Sawyer, A.M., Dhillon, A.P. *et al.* 1989: Pathogenesis of Crohn's disease: multifocal gastrointestinal infarction. *Lancet* **334**, 1057–62.

Warren, B.F., Shepherd, N.A., Bartolo, D.C.C. and Bradfield, J.W.B. 1993: Pathology of the defunctioned rectum in ulcerative colitis. *Gut* **34**, 514–6.

Winslet, M.C., Allan, A., Poxon, V., Youngs, D. and Keighley, M.R.B. 1994: Faecal diversion for Crohn's colitis: a model to study the role of faecal stream in the inflammatory process. *Gut* **35**, 236–42.

Wright, J.P., Young, G.O. and Tigler-Wybrandi, N. 1987: Predictors of acute relapse of Crohn's disease: a laboratory and clinical study. *Digestive Diseases and Sciences* **32**, 164.

Yang, H., McElree, C., Roth, M.-P., Shanahan, F., Targan, S.R. and Rotter, J.I. 1993: Familial empirical risks for inflammatory bowel disease: differences between Jews and non-Jews. *Gut* **34**, 517–24.

Zelas, P. and Jagelman, D.G. 1980: Loop ileostomy in the management of Crohn's colitis in the debilitated patient. *Annals of Surgery* **191**, 164–8.

Zwiren, G.T., Andrews, H.G. and Caplan, D.B. 1981: Total colectomy with ileo-endomuscular pull-through in the treatment of ulcerative colitis in children. *Journal of Pediatric Surgery* **16**, 174–9.

CHAPTER 41

Gastrointestinal duplication

D.M. BURGE

Introduction   Anatomical types
Embryology and pathology   Results
Clinical features   References

Introduction

Congenital duplication of the gastrointestinal tract can take many forms, occur in any part of the enteric system from mouth to anus and present in very many different ways. Although the term duplication cyst is commonly used, 10–20% are tubular structures (Pinter *et al.*, 1992) which can communicate at either or both ends with the gut lumen. The spectrum of the condition includes small cysts within the wall of the bowel or within other organs such as pancreas, large tense cysts on the mesenteric border of the bowel causing luminal obstruction by stretching and long tubular duplication or triplication of entire sections of the gastrointestinal tract. Symptoms produced by duplications vary according to their position, size, type and histology. Features common to all duplications are attachment to the gastrointestinal tract, a well-developed smooth muscle coat and an epithelial lining of gastrointestinal origin. Multiple duplications can occur in the same patient and other congenital anomalies may be present (Narasimharao and Mitra, 1987; Olsen *et al.*, 1992).

Embryology and pathology

Given that duplication anomalies are a heterogeneous group it is unlikely that they have a common embryological cause. Some enteric duplications are densely adherent to the spinal column, are associated with hemivertebrae, have a cystic intraspinal component or open as an enteric fistula on the skin of the back (Bentley and Smith, 1966). A concept that explains these less common, but clinically important, variants is that of the split notocord (Faris and Crowe, 1975). The notocord is a structure that develops in the midline of the embryo during the third week. It is destined to remain in part as the nucleus pulposus of the intravertebral discs but in early embryonic life plays a vital role in organizing the symmetry of the embryo and in the development of the spine. Its presence separates developing endoderm (destined to be intestine) from ectoderm (destined to be skin). If a longitudinal split develops in the notocord, endoderm and ectoderm can connect. This connection may result in a complete fistula from bowel to skin, which passes through the spinal cord and column (Singh and Singh, 1982). Variations include intraspinal cysts that can enlarge and cause spinal compression with neurological signs (Velasco-Siles *et al.*, 1986).

The histology of enteric duplications usually reflects that of the neighbouring gastrointestinal tract. Thus in foregut lesions gastric epithelium predominates whilst cysts farther down the gastrointestinal tract will contain small and/or large bowel mucosa. However different types of lining can be found in cysts at any site and even pancreatic tissue and neural tissue can be present. The lesions have a full intestinal muscle wall that may merge with the wall of neighbouring bowel.

Clinical features

Clinical features arising from duplications vary with their site and are dealt with below. About 30% present in the neonatal period (Holcomb *et al.*, 1989) and most have presented by the age of 10 years. The diagnosis can be made on prenatal ultrasound (Goyert *et al.*, 1991; Duncan *et al.*, 1992). Preoperative diagnosis of the exact nature of thoracic or abdominal cystic lesions is not always possible. The presence of a vertebral anomaly on plain X-ray is indirect evidence that the associated lesion may be a foregut duplication cyst (Fig. 41.1). The ultrasound appearance of abdominal duplications may clearly show the inner mucosal layer and outer muscle wall coats (Barr *et al.*, 1990) (Fig. 41.2). Cross-sectional imaging using computerized tomography or magnetic resonance imaging may give valuable information and is essential if an intraspinal component is suspected. Gastrointestinal contrast studies may yield useful information particularly about the extent of hindgut tubular duplications (Fig. 41.3). The presence of ectopic gastric mucosa, which is found in 35% of duplications (Idstad *et al.*, 1988) may be demonstrated by ^{99m}Tc-pertechnetate radionuclear scan (Fig. 41.4).

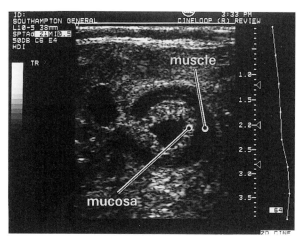

Fig. 41.2 Ultrasound scan of an intra-abdominal duplication demonstrating the mucosal and muscle layers.

Anatomical types

THORACIC DUPLICATIONS

Approximately 20% of duplications arise from the oesophagus (Holcombe *et al.*, 1989). Presentation is usually in the neonatal period with respiratory distress from birth or within the first few days as the lesion continues to fill with secretions produced by its lining mucosa, and compresses the lung hilum (Fig. 41.5). A

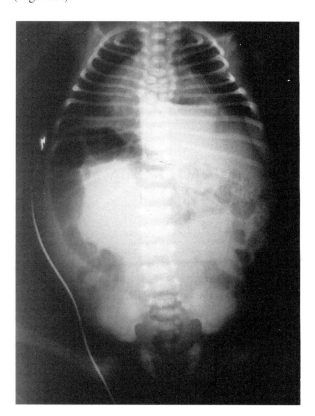

Fig. 41.1 Radiograph of an infant showing thoracic vertebral anomalies associated with an abdominal space-occupying lesion which was a cystic small bowel duplication.

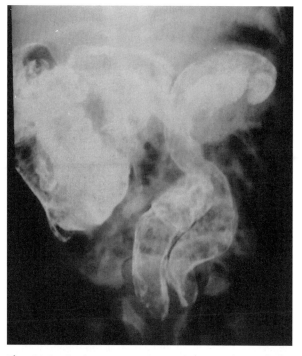

Fig. 41.3 Barium enema in an infant with a tubular rectal duplication.

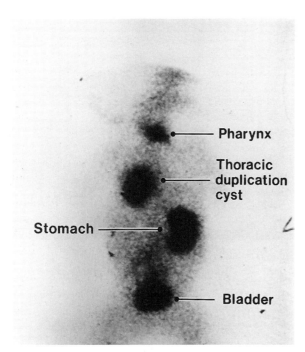

Fig. 41.4 ^{99m}Tc-pertechnetate radionuclear scan showing thoracic uptake of radionuceotide by a thoracic duplication cyst.

high proportion of these lesions contains gastric mucosa which can cause ulceration into the oesophagus or trachea producing gastrointestinal bleeding or haemoptysis (Burgner *et al.*, 1994).

Thoracic lesions may extend across the diaphragm

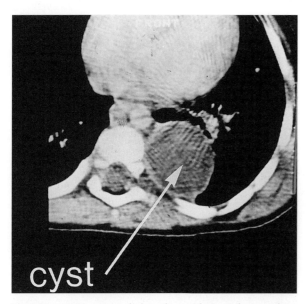

Fig. 41.5 CT scan of the chest of an infant with a thoracic duplication cyst causing deviation of the ipsilateral mainstem bronchus.

(Sonoda *et al.*, 1987) and in some cases the bulk of the duplication is intra-abdominal. For this reason careful abdominal imaging should be undertaken. Once the lesion has been confirmed as cystic the main differential diagnosis is bronchogenic cyst or cystic teratoma. It is this group of duplications that the presence of vertebral anomalies and abnormal uptake on ^{99m}Tc-pertechnetate radionuclear scan may help in preoperative diagnosis.

Treatment is by thoracotomy and excision. Particular care must be taken if the cyst is within the wall of the oesophagus or densely adherent to the trachea or lung hilum. Large lesions may involve extensive dissection. Thoracoabdominal lesions can be removed by staged surgery, approaching the end causing the presenting symptoms in the first instance (Nayar and Freeman, 1994).

GASTRODUODENAL DUPLICATIONS

Gastric duplications usually arise from the greater curve of the stomach (Fig. 41.6). Large lesions may present as

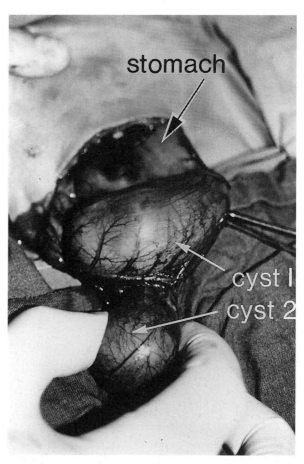

Fig. 41.6 Two duplication cysts arising from the greater curvature of the stomach. The upper cyst, which was within the muscle wall of the stomach, was excised without breaching the gastric mucosa.

an abdominal mass, as an acute abdomen (Sieunarine and Marimohansingh, 1989) or with gastrointestinal bleeding. Smaller lesions may present with pancreatitis (see below).

Pyloric and duodenal duplications usually present by causing obstruction to the intestinal lumen (Bailey *et al.*, 1993; Bergman and Jacir, 1993) or pancreatitis. These lesions are usually quite small. Those sited in the duodenum are located on its posteromedial border. This can make them hard to find at surgery especially if peptic irritation or pancreatitis has occurred.

Acute pancreatitis, sometimes recurrent or associated with pseudocyst formation, has been reported as a presenting feature of duplications (Soundarajan and Subramaniam, 1988; Wold *et al.*, 1988; Lavine *et al.*, 1989; Alessandrini and Derlon, 1991; Okuyama *et al.*, 1992). Such lesions may contain ectopic pancreatic tissue and an accessory duct connection with the main pancreatic duct system (Lavine *et al.*, 1989).

The most helpful investigations in this group of duplications are ^{99m}Tc-pertechnetate radionuclear scanning and cross-sectional imaging. Endoscopic retrograde cholangiopancreatography (ERCP) may demonstrate abnormal pancreatic duct anatomy in some cases with pancreatitis. Surgical excision is the treatment of choice. With some gastric duplications this can be accomplished without breaching the mucosa of the stomach (Lima *et al.*, 1992).

INTRA-ABDOMINAL CYSTIC DUPLICATIONS

Most abdominal cystic duplications originate in the small bowel (Holcomb *et al.*, 1989). They arise from the mesenteric border and the muscle coats merge with those of the adjoining bowel, with which they share a blood supply (Fig. 41.7). The most common presentation in neonates is with a large abdominal mass. More recently, these lesions have been detected on prenatal ultrasound (Balen *et al.*, 1993). They may also present acutely in older children as abdominal pain simulating appendicitis (Idstad *et al.*, 1988), as intussusception with the duplication as the lead point (Idstad *et al.*, 1988; Stringer *et al.*, 1992), as intestinal obstruction due to stretching of the adjacent bowel or volvulus, or with perforation (Royle and Doig, 1988).

Lesions in this site are less likely to be associated with vertebral anomalies and the presence of ectopic gastric mucosa. They will be identified as a cystic mass on ultrasound scanning. The differential diagnosis includes mesenteric (lympangiomatous) cyst, choledochal cyst and, in the female, ovarian cyst. A skilled ultrasonologist will often be able to give a precise diagnosis (Barr *et al.*, 1990). It is advisable to obtain a chest X-ray in such cases as thoracic duplications may coexist.

Treatment is by surgical excision. This usually requires the removal of the adjacent small bowel, although occasionally this can be preserved without damage to its blood supply (Balen *et al.*, 1993).

TUBULAR DUPLICATION

This is the most common type of duplication to affect the colon (Fig. 41.8), although small bowel tubular duplications occur. Presentation depends to some extent on anatomy and on the type of lining epithelium. Tubular duplications that communicate with the intestinal lumen proximally but not distally may present as an abdominal mass owing to ballooning of the distal blind end with intestinal contents. Abdominal pain or gastrointestinal bleeding is the likely mode of presentation

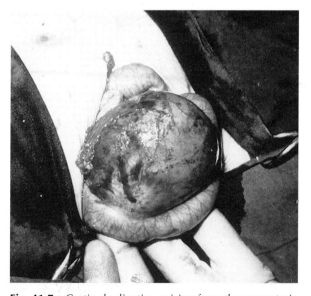

Fig. 41.7 Cystic duplication arising from the mesenteric border of the small bowel.

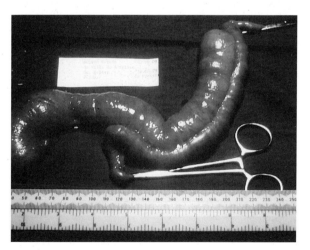

Fig. 41.8 Tubular duplication of the transverse colon.

when ectopic gastric mucosa is present. Colonic tubular duplications may open in the perineum with anal duplication (Pieretti and Lago, 1994) or be associated with other obvious external abnormality (Azmy, 1990).

In many cases the exact nature and extent of tubular duplications will not be appreciated until laparotomy. If the diagnosis is anticipated by external signs, contrast enema studies may aid the planning of surgery.

The surgical treatment of tubular duplications may be very difficult. If a long segment of small bowel is involved, simple excision of the duplication and adjacent bowel may risk short bowel syndrome. In such cases it is possible to incise the muscle coat, strip out the mucosal lining and close the points of communication with the bowel lumen. Long colonic duplications will often require temporary colostomy with subsequent detailed radiological investigation of the anatomy before final corrective surgery (Nayer and Freeman, 1994).

RECTAL DUPLICATIONS

This rare variety of duplication (La Quaglia *et al.*, 1990) is worth a special description as its methods of presentation may mimic other conditions. It may present as a retrorectal mass causing constipation and be confused with sacrococcygeal teratoma or anterior meningocele, as a cause of rectal bleeding (Bar-Maor and Ben-David, 1994) or be mistaken for a simple anal fistula (Narasimharao *et al.*, 1987). Excision is best achieved via a posterior sagittal approach.

Results

The majority of children with gastrointestinal tract duplications will survive without long-term morbidity (Holcomb *et al.*, 1989). At most risk are those with intraspinal involvement and those with long small bowel tubular duplications. Complete excision of the entire lesion, or at least its mucosal lining, is essential to prevent recurrent cyst formation or complications arising from ectopic gastric mucosa. Malignant tumours, including carcinoid (Rubin *et al.*, 1981; Horie *et al.*, 1986), adenocarcinoma (Chnang *et al.*, 1981) and squamous cell carcinoma (Hickey and Corson, 1981), have been reported in a number of duplications.

References

Alessandrini, P. and Derlon, S. 1991: Gastric duplication communicating with an aberrant pancreas. *European Journal of Pediatric Surgery* **1**, 309–11.

Azmy, A.F. 1990: Complete duplication of the hindgut and lower urinary tract with diphallus. *Journal of Pediatric Surgery* **25**, 647–9.

Bailey, P.V., Tracy, T.F., Jr, Connors, R.H., Mooney, D.P., Lewis, J.E., Weber, T.R. 1993: Congenital duodenal obstruction: a 32-year review. *Journal of Pediatric Surgery* **28**, 92–5.

Balen, E.M., Hernandez-Lizoain, J.L., Pardo, F., Longo, J.M., Cienfuegos, J.A.A., V 1993: Giant jejunoileal duplication: prenatal diagnosis and complete excision without intestinal resection. 1993: *Journal of Pediatric Surgery* **28**, 1586–8.

Bar-Maor, J.A. and Ben-David, S. 1994: Duplication of the rectum presenting as perforating peptic ulcer. *Paediatric Surgery International* **9**, 214–15.

Barr, L.L, Hayden, C.K.J. and Stausberg, S.D., *et al.* 1990: Enteric duplication cysts in children: are the ultrasonographic wall characteristics diagnostic? *Pediatric Radiology* **20**, 326–8.

Bentley, J.F.R. and Smith, J.R. 1960: Developmental posterior enteric remnants and spinal malformations. *Archives of Disease in Childhood* **35**, 76–86.

Bergman, K.S., Jacir, N.N. 1993: Cystic duodenal duplication: staged management in a premature infant. *Journal of Pediatric Surgery* **28**, 1584–5.

Burgner, D.P., Carachi, R. and Beattie, T.J. 1994: A thoracic foregut duplication cyst presenting with neonatal respiratory distress and haemoptysis. *Thorax* **49**, 287–8.

Chnang, M.T., Barba, F.A., Kaneko, M. and Tiersrein, A.S. 1981: Adenocarcinoma arising in an intrathoracic duplication of foregut origin: a case report and review of the literature. *Cancer* **47**, 1887–90.

Duncan, B.W., Adzick, N.S. and Eraklis, A. 1992: Retroperitoneal alimentary tract duplications detected in utero. *Journal of Pediatric Surgery* **27**, 1231–3.

Faris, J.C. and Crowe, J.E. The split notocord syndrome. 1975: *Journal of Pediatric Surgery* **10**, 467

Goyert, G.L., Blitz, D., Gibson, P., *et al.* 1991: Prenatal diagnosis of duplication cyst of the pylorus. *Prenatal Diagnosis* **11**, 483–6.

Hickey, F.W. and Corson, J.M. 1981: Squamous cell carcinoma arising in a duplication of the colon. *Cancer* **47**, 602–9.

Holcomb, G.W., Gheissari, A. O'Neill, J.A., *et al.* 1989: Surgical management of alimentary tract duplications. *Annals of Surgery* **209**, 167–74.

Horie, H., Iwasaki, I. and Takahashi, H. 1986: Carcinoid in a gastrointestinal duplication. *Journal of Pediatric Surgery* **21**, 902–4.

Idstad, S.T., Tollerud, D.J., Weiss, R.G., Ryan, D.P., McGowan, M.A. and Martin, L.W. 1988: Duplications of the alimentary tract. Clinical characteristics, preferred treatment, and associated malformations. *Annals of Surgery* **208**, 184–9.

La Quaglia, M.P., Feins, N., Eraklis, A. and Hendren, W.H. 1990: Rectal duplications. *Journal of Pediatric Surgery* **25**, 980–4.

Lavine, J.E., Harrison, M. and Heyman, M.B. 1989: Gastrointestinal duplications causing relapsing pancreatitis in children. *Gastroenterology* **97**, 1556–8.

Lima, M., Grandi, M., Ruggeri, G., Caccian, A., Domini, M., and Tani, G. 1992: Gastric duplication cyst in a child treated by extramucosal excision. *Paediatric Surgery International* **7**, 206–8.

Narasimharao, K.L., Patel, R.V., Malik, S.K. *et al.* 1987: Chronic peri-anal fistula. Beware of rectal duplication. *Postgraduate Medical Journal* **63**, 213–14.

Narasimharao, K.L. and Mitra, S.K. 1987: Esophageal atresia associated with esophageal duplication cyst. *Journal of Pediatric Surgery* **22**, 984–5.

Nayar, P.M. and Freeman, N.V. 1994: Gastrointestinal duplications. In Freeman, N.V., Burge, D.M., Griffiths, D.M., and Malone, P.S., (eds), *Surgery of the newborn*. Edinburgh: Churchill Livingstone, 255–66.

Okuyama, H., Matsuo, Y., Fukui, Y., Imura, K., Kamata, S. and Okada, A. 1992: Intrahepatic duodenal duplication associated with pancreatic pseudocysts. *Journal of Pediatric Surgery* **27**, 1573–7.

Olsen, L., Anneren, G., Henze, A., Lundkvist, K. and Lonnerholm, T. 1992: Multiple intestinal duplications in a child with thoracic myelomeningocele and hydrocephalus. *European Journal of Pediatric Surgery* **2**, 45–8.

Pieretti, R.V. and Lago, J. 1994: Complete tubular side-by-side duplication on the colon and ileum. *Paediatric Surgery International* **9**, 127–8.

Pinter, A.B., Schubert, W., Szemledy, F., Gobel, P., Schafer, J. and Kustos, G. 1992: Alimentary tract duplications in infants and children. *European Journal of Pediatric Surgery* **2**, 8–12.

Royle, S.G. and Doig, C.M. 1988: Perforation of the jejunum secondary to a duplication cyst lined with ectopic gastric mucosa. *Journal of Pediatric Surgery* **23**, 1025–6.

Rubin, S.Z., Mancer, J.F.K. and Stephemns, C.A. 1981: Carcinoid in a rectal duplication: a unique pediatric surgical problem. *Canadian Journal of Surgery* **24**, 351–2.

Sieunarine, K. and Manmohansingh, E. 1989: Gastric duplication cyst presenting as an acute abdomen in a child. *Journal of Pediatric Surgery* **24**, 1152.

Singh, A. and Singh, R. 1982: Split notocord syndrome with dorsal enteric fistula. *Journal of Pediatric Surgery* **17**, 412–13.

Sonoda, N., Takaya, J., Okamoto. K., Taniuchi, S., Iwase, S., Kobayashi, Y., Uetsuji, S., Yamada, T. and Ogura, M. 1987: Transdiaphragmatic duodenal duplication in a premature infant. *Journal of Pediatric Surgery* **22**, 372–3.

Soundararajan, S. and Subramaniam, T.K. 1988: Gastropancreatic duplications. *Paediatric Surgery International* **3**, 288–9.

Stringer, M.D., Capps, S.N.J. and Pablot, S.M. 1992: Sonographic detection of the lead point in intussusception. *Archives of Disease in Children* **67**, 529–30.

Velasco-Siles, J.M., Paredes, E., Escanero, A. and Alcala, H. 1986: Spinal cord compression due to cystic duplication of the primitive digestive tract. *Child's Nervous System* **2**, 159.

Wold, M., Callery, M. and White, J.J. 1988: Ectopic gastric-like duplication of the pancreas. *Journal of Pediatric Surgery* **23**, 1051–2.

CHAPTER 42

Acute abdominal pain

R. SURANA AND B. O'DONNELL

Prologue
Introduction
Clinical features
Management
Physical examination
Active observation
Acute non-specific abdominal pain
Acute appendicitis
Management of childhood appendicitis

Laparoscopic appendicectomy
Management of appendix mass
Differential diagnosis
Acute abdominal pain in infants
and toddlers
Appendicitis in the young child
References
Further reading
Appendix

Prologue

Acute abdominal pain and recurrent abdominal pain in childhood are separate and distinct problems. Both are completely different from acute and recurrent abdominal pain in adults.

In temperate climates over 95% of children between the ages of 2 and 14 years with acute abdominal pain of less than 7 days' duration will have one of two problems. The child will have either acute non-specific abdominal pain (ANSAP) or appendicitis.

Of those requiring urgent surgery in 99% of boys and 98% of girls the surgery will be for appendicitis. Only 1% will have a complication of Meckel's diverticulum or another rarity and 1% of girls requiring urgent surgery will have a complication of an ovarian cyst or fallopian tube.

Our hospital admission figures over the last 15 years show an almost equal split between ANSAP and appendicitis but ANSAP is really much more common as most patients with ANSAP are not admitted to hospital and are either never seen at a hospital or if seen as out-patients, are sent home.

In recurrent abdominal pain, that is any abdominal pain of more than 7 days' duration, or any recurrent abdominal pain of any duration or any number of attacks, without any history of wetting or chronic diarrhoea, the cause will be psychogenic in 19 out of 20 patients (95% or more). The more severe the recurrent pain the more likely it is to be psychogenic in origin.

Introduction

Acute abdominal pain, for practical purposes, is defined as abdominal pain of less than 7 days' duration. This is a commonly encountered problem in paediatric practice and constitutes about 5% of the total hospital admissions and about 20% of the total general surgical admissions. The diagnosis and management of such a large group is at once easier and more difficult with children than the adults. It is easier because of a much narrower range of diagnostic possibilities in children than in adults (Table 42.1). But it is more difficult because of communication difficulties and atypical presentations in younger children (Surana *et al.*, 1995b).

Table 42.1 Diagnosis of admissons with acute abdominal pain

Diagnosis	Study		
	Our Lady's Hospital for Sick Children (%)	Sheffield[a] (%)	Europe[b] (%)
Acute non-specific abdominal pain	54.8	61.2	63.1
Appendicitis	39.4	21.9	32.7
Urinary infection	1.0	1.9	2.6
Others	4.8	6.8	1.6

[a]Surana and O'Donnell (unpublished data).
[b]Dickson *et al.* (1988).

Clinical features

INCIDENCE

It is difficult to establish the precise incidence of abdominal pain in a population but it is likely that almost all children under 15 years of age experience acute abdominal pain at some time. Most of these attacks are dealt with by the parents at home. Some children are seen and managed by general practitioners. A third group of children is referred to the hospital because they are ill or the nature of the problem is uncertain. Cases of abdominal pain constitutes 4% of the patients seen in accident emergency department. Of these, possibly half of the patients are sent home from the emergency department by someone who frequently sees such a problem and the remaining half of the patients will be admitted (Surana and O'Donnell, unpublished data).

CAUSES

The range of possibilities in children with acute abdominal pain is narrower than in adults. Table 42.1 shows the breakdown of admissions with acute abdominal pain in children. The two most common causes of acute abdominal pain are ANSAP, followed in frequency by acute appendicitis (Table 42.1). It is obvious that the most common indication for surgery in patients with acute abdominal pain is appendicitis. Other causes that require operation, urgently or electively, are uncommon, and occur in about 1% of cases between the ages of 2 and 14 years.

Management

As shown in Table 42.1, the most common cause of acute abdominal pain is ANSAP. This recognition of ANSAP as a common cause of pain along with the better definition and delineation of ANSAP, has improved the management of these children. It has also helped to change the approach from look and see to wait and see, thus avoiding unnecessary laparotomies. Once the concept of ANSAP is firmly established, the management of children with acute abdominal pain is simpler. The questions that need to be answered after seeing a child is whether he or she needs an operation, and if an operation is not indicated, whether it is safe to discharge the patient. If it is decided that surgery is not warranted and it is not advisable to discharge the patient, the practice of active observation is undertaken.

CONSULTATION

Children and parents consulting a hospital doctor are usually concerned, anxious and worried and more so when faced with an emergency situation where the nature of the problem is uncertain. It is important that the doctor in question creates confidence in them. To begin with, it is necessary to create an atmosphere in which a diagnosis can be made. A crying child, worried parent and a brusque, harassed doctor, all standing up and hardly listening to one another will combine to produce an atmosphere in which a diagnosis may be impossible.

It is preferable to obtain some information about the child and parents before the interview. It is better to start with 'hello John/Mary' (it is important to get the gender right), and introducing yourself by saying 'my name is John Hunter and I am the casualty officer', or whatever. Ask parents to sit down and the child to lie down, and then make yourself seated. Give the impression that you have all the time in the world to solve the problem at hand. If you begin with personal details, the parents and child feel that you really want to know everything. Getting straight to the point will not pay off in these circumstances. Patience, tact and the appearance of not being in a hurry will yield the best results.

HISTORY

It is better to let the story be unfolded on its own. You may need to modulate the time-scale of the present episode. Try to keep 'pain' out of the conversation.

The nature of the presenting problem needs to be established. How and when did it start? Was there any history of trauma and did it wake the child up? Did it start in the school? Where did it start and where is it now? Has it got better or worse? Does anything make it better or worse? Has anything been tried to make it better?

Vomiting is quite usual. The nature, contents, frequency and volume are important. Bilious vomiting in children is ominous and should raise the possibility of organic pathology. An idea of fluid loss can be obtained from the history.

Anorexia is a usual accompaniment. A child who is hungry and asking for food is unlikely to have advanced disease.

Some information should be obtained regarding the bowel movements. The child may not understand the nature of enquiry and the parents' help should be sought to find out the household term used for bowel movement (e.g. big job/poo poo). Diarrhoea may be a presenting feature of a perforated appendix, especially in preschool children (Surana *et al.*, 1995b).

Any change in the pattern of micturition (or wee wee/pee pee/passing water or urine) should be specifically noted and further details such as dysuria, haematuria and wetting frequency be obtained.

A history of recent illnesses such as upper respiratory tract infections and analgesic or antibiotic use should be sought as it may change the clinical findings. Previous attacks are usually uncommon in children with appendicitis.

Physical examination

The cardinal rule of physical examination, 'look and feel', should be adhered to. Examination of young children needs patience and tact. Pyrexia is present in most of the patients with appendicitis but a normal temperature does not exclude a complicated appendicitis. Similarly mild pyrexia may be found in patients with ANSAP. A temperature of 38.5°C or more with definite abdominal signs usually means a perforated appendix. Persistent or progressive tachycardia is significant and may be a sign of peritonitis. It also indicates the need for preoperative fluid therapy in patients with appendicitis. Signs of other conditions such as upper respiratory tract infection, otitis media and Henoch–Schönlein purpura should be looked for.

EXAMINATION OF THE ABDOMEN

Abdominal examination should be slow, meticulous and gentle. Parents should be encouraged to stay close and even to hold the child's hand, which will create confidence in the child. It is essential to have the abdomen in full view but sometimes in a toddler it may be wise to slip a hand in under the clothes to palpate the abdomen. A note is made of whether the abdomen is distended and whether it moves with respiration.

Before starting to palpate the abdomen, the child is asked to point to the spot of maximum tenderness with his or her left hand. The examinination starts from the furthest point of tenderness, taking the area of maximum pain last. The groins are examined for evidence of hernia and scrotum for fully descended, untorted testes.

Examination of the abdomen is done with the palm of the hand and not by poking with the fingers. The child should be distracted from the examination and the doctor should always look at the child's face for evidence of pain rather than asking him or her whether it hurts. The area of tenderness is mapped precisely. Guarding in a relaxed child a valuable finding. Rebound tenderness is not really a useful sign. It may be worth going around the abdomen to confirm or alter initial findings. In an ill, apprehensive child, it may be better to re-examine the abdomen with sedation.

Auscultation of the abdomen is not often useful. Normal bowel sounds do not indicate absence of abdominal pathology but absence of bowel sounds is a significant finding. The stethoscope may be used to press the tender area gently to confirm earlier findings and then auscultate the chest. A note is made if it is difficult for the child to sit up.

If the child is not obviously critically ill, then it may be worthwhile to ask him or her to get out of the bed and walk a few paces or jump up and down to give the examiner a better idea of the problem.

RECTAL EXAMINATION

In a child with definite abdominal findings, it is usually unnecessary to perform a rectal examination as it is unpleasant and may be quite traumatic to children. Rectal examination is, however, occasionally helpful in patients with pelvic appendicitis. When necessary it should be performed with utmost gentleness using a well-lubricated glove.

PROVISIONAL DIAGNOSIS

At this point it is possible to reach a provisional diagnosis and three categories should be kept in mind: (i) acute non-specific abdominal pain or possibly appendicitis but no surgery indicated at that point, (ii) acute appendicitis with surgery required or (iii) other uncommon causes.

If the diagnosis is uncertain, which may happen in 50–70% of the patients with acute abdominal pain at initial assessment, active observation is a useful approach to resolve the uncertainty.

Active observation

The objective of active observation is to achieve a more accurate diagnosis and avoid unnecessary surgery. As appendicitis is an evolving process, the definite diagnosis may not be possible at the time of initial presentation. Therefore, in patients with uncertain diagnosis a conscious decision is taken to keep the patient under surveillance until the pain has gone or almost gone or intervention is required. Active observation differs from the other types of observation in that a doctor is committed to visiting the patient within a specific predetermined interval, without waiting to be called to the patient because of a change in the patients' condition. This interval is determined depending on the clinical condition of the patient and the likelihood of surgery being necessary.

Active observation entails admission to the hospital and a serial monitoring of vital signs. The temperature and pulse are taken at hourly, 2- or 4-hour intervals depending on the patients' condition. The interval of revisiting the patient should be determined at the preceding visit. An interval of less than 2 hours is not likely to make any significant difference. At every visit, parental and nursing report should be obtained and the pulse and temperature chart carefully scrutinized before examining the child. Features of the history are recapitulated and complete re-evaluation is undertaken. In a hospital setting, another doctor may be seeing the patient so the present history and clinical finding should be carefully documented by each person at each visit.

It may not be possible to reach a definite diagnosis at the second visit, in which case a third visit is planned and so on. An effort is made to reach and establish a diagnosis at each visit. A clear explanation should be given to the parents every time the child is seen.

If active observation is a part of the hospital policy, it rests in part on being able to move the child to the operating theatre when required. Conversely, the attitude that it is better to 'look and see', as may be encountered in many hospitals, is not a scientific attitude. The objections to this policy come from the fear that the delay in surgery will lead to increased incidence of perforation and postoperative morbidity. Although it is possible that in a small number of patients this practice will allow appendicitis to advance, our data have shown that there was no real increase in the number of perforations in patients who underwent appendicectomy after active observation and certainly the morbidity was no worse in these patients (Surana *et al.*, 1995a). The advent of better antimicrobial agents and intravenous therapy has certainly minimized the effect of the delay.

INVESTIGATION

In the majority of the patients, a careful physical examination is all that is necessary to arrive at a diagnosis. Laboratory and radiological investigations are neither sensitive nor specific. The spectrum of the possible diagnosis in children is so narrow that the approach adopted in adults is unnecessary. The question that is pertinent in children with acute abdominal pain remains 'is it appendicitis or not?'

WHITE CELL COUNT

Leucocytosis, with an increase in neutrophil count, has been considered to be of significance in patients with an acute abdomen. However, it is unlikely that a doctor will remove the appendix just because there is a leucocytosis and not operate because the white cell count is normal. It has to be considered in perspective, since leucocytosis may be seen in patients who do not have appendicitis and a normal leucocyte count has been present in patients with perforation and peritonitis.

OTHER BLOOD TESTS

Serum amylase estimation, which is a routine practice in adults, is totally unnecessary in children. Urea and electrolytes may occasionally be required in very sick, dehydrated children. C-reactive protein has been used in differentiating patients with acute appendicitis from others and a specificity up to 76% has been reported.

URINE ANALYSIS AND CULTURE

Two per cent of girls admitted with acute abdominal pain will have bacteriologically proven urinary infection. Urinary infection is much more common in girls than in boys unless predisposed by some known kidney or bladder disease. It is distinctly uncommon to have significant urinary infection without urinary symptoms. If urine is infected, it should be further confirmed by another midstream urine culture and treated appropriately. Further investigation, such as renal ultrasound should be undertaken.

RADIOLOGY

Plain radiographs rarely help to establish the diagnosis of acute abdominal pain. A radiopaque calculus may occasionally be seen. The non-specific features of appendicitis include scoliosis, faecolith, blurring of the right psoas margin and abnormal gas pattern in the right lower quadrant and/or air–fluid levels.

Barium enema is a useless investigation in the diagnosis of acute appendicitis and yields considerable false-positive and false-negative results.

ULTRASONOGRAPHY

With the advent of real-time imaging, there has been increasing interest in using ultrasonography as a tool in the diagnosis of acute abdominal pain. Sonography is a quick, non-invasive and well-tolerated investigation. It also has advantages of detecting other abnormalities such as ovarian pathology, ureteric dilatation and hydronephrosis, but this requires experience, knowledge of basic technology and sonographic anatomy. False-negative results may be obtained in as many as 16% of the patients in experienced hands and may contribute to the delay in diagnosis and treatment. Therefore a judicious use of ultrasonography is necessary and it does not substitute for the proper, thorough clinical examination. Ultrasonographically, the appendix is considered inflamed if its diameter is more than 6 mm. Other signs of appendicitis include decreased echogenicity of the surrounding fat or the presence of a poorly defined hypoechoic round or oval structure adjacent to the caecum and independent of loops of bowel. Criteria for appendicular rupture are clear asymmetry in the wall thickness with indistinctness of the wall layer or the presence of air–fluid collection around the appendix.

RADIONUCLEOTIDE-LABELLED LEUCOCYTE SCAN

This may be useful in patients with uncertain diagnosis. Indium III and technetium-^{99m}Tc leucocyte scans have been reported to be useful (Henneman *et al.*, 1990). The ^{99m}Tc scan takes 4 hours and the indium III scan up to 17–24 hours. A sensitivity of 100% and an accuracy of 92% have been reported, with a positive predictive value of 78% and negative predictive value of 100%. In a quarter of cases it is indeterminative and entails a dose of radiation, however low.

LAPAROSCOPY

Laparoscopy is a unique procedure which has been used as a diagnostic and therapeutic tool, but the disadvantages include the necessity of a general anaesthetic in children, potential complications associated with the procedure and the temptation of removing a normal appendix. A computed tomography (CT) scan or magnetic resonance imaging (MRI) is usually unnecessary in the management of the patients with acute abdominal pain.

Acute non-specific abdominal pain

ANSAP is defined as abdominal pain of short duration (less than 7 days) with no identifiable cause. This descriptive term, although not a diagnosis in itself, is used to include those patients who do not have a convincing, acceptable, alternative explanation. The diagnosis is often retrospective but can be made prospectively if the possibility is considered carefully.

PATHOPHYSIOLOGY

Although ANSAP is useful in planning the management of the patients with acute abdominal pain, it actually means that it is not known what exactly is the matter with the patient. What is known is that the patient does not require surgery at that time. The precise pathophysiology of ANSAP is not known. Various hypotheses from viral origin to bowel motility disorder have been put forward.

NATURAL HISTORY OF ANSAP

The pain usually lasts for 12–48 hours. The patient will typically have a nights' sleep and wake up to find the pain gone. If the pain lasts for more than 48 hours or so and is getting worse, possibilities other than ANSAP should be seriously considered. The patient must be kept under surveillance until the pain has gone or an alternative satisfactory explanation for the pain is discovered.

PRESENTATION

Abdominal pain often begins in the centre of the abdomen and does not tend to radiate to the iliac fossa but occasionally it may involve the hypogastrium or right lower quadrant. The onset of the pain is gradual and it may come and go. The important feature of the pain is that it does not usually worsen with the movements or coughing. Nausea and vomiting, although not common, do not mean that the patient does not have ANSAP. There may be loss of appetite. Constipation is certainly not a feature.

The temperature may be normal or slightly raised. A high temperature makes the diagnosis of ANSAP unlikely. The pulse rate at admission is unreliable as the child may be apprehensive, but progressive tachycardia usually indicates other possibilities. The tongue is normal and there is no halitosis. The central abdomen may be tender or tenderness may be diffuse. Rarely there is a guarding. Focal tenderness and guarding in the right iliac fossa make ANSAP unlikely.

MANAGEMENT

Patients with acute abdominal pain where a diagnosis other than ANSAP cannot be ruled out should be admitted to the hospital for active observation. Explanation and reassurance to parents and children is a vital part of the management. Once it is decided that the child does not have evidence of appendicitis, then the parents must be told that the examination shows that the child does not require surgery or additional tests at that point, but that he or she will need to be observed in hospital. Parents are usually satisfied once they realize that an unnecessary operation on their child is being avoided. Once the symptoms have resolved, the parents and child are reassured about the innocent and transient nature of the condition.

Acute appendicitis

Acute appendicitis is the most common surgical emergency in paediatric practice. Ninety-eight per cent of operations required for abdominal pain will have surgery for suspected appendicitis. The diagnosis of appendicitis may be straightforward or impossible depending on the exact nature of the process at the time when the patient is seen and on the age of the patient.

PATHOLOGY

The most important factor in the pathogenesis of the appendicitis is luminal obstruction of the appendix. The obstruction may be complete or incomplete, and incomplete obstructions may become complete owing to inflammatory swelling of the surrounding tissue.

FOCAL APPENDICITIS

In about 10% of appendicectomies, routine histological examination does not show submucosal or transmural inflammation but neutrophils and pus are seen in the lumen with superficial foci of mucosal inflammation, ulceration and an occasional crypt abscess. Whether such findings are the cause of the symptoms may be debated.

ACUTE APPENDICITIS

The typical acutely inflamed appendix is congested and oedematous with submucosal or transmural neutrophil infiltration. Serosal exudate is not present.

ACUTE SUPPURATIVE APPENDICITIS

The appendix is turgid and congested, the peritoneal surface is extensively coated with a yellow–white fibrinopurulent exudate, luminal obstruction is usually evident and there is marked turbid, purulent, peritoneal fluid. The wall of the appendix is inflamed through its full thickness. Foci of suppuration are present, associated with destruction of the mucosa and underlying lymphoid tissue. On the peritoneal surface, there is a marked reactive swelling of the mesothelial cells.

GANGRENOUS APPENDICITIS

In more advanced stages, ischaemia causes grey–green or blackish areas of gangrene in the wall of the appendix. The lumen may contain pus. Peritoneal fluid is increased and is usually purulent. Histologically, there is a loss of normal tissue architecture.

PERFORATED APPENDICITIS

The wall of the appendix has perforations that are usually on antimesenteric border with escape of the organisms to the peritoneal cavity. The peritonitis may initially be local or may be localized because of the anatomical position such as the paracoloic gutter or pelvis. In other situations the peritonitis may be generalized. Rarely, infective thrombi may travel along the portal system and cause portal pyemia. Perforated appendicitis is more common in younger children: 50% of preschool children were found to have perforation as compared to 16.6% in all children treated in our hospital (Surana *et al.*, 1995b).

APPENDIX MASS

This includes the inflammatory mass and abscess. The appendiceal inflammatory mass is formed by the localization process and usually consists of the appendix surrounded by small bowel and/or omentum. This mass may contain thick fetid pus. Although it is generally believed that young children have a limited ability to form an appendix mass because of the thin-walled appendix and short omentum, in our series half of patients under 2 years, one-third of patients under 3 years and one-fifth of patients under 5 years had progressed to develop appendix mass (Puri and O'Donnell, 1978, 1989; Puri *et al.*, 1981; Surana *et al.*, 1995b).

An analysis of the pathological findings of 954 patients with appendicitis in these two age groups (i.e. preschool children and others) treated in Our Lady's Hospital for Sick Children is shown in Table 42.2.

Table 42.2   Analysis of appendicitis patients (*n* = 954)

Diagnosis	Preschool children		Other children	
	n	(%)	*n*	(%)
Acute appendicitis	14	(22.2)	597	(66.8)
Perforated appendix	35	(55.6)	124	(13.9)
Appendix mass	12	(19.0)	74	(8.3)
Histologically normal appendix	2	(3.2)	98	(11.0)
Total	63	(100.0)	893	(100.0)

HISTORY

The classical triad of appendicitis symptoms is pain, vomiting and fever. The presenting symptom in the majority of the patients is pain in the right lower quadrant. It may have begun around the umbilicus. The pain is often steady and griping in nature rather than colicky, and is not usually severe. The pain associated with appendicitis improves with rest but is aggravated by movement. Toddlers between 1 and 5 years old may not actively complain of pain but instead show increasing irritability and disinclination to move about. The duration of pain is of considerable significance. The duration of symptoms in preschool children in our series varied according to the pathology. The mean duration of symptoms for acute appendicitis was 39.8 hours, perforation 52.6 hours and appendix mass 87.7 hours (Surana *et al.*, 1995b).

Typically, the child with appendicitis is not hungry and may actually have gone off food. Nausea and vomiting are typically present but the usual story is of one or two non-bilious vomits. Constipation is not a common feature, but diarrhoea, if present, is of significance. Twenty per cent of preschool children complain of diarrhoea at presentation. Similarly, gastroenteritis may simulate appendicitis.

A past history of similar attacks of pain is rarely of significance in childhood. Indeed, few patients with proven appendicitis have a previous history of abdominal pain. Other associated symptoms such as dysuria, wetting, frequency, cough and nasal discharge are uncommon in older children but may be present in preschool children.

PHYSICAL EXAMINATION

It is better to examine a child in a lying down position with a parent in close attendance to reduce anxiety. The child should be stripped down to the middle of the thighs so that a valid inspection may be carried out. The child is rarely flushed unless the condition is complicated. The temperature may be normal in an older child unless the appendix is perforated but it is elevated in two-thirds of preschool children with uncomplicated appendicitis. The temperatures are usually in the range of 38–38.5°C. Temperatures of 39°C or over suggest an appendix complicated by perforation and peritonitis or abscess formation or alternatively and much more likely, a non-surgical condition.

Tachycardia at admission is not a reliable sign as it may be caused by anxiety, but persistent or progressive tachycardia of more than 120 beats/min suggests peritonitis and these patients will usually require some preparation with intravenous fluids before surgery. The mouth may be dry and halitosis may be noticeable. Enlarged cervical lymph nodes are common in children with viral infections. Respiratory signs may be obvious on inspection and auscultation. Active alae nasi, tachypnoea, dyspnoea or cough may suggest extra-abdominal pathology.

ABDOMINAL EXAMINATION

It is frequently useful to ask the child to point to the area of maximum tenderness ('where is it sore?'). The child should be encouraged to outline the area of maximum tenderness. The examination of the abdomen should begin away from the site of pain, at the left upper quadrant, then the left lower quadrant, then the right upper quadrant and finally the right lower quadrant. The examination should be as delicate as possible. Guarding over the tender area is common in patients with appendicitis. The silver dollar sign is a reliable sign where the area of tenderness can be covered with a US silver dollar (diameter of 3.5 cm). Rebound tenderness is a subjective sign and should not be used in children. McBurney's point is the point that lies one-third of the way along the line from the anterior superior iliac spine to the umbilicus. It is the best guide to the base of the appendix but it must be remembered that the tip of the appendix may be inflamed and may commonly be retrocaecal, less commonly in the pelvis and least commonly along the ileum.

The pelvis in the young child is shallow, so that even if the appendix lies in the pelvis, it may be possible to elicit the tenderness of a pelvic appendicitis in the lower abdomen. If the bladder is full, which may be due to the bladder spasm because of surrounding inflammation of the appendix, it may be necessary to pass a fine catheter to empty the bladder if the child cannot empty it with encouragement or running a tap.

Sometimes it is necessary to repeat the examination while distracting the child from the real object of investigation to confirm or refute the degree of tenderness.

RECTAL EXAMINATION

It is usually unnecessary to perform rectal examination in children, especially if the definitive signs of appendicitis are elicited on the abdominal examination. However, if the history is longstanding and the child is ill, the pelvic appendix may only be detected by gentle rectal examination.

FINDINGS IN COMPLICATED APPENDICITIS

The complications of appendicitis are due to perforation causing local or general peritonitis or appendix mass (abscess). The history and clinical findings may be modified by any of these events. The history is likely to be longer but not invariably so. Perforations may occur in patients with few hours of history but this is distinctly uncommon. Appendix mass, in contrast, has an ill-defined history going back at least 3–5 days.

The child with a perforated appendicitis is usually iller, may have vomited more frequently, is not anxious for food and probably has pyrexia of more than 38.5°C and persistent tachycardia of 120 beats/min or more. The tenderness is more marked and widespread.

The history in patients with appendix mass is usually longer. The mass may be difficult to palpate in unsedated children, particularly in preschool children in whom it is most common. There may be vague tenderness in the right lower quadrant. It may not be possible to delineate the mass until the child is sedated and sometimes it may not be possible to diagnose an appendix mass unless the child is anaesthetized. The mass may vary from 5 to 12 cm in diameter.

In the appendix mass, the small bowel is involved in the marking-off process and it may be distended with gas. The whole abdomen may become slightly distended and may give the false appearance of generalized peritonitis.

The distinction between appendix mass and perforation with peritonitis is important from the therapeutic point of view as the management of a patient with peritonitis is a removal of the appendix following preoperative preparation while the appendix mass is initially treated vigorously with antibiotics. If the child cannot be examined satisfactorily without sedation, then the dose of sedative must be tailored so as to enable proper examination. Although, in our experience, it was not possible to diagnose the appendix mass without a general anaesthetic in more than 50% of the patients, every effort should be made to establish the diagnosis before that point.

EXTRA TESTS IN DOUBTFUL CASES

It is helpful to observe the manner in which the child approaches the bed. The child may walk with a tendency to tilt to the right side. When the child is lying, he or she may sit up slowly and gingerly because of the inflammatory process.

On being asked to 'hop out of bed' a child with a definite appendicitis will begin this slowly and carefully. This may be so obvious as to make it unnecessary to go through with it to establish the cause of the pain. Conversely, a child who may have been tender on examination may readily jump in and out of bed providing, another morsel of information.

The child is asked to jump up and down three to four times, and to go higher each time. If this does not cause pain, the child is unlikely to have complicated appendicitis.

Management of childhood appendicitis

The treatment of appendicitis is appendicectomy. The surgery should be undertaken as soon as possible. How-ever, if a perforated appendicitis is diagnosed preoperatively, the child will need preparation of up to 12 hours before surgery. It is not usually necessary to perform appendicectomy in the middle of the night (Surana *et al.*, 1993). If the child has acute appendicitis, the chances of the condition progressing to complicated appendicitis are minimal with the use of antibiotics, but it may be difficult to prove this. If the child has perforation, he or she will most certainly need preoperative preparation with fluids and antibiotics before surgery is undertaken. Routine delay in operation is not advocated.

Early complications such as wound infection or pelvic abscess are now uncommon. Peritonitis and pelvic abscess have been shown not to be significant causes of infertility in girls (Puri *et al.*, 1984).

If the theatre is made available during the daytime, one-third of nocturnal operations will be avoided and junior staff will not be forced to operate on the 'doubtful abdomen' (Sherlock *et al.*, 1984; Commission on the Provision of Surgical Services, 1988).

PREPARATION

In an unperforated appendicitis, little preparation is required other than the appropriate anaesthetic premedication. If there is an evidence of perforation, such as generalized tenderness, abdominal distension, tachycardia, pyrexia above 38.5°C or dehydration, the operation should be deferred until the pyrexia is controlled. Antibiotics against Gram-negative bacilli and anaerobes are commenced and intravenous fluids administered to correct the deficit with Ringer's lactate solution. The patient should be properly hydrated and the temperature and pulse brought under control. If uncontrolled, the induction of anaesthetic may accelerate the pulse further and may even cause peripheral circulatory failure while the temperature may rise steeply to hyperpyrexia. If the patient looks very ill and dehydrated, a urethral catheter is passed to monitor the response to hydration.

EXAMINATION UNDER ANAESTHESIA

Before proceeding to incision, the abdomen should be properly examined under anaesthesia to make absolutely certain that an appendix mass is not present. If an appendix mass is more than 6 or 7 cm in diameter and is fixed, then it is better to defer surgery.

INCISION

Once an appendix mass has been ruled out, the incision is accurately placed. The incision is based on the McBurney's point, which is one-third of the way from the anterior superior iliac spine to the umbilicus. The incision is almost transverse, with two-thirds of the incision lateral to the McBurney's point and one-third medial. The incision should be clear of the anterior superior iliac spine and should not be too low or too medial.

PROCEDURE

The skin and subcutaneous fascia are divided, and then the external oblique muscle and aponeurosis are divided in the line of the fibres. The internal oblique muscle fibres are separated by blunt-tipped scissors or artery forceps. Transversus muscle fibres are also separated along with this layer. The muscle fibres are then pulled apart. The peritoneum is grasped with artery forceps and lifted upwards, making sure to avoid the bowel and another artery forceps applied 5 mm away. The peritoneum is then incised transversely with a knife and the opening enlarged with the scissors.

If free pus or peritoneal fluid is encountered, a specimen is obtained for bacteriological examination and then the pus removed by sump suction, avoiding trauma to the bowel.

The caecum is then gently delivered out of the wound. If the caecum is adherent to the posterior abdominal wall because of either congenital band or inflammatory adhesions, then the lateral peritoneal fold is divided by fingers. The difficulties in this step may be compounded by inadequate or wrong placement of the incision. If necessary, the incision may be enlarged by cutting the muscles upwards and laterally. If further enlargement is necessary, then these muscles are divided medially and inferiorly. Alternatively, the wound may be enlarged by cutting the anterior and posterior rectus sheath, securing the inferior epigastric vessels and then retracting the rectus muscle medially.

A haemostat is placed on the mesoappendix, which is then divided between haemostats. The vessels are ligated. Once freed from the mesoappendix, a haemostat is applied to the base of the appendix about 8 mm from its junction with the caecum. A purse-string suture is placed in the seromuscular layer of the caecum. The appendix is then ligated with 3/0 chromic catgut proximal to the haemostat. The appendix is cut with a knife close to the haemostat. The appendix stump is then buried in the caecal wall. All free pus is carefully mopped with swabs soaked in saline or antibiotics. The caecum is then carefully replaced in the abdominal cavity. This may be the most difficult part of the operation.

If the appendix is normal, terminal ileum, the mesentery is carefully inspected and a search made for the Meckel's diverticulum. In girls, the fallopian tube and ovaries are palpated to ensure that there is no pathology.

CLOSING THE WOUND

The peritoneum is closed first with a continuous absorbable suture. The fibres of transverse abdominis and internal oblique are approximated with two or three interrupted sutures. The external oblique is closed with a continuous absorbable suture such as 3/0 Vicryl® or Dexon®. The subcutaneous layer is approximated with 4/0 Vicryl® or Dexon® The skin is closed with a subcuticular 5/0 Dexon® or Vicryl® with no increase in complications (Surana and Puri, 1994). Intraperitoneal drains or delayed primary wound closure will be unnecessary, even in patients with perforation and gross contamination, if the proper technique is adhered to. Although not necessary, a dressing will probably reduce the child's fear and his or her temptation to interfere with the wound.

POSTOPERATIVE CARE

Antibiotics are started preoperatively or at induction and may be continued for 5–7 days in patients with perforation. These should include agents against Gram-negative bacilli and anaerobes, especially bacteroides.

Analgesics are prescribed for at least the first 24–48 hours and administered at 6-hour intervals, or more frequently if required.

A nasogastric tube is rarely required in children. Patients with acute appendicitis are usually ready to start oral fluids 12–24 hours after the operation, while those with gross peritonitis may require intravenous fluids. Intravenous fluid requirements are assessed daily and discontinued as soon as possible.

POSTOPERATIVE COURSE AND FOLLOW-UP

Most patients are ready to go home within 48–72 hours and the majority only require an overnight stay. All these children are followed up a week later to check on the histology and make sure that they have no postoperative infective complications such as wound infection or intra-abdominal abscess. At discharge, parents are advised about the possibility of wound infection and intra-abdominal abscess presenting as redness of the wound, discharge from the wound, pyrexia, vomiting, diarrhoea or abdominal distension.

POSTOPERATIVE COMPLICATIONS

With the advent of better antimicrobial agents, especially against anaerobes, the incidence of postoperative complications has decreased. The incidence of complications in our series was 4.4% (Table 42.3).

WOUND INFECTION

Wound infection occurred in 1.8% of the patients in our series and included patients who developed wound infection after discharge. All of these patients could be managed with incision or aspiration, drainage and antibiotics. Complications such as necrotizing fasciitis develop very rarely and any need for debridement and resuturing is unusual.

Table 42.3 Postoperative complications (*n* = 870)

Complications	Number	Percentage
Wound infection	16	1.8
Scrotal inflammation	1	0.1
Intra-abdominal abscess	14	1.6
Adhesive obstruction	6	0.7
Total No. of complications	37	4.2

SCROTAL INFLAMMATION

In young patients, when processus vaginalis is patent, inflammation may track down to the scrotum.

INTRA-ABDOMINAL ABSCESS

Postoperative intra-abdominal abscesses occurred in 1.6% of our patients. Common sites are the pelvis and paracolic region and rarely the subphrenic region. With aggressive use of antibiotics, most of the intra-abdominal abscesses resolve and can be easily monitored by clinical course and serial ultrasound scan (Surana *et al.*, 1993; Suranan and Puri, 1994). Abscesses that fail to respond need drainage. Well-localized intra-abdominal abscesses may be drained percutaneously under ultrasound control. Pelvic abscesses should be allowed to drain per rectum. Only rarely are laparotomy and drainage required.

FEMALE INFERTILITY

It is still stated in some texts that infertility is common following pelvic or intra-abdominal abscess complicating appendicitis. This is misleading. Pelvic tuberculosis in the past and pelvic inflammatory disease at present undoubtedly cause infertility. The evidence about complicated appendicitis goes against this belief. Two careful follow-ups of women at risk showed that it has little basis in practice, and patients and parents can be reassured that prepubertal pelvic abscess will not result in diminished fertility (Puri *et al.*, 1984; 1989).

MORTALITY

Death due to childhood appendicitis is rare and should be less than one per 3000. Such deaths are usually due to inadequate preparation of the patient or an over-dependence on antibiotics in those who need post-appendicectomy drainage.

Laparoscopic appendicectomy

The first reported case of an appendix removed laparoscopically was by Semm in 1983. Implementation of this method in childhood has been rather slow but is gathering momentum and its advantages over open appendicectomy have not been universally accepted. Early discharge following appendicectomy by the open method has been practised for many years (Buicke *et al.*, 1985) and the small skin crease incision closed with a subcuticular suture is rarely a cosmetic embarrassment.

Laparoscopic appendicectomy carried out by a well-trained and experienced surgeon is a safe procedure provided the Hassan technique for insertion of the first trocar is used. It does have a small cosmetic advantage and the 10–12 mm trocar at the umbilicus and two other 5 mm trocars are required. The scars are hardly noticeable. Appendicectomy by this method is definitely easier in the obese patient. The ability to explore the whole abdominal cavity, particularly if the appendix looks normal, is an advantage, and for the same reason, cleansing the abdominal cavity can be more effective. Furthermore, this may result in a reduction in the incidence of intraperitoneal abscesses and postoperative adhesions (El Ghoneimi *et al.*, 1994).

Laparoscopic appendicectomy is a more expensive method of removing the appendix, but in some units hospital stay has been reduced, thus decreasing the differential (Gilchrist *et al.*, 1992). Laparoscopy is here to stay.

Management of appendix mass

The management of the appendix mass is controversial. Conventional thinking is to treat preoperatively diagnosed appendix masses with intravenous fluids, antibiotics and delayed appendicectomy. However, a dilemma may occur when the diagnosis is made under anaesthesia (50%). Continuation of conservative management is to be advocated. Of 29 preschool children with appendix mass treated in our hospital over 5 years, only two patients failed to respond to this approach and required drainage of an appendix abscess. In our experience, 90% of the patients respond to this approach and drainage of abscess is required in only 10% of the patients. An interval appendicectomy is then undertaken at an interval of 4–6 weeks. Complications occurred in two of 29 patients with this approach, a wound infection in one and an intra-abdominal abscess in the other. Some authors advocate early appendicectomy at the same admission.

Differential diagnosis

URINARY INFECTION

Urinary tract infection (UTI) is an uncommon cause of acute abdominal pain in childhood, especially if not accompanied by urinary symptoms such as dysuria, wetting, frequency or haematuria. It is an uncommon cause of abdominal pain in girls and it is an even less common cause in boys. Constitutional symptoms such as fever, vomiting and anorexia are not unusual. If the patient had previously proven urinary infection or has a congenital urinary tract anomaly, then the possibility of UTI should be considered. The diagnosis of urinary infections in other patients in the absence of urinary symptoms is unwise.

However, it must be remembered that about 2% of schoolgirls will have covert bacteriuria. A pelvic appendicitis may cause an infected urine, but the clinical features should be clear on abdominal or rectal examination. The diagnosis of urinary infection must be based on bacteriological evidence. The presence of albumin in the urine is unreliable but white cells in the urine are a useful indicator. In a patient with urinary infection, another specimen of urine is preferable and should always be taken before commencing antimicrobial therapy. All children with bacteriological evidence of urinary infection must be investigated further to confirm or rule out congenital genitourinary anomalies. Renal ultrasound is a simple, non-invasive modality but lesser grades of reflux may only be picked up by a micturating cystourethrogram. Radionuclide scans are necessary to identify scarring and for estimating differential function of the two kidneys.

The treatment of urinary infection is with appropriate antibacterial agents. If the patient is febrile and has a previous history of urinary infection, antibiotics may be started after getting the clean specimen of urine, but if the patient has had no previous urinary infection and is afebrile, the treatment may be deferred until a definite diagnosis is made. It is unlikely that this will cause significant parenchymal damage but will avoid irrational use of antibiotics, unnecessary labelling of diagnosis of UTI and emergence of the resistant bacteria. Symptomatic improvement may be achieved by drinking large quantities of fluids.

MESENTERIC ADENITIS

Occasionally at operation there may be enlargement of the mesenteric lymph nodes with a normal appendix. These patients are labelled as having mesenteric lymphadenitis. As the percentage of normal appendicectomy goes down, the incidence of mesenteric lymphadenitis decreases. There is no evidence that the enlarged lymph nodes are a cause of pain.

Clinically these patients present with abdominal pain and pyrexia (39°C or more). Vomiting is not common and appetite may be normal. There is often an upper respiratory infection with enlargement of the neck lymph nodes. The tenderness is usually medial to the lateral border of the rectus abdominus muscle and guarding is not a feature.

The condition usually settles within 24–48 hours and the abdominal pain disappears. Recurrence is uncommon.

CONSTIPATION

Although frequently considered as a differential diagnosis of acute abdominal pain, it is doubtful whether constipation of 2–3 days' duration is a frequent cause of acute abdominal pain. The diagnosis is more likely if the pain is relieved by a suppository or an enema.

MECKEL'S DIVERTICULITIS

Although rare, Meckel's diverticulitis may present with acute abdominal pain indistinguishable from acute appendicitis. One-third of patients with diverticulum may have perforation and peritonitis. These patients usually present with periumbilical pain and tenderness is usually medial but may be anywhere in the lower abdomen. The treatment is laparotomy with resection of diverticulum. Less than 1% of surgery for the acute abdomen in childhood is for complications of Meckel's diverticulum.

CHOLECYSTITIS

Gallbladder inflammation may occur in patients with cholelithiasis of haemolytic or non-haemolytic origin. Acalculous cholecystitis is being diagnosed with increasing frequency in recent years. Usually these patients present with right upper quadrant pain, nausea, vomiting and jaundice with right upper quadrant tenderness. Ultrasonography is the investigation of choice and shows a thickened gall bladder wall, diminished contactility and echogenic debris. An oral cholecystogram or intravenous cholangiography may occasionally be necessary. Mild forms of cholecystitis are managed by nasogastric suction, intravenous fluids and antibiotics. Cholecystectomy, usually laparoscopic, is indicated in patients with severe deterioration in their clinical condition.

OMENTAL DISEASE

Rarely, the omentum may be the cause of abdominal pain. This may be due to idiopathic torsion, infarction or omental cysts. The clinical features are indistinguishable from acute appendicitis and preoperative diagnosis is unlikely. The treatment is laparotomy and resection of the involved omentum.

GASTROENTERITIS

This may rarely occur in association with appendicitis. Similarly, diarrhoea may be a presenting feature of acute appendicitis. Copious diarrhoea and hyperactive bowel sounds without localizing signs are indicative of gastroenteritis.

VIRAL HEPATITIS

Hepatitis may cause acute abdominal pain, usually in the right upper quadrant. Jaundice is preceded by a prodromal illness with anorexia, nausea and vomiting. The urine is dark coloured and there is usually soft, tender hepatomegaly. There may be a local epidemic.

PERIODIC SYNDROME

There is usually a history of previous episodes of abdominal pain, headache, pallor and severe vomiting with occasional dehydration. These attacks may recur three or four times a year and last for 3–4 days. Dehydrated patients require admission and intravenous fluids.

OVARIAN PATHOLOGY

The ovarian cyst *per se* rarely causes abdominal pain but haemorrhage into the cyst, torsion of the cyst or normal adenxa can present with acute abdominal pain. Occasionally, ovulation-induced haemorrhage causing localized peritonitis can cause abdominal pain and is termed Mittelschmerz. The abdominal pain secondary to ovarian pathology usually occurs in peripubertal girls. The pain is in a lower quadrant or the hypogastrium and may be associated with nausea and vomiting. Ultrasound is helpful in detecting ovarian pathology. The treatment for patients with torsion is early laparotomy to salvage the ovary and remove the cyst. Oophorectomy is rarely necessary and should be avoided if at all possible. In these patients, with torsion of normal adnexa, contralateral oophoropexy should be performed as predisposing factors such as excessive mobility and hormonal activity may cause similar problems on the other side.

HENOCH–SCHÖNLEIN PURPURA

This is systemic vasculitis of unknown origin and probably related to autoimmune phenomena. Two-thirds of the patients present with abdominal pain. Associated features include nausea, vomiting, bloody stools, nephritis and occasionally scrotal inflammation. These symptoms are due to haemorrhage into the bowel wall or complications such as intussusception, obstruction and perforation. The rash is a pathognomic feature and is initially urticarial eventually becoming haemorrhagic involving the ankles, buttocks and perineal areas. Ultrasound is a valuable tool in these patients to distinguish complications requiring surgery from intramural haemorrhages. Intussusceptions in these patients can be monitored by ultrasound scan with resolution in the majority of the patients. Corticosteroids lead to symptomatic improvement but do not alter the progress of the disease.

DISCITIS

This is a rare condition causing acute abdominal pain in children, in which an inflammatory lesion affects the intervertebral disc. The common manifestations are back pain, fever and high erythrocyte sedimentation rate. Clinical signs include tenderness over the back, difficulty in sitting up and limitation of straight leg raising. The aetiology is unknown. X-rays may not be diagnostic but radionuclide bone scans show an increased uptake at the affected space. Treatment consists of immobilization and appropriate antibiotics.

INGUINAL HERNIA: TORSION OF THE TESTIS

Obstructed inguinal hernia and torsion of testis may present with lower abdominal pain but exposure of the body to the midthighs and careful examination will point to the obvious cause.

NON-ABDOMINAL CAUSES

Right-sided basal pneumonia may present as an acute abdomen, and acute subhepatic appendicitis may cause sympathetic pleural effusion. The diagnosis is usually based on the abdominal and chest findings. X-ray will demonstrate the consolidation. Appendicitis can occur in the presence of pneumonia.

Acute abdominal pain in infants and toddlers

Abdominal pain at this age is almost always due to organic causes. The presenting feature may be the irritability of a milder pain at an earlier point of the disease. At this age, there are three common causes of abdominal pain: intussusception (see Chapter 37), appendicitis and acute non-specific abdominal pain.

Appendicitis in the young child

Appendicitis in young children is a different matter. The majority of the patients have progressed to complicated disease. Of 35 patients under 3 years treated over a 5-year spell, 12 patients had developed appendix mass, 18 patients had macroscopic or microscopic perforation and two patients had a gangrenous appendix. This was probably due to communication difficulties leading to delay in seeking medical advice, atypical presentation and failure to suspect appendicitis. There may be a history of diarrhoea, irritability and cough in a significant number of patients. The patient may well have pyrexia and tachycardia. It is usually difficult to assess the abdomen without adequate sedation. If a mass is felt, intravenous antibiotics, aminoglycoside and anti-anaerobic agents should be started until the mass and tenderness resolve. Electively appendicectomy is then performed after

4–6 weeks. However, over 50% (seven of 12) of the appendix masses may be palpable only under anaesthetic. If a mass is palpated, a conservative management is undertaken with no operation at that stage. Only one of the 12 patients failed to respond to this approach and required preoperative drainage of the pus.

Computer-aided differential diagnosis of acute abdominal pain in children is unnecessary. A proforma directed specifically towards the problem in children will provide all of the information required for a decision (see Appendix).

References

Buick, R.G., Fitzgerald, R.J. and Courtney, D. 1985: Early discharge following appendicectomy in children. *Annals of the Royal College of Surgeons of England* **67**, 105–6.

Commission on the Provision of Surgical Services 1988: Report of the working party on the composition of the surgical team. *General Surgery, Orthopaedics and Otolaryngology.* London: Royal College of Surgeons of England.

Dickson, J.A.S., Jones, A. Telfer, S. and de Dombal, F.T. 1988: Acute abdominal pain in children. *Scandinavian Journal of Gastroenterology* **144**, 43–6.

Dombal, F.T. de 1988: The OMGE acute abdominal pain survey. Progress Report 1986. *Scandinavian Journal of Gastroenterology* **144**, 35–42.

El Ghoneimi, A., Valla, J.S. and Limonne, B. *et al.* 1994: Laparoscopic appendicectomy in children: report of 1,379 cases. *Journal of Pediatric Surgery* **29**, 786–9.

Gilchrist, B.F., Lobe, T.E., Kurt, P. *et al.* 1992: Is there a role for laparoscopic appendectomy in pediatric surgery? *Journal of Pediatric Surgery* **27**, 209–14.

Henneman, P.L., Marcus, C.J., Inkelis, S.H., Butler, J.A. and Baugartner, F.J. 1990: Evaluation of children with possible appendicitis using technetium[99m] leukocyte scan. *Pediatrics* **85**, 838–43.

Puri, P. and O'Donnell, B. 1978: Appendicitis in infancy. *Journal of Pediatric Surgery* **13**, 173–4.

Puri, P., Guiney, E.J., O'Donnell B. *et al.* 1984: Effects of perforated appendicitis in girls on subsequent fertility. *British Medical Journal* **288**, 25–6.

Puri, P., McGuinness, E.P.J. and Guiney, E.J. 1989: Fertility following perforated appendicitis in girls. *Journal of Paediatric Surgery* **24**, 547–9.

Puri, P., O'Donnell, B. 1989: Management of appendiceal mass in children. *Pediatric Surgery International* **4**, 306–8.

Purim, P., Boyd, E., Guiney, E.J. and O'Donnell, B. 1981: Appendix mass in the very young child. *Journal of Pediatric Surgery* **16**, 55–7.

Semm, K. 1983; Endoscopic appendicectomy. *Endoscopy* **15**, 59–64.

Sherlock, D.J., Randle, J. Playforth, M., Cox, R. and Holl-Allen, R.T.J. 1984: Can nocturnal emergency surgery be reduced? *British Medical Journal* **289**, 170–1.

Surana, R., O'Donnell, B. and Puri, P. 1995a: Appendicitis diagnosed following active obstruction does not increase morbidity in children. *Pediatric Surgery International* **10**, 76–8.

Surana, R., Quinn, F., Puri, P. 1995b: Appendicitis in preschool children. *Pediatric Surgery International* **10**, 68–70.

Surana, R., Quinn, F.M.J. and Puri, P. 1993: Is it necessary to perform appendicectomy in the middle of the night in children? *British Medical Journal* **306**, 1168.

Surana. R., Puri, P. 1994: Primary wound closure following perforated appendicitis. *British Journal of Surgery* **81**, 440.

Further reading

Dombal, F.T. de 1990: *Diagnosis of acute abdominal pain.* London: Churchill Livingstone.

O'Donnell, B. 1985: *Abdominal pain in children.* Oxford: Blackwell Scientific.

Appendix

ACUTE ABDOMINAL PAIN (OF LESS THAN 7 DAYS' DURATION) QUESTIONNAIRE

Family name:
Given name:
Hospital no.:
Age (years):
Sex: M/F
Today's date:
Time:

Pain

Where did it start?: Umbilicus/epigastrium/hypogastrium/ RIF/LIF/Rt lumbar/Lt lumbar/hypochondrium R/L/other. (Diagram)
Where is it now?:
When did it start day/hour?:
Duration in hours?: 6/6–12/12–18/18–24/24–36/36–48/48+ (how long?)
Severity: Nil/mild/moderate/severe/incapacitating/crying with pain
Type: Dull/sharp/comes and goes/steady/?other
Made worse by: Coughing/passing urine/eating/getting out of bed/walking
Made better by: ?Anything – specify
How is the pain now: Worse/better/the same

Other symptoms

?Anorexia/nausea/vomiting
What was vomited?
How often?
?Headache/neck pain/limb pain/flu/cough/other
Bowels: Normal/unformed (diarrhoea)/constipation/other
Micturition: Normal/frequency/dysuria (pain on p.u.)/ wetting/other
Female menarche?: yes/no
Further information about present (or past) episodes:

Past medical history

Previous hospital admissions: Where/when/for what/how long/nil
Previous severe illness (name it):
Previous similar pain?
Recurrent abdominal pain?
Any recent medication?
Any serious problems in siblings?
Allergies?

Physical examination

Mood: Normal/distressed/anxious/other
Temperature:
Pulse:
Respirations:
Any respiratory infection now?

Abdominal examination

Movement: Normal/decreased: distension/no distension
Tenderness (indicate on diagram): Diffuse/localized
Guarding: yes/no
Rigidity: yes/no
Rebound: yes/no
Bowel sounds: Normal/decreased/increased
Rectal examination (if advisable):
Investigation (if advisable): urine/abdominal X-ray/blood count
Provisional diagnosis: Acute non-specific abdominal pain (ANSAP) (50%)
Appendicitis (40%)
Other (name it) (10%)
If appendicitis: ?Acute/suppurative/gangrenous/peritonitis/appendix mass

Management

1) Active observation
2) For theatre: requires i.v. yes/no/?
   pre-operative antibiotics yes/no
3) Other
Signed ....

Active observation

No i.v. (unless significant dehydration)/no antipyretics/no antibiotics. May have up to 60 ml clear fluid/2 h. Temperature, pulse and respirations every 2 h and then every 4 h. Revisit patient by arrangement in ?2 h/4 h/8 h.

Revisit

Date:
Time:
Initials:
Taking fluids: yes/no
Vomiting:
Hungry: yes/no
Thirsty: yes/no
Pain: better/worse/same
Tenderness: better/worse/same/diffuse/localized
Provisional diagnosis: ANSAP/appendicitis/other
Management: If ANSAP ?mixed measured fluids ?light diet ?full diet ?discharge
If appendicitis: for theatre ?preop antibiotics.

Revisit

Date:
Time:
Initials:
Taking fluids: yes/no
Vomiting:
Hungry: yes/no
Thirsty: yes/no
Pain: better/worse/same
Tenderness: better/worse/same/diffuse/localized
Provisional diagnosis: ANSAP/appendicitis/other
Management: If ANSAP ?mixed measured fluids ?light diet ?full diet ?discharge
If appendicitis: for theatre ?preop antibiotics.
Date:
Time:
Ward:

Additional information and progress

Discharge diagnosis: ANSAP/appx/other
Follow up in 7 days or less in SOP/PPC/where/when
Signed ....

CHAPTER 43

Recurrent abdominal pain

R. SURANA AND B. O'DONNELL

Incidence	Organic causes
Causes of recurrent abdominal pain	Results
Clinical features	References
Management	Further reading
Psychogenic causes	Appendix 1
Domestic causes	Appendix 2

Recurrent abdominal pain (RAP) is a common problem for those engaged in the care of children. It is often regarded as a taxing ordeal for the doctor and the child. Most milder episodes are dealt with by parents or family doctors, while some are referred to paediatricians and as a last resort to a surgeon. There may be a feeling that something is being missed and this may outweigh the solid, positive evidence of a strong emotional basis. The referring letter also usually seeks an organic cause: 'there must be something there ... the child isn't imagining the pain' and rarely hints at domestic or personal issues. In such patients, the pursuit of organic causes becomes in itself a barrier to correct diagnosis – usually not organic – and management. The mainstay of management is a commitment to help based on an organized approach.

Incidence

It is difficult to estimate the incidence of RAP because so much depends on definitions. The word 'pain' derives from the Greek 'paine' which means punishment or penalty. A practical definition is three well-remembered attacks of pain over a 3-month period. Various studies have estimated that between 8 and 15% of school children experience RAP at some point.

Causes of recurrent abdominal pain

Causes are usually grouped into psychogenic and organic. The great majority are psychogenic and related to anxiety due to psychosocial or emotional stress: 'Fear is the dominant emotion of childhood' (Graham Greene).

Clinical features

THE CONSULTATION

Parents and patients expect doctors to take their problems seriously. Doctors have to demonstrate their commitment by preparing themselves for the consultation and by allotting it enough time. The initial interview with the patient and the parent or parents is the most important step, not only in the diagnosis but in the total management of the condition. It is important to be organized and it is routine for the doctor to fill out a proforma (see Appendix). The worst thing that can happen at a consultation is that the doctor runs out of questions and begins to 'investigate'.

CLINICAL HISTORY

The history is the most important aspect of the consultation. It is taken not only to obtain the details but also to allow the child and parents to absorb the implications of the questions and the answers.

Pain

The details of the pain should be made clear and include: when and how it began, frequency, time when the pain comes, site, radiation, nature of the pain, severity, relieving or aggravating factors, etc. Most emotional pains are central and few organic pains are severe. Two useful questions are, 'do you have to lie down with the pain?' (index of severity) and 'do you ever cry with the pain?' (emotional response).

Associated features of the attack

The most common description is: he/she goes pale when he/she gets the pain. Nausea without vomiting is very much a feature but the occasional vomit is quite common. Other associated features such as headache, fever, dizziness, weakness and fainting all point to a psychosomatic cause. Constipation or diarrhoea are unusual. Urinary complaints should be noted. Ask the parents and child to describe the personality type of the patient. Learned response patterns and personality patterns have an impact in that youngsters vary in their mechanisms to deal with discomfort or stress. Some children somatize, allowing stress to manifest in physical complaints as the child learns that the somatization is rewarding, offering sympathy and benefits.

Does this pain disrupt the lifestyle of the child or family? Previous hospitalization, prolonged illness and investigations should be reviewed. It is well to build up a picture of the household – any long-term illness in the family, stressful life events, recent changes – home, school, teachers, friends, etc. The question regarding school performance should be asked: level at school, dislike for any subject and extracurricular activities are enquired into. Later in the interview it may be useful to ask whether the patient or parents feel that any important points have been omitted so far and to enquire what they consider to be the cause of the problem.

Physical examination

Regardless of how obvious the positive evidence of psychological cause is, it is vital that physical examination be carried out thoroughly. Weight should be recorded for objective evidence of the weight loss. The head, neck and mouth are examined first. Before abdominal examination proceeds, it is better to ask the child to point to the area of the pain. Examination begins as far away from the area of pain as possible. One should palpate the abdomen while distracting the child with some conversation and observing his or her face for evidence of tenderness. The groin should be examined for the evidence of hernia and normally located testes. It is rather unusual to find a positive physical sign on examination in a patient whose primary complaint is RAP.

Nevertheless, physical examination should be thorough if the doctor's opinion is to be taken seriously, and rarities do occur.

Investigation

By now, the parents and child often suspect that the problem is psychogenic but need reassurance that there is no organic cause. Ordering a test or battery of tests can undermine this belief and would actually hinder the effective management. The feeling may grow that there may be another test that could detect the problem.

The investigations are required only if there is positive evidence to suggest an organic cause, e.g. with urinary symptoms or other evidence to suggest urological problems.

Management

Management of the problem begins not at the end of the examination but at the very beginning. It may be helpful to state that there is plenty of evidence to suggest that anxiety is causing a problem and that there is no evidence of any organic disease. It is important to stress that the child's pain is real and to reassure them the pain associated with anxiety is not imaginary. Once the child and parents realize this concept then analysing the problem with possible treatment options is not difficult.

Psychogenic causes

By far the most common cause of RAP lies in the psychogenic category. The psychogenic theory assumes that the stress in some way induces the pain.

Domestic causes

Parental depression, separation of parents, financial problems and serious illness in the house are all proven triggers of RAP. Three other areas contribute to anxiety in children.

THE STRIVER

This is the ambitious, perfectionist, over-achieving child who may well have a crowded curriculum at school and a number of competitive pastimes as well. The child's ambition usually comes from within himself or herself, but sometimes the child is trying to live up to the expectations of ambitious parents. Management of the anxiety depends on building up the confidence through reassurance, hard work and experience.

CURRICULUM PROBLEMS

Difficulties coping with school in general are less common in children with recurrent abdominal pain, but they may have difficulties specifically with one or more subjects combined with an unsympathetic teacher. It is important to establish the baseline of the child's abilities.

THE OVERWEIGHT CHILD

This is a distinct group that may present with RAP. Although some chubby children are genuinely happy, children who are seriously overweight are usually made conscious of their appearance and have a limited participation in social activities. The child complains of pain in the abdomen due to his or her anxiety and the parents are often sympathetic and genuinely sorry for the child. The mentally handicapped comprise another group who cause anxiety.

Organic causes

This group constitutes under 2% of the total patients with RAP.

GASTROINTESTINAL CAUSES

Constipation

Constipation is one of the most commonly cited gastrointestinal causes of abdominal pain. The prominent symptoms are infrequent passage of stools, down to one bowel motion every couple of weeks. Misuse of laxatives can cause abdominal colic; therefore, when constipation is suggested as a cause of RAP, a detailed history of the laxatives and purgatives used should be taken.

Malrotation

A history of bilious vomiting and recurrent attacks of pain is typical of malrotation. The condition may be missed unless great care is taken to elucidate the history. Malrotation causes duodenal obstruction by Ladd's bands or intermittent volvulus because of short mesentery or around a band. This is probably the only indication to undertake a barium meal. Nowadays, most cases of malrotation are diagnosed in the first year of life.

Inflammatory bowel disease

Crohn's disease and ulcerative colitis may present and continue to cause recurrent abdominal pain. In Crohn's disease, the pain is usually in the right quadrant and may begin as a diffuse, vague abdominal discomfort. In the majority, abdominal pain is minimal or overshadowed by a failure to thrive and other characteristic symptoms. Clinical anaemia or persistent upset of bowel habit with a right-quadrant sausage-like mass

may be a pointer. Ulcerative colitis does not usually present with abdominal pain but is more likely to present with diarrhoea, blood in stools and failure to thrive.

Peptic ulcer disease

Peptic ulcer disease is uncommon in children and the incidence of the disease is diminishing. There is an increased familial incidence in the paediatric age group. Patients are usually of school age and boys are more commonly affected than the girls. They may also present with haematemesis, melaena, anaemia and vomiting. Physical examination is not particularly helpful in the diagnosis of peptic ulcer disease in children. Epigastric tenderness is infrequent but anaemia may be noted. Duodenal ulcer is more common than gastric ulcer. Endoscopy may be preferred over contrast studies. As bleeding is not uncommon, attention should be paid to ruling out anaemia. The Zollinger–Ellison syndrome is extremely rare in childhood and therefore, unless the history is suggestive, serum gastrin levels are not required as a part of a routine diagnosis. The management of peptic ulceration in childhood is by the use of H_2 antagonists such as cimetidine or ranitidine, or a Na/K-ATPase inhibitor such as omeprazole, with appropriate antibodies if *Helicobacter pylori* is considered or proven as a factor. Surgery is rarely indicated.

Helicobacter pylori

There has recently been increased interest in *H. pylori* infection as a causative factor of RAP; however, a large, prospective study showed that although 8.5% of the patients with RAP had antibodies to *H. pylori*, there was a similar incidence in control groups.

Uropathy

Uropathy is one of the organic causes that dominates thinking on the subject. Although it is one of the causes of RAP, these children usually have other features such as urinary complaints, urinary infection or a mass. Urolithiasis is usually associated with urinary infection and/or haematuria, although some calculi are painless. The greatest concern is the possibility of missing hydronephrosis. In a review of 58 patients with pelviureteric junction obstruction, 18 patients presented with abdominal pain and five with haematuria and/or urinary infection. Only two of these 18 children had RAP and one of them had another leading feature, a mass. Thus RAP is an uncommon feature of pelviureteric junction obstruction. Intravenous urography may show up the presence of an anatomical variation such as uncomplicated duplex system or pelvic kidney, which may not be related to the pain. Ultrasonography is a better option to rule out any upper urinary tract abnormality as it is quick, easy and non-invasive and does not involve radiation, but the significant positive findings will be few and far between.

Gynaecological pathology

Gynaecological conditions that may cause RAP include endometriosis, pelvic inflammatory disease, dysmenorrhoea and, most importantly, ovarian cyst. With the more widespread use of ultrasonography increasing numbers of ovarian cysts are diagnosed which may be physiological, but the larger cysts carry a risk of acute or intermittent torsion.

Neoplasia

The most serious, and fortunately rare, cause of RAP is neoplasms and this is often an unspoken worry among the parents. Lymphoma, neuroblastoma and Wilm's tumour may cause abdominal pain but associated features such as unexplained weight loss, other constitutional symptoms and mass should raise this possibility.

Results

Seventy-four children with RAP were managed over a 4-year period. The male-to-female ratio was 1:2 (25 males: 49 females). The man age at onset of abdominal pain was 8 years. The majority of these children had recurrent abdominal pain for less than 12 months (Table 43.1). Associated symptoms included pallor, nausea, occasional vomiting, headache, dizziness, anorexia, weight loss and urinary symptoms. Forty per cent of these patients had central abdominal pain, 24% had upper abdominal pain, 26% had lower abdominal pain and 10% had pain that was generalized, radiating or in different regions.

Table 43.1 Duration of abdominal pain

Duration	n	Percentage
< 6 months	35	47.3
6–12 months	12	16.2
1–2 years	8	10.8
> 2 years	15	20.3
Unknown	4	5.4

Table 43.2 Domestic problems

Problem	n
Death in family	4
Unemployment	5
Change of house	6
Alcoholism	2
Marital conflicts	2

Table 43.3 Medical problems in the family

Problem	n
Migraine	10
Hypertension	7
Recurrent abdominal pain	7
Depression	5
Peptic ulcer	4
Appendectomy	5
Other	13

Table 43.4 Problems at school (n = 30)

Problem	n
Not happy	6
Change of school	4
Change of teacher	3
Problems with teacher	4
Bullying	2
Problems with subjects	16

The history of domestic problems was obtained in 19 children with RAP and is illustrated in Table 43.2. Table 43.3 shows medical problems in the family of these children with RAP. Most of the children were happy at school but, on further enquiries, 30 children had some problems at school (Table 43.4).

Only 13 (21%) children were described as normal or average. Of the remaining 61 children, 24 children were labelled as strivers, fussy or perfectionists. Anxiety was a feature in 12 children and nine children were moody.

Twenty-eight investigations were undertaken in 19 of these 74 children (excluding full blood count and urine examination) and included ultrasound, plain X-ray abdomen, barium meal and/or enema, intravenous pyelography, micturating cystourethrogram, cytoscopy, sigmoidoscopy, stool examination and ESR. None of these investigations revealed any abnormality.

OUTCOME

The majority (78%) of the children improved over a 2-year period. An improvement was seen in 88% of the children who were followed up over 5 years. On an attempt to follow-up over 10 years, 38 patients (mean age 20 years) responded. Eight of these patients had appendectomy performed in the intervening period. One patient has recurrent abdominal pain two or three times a year but no cause has been found. All other patients (with or without appendectomy) have improved with no more episodes of abdominal pain.

References

Asborn, M., Maki, M., Ruuska, T. *et al.* 1993: Upper gastro-intestinal endoscopy in recurrent abdominal pain in childhood. *Journal of Pediatric Gastroenterology and Nutrition* **16**, 273–7.

Carber, J., Zeman, J. and Walker, L.S. 1990: Recurrent abdominal pain in children: psychiatric diagnosis and parenteral psychopathology. *Journal of American Academy of Child and Adolescent Psychology* **29**, 648–56.

Levine, M.D. and Rappaport, L.A. 1984: Recurrent abdominal pain in school children: the loneliness of the long distance physician. *Pediatric Clinics of North America* **31**, 969–91.

Van der Mear, S.B., Forget, P.P., Loffeld, R.J., Stobberingh, E., Kuijten, R.H. and Arends, J.W. 1992: The prevalence of *Helicobacter pylori* serum antibodies in children with recurrent abdominal pain. *European Journal of Pediatrics* **151**, 799–801.

Further reading

O'Donnell, B. 1985: *Abdominal pain in children.* Oxford: Blackwell Scientific.

Appendix 1

STRUCTURED HISTORY AND PHYSICAL EXAMINATION

We have used a form for a structured history and physical findings of both acute abdominal pain and recurrent abdominal pain for more than 15 years. As the conditions are completely different we use a colour-coded form for each one. The form for acute abdominal pain is green and the form for recurrent abdominal pain is yellow ... but they can be any colour. The important issue is that each relevant patient has their key data in a readily accessible and fixed order. There is absolutely no need for a computer at the time of admission or at the time of decision. It seems reasonable that any institution dealing with more than 20 patients with these problems in each year should have some baseline of vital facts. The argument is as strong for those seeing the problem every day as for those seeing it occasionally.

A structured history and physical examination improves the management of these patients for all grades of staff.

Appendix 2

RECURRENT ABDOMINAL PAIN (RAP) QUESTIONNAIRE (CIRCLE REPLIES)

Addressograph or
Name (Family name first):
Sex: M/F
Address:
Date of 1st consultation:
Hospital number:
Age at consultation:
Date of birth:
Mode of referral: GP Consultant/Hospital Inpatient/Casualty/Parents
Siblings and place in family: 1, 2, 3, 4, 5, 6, more ?adopted
Place of birth:
Birth weight:
Previous illnesses: Hospitalization/eye problems?
Immediate reason for consultation:
How many times have you seen your doctor(s)?:
Total duration of symptoms (months):
Age at onset: 1, 2, 3, 4, 5, 6, 7, 8, 9, 10, 11, 12, 13, 14
Age at presentation: 1, 2, 3, 4, 5, 6, 7, 8, 9, 10, 11, 12, 13, 14
Frequency of attacks: ?/hour/day/week/month/all the time/other
Duration of attacks: 1/5/30/60 mins/hours/day/days
Site of pain: Periumbilical/loins/epigastrium/hypogastrium/RIF/LIF/other
Type and severity: Mild/moderate/severe/incapacitating/crampy/dull/sharp/knife-like/do you have to lie down – sit down?/do you ever cry with the pain?
Does the pain move or radiate?: Yes/No
Time when pain is worst: Morning/mid-day/night/weekends/other/no particular time
Is problem getting: Better/worse/just the same. Does anything make it better?
Have you tried anything?
Does anything make it worse?
Is it worse on micturition (peeing)?
Is it worse on defecation (big jobbie)?
Associated features of attack: Pallor/headache/nausea/vomiting/fever/constipation/diarrhoea/dizziness/weakness/fainting/lightheadedness/others – specify/none
Special foods bring it on?: Chocolate/eggs/milk/others
Urinary symptoms: Wetting/frequency/dysuria (pain on passing urine)/scalding (burning)/other/no urinary symptoms/eneuresis (bedwetting)?
Other complaints: Aches or pains in back/chest/legs/pins and needles?/loss of weight/anorexia/fatigue/insomnia/nightmares/is the child a good sleeper?/others – specify
Impact of the pain on the child:
Does the pain significantly disrupt the lifestyle of the child or the family, in relation to: School/recreation/sleep/behaviour in home with friends
Household members: Total number:
/Mother/Father/others.
Medical problems in other members of the family: Hypertension/peptic ulcer/migraine/recurrent abdominal pain/depression/allergies/operations/others/worries about specific diseases?/Is anyone on medication for anything?

Mother's and father's health (past and present) Details:
Father's occupation:
Mother's occupation:
Family problems: Death/alcoholism/unemployment/job strain/financial problems/marital conflict/housing/change of address/born abroad
School performances: Position in class/number in class/ change of school/school reports/upper third/middle third/ last third/school absences or sent home/kept home/change of teacher/any bullying/problems with specific subject/ ?Irish/?Maths
Attitude to: School/homework/teachers/peers/mother/father
Extracurricular activities: Games/gymnastics/(physical education)/music/drama/dancing/swimming/languages/others
Career intentions:
Parents' opinion on cause of pain:

Personality type

1. Normal/average/casual/easygoing/happy/outgoing/ smiling
2. Worrier/anxious/striver/achiever/fussy/highly strung/tidy/perfectionist
3. Moody/shy/excitable/no patience/a temper/clinging/ sensitive/emotional
4. One word to describe yourself/him/her:

Physical examination

Weight:
Height:
Tense/relaxed/dermatographia – yes/no
Examination – easy/difficult/impossible
Investigations: Yes/No
Hb/MSU/U/S/Ba. meal/EEG/other
?any value?inpatient/?outpatient
Diagnosis: Explanation/drugs/diet/operation/admission/ readmission
Signed . . . .

Revisit:
Involvement of: Social worker/psychologist/child psychiatrist
Follow-up: Yes/How long?/No
Symptoms: Better/same/worse/cured
School absences: worse/same/better
Lost to follow-up: Yes/no
Date when last seen:
Findings if operation: ?Appendix/if appendix ?histology
Post-op course: Improved/same/worse
Additional information and progress

CHAPTER 44

The gallbladder and pancreas

M. DAVENPORT AND E.R. HOWARD

Diseases of the gallbladder
Diseases of the pancreas

References
Further reading

Diseases of the gallbladder

CONGENITAL ANOMALIES OF THE GALLBLADDER

Most developmental anomalies of the gallbladder are incidental findings. Robert Gross (1936) recorded several anatomical variants in an extensive literature review and described bilobar gallbladders as well as examples of duplication and diverticula. The gallbladder may also vary in position and has been recorded on the left side of the liver and within the liver substance (intrahepatic). Most of these anomalies have been identified in adults and have only rarely been associated with symptoms during childhood (Ternberg and Keating, 1975).

Gallbladder agenesis can occur as a single anomaly but is usually found in association with biliary atresia or with duodenal atresia (Coughlin *et al.*, 1992). Incomplete vacuolation of the lumen during development is believed to be the cause of a septate or multiseptate gallbladder and the septa may include muscle fibres in their structure. This anomaly may be complicated by stone formation secondary to bile stasis (Esper *et al.*, 1992). Multiseptate gallbladders have been described in association with congenital cystic disease of the bile ducts (Tan *et al.*, 1993).

ACUTE HYDROPS

Acute, symptomatic, distension of the gallbladder can occur in the absence of inflammatory change, calculi or any congenital anomaly. The aetiology is not clear, although the condition frequently follows upper respiratory tract infections and non-specific viral illness (Rumley and Rodgers, 1983). Mesenteric adenitis and Kawasaki disease (mucocutaneous lymph node syndrome: Maglavy *et al.*, 1978) have been reported as associated conditions. Chamberlain and Hight (1970) reviewed 29 cases and found a mean age at presentation of 5 years with a preponderance of boys. The presenting symptoms included abdominal pain, vomiting, tenderness in the right hypochondrium and a palpable gallbladder in about half of all cases. Hydrops is commonly misdiagnosed as appendicitis or intussusception, although a correct diagnosis can be made without difficulty with ultrasonography. Conservative treatment may be successful although the treatment of cases diagnosed at laparotomy has often consisted of either cholecystectomy or cholecystostomy (Maglavy *et al.*, 1978). Function does return in gallbladders left *in situ*.

ACUTE ACALCULOUS CHOLECYSTITIS

Acalculous cholecystitis may occur without a history of any preceding illness but more usually it is a complication of trauma or sepsis (Ternberg and Keating, 1975). Associated illnesses have included leptospirosis, scarlet fever and burn wound infection with *Pseudomonas* and *Salmonella typhimurium* (Roca *et al.*, 1988). Septicaemia and fever are typical and a mass in the right hypochondrium may be palpable. Jaundice occurs in approximately one-third of the cases associated with another illness. A laparotomy may be indicated either because of difficulty in diagnosis or because of failure of resolution with antibiotic therapy. A tube cholecystostomy is all that is needed for the majority of cases, although on occasion cholecystectomy may be indicated (Ternberg and Keating, 1975). This condition can occur in the neonatal period when it is usually confused with necrotizing enterocolitis (Fernandes *et al.*, 1989).

A rare variant of gallbladder inflammation in children, xanthogranulomatous cholecystitis, has been described (Ayling *et al.*, 1993) in a 10-year-old child who presented with a 5-month history of abdominal pain complicated by jaundice. The jaundice was secondary to involvement of the common bile duct in the inflammatory process. Cholecystectomy was performed and histological examination showed the typical features of chronic inflammation and nodules of lipid-laden macrophages.

ACUTE CHOLECYSTITIS AND CHOLELITHIASIS

Although cholelithiasis is unusual in children, an ultrasound screening programme of children between 6 and 15 years revealed a prevalence of 0.13%. This suggests that the diagnosis should be considered in cases of recurrent abdominal pain in childhood. Pigment stones are more prevalent in this age group, although cholesterol stones may be found. The more common underlying disorders include haemolytic anaemias such as spherocytosis, thalassaemia and sickle cell disease, and congenital anomalies of the biliary tract. One study (Reif *et al.*, 1991) identified 50 children with gallstones over a 10-year period, with a mean age of 12 years and a small female preponderance (3:2). There was no obvious underlying cause in 20% of this series.

Any chronic haemolytic process may cause the development of pigment stones in children. The prevalence may be as high as 60% in congenital spherocytosis, but is somewhat lower in homozygous sickle cell disease, ranging from 13 to 37% of cases (Flye and Silver, 1972; Webb *et al.*, 1989). The diagnosis of cholelithiasis in sickle cell patients is often difficult because recurrent jaundice, fever and leucocytosis do occur in sickling crises and the concomitant changes in liver function are often similar to those seen with biliary tract obstruction. Ultrasonography and biliary tract scintigraphy are useful for differentiating sickling crises from gallstone-induced abdominal pain, although a low predictive value was found for either test when used alone (Serafini *et al.*, 1987).

Complications, particularly chest infections and haemolytic problems, are not infrequent after surgery in sickle cell children, and preoperative transfusion regimens to reduce the levels of haemoglobin S are now in routine use. Preoperative hydration, meticulous intra-operative oxygenation and prevention of acidosis are also important in the management of the sickle patient (Banerjee *et al.*, 1991).

A preoperative ultrasound scan of the gallbladder should be performed if splenectomy is being considered for haemolytic disorders to detect gallstones in these children and concomitant cholecystectomy has been recommended even for asymptomatic stones (Pappis *et al.*, 1989).

Cholelithiasis in the neonatal period has been noted with increasing frequency and has been attributed to the increased use of total parenteral nutrition (TPN) and to more accurate diagnosis with improved ultrasound techniques. The formation of TPN-related gallstones is unclear but may include alterations in bile due to the amino acid infusion (Presig and Rennert, 1977) or to a lack of enteral stimulation. Biliary sludge appears to predate true stones and has been identified in approximately 40% of neonates receiving TPN (Matos *et al.*, 1987). Spontaneous resolution of cholelithiasis in infants has been reported (Keller *et al.*, 1985; Holgerson *et al.*, 1990), particularly if the stones were not calcified, and a conservative policy is now justified (St-Vil *et al.*, 1992), although complications can occur.

Heaton *et al.* (1991) reported nine infants with an obstructed biliary tree, caused by bile and sludge in seven infants aged 2–12 weeks, and by gallstones in two infants aged 4 and 6 months. Underlying factors such as prematurity or haemolysis were not present in most of these infants but there was a high incidence of congenital anomalies of the biliary tree.

Gallstones, predominantly pigment in composition, may be associated with ileal resection or disease. These are caused by a disturbance of the enterohepatic re-cycling of bile salts and an increased lithogenicity of bile (Pellerin *et al.*, 1975; Heuti *et al.*, 1982).

Outside the neonatal period, most authors recommend removal of gallstones, particularly if they are calcified. The standard procedure used to be cholecystectomy through a right subcostal incision, but recently this has been replaced in many centres by the technique of laparoscopic cholecystectomy. This has proved beneficial, particularly to children with sickle cell disease, because of a reduced morbidity from respiratory complications (Newman *et al.*, 1991; Holcombe *et al.*, 1991).

SPONTANEOUS PERFORATION OF THE COMMON BILE DUCT IN INFANCY

Spontaneous perforation of the common bile duct occurs typically during the first 2 months of life and over 80 cases have now been described. In all six cases seen at King's College Hospital, London (Davenport *et al.*, 1991), the perforation occurred at the junction of the cystic duct and common hepatic duct (Fig. 44.1). It has been suggested that this is a site of intrinsic weakness in the wall of the bile duct and that the perforation occurs during a transient duct obstruction and an elevation of intraduct pressure.

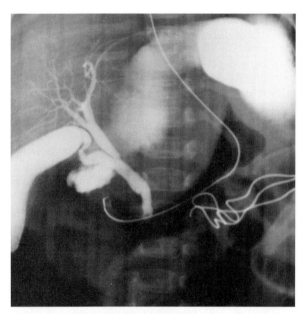

Fig. 44.1 Operative cholangiogram demonstrating a spontaneous perforation of the common bile duct at the junction with the cystic duct. This 3-month-old boy presented with mild jaundice and biliary ascites.

The clinical presentation is rarely acute. More usually the infant is noted to have progressive abdominal distension, jaundice and failure to thrive due to an accumulation of bile ascites. Bile-stained hydroceles or herniae are rare but are pathognomonic signs. Abdominal ultrasound shows either a complex heterogeneous mass in the right upper quadrant or a cystic collection of fluid with ascites. The ultrasound findings may be confused with a diagnosis of choledochal cyst. Intrahepatic biliary dilatation is unusual. Radioisotope hepatobiliary scans are useful in confirming the biliary nature of the ascites.

Surgical treatment is mandatory. Peritoneal lavage and simple drainage of the area of perforation may be successful in many cases (Lilly *et al.,* 1974), but an operative cholangiogram should first be performed through the gallbladder to confirm the diagnosis and allow assessment of the distal common bile duct. A congenital stricture of the duct will occasionally be identified (Davenport *et al.,* 1991). In many cases it is possible to insert a small T-tube (6 Fg) into the site of the perforation duct which allows the formation of a controlled fistula and a safe, rapid resolution of symptoms.

RHABDOMYOSARCOMA OF THE BILE DUCTS

Although this is the most common primary tumour of the biliary tree it accounts for less than 1% of all rhabdomyosarcomas (Ruyman *et al.,* 1985). The peak age of occurrence is 5 years and it affects boys and girls equally. The usual presentation is one of a painless,

obstructive jaundice. Ultrasound, computed tomography (CT) and magnetic resonance imaging (MRI) may allow a correct preoperative diagnosis by showing solid material within dilated intrahepatic and extrahepatic ducts, but laparotomy is usually indicated, if only for histological confirmation. The commonest site of origin is the region of the junction of common hepatic with the cystic duct and macroscopically the tumour appears as intraluminal polypoid masses and a plate-like thickening of the duct wall (Lack *et al.,* 1981). It infiltrates beneath duct epithelium into the liver substance and invades adjacent organs early, often limiting complete surgical resection. Metastases may be seen in up to 40% of children at presentation. Histologically, these tumours are embryonal rhabdomyosarcomas with botryoid features.

Currently, the aim of management of these aggressive tumours is to resect surgically as much of the tumour as possible and restore biliary continuity with a hepatico-jejunostomy. Cytotoxic chemotherapy, using agents such as actinomycin D, vincristine and cyclophosphamide, is then initiated and may be combined with local radiotherapy. The prognosis of such tumours is not good, despite advances in chemotherapy regimes, as there have been only 11 survivors from 66 reported cases in a recent review of the world literature (Heaton and Howard, 1991).

Diseases of the pancreas

DEVELOPMENTAL ANOMALIES

Complete agenesis of the human pancreas is rare and probably incompatible with life (Lemons *et al.,* 1979) although one case (Howard *et al.,* 1980) of survival to 26 months was reported with functional agenesis of the pancreas. Anatomical details in this case were, however, lacking. Hypoplasia and dysplasia leading to exocrine pancreatic insufficiency are associated with a number of usually hereditary syndromes such as the Schwachman–Diamond (1964) and the Johanson–Blizzard (1971) syndromes.

Embryology of the pancreas

The normal pancreas develops as two glandular structures arising from the primitive gastrointestinal tract at the junction of foregut and midgut (Fig. 44.2). The two portions arise from opposite sides of the duodenum but the ventral portion rotates clockwise (looked at from above) around the duodenal axis to converge and coalesce with the dorsal portion on the left side. The superior mesenteric vessels therefore become surrounded by glandular tissue. The distal portion of the main pancreatic duct (of Wirsung) is composed of the embryological dorsal duct but the proximal portion represents the original ventral duct. The accessory pancreatic duct (of

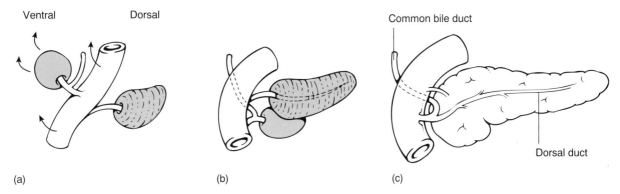

Fig. 44.2 A diagrammatic illustration of the embryological development of the pancreas. (a) Ventral and dorsal out-growths from the foregut; (b) the ventral portion of gland rotates clockwise around the duodenum; (c) fusion of the two duct systems to form the main pancreatic duct of Wirsung and the accessory duct of Santorini.

Santorini) is the original proximal portion of the dorsal duct. This coalescence of the two duct systems occurs at around 6 weeks' gestation.

Anomalies of this complex pattern of development can result in important clinical conditions such as annular pancreas and pancreas divisum.

Annular pancreas (see also Chapter 18)

At least two hypotheses have been suggested for the development of this condition. In 1910 Lecco proposed that the tip of the rotating ventral anlage remained fixed to the ventral duodenum and therefore persisted along the right side of the duodenum as rotation occurred. Previously, in 1901, Tieken suggested that the ventral anlage consisted of right and left elements and that as rotation occurs the left half persists and is drawn around the duodenum as a tongue (Tieken, 1901). A genetic basis for the anomaly has been inferred from the reports of familial annular pancreas (Jackson and Apostolides, 1978).

The annular pancreas is usually integral to the muscularis of the duodenal wall itself and most authors consider it to be related to abnormalities of duodenal development such as stenosis or atresia. Most large reports of intrinsic duodenal obstructions record the presence of an annular pancreas in up to one-third of cases.

Just over half of all cases of annular pancreas are recognized during childhood. Over 80% of the children present in the neonatal period (Kiernan *et al.*, 1980) and the usual clinical feature is of upper gastrointestinal obstruction with bile-stained vomiting. There may be a history of maternal polyhydramnios and 'meconium-stained' liquor due to prenatal vomiting. The classical double-bubble appearance on a plain radiograph may suffice for diagnosis in neonates, although contrast studies are usually required in later life. A relationship with pancreatitis has been noted in both adults (Drey, 1957) and in children (Crombleholme *et al.*, 1990; Tagge *et al.*, 1991).

Surgical treatment is directed towards the underlying duodenal pathology and a duodeno-duodenostomy is usually performed. Direct division of the annulus has a high complication rate, usually due to inadvertent pancreatic duct damage (Ravitch and Woods, 1950). No treatment is advised if an annulus is found incidentally, although a radiological evaluation of the duodenum should be performed.

Pancreas divisum

This term refers to a condition where a morphologically normal pancreas is composed of two independently drained glandular structures which retain their embryological drainage pattern. The body and tail of pancreas drain through the much smaller accessory duct owing to a failure of coalescence between the two primitive duct systems. Incomplete communication between the duct systems and a complete absence of the ventral duct are related anomalies. The term dominant dorsal duct syndrome has been used to encompass all these variants and implies that most of the pancreatic secretion occurs via the accessory or dorsal duct (Warshaw *et al.*, 1990).

Pancreas divisum is a common abnormality, that occurs in 6–10% (Cotton, 1980; Warshaw *et al.*, 1990) of the population. Although its presence has been related to acute and chronic pancreatitis it seems unlikely that such a common anomaly is responsible in itself for the complication. It has been suggested that the precipitating factor is an associated accessory duct stenosis. Although pancreas divisum is a congenital abnormality, it usually presents in adult life and the condition was not recorded in two large series of cases of pancreatitis in children (Syan *et al.*, 1987; Vane *et al.*, 1989). However, we now recommend that an endoscopic retrograde cholangiopancreatography (ERCP) examination be performed in children who present with 'idiopathic' acute pancreatitis to exclude both this and other congenital ductal anomalies (Wagner and Golladay, 1988; Adzick *et al.,* 1989). ERCP is now a practical procedure for all age groups, including infants (Wilkinson *et al.,* 1991).

The combination of pancreatic ultrasonography and secretin stimulation has been used in a series of 100 adults with pancreas divisum to demonstrate functional accessory duct obstruction and by implication those who might benefit from a duct drainage procedure (Warshaw *et al.,* 1990). Reports of surgical intervention in children have usually been favourable (Adzick *et al.,* 1989; Crombleholme *et al.,* 1990). Endoscopic sphincterotomy has been used in adults, often without success (Russell *et al.,* 1984), and if treatment is indicated, a formal transduodenal sphincterotomy or sphincteroplasty is probably the procedure of choice (Russell *et al.,* 1984; Adzick *et al.,* 1989; Tagge *et al.,* 1991).

PANCREATITIS IN CHILDHOOD

Acute pancreatitis

Pancreatitis in children has many features in common with the adult disease; however, some points are peculiar to children.

Acute pancreatitis is an uncommon cause of acute abdominal pain in childhood. Severe epigastric pain and persistent vomiting are typical and abdominal ultrasonography and a serum amylase estimation should be diagnostic. Other biochemical tests such as raised serum trypsin and lipase may be useful in some cases. Awareness of the condition in childhood is all important in diagnosis.

There are many aetiological factors in this age group (Table 44.1). The most common causes include secondary effects of drugs (particularly cytotoxic chemotherapy), blunt abdominal trauma (e.g. seat belts and child abuse) and congenital anomalies of the pancreatic duct (e.g. stenosis and common pancreatobiliary channel) (Synn *et al.,* 1987; Weizman and Durie, 1988). Gallstone-induced pancreatitis may be seen at times, particularly in sickle cell anaemia and spherocytosis (Synn *et al.,* 1987), and acute pancreatitis may complicate multisystem diseases such as the Reye syndrome and the haemolytic uraemic syndrome (Weizman and Durie, 1988). In the Reye syndrome, for instance, pancreatitis has been recorded in up to two-thirds of cases but the neurological manifestations, particularly encephalopathy, may mask abdominal symptoms and specific tests such as a serum amylase level become very important. Pancreatitis, although rare in childhood, is an occasional complication of mumps (Kobayashi *et al.,* 1989), but in this condition a raised serum amylase may also be secondary to an associated parotitis.

Pancreatitis may be induced by blockage of the pancreatic duct and, world-wide, the most common cause is

Table 44.1   Causes of acute pancreatitis in childhood

Anatomical or structural	Common channel (Tagge *et al.,* 1991) (especially with choledochal cyst)
	Pancreas divisum (Cotton, 1980) Anomalous entry of pancreatic duct (Doty *et al.,* 1985) Duplication cyst (Akers *et al.,* 1972) Annular pancreas (Tagge *et al.,* 1991) Stenosis of ampulla
Drug induced	Steroids Azathioprine L-Asparaginase
Duct occlusion	Gallstones (e.g. sickle cell disease) Ascariasis (Khuroo *et al.,* 1990, 1992) Foreign body
Viral	e.g. Mumps (Kobayashi *et al.,* 1989)
Trauma	Blunt (e.g. seat belt, child abuse) Post-ERCP
Multisystem or metabolic	Reye syndrome Haemolytic uraemic syndrome Wilson's disease Cystic fibrosis Hypercalcaemia Hyperlipidaemia (types I, IIa and IV)

the roundworm *Ascaris lumbricoides* (Khuroo *et al.*, 1990, 1992). The parasite inhabits the upper gastrointestinal tract and may migrate through the duodenal ampulla into the biliary or pancreatic ducts causing biliary colic, cholangitis or acute pancreatitis. A report from Kashmir of 500 children and adults with documented hepatobiliary and pancreatic ascariasis included 31 who presented with acute pancreatitis (Khuroo *et al.*, 1990). ERCP has a therapeutic role in the management of these patients and successful removal of worms from the ampulla and ducts during episodes of acute pancreatitis has been reported using biopsy forceps and endoscopic baskets. Standard anti-helminthic therapy (e.g. mebendazole) is also required.

Pancreatitis may follow direct surgical or endoscopic trauma to the duct system and may follow an ERCP examination, for instance and has also been reported after open-heart surgery. A high prevalence of a raised serum amylase and acute pancreatitis was described in 54 children after cardiac procedures (Leijala and Louhimo, 1988).

A high incidence of pancreatitis has been noted in the group of children with mental retardation and cerebral palsy and an association with gastric fundoplication was described in these patients (Ravitch and Woods, 1950). The reason for the relationship remains unclear.

The principles of management in the acute phase include intravenous fluid support, effective analgesia, restriction of oral intake and anticipation of complications. It is important to point out that childhood acute pancreatitis is not a benign disease and once diagnosed it demands observation and management identical with that recommended in the adult patient. Significant mortality rates of 17–21% have been reported (Synn *et al.*, 1987; Weizman and Durie, 1988), although many of the deaths may be attributed to the underlying multisystem disease. The operative treatment and investigation of recurrent acute pancreatitis is detailed below.

Typical early complications, such as hypoglycaemia and hypocalcaemia, experienced in adults with acute pancreatitis may occur in children. The most commonly reported late complication is pseudocyst formation which may present with abdominal pain and vomiting caused by gastric outlet obstruction. The outcome is variable and in a series of 25 children who developed the complication one-third were managed conservatively, half had a cystogastrostomy and the remainder a cystojejunostomy-en-Roux (Millar *et al.*, 1988).

Chronic pancreatitis

This is probably underrecognized as a cause of chronic abdominal pain in children and adolescents (Fig. 44.3). It may also present as food avoidance, weight loss, growth retardation and even developmental delay before overt pancreatic exocrine and endocrine failure becomes apparent. Obstructive jaundice may be caused

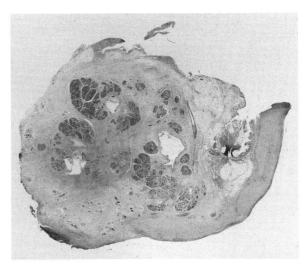

Fig. 44.3 Histological section from the distal pancreas of an 11-year-old boy with a long history of idiopathic chronic pancreatitis. The resected distal pancreas shows a reduced number of pancreatic acini surrounded by fibrous tissue. Dilated ducts are also seen. This segment of pancreas was surrounded by a pseudocyst.

by stenosis of the common bile duct (Wheatley and Coran, 1988).

Hereditary pancreatitis usually presents in childhood and is inherited as an autosomal dominant disease with variable penetrance. A defect in cellular cytochrome coxidase activity may be identified in a few cases (Kato *et al.*, 1990). The usual age of onset is 10 years and approximately 80% of cases have developed symptoms by 20 years. It is important to exclude other hereditary metabolic disorders such as alpha-1-antitrypsin deficiency, hyperparathyroidism with hypercalcaemia and hyperlipaemia prior to diagnosing hereditary pancreatitis. In

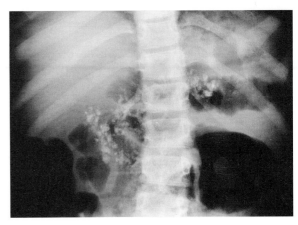

Fig. 44.4 Plain abdominal X-ray from a 10-year-old girl who had a long history of idiopathic relapsing pancreatitis. Calcification is seen throughout the head and body of the gland.

some of these patients pancreatic calcification may be seen on plain abdominal radiographs (Fig. 44.4) and abnormally dilated ducts and occasionally strictures may be found on ERCP, although it may be difficult to decide whether these are primary or secondary lesions. In 42 patients with hereditary pancreatitis it was suggested that surgical intervention should be restricted to those with demonstrable duct anomalies (Moir *et al.*, 1992).

Congenital ductal anomalies should be identified with ERCP or intraoperative cholangiopancreatography (Jackson and Apostolides, 1978; Cotton, 1980; Scott *et al.*, 1984). A common pancreatobiliary channel, particularly in association with a choledochal cyst, should be treated by pancreatobiliary disconnection and biliary drainage into a Roux loop (see Chapter 22) (Figs 44.5 and 44.6). Main or accessory duct drainage procedures such as sphincteroplasty or sphincterotomy may be indicated for ampullary stenoses and retrograde drainage procedures [e.g. Puestow's longitudinal pancreatojejunostomy (Scott *et al.*, 1984; Crombleholme *et al.*, 1990) or distal pancreatojejunostomy] are useful for more distal strictures and dilated pancreatic ducts.

HYPERPLASTIC, NEOPLASTIC AND ALLIED DISORDERS OF THE PANCREAS

Nesidioblastosis (Greek: nesidion – islet)

This condition is characterized clinically by persistent hypoglycaemia and symptoms are commonly noted in the neonatal period. It accounts for approximately 1% of cases of hypoglycaemia in early infancy (Spitz *et al.*,

1992). Although it is usually an isolated, sporadic condition it may occur as part of the multiple endocrine neoplasia syndrome (Vance *et al.*, 1972; Thompson *et al.*, 1989) and can be familial (Moreno *et al.*, 1989). Pathologically it is divisible into two types, focal and diffuse, which occur with equal frequency (Goossens *et al.*, 1989). Classical nesidioblastosis, islet cell hyperplasia and other allied adenomatoses, including islet cell adenoma, may be thought of as a spectrum of disease and the term islet cell dysmaturation syndrome has been applied to the whole group (Bjerke *et al.*, 1990).

Most infants have a high birth weight and demonstrable hepatomegaly due to excess glycogen deposition. The diagnosis is of some urgency as cerebral damage and mental retardation are a consequence of poorly treated neonatal hypoglycaemia. Rapid correction, often with large amounts of glucose (e.g. 10–25 mg/kg/min), via a central venous line is mandatory if the diagnosis is considered. Inappropriate hyperinsulinaemia in the presence of hypoglycaemia confirms the diagnosis.

Radiological imaging is not usually helpful, although occasionally an adenoma may be demonstrated. Medical

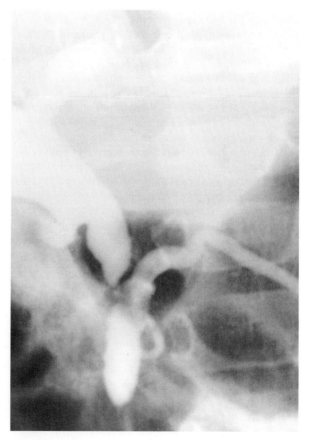

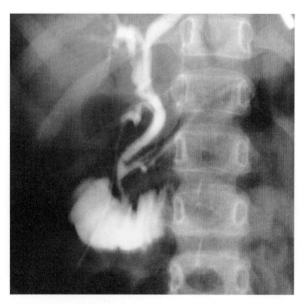

Fig. 44.5 Operative cholangiogram showing a long common pancreaticobiliary channel without associated choledochal cyst. This 7-year-old girl presented with pancreatitis and was cured by hepaticojejunostomy.

Fig. 44.6 Operative cholangiogram showing a long common pancreaticobiliary channel, in association with a fusiform choledochal cyst, in a 6-year-old girl with pancreatitis.

therapy includes diazoxide, glucagon and the somato-statin analogue octreotide (Battershill and Clissold, 1989). Surgery is recommended if medical treatment fails. It is unusual to find a macroscopic abnormality at laparotomy and therefore the surgeon must be prepared to perform a near-total pancreatectomy. The amount of pancreatic tissue to be removed in nesidioblastosis has been controversial. Subtotal (approximately 75%) resection is associated with a failure rate of at least 50% and a near-total pancreatectomy is now recommended (Harken *et al.*, 1971). Approximately 95% of the pancreas, including the uncinate process, is removed but a thin rim of tissue is conserved to protect the common bile duct and duodenal vascular arcade (Warden *et al.*, 1988). The spleen is preserved whenever possible. Exocrine and endocrine failure have been recorded after this operation but it is uncommon. Clinical exocrine failure was recorded in only one of seven, following near-total pancreatectomy, although impaired enzyme and bicarbonate secretion could be demonstrated in about half of the remainder (Dunger *et al.*, 1988).

Islet cell adenomas

Functioning insulin-secreting islet cell adenomas occur in an older age group and present with hypoglycaemic episodes. The features of Whipple's triad are diagnostic when symptoms occur during a period of fasting in association with hypoglycaemia and are relieved by the administration of glucose. Precise preoperative localization of the tumour should be attempted with selective arteriography and venous insulin sampling, as limited pancreatic resections are adequate. Adenomas arise in the body and tail of the pancreas in approximately 75% of cases and multicentric tumours are found in about 14%. At operation a typical islet cell tumour is usually pink and well-encapsulated. Enucleation or distal pancreatectomy may be all that is required although

rebound hyperglycaemia may follow. If a rapid insulin assay is available then this should be used to confirm the completeness of the operation.

Islet cell tumours producing other hormones have been recorded in childhood, for example vasoactive polypeptide (VIP)-producing tumours, although in contrast with adult patients the majority are found in association with neurogenic tumours such as ganglioneuromas and neuroblastomas (Grosfeld *et al.*, 1990). Two have been recorded arising from pancreas – one in a non-beta cell adenoma in the tail of the pancreas (Brenner *et al.*, 1986) and one associated with generalized islet cell hyperplasia (Ghishan *et al.*, 1979). No cases of somatostatinoma or glucagonoma have been reported in children.

The Zollinger–Ellison syndrome of resistant peptic ulceration due to hypergastrinaemia may occur in children and of the 44 cases in the US Childhood Disease Registry (Tudor, 1988), 38 were in boys, with a mean age at presentation of 11 years (Grosfeld *et al.*, 1990). Forty-one cases were due to a pancreatic gastrinoma, of which 65% were malignant.

Cystic lesions of the pancreas

Pancreatic cysts are uncommon in childhood and the usual cause is a pseudocyst following blunt abdominal trauma. Table 44.2 is a representative classification based on the type of epithelial lining and whether the cyst is congenital or acquired (Howard, 1989). Developmental or congenital cysts are lined by epithelium with a deeper layer of acinar tissue. Although these are usually asymptomatic and confined to the body or tail of the pancreas they can cause obstructive jaundice (Pilot *et al.*, 1964). Intrapancreatic gastric duplication cysts (Akers *et al.*, 1972) are often small but may cause symptoms (e.g. recurrent pancreatitis). Careful resection after identification of any ductal communication is indicated (Welch, 1986). Multiple pancreatic cysts may

Table 44.2 Classification of pancreatic cysts

Congenital	Single true cyst
	Polycystic disease:
	    (a) pancreas alone
	    (b) as part of systemic disorder
	        (e.g. von Hippel–Lindau, polycystic kidney, cystic fibrosis)
	Dermoid cyst (Assawamatiyanont and King, 1977)

Neoplastic	Serous cystadenoma Mucinous cystadenoma – cystadenocarcinoma Papillary–cystic neoplasm (Todani *et al.*, 1988)
Acquired	Parasitic (e.g. hydatid disease) Retention cysts (Welch, 1986) Tropical fibrocalcareous disease (Olurin, 1971)
Pseudocysts	Trauma (Ford *et al.*, 1990) Acute and chronic pancreatitis

occur as part of a multisystem disorder such as the von Hippel–Lindau syndrome (an association of retinal haemangiomas, cerebellar cysts or tumours and pheochromocytomas), polycystic kidney disease and cystic fibrosis. Most of these cysts are asymptomatic. Rare cases of pancreatic dermoid cysts have been recognized, typically containing thick sebaceous material, teeth and cartilage (Assawamatiyanont and King, 1977). Protein-calorie malnutrition in developing countries may also produce fibrocalcareous changes in the pancreas leading to cyst formation (Olurin, 1971).

Although proliferative and neoplastic cysts rarely present in childhood, a few cases, particularly of mucinous cystadenoma, have been reported (Gunderson and Javis, 1969). These cysts are found more commonly in girls and are slow growing, insidious and often located in the body and tail of the pancreas. It is possible to treat large lesions by internal drainage but most authors (Grosfeld *et al.*, 1990) advocate total excision wherever possible because of the risk of malignant change (Tsukimoto *et al.*, 1973; Hodgkinson *et al.*, 1978).

Malignant lesions of the pancreas

Malignant tumours of the pancreas are rare in children. Histologically they are either adenocarcinoma of acinar cell rather than ductal cell origin or islet cell carcinoma (Lack *et al.*, 1983; Tersigni *et al.*, 1984). Acinar cell tumours have periodic acid-Schiff (PAS)-positive granules and zymogen granules within the cytoplasm. A few cases of rhabdomyosarcoma have also been reported (Vane *et al.*, 1989). Adenocarcinoma tends to present late with advanced local disease and in the 12 cases reviewed by Welch (1986) all were dead within 10 months of presentation despite a variety of treatment modalities. The Japanese experience with this tumour was similarly bleak and just under half had metastases or were unresectable from local spread at the time of presentation (Tsukimoto *et al.*, 1973). Where complete surgical resection was not possible neither chemotherapy nor radiotherapy had any effect on survival.

The term pancreatoblastoma has been used to describe tumours arising in infants and young children with features of a more differentiated histological pattern which typically includes an organoid and rosette pattern formation (Horie *et al.*, 1977). An increase in plasma α-fetoprotein has been reported (Morohoshi *et al.*, 1990; Inomata *et al.*, 1992). These lesions are usually encapsulated and long-term survival has been seen after complete resection (Horie *et al.*, 1977) or, in one report, after chemotherapy (Inomata *et al.*, 1992). Certain syndromes such as the Beckwith–Wiedemann syndrome seem to have an association not only with the development of hepatoblastoma and nephroblastoma but also with pancreatoblastoma (Drut and Jones, 1988).

Papillary–cystic tumour of the pancreas (Frantz's tumour) is an unusual low-grade neoplasm which occurs almost exclusively in young women and girls. In a series of 116 cases with this tumour half were under 19 years at presentation and only two occurred in males (Todani *et al.*, 1988). Most of the tumours presented with slowly growing abdominal masses with calcification on the abdominal radiograph. The typical operative findings were of a well-demarcated pancreatic mass with a thick capsule, calcification and a mixed solid and cystic appearance (Todani *et al.*, 1988; Matsunou and Konishi, 1990; Ward *et al.*, 1993). The origin is thought to be from totipotent primordial pancreatic cells capable of differentiating along exocrine or endocrine lines (Todani *et al.*, 1988). Oestrogen or progesterone receptors have occasionally been demonstrated on some of the cell lines (Ladanyi *et al.*, 1987). Most authors have reported long-term survival and cure in adequately resected tumours (Lack *et al.*, 1983; Todani *et al.*, 1988; Jaksic *et al.*, 1992; Ward *et al.*, 1993).

PANCREATIC TRAUMA

Pancreatic trauma in children is usually due to certain well-defined injuries. Thus bicycle handlebar injury (45%) and child abuse (18%) were the most common causes of blunt pancreatic trauma requiring laparotomy in one series from the USA (Smith *et al*, 1988). CT, ultrasound and ERCP are useful investigations for demonstrating major pancreatic duct damage, which is the single most important prognostic factor (Fig. 44.7). However, clinical experience has shown that this is still often difficult to achieve with any degree of sensitivity or specificity. A rising serial serum amylase has also been used to differentiate major from minor pancreatic trauma (Smith *et al.*, 1988).

The diagnosis of major duct damage indicates the need for early laparotomy (Syn *et al.*, 1987). If there has been distal duct disruption then a formal distal pancreatectomy with splenic preservation should be performed (Smith *et al.*, 1988). More proximal duct damage may require distal pancreaticojejunostomy-en-Roux to try to preserve functioning tissue.

A pseudocyst may occur as a later complication or may be the presenting feature if the original injury was masked or trivial. Spontaneous resolution of traumatic pseudocysts occurs in about half of the cases reported (Bass *et al.*, 1988). For the remainder there are a number of options such as percutaneous drainage of pseudocysts in children. Failure of resolution in three of four cases with percutaneous drainage has been reported (Rescorla *et al.*, 1990), whilst others had complete success in three of their children where this method was used (Bass *et al.*, 1988).

The critical diagnostic question is whether or not there has been major duct disruption and, although CT scans are useful (Bass *et al.*, 1988), ERCP remains the most satisfactory investigative tool (Rescorla *et al.*, 1990). Laparotomy and internal drainage still have a

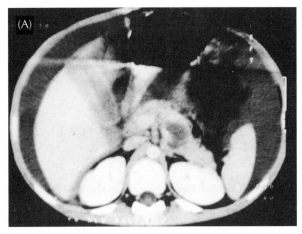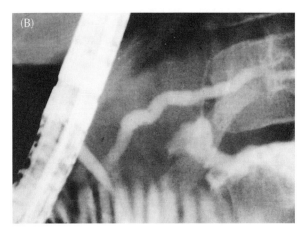

Fig. 44.7 (A) CT scan of the pancreas in a 10-year-old boy who had suffered an abdominal injury and subsequent pancreatitis and ascites. A cystic area is seen at the junction of the head and body of the gland. (B) ERCP examination in the same boy showing a leak of contrast from the main pancreatic duct. The injury healed after 1 month of conservative treatment.

place in the management of pseudocysts although it is uncertain whether this should be reserved for failed percutaneous drainage. Ford *et al.* (1990) have suggested that these cysts mature at an earlier stage than in adults and that internal drainage may be performed at about 3–4 weeks, compared with 5–6 weeks in adults. Eight of 16 children in this series underwent cystgastrostomy without complication.

References

Adzick, N.S., Shamberger, R.C., Winter, H.S. and Hendren, W. H. 1989: Surgical treatment of pancreas divisum causing pancreatitis in children. *Journal of Pediatric Surgery* **24**, 54–8.

Akers, D.R., Favara, B.E., Franciosi, R.A. and Nelson, J.M. 1972: Duplication of the alimentary tract. Report of three unusual cases associated with the bile and pancreatic ducts. *Surgery* **71**, 817–23.

Assawamatiyanont, S. and King, A.D., Jr 1977: Dermoid cysts of the pancreas. *American Surgeon* **43**, 503–4.

Ayling, R.M., Heaton, N.D., Davenport, M., Driver, M. and Howard, E.R. 1993: Xanthogranulomatous cholecystitis in a 10 year old boy. *Pediatric Surgery International* **8**, 170–2.

Banerjee, A.K., Layton, D.M., Rennie, J.A. and Bellingham, A.J. 1991: Safe surgery in sickle cell disease. *British Journal of Surgery* **78**, 516–17.

Bass, J., Di-Lorenzo, M., Desjardins, J.G., Grignon, A. and Ouimet, A. 1988: Blunt pancreatic injuries in children: the role of percutaneous external drainage in the treatment of pancreatic pseudocysts. *Journal of Pediatric Surgery* **23**, 721–4.

Battershill, P.E. and Clissold, S.P. 1989: Octretide. A review of pharmacokinetic properties and therapeutic properties and therapeutic potential in conditions associated with excessive secretion. *Drugs* **38**, 658–702.

Bjerke, H.S., Kelly, R.E., Geffner, M.E. and Fonkalsrud, E.W. 1990: Surgical management of islet cell dysmaturation syndrome of young children. *Surgery, Gynecology and Obstetrics* **191**, 321–5.

Brenner, R.W., Sank, L.I., Kerner, M.B. *et al.* 1986: Resection of a vipoma in a 15 year old girl. *Journal of Pediatric Surgery* **21**, 983–5.

Chamberlain, J.W. and Hight, D.W. 1970: Acute hydrops of the gallbladder in childhood. *Surgery* **68**, 899–905.

Cotton, P.B. 1980: Congenital anomaly of pancreas divisum as cause of obstructive pain and pancreatitis. *Gut* **21**, 105–14.

Coughlin, J.P., Rector, F.E. and Klein, M.D. 1992: Agenesis of the gallbladder in duodenal atresia: two case reports. *Journal of Pediatric Surgery* **27**, 1304.

Crombleholme, T.M., deLorimier, A.A., Way, L.W., Adzick, N.S., Longaker, M.T. and Harrison, M.R. 1990: The modified Puestow procedure for chronic relapsing pancreatitis in children. *Journal of Pediatric Surgery* **25**, 749–54.

Davenport, M., Heaton, N.D. and Howard, E.R. 1991: Spontaneous perforation of the bile duct in infancy. *British Journal of Surgery* **78**, 1068–70.

Doty, J., Hassall, E. and Fonkalsrud, E.W. 1985: Anomalous drainage of the common bile duct into the 4th part of the duodenum. *Archives of Surgery* **120**, 1077–9.

Drey, N.W. 1957: Symptomatic annular pancreas in the adult. *Annals of Internal Medicine* **46**, 750–72.

Drut, R. and Jones, M.C. 1988: Congenital pancreatoblastoma in Beckwith–Wiedemann syndrome: an emerging association. *Pediatric Pathology* **8**, 331–9.

Dunger, D.B., Burns, C., Ghale, G.K., Muller, D.P.R., Spitz, L. and Grant, D. Pancreatic exocrine and endocrine function after subtotal pancreatectomy for nesidioblastosis. *Journal of Pediatric Surgery* **23**, 112–15.

Esper, E., Kaufman, D.B., Crary, G.S., Snover, D.C. and Leonard, A.S. 1992: Septate gallbladder with cholelithiasis: a cause of chronic abdominal pain in a 6 year old child. *Journal of Pediatric Surgery* **27**, 1560–2.

Fernandes, E.T., Hollabaugh, R.S., Boulden, T.F. and Angel, C. 1989: Gangrenous acalculous cholecystitis in a premature infant. *Journal of Pediatric Surgery* **24**, 608–9.

Flye, M.W. and Silver, D. 1972: Biliary tract disorders and sickle cell disease. *Surgery* **72**, 361–7.

Ford, E.G., Hardin, W.D., Jr, Mahour, G.H. and Wooley, M.M. 1990: Pseudocyst of the pancreas in children. *Annals of Surgery* **56**, 384–7.

Ghishan, F.K., Soper, R.T., Nassif, E.G. *et al.* 1979: Chronic diarrhoea of infancy: non-beta cell hyperplasia. *Pediatrics* **64**, 46–9.

Goossens, A., Gepts, W., Saudubray, J.M. *et al.* 1989: Diffuse and focal nesidioblastosis. A clinicopathological study of 24 patients with persistent hyperinsulinaemic hypoglycemia. *American Journal of Surgical Pathology* **13**, 766–75.

Grosfeld, J.L., Vane, D.W., Rescorla, F.J., McGuire, W. and West, K.W. 1990: Pancreatic tumours in childhood: analysis of 13 cases. *Journal of Pediatric Surgery* **25**, 1057–62.

Gross, R. E. 1936: Congenital anomalies of the gallbladder: a review of 148 cases, with report of a double gallbladder. *Archives of Surgery* **32**, 132–62.

Gunderson, A.K. and Javis, J. F. Pancreatic cystadenoma in childhood. *Journal of Pediatric Surgery* **4**, 478–81.

Harken, A.H., Filler, R.M., AvRuskin, T.W. and Crigler, J.F. 1971: The role of total pancreatectomy in treatment of unremitting hypoglycemia. *Journal of Pediatric Surgery* **6**, 284–9.

Heaton, N.D. and Howard, E.R. 1991: Tumours of the extrahepatic bile ducts. In Howard, E.R. (ed.), *Surgery of liver disease in childhood*. Oxford: Butterworth-Heinnemann, 107–12.

Heaton, N.D., Davenport, M. and Howard, E.R. 1991: Intraluminal biliary obstruction. *Archives of Disease in Childhood* **66**, 1395–8.

Heubi, J.E., Soloway, R.D. and Balisteri, W.F. 1982: Biliary lipid composition in healthy and diseased infants, children and young adults. *Gastroenterology* **82**, 1295–9.

Hodgkinson, D.J., ReMine, W.H. and Weiland, L.H. 1978: A clinicopathological study of 21 cases of adenocarcinoma. *Annals of Surgery* **188**, 679–84.

Holcombe, G.W., Olsen, D.O. and Sharp, K.W. 1991: Laparoscopic cholecystectomy in the pediatric patient. *Journal of Pediatric Surgery* **26**, 1186–90.

Holgerson, L.O., Stolar, C., Berdon, W.E., Hilfer, C. and Levy, J.S. 1990: Therapeutic implications of acquired choledochal obstruction in infancy: spontaneous resolution in three infants. *Journal of Pediatric Surgery* **25**, 1027–9.

Horie, A., Yano, Y., Kotoo, Y. and Miwa, A. 1977: Morphogenesis of pancreatoblastoma, infantile carcinoma of the pancreas. Report of two cases. *Cancer* **39**, 247–54.

Howard, C.P., Go, V.L.W., Infante, A.J., Perrault, J., Gerrich, J.E. and Haymond, M.W. Long-term survival in a case of functional pancreatic agenesis. *Journal of Pediatrics* **97**, 786–9.

Howard, J.M. 1989: Cystic neoplasms and true cysts of the pancreas. *Surgical Clinics of North America* **69**, 651–65.

Inomata, Y., Nishizawa, T., Takasan, H., Hayakawa, and Tanaka K. 1992: Pancreatoblastoma resected by delayed primary operation after effective chemotherapy. *Journal of Pediatric Surgery* **27**, 1570–2.

Jackson, L.G. and Apostolides, P. 1978: Autosomal dominant inheritance of annular pancreas. *American Journal of Medical Genetics* **1**, 319–21.

Jaksic, T., Yaman, M., Thorner, P., Wesson, D.K, Filler, R.M. and Shandling, B. 1992: A 20 year review of pediatric pancreatic tumors. *Journal of Pediatric Surgery* **27**, 1315–17.

Johanson, A. and Blizzard, R. 1971: A syndrome of congenital aplasia of the alae nasi, deafness, hypothyroidism, dwarfism, absent permanent teeth and malabsorption. *Journal of Pediatrics* **79**, 981–7.

Kato, S., Miyabayashi, S., Ohi, R. *et al.* 1990: Case report: chronic pancreatitis in muscular cytochrome c oxidase deficiency. *Journal of Pediatric Gastroenterology and Nutrition* **11**, 549–52.

Keller, M.S., Markle, B.M., Laffey, P.A. *et al.* 1985: Spontaneous resolution of cholelithiasis in infants. *Radiology* **157**, 345–8.

Khuroo, M.S., Zargar, S.A., Yattoo, G.N., Koul, P., Khan, B. A., Dar, M.Y. and Alai, M.S. 1992: Ascaris-induced acute pancreatitis. *British Journal of Surgery* **79**, 1335–8.

Khuroo, M.S., Zargar, S.A. and Mahajan, R. 1990: Hepatobiliary and pancreatic ascariasis in India. *Lancet* **335**, 1503–6.

Kiernan, P.D., ReMine, S.G., Kiernan, P.C. and ReMine, W.H. 1980: Annular pancreas: Mayo clinic experience from 1957 to 1976 with review of the literature. *Archives of Surgery* **115**, 46–50.

Kobayashi, A., Tatsumo, K., Takagi, Y. and Sakoh, A. 1989: Exocrine function in children with mumps pancreatitis. *Acta Paediatrica Scandinavica* **78**, 129–30.

Lack, E.E., Cassady, J.R., Levey, R. and Vawter, G.F. 1983: Tumors of the exocrine pancreas in children and adolescents. *American Journal of Surgical Pathology* **7**, 319–27.

Lack, E.E., Perez-Atayde, A.R. and Shuster, S.R. 1981: Botryoid rhabdomyosarcoma of the biliary tree. *American Journal of Surgical Pathology* **5**, 643–52.

Ladanyi, M., Mulay, S., Arsenau, J. *et al.* 1987: Estrogen and progesterone receptor determination in the papillary cystic neoplasm of the pancreas with immunohistochemical and ultrastructural observations. *Cancer* **60**, 1604–11.

Lecco, T.M. 1910: Zur Morphologie des Pankreas Annulare. *Sitzungsb Akad Wissensch* **119**, 391–406.

Leijala, M. and Louhimo, I. 1988: Pancreatitis after open-heart surgery in children. *European Journal of Cardiovascular Surgery* **2**, 324–8.

Lemons, J.A., Ridenour, R. and Orsini, E.N. 1979: Congenital absence of the pancreas and intrauterine growth retardation. *Pediatrics* **64**, 255–7.

Lilly, J.R., Weintraub, W.H. and Altman, R.P. 1974: Spontaneous perforation of the extrahepatic bile ducts and bile peritonitis in infancy. *Surgery* **75**, 664–73.

Maglavy, D.B., Speert, P. and Siver, T.M. 1978: Mucocutaneous lymph node syndrome, report of 2 cases complicated by acute hydrops and diagnosed by ultrasound. *Pediatrics* **61**, 699–702.

Matos, C., Avni, E.F., Van Gausbeke, D. *et al.* 1987: Total parenteral nutrition and gallbladder disease in neonates. *Journal of Ultrasound Medicine* **6**, 243–8.

Matsunou, H. and Konishi, F. 1990: Papillary-cystic neoplasm of the pancreas. A clinicopathological study concerning the tumor aging and malignancy of nine cases. *Cancer* **65**, 283–91.

Millar, A.J.W., Rode, H., Stunden, R.J. and Cywes, S. 1988: Management of pancreatic pseudocysts in children. *Journal of Pediatric Surgery* **23**, 122–7.

Moir, C.R., Konzon, K.M. and Perrault, J. 1992: Surgical therapy and long-term follow-up of childhood hereditary pancreatitis. *Journal of Pediatric Surgery* **27**, 282–7.

Moreno, L.A., Turck, D., Gottrand, F. *et al.* 1989: Familial hyperinsulinism with nesidioblastosis of the pancreas: further evidence for autosomal recessive inheritance. *American Journal of Medical Genetics* **34**, 584–6.

Morohoshi, T., Sagawa, F. and Mitsuya, T. 1990: Pancreatoblastoma with marked elevation of serum alpha fetoprotein. *Virchows Archives* **416**, 265–70.

Newman, K.D., Marmon, L.M., Attorri, R. and Evans, S. 1991: Laparoscopic cholecystectomy in pediatric patients. *Journal of Pediatric Surgery* **26**, 1184–5.

Olurin, E.O. 1971: Pancreatic cysts: a ten year review. *British Journal of Surgery* **58**, 502–8.

Pappis, C.H., Galanski, S., Moussatos, G., Keramidas, D. and Kattamis, C. 1989: Experience of splenectomy and cholecystectomy in children with chronic hemolytic anaemia. *Journal of Pediatric Surgery* **24**, 543–6.

Pellerin, D., Bertin, P., Nihoul-Fekete, C.L. and Racour, C.L. 1975: Cholelithiasis and ileal pathology in childhood. *Journal of Pediatric Surgery* **10**, 35–41.

Pilot, L.M., Gooselaw, J.G. and Issacson, P.G. 1964: Obstruction of the common bile duct by a pancreatic cyst. *Lancet* **84**, 204.

Presig, R. and Rennert, O. 1977: Biliary transport and cholestatic effects of amino acids. *Gastroenterology* **73**, 1240.

Ravitch, M.M. and Woods, A.C. 1950: Annular pancreas. *Annals of Surgery* **132**, 1116–27.

Reif, S., Sloven, D.G. and Lebenthal, E. 1991: Gallstones in children. Characterization by age, etiology and outcome. *American Journal of Gastroenterology and Nutrition* **145**, 105–8.

Rescorla, F.J., Cory, D., Vane, D.W., West, K.W. and Grosfeld, J.L. 1990: Failure of percutaneous drainage in children with traumatic pancreatic pseudocysts. *Journal of Pediatric Surgery* **25**, 1038–42.

Roca, M., Sellier, N., Maensire, A. *et al.* 1988: Acute acalculous cholecystitis in *Salmonella* infection. *Pediatric Radiology* **18**, 421–3.

Rumley, T.O. and Rodgers, B.M. 1983: Hydrops of the gallbladder in children. *Journal of Pediatric Surgery* **18**, 138–40.

Russell, R.C., Wong, N.W. and Cotton, P.B. 1984: Accessory sphincterotomy (endoscopic and surgical) in patients with pancreas divisum. *British Journal of Surgery* **71**, 954–7.

Ruymann, F.B., Raney, R.B., Crist, W.M., Lawrence, W., Lindberg, R.D. and Soule, E.H. 1985: Rhabdomyosarcoma of the biliary tree in childhood. A report of the intergroup rhabdomyosarcoma study. *Cancer* **56**, 575–81.

Schwachman, H., Diamond, L.K., Oski, F.A. and Khaw, K.T. 1964: The syndrome of pancreatic insufficiency and bone marrow dysfunction. *Journal of Pediatrics* **64**, 645–63.

Scott, H.W., Jr, Neblett, W.W., O'Neil, J.A., Jr *et al.* 1984: Longitudinal pancreaticojejunostomy in chronic pancreatitis with onset in childhood. *Annals of Surgery* **199**, 610–22.

Serafini, A.N., Spoliansky, G., Sfakianskis, G.N., Montalvo, B. and Jensen, W.N. 1987: Diagnostic studies in patients with sickle cell anaemia and acute abdominal pain. *Archives of Internal Medicine* **147**, 1061–2.

Smith, S., Nakayama, D.K., Gantt, N., Lloyd, D. and Rowe, M. 1988: Pancreatic injuries in childhood due to blunt trauma. *Journal of Pediatric Surgery* **23**, 610–14.

Spitz, L., Bhargava, R.K., Grant, D.B. and Leonard, J.V. 1992: Surgical treatment of hyperinsulinaemic hypoglycaemia in infancy and childhood. *Archives of Disease in Childhood* **67**, 201–5.

St-Vil, D., Yazbeck, S., Luks, F.I., Hancock, B.J., Filiatrault, D. and Youssef, S. 1992: Cholelithiasis in newborns and infants. *Journal of Pediatric Surgery* **27**, 1305–7.

Synn, A.Y., Mulvihill, S.J. and Fonkalsrud, E.W. 1987: Surgical management of pancreatitis in childhood. *Journal of Pediatric Surgery* **22**, 628–32.

Tagge, E.P., Smith, S.D., Raschbaum, G.R., Newman, B. and Wiener, E.S. 1991: Pancreatic ductal abnormalities in children. *Surgery* **110**, 709–17.

Tan, C.E.L., Howard, E.R., Driver, M. and Murray-Lyon, I.M. 1993: Noncommunicating multiseptate gallbladder and choledochal cyst: a case report and review of the literature. *Gut* **34**, 853–6.

Ternberg, J.L. and Keating, J.P. 1975: Acute acalculous cholecystitis: complication of other illnesses in childhood. *Archives of Surgery* **110**, 543–7.

Tersigni, R., Arena, L., Alessandroni, L. *et al.* 1984: Pancreatic carcinoma in childhood: case report of long survival and review of the literature. *Surgery* **96**, 560–6.

Thompson, N.W., Bondeson, A.G., Bondeson, L. and Vinik, A. 1989: The surgical treatment of gastrinoma in MEN I syndrome patients. *Surgery* **106**, 1081–6.

Tieken, T. 1901: Annular pancreas. *American Journal of Medicine* **2**, 826.

Todani, T., Shimada, K., Watanabe, Y., Toki, A., Fujii, T. and Urushihara, N. 1988: Frantz's tumor: a papillary and cystic tumor of the pancreas in girls. *Journal of Pediatric Surgery* **23**, 116–21.

Tsukimoto, I., Watanabe, K., Lin, J.B. and Nakajima, T. 1973: Pancreatic carcinoma in children in Japan. *Cancer* **31**, 1203–7.

Tudor, R.B. 1988: Childhood Disease Registry. Bismarck, ND.

Vance, J.E., Stoll, R.W., Kitabachi, A.K., Buchanan, K.D., Hollander, D. and Williams, R.H. 1972: Familial nesidioblastosis as the predominant manifestation of multiple endocrine adenomatosis. *American Journal of Medicine* **52**, 211–27.

Vane, D.W, Grosfeld, J.L., West, K.W. and Rescoria, F.J. 1989: Pancreatic disorders in infancy and childhood: experience with 92 cases. *Journal of Pediatric Surgery* **24**, 771–6.

Wagner, C.W. and Golladay, E.S. 1988: Pancreas divisum and pancreatitis in children. *American Surgeon* **54**, 22–6.

Ward, H.C., Leake, J. and Spitz, L. 1993: Papillary cystic cancer of the pancreas: diagnostic difficulties. *Journal of Pediatric Surgery* **28**, 89–91.

Warden, M.J., German, J.C. and Buckingham, B.A. 1988: The surgical management of hyperinsulinism in infancy due to nesidioblastosis. *Journal of Pediatric Surgery* 1988; **23**, 462–5.

Warshaw, A.L., Simeone, J.F., Schapiro, R.H. and Flavin-Warshaw, B. 1990: Evaluation and treatment of the dominant dorsal duct syndrome (pancreas divisum redefined). *American Journal of Surgery* **159**, 59–66.

Webb, D.K., Darby, J.S., Dunn, D.T., Terry, S.I. and Serjeant, G.R. 1989: Gallstones in Jamaican children with homozygous sickle cell disease. *Archives of Disease in Childhood* **89**, 693–6.

Weizman, Z. and Durie, P.R. 1988: Acute pancreatitis in childhood. *Journal of Pediatrics* **113**, 24–9.

Welch, K.J. 1986: The pancreas. In Welch, K.C., Randolph, J.G., Ravitch, M.M., O'Neil, J.A. and Rowe, M.I. (eds), *Pediatric surgery* , 4th ed. Chicago; IL: Year Book Medical Publishers; 1086–106.

Wheatley, M.J. and Coran, A.G. 1988: Obstructive jaundice secondary to chronic pancreatitis in children: report of two cases and review of the literature. *Surgery* **104**, 863–9.

Wilkinson, M.L., Mieli-Vergani, G., Ball, C., Portmann, B. and Mowat, A.P. 1991: Endoscopic retrograde cholangio-pancreatography in infantile cholestasis. *Archives of Disease in Childhood* **66**, 121–3.

Further reading

Davenport, M. and Howard, E.R. 1991: Surgical treatment of pancreatic disease in childhood. In Johnson, C.D. and Imrie, C.W. (eds), *Pancreatic disease: progress and prospects*. London: Springer, 333–50.

Howard E.R. 1991: *Surgery of liver disease in children*. London: Butterworth-Heinemann.

CHAPTER 45

Constipation

D.M. GRIFFITHS

Introduction   Clinical features
Definition   Neurogenic bowel
Anatomy   References
Physiology

Introduction

All paediatric surgical trainees need to be aware that the family of a child who is 'only' constipated may be just as worried and anxious as the family of a child with a more obvious surgical disease. In fact, they may be even more worried, as they have probably been struggling for months with a screaming, miserable, intermittently anorexic child, whose bowel habit has become more important than anything else at home and the main topic of long distance phone calls, if a family member is away from home. In addition, the family may be fed up with unhelpful professionals who have been dismissive of their problem.

Although the vast majority of children with constipation should be managed by the general practioner and health visitor, with support from the paediatric community district nurse, many families are seen in hospital by paediatricians. A few come to paediatric surgeons, either for exclusion of major pathology (e.g. Hirschsprung's disease) or because of complications (e.g. prolapse and piles). Thus, although there may appear to be many constipated children in the surgical clinic or in hospital as emergency admissions, many more are treated by more appropriate doctors in the community or in medical departments.

There are no miracle cures for constipated children. Most children have had their problem for months before medical advice is sought and this results in a distended atonic bowel. It will take months or even a year for the bowel to work normally again and the parents need to accept this at the start.

Definition

Not only parents differ about what they mean by constipation, so do doctors, even gastroenterologists who deal with the problem every day.

The present author prefers the definition 'difficulty or delay in the passage of stools', (not a description of the hardness of the stool, although this is often but not always associated; Clayden and Agnarsson, 1991), to that of 'constipation is defined by the consistency of the stool, not the frequency of defecation ... A constipated stool is in a small ball or partially segmented with a hard leading end' (Jones and Woodward, 1986). Parents can mean either, but the first definition has the advantage of including children who have a colon, sigmoid and rectum full of stools, who pass them daily, but who have no control because the rectum is always full.

Anatomy

Traditional anatomists describe multiple pelvic floor muscles as if they are isolated entities similar to limb muscles, associated with a separate anal sphincteric complex, with an internal sphincter of smooth muscle and a striated external sphincter. These pelvic floor muscles (ischiococcygeus, puborectalis, pubococcygeus, rectourethralis, etc.) are all neatly delineated and labelled with great care. They are separate from the anus, although the fibres of one muscle (pubococcygeus) are located between the subdivisions of the external sphincter, and the puborectalis sling is attached to the top of the anal canal to create the anorectal angle. The internal sphincter is a thickening of the circular smooth muscle fibres of the rectum and appears obvious in the diagrams. The external sphincter is similarly clearly divided into three parts (subcutaneous, superficial and deep), all with a different cross-sectional shape.

Surgically, the situation is rather different (Pena, 1986). The entire pelvic floor and external sphincter consists of a continuous sheet of voluntary muscle which is funnel shaped. It is attached anteriorly to the pubis, posteriorly to the coccyx and laterally to the pelvis and ischiae. This muscle sheet is attached medially to the rectum at its junction with the anus and becomes cylindrically shaped around the anal canal as the external sphincter. The anatomical separation is not at all obvious. However, the anterior fibres from the pubis, when contracting, will tend to pull the anus forwards and other, more vertical, fibres will tend to pull the anus up, i.e. the levator ani effect.

Unlike the pylorus, the cylindrical extension of the muscular funnel around the anal canal consists not of circular muscle, but of two bundles of fibres on either side of the anus, enclosing one half each, and merging anteriorly and posteriorly enough to mimic a completely circular muscle. They continue as paramedian or parasagittal fibres, running posteriorly to the coccyx and anteriorly to the perineal body (Figs 45.1 and 45.2).

The internal sphincter is indistinguishable from the circular muscle of the rectum and is not an obviously separate structure. Physiologically, although an increased tone in the anal canal exists, it is possibly due not only to the all-powerful internal sphincter, but to all of the anal muscles, including the voluntary external sphincter and the lower part of the pelvic floor.

Physiology

CONTINENCE

Normally the rectum is empty, with the faecal mass in the sigmoid colon. The faeces are not passed because of the very sophisticated anorectal continence mechanisms that can distinguish between solid, liquid and gas, allowing the latter to pass at times when the solid or liquid faeces must be retained.

The valves of Houston and the anorectal angle physically impede the faeces. The anorectal angle is 80–90° at rest and becomes more obtuse (100–105°) during defaecation. The valves cause the rectum to be kinked with a major kink at the anorectal angle. Any rise in intra-abdominal pressure causes a flap-valve collapse of the rectum and a flutter-valve collapse of the anorectum.

The longitudinal mucosal folds of the anus come together even when the internal sphincter is partially relaxed.

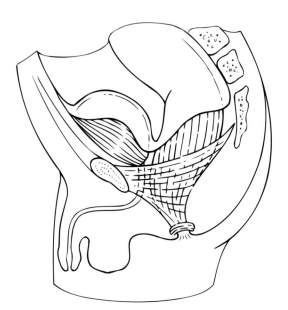

Fig. 45.1 Normal male anatomy, sagittal view (relaxation). (After Pena, Surgical management of anorectal malformations, New York: Springer, 1990.)

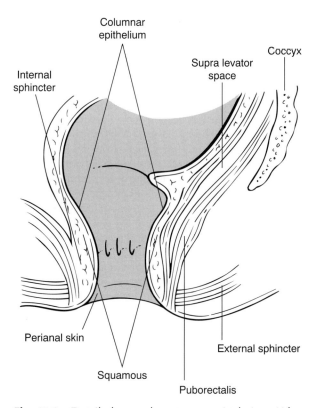

Fig. 45.2 Detailed normal anatomy, sagittal view. (After Pena, Surgical management of anorectal malformations, New York: Springer, 1990.)

Both the involuntary internal sphincter and the voluntary external sphincter have a resting tone. This anal tone of about 30–40 mmHg will normally protect against soiling. The external sphincter fatigues rapidly when maximally contracted (about 30 s in children).

The sensory innervation of the rectum (via stretch receptors) and anus (via touch receptors) allow the brain to exert voluntary control over the passage of faeces.

DEFECATION

The physiology of defecation is straightforward, but requires a correct, continuous sequence of motor and sensory nervous messages to produce the results that the child and the parent desire. By definition, therefore, there are many ways in which the sequence can go wrong. The normally empty rectum fills due to sigmoid contractions. Distension of the rectum activates its stretch receptors, causing contraction of the rectal and right colonic smooth muscle and inhibition of the internal and external anal sphincters (the anorectal reflex). The sensation of the desire to defecate grows ever greater as the stool descends towards the anal canal. The pelvic floor descends because the levator ani and funnel relax, straightening the anorectal angle and allowing the stool to descend on to the sensory zone of the anorectal canal. As the anus becomes directly stimulated, the external sphincter contracts, causing a further increase in rectal pressure and contraction, producing an urgent desire to defecate and relaxation of the external sphincter. By increasing the intra-abdominal pressure, straining aids expulsion of the faeces through the anus.

As the rectum empties, the internal and external sphincters recover their resting tone and the child experiences relief from the desire to defecate, reinforced by parental acclaim.

The physiological events (rectal filling, distension, sensation, contraction and anal relaxation) and the psychological events (perception of the sensation of rectal filling, voluntary sphincter relaxation, social and learned responses) all inter-relate to an extreme degree which is not present in, say, swallowing food. Thus any family with a child who has problems with defecation needs to have both the physical and psychological parts of the problem treated, whether the initial cause is physical or psychological.

Clinical features

BABIES

Medical

The bowel habit of babies depends on whether they are breastfed or bottle-fed. Breastfed babies exhibit huge variation in stool frequency, from ten times per day to once every 10 days, whilst bottle-fed babies usually go once or twice a day. Constipation in babies is usually acute, of short duration and dramatically affected by simple measures such as increasing the fluid intake or adding fruit juice (especially orange juice) or brown sugar to the feed.

Surgical

Ninety-five per cent of normal babies pass meconium within the first 24 hours. Any baby not passing meconium by then should be thoroughly examined for obvious anatomical abnormalities, e.g. anorectal anomalies, or more subtle anomalies which require a rectal examination, such as anal or rectal stenosis.

Mild degrees of anterior ectopia are said to be associated with an increased incidence of constipation and may require surgical treatment (Hendren, 1978). Not all paediatric surgeons would agree with this, although it is true that obvious low anomalies have a lifetime tendency to constipation.

Hirschsprung's disease will present in neonates with failure to pass meconium, bile-stained vomiting and distension. Depending on the length of aganglionic bowel and the physiological function of the remainder, the baby or older child may present at any age with constipation. If there are faeces down to the anus, then Hirschsprung's disease is very unlikely, and an acquired cause needs to be treated.

Children with high anorectal anomalies are more likely to be incontinent than constipated. Those with low anorectal anomalies have a lifetime tendency to constipation and should never be allowed to wait for more than 48 hours without opening their bowels. As the problem is at the extreme end of the bowel, common sense suggests that this tendency to constipation is best treated not by oral laxatives, but by suppositories.

TODDLERS

Medical

The diet of toddlers and infants is often lacking in anything that is good for them, especially any form of fibre. This may result in hard motions which are infrequently passed and can be managed by attempting to improve the diet.

The standard 'drugs' used are lactulose and senakot. Lactulose is a modified sugar which is not absorbed, but causes the colonic flora to multiply, thus producing larger, softer stools. It is given twice or three times daily and the dose is increased until the stools are soft. Toddlers love it because it is sweet, but it will dissolve teeth and these need to be brushed after medication.

Senakot can be given as tablets, granules or elixir, and is made from senna pods. The pharmacological action is the same as with figs and prunes. It is absorbed from the stomach and secreted into the colon where it stimulates colonic contractions 8–10 hours later. Thus, it is best given at night to take advantage of the gastro-colic reflex after breakfast. Again, the dose needs to be increased from 5 ml of elixir nightly until the child is opening his or her bowels consistently, after which the dose needs to be reduced slightly.

Once the child's bowel is under the parents' control and can be made to function on a regular basis, the worst scenario is for the laxatives to be stopped suddenly. The constipation, which has taken weeks or months to develop, will instantly recur and the whole family becomes dispirited. This disaster occurs because the bowel, which is full of faeces and has emptied poorly for a long time, has become dilated and poorly motile. As the lactulose and senakot ensure regular emptying, the size and motility return to normal, but this may take months, so the parents need to be warned of this at the outset. The laxatives therefore need to be reduced very slowly, in the knowledge that if the stool consistency or frequency falters the doses can be increased once again (increase the lactulose to soften the stool and increase the senakot to ensure its evacuation).

Surgical

Anal fissures

These are common in toddlers and cause painful, bright red bleeding on defecation. Unlike fissures in adults, they are usually anterior and heal without any surgical intervention. The dietary vagaries of the toddler produce a hard motion which tears the delicate anal mucosa. This bleeds, is painful and causes anal spasm. Next time the urge to defecate arises, the toddler remembers the pain and deliberately hangs on, producing another hard motion which tears the anal mucosa again. This vicious cycle is terrible for both the child and the parents. Treatment with enough lactulose (to make the motions soft), senakot (to make the child go regardless), and 5% xylocaine (to anaesthetize the anus), breaks the cycle in three places and allows healing to occur. Simultaneously, the diet needs to be improved. The laxatives must be continued until the bowel is working normally and the toddler is no longer hanging on because of the memory that defecation used to hurt.

Giving a suppository to a child with an anal fissure is cruel. As a last resort, an anal stretch may still be justifiable in a child, though the long-term results are unknown. Lateral internal sphincterotomy may be more physiological. Both probably work by making the child incontinent long enough for the fissure to heal.

Rectal prolapse

A prolapse is a concentric, dark red, shiny, moist lump protruding from the anus which may bleed. It may occur in two groups of toddlers. It is usually associated with persistent, sustained straining to pass a large hard faecal mass which, at this age, is usually performed whilst squatting on a potty. Some feel that this position may make a prolapse more likely. Alternatively, prolapse occurs with profuse diarrhoea, as in malnutrition or malabsorption (1% of children with cystic fibrosis present with prolapse).

If a child's rectum prolapses the parent will be terrified and require reassurance that their child will usually recover without surgery. They need to be taught to lie the child down on a bed or sofa, when most prolapses will spontaneously reduce. If not, gentle pressure will reduce it, but this may be more than some parents, usually mothers, are prepared to do. Wearing a rubber glove makes it slightly easier, but thick kitchen paper may be more convenient.

Children over 18 months old can be taught to 'pant like a dog' instead of straining abdominally during defecation. This mimics a midwife's advice during the second stage of labour.

The cause should be treated, either by laxatives or by investigation of the diarrhoea. The parents need constant reassurance that the prolapse will usually stop recurring by itself, but that this may take months.

A few recalcitrant prolapses require surgical assistance and fixation can be hastened by the injection of 5% phenol in almond oil circumferentially above the anal valves as a day case under general anaesthetic. Only in the most unusual cases will a surgical operation be necessary.

OLDER CHILDREN

Medical

The older child is more likely to have a psychological cause for constipation, once the obvious dietary and surgical causes have been excluded. This may be a problem at home with parental toileting pressure, or sibling rivalry or bullying at school. Although the primary problem may be psychological, the resulting constipation requires just as much active, medical, laxative management as any other child with constipation, whilst the underlying cause is resolved.

Surgical

Faecaloma

After many weeks of inefficient bowel action, some children develop a faecal mass or faecaloma in the rectum, which may be palpable abdominally. This may cause continuous soiling, either from spurious diarrhoea as liquid faeces flow around the faecaloma, or as the child passes small portions of the mass through a half-open anus. Rectal sensation is usually absent and the child is unaware of the presence of the mass, although older children may be able to palpate their own mass abdominally and complain of it.

Opinions differ as to how to treat the faecaloma. Huge doses of liquid paraffin (Parachoc®) will emulsify it, but this treatment is not available in the UK. Other oral laxatives are ineffective when faced with a huge mass of this sort. Therefore the kindest treatment is a manual evacuation under general anaesthetic. This is not a procedure to be delegated to a very junior trainee, as they may be less than thorough at emptying absolutely all possible faeces from the rectum and colon. The anus is stretched as part of the procedure and this may be therapeutic if there has been a fissure as well. Intensive medical management of the underlying constipation is vital to prevent a relapse.

External haemorrhoidal veins

Some children present with a lump beside the anus due to a varicosity of the external haemorrhoidal plexus of veins. This differs from a prolapse as it is purple, is not moist, and is to one side of the anus, but it may bleed. Sometimes the dilated veins completely surround the anus, producing a spectacular effect. Unlike piles in adults, which arise from the internal haemorrhoidal plexus, these dilated veins usually resolve with time and the family should be given firm reassurance. However, sometimes the anxiety generated is best treated by an active manoeuvre and the veins can be sclerosed with 5% phenol in almond oil (or even excised) as a day case under a general anaesthetic.

'Soggy bottom'

A moist, sore anus with multiple radial fissures on to the perianal skin, bright red bleeding and painful defecation is due to a group A streptococcal infection. Any secondary constipation should be treated and either oral penicillin V and adjuvant fucidin or Timodene ointment applied to the anus for 3 weeks. Recurrence is possible.

Rectal polyp

A juvenile polyp may present at any age with painless bright red rectal bleeding, but is rare in neonates and toddlers. It is a hamartoma, is usually solitary and 80% are within the view of a sigmoidoscope. They may autoamputate and the stump may then become a form of pyogenic granuloma with persistent painless rectal bleeding. A rectal examination is unnecessary in outpatients because the history will make a sigmoidoscopy necessary as a day case under a general anaesthetic. Low polyps may prolapse through the anus and cause diagnostic confusion with rectal prolapse and external haemorrhoidal veins, as well as being easy to miss with a sigmoidoscope if the low rectum is not examined carefully. There is no increased risk of carcinoma and, if anything, the presence of juvenile polyps is associated with an increased life expectancy.

Neurogenic bowel

The denervated colon has a very slow rate of spontaneous motility, which allows the extra efficient absorption of faecal water, resulting in hard motions which are infrequently passed. There may be associated spurious diarrhoea, so that the ensuing faecal incontinence may be for both solid and liquid faeces. In adolescence, this will lead to low self-esteem and depression.

As with the neurogenic bladder, much has been made of the difference between high and low lesions, but it has become apparent that since the spinal lesion can be patchy and asymmetric, the clinical presentation may be far from clear cut. Thus, treatment regimes that hinge on the presence or absence of the anocutaneous reflex are unreliable (stroking the perianal skin with an orange stick to elicit contraction of the external sphincter).

In spina bifida, most children have no rectal sensation, or voluntary external sphincter and many have no ability to strain abdominally. Some have large faecal masses with long transit times which are suddenly expelled with no warning. Others may have a little rectal sensation but no efficient retention mechanism and their tendency to incontinence may be exacerbated by the fact that they have limited mobility. There is no correlation between the extent of limb paralysis, bladder control and bowel control. This will depend on the medical and physical capabilities of the child and the family.

MEDICAL TREATMENT

Diet, fluids and toileting routines

If the child can be persuaded to eat a high-fibre diet, with plenty of fluid, this may make the stools less hard, but if it makes them too soft then the incontinence may become worse.

Regular visits to the toilet after meals to catch the gastrocolic reflex may suggest some form of control, but the time involved may be counterproductive.

Biofeedback

This involves training the child to recognize that they are about to defecate, enabling them to withhold the stool long enough to pass it into the toilet. However, it has not been shown to be any more useful than regular toilet visits.

Manual evacuation

For many younger children this is the mainstay of continence. Firm motions are easily removed once or twice a day by the parents, and the child may well be completely clean in between, especially if sedentary. However, those who can walk usually find this method inadequate.

Oral medications

As with a high-fibre diet, stool softeners may help or hinder the child by producing softer motions that may leak more easily. Stimulant laxatives are unpredictable, and unless there is rectal sensation will tend to contribute little. A very few children with neurogenic bowel have a tendency to diarrhoea and they may be helped by codeine or Imodium (loperimide).

Suppositories and enemata

The fundamental problem with both these forms of treatment is the lack of a competent sphincter. This usually allows the suppository or enema to be expelled long before it has been useful, although enough may be retained to allow partial evacuation. Stimulant suppositories, e.g. Dulcolax (Bisacodyl), or enemata, e.g. Fletcher's phosphate enema, are the most successful.

The Shandling tube

This instrument was designed to avoid the problem of the lack of a competent sphincter (Shandling and Gilmour, 1987). The tube is essentially a modified Foley catheter with a T-bar to prevent overinsertion. With the balloon fully inflated, there is a seal at the anus. The colonic lavage (20 ml 0.9% sodium chloride/kg) is retained and mechanical flushing of the colon is achieved.

Once the child and their parents overcome their initial horror at the physical size and appearance of the tube, an encouraging specialist nurse can achieve excellent results with continence, cleanliness and psychological improvement. However, it is technically quite awkward to use and older children who wish to become independent can find it too difficult, unless they have good co-ordination and are determined to succeed.

Surgical

MACE (Malone antegrade continence enema)

This is a combination of two well-established ideas: on-table colonic lavage through the appendix stump and the Mitrofanoff principle (Griffiths and Malone, 1995). One end of the appendix on its blood supply is re-implanted into the caecum and the other brought out to the skin, preferably at the umbilicus. This allows a phosphate enema and lavage to be given directly into the caecum, resulting in a complete colonic evacuation, often within 30–40 min.

This operation works best in children with a neurogenic bowel, although it can also work in children with high anorectal anomalies, Hirschsprung's disease and severe constipation. In children with a neurogenic bowel the success rate approaches 80%, and can allow a motivated adolescent to become independent of their carers, which is an important psychological step.

As with all operations there is a complication rate, which is not true of suppositories. The most common problems are stomal, with breakdown and stenosis occurring in a percentage of cases. The percutaneous insertion of a caecostomy has been shown to be efficient and avoids a laparotomy (Shandling *et al.*, 1996).

A major advantage of the operation is that, unlike some reconstructive procedures, the fallback operation, colostomy, is still possible if the MACE fails.

Colostomy

Before embarking on a colostomy in a child, the parents and child need to be seen and assessed by the paediatric stoma nurse, who can discuss the rights and wrongs, advantages and disadvantages, and ins and outs of stomas with them. Some families benefit from meeting another child with a stoma, before this discussion or at least preoperatively.

In the child who is faecally incontinent, or has constipation that is totally resistant to everything, a colostomy is not a disaster but a miracle. It can allow a child who is completely worn out by enemata, lavage and operations to regain some control and lead a more normal life. Freedom from other people attacking their anus, the lack of soiling and the absence of colic induced by phosphate enemata are all positive advantages of colostomies.

Before resorting to surgery, every child will have jumped through all of the medical hoops and still be constipated. These children and their families are desperate and want a success first time. Most will not initially countenance a colostomy, so a MACE is a more appropriate operation. But if the MACE fails, either because the child cannot be made clean or because they cannot cope with the MACE regime, then a colostomy will not be a retrograde step at all.

A right transverse/hepatic flexure end colostomy is easier to manage than an ileostomy because the effluent is a sludge rather than a slurry. The position of the bag is critical and will depend on many factors, including the mobility of the child and any previous surgery.

The residual colon can be oversewn and left *in situ*, thus minimizing the operation, but if defunctioned colitis is a problem with a bloody, mucous discharge, then colonic lavage with short-chain fatty acids may help. If necessary, the residual bowel may have to be removed, leaving just a rectal stump.

Most complications related to the stoma bag can be solved by the paediatric stoma care nurse, but a poorly constructed stoma may need revision. The most common surgical complications are prolapse, retraction, stenosis and bleeding.

- Prolapse: This is not usually a mucosal prolapse, as occurs at the anus, but an intussusception of redundant proximal bowel. This can be avoided by ensuring that the bowel is unable to intussuscept. A left iliac fossa colostomy can usually be made extraperitoneally, but this is awkward in the right upper quadrant. Some surgeons attach the colon to the anterior abdominal wall, but leaving the right colon attached to the posterior abdominal wall and only mobilizing enough to construct the stoma should be more successful. The surgeon can attempt to ignore minor prolapses, although the patient may be very aware of the bulky stoma and expect one as flush as the one they started with. Major prolapses require revision. Some families will go to enormous lengths to avoid reoperation, including bandaging the abdomen with crepe bandages for years, but revision is inevitable. These families need to be aware of the risk of strangulation of the prolapsed bowel. Usually the prolapse will reduce spontaneously on lying down and resting, but some come to reduction under a general anaesthetic. This is usually an out-of-hours emergency and revision should be delayed to an elective list. This allows time for the oedema to settle and for a full rediscussion of the need for a stoma with the parents and child.

- Retraction: This is usually due to ischaemia and associated with stenosis. It requires revision.
- Stenosis: This may be of the bowel, due to ischaemia, or at the level of the rectus sheath hole if this is not initially of adequate size. Dilatation is usually a waste of time and revision is required.

- Bleeding: This is usually due to major prolapse and very distressing to the child and family. The bleeding does not warrant treatment as such, but the prolapse does.

References

Clayden, G. and Agnarsson, U. 1991: *Constipation in childhood*. Oxford: Oxford Medical Publications.

Griffiths, D.M. and Malone, P.S. 1995: The Malone antegrade continence enema. *Journal of Paediatric Surgery* **30**, 68–71.

Hendren, W. H. 1978: Constipation caused by anterior location of the anus and its surgical correction. *Journal of Paediatric Surgery* **13**, 505–12.

Jones, P.G. and Woodward, A.A. (eds) 1986: *Clinical paediatric surgery*, 3rd ed. Oxford: Blackwell Scientific.

Pena, A. 1986: Anatomical considerations relevant to faecal continence. *Seminars in Surgical Oncology* **3**, 141–5.

Shandling, B and Gilmour, R.F. 1987: The enema continence catheter in spina bifida: successful bowel management. *Journal of Paediatric Surgery* **22**, 271–3.

Shandling, B., Chait, P.G. and Richards, H.F. 1996: Percutaneous cecostomy: a new technique in the management of fecal incontinence. *Journal of Pediatric Surgery* **31**, 534–7.

CHAPTER 46

Portal hypertension

H. RODE

Introduction
Pathophysiology
Aetiology
Classification

Consequences of portal hypertension
Clinical features
Management
References

Introduction

Portal hypertension is defined as impairment of venous outflow from the portal tract with pressures exceeding 11 mmHg in the portal system or a splenic pulp pressure exceeding 16 mmHg (Whitington, 1985).

The obstruction to portal venous flow is either pre-hepatic, intrahepatic or suprahepatic and this distinction has important practical implications regarding aetiology, clinical presentation, complications, management and outcome. Portal hypertension and resultant compensatory portosystemic shunting and hepatic parenchymal function are particularly responsible for many of the important complications. In general terms, the following assumptions can be made. Varices are usually the result of portal hypertension, variceal bleeding is usually well tolerated in children and sclerotherapy has largely replaced portosystemic shunts. Ascites is well controlled with nutritional care and diuretics, splenic embolization is preferred to splenectomy and liver transplantation is a very valuable therapeutic alternative for children with end-stage liver disease and portal hypertension. The underlying disease process will determine the ultimate prognosis.

Pathophysiology

Portal hypertension results from a complex interplay of events within the mesenteric–portohepatic circuit. The normal valveless portal venous system has the capacity to accommodate large changes in portal blood flow. The direction of flow is determined by pressure gradients and vessel patency. Two theories have been proposed: the 'backward/resistance' theory, where portal hypertension is attributed to increased resistance in portal venous flow (hepatofugal) and the 'forward-flow' theory in which increased splanchnic inflow into the portal circulation (hepatopetal) maintains high portal pressures, despite the run-off through portosystemic collaterals (Witte *et al.*, 1974; Benoit *et al.*, 1985; Sikuler and Groszman, 1986; Rikkers, 1990).

In cirrhotic portal hypertension the architecture of the liver is distorted principally at sinusoidal level by cirrhosis, fibrosis and regenerating liver nodules causing resistance to flow and elevated portal pressures with further damage to the hepatic parenchyma. Recent studies have shown a dynamic vascular component to flow resistance based on perivenular and perisinusoidal myofibroblast mediators (Bhathol and Grosman, 1985). Porto-collateral smooth muscle vasculature can also play a dynamic role within the resistance theory (Garcia-Tsao and Groszman, 1987). The backward theory therefore has two components, i.e. fixed and dynamic.

The 'forward-flow' theory is based on hyper-dynamic splanchnic circulation (Rikkers, 1990). It is presumed to act as a compensatory protective homeostatic mechanism to maintain hepatic perfusion and functions through increased cardiac output, reduced peripheral vascular resistance and splanchnic hyperaemia (Karrer,

1992). Although the mechanisms of these changes are not clearly understood, factors such as an expanded plasma volume, portosystemic shunting, an increase in humoral vasodilators (glucagon), decreased sensitivity to vasoconstrictors or aberrant autonomic control may be involved (Okumura *et al.*, 1989; Rikkers, 1990; Karrer, 1992).

The disturbed haemodynamic pathway within the portal system and the resultant compensatory portosystemic shunting are responsible for many of the important complications. Obstruction proximal to the hepatic sinusoids is seen more commonly in children, hepatic cellular function is usually better preserved, ascites and coagulopathy are rare, general nutrition is satisfactory, bleeding episodes are easier to control and the prognosis is improved. The outcome of obstruction distal to the sinusoids (cirrhosis) is poorer, hepatic function is often compromised and progressively deteriorating and complications are worse, with more ascites, coagulopathy and bleeding (Karrer, 1992).

Longstanding portal hypertension is also associated with portal hypertensive intestinal vasculopathy most often involving the stomach (gastropathy) and can be a common source of bleeding. The significance of small bowel involvement (enteropathy) is unclear and colonic involvement (colopathy) can simulate inflammatory bowel disease. Surgical decompression can prevent both acute and chronic rebleeding and has shown reversibility of endoscopic and histological changes (Viggiano and Gostout, 1992).

Aetiology

The causes of portal hypertension are usually divided into presinusoidal, sinusoidal and postsinusoidal, depending on the anatomical site of increased resistance to flow. This does not account for the considerable overlap between the presinusoidal and sinusoidal components of portal hypertension in different types of cirrhosis and whether the hepatic parenchyma *per se* is subject to high pressures or not. Non-cirrhotic portal hypertension is nearly always due to increased vasculature resistance. A schematic presentation of common causes for portal hypertension in children is shown in Table 46.1.

Classification

PREHEPATIC OBSTRUCTION

In the paediatric age group, prehepatic obstruction is most commonly the result of portal vein obstruction. Portal vein thrombosis may result from perinatal omphalitis, intra-abdominal sepsis, umbilical vein catheterization or severe neonatal illness and dehydration. The thrombosis may involve the main portal vein and bifurcation or extend into the distal intrahepatic branches (Howard, 1991). In over 50% of children no definitive aetiology can be identified (Galloway and Henderson, 1990). Other causes, such as congenital

Table 46.1 Common causes of portal hypertension

Anatomical site		Causes
Suprahepatic		Budd–Chiari syndrome Veno-occlusive disease Constrictive pericarditis Congestive heart failure

Intrahepatic	Postsinusoidal
	  Hepatic function impaired
	  Prognosis poor
	  More severe complications
		Liver cirrhosis/fibrosis
		  Biliary atresia
		  Cystic fibrosis
		
		  α_1-Antitrypsin deficiency
		  Viral hepatitis with postnecrotic cirrhosis
		  Wilson's disease

	Presinusoidal
	  Hepatic function preserved
	  Better prognosis
	  Fewer complications
		Congenital hepatic fibrosis
		Primary biliary cirrhosis
		Hepatosplenic schistosomiasis

Prehepatic		Portal vein thrombosis Idiopathic portal hypertension ±50% Increased splanchnic inflow

intrahepatic fistula, portal vein atresia, trauma and tumour compression, are exceptional. Occlusion of the splanchnic veins may indicate an underlying hematological disease (Heaton *et al.*, 1990).

INTRAHEPATIC OBSTRUCTION

Many liver diseases resulting in liver cirrhosis or fibrosis will cause portal hypertension. Biliary atresia is the single most important cause in children. Other causes include cystic fibrosis, α_1-antitrypsin deficiency, viral hepatitis with postnecrotic cirrhosis, and in specific regions schistosomiasis due to the deposition of ova, granulation formation and portal tract fibrosis. Idiopathic non-cirrhotic hepatic fibrosis is an uncommon cause (Okuda *et al.*, 1982; Howard, 1991). The disease presents predominantly in children and adolescents and has an autosomal recessive inheritance. Progressive fibrotic compression and hypoplasia of the intrahepatic branches of the portal vein results in presinusoidal obstruction. The disease either manifests with hepatosplenomegaly or is associated with multiple forms of kidney disease.

Portal hypertension associated with acute viral hepatitis, fulminating hepatitis and drug induced-hepatitis is rarely of clinical significance in children.

SUPRA-HEPATIC OBSTRUCTION

Most lesions resulting in the Budd–Chiari syndrome can be divided into one of three categories: non-thrombotic veno-occlusive disease of the liver, thrombotic occlusion of the hepatic veins or suprahepatic vena cava, or membranous obstruction of the suprahepatic inferior vena cava. Predisposing factors implicated are polycythaemia, blood dyscrasias, systemic lupus erythematosus, malignancy, chemotherapy and oral contraceptives. A specific cause for the Budd–Chiari syndrome can be found in more than 70% of cases. The disease runs a variable clinical course ranging from an acute, rapid fatal illness to a more chronic condition characterized by progressive cirrhosis, portal hypertension, ascites and wasting.

Consequences of portal hypertension

The underlying primary disease process and status of hepatic function will have a profound influence on the clinical presentation, progression and consequences of portal hypertension.

COLLATERAL CIRCULATION AND OESOPHAGEAL VARICES

Because of the disturbed haemodynamic pathway within the portal system, portosystemic collaterals and increased lymph production develop in an attempt to decompress the portal system. These sites are predominantly around the lower end of the oesophagus, falciform ligament, haemorrhoidal plexus, posterior abdominal wall, draining into the inferior vena cava, left kidney, pulmonary vein and extraperitoneal surfaces of abdominal organs. These collateral channels dilate and multiply to accommodate the increased blood flow.

The normal venous anatomy of the lower oesophagus consists of five distinct components (Kitano *et al.*, 1986):

- intraepithelial channels running radially within the epithelial layer, draining the capillary network of this area and joining the superficial venous plexus
- superficial venous plexus (SVP) forming a rich network in the submucosal layer and communicating with the deep intrinsic veins
- deep intrinsic veins (DIV) consisting of three to five main trunks:

both the SVP and the DIV communicate freely with their counterpart veins in the stomach

- adventitial veins consisting of numerous veins in the perioesophageal area
- perforating veins connecting the deeper venous plexuses with the adventitial veins predominantly in the area above the gastro-oesophageal junction.

All of these channels are dilated in patients with portal hypertension (Kitano *et al.*, 1986). The massively enlarged and tortuous deep intrinsic veins constitute the variceal channels with few vascular communications with one another, but link up with the superficial venous plexus and, in established portal hypertension, displace the superficial venous plexus and come to lie immediately below the epithelial surface constituting the main variceal channels seen on endoscopy. Portal hypertension is a prerequisite for the development of varices and variceal haemorrhage rarely occurs with portal pressures below 12 mmHg (Viallet *et al.*, 1975). Two main theories have been advanced to explain variceal bleeding, i.e. erosive and eruptive: varic size, portal pressure, peptic erosion, ingestion of salicylates, upper respiratory tract infection, the overlying mucosa and connective tissue and delicate haemodynamic changes within the portosystemic vascular bed are all factors determining the potential for variceal rupture (Lebrec *et al.*, 1980; Garcia Tsao and Groszman, 1987). It is postulated that variceal bleeding occurs as a result of rupture or erosion of one of these dilated deep intrinsic variceal channels, which has come to lie adjacent to the epithelial surface. Another source may be a branch of the superficial venous plexus at or near the point of direct communication with a large varix. Minor variceal bleeding with spontaneous cessation of bleeding can arise from a ruptured branch of the SVP or from dilated intraepithelial channels (Kitano *et al.*, 1986). Prerupture of these branches is represented by cherry-red spots or red weal markings. Ectopic varices may develop throughout the gastrointestinal tract, biliary tree, bladder, vagina and perineum.

The venous communication across the four main components could explain the success of intravariceal sclerotherapy as well as the difficulty in eradicating varices in some patients (persistence of variceal veins, recanalization of deep vascular channels, enlargement of veins in the superficial venous plexus) and variceal recurrence in others (McCormack *et al.*, 1983). Paravariceal sclerotherapy, however, may function by venous thrombosis of smaller veins and plexuses and fibrotic thickening and reinforcement of the overlying mucosa (Paguet, 1985; Kitano *et al.*, 1986; Terblanche *et al.*, 1990). Following injection, thrombosis and tissue necrosis are evident histologically within 24 hours, ulceration within 7 days and fibrosis by 1 month. Sclerotherapy accelerates the development of collateral venous channels at sites that tend not to bleed.

ASCITES

The development of ascites is a sign of moderate or severe disease, and is more common in parenchymal portal hypertension. Ascites may present acutely or later with deteriorating liver function or following gastrointestinal haemorrhage. Ascitic fluid arises from an increase in hepatic–sinusoidal pressure and low serum albumin. The resultant fluid shift into the extravascular space exceeds the capacity of the lymphatic drainage system and fluid exudes through the liver capsule and serosal surfaces of the gut into the peritoneal cavity. Ascites is often chronic and progressive, can interfere with respiration and feeding, and can be a focus of primary infection.

SPLENOMEGALY AND HYPERSPLENISM

Splenomegaly is an important clue to portal hypertension and in a quarter of children could be the first manifestation. Splenic size does not correlate with the level of obstruction, portal pressure or duration of disease (Karrer, 1992). The spleen is subject to an increased risk of rupture and can cause a dragging sensation or pain in the upper quadrant.

Clinical features

Because of the aetiological heterogenicity, the clinical presentation will largely be determined by the evolution of the primary disease, level of vascular obstruction, adequacy of the collateral circulation and complications of portal hypertension. A distinction must be made between presinusoidal obstruction with predominantly normal liver function and manifestations of portal hypertension,

i.e. collateral circulation with oesophageal varices and splenomegaly and postsinusoidal obstruction with impaired liver function and portal hypertension.

Bleeding from oesophageal varices is the most common manifestation (70%) of portal hypertension in children. Bleeding is typically of sudden onset and profuse, can cease spontaneously and has few identifiable precipitating causes. Children with extrahepatic portal vein obstruction generally bleed at an earlier age (mean 4.3 years) than those with intrahepatic disease (mean 8.5 years) and 73% of all children will bleed before the age of 10 years (Hill and Bowie, 1991). Having bled once, all children are at risk of further episodes. Bleeding often follows an upper respiratory tract infection treated with aspirin. Occasionally, the bleeding is more insidious with iron-deficient anaemia, melaena or occult-positive stools.

A child with portal vein thrombosis typically presents with oesophageal haemorrhage, no clinical or biochemical stigmata of liver failure, splenomegaly and no growth impairment. Conversely, children with liver disease and portal hypertension have a contrasting history and clinical presentation. Manifestations of the primary disease, i.e. cystic fibrosis or biliary atresia, and of chronic liver disease, i.e. jaundice, ascites, splenomegaly, bleeding tendency, poor nutritional status and caput medusa, are often present long before haemorrhage becomes apparent. Hepatomegaly or a small nodular and hard liver may be of equal importance. Ascites are not always easy to detect clinically and can be of sudden or protracted onset. Longstanding splenomegaly, a constant sign of portal hypertension, can be complicated by hypersplenism and although pancytopenia may be prominent it seldom requires therapy (Spence *et al.*, 1984a). All of these manifestations of liver failure are variable and depend on the degree of decompensation.

Management

DIAGNOSIS

Diagnostic investigations should be directed towards establishing the cause, the anatomy of the mesenteric–portohepatic vascular system and collaterals, and the complications.

The evaluation of liver functions requires the rational combination of clinical examination, laboratory tests, radiological imaging and histology. Liver function tests may be normal in congenital hepatic fibrosis and portal vein thrombosis, minimally abnormal in the Budd–Chiari syndrome and grossly abnormal in biliary atresia. Hepatic insufficiency is characterized by hyperbilirubinaemia, hypoalbuminaemia, elevated liver enzymes, coagulopathy and hyperammonia. The grading of liver disease in a child is not an important factor in predicting variceal haemorrhage.

Liver biopsy with confirmation of normal or abnormal hepatic morphology is an essential component to document.

A plain abdominal roentgenogram should be carried out as a routine and will reveal indirect evidence of visceromegaly, organ displacement, presence of collateral circulation and ascites.

The most readily available and useful screening modality is ultrasonography. It allows visualization of the parenchyma of the liver and spleen, the portal vein and main tributaries, the hepatic veins and intrahepatic and suprahepatic vena cava and other collaterals. Non-invasive methods for the determination of portal vein and hepatic arterial flow, direction and velocity are available (Moriyasu *et al.*, 1984).

The portal venous system can be mapped through arterioportography following selective celiac axes and superior mesenteric arterial angiography. Digital splenoportography is an alternative method in children with improved visualization of the portal venous system and collateral anatomy (Balkanci *et al.*, 1991). Direct portography may not provide detailed information regarding the portal vein and collateral circulation in the presence of hepatofugal flow in patients with portal hypertension.

Portal venous pressure measurements can be made by several invasive methods, i.e. laparotomy, splenoportography and wedge hepatic venous pressure, but these are no longer conducted routinely.

Upper gastrointestinal fibre-optic endoscopy, usually carried out under general anaesthesia, is the preferred method of confirming the diagnosis of oesophageal varices. Varices usually affect the lower 3–5 cm of the oesophagus and may extend into the fundus of the stomach (Millar *et al.*, 1991). Endoscopy will exclude other possible causes of haemorrhage and has therapeutic implications. Endoscopic signs of impending variceal rupture have been proposed, including variceal size and colour (white or blue), cherry-red spots, red weal markings, subepithelial blood-filled channels and erosion of the epithelium by a large branch of the superficial venous plexus (Beppu *et al.*, 1981; Spence *et al.*, 1984b; Kitano *et al.*, 1987).

Intravariceal pressure can also be measured and used as a predictor of variceal haemorrhage (Lebrec, 1992). Barium oesophagogastroduodenography is an alternative method of assessing the anatomy of the foregut.

TREATMENT

The underlying cause and complications of portal hypertension will determine the treatment strategies. Children generally have a better prognosis, especially those with extrahepatic biliary atresia. Deterioration of cirrhotic liver disease is more gradual in children than in adults, and they can outgrow the effects of portal hypertension with the formation of more effective collaterals with time (Webb and Sherlock, 1979). Shunt surgery is generally not favoured in children and the efficacy of either transvariceal or paravariceal sclerotherapy or both has been shown to control haemorrhage and to eradicate varices. The gastric fundal varix is a hidden cause of ongoing bleeding and rebleeding occurs in approximately one-third of children during the period of variceal obliteration (Millar *et al.*, 1991). Liver transplantation remains a viable option for end-stage liver disease.

Oesophageal variceal haemorrhage

There are three considerations: the emergency management of acute variceal bleeding, long-term management of patients following a variceal bleed including the use of repeated sclerotherapy, shunts and β-blockers, and prophylactic management of varices that have not bled before (Table 46.2).

Children with decompensated hepatic function, encephalopathy, coagulopathy, ascitis, malnutrition and infections are at risk for intervention, and non-surgical measures and nutritional support are cornerstones of initial management. Most variceal bleeding, however, responds to bed rest, blood transfusions and vasopressin infusions. It is important that these children avoid aspirin-containing medications.

Acute variceal haemorrhage

Initial measures

All patients require intensive care, and standard methods of resuscitation should be instituted including crystalloids, colloid solutions, fresh blood or blood components, nasogastric decompression (gastric evacuation of blood, assessment of ongoing bleeding and cold gastric lavages), and ongoing monitoring. Over transfusion should be avoided and albumin transfusions may help to prevent postoperative ascites. Although bleeding may cease in approximately 60% of children, it is impossible to predict who will continue to bleed and who will require further emergency therapy (Terblanche *et al.*, 1989).

Endoscopy

Immediate fibre-optic endoscopy is essential. It will confirm the presence of oesophageal varices and the source of bleeding. The majority of patients will fall into one of three groups: those with active bleeding varices, those with varices that have stopped bleeding (endoscopy fails to identify any other source and the varix, or varices, has an adherent clot overlying it) and those with another source of bleeding.

Once variceal bleeding has been confirmed, therapy should be instituted henceforth. Three methods are used in conjunction with each other to control variceal haemorrhage initially, i.e. intravenous vasopressin, sclerotherapy and balloon tamponade.

Table 46.2   Algorithm for oesophageal variceal bleeding

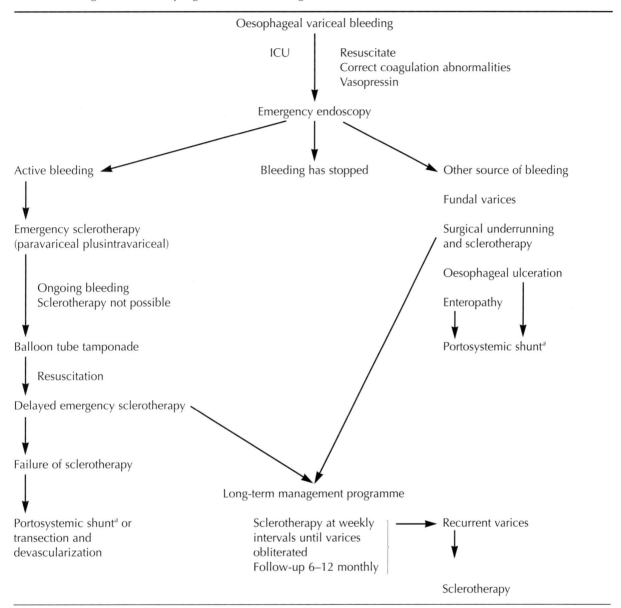

[a]Indications for portosystemic shunts: sclerotherapy failure; unsuitable for liver transplantation; bleeding from some source distal to oesophagus; isolated portal vein thrombosis; lack of compliance, inadequate long-term care.
Prophylactic sclerotherapy not recommended; long-term pharmacological agents – experimental.

Vasopressin

The continuous intravenous infusion of vasopressin at a dose of 0.2–0.4 U/1.73 m^2/min (or 0.4 U/min), has an overall efficacy of approximately 50% and should be started when variceal bleeding is suspected (Hussey, 1985; Terblanche *et al.*, 1989; Hill and Bowie, 1991; Howard, 1991). It functions by generalized vasoconstriction, diminished portal blood flow and reduced portal hypertension. Vasopressin combined with nitro-

glycerin is not utilized in children. Cardiac complications, plasminogen activator and factor VIII, release may potentially limit the use of vasopressin (Bornman *et al.*, 1994). The value of alternative drugs including somatostatin, terlipressin, metoclopramide, prostaglandins, propranolol and cisapride is as yet unproven and cannot be recommended in the treatment of acute variceal bleeding (Grose and Hayes, 1992).

Emergency sclerotherapy

Emergency sclerotherapy is as effective in controlling acute bleeding as balloon tamponade and is the treatment of choice, once adequate venous access has been established and hypovolaemia resolved. In the small child general anaesthesia and endotracheal intubation are required, which will allow for airway protection and a good-quality and safe procedure.

Variceal bleeding usually originates from an area 1–2 cm above the gastro-oesophageal junction or from gastric fundal varices (Sarin and Kamer, 1989; Millar *et al.*, 1991). Active bleeding may obscure the site of bleeding and vigorous lavage may be required for visualization of the bleeding point. Blind attempts at injection should be guarded against. The most efficacious injection method is a combination of paravariceal and transvariceal sclerotherapy using a flexible endoscope (Terblanche *et al.*, 1989; Maksoud *et al.*, 1991).

Initial paravariceal submucosal injection is made immediately adjacent to the bleeding site using 0.5–1 ml of 5% etanolamine oleate or 0.5–1 ml of 0.5–1% pilodocanol (Paguet, 1982; Howard *et al.*, 1988; Terblanche *et al.*, 1989, 1990). Alternatively, TES (tetradecylsulphate, ethanol and saline in equal proportions, dose 0.5–3 ml per varix, with a maximum of 0.8 ml/kg per session) can be used (Bornman *et al.*, 1994). The amount instilled at each site should be enough to produce visible blanching and swelling of the mucosa (±1–3 ml). This is then followed by transvariceal sclerotherapy into each variceal channel commencing at the gastro-oesophageal junction and proceeding proximally in a helical fashion for 5–7 cm (Lilly, 1981; Paguet, 1982; Terblanche *et al.*, 1990; Hill and Bowie, 1991). It is neither necessary nor advisable to obliterate more proximal varices.

Any additional or residual bleeding from a varix or needle puncture site should be controlled by further paravariceal injections. The combined three-part sclerotherapy method of Kitano *et al.* (1987) may be hazardous and is not recommended as standard practice. If bleeding recurs in the early postinjection period the patient should be re-endoscoped and the bleeding varix injected.

The child is then observed in an intensive care unit (ICU) and oral fluids are allowed within the first 24 hours. Sclerotherapy controls acute bleeding in 80–100% of patients (Webb and Sherlock, 1979; Paguet, 1982; Spence *et al.*, 1884b; Maksoud *et al.*, 1991) (Table 46.3).

Balloon tamponade

A Sengstaken–Blakemore tube or a 4 lumen Minnesota balloon tube is very effective in temporarily controlling acute variceal haemorrhage. It also allows time for resuscitation and planning of further management. The tube should be positioned carefully, and not left for longer than 6–12 hours. Pulmonary aspiration, laryngeal and tracheal obstruction are the most serious complications. Repeat endoscopy and sclerotherapy should then be performed because of the 50% chance of recurrent bleeding (Panes *et al.*, 1988). This approach has a success rate of up to 80–96.5% in arresting bleeding from gastro-oesophagoeal varices (Paguet and Lazar, 1994).

Prevention of recurrent variceal bleeding

Repeat flexible endoscopy and sclerotherapy is then performed every 1–2 weeks until all varices have been eradicated or converted into thrombosed cords. In the presence of sloughing or ulceration of the oesophageal mucosa, repeat injection should be delayed for 1 week until healing has occurred (Terblanche *et al.*, 1989; Hill and Bowie, 1991). The administration of omeprazole or ranitidine may accelerate healing. With further variceal bleeding the same programme is repeated after haemodynamic stability has been achieved. Once all varices have been sclerosed, endoscopy is repeated at 3, 6, 9 and 12 months and every 6–12 months thereafter. On average five to nine injections are required to eradicate varices (Stellan and Lilly, 1985; Hill and Bowie, 1991). Recurrence of varices, usually single, can occur in 12–33% of children within 1–3.5 years following initial eradication and long-term surveillance is mandatory (Paguet, 1985; Howard *et al.*, 1988; Hill and Bowie, 1991). Fortunately, recurrent variceal bleeding episodes are usually minor and self-limiting.

Complications of sclerotherapy are common (54%) and though mostly minor include mild pyrexia, retrosternal discomfort, tachycardia, transient dysphagia, oesophageal ulceration, stricture, oesophageal perforation and rebleeding (Heaton and Howard, 1991; Hill and Bowie, 1991). Rigid endoscopy, repeated injections into the same bleeding varix, the use of highly sclerosing agents and large total volumes may predispose to these complications.

Gastric varices

Bleeding from these varices is usually more severe and carries a higher morbidity. In up to one-third of patients variceal bleeding arises from gastric varices (Stellan and Lilly, 1985 Sarin and Kamar, 1989; Hill and Bowie, 1991; Millar *et al.*, 1991). Those situated within the gastro-oesophageal junction or lesser curvature may be managed by sclerotherapy, and often disappear following oesophageal sclerotherapy. Active bleeding from fundal varices can best be controlled through a high anterior gastrostomy and underrunning with an absorbable suture, followed by oesophageal variceal endosclerosis at a later date (Miller *et al.*, 1991).

Table 46.3 Surgical modalities of management and results

(a) Sclerotherapy

Author	Number (%)	Obliteration of varices (%)	Rebleeding (%)	Number of sessions (%)	Recurrent oesophageal varices (%)	Serious complications (%)	Follow-up (years)	Mortality (%)
Paguet (1982)	59	100	3.4	3	0	10	< 10	0
Stellen and Lilly (1985)	25	88	0	3	12	8	< 2.6	4
Howard *et al.* (1988)	108	80	35	6	11	45	2.9	1
Hill and Bowie (1991)	33	94	36	5	33	30	2.7	0
Maksoud *et al.* (1991)	62	85.4	45	3.6	–	3.2	2.4	4.8
Heaton and Howard (1993)	252	95	39	6	12	–	3.4	0

(b) Portosystemic shunts

	Number	Shunt patency (%)	Blocked shunt (%)	Recurrent oesophageal bleeding (%)	Follow-up (years)	Mortality (%)
H-Type shunt (Gauthier *et al.*, 1989)	84	93	7	4.7	± 3	0
Splenorenal side-to-side shunt (Mitra *et al.*, 1993)	104	87	13	10	4.5	1
Distal splenorenal shunt (Maksoud *et al.*, 1991)	39	95	5	5	11	0
Mesocaval (Bismuth *et al.*, 1980)	19	100	0	0	4.2	0
Splenorenal (Bismuth *et al.*, 1980)	59	93	7	3.4	4.2	0
Portacava1 (Bismuth *et al.*, 1980)	11	91	0	9	4.2	0

(c) Partial splenic embolization (PSE)

	Number	Annual number of episodes of variceal bleeding		Follow-up (years)	Mortality (%)
		Pre-PSE	Post-PSE		
Brandt *et al.* (1989)	12	1.8	0.5	3.3	0

(d) Oesophageal transection and devascularization

	Number	Ablation of oesophageal variceal bleeding (%)	Recurrent oesophageal bleeding (%)	Complications (%)	Mortality (%)
Superiua *et al.* (1983)	8	100%	0	50	0

ALTERNATIVE THERAPY

The main alternatives to sclerotherapy are pharmacotherapy, endoscopic variceal ligation, portosystemic shunts, transection and devascularization operations, and hepatic transplantation.

Long-term pharmacological therapy is an appealing alternative to surgical therapy. Most experience has been gained with the non-selective β-receptor antagonist propranolol. This drug reduces cardiac output, reduces portal venous inflow, constricts the splanchnic arterial bed, and currently is the only drug indicated for the prophylaxis of variceal bleeding. The most useful indication is for a highly selected group of patients who are unable to undergo sclerotherapy. Survival is not improved and with β-blockage difficulties may be encountered with vasomotor control during resuscitation, the risk of bleeding on withdrawal is increased and it may aggravate encephalopathy (Terblanche *et al.*, 1989). Calcium channel blockers, serotonin antagonists and nitrates are under investigation. There are no firm data on children to justify the routine use of any of these drugs (Hassall, 1994).

Endoscopic variceal ligation

The novel technique of endoscopic variceal ligation (EVL) could be an effective alternative to endoscopic sclerotherapy. Varices are mechanically ensnared with small elastic O-rings, causing necrosis within 4–7 days followed by re-epithclialization and scar formation. Experience has shown successful bleeding control and eradication of varices and merits further evaluation (Van Stiegman and Goff, 1988). Initial EVL of large varices followed by sclerotherapy may ultimately prove the best way to eradicate varices expeditiously (Hayes, 1996).

Portosystemic shunts

Emergency portosystemic shunts can effectively reduce variceal bleeding and prevent recurrent bleeding but are seldom indicated in children (Maksoud and Mies, 1982; Cello *et al.*, 1987; Terblanche *et al.*, 1989; Heaton and Howard, 1993). Shunts can be constructed successfully with a vessel size as small as 5 mm in diameter. Unfortunately, these shunts partially or completely divert hepatotrophic blood away from the liver.

Shunts are indicated in children under the following circumstances (Table 46.3):

- continual oesophageal variceal bleeding following failed emergency sclerotherapy
- bleeding from ectopic variceal sites not accessible to sclerotherapy
- uncontrollable or continued bleeding from oesophageal ulceration following sclerotherapy
- isolated portal vein thrombosis
- patients with variceal haemorrhage who are not suitable for liver transplantation

- technical expertise for sclerotherapy not available and in children where long-term care cannot be assured.

Disadvantages of shunt procedures are the unpredictable occurrence of postoperative encephalopathy, the high failure rate of shunts in small children (younger than 10 years) because of technical difficulties, thrombosis and a rebleeding rate of 2–47%, accelerated liver failure because of diversion of portal blood flow, concern about major surgery in patients who may stop haemorrhaging spontaneously, the development of effective spontaneous portosystemic shunts with time (48%), a surgical procedure that could compromise future liver transplantation and a 4.2% (range 0–11%) mortality (Voorhees *et al.*, 1973; Webb and Sherlock, 1979; Bismuth *et al.*, 1980; Maksoud and Mies, 1982; Spence *et al.*, 1984b; Paguet, 1985; Alagille *et al.*, 1986; Howard *et al.*, 1988; Brems *et al.*, 1989; Maksoud *et al.*, 1991; Paguet and Lazar, 1994).

Emergency shunts are indicated in approximately 4–10% of patients who do not respond to sclerotherapy (Cello *et al.*, 1987; Heaton and Howard, 1993). These shunts are associated with significant morbidity and mortality of 0–22% and rebleeding rates from 2 to 47% (Howard *et al.*, 1988).

The distal splenorenal shunt is usually reserved for elective surgery (Bismuth *et al.*, 1980; Heaton and Howard 1993). The shunt decompresses the oesophagogastric and splenic vascular bed and maintains portal hepatic perfusion (Bismuth *et al.*, 1980; Maksoud and Mies, 1982; Terblanche *et al.*, 1989; Maksoud *et al.*, 1991; Heaton and Howard, 1993). Long-term shunt patency is 95% (10-year follow-up) and shunt closure is characterized by the early reappearance of varices, abdominal pain and rapid splenomegaly, which is a very difficult situation to handle (Maksoud *et al.*, 1991). The shunts can, however, progressively lose their selectivity within 3 months, with a decrease in the high pressure portal perfusion due to collaterals developing between the portomesenteric and the gastrosplenic system or advancing liver disease (Bismuth *et al.*, 1980; Warren *et al.*, 1980; Belghiti *et al.*, 1981). However, modification of the shunt, preventing deviation of blood away from the liver via the pancreatic siphon, appears to preserve portal perfusion and stabilize hepatic mass (Warren *et al.*, 1984, 1986; Inokuchi and Sugimachi, 1990). Alternatively, the H-type superior mesojugular-caval shunt, using an internal jugular vein graft, appears to offer the best long-term patency and lowers the rebleeding rate (Belghiti *et al.*, 1981; Gauthier *et al.*, 1989; Sahni *et al.*, 1990). This H-type shunt may also be the choice in patients who are candidates for liver transplants (Brems *et al.*, 1989). In developing countries a primary splenorenal shunt should be considered as primary procedure and sclerotherapy be reserved for unsuitable veins for surgery or rebleeding after a shunt procedure (Belghiti *et al.*, 1981; Gauthier *et al.*, 1989; Sahni *et al.*, 1990). Side-to-side splenorenal shunt without splenectomy for non-cirrhotic portal hypertension effectively reduces the size of oesophageal varices with no further rebleeding, ameliorates hypersplenism, remains patent in 87% of children and does not increase the risk of portosystemic encephalopathy. This shunt should be seriously considered if compliance with medical care cannot be assured or if care is not readily available (Mitra *et al.*, 1993).

Angiographic portosystemic shunt

Transjugular intrahepatic portosystemic shunt (TIPS) is a novel idea and is indicated for variceal haemorrhage refractory to sclerotherapy and for patients awaiting liver transplantation (Richter *et al.*, 1990). The technique involves the placement of a flexible and expandable wire-mesh stent to create a channel between hepatic and portal veins within the liver substance. TIPS functions as a side-by-side shunt and maintains hepatopetal and sinusoidal perfusion.

Limited clinical experience has shown substantial control of variceal bleeding, resolution of ascites and the absence of encephalopathy. The safety and efficacy of the procedure still have to be confirmed.

OTHER METHODS

Although oesophageal transection and devascularization procedures are seldom performed in children, they would seem to be the preferred procedures if portosystemic shunting is not feasible (Heaton and Howard, 1991, 1993). Their main role is in the emergency management of variceal bleeding, in patients in whom repeated sclerotherapy has failed, in younger children where shunts are not feasible and when sclerotherapy is not available (Superima *et al.*, 1983; Terblanche *et al.*, 1989; Idezuki *et al.*, 1990; Orozco *et al.*, 1992). Technical considerations include either thoracoabdominal or transabdominal portoazygos devascularization of the upper half of the stomach and lower third of the oesophagus, with splenic preservation and oesophageal transection. The procedure maintains portal flow but is associated with a rebleeding rate of 10% (Superima *et al.*, 1983; Idezuki *et al.*, 1990; Orozco *et al.*, 1992).

Most other emergency procedures either have been abandoned (e.g. percutaneous transhepatic obliteration of varices), remain to be proven or are not indicated in children, for example, partial oesophagogastrectomy with colonic interposition, splenic transposition, (Terblanche *et al.*, 1989) or electrocautery and colonic exclusion to reduce the incidence of postshunt encephalopathy (Heaton and Howard, 1991; Orozco *et al.*, 1992).

Hepatic transplantation is the only available therapy that prevents recurrent variceal bleeding and resolves the underlying liver disease, and this is the accepted treatment for otherwise healthy patients who have end-stage liver disease (Hobbs, 1987; Bismuth *et al.*, 1990; Muzzaferro *et al.*, 1990).

Prophylactic management of varices

Varices will always predispose a patient to the risk of bleeding (Maksoud *et al.*, 1991), which can be as high as 42%. Although raised portal pressure (>12 mmHg), large varices, varices with erosion and/or poor coagulation factors, poor liver function, and endoscopic findings of cherry-red spots or red weal markings (Lebrec *et al.*, 1980; Garcia-Tsao *et al.*, 1985; Kitano *et al.*, 1986; North Italian Endoscopic Club, 1988) are associated with an increased risk of bleeding, the magnitude and timing of this risk is unpredictable. Prophylactic sclerotherapy or shunts are therefore not advocated. Children living in remote areas or with large extensive varices may be candidates for prophylactic variceal injection (Stringer *et al.*, 1989). Elective shunt procedures for recurrent haemorrhage despite repeated sclerotherapy may be required for 10% of children (Paguet and Lazar, 1994).

Hypersplenism

Splenectomy is not advocated as a procedure of choice for symptomatic hypersplenism, as it may increase the incidence of infection, precipitate portal vein thrombosis, preclude specific shunt procedures and fail to reduce the incidence of variceal bleeding. In contrast, selective splenic embolization fulfils all the criteria of effectively controlling hypersplenism, reducing the incidence of rebleeding from 2.4 to 0.8 episodes per year, conserving splenic immune function, reducing the size and maintaining portal venous flow. The aim of the procedure is to infarct 70–80% of splenic tissue. It must be done in conjunction with pneumococcal vaccination and possibly long-term antibiotic prophylaxis to the age of 6 years. Immediate morbidity rates are high, with all patients experiencing transient but significant complications (Brandt *et al.*, 1989). Splenectomy may be indicated for isolated portal vein thrombosis with recurrent or life-threatening haemorrhage and a massive spleen, but should be deferred in patients with minimal transfusion requirements or prior episodes of gastrointestinal bleeding (Loftus *et al.*, 1993).

Ascites

Most patients with mild to moderate ascites can be managed with the rational use of salt restriction and diuretics. Those patients with tense ascites, respiratory impairment, infection, renal impairment or hepatic encephalopathy should receive additional measures such as bed rest, fluid restriction, spironolactone in combination with flurosemide and salt-poor human albumin infusions. Medically, refractory ascites should be treated with large-volume paracentesis and albumin or plasma transfusions. These patients should be considered for liver transplantation. Peritoneovenous shunts will relieve ascites but are associated with a high rate of complications, including blockage, bacterial infections, intravascular coagulopathy, pulmonary oedema and gastrointestinal haemorrhage. These shunts should be limited to a very selected group where the benefits outweigh the risks.

In summary, sclerotherapy is the definitive treatment for children with extrahepatic portal hypertension, with surgical shunts being reserved for sclerotherapy failure. Partial splenic embolization is seldom carried out, and endoscopic varix ligation may supersede sclerotherapy in the future. The prognosis for children with intrahepatic portal hypertension will depend on the primary liver condition, and sclerotherapy may successfully temporize bleeding episodes. Liver transplantation is indicated for those patients with deteriorating liver function and bleeding varices. Non-compliant patients or those from remote geographical areas should receive prophylactic sclerotherapy or selective shunt procedures.

References

Alagille, D., Carlier, J.C., Chiva, M., Ziadel, R., Ziader, M. and Moy, F. 1986: Long term neuropsychological outcome in children undergoing porto-systemic shunts for portal vein obstruction without liver disease. *Journal of Pediatric Gastroenterology and Nutrition* **5**, 861–6.

Balkanci, F., Farid, H., Guram, S., Senanti, S., Atique, M.H. and Yuce, A. 1991: A high incidence of spontaneous splenorenal shunting shown by digital splenoportography. *Pediatric Radiology* **21**, 145–7.

Belghiti, J., Grenier, P., Nouel, O., Nahum, H. and Fekete, F. 1981: Long-term loss of Warren's shunt selectivity. *Archives of Surgery* **116**, 1121–4.

Benoit, J.N. Wocmack, W.A, Hernandez, L. and Granger, D.N. 1985: Forward and backward flow mechanisms of portal hypertension. *Gastroenterology* **89**, 1096–9.

Beppu, K., Inokuchi, K., Koyanayi, N. *et al.* 1981: Prediction of variceal hemorrhage by esophageal endoscopy. *Gastrointestinal Endoscopy* **27**, 213–8.

Bhathol, P. and Grossman, H. 1985: Reduction of the increased portal vascular resistance of the isolated perfused cirrhotic rat liver by vasodilators. *Journal of Hepatology* **1**, 325–7.

Bismuth, H., Adam, R., Mathar, S. and Sherlock, D. 1990: Options for elective treatment of portal hypertension in cirrhotic patients in the transplantation era. *American Journal of Surgery* **160**, 105–10.

Bismuth, H., Franco, D. and Alagille, D. 1980: Portal diversion for portal hypertension in children. The first ninety patients. *Annals of Surgery* **192**, 18–24.

Bornman, P.C., Krige, J.E.J. and Terblanche, J. 1994: Management of oesophageal varices. *Lancet* **343**, 1079–84.

Brandt, C.T., Rothbarth, L.G., Kampe, D., Karrer, F.M. and Lilly, J.R. 1989: Splenic embolization in children. Long-term efficacy. *Journal of Pediatric Surgery* **24**, 642–5.

Brems, J.J., Hiatt, J.R., Klein, A.S. *et al.* 1989: Effect of a prior portasystemic shunt on subsequent liver transplantation. *Annals of Surgery* **209**, 51–6.

Cello, J.P., Grendell, J.H., Grass, R.A., Weber, T.E. and Trunkey, D.D. 1987: Endoscopic sclerotherapy versus portacaval shunt in patients with severe cirrhosis and acute variceal hemorrhage: long-term follow-up. *New England Journal of Medicine* **316**, 11–15.

Galloway, J.R. and Henderson, J.M. 1990: Management of variceal bleeding in patients with extrahepatic portal vein thrombosis. *American Journal of Surgery* **160**, 122–7.

Garcia Tsao, G., Groszmann, R.J., Fisher, R.L., Conn, H.O., Atterbury, C.E. and Glockman, M. 1985: Portal pressure, presence of gastro-esophageal varices and variceal bleeding. *Hepatology* **5**, 419–24.

Garcia-Tsao, G. and Groszman, R.J. 1987: Portal haemodynamics during nitroglycerin administration in cirrhotic patients. *Hepatology* **7**, 805–9.

Gauthier, F., De Drenzy, O., Valayer, J. and Montupet, P.H. 1989: H-type shunt with autologous venous graft for treatment of portal hypertension in children. *Journal of Pediatric Surgery* **24**, 1041–3.

Grose, R.D. and Hayes, P.C. 1992: The pathophysiology and pharmacological treatment of portal hypertension. *Alimentary Pharmacology and Therapeutics* **6**, 521–40.

Hassall, E. 1994: Nonsurgical treatments for portal hypertension in children. *Pediatric Endoscopy* **4**, 223–58.

Hayes, P.C. 1996: The coming of age of band ligation for oesophageal varices? *British Medical Journal* **312**, 1111–12.

Heaton, N.D. and Howard, E.R. 1991: Complications of portal hypertension. In Howard, E.R. (ed.), *Surgery of liver disease in children.* Oxford: Butterworth-Heinenann, chapter 18, 181–90.

Heaton, N.D. and Howard, E.R. 1993: Surgical intervention in children with portal hypertension. *Pediatric Surgery International* **8**, 306–9.

Heaton, N.D., Karani, J. and Howard, E.R. 1990: Portal vein thrombosis in myeloproliferative disease. *British Medical Journal* **300**, 945.

Hill, I.D., and Bowie, M.D. 1991: Endoscopic sclerotherapy for control of bleeding varices in children. *American Journal of Gastroenterology* **86**, 472–6.

Hobbs, K.E. 1987: Liver transplantation: a review. *Journal of Hepatology* **4**, 148–53.

Howard, E.R. 1991: Aetiology of portal hypertension and anomalies of the portal venous system. In Howard, E.R. (ed.), *Surgery of liver disease in children.* Oxford: Butterworth-Heinemann, chapter 15, 151–60.

Howard, E.R., Stringer, M.D., Mowat, A.P. 1988: Assessment of injection sclerotherapy in the management of 152 children with oesophageal varices. *British Journal of Surgery* **75**, 404–8.

Hussey, K.P. 1985: Vasopressin therapy for upper gastrointestinal tract hemorrhage: has its efficacy been proven? *Archives of Internal Medicine* **145**, 1263–7.

Idezuki, Y., Sanjo, K., Bandai, Y., Kawasaki, S. and Ohashi, K. 1990: Current strategy for esophageal varices in Japan. *American Journal of Surgery* **160**, 98–104.

Inokuchi, K. and Sugimachi, K. 1990: The selected shunt for variceal bleeding: a personal perspective. *American Journal of Surgery* **160**, 48–53.

Karrer, F.M. 1992: Portal hypertension. *Seminars in Pediatric Surgery* **1**, 134–44.

Kitano, S., Koyanagi, N., Iso, Y., Higashi, H. and Sugimachi, K. 1987: Prevention of recurrence of esophageal varices after endoscopic injection sclerotherapy with ethanolamine oleate. *Hepatology* **7**, 810–15.

Kitano, S., Terblanche, J., Kahn, D. and Bornman, P.C. 1986: Venous anatomy of the lower oesophagus in portal hypertension: practical implications. *British Journal of Surgery* **73**, 525–31.

Lebrec, D. 1992: Methods to evaluate portal hypertension. *Gastro-enterological Clinics of North America* **21**, 41–59.

Lebrec, D., DeFleury, P., Rueff, B., Nahum, H. and Benhamoa, J.P. 1980: Portal hypertension, size of esophageal varice and risk of gastro-intestinal bleeding in alcoholic cirrhosis. *Gastroenterology* **79**, 1139–44.

Lilly, J.R. 1981: Endoscopic sclerosis of esophageal varices in children. *Surgery, Gynecology and Obstetrics* **152**, 513–14.

Loftus, J.P., Nagorney, D.M. and Ilstrup Kunsdman, A.R. 1993: Sinistral portal hypertension. Splenectomy or expectant management. *Annals of Surgery* **217**, 35–40.

Maksoud, J.G. and Mies, S. 1982: Distal splenorenal shunt (DSS) in children. Analysis of the first 21 consecutive cases. *Annals of Surgery* **195**, 401–5.

Maksoud, J.G., Goncalves, M.E.P., Porta, G., Miura, I. and Velhote, M.C.P. 1991: The endoscopic and surgical management of portal hypertension in children: analysis of 123 cases. *Journal of Pediatric Surgery* **26**, 178–81.

McCormack, T.T., Rose, J.D., Smith, P.M. and Johnson, A.G. 1983: Perforating veins and blood flow in oesophageal varices. *Lancet* **ii**, 1442-4.

Millar, A.J.W., Brown, R.A., Hill, I.D., Rode, H. and Cywes, S. 1991: The fundal pile: bleeding gastric varices. *Journal of Pediatric Surgery* **26**, 707–9.

Mitra, S.K, Rao, K.L.N, Narasimhan, K.L. *et al.* 1993: Side-to-side lieno-renal shunt without splenectomy in noncirrhotic portal hypertension in children. *Journal of Pediatric Surgery* **28**, 398–402.

Moriyasu, F., Ban, H., Nishida, O. *et al.* 1984: Quantitative measurement of portal blood flow in patients with chronic liver disease using an ultrasonic duplex system composed of a pulsed doppler flowmeter and B-mode electro scanner. *Gastroenterologia Japonica* **19**, 529–36.

Muzzaferro, V., Todo, S., Tzakis, A.G., Stieber, A.C., Makowka, L. and Starzyl, T.E. 1990: Liver transplantation in patients with previous portasystemic shunt. *American Journal of Surgery* **160**, 111–16.

North Italian Endoscopic Club for the Study and Treatment of Esophageal Varices 1988: Prediction of the first variceal hemorrhage in patients with cirrhosis of the liver and esophageal varices: a prospective multicenter study. *New England Journal of Medicine* **319**, 983–9.

Okuda, K., Nakashima, T., Okudaira, M., Kage, M. and Aida, Y. 1982: Liver pathology of idiopathic portal hypertension: comparison with non-cirrhotic portal fibrosis of India. *Liver* **ii**, 176–92.

Okumura, H., Aramaki, T. and Katsuta, Y. 1989: Pathophysiologic and epidemiology of portal hypertension. *Drugs* **37**, 2–12.

Orozco, H., Mercado, M.A., Takahashi, T., Hernandez-Ortiz, J., Capellan, J.F. and Garcia-Tsao, G. 1992: Elective treatment of bleeding varices with the Suguira operation over ten years. *American Journal of Surgery* **163**, 585–9.

Paguet, K.J. 1982: Prophylactic endoscopic sclerosing treatment of the esophageal wall in varices – a prospective controlled randomized trial. *Endoscopy* **14**, 4–5.

Paguet, K.J. 1985: Ten years experience with para-variceal injection sclerotherapy of esophageal varices in children. *Journal of Pediatric Surgery* **20**, 109–12.

Paguet, K.J. and Lazar, A. 1994: Current therapeutic strategy in bleeding esophageal varices in babies and children and long-term results of endoscopic paravariceal sclerotherapy over twenty years. *European Journal of Pediatric Surgery* **4**, 165–72.

Panes, J., Teres, J., Bosch, J. and Rodes, J. 1988: Efficacy of balloon tamponade in treatment of bleeding gastric and esophageal varices. Results in 151 consecutive episodes. *Digestive Diseases and Sciences* **33**, 454–9.

Richter, G.M., Noeldge, G., Palmaz, J.C. *et al.* 1990: Transjugular intrahepatic portacaval stent shunt. Preliminary clinical results. *Radiology* **174**, 1027–130.

Rikkers, L.F. 1990: New concepts of pathophysiology and treatment of portal hypertension. *Surgery* **107**, 481–8.

Sahni, P., Pande, G.K. and Nundy, S. 1990: Extrahepatic portal vein obstruction. *British Journal of Surgery* **77**, 1201–2.

Sarin, S.K. and Kamar, A. 1989: Gastric varices: profile, classification and management. *American Journal of Gastroenterology* **84**, 1244–49.

Sikuler, E. and Groszman, R.J. 1986: Interaction of flow and resistance in maintenance of portal hypertension in a rat model. *American Journal of Physiology* **250**, G205–12.

Spence, R.A.J, Johnson, G.W., Odling-Smee, G.W., and Rodgers, H.W. 1984a: Bleeding oesophageal varices with long term follow up. *Archives of Disease in Childhood* **59**, 336–40.

Spence, R.A.J., Sloan, J.M. and Johnson, G.W. 1984b: Histologic factors of the esophageal transection ring as clues to the pathogenesis of bleeding varices. *Surgery, Gynecology and Obstetrics* **159**, 253–9.

Stellen, G.P. and Lilly, J.R. 1985: Esophageal endosclerosis in children. *Surgery* **89**, 970–5.

Stringer, M.D., Howard, E.R. and Movat, A.P. 1989: Endoscopic therapy in the management of oesophageal varices in 61 children with biliary atresia. *Journal of Pediatric Surgery* **24**, 438–42.

Superima, R.A., Weber, J.L. and Shandling, B. 1983: A modified Suguira operation for bleeding varices in children. *Journal of Pediatric Surgery* **18**, 794–9.

Terblanche, J., Burroughs, A.K. and Hobbs, K.E.F. 1989: Controversies in the management of bleeding esophageal varices. Parts I and II. *New England Journal of Medicine* **320**, 1393–98 and 1469–75.

Terblanche, J., Krige, J.E.J. and Bornman, P.C. 1990: Endoscopic sclerotherapy. *Surgical Clinics of North America* **70**, 341–59.

Van Stiegman, G. and Goff, J.S. 1988: Endoscopic esophageal varix ligation. Preliminary clinical experience. *Gastrointestinal Endoscopy* **34**, 113–17.

Viallet, A., Marleau, D., Huet, P.M., Martin, F., Farley Villeneuve, J.P., and Lavoie, P. 1975: Hemodynamic evaluation of patients with intrahepatic portal hypertension. relationship between bleeding varices and the porto-hepatic gradients. *Gastroenterology* **69**, 1297–300.

Viggiano, T.R. and Gostout, C.J. 1992: Portal hypertensive intestinal vasculopathy: a review of the clinical, endoscopic and histopathologic features. *American Journal of Gastroenterology* **87**, 944–54.

Voorhees, A.B., Chaitman, E., Schneider, S., Nicholson, J.F., Kornfeld, D.S. and Price, J.B. 1973: Portal-systemic encephalopathy in the non-cirrhotic patient. *Archives of Surgery* **107**, 659–63.

Warren, W.D., Millikan, W.J., Henderson, J.M. *et al.* 1986: Splenopancreatic disconnection: improved selectivity of distal splenorenal shunt. *Annals of Surgery* **204**, 346–55.

Warren, W.D., Millikan, W.J., Henderson, J.M., Rasheed, M.E. and Salam, A.A. 1984: Selective variceal decompression after splenectomy or splenic vein thrombosis. *Annals of Surgery* **199**, 694–701.

Warren, W.D., Millikan, W.J., Smith, R.B., Rypins, E.B. *et al.* 1980: Noncirrhotic portal vein thrombosis. Physiology before and after shunts. *Annals of Surgery* **192**, 341–9.

Webb, L.J., and Sherlock, S. 1979: The aetiology, presentation and natural history of extra-hepatic portal venous obstruction. *Quarterly Journal of Medicine* **192**, 627–39.

Whitington, P. 1985: Portal hypertension in children. *Pediatric Annals* **14**, 494–9.

Witte, C.L., Witte, M.H., Bair, G., Mobley, W.P. and Morton, D. 1974: Experimental study of hyperdynamic vs stagnant mesenteric blood flow in portal hypertension. *Annals of Surgery* **179**, 304–10.

CHAPTER 47

Deformities of the chest wall

J.C. MOLENAAR

Pectus excavation (funnel chest)
Pectus carinatum (pigeon chest)
Congential fissure of the sternum
(congenital cleft sternum)

Congenital absence of ribs
Poland syndrome
References

Pectus excavatum (funnel chest)

Pectus excavatum is the most common chest wall deformity in childhood. Its operative treatment goes back to the beginning of this century when large extrapleural resections of deformed cartilages were carried out, leading to paradoxical respiration and, if the pleura were opened, to even more respiratory difficulty. Nissen was the first to suggest the idea of transecting cartilages from the sternum, thus allowing the sternum to be lifted into a normal position. This idea was initially used by Sauerbruch (Bier *et al.*, 1934) and formed the basis of modern operative treatment of this condition (Ravitch, 1968; Haller *et al.*, 1989).

CLINICAL FEATURES

A newborn rarely presents with pectus excavatum. The abnormality develops over the first years of infancy and childhood and then becomes an increasing worry for the parents. Its cause is entirely unknown and its occurrence is sporadic but there is a familial incidence.

Apart from the unsightly appearance of the anomaly the patients are usually symptom free. If there are symptoms, of either respiratory or cardiac origin, these may be caused by associated anomalies of the heart or lungs, and further investigations are required. In asymmetrical pectus excavatum there are secondary changes on the spine resulting in vertebral torsion and scoliosis.

In the healthy-looking boy or girl with a normal posture the chest deformity (Fig. 47.1) causes anxiety, hence the request for treatment. In the teenager with a pubertal growth spurt, increasing height and bad posture the effects are even more striking (Fig. 47.2). Marfan's syndrome may be associated with pectus excavatum.

MANAGEMENT

Conservative treatment

There have been reports in the literature of conservative treatment (Hage and Bowen, 1992), but there is general agreement that surgical correction is required in the severe case. Less agreement exists about the age for recommending operative correction.

Except for cosmetic reasons there are no absolute criteria for operative intervention. Patients with pectus excavatum have smaller thoracic cavities and lower total lung capacity, but there is no scientific proof that pulmonary or cardiac function will improve after surgery (Shamberger and Welch, 1988). Interestingly enough, there are no psychological data to prove that surgical treatment has a positive effect on self-image and it is possible that patients who choose operative treatment are less able to accept and deal with their deformity (Wynn *et al.*, 1990; Kagaraoka *et al.*, 1992; Asness, 1992).

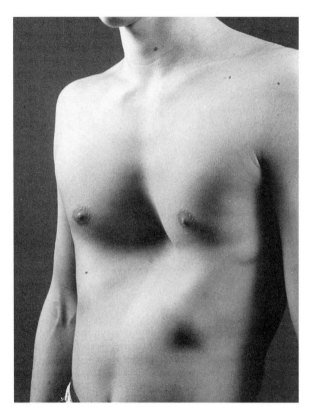

Fig. 47.1 Pectus excavatum.

Surgical treatment

For these reasons it seems that operative treatment should only be offered at an age when the child can take part in the decision and is able to understand the operation and postoperative events.

The operative technique is based on the principle, first suggested by Nissen, of transecting the cartilage from the sternum and lifting the sternum. To keep the sternum in this position essential additions to this principle have been made (Ochsner and Debakey, 1938; Brown, 1939). The main steps of the operation are described by Haller *et al.* (1989) and are as follows.

A transverse skin incision is made below the nipples (submammary in girls) and centred, if possible, over the deepest part of the concavity. Skin flaps are then lifted at the level of the pectoral fascia using electrocoagulation to minimize blood loss. The pectoral muscles are reflected by incising the fascia in the midline and sweeping the muscle flaps laterally with an inferior transverse relaxing incision along the seventh rib. All abnormal costal cartilages are removed subperiochondrally, thus preserving the perichondrium (usually the fourth to seventh rib bilaterally). A subxiphoid incision is made with finger mobilization of the substernal space. Care must be taken to avoid opening the pleural cavities. The intercostal muscle bundles are then divided from the sternum, thus allowing full mobilization of the sternum.

The lowest normal rib (third or fourth) is then obliquely transected from the medial and lateral of the associated costal cartilage. A transverse (wedge) osteotomy of the sternum is performed above the lowest normal rib. The sternum is elevated and fixed with non-absorbable mattress sutures through the periosteum at the site of the osteotomy. With this sternal elevation, the medial part of the transected cartilage lies on and is supported by its lateral partner and is then fixed with a single suture. The sternal fixation and bilateral sternal support constitute the internal dynamic tripod suspension and there is no need for additional hardware support. In children over 10 years of age and adults a temporary stainless-steel strut beneath the sternum is required and is fixed bilaterally to the fifth or sixth ribs.

A soft plastic chest drain is left in the substernal space. The pectoralis muscle fascia is closed in the midline and small silastic drainage catheters are left beneath the skin flaps. The skin is closed with a subcuticular suture.

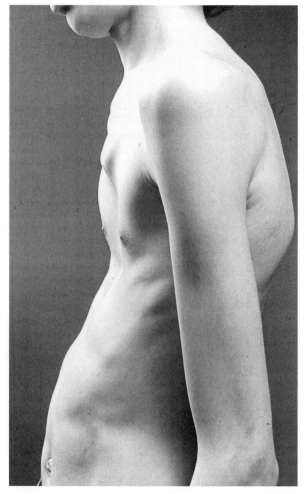

Fig. 47.2 Pectus excavatum in combination with bad posture.

There are modifications of this technique, but the principle in all remains the same.

The reported results of the surgical treatment of pectus excavatum have been variable, ranging from excellent to poor. In patients with Marfan's syndrome there is a higher risk of recurrence. Recurrence in patients with isolated pectus excavatum may be due to an underlying hereditary disorder of connective tissue (Am *et al.*, 1989).

Pectus carinatum (pigeon chest)

Pectus carinatum is the second most common anomaly of the chest wall. Its incidence varies depending on the published series, but does not account for more than 20% of chest wall malformations (Welch and Vos, 1973; Robicsek *et al.*, 1979). The pathogenesis is unknown, but it is thought that the primary cause lies in the costal cartilages rather than in the sternum.

CLINICAL FEATURES

Three forms of pectus carinatum are described: the lower, chondrogladiolar form (Fig. 47.3), the higher chondromanubrial arcuate form (Fig. 47.4) and the asymmetrical lateral pectus carinatum (Fig. 47.5). The cosmetic aspects dominate the symptomatology but the rigid expiratory position of the chest wall may interfere with respiration and lead to chronic, non-specific respiratory symptoms.

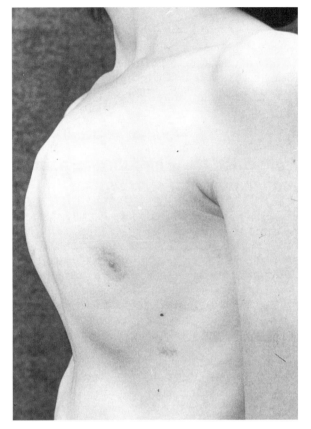

Fig. 47.4 Chondromanubrial pectus carinatum.

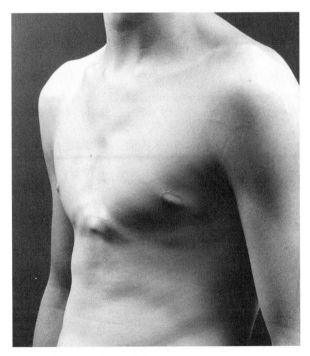

Fig. 47.3 Chondrogladiolar pectus carinatum.

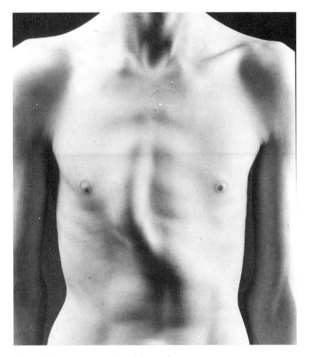

Fig. 47.5 Asymmetrical lateral pectus carinatum.

MANAGEMENT

Operative correction is the treatment of choice. The technique is similar in its access to the sternum and excision of costal cartilages, but here the sternum is not lifted, but brought down by applying one or two osteotomies depending on the type of malformation. The cosmetic results are usually very satisfactory.

Congenital fissure of the sternum (congenital cleft sternum)

The pathoembryology of this rare anomaly has been described extensively (Eijgelaar and Bijtel, 1970). The first mesenchymal anlage of the sternum becomes visible at the sixth week of embryonic development and fusion starts in a craniocaudal direction and finishes by the tenth week. Ossification centres appear first in the manubrium sterni at the sixth month of development and develop in the same direction during the following months. Ossification is not completed until after puberty, but bony fusion between the manubrium, the body of the sternum and the xyphoid process rarely occurs. When fusion of sternal bands fails to occur, the sternum does not develop (bifid sternum), whereas when the fusion process is interrupted, an upper or a lower cleft develops (cleft sternum: cranial or caudal).

Partial clefts of the sternum (usually cranial) are more common than complete clefts. A caudal cleft is often associated with other congenital anomalies such as ectopia cordis, diaphragmatic hernia, omphalocele and a communicating pericardial and peritoneal cavity (pentalogy of Cantrell; Cantrell *et al.*, 1958).

CLINICAL FEATURES

The anomaly is usually immediately apparent at birth (Fig. 47.6). From the distal end of the cleft in the midline there is often a linear mark of scar-like tissue.

In the simple cleft, symptoms are limited to paradoxical respiratory movements of the defect in the chest wall. Breathlessness and cyanosis are rare and should raise the suspicion of an associated cardiac defect. In ectopia cordis the heart is situated uncovered in front of and outside the incompletely fused lower chest and upper abdominal wall, and there are associated congenital cardiac defects. The baby is otherwise normal, without concomitant anomalies of the skeleton or other organs such as the lungs, kidneys or intestinal tract.

MANAGEMENT

The simple asymptomatic sternal cleft is not a vital indication for surgical treatment. Adults have been

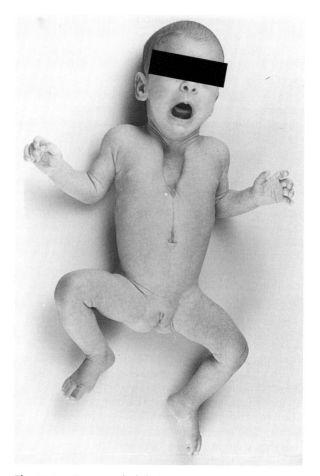

Fig. 47.6 Congenital cleft sternum.

described with sternal clefts who are free of symptoms, and the need for operative correction is therefore a debatable point. The deformity is unsightly and the heart's pulsations are alarmingly visible, causing highly understandable reasons for closing the defect. The surgeon who plans surgical correction should be aware that the indication is purely cosmetic. Surgical correction is most appropriate in the neonatal period when the defect is more easily closed than at a later stage in life.

Surgical correction can best be performed using Sabiston's (1958) technique (Fig. 47.7). Excision of a wedge in the distal fused part of the sternum is essential for good mobilization and approximation of the two sternal bars. In the neonate, incision and subsequent sliding of the costal cartilages is not necessary to approximate the two sternal halves, but this technique is easy to perform and provides remarkable enlargement of the thoracic volume and lessening of tension in the closure of the cleft. To prevent the later occurrence of cervical lung hernia, approximation and fixation with a few stitches of the sternal ends of the

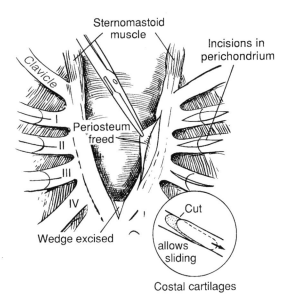

Fig. 47.7 Sabiston's technique for correction of cleft sternum.

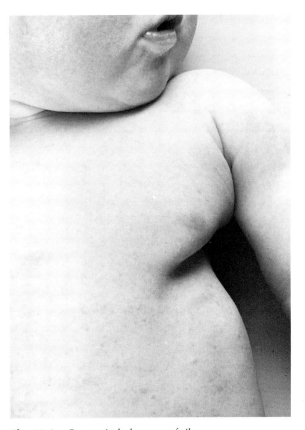

Fig. 47.8 Congenital absence of ribs.

sternocleidomastoid muscles has been recommended (Daum and Heiss, 1970).

The closure of complicated clefts has a clear medical indication. In the Cantrell syndrome the omphalocele has to be managed first and prior to definitive surgery the cardiac condition must be investigated.

Surgical correction of the sternal defect can usually be done in a one-stage procedure depending on the cardiac condition. If the gap is too large and cannot be closed primarily then a variety of techniques can be applied using marlex mesh (Hoffman, 1965), stainless-steel mesh (Ravitch, 1977) or autogenous cartilage grafts (Ravitch, 1968).

Congenital absence of ribs

This again is a rare abnormality unless associated with spina bifida. There is an association of partial absence of a few upper ribs, asymmetric or absent breast and nipple and partial absence of the pectoralis muscle. The aetiology of this anomaly is unknown.

CLINICAL FEATURES

The defect is obvious at birth (Fig. 47.8). There may be an associated congenital scoliosis which is apparent at this stage or may be a later development. Sometimes the breast and pectoralis major muscle is absent, but this is not constant. In larger defects there is always paradoxical respiration but respiratory symptoms are usually mild or absent.

MANAGEMENT

If surgical treatment is required it should be performed early after birth, as the defect is smaller in size and less rigid. Satisfactory results can be achieved by using a rib graft taken from the normal contralateral side. Sometimes an abnormal rib, being a part of the abnormality, can be used for this purpose by adapting it to fill and close the defect (Ravitch, 1961). On long-term follow-up one should always be aware of the possibility of the development of a progressive scoliosis.

Poland syndrome

This extremely rare syndrome, first described by Alfred Poland, shows a variety of anomalies. The classical findings in this syndrome are absence or malposition of nipple and breast, absence of the pectoralis minor and part of the major pectoralis, absence of a few ribs and cartilages and a malformation of the hand on the same side. Operative treatment follows the same principle as in congenital absence of ribs, but for the muscular defect other techniques such as pedicled grafts of latissimus muscle may be used.

ACKNOWLEDGEMENT

I thank Mr L.K.R. Shanbhogue, ChM, FRCS, for reading the manuscript, and J. Hagoort, MA, for editorial assistance.

References

Arn, P.H., Scherer, L.R., Haller, J.A., Jr and Pyeritz, R.E. 1989: Outcome of pectus excavatum in patients with Marfan syndrome and in the general population. *Journal of Pediatrics* **115**, 954–8.

Asness, R.S. 1992: Lessons from an adolescent with pectus excavatum [Letter]. *Pediatrics* **89**, 979.

Bier, Braun, and Kummel 1934: *Chirurgische Operationslehre*, band II. Leipzig: Verlag von Johann Ambrosius Barth.

Brown, A.L. 1939: Pectus excavatum (funnel chest). *Journal of Thoracic Surgery* **9**, 164–9.

Cantrell, J.R., Haller, J.A. and Ravitch, M.M. 1958: A syndrome of congenital defects involving the abdominal wall, sternum, diaphragm, pericardium and heart. *Surgery, Gynecology and Obstetrics* **107**, 602–14.

Daum, R. and Heiss, W. 1970: Zur operativen korrektur angeborener sternumspalten. *Thoraxchirurgie* **18**, 432–6.

Eijgelaar, A. and Bijtel, J.H. 1970: Congenital cleft sternum. *Thorax* **25**, 490–8.

Hage, S.A. and Bowen, J.R. 1992: Preliminary results of orthotic treatment of pectus deformities in children and adolescents. *Journal of Pediatric Orthopedics* **12**, 795–800.

Haller, J.A., Jr, Schere, L.R., Turner, C.S. and Colombani, P.M. 1989: Evolving management of pectus excavatum based on a single institutional experience of 664 patients. *Annals of Surgery* **209**, 578–83.

Hoffman, E. 1965: Surgical correction of bifid sternum. *Archives of Surgery* **90**, 76–80.

Kagaraoka, H., Ohnuki, T., Itaoka, T., Kei, J., Yokoyama, M. and Nitta, S. 1992: Degree of severity of pectus excavatum and pulmonary function in preoperative and postoperative periods. *Journal of Thoracic and Cardiovascular Surgery* **104**, 1483–8.

Ochsner, A. and Debakey, M. 1938: Chone-chondrosternon. *Journal Thoracic Surgery* **8**, 469–75.

Ravitch, M.M. 1961: Operative treatment of congenital deformities of the chest. *American Journal of Surgery* **101**, 588–97.

Ravitch, M.M. 1968: The chest wall. In Welch K.J., Randolph, J.G., Ravitch, M.M., O'Neill, J.A., Jr and Rowe, M.I. (eds), *Pediatric surgery*, 4th ed. Chicago, IL: Year Book Medical.

Ravitch, M.M. 1977: *Congenital deformities of the chest wall and their operative correction*. Philadelphia, PA: W.B. Saunders.

Robicsek, F., Cook, J.W., Daugherty, H.K. and Selle, J.G. 1979: Pectus carinatum. *Journal of Thoracic and Cardiovascular Surgery* **78**, 52–61.

Sabiston, D.C. 1958: The surgical management of congenital bifid sternum with partal ectopia cordis. *Journal of Thoracic Surgery* **35**, 118–22.

Shamberger, R.C. and Welch, K.J. 1988: Cardiopulmonary function in pectus excavatum. *Surgery, Gynecology and Obstetrics* **166**, 383–91.

Welch, K.J., and Vos, A. 1973: Surgical correction of pectus carinatum. *Journal of Pediatric Surgery* **8**, 659–67.

Wynn, S.R., Driscoll, D.J., Ostrom, N.K. *et al.* 1990: Exercise cardiorespiratory function in adolescents with pectus excavatum. *Journal of Thoracic and Cardiovascular Surgery* **99**, 41–7.

CHAPTER 48

Head and neck

D.P. DRAKE

Cystic hygroma
Teratomas
Lymphadenopathy
Thyroid
Thyroglossal cysts
Branchial anomalies
Parotid

Other salivary glands
Preauricular sinus
Torticollis
Dermoid cysts
Midline skin fusion defect
Miscellaneous
References

Cystic hygroma

Cystic hygromas are thin-walled cysts filled with clear fluid that arise in the neck and axillae. They result from maldevelopment of the lymphatic jugular sacs in the first trimester and may be demonstrated on ultrasound scanning in the second trimester of pregnancy (Langer *et al.*, 1990). These have a high incidence of associated fetal hydrops, cardiac and chromosomal anomalies, most often Turner's syndrome, and the prognosis for survival is poor. By contrast, diagnosis in the third trimester is rarer but carries the same prognosis as those presenting postnatally.

Their incidence is 1 in 12 000 live births, with many being detected at birth and 90% appearing in the first 2 years of life. They are soft fluctuant masses which transluminate brightly and distort local anatomy (Bill and Sumner, 1965). Some are discreet but many transgress tissue planes involving skin, subcutaneous tissue, muscle and the structures of the pharynx and larynx. Extension into the mediastinum can occur.

Lesions involving the tongue, pharynx or larynx may present with upper airway obstruction. Infection may be the initial presentation.

Investigations should include radiography of the neck and chest to demonstrate displacement of the upper airway and mediastinal involvement. Sonography confirms the presence of multiple cystic lesions (Sheth *et al.*, 1987) and magnetic resonance imaging scans (MRI) will give more detailed definition of the extent of the lesion and the disruption of normal anatomy (Siegal *et al.*, 1989). There is seldom difficulty in making the diagnosis, except in the floor of the mouth, where they can be confused with retention cysts of the salivary glands.

Surgical excision is the treatment of choice and there is little advantage in delaying this once the diagnosis is made. Resolution of the cysts, either spontaneously or following infection, is rare (Merriman *et al.*, 1992). Respiratory difficulties are an indication for urgent treatment, often requiring a tracheostomy. Total excision is the ideal but is impossible for extensive lesions involving all structures from the skin to the larynx and for those in the floor of the mouth and tongue. Mutilating surgery is not justified as these are benign lesions, and suction drainage and prophylactic antibiotics are indicated.

Laser surgery is indicated for cysts involving the pharynx, larynx and trachea (Cohen and Thompson, 1986).

Sclerotherapy should be considered for lesions not amenable to surgical excision. Good results have been reported with bleomycin (Tanaku *et al.*, 1990) but this carries the small risk of pulmonary fibrosis, which can be fatal. The Japanese have reported excellent results with OK432, which is a streptococcal extract (Ogita *et al.*, 1991). Cyst aspiration and injection may be performed under ultrasound control and repeated at intervals.

Cystic hygromas are associated with much morbidity, including recurrent infection, accumulation of fluid in postoperative wounds and growth of residual cysts. When tracheostomies are indicated, it can be several years before the patient is successfully decannulated. Lesions extending into the mediastinum and involving the airways are associated with a small but persistent mortality (Hancock *et al.*, 1992). Nerves are at risk of injury during neck dissections.

Teratomas

Cervical teratomas represent less than 10% of neonatal teratomas and presentation later in childhood is very rare. They are thought to arise from totipotential cells found in the embryonic thyroid anlage (Roediger *et al.*, 1974). All three germ layers are represented. Although the majority are benign, malignancy with distal metastases to the lung and liver has been described (Jordan and Ganderer, 1988).

Large cervical teratomas are associated with maternal polyhydramnios and may cause dystocia. Antenatal intervention with drainage of large cysts in the teratoma has been described with a successful outcome (Roodhooft *et al.*, 1987). Postnatally, they present with a solid embossed swelling in the neck, crossing the midline anteriorly. The mass may extend into the superior mediastinum and it does not transilluminate. Some are associated with airway obstruction.

Plain radiography may demonstrate spicules of calcification within the tumour and tracheal compression or deviation. Sonography demonstrates that the lesion has solid and cystic elements. Radioisotope thyroid scanning is indicated in the older child but is of no preoperative value in the neonate.

Treatment consists of surgical excision through a transverse cervical incision. The teratoma may be adjacent to the thyroid gland or firmly attached to it and total excision may involve a partial thyroidectomy. On occasions the thyroid gland is unrecognizable because of compression and displacement. Adjacent enlarged lymph nodes should be excised.

Postoperatively thyroid function is normal. Benign teratomas including those with immature histology are cured by surgical excision (Dehner *et al.*, 1990) and spread to local lymph nodes also carries an excellent prognosis. The majority of the mortality is related to still births and difficulties with airway management immediately after delivery. The rare malignant teratoma with distal metastases will require chemotherapy.

Oropharyngeal teratomas, which include the epignathus containing recognizable organs, are exceedingly rare (Hatzihaberis *et al.*, 1978). They are more common in females and may be associated with a cleft palate. The priority at birth is to establish an airway. Surgical excision is the definitive treatment, with incomplete dissection being preferable to mutilating surgery, as malignant dissemination is very rare (Valente *et al.*, 1985).

Lymphadenopathy

Most children with cervical lymphadenitis have a self-limiting illness or resolution following a short course of antibiotics. Referral for a surgical opinion is appropriate if a mass of enlarged matted nodes, measuring more than 3 cm in maximum diameter, is present for more than 3 weeks (Scobie, 1969). Table 48.1 indicates the differential diagnoses that should be considered.

A full history should give important clues and investigation will include a full blood count for all patients, a chest radiograph and skin testing when tuberculosis is suspected. Serology may be requested for suspected infectious mononucleosis. Needle aspiration using a

Table 48.1 Differential diagnoses for cervical lymphadenitis

Type	Cause	
Acute	Bacterial	Streptococcus
		Staphylococcus
	Viral	
Subacute	Bacterial	Actinomycosis
		Cat scratch fever
	Protozoa	Toxoplasmosis
	Viral	Ebstein–Barr (infectious mononucleosis)
Chronic	Bacterial	*Mycobacterium tuberculosis*
		Mycobacterium avium-intracellulare scrofulaceum
	Viral	HIV

wide-bore needle may obtain useful material for microbiology but the procedure requires local anaesthesia and sedation.

Acute lymphadenitis is secondary to viral or bacterial infections of the upper respiratory tract. Penicillin-resistant staphylococci and group A β-haemolytic streptococci are the common organisms isolated, staphylococci predominating in younger children and leading to suppuration. Prompt treatment with a β-lactamase resistant antibiotic may resolve the infection but, when suppuration has occurred, incision and drainage under antibiotic cover is recommended. When dental disease is present, antibiotic treatment should include anaerobic cover.

Tuberculous adenitis as a manifestation of systemic infection is diagnosed in older children, many from less developed countries and usually following contact with a known carrier. A purified protein derivative (PPD) skin test is strongly positive and a chest radiograph should be requested. Treatment is with chemotherapy, for example rifampicin and isoniazid for 12–18 months, and an excision biopsy is often not required to confirm the diagnosis, so long as the response to therapy is satisfactory. In children aged 1–5 years, non-tuberculous or *Mycobacterium avium-intracellulare scrofulaceum* is a more common cause of chronic lymphadenitis and, when present for several weeks, leads to a purplish discoloration of the overlying skin. Sinus formation can occur with delay in treatment. Systemic symptoms are mild or absent and skin testing for *Mycobacterium tuberculosis* is negative. Treatment is excision biopsy of caseating nodes and chemotherapy is not indicated (White *et al.*, 1986). However, biopsy material must be sent for mycobacterial culture and histology to confirm the diagnosis and aid in the management of the very rare recurrences.

Cat scratch disease can present as subacute lymphadenitis some weeks after the 'forgotten' scratch. Although the disease is self-limiting, excision biopsy is often undertaken when there is diagnostic uncertainty. Histologically, there is a non-caseating granulomatous reaction. The causative organism is variable, a pleomorphic Gram-negative bacillus has been identified (English *et al.*, 1988) and more recently *Rochalimaea henselae* has been incriminated (Tompkins and Steigbigel, 1993).

Malignant disease can present as enlarged cervical lymph nodes, lymphomas from the age of 5 years and leukaemia in all age groups. Rhabdomyosarcoma, neuroblastoma and a metastasis of papillary carcinoma of the thyroid are other rare causes of cervical lymphadenopathy.

Thyroid

The thyroid gland originates as an outpouching of the primitive pharyngeal floor at a site represented by the foramen caecum. It descends in the neck to be joined by lateral elements from the fourth and fifth branchial pouches, taking up its adult position anterior to the trachea and the developing parathyroid glands in the fifth and sixth weeks of development.

Complete failure of this descent results in a lingual thyroid gland. This is a rare clinical finding but may present with dysphagia. Treatment with thyroxine will reduce the size of the gland but surgical excision may be required. Transplanting thin slices of excised thyroid tissue to the thigh has maintained a child euthyroid for many years (Danis, 1973).

Ectopic thyroid tissue should be in the differential diagnosis of a midline swelling adjacent to the hyoid bone. When encountered at operation, this is a solid organ with a rich blood supply. The recommended management is a biopsy and thyroid replacement therapy to reduce the bulk of the ectopic thyroid.

Paediatric thyroid cancers were rare before 1950, when there was a marked increase in incidence related to exposure to ionizing radiation for the treatment of benign conditions of the neck (Wilson *et al.*, 1958). The incidence has since fallen but tumours of the thyroid are described uncommonly after irradiation for lymphoma (Hawkins *et al.*, 1987). Nuclear fall-out carries a higher risk to both young children and the fetus (Beverstock *et al.*, 1992). Thyroid cancer is more common in girls and children with pre-existing thyroid disease.

Papillary carcinoma is the most common paediatric thyroid malignancy, presenting as a palpable nodule in the thyroid or an adjacent lymph node. Follicular carcinoma is less common but spreads via the bloodstream to the lungs, bone and liver.

The rare anaplastic tumours spread locally through the thyroid capsule. Medullary cell carcinomas arise from the C cells and are mostly familial, being associated with multiple endocrine neoplasia type 2A. They have an autosomal dominant inheritance and can occur in children as young as 2 years (Telander *et al.*, 1989).

Patients with suspected tumours should be investigated with a technetium isotope scan, ultrasound scan and plain radiography to assess tracheal compression. Thyroid function should be measured and auto-antibodies assayed, if there is a multinodular thyroid suggesting thyroiditis. Fine needle aspiration is of value, as cysts that are impalpable following aspiration do not require exploration and operation may be deferred if cytology of aspirated material suggests a benign disease.

All solitary nodules should be excised with a margin of thyroid tissue. Papillary carcinomas may be multicentric and a subtotal thyroidectomy is recommended, leaving only a posterior rim of the contralateral lobe to protect the contralateral parathyroid glands and recurrent laryngeal nerve. Ipsilateral lymph nodes should be sampled but a block dissection is not indicated. Postoperatively, thyroxine is given to inhibit secretion of thyroid-stimulating hormone and metastases may be treated with [131]I. As the prognosis is excellent, with 90% of children surviving over 30 years, radical and potentially mutilating surgery should be avoided (Zimmerman *et al.*, 1988).

For a follicular carcinoma, all thyroid tissue should be excised and radioiodine scanning performed post-operatively to detect metastases, which are treated with [131]I.

Medullary carcinoma of the thyroid may present as a nodule or be identified by screening at-risk families, estimating plasma immunoreactive thyrocalcitonin (ICT) following pentagastrin stimulation. Medullary cancer is multicentric and spreads via lymphatics. The surgical treatment consists of a total thyroidectomy and sampling of adjacent lymph nodes. When the tumour is palpable, extrathyroid spread is invariable. Radical neck dissection offers no advantage and metastases are neither radiosensitive nor chemosensitive. Therefore cure can best be effected by a total thyroidectomy when the tumour is impalpable and screening of at-risk children should be performed in infancy (Telander *et al.*, 1986).

Thyroglossal cysts

The thyroglossal duct connects the foramen caecum in the tongue to the pyramidal lobe or isthmus of the thyroid. Although the majority of the duct regresses, the midportion remains as a discontinuous microscopic tube of undifferentiated epithelium adjacent to the hyoid bone (Stayl and Lyall, 1954). Secretory activity may be induced in this epithelium postnatally at any age, even in late adult life. Thyroglossal cysts are more common than branchial cysts but are rare in the newborn period.

Thyroglossal cysts present as midline swellings in the neck, most often adjacent to the hyoid bone. Less commonly the swelling may be to the left of the midline, lower in the neck or within the tongue. The swelling rises in the neck with swallowing or protrusion of the tongue. The initial presentation may be of an infected cyst, which is tender with erythema of the overlying skin. The differential diagnoses include an aberrant thyroid gland, a dermoid cyst or lymphadenitis. When there is clinical suspicion of hypothyroidism, thyroid function tests and a radioisotope thyroid scan should be performed.

The treatment is surgical excision of the cyst and its associated duct (Sistrunk, 1920). The cyst is dissected from the adjacent strap muscles and the central 1.5 cm of hyoid bone is excised. A midline core of tissue, passing cranially from the hyoid bone towards the tongue, is dissected in continuity with the cyst and the segment of bone. It is not advisable to take the dissection as far as the foramen caecum (Horisawa *et al.*, 1992) and placing a finger within the mouth to displace the tongue down-

wards and forwards is not necessary. The muscles are repaired with absorbable sutures and good haemostasis makes routine drainage of the wound unnecessary.

The most important postoperative complication is a recurrent cyst or sinus, which is more common if there has been infection before the first operation (Athow *et al.*, 1989). A recurrence follows inadequate excision of the thyroglossal duct, most probably related to the horizontally branching ducts at the level of the hyoid bone. Adequate excision of the midportion of the hyoid is crucial (Ein *et al.*, 1984). Surgery for recurrence should be delayed for several weeks and follows the same principles as the original operation.

Papillary carcinoma, presenting in adults, has been described in remnants of the thyroglossal duct (Maziak *et al.*, 1992).

Branchial anomalies

During the fourth week after fertilization, the embryo develops five pairs of endodermal pharyngeal pouches, followed by four pairs of ectodermal branchial clefts. The dorsal aspect of the first branchial cleft becomes the external auditory canal and the other three pairs of branchial clefts normally disappear. The pharyngeal pouches give rise to a number of important structures (Table 48.2).

Anomalies of the first branchial cleft are uncommon but include a cyst in the retroaural crease or a sinus, lined by stratified squamous epithelium, passing from the external auditory canal to open on the skin posterior to the angle of the mandible (Work, 1972). Cysts within the parotid fascia can be of first branchial cleft origin.

Table 48.2 Derivatives of branchial pouches

Pharyngeal pouch	Derivatives
First	Eustachian tube Middle ear, mastoid ear cells
Second	Palatine tonsil Supratonsillar fossa
Third	Pyriform fossa Inferior parathyroids Thymus
Fourth	Pyriform fossa Superior parathyroids Lateral anlage of thyroid gland (Thymus)
Fifth	Ultimobranchial body Lateral anlage of thyroid gland

The most common presentation is of an inflammatory swelling, with a chronic discharging sinus following incision and drainage. The definitive treatment is surgical excision of the cyst or sinus, when it is quiescent. Great care must be taken to identify and preserve the facial nerve, which lies adjacent and usually superficial to the sinus (Millar *et al.*, 1984). Dissection must be continued up to the external auditory canal, where the sinus may be in communication with its lumen.

Most branchial anomalies are associated with the second branchial cleft, which may persist as a sinus opening on the skin at the anterior border of the sternomastoid muscle or, less commonly, as a fistula communicating with the tonsillar fossa (Ford *et al.*, 1992). Ten per cent are bilateral. Branchial cysts are well described in older children and young adults; these are not attached to the skin but may communicate with the pharynx. Subcutaneous cartilagenous rests, usually overlying the anterior border of the sternomastoid muscle, are also branchial remnants.

The clinical presentation of a branchial sinus is in infants with an intermittent discharge of mucoid fluid. Infection is a risk and early surgical excision is recommended. The sinus may be cannulated with a ureteric catheter or intravenous cannula to demonstrate its length and course in the neck, as it passes cranially deep to the sternomastoid muscle and medially between the bifurcation of the carotid artery. It passes over the hypoglossal and glossopharyngeal nerves. A short sinus may be excised with an ellipse of skin at the exit site but a longer sinus or fistula is best dissected through a higher neck incision with a smaller ellipse at the exit site. All dissection must stay close to the tract to avoid damage to adjacent vessels and nerves. Histologically, the sinus is lined by a combination of squamous and respiratory epithelium.

Branchial cysts present as fluctuant swellings in the upper third of the neck deep to the sternomastoid muscle. An ultrasound scan will confirm that the lesion contains fluid. Surgical excision of the cyst should include any deep communication with the pharynx when present and great care must be taken to avoid damage to the hypoglossal nerve.

Sinuses or cysts of third or fourth pharyngeal pouch origin arise adjacent to the pyriform fossa and are invariably left-sided. These are rare but should be considered in a child presenting with recurrent abscesses involving the left lobe of the thyroid gland. A large infected cyst may compromise the upper airway, presenting with stridor in an infant (Burge and Middleton, 1983). A barium swallow may demonstrate the sinus arising in the pyriform fossa and a plain radiograph of the neck may outline air in a cyst which communicates with the pharynx. An isotope scan of the thyroid gland may show reduced uptake in the left lobe. Antibiotics should be used for acute infections, followed by surgi-

cal excision when the tissues are quiescent. The dissection will include the left lobe of the thyroid, which should be excised if involved in the inflammatory process (Miller *et al.*, 1983). A third pouch sinus passes cranial to the superior laryngeal nerve and the inferior constrictor muscle of the pharynx; and a fourth pouch passes caudal to these structures (Bavetta *et al.*, 1992). The recurrent laryngeal nerve is adjacent to the fourth pouch sinus as it enters the inferior constrictor muscle and it should be identified and preserved.

Parotid

Recurrent painful swelling of the parotid gland is a condition of unknown aetiology, possibly related to a secretary IgA deficiency in saliva (Cohen *et al.*, 1992). Most episodes of acute parotitis are unilateral and can be modified with the use of antibiotics and analgesia. Attacks become less frequent for most children as they approach puberty. Chewing gum stimulates the flow of serous saliva and may have a prophylactic effect. Surgery is rarely required and only when the attacks persist into adolescence or the gland suppurates. Although a sialogram demonstrates sialectasis, thus confirming the clinical diagnosis, the information gained from this uncomfortable investigation does not alter the management of the disorder and is rarely justified.

Lymphadenitis of the preparotid lymph glands, secondary to infections such as atypical mycobacterium or cat scratch fever, has to be distinguished from parotid swellings (Carnacho *et al.*, 1989) and a computed tomography (CT) scan is valuable in defining the relationship of the swelling to the parotid fascia.

TUMOURS OF THE PAROTID

Tumours of the parotid gland represent 5% of all paediatric tumours. Ultrasound scanning is useful in making the diagnosis and relationships to the facial nerve are best delineated by MRI scans. Haemangiomas, which may be accompanied by a cutaneous capillary naevus, and lymphangiomas are benign swellings in the parotid region. Most haemangiomas will resolve spontaneously by the age of 5 years and run an intermittent course (William, 1975). They are more common in girls. Observation and reassurance are the key to management, as any surgical intervention is very hazardous to the facial nerve and intralesional injections are of doubtful benefit. Lymphangiomas do not regress spontaneously and surgical excision may be indicated after a period of observation.

The benign mixed parotid tumour has been described in older children and more rarely in infants (Bianchi and Cudmore, 1978). Wide excision with a margin of parotid tissue is essential to avoid local recurrence and a superficial parotidectomy, with identification of the facial nerve and its branches, is recommended for tumours in the superficial lobe.

Mucoepidermoid carcinomas account for half of the malignant tumours of the parotid gland (McKelvie, 1989), with the rarer acinic cell and undifferentiated carcinomas, adenocarcinomas and rhabdomyosarcomas. Wide surgical excision, which may include branches of the facial nerve, is indicated and both radiotherapy and chemotherapy should be considered in the management of these rare and often resistant tumours.

Other salivary glands

Swellings of the submandibular gland are most often related to sialadenitis, which may be secondary to a calculus in the submandibular duct. A plain radiograph is indicated and a calculus, accessible in the floor of the mouth, should be removed from the duct. Persistent or recurrent and painful swelling of the gland is best managed by excision, taking care to preserve the mandibular branch of the facial nerve and the lingual and hypoglossal nerves, which are adjacent to the deep surface of the gland.

A ranula is a cystic swelling presenting in the floor of the mouth, adjacent to the submandibular duct and displacing the tongue. It represents extravasation of saliva from the sublingual gland and can grow to a large size, interfering with speech and swallowing (Batsakis and McClatchey, 1988). Marsupialization is recommended, preserving the submandibular duct and suturing the lining of the cyst to the floor of the mouth with a fine continuous absorbable suture. Excision of the ranula should be avoided as control of the ensuing haemorrhage may damage adjacent nerves and ducts and predispose to recurrent cysts. A plunging ranula does not present orally but as a swelling in the submental region below the mylohyoid muscles. These cannot be marsupialized and are best excised along with the sublingual gland (Parekh *et al.*, 1987).

Preauricular sinus

The external ear forms from a number of tubercles and a failure of fusion can result in a sinus, opening on to the ear or immediately anterior to it. The sinus does not communicate with the external auditory canal but is adjacent to the cartilage of the pinna. Other members of the family may be affected and many sinuses will remain asymptomatic throughout life. Infection is the indication for surgical intervention.

The operation should be performed under antibiotic cover, when the sinus is not clinically infected. Infiltration with local anaesthetic and adrenaline reduces bleeding from skin edges but injection of dye into the sinus cannot be recommended. Through a racket-shaped preauricular incision, skin flaps are elevated and the sinus with its branches dissected, using a needle-point diathermy (Wright 1994). Anteriorly the superficial temporal vessels are identified and preserved, while posteriorly a shaving of cartilage may be taken with the sinus and inferiorly the external auditory canal marks the limit of dissection. Although prior infection makes the operation more difficult, asymptomatic sinuses should not be subjected to surgery.

Wound infections should be managed with drainage and appropriate antibiotics, but recurrent postoperative infections are an indication to re-explore and excise remnants of the sinus.

Torticollis

Torticollis presenting at the age of a few weeks is most often associated with a palpable tumour of the sternomastoid muscle and limitation of neck rotation towards the side of the tumour. Thirty per cent of these infants are born by breech delivery, suggesting that the abnormality has a prenatal aetiology, although others favour birth trauma causing haemorrhage and fibrosis in the muscle (MacDonald, 1969). The parents should be taught passive stretching exercises to rotate the head ten times in the direction of the tumour, as far as the infant will permit. These should be repeated twice a day over 2 months and the range of neck movement reassessed. When full neck movement is achieved, the exercises should continue daily until approximately 9 months of age. With adequate supervision, open surgery can be avoided in these infants (Cameron *et al.*, 1994).

However, children presenting later than 3 months of age have an increasing failure rate for passive stretching exercises and a proportion will require open division of the sternomastoid muscle and its associated fascia. Many of these children will have a degree of hypoplasia of the ipsilateral face. The myotomy must be followed by adequate physiotherapy to maintain full correction of posture and neck movement.

Secondary torticollis may be related to underlying vertebral or ocular pathology and should be managed by the appropriate specialists.

Dermoid cysts

Dermoid cysts occur along embryological fault lines where tissue can be sequestered between growing plates of ectoderm. Their lining includes epidermoid structures such as sebaceous glands and hair follicles and they contain keratinous material.

The most common example in the head and neck is the external angular dermoid, which occurs at the lateral limit of the eyebrow. These are hard swellings, not attached to skin but are firmly sited in a depression of the periosteum and outer table of the frontal bone. They usually present in the first 6 months of life and can grow to a diameter of 3 cm. Very rarely, extension through the orbital bone has been described. Excision is recommended through a small overlying incision but the eyebrow should not be shaved. Dermoids may also occur posteriorly to this site in the frontotemporal region overlying the coronal sulcus.

Midline scalp dermoids are found at two sites, those over the anterior fontanelle being immediately superficial to the dura and sagittal sinus, but those at the posterior fontanelle may extend intracranially to the roof of the third ventricle. Preoperative evaluation with CT scanning is recommended.

A midline pit at the bridge of the nose, with a protruding hair and subcutaneous swelling, is a dermoid sinus, which may communicate with an intracranial cyst through the cribriform plate of the frontal bones. This represents a failure of obliteration of the embryological tract from the foramen caecum to the nasal tip. Dermoid cysts and sinuses at the bridge of the nose, with nasal gliomas and encephaloceles, form a continuum of lesions and should all be investigated with CT scanning to identify any intracranial extension or skull defects. Excision of purely extracranial lesions can be achieved through a midline nasal incision but those with an intracranial component require a craniofacial approach (Penster *et al.*, 1988).

Dermoid cysts may also occur in the midline of the neck, either in the supra-sternal notch or adjacent to the hyoid bone, where they may be indistinguishable preoperatively from a thyroglossal cyst.

Midline skin fusion defect

This is a peculiar, congenital and depressed scar in the midline of the neck, where dermal structures are missing. There may be a sinus from the inferior limit of the scar to the sternal notch. The lesion should be excised and the defect closed with a Z-plasty, to avoid reproducing a midline scar.

Miscellaneous

PILOMATRIXOMA

These calcified epitheliomas are hamartomas of hair follicles and occur on the head and neck and the upper limbs, being more common in girls and described in children, adolescents and young adults. They are attached to skin and have a hard irregular edge. There may be a history of recurrent inflammation and pain leading to ulceration of the overlying skin. Malignant change has been reported but it is extremely rare.

Treatment is by simple excision with the overlying skin, local recurrence is very uncommon and multiple lesions have been described (Bingul *et al.*, 1962).

SEBACEOUS NAEVUS

This is a congenital hamartoma of sebaceous glands presenting as a salmon-pink, raised and hairless lesion of the scalp or face. It thickens with age and may be associated with discharge at puberty. As neoplastic change to basal cell carcinoma is described in adults, total excision during childhood is recommended (Kaplan and Nickoloff, 1987).

FRAENUM

When a tight lingual fraenum or tongue tie is a thin transparent band of tissue, this may resolve spontaneously, probably from laceration on the lower incisor teeth once these have erupted. Thicker bands of tissue persist with tethering of the tip of the tongue to the floor of the mouth and surgical division is justified, as untreated these may cause a lisp and difficulty licking ice cream from the upper lip! The operation is recommended after the age of 6 months and is best achieved with bipolar diathermy, the child having a general anaesthetic and the airway being protected either by endotracheal intubation or by a laryngeal mask.

An upper lip fraenum passes between the upper incisors and tethers the upper lip, causing ugly distortion when smiling. This fraenum should be excised with the underlying fibrous cord to allow normal development of the teeth.

CONGENITAL EPULIS

This is a rare, soft-tissue tumour attached to the maxillary alveolus, usually occurring in girls. It is a benign lesion of mesenchymal origin and does not grow postnatally. It should be excised locally, taking care not to damage the adjacent tooth buds. Recurrence is not described (Cussen and MacMahon, 1975).

THYMIC REMNANTS

The thymus gland is derived from the third branchial pouches and fuses in the midline of the neck in the eighth week of gestation, before descending into the superior mediastinum. A remnant may remain in the neck, presenting as a soft and poorly defined swelling deep to the strap muscles. Ectopic thymic tissue can cause respiratory distress by tracheal compression (Spigland *et al.*, 1990). The diagnosis is rarely made preoperatively, surgical excision being recommended for a mass of uncertain origin. The presence of Hassall's corpuscles confirms the diagnosis histologically and cystic change may be present.

References

Athow, A.C., Fagg, N.C.K. and Drake, D.P. 1989: Management of thyroglossal cysts in children. *British Journal of Surgery* **76**, 811–14.

Batsakis, T.G. and McClatchey, K.D. 1988: Cervical ranulas. *Annals of Otology, Rhinology and Laryngology* **97**, 561–2.

Bavetta, S., Hall, C.M. and Drake, D.P. 1992: Recurrent neck abscess caused by a fourth pharyngeal pouch sinus. *Journal of the Royal Society of Medicine* **85**, 757–8.

Beverstock, K., Egloff, B. and Pinchera, A. 1992: Thyroid cancer after Chernobyl. *Nature* **359**, 21–2.

Bianchi, A. and Cudmore, R.E. 1978: Salivary gland tumours in children. *Journal of Pediatric Surgery* **13**, 519–21.

Bill, A.H.J. and Sumner, D.S. 1965: A unified concept of lymphangioma and cystic hygroma. *Surgery, Gynaecology and Obstetrics* **120**, 79–86.

Bingul, O., Graham, J.H., Helwig, E.B. 1962: Pilomatrixoma (calcifying epithelioma) in children. *Pediatrics* **30**, 233–40.

Burge, D. and Middleton, A. 1983: Persistent pharyngeal pouch derivatives in the neonate. *Journal of Pediatric Surgery* **18**, 230–4.

Cameron, B.H., Langer, J.C. and Cameron, G.S. 1994: Success of non-operative treatment for congenital muscular torticollis is dependent on early therapy. *Pediatric Surgery International* **9**, 391–3.

Carnacho, A.E., Goodman, M.L. and Eavery, R.D. 1989: Pathological correlation of the unknown solid parotid mass in children. *Otolaryngology, Head and Neck Surgery* **101**, 566–71.

Cohen, H.A., Gross, S., Nussinovitch, M., Frydman, M. and Varsano, I. 1992: Recurrent parotitis. *Archives of Disease in Childhood* **67**, 1036–7.

Cohen, S.R. and Thompson, J.W. 1986: Lymphangiomas of the larynx in infants and children. A survey of pediatric lymphangioma. *Annals of Otology, Rhinology and Laryngology* **127** (Suppl.), 1–20.

Cussen, L.J. and MacMahon, R.A. 1975: Congenital granular-cell myoblastoma. *Journal of Pediatric Surgery* **10**, 249–53.

Danis, R.K. 1973: An alternative in management in lingual thyroid: excision with implantation. *Journal of Pediatric Surgery* **8**, 869–70.

Dehner, L.P., Mills, A., Talerman, A. *et al.* 1990: Germ cell neoplasms of head and neck soft tissues: a pathologic spectrum of teratomatous and endodermal sinus tumors. *Human Pathology* **21**, 309–18.

Ein, S.H., Shandling, B., Stephens, C.A. and Mancer, K. 1984: The problem of recurrent thyroglossal duct remnants. *Journal of Pediatric Surgery* **19**, 437–9.

English, C.K., Wear, D.J., Margileth, A.M., Lissner, C.R. and Walsh, G.P. 1988: Cat scratch disease: isolation and culture of the bacterial agent. *Journal of the American Medical Association* **259**, 1347–52.

Ford, G.R., Balakrishnan, A., Evans, J.N.G. and Bailey, C.M. 1992: Branchial cleft and pouch anomalies. *Journal of Laryngology and Otology* **106**, 137–43.

Hancock, B.J., St-Vil, D., Luks, Fl., Di Lorenzo, M. and Blanehard, H. 1992: Complications of lymphangiomas in children. *Journal of Pediatric Surgery* **27**, 220–6.

Hatzihaberis, F., Stamatis, D. and Staurinos, D. 1978: Giant epignathus. *Journal of Pediatric Surgery* **13**, 517–18.

Hawkins, M.M., Draper, G.J. and Kingston, J.E. 1987: Incidence of second primary tumours among childhood cancer survivors. *British Journal of Cancer* **36**, 339–47.

Horisawa, M., Niinomi, N. and Ito, T. 1992: What is the optimal depth for core out toward the foramen caecum in the thyroglossal duct operation? *Journal of Pediatric Surgery* **27**, 710–13.

Jordan, R.B. and Ganderer, M.W.L. 1988: Cervical teratomas: an analysis, literature review and proposed classification. *Journal of Pediatric Surgery* **23**, 583–91.

Kaplan, E. and Nickoloff, B.J. 1987: Clinical and histological features of nevi with emphasis on treatment approaches. *Clinical Plastic Surgery* **14**, 277–85.

Langer, J.C., Fitzgerald, P.G., Desa, D., Filly, R.A., Golbus, M.G., Adzick, N.S. and Harrison, M.R. 1990: Cervical cystic hygroma in the fetus; clinical spectrum and outcome. *Journal of Pediatric Surgery* **25**, 58–62.

MacDonald, D. 1969: Sternomastoid tumour and muscular torticollis. *Journal of Bone and Joint Surgery* **51B**: 432–43.

Maziak, D., Borowy, Z.J., Deitel, M. *et al.* 1992: Management of papillary carcinoma arising in thyroglossal duct anlage. *Canadian Journal of Surgery* **35**, 522–5.

McKelvie, P.A. 1989: Salivary gland tumours in children. *Pediatric Surgery International* **4**, 21–4.

Merriman, T., Davidson, P.M. and Myers, N.A. 1992: The spectrum of cervical cystic hygroma. *Pediatric Surgery International* **7**, 253–5.

Millar, P.D., Corcoran, M. and Hobsley, M. 1984: Surgical excision of first cleft branchial fistulae. *British Journal of Surgery* **71**, 696–7.

Miller, D., Hill, J.L., Sun, C.C., O'Brien, D.S. and Haller, J.A. 1983: The diagnosis and managent of pyriform sinus fistulae in infants and young children. *Journal of Pediatric Surgery* **18**, 377–81.

Ogita, S., Tsutu, T., Dejuchi, E. *et al.* 1991: OK-432 therapy for unresectable lymphangiomas in children. *Journal of Pediatric Surgery* **26**, 263–70.

Parekh, D. Stewart, M., Joseph, C. and Lawson, H.H. 1987: Plunging ranula: a report of three cases and review of literature. *British Journal of Surgery* **74**, 307–9.

Pensler, J.M., Bauer, B.S. and Naidich, T.P. 1988: Craniofacial dermoids. *Plastic and Reconstructive Surgery* **82**, 953–8.

Roediger, W.E., Spitz, L. and Schmaman, A. 1974: Histogenesis of benign cervical teratomas. *Teratology* **10**, 111–18.

Roodhooft, A.M., Delbeke, L. and Vaneerdeweg, W. 1987: Cervical teratoma: prenatal detection and management in the neonate. *Pediatric Surgery International* **1**, 181–4.

Scobie, W.G. 1969: Acute suppurative adenitis in children. A review of 964 cases. *Scottish Medical Journal* **14**, 352–8.

Sheth, S., Nussbaum, A.R., Hutchins, G.M. and Sanders, R.C. 1987: Cystic hygromas in children: sonographic–pathological correlation. *Radiology* **162**, 821–4.

Siegel, M.J., Glazer, H.S., St Amour, T.E. and Rosenthal, D.D. 1989: Lymphangiomas in children: MR imaging. *Radiology* **170**, 467–70.

Sistrunk, W.E. 1920: Surgical treatment of cysts of the thyroglossal tract. *Annals of Surgery* **71**, 121–4.

Spigland, N., Bensoussan, A.L., Blanchard, H. and Russo, P. 1990: Aberrant cervical thymus in children; three case reports and a review of the literature. *Journal of Pediatric Surgery* **25**, 1196–9.

Stahl, W.M. and Lyall, D. 1954: Cervical cysts and fistulae of thyroglossal tract origin. *Annals of Surgery* **139**, 123–8.

Tanaku, K., Inomata, Y., Utsonomiya, H. *et al.* 1990: Sclerosing therapy with bleomycin emulsion for lymphangiomas in children. *Pediatric Surgery International* **5**, 270–3.

Telander, R.L., Zimmerman, D., Sizemore, G.W. *et al.* 1989: Medullary carcinoma in children. *Archives of Surgery* **124**, 841–3.

Telander, R.L., Zimmerman, D., van Heerden, J.A. *et al.* 1986: Results of early thyroidectomy for medullary carcinoma in children with multiple endocrine neoplasia type II. *Journal of Pediatric Surgery* **21**, 1190–4.

Tompkins, D.C. and Steigbigel, R.T. 1993: Rochalimea's role in cat scratch disease and bacillary angiomatosis. *Annals of Internal Medicine* **118**, 338–90.

Valente, A., Grant, J.D. and Brereton, R.J. 1988: Neonatal tonsillar teratoma. *Journal of Pediatric Surgery* **23**, 364–6.

White, M.P., Bangash, H., Goel, K.M. and Jenkins, P.A. 1986: Non-tuberculous mycobacterial lymphadenitis. *Archives of Disease in Childhood* **61**, 368–71.

William, H.G. 1975: Hemangioma of the parotid gland in children. *Plastic and Reconstructive Surgery* **56**, 19–34.

Wilson, J.M., Kilpatrick, R., Eckert, H. *et al.* 1958: Thyroid neoplasms following irradiation. *British Medical Journal* **2**, 929–34.

Work, W.P. 1972: Newer concepts of first branchial cleft defects. *Laryngoscope* **82**, 1581–93.

Wright, J.E. 1994: Pre-auricular sinus in children: personal series and surgical technique. *Pediatric Surgery International* **9**, 323–4.

Zimmerman, D., Hay, I.D., Gough, I.R. *et al.* 1988: Papillary thyroid carcinoma in children and adults: long-term follow up of 1039 patients conservatively treated at one institution during 3 decades. *Surgery* **104**, 1157–66.

PART IV

Paediatric urology

CHAPTER 49

Urinary infection: principles

J.M. SMELLIE

Introduction
Significance
Aetiology
Factors predisposing to urinary tract infection
Diagnosis

Management
Special situations
Conclusions
References
Further reading

Introduction

Urinary tract infection (UTI) is a common and recurrent condition in infancy and childhood. It tends to be over-looked because of its non-specific symptoms and over-diagnosed if only local symptoms without urine culture are relied on. Epidemiological studies have indicated an overall prevalence of significant bacteriuria in school-children of about 2% in girls and less than 1% in boys, although the genders are equally affected in the first year of life, boys more often than girls in the first 6 months. Estimates have been made of the incidence of symptomatic urinary infection but these have varied because they have depended on referral practice and hospital admission policies. A survey of Swedish 7-year-old children at school entry showed that 8.5% of girls and 1.4% of boys had a past history of bacterio-logically proven symptomatic UTI (Hellström *et al.*, 1991), and the urinary tract remains one of the most common sites of bacterial infection in childhood. Although the renal outcome in the majority is benign, it may be serious in up to a quarter of infected children, particularly those with vesicoureteric reflux (VUR) or obstructive uropathy.

Infection of the urinary tract may be the mode of presentation of infants or children with underlying structural or functional abnormalities of the urinary tract, it may complicate surgical procedures either preoperatively or postoperatively; and it may be discovered on routine urine culture or on screening programmes [asymptomatic bacteriuria (ASB)] (Verrier-Jones *et al.*, 1986). This screening bacteriuria will not be considered further in this chapter.

In the unobstructed urinary tract, reinfection with a fresh organism or species frequently occurs. Less commonly, infection with the same organism may persist or relapse where there is sluggish or obstructed flow of urine. Any renal consequence of a defect in the normal function of ureter, bladder or urethra is considerably augmented if complicated by infection.

An understanding of the aetiology and mechanisms involved in urinary tract infection is thus essential for its effective practical management.

Significance

Urinary tract infection can cause illness or fever or unpleasant symptoms, which may or may not affect the kidneys, but of fundamental importance is the causative relationship between urinary tract infection, VUR and the renal scarring of chronic atrophic pyelonephritis or reflux nephropathy. This renal scarring is found in 5–25% of children with UTI, the proportion increasing with age and presumably the longer risk of exposure to recurrent infection (Smellie and Prescod, 1986). In children it is almost invariably associated with VUR (Smellie *et al.*, 1975, 1981; Smellie and Prescod, 1986). In documented clinical examples of new radiological scars that had developed either in a structurally normal kidney or in a normal segment of an already scarred kidney, both VUR and UTI were almost always present (Smellie *et al.*, 1985) and these associations have been demonstrated in experimental models (Hodson *et al.*, 1975; Ransley and Risdon, 1978). Functional defects of renal uptake of ^{99m}Tc DMSA are also well documented during or following acute UTI. Particularly in infants, these renal defects have sometimes been reported without demonstrable reflux (Rushton and Majd, 1992; Jakobsson *et al.*, 1992) but their clinical significance remains to be determined on long-term clinical and radiological follow-up.

Experimentally, renal damage associated with sterile reflux has been confined to kidneys exposed to prolonged high renal pelvic pressure secondary to partial urethral obstruction.

Aetiology

The urinary tract is normally sterile from the kidney to the external urethral orifice, although there may be bacterial colonization of the periurethral area in girls and the preputial sac in boys. This state is maintained by the normal bladder defence mechanisms, which mainly consist of the washout process. Urine, which is formed continuously by the kidneys, collects in the bladder from which it is emptied completely and at regular intervals. The characteristics of the bladder mucosa (the transitional epithelium and IgA content) and the general body immunity also contribute to the defence against bladder invasion and colonization. The external and internal urethral sphincters and the vesicoureteric junction also serve to exclude or compartmentalize bacterial invaders.

Infection of the urinary tract results from an imbalance between host and pathogen. There is either a fault in the normal bladder defences or the urinary pathogen has particular invasive qualities of motility (e.g. *Bacillus proteus*), adhesiveness (e.g. p-fimbriated *Escherichia coli*), or resistance to antibacterial agents. In the infant and child, UTI usually results from defects of host defences rather than from bacterial virulence so that when infection occurs at this age an underlying cause should be sought.

Factors predisposing to urinary tract infection

These are set out in Table 49.1. The main cause of UTI is urinary stasis and an increase in the volume of bladder residual urine. This may result from mechanical obstruction by stones or by structural narrowing of tubes, from saccules and diverticula of the bladder or from impairment of the normal bladder-emptying mechanisms secondary to a neurological (e.g. spinal dysraphism or injury) or functional (e.g. detrusor sphincter dyssyner-

Table 49.1 Factors predisposing to urinary tract infection

Urinary stasis	
Obstruction to flow	Mechanical
	Neuropathic
VUR	
Constipation	
Incomplete or hurried voiding	
Infrequent micturition	
Low fluid intake	
Dysfunctional voiding/unstable bladder	
Irritation of bladder mucosa	
Stones/gravel	
Chemical irritants	
Inflammation secondary to infection	
Reduced immunity	Local
	General

gia) abnormality. The volume of residual urine will also be increased when refluxed urine returns from the ureter to the bladder after micturition, when voiding is hurried or incomplete (as in the newly toilet-trained toddler), or from constipation when the loaded colon or rectum can interfere mechanically with bladder emptying (O'Regan *et al.*, 1985; Dohil *et al.*, 1994). Neurological defects will affect both bowel and bladder function. A reduced urine flow will lead to infrequent micturition and a greater risk of bacterial invasion of the bladder, so that infrequent drinks and dehydration in infancy can also increase the risk of UTI. Inflammation and irritation of the bladder mucosa by stones, 'gravel', concentrated urine, antiseptics added to the bath or swimming pool water, viral bladder infections and recent bacterial infection can also encourage bladder colonization.

Invasion of the urethra and bladder by the ascending route is probably a common occurrence, assisted by bacterial characteristics, external colonization and surface-tension lowering agents such as bubble bath but colonization of the bladder is usually prevented by the defence mechanisms outlined above.

Table 49.2 Radiological findings in children with symptomatic infection investigated by intravenous urogram and contrast micturating cysto-urethrogram (MCU)

Result	Percentage
No structural abnormality	60
VUR (31% with renal scarring)	35
Renal scarring (92% with VUR)	12
Stones/obstruction	4
Duplex, horseshoe and anomalies, with or without VUR, without obstruction	8

Table 49.2 sets out the findings on investigation of children with symptomatic UTI. This shows VUR to be the most common abnormality, seen in about one-third: overall about 30% of the children with reflux are found to have scarred kidneys on presentation. Stones and obstructive lesions occur infrequently. Although no structural abnormality may be seen in over half the children investigated, they will often be found to have an increased bladder residue, a loaded large bowel or a clinical history of bladder instability (Smellie *et al.*, 1981; Smellie and Prescod, 1986).

Diagnosis

DEFINITION

UTI is defined as a state in which organisms are actively multiplying within the urinary tract, usually producing an inflammatory response. The diagnosis thus depends on the demonstration of a significant number of organisms in the bladder urine. Significant bacteriuria (a pure growth of 10^5 or more organisms per millilitre on culture of a clean, fresh specimen of urine passed per urethram, or any growth from direct bladder aspirate) may precede symptomatic infection. This is usually accompanied by significant pyuria, i.e. more than 10 white blood cells (WBC)/mm^3 of uncentrifuged fresh urine, indicating an inflammatory response.

Thus the diagnosis is critically dependent on the technique of urine collection, preliminary testing, storage and transport and the results will be invalid if the greatest care is not taken at each of these stages.

It is essential to collect a sample of urine suitable for culture before the introduction of antibacterial treatment. The method of collection depends on the age, gender and hydration of the child, and his or her ability to co-operate and on the presence of urinary diversion, or functional obstruction or malformation of the urethra.

COLLECTION OF URINE SAMPLE (TABLE 49.3)

Urine passed per urethram can be collected by a midstream or clean-catch technique (for continent toddlers, older children and infant boys) or by the careful use of a perineal bag. The bag should be applied after local cleaning with water, but not with antiseptic as this could falsify results. The infant or toddler is kept upright so that urine, when passed, collects in the dependent bag and is not in contact with the perineum. The bag can be removed immediately and the sample transferred to a sterile container through a snipped lower corner, thereby reducing the risk of perineal contamination. A negative result is valuable in excluding the diagnosis when

Table 49.3   Methods of urine collection

Per urethram	Midstream or clean catch
	Perineal bag
	Catheter
Bladder	Suprapubic aspiration
	Suprapubic catheter
Ureteric catheter	
Stoma of urinary diversion	
Renal pelvis	Needle aspiration

this is only a possibility, whereas a pure bacterial growth in significant numbers with pyuria is diagnostic. Concerned parents can be relied on to carry out these techniques meticulously if details are carefully explained, whereas busy ward staff cannot always spare the time to keep the child under observation. Catheter specimens can be collected by urethral catheter or by a suprapubic catheter if *in situ*. The catheter is useful in the sick infant who is dehydrated or in whom the bladder is impalpable and suprapubic aspiration inappropriate, or during procedures such as cystography, but is undesirable if the bladder is distended, suggesting lower tract obstruction. Using a fine, polythene infant-feeding catheter the risk of iatrogenic cystitis is minimal. The urine collected by catheter should normally be sterile. Collection of urine by direct needle puncture of the bladder [suprapubic aspiration (SPA)] is the method of choice in the sick infant. In experienced hands and with a palpable bladder the technique is simple and uncomplicated, the needle passing through midline extraperitoneal bloodless tissue. A high success rate can be achieved by ultrasononic guidance (Buys *et al.*, 1994). Any bacterial growth from bladder aspirate is significant provided urine is collected at the maximum depth penetrated by the needle. If the needle is inserted and then withdrawn, the tip may be contaminated by faecal organisms which would be likely to have the same identity as possible urinary pathogens.

The results of culture of urine collected in more complex situations require individual consideration and some reliance on coincidental clinical features, as for example from the stoma of a urinary diversion, when a mixed growth of doubtful pathological significance may be obtained.

PRELIMINARY TESTING

Rapid treatment of any symptomatic UTI is essential if the risk of permanent renal damage is to be reduced. There is clinical evidence that delay in treatment is an important factor in the acquisition of new scars (Winberg *et al.*, 1982; Smellie *et al.*, 1985). Although the diagnosis may remain in doubt in some instances, the history, taken together with preliminary examination of

Table 49.4 Preliminary testing for urinary tract infection

Urinoscopy
Nitrite dipstick
Leucocyte esterase dipstick
Microscopy

the urine, will usually allow treatment to be started, pending the result of formal culture. Methods currently in use are listed in Table 49.4.

A bacterial count of $>10^7$/ml will normally produce detectable cloudiness of freshly passed urine on urinoscopy or direct observation, as will 10^5/ml with pyuria (K. Verrier-Jones, personal communication). The nitrite dipstick test has a high sensitivity and specificity, but a false-negative result will be obtained: (i) when the bladder has been emptied recently or there is increased frequency of micturition so that the period of contact between organism and urinary nitrate in the bladder is insufficient for the conversion of nitrate to nitrite to occur; (ii) if the infecting organism is not a nitrate converter (e.g. *Streptococcus faecalis*); and (iii) occasionally when a heavy mixed growth of organisms infects an obstructed urinary tract.

The leucocyte esterase dip test for pyuria is helpful and a positive result is usually evident within 1 min. A combined nitrite and leucocyte esterase stick has a high sensitivity and specificity (Multistix, Bayer).

Microscopy of the uncentrifuged fresh sample will rapidly demonstrate both organisms and pus cells.

STORAGE AND TRANSPORT

The immediate care and transport of the freshly passed sample are crucial if a reliable result is to be obtained. Methods used to prevent the growth of contaminants include immediate chilling to 4°C and later transfer to the laboratory in a cooled container, or the use of borate tubes (provided that the correct volume of urine is added to the tube to avoid both false-negative and false-positive results), or using a dipslide which is then incubated or posted to the laboratory, after either being dipped in the sample or held in the urinary stream. A urine sample refrigerated immediately can be kept at 4°C for several days before culture, but any pus cells will be distorted after 12–24 hours (Table 49.5).

Table 49.5 Urine storage and transport

Chilled to 4°C
Borate tube
Dipslide (for culture only)

CLINICAL FEATURES

Infants and children can present with a wide range of symptoms. Fever is the most common but not always present. Infants may have any of the symptoms common in this age group, from feeding problems, irritability and weight loss to alimentary disturbances or convulsions. In the toddler there may be delay in the normal control of bladder function; and dysuria is as often caused by external irritation, e.g. threadworms, as by a urinary infection. The older child is more likely to complain of localizing symptoms or signs, abdominal or loin pain, dysuria, frequency, haematuria or offensive urine.

The full history should include details of bowel, micturition and drinking habits. There is often a difference of opinion between parent and child regarding both bowel and voiding habits, and keeping a diary of bowels may be useful. In the older child it may be found that drinks at breakfast are omitted, the use of school toilets is minimized and there may be no lunchtime drink available at school. Previous similar episodes and any family history of renal problems, UTI and hypertension should be noted.

On examination, special attention should be directed to somatic size and growth, bladder palpability, blood pressure, spinal abnormalities, perineal and lower limb sensation and reflexes, and the urinary stream in boys.

Management

Management objectives are to eradicate the presenting infection, identify the cause, and correct, alleviate or modify this in order to prevent recurrence of infection and renal damage. Table 49.6 outlines how these aims may be achieved.

ACUTE INFECTION

Timing

Since there is good clinical evidence that delay in effective treatment is an important factor in infective renal damage (Winberg *et al.*, 1982; Smellie *et al.*, 1985) and

Table 49.6 Management of urinary tract infection in infants and children

Think of the diagnosis
Urine collection to establish diagnosis
Rapid antibacterial treatment
Low-dose antibacterial prophylaxis until investigation
Surgical treatment of obstruction and stones
Explain problem to parents and child
Prevent further recurrence
Follow-up

also experimental evidence that rapid treatment can modify or prevent the development of scars (Ransley and Risdon, 1981; Wikstad *et al.*, 1990), speedy introduction of antibacterial treatment is essential.

Choice of drug

The diagnosis has therefore to be made without delay, and with the help of preliminary testing of the urine sample, the 'best guess' antibacterial agent can be given immediately. Drug resistance patterns vary between hospital and domiciliary practice and among different geographical localities and are also influenced in the individual by any recent preceding antibacterial therapy (Grüneberg *et al.*, 1975). Recent amoxycillin, for example, would have increased the ampicillin resistance of the faecal coliform flora and the likelihood of a urinary pathogen being amoxycillin resistant. Discussion with the microbiologist and a careful history will help in making an appropriate choice.

If there is no response to treatment within 48 hours, either the wrong drug has been prescribed or there is an element of obstruction to urinary outflow. By this time, the result of the urine culture and organism sensitivity should be available, allowing a change in antibiotic or chemotherapy to be made if necessary.

Duration

For a first known symptomatic or febrile infection in a child previously uninvestigated, so that the renal status and the presence or absence of VUR, stones or obstruction is unknown, a 5–7-day course of antibacterial treatment is advisable. It is also recommended for a recurrence of UTI in a child with reflux or renal scarring. A single dose or 24 hours of treatment can be sufficient in the older child known to have a structurally normal urinary tract, if a good fluid intake, attention to bowels and regular complete voiding are also instituted.

If eradication of the acute infection is successful, a low dose of a suitable antibacterial drug should immediately be given prophylactically to prevent further infection until investigation has been carried out. If the infection persists in spite of appropriate treatment, then investigation should be undertaken urgently to exclude an obstructive lesion.

INVESTIGATION

The purposes for which investigation is undertaken are shown in Table 49.7. The methods available include laboratory and imaging methods, urodynamics and cystoscopy.

Laboratory

A raised estimate of C-reactive protein, erythrocyte sedimentation rate (ESR) and WBC count are non-

Table 49.7 Purpose of investigation

Discovery of cause, in order to prevent recurrence

Identification of underlying abnormalities, e.g. VUR, obstruction, stones

Determination of renal status and the presence or risk of renal scarring

specific indicators of inflammation. The desmopressin water concentration test relates to renal function but is not applicable in infancy and early childhood, the age group in which rapid diagnosis and treatment are most important. Useful information is gained from the identity and sensitivity pattern of the urinary organism.

E. coli is the most common urinary pathogen and is found in over 90% of first known infections. *B. proteus* occurs particularly in boys and may be associated with calculi (Ghazali *et al.*, 1973). *Pseudomonas* species suggest previous surgery, instrumentation or a contaminated specimen. *Staphylococcus epidermidis* can occur as a urinary pathogen in adolescent girls. The report of a 'mixed growth of doubtful significance' requires repetition but a significant growth of two distinct organisms merits treatment and investigation. It may be found where there are renal, ureteric or bladder stones.

Highly resistant organisms usually indicate serious stasis and previous attempts to eradicate infection by repeated changes of antibiotic.

Abacterial pyuria is classically due to tuberculous renal infection, now very rarely seen, but can also result from even a single dose of antibiotic being taken before the urine is collected from a child with a non-tuberculous bacterial UTI. Pyuria has also been reported in febrile children without UTI.

Proteinuria may occur during a febrile illness and is not diagnostic of UTI. The urine should be retested later. In a child known to have had recurrent infections, however, proteinuria may have serious import and will require follow-up and further study. Estimates of plasma urea, creatinine and electrolytes should be made in any child with UTI who is sufficiently ill to need hospital admission and also in those known or found to have renal involvement.

Imaging

The radiological findings based on 746 children aged 0–12 years with symptomatic UTI (Smellie *et al.*, 1981; Smellie and Prescod, 1986), set out in Table 49.2 give an indication of the distribution of abnormal findings. With the development of new imaging methods and concern to reduce procedures that are invasive or involve radiation of children, a number of different schemes of investigation has been suggested, though there is no agreed plan (Report of the Royal College of Physicians, 1991; Haycock, 1991; Koff, 1991; Rickwood *et al.*, 1992). It has become clear that at present there is no single imaging modality for investigating the child's urinary tract following UTI which will alone provide all the necessary information for management or the prediction of prognosis. It is also clear that the choice of combination of imaging methods is affected by the age and clinical history of the child and the availability of suitable equipment and expertise in interpretation of the results. For example, ultrasonography, which has the advantage of being non-invasive and without radiation, is observer dependent and difficult to reproduce serially for follow-up purposes. It is valuable for the diagnosis of obstructive surgical conditions but currently unreliable in identifying VUR renal inflammation or renal scarring (Stokland *et al.*, 1994; Smellie *et al.*, 1995), information essential in planning the management of a child with infection of the unobstructed urinary tract. The imaging methods currently available, with their particular strengths and shortcomings, are listed briefly in Table 49.8.

The medical and surgical demands of investigation differ, the surgeon being particularly interested in VUR, obstructive lesions and stones. Obstructive hydronephrosis is well demonstrated by ultrasonography while radiopaque stones can be seen on a plain abdominal film (Hanbury *et al.*, 1989). The physician would expect the diagnosis of most obstructive lesions to be made in infancy on follow-up of fetal renal tract dilatation, and stones are found in only a very small proportion of children presenting to a medical clinic with urinary infection (Smellie *et al.*, 1981; Smellie and Prescod, 1986). Of greater concern are the detection of renal inflammation and renal scars, which require reliable renal imaging, and the demonstration of VUR and its severity. For this, either a ^{99m}Tc DMSA scan or a limited intravenous urogram and a voiding cystonurethrogram are necessary. Direct isotope cystography considerably reduces the radiation dosage but does not visualize the urethra or allow grading of the severity of reflux. Indirect isotope (MAG3 or DTPA) cystography can be used in the follow-up study of VUR and to assess proportionate renal function, but lesser grades of reflux can be overlooked.

Urodynamics, cystoscopy and DTPA renography are not first-line investigations.

SURGICAL INTERVENTION

UTI is essentially a medical condition requiring treatment, investigation and often prolonged follow-up to ensure that further infections are either prevented or suitably managed. If there is persistent infection despite appropriate antibacterial treatment, or resistant urinary pathogens emerge, surgical consultation is urgently needed. There is no point in making repeated changes of antibacterial drug, which will increase bacterial resistance and thereby reduce the choice of effective agents that may be needed in the perioperative period. Surgical consultation is also needed if there is dilatation of any section of the urinary tract, or if there are stones, bladder diverticula or large paraureteric saccules. The management of the child with gross reflux with or without a hypoplastic or dysplastic kidney needs joint discussion between the paediatric nephrologist and the urologist.

Further management and follow-up will be determined by local circumstances and by the availability of family doctor and laboratory support and parental compliance.

PREVENTION OF RECURRENT UTI

The most important factor in predisposing to UTI is urinary stasis with the accumulation of residual bladder urine (Lidefelt *et al.*, 1989) and antibacterial treatment will only be effective if there is adequate urinary drainage. Structural obstruction requires surgical correction – the management of children with functional obstruction is dealt with in the section on the neuropathic bladder. Other approaches to the prevention of recurrent infection are listed in Table 49.9.

Reduction of residual urine

After taking a careful history of the daily routine, appropriate adjustments can be made to ensure that the infant or child has an early morning drink and regular drinks throughout the day at intervals not exceeding 3 hours (a bedtime drink may have to be omitted if the child is suffering from nocturnal enuresis). A habit of voiding every 2–3 hours should also be established and, in the older child, the parent should discuss the school toilet facilities with the schoolteacher or school doctor. Double micturition at bedtime is also useful, even in those without VUR. A routine can be set up of the child voiding on preparing for bed, then taking the dose of prophylactic if this is prescribed, followed by teethbrushing and then a second void after a few minutes. This helps to ensure that the bladder is empty on retiring and that the antibacterial agent is taken to cover the long period overnight with no voiding. Constipation can be corrected by a regular dose of a laxative such as senna or lactulose, taken daily until a regular motion is achieved. The dose can then be reduced over the course of a month while a diary is maintained, thus ensuring that the bowels continue to be opened regularly. Holidays spent camping or in hot countries are notoriously associated with recurrence of urinary infection and parents should be warned that adequate drinks, regular voiding and bowel habits should be maintained in these unusual circumstances.

Table 49.8 Investigation: imaging methods

Imaging technique	Advantage	Disadvantage
IVU (Intravenous urography)	Gives comprehensive structural assessment of renal tract. Confirms suspected renal scarring. Differentiates duplex and other malformations. Allows serially reproducible measurement of kidneys and parenchyma; assessment of ureteric calibre, bladder size and postmicturition residue, faecal bowel loading, spinal defects, and radiopaque and metabolic stones. Number of exposures can be limited to reduce radiation.	Radiation dose, which is related to the number of films exposed. Possibility of reaction to contrast media (less likely with non-ionic compounds and in children).
MCU (Contrast micturating cysto-urethrogram)	Reliable demonstration of VUR with grading of severity indicates bladder size, thickness and function, shape, irregularities and diverticula. Visualizes bladder neck and urethra.	Radiation dose. Involves catheterization. Needs careful preparation of parent and child.
DMSA (^{99m}Tc dimercapto-succinic acid study)	Defects of isotope uptake seen during or after acute UTI give early indication of those at risk of renal damage needing treatment and follow-up. Measures proportionate renal function Persistent defects of isotope uptake correlate fairly closely with scarring on IVU.	Abnormal images indicate non-specific defects of tubular function. Involves injection of radioisotope; radiation dose depends on dose of isotope injected.
Direct isotope cystography	Lower radiation dose than contrast cystography. Bladder capacity and residue can be calculated.	Involves catheterization. Urethra and bladder neck not visualized. Reflux grading not usually possible.
Indirect cystography DTPA, MAG3 renography	Detects moderate to severe VUR and obstruction to flow. Estimates percentage contribution from each kidney to total glomerular filtration rate.	Involves injection. Secondary investigation of suspected obstruction. Indirect isotope cystography limited by age and acquisition of bladder control.
Ultrasonography	Non-invasive. No radiation. Can identify hydronephrosis, ureteric dilatation and bladder enlargement. In older child, bladder capacity and residual urine may be calculated. Relatively inexpensive. Antenatal studies may detect fetal urinary tract abnormalities.	Observer dependent. Unreliable for detection of renal inflammation, VUR, stones, renal scarring; also assessment of bladder capacity in uncooperative young child. Positive findings need further investigation. A negative result may give false reassurance. Serial renal size measurements not usually comparable.

Table 49.9 Prevention of recurrent urinary tract infection

Reduce residual bladder urine
Exclude/relieve mechanical obstruction
Regular, frequent, complete voiding
Double micturition at bedtime
Correction of constipation
Drinks at regular intervals

Low-dose antibacterial prophylaxis

Discourage use of surface-tension lowering agents and disinfectants in bath water

Prevent local irritation
Treat threadworms and other external irritants
Avoid tight clothes and heavily chlorinated swimming pool water (or apply barrier cream)

Explain rationale to parents and child

Prophylaxis

The purpose of prophylaxis is to prevent reinfection of a susceptible urinary tract after the presenting UTI has been eradicated. It is contraindicated where there is obstruction to urine flow because resistant urinary pathogens will be generated. Prophylaxis should always be accompanied by methods of reducing urinary stasis and the volume of residual bladder urine.

A suitable antibacterial drug for prophylaxis should be effective against urinary pathogens, excreted in high concentration in the urine, free from side-effects and palatable so that compliance is good. It should not induce bowel flora resistance as urinary pathogens mainly originate from the faecal flora, and should be given in the lowest effective dose (a quarter to half the therapeutic dose), in a single dose taken each evening to cover the longest interval between bladder emptyings. Drugs that have been found to fulfil these requirements include trimethoprim, either alone or in combination with sulphamethoxazole, and nitrofurantoin. A dose of 1 mg/kg/day of either nitrofurantoin or trimethoprim (TMP) is adequate and no serious side effects have been encountered (Smellie *et al.*, 1988) using such small doses.

The length of time for which prophylaxis is necessary is empirical and the suggested duration is mainly based on clinical experience. A controlled trial in children with structurally normal urinary tracts showed that 6–12 months prevented recurrence during prophylaxis and significantly reduced the recurrence rate after its cessation, compared with children receiving no prophylaxis (Smellie *et al.*, 1978). When good voiding and bowel habits are established, prophylaxis can be unnecessary.

If UTI recurs during a period of prophylaxis, the sensitivity of the infecting organism provides a clue. If sensitive to the prescribed antibacterial prophylactic, the child is likely to be non-compliant or the dose has been reduced too low. If the organism is resistant to the prescribed antibiotic, it is most likely that too high a dose has been prescribed. Alternatively, there may be urinary stasis because of obstruction which has been overlooked or an unstable bladder and failure to comply in a bladder-emptying regimen.

FOLLOW-UP

Follow-up involves reinforcement of therapeutic measures, the culture of a urine sample if there are suspicious symptoms, and reintroduction of treatment and appropriate reinvestigation as necessary, as well as the recording of blood pressure and renal function in those with scarred kidneys. Its duration is a matter for individual consideration and the following guidelines are suggested: continued supervision is advisable for a minimum of 1 year for any child with UTI (after which the risk of recurrence is much reduced), for as long as VUR persists, until risks of post-operative infection or obstruction have been excluded, and for life in children who have renal scarring.

In children with even one UTI a period of follow-up is necessary because of the tendency for UTI to recur and to reinforce measures to reduce this risk. Without supervision from birth, the possibility of earlier UTI cannot be excluded with certainty.

Special situations

NEWBORN AND INFANTS

The diagnosis of UTI in a sick infant is ideally made on culture of bladder aspirate (SPA) or of a catheter specimen of urine. In this age group it can be excluded by negative culture and microscopy of a carefully collected 'bag' urine. A septicaemic illness due to a coccal infection may be complicated by renal abscesses; conversely, a coliform infection of a refluxing urinary tract can be accompanied by coliform bacteraemia or septicaemia.

Parenteral treatment is usually indicated in the newborn in line with the current antibacterial regimen in local use. Speed in diagnosis and treatment is particularly important because the rapidly growing kidney appears to be especially vulnerable. Investigation should concentrate on identifying obstruction, reflux and any evidence of renal abnormality.

VESICOURETERIC REFLUX

VUR, the most common abnormal finding on investigation of infants and children with UTI (approximately

35%), varies in severity, outcome and renal associations. The return of refluxed urine into the bladder increases the residual urine and so encourages persistence or recurrence of UTI. An incompetent vesicoureteric junction (VUJ) allows the easy ascent of organisms from the bladder to the renal pelvis and exposes the renal papillae to bladder voiding pressures. There is conflicting evidence concerning the role of infection in promoting VUJ incompetence.

The objective of surgical treatment is to stop reflux, and that of medical management is to prevent recurrence of UTI by reducing residual urine combined with continuous low-dose antibacterial prophylaxis. Medical management is very effective in children with reflux without severe dilatation (international grade I–III), the substantial majority. In over 75% of cases, infection is prevented or well controlled and reflux is self-limiting, so that this is generally the management of first choice. If after several years there is good compliance in eliminating residual urine, it may be unnecessary in the older child to continue antibacterial prophylaxis when the kidneys will be less susceptible to damage. This is on condition that (i) the family is sensible and understands the problem, and is provided with a sterile container for urine sample collection and a small supply of a suitable antibacterial tablet in case of a recurrence, and (ii) the management regimen is reinforced with regular supervision. (As part of a research protocol, the author has usually continued antibacterial prophylaxis until adolescence or until reflux ceases, whichever occurs first.)

In children with International reflux grade III or IV, neither medical nor surgical management has been shown to be superior in terms of renal growth or renal scarring (Birmingham Reflux Study Group, 1987; International Reflux Study Group, 1992). In infant boys with severe reflux spontaneous resolution has frequently been observed (Bailey, R.R., second C.J. Hodson Symposium, 1991).

In children with gross reflux and hypoplastic or dysplastic kidneys, there is little difference in outcome between medical and surgical treatment.

Any child with VUR treated surgically with or without renal scarring needs to be followed postoperatively, with urine checks. This is to prevent recurrent infection if VUR persists and to detect any early or delayed postoperative obstruction.

RENAL SCARRING

Whether or not there is demonstrable reflux it is thought that the child with radiological renal scarring should have lifelong supervision, to prevent recurrent UTI during childhood and to check the blood pressure at regular intervals, as well as the renal function if both kidneys are involved. Advice on potential complications of pregnancy and the investigation of offspring for VUR is also necessary.

NEUROPATHIC BLADDER

In the child with a neuropathic bladder, urinary infection is a common complication. The risk of renal damage is greater where there is a small thick-walled bladder with high-pressure reflux than where the bladder is thin-walled and large. In either situation, the unnecessary use of antibiotics should be avoided and prophylaxis should be deferred until a good bladder-emptying pattern is established (by intermittent catheterization or other means). Effective antibacterial treatment would then be available if symptomatic infection should develop.

UNSTABLE BLADDER

Impaired bladder function is being increasingly recognized clinically as a factor in children with recurrent UTI (O'Regan *et al.*, 1985; Koff, 1992). Where there is a problem with day wetting after 5 years of age a careful MCU, or urodynamic study may be needed. Many children who have a past history of squatting or of urgency, frequency, constipation and recurrent infection may benefit from a small dose, e.g. 2.5 mg o.m. or b.d., of oxybutynin.

URINARY TRACT INFECTION COMPLICATING SURGERY

The principles outlined earlier also apply to infection preceding or following any surgical procedure: (i) if possible, an uncontaminated sample should be obtained for culture and, particularly if the child is already on an antibiotic drug, examined microscopically; (ii) adequate drainage of the infected site is an essential concomitant of antibacterial treatment; and (iii) obstruction to urine flow from the kidney will increase the risk of renal damage. For example, it was thought by the Stanford group that new radiological renal sears observed postoperatively in previously normal kidneys might have resulted from surgery being undertaken too soon after an acute infection so that any potential renal damage could have been aggravated by transient postoperative oedema and VUJ narrowing (Filly *et al.*, 1974; Govan, D., personal communication).

Conclusions

The urinary tract is normally sterile and when it becomes infected there is some underlying cause. This should be sought, identified and corrected. This involves a full clinical history and examination and appropriate investigation. Good drainage or a free urinary flow must be ensured, by surgery or by bladder and bowel training as appropriate, and by low-dose antibacterial prophylactic cover while the urinary tract remains susceptible to infection. Because of the tendency for UTI to recur, children should be followed-up to detect or prevent recurrence and the later complications of damaged kidneys.

References

Birmingham Reflux Study Group 1987: Prospective trial of operative versus non-operative treatment of severe vesico-ureteric reflux in children: 5 years' observation. *British Medical Journal* **295**, 237–41.

Buys, H., Pead, L., Hallett, R. and Maskell, R.M. 1994: Suprapubic aspiration under ultrasound guidance in children with fever of undiagnosed cause. *British Medical Journal* **308**, 690–2.

Dohil, R., Roberts, E., Verrier-Jones, K. and Jenkins, H.R. 1994: Constipation and reversible urinary tract abnormalities. *Archives of Disease in Childhood* **70**, 56–7.

Filly, R., Friedland, G.W., Govan, D.E. and Fair, W.R. 1974: Development and progression of clubbing and scarring in children with recurrent urinary tract infections. *Radiology* **113**, 145–53.

Ghazali, S., Barratt, T.M. and Williams, D.I. 1973: Urolithiasis in Britain. *Archives of Disease in Childhood* **48**, 286–95.

Grüneberg, R.N., Leakey, A., Bendall, M.J. and Smellie, J.M. 1975: Bowel flora in urinary tract infection: effective chemotherapy with special reference to co-trimoxazole. *Kidney International* **8**, S122–9.

Hanbury, D.C., Whitaker, R.H., Sherwood, T. and Farman, P. 1989: Ultrasound and plain X-ray screening in childhood urinary tract infection. *British Journal of Urology* **64**, 638–40.

Haycock, G.B. 1991: A practical approach to evaluating urinary tract infection in children. *Pediatric Nephrology* **5**, 401–2.

Hellström, A., Hanson, E., Hansson, S., Hjälmös, K., and Jodal, U. 1991: Association between urinary symptoms at 7 years old and previous urinary tract infection. *Archives of Disease in Childhood* **66**, 232–4.

Hodson, C.J., Maling, T.M.J., McManamon, P.J. and Lewis, M.G. 1975: The pathogenesis of reflux nephropathy. *British Journal of Radiology* **13** (Suppl.), 1–26.

International Reflux Study Group in Children, European Branch 1992: 5 year study of medical or surgical treatment in children with severe reflux: radiological renal findings. *Pediatric Nephrology* **6**, 223–30.

Jakobsson, B., Nolstedt, L., Svensson, L., Söderlundh, S. and Berg, U. 1992: 99m technetium dimercaptosuccinic acid scan in the diagnosis of acute pyelonephritis in children: relation to clinical and radiological findings. *Pediatric Nephrology* **6**, 328–34.

Koff, S.A. 1991: A practical approach to evaluating urinary tract infection in children. *Pediatric Nephrology* **5**, 398–400.

Koff, S.A. 1992: Relationship between dysfunctional voiding and vesicoureteric reflux. *Journal of Urology* **148**, 1703–5.

Lidefelt, K.J., Erasmie, U. and Böllgren, I. 1989: Residual urine in children with acute cystitis and in healthy children: assessment by sonography. *Journal of Urology* **141**, 916–17.

O'Regan, S., Yazbeck, S. and Schick, E. 1985: Constipation, bladder instability, urinary tract infection syndrome. *Clinical Nephrology* **23**, 152.

Ransley, P.G. and Risdon, R.A. 1978: Reflux and renal scarring. *British Journal of Radiology* **14** (Suppl.), 1–35.

Ransley, P.G. and Risdon, R.A. 1981: Reflux nephropathy: effects of antimicrobial therapy on the evolution of the early pyelonephritic scar. *Kidney International* **20**, 733–42.

Report of a Working Group of the Royal College of Physicians 1991: Guidelines for the management of acute urinary tract infection in childhood. *Journal of Royal College of the Physicians of London* **25**, 36–43.

Rickwood, A.M.K., Carty, H.M., McKendrick, T. *et al.* 1992: Current imaging of childhood urinary infections: prospective survey. *British Medical Journal* **304**, 663–5.

Rushton, H.G. and Majd, M. 1992: Dimercaptosuccinic acid renal scintigraphy for the evaluation of pyelonephritis and scarring: a review of experimental and clinical studies *Journal of Urology* **148**, 1726–32.

Smellie, J.M. and Prescod, N. 1986: Natural history of overt urinary infection in childhood. In Asscher, A.W. and Brumfitt, W. (eds), *Microbial disease in nephrology*. Chichester: John Wiley, 243–55.

Smellie, J.M., Edwards, D., Hunter, N., Normand, I.C.S. and Prescod, N. 1975: Vesico-ureteric reflux and renal scarring. *Kidney International* **8**, S65–S72.

Smellie, J.M., Grüneberg, R.N., Bantock, H.M. and Prescod, N. 1988: Prophylactic co-trimoxazole and trimethoprim in the management of urinary tract infection in children. *Pediatric Nephrology* **2**, 12–17.

Smellie, J.M., Katz, G. and Grüneberg, R.N. 1978: Controlled trial of prophylactic treatment in childhood urinary tract infection. *Lancet* **ii**, 175–8.

Smellie, J.M., Normand, I.C.S. and Katz, G. 1981: Children with urinary infection: a comparison of those with and those without vesico-ureteric reflux. *Kidney International* **20**, 717–22.

Smellie, J.M., Ransley, P.G., Normand, I.C.S., Prescod, N. and Edwards, D. 1985: Development of new renal scars: a collaborative study. *British Medical Journal* **290**, 1957–60.

Smellie, J.M., Rigden, S.P. and Prescod, N.P. 1995: Urinary tract infection: a comparison of four methods of investigation. *Archives of Disease in Childhood* **72**, 247–50.

Stokland, E., Hellström, M., Hansson, S., Jodal, U., Odén, A. and Jacobsson, B. 1994: Reliability of ultrasonography in identification of reflux nephropathy in children. *British Medical Journal* **309**, 235–9.

Verrier-Jones, K., Verrier-Jones, E.R. and Asscher, A.W. 1986: Covert urinary tract infections in children. In Asscher, A.W. and Brumfitt, W. (eds), *Microbial disease in nephrology*. Chichester: John Wiley, 225–37.

Wikstad, I., Hannerz, L., Karlsson, A., Eklöf, A-C., Olling, S. and Aperia, A. 1990: 99m technetium dimercaptosuccinic acid scintigraphy in the diagnosis of acute pyelonephritis in rats. *Pediatric Nephrology* **4**, 331–4.

Winberg, J., Bollgren, I., Källenius, G., Möllby, R. and Svensson, S.B. 1982: Clinical pyelonephritis and focal renal scarring. *Pediatric Clinics of North America* **29**, 801–13.

Further reading

International Workshop on Reflux and Pyelonephritis 1992: *Journal of Urology* **148**, 1639–758.

Postlethwaite, R.J. (ed.) 1994: *Clinical paediatric nephrology*, 2nd ed. Oxford: Butterworth Heinemann.

Rushton, H.G. 1997: Urological review: the evaluation of acute pyelonephritis and renal scarring with technetium 99m-dimercaptosuccinic acid renal scintigraphy. *Pediatric Nephrology* **11**, 108–20.

Smellie, J.M. 1991: AUA Lecture: Reflections on 30 years of treating children with urinary tract infections. *Journal of Urology* **146**, 665–8.

Smellie, J.M. and Normand, I.C.S. 1985: Urinary infections in children, 1985. *Postgraduate Medical Journal* **61**, 895–905.

Smellie, J.M. and Normand, I.C.S. 1992: Urinary tract infection. In Campbell, A.G.M. and McIntosh, N. (eds), *Forfar and Arneil's Textbook of paediatrics*, 4th ed. Edinburgh: Churchill Livingstone. 1031–46.

Tamminen-Möbius, T., Olbing, H. and Smellie, J.M. 1993: Management of children with severe vesico-ureteric reflux: overview, including the 5-year results of the European Branch of the International Reflux Study in Children. In Andreucci, V.E. and Fine, L.G. (eds), *International yearbook of nephrology, dialysis and transplantation*, Chapter 8. Oxford: Oxford University Press, 85–96.

Verrier-Jones, K. and Asscher, A.W. 1992: In Edelmann, C.M., Bernstein, J., Meadow, R., Spitzer, A. and Travis, L. (eds), *Urinary tract infection in paediatric kidney disease,* 2nd ed. Boston, MA: Little Brown, vol. 2, 1943–91.

White, R.H.R. 1987: Management of urinary tract infection. *Archives of Disease in Childhood* **62**, 421–7.

CHAPTER 50

Renal failure

S.P.A. RIGDEN

ACUTE RENAL FAILURE
Introduction
Aetiology and pathophysiology of
acute renal failure
Management
Outcome and the future

CHRONIC RENAL FAILURE
Introduction
Organization of services

Incidence
Causes of chronic renal failure
Progression of renal failure
Clinical features
Investigations
Management of preterminal renal failure
Management of end-stage renal failure
Treatment
References
Further reading

ACUTE RENAL FAILURE

Introduction

Acute renal failure (ARF) is defined as a sudden decline in renal function resulting in failure of body homeostasis. ARF is usually reversible, but, despite significant advances in supportive care, is still associated with a mortality of 10–60%, depending on the cause. The causes of ARF in childhood are diverse: in some cases the cause is obvious, but in others considerable clinical and investigative skills are required to determine the aetiology. All children with ARF require careful and sometimes complex management, and often close collaboration between the paediatric nephrologist, urologist and radiologist as well as specialized paediatric nursing and dietetic services.

ARF is usually, although not invariably, accompanied by oliguria, or a urine output of <300 ml/m^2 body surface area/24 hours. In children this is more usefully defined as a urine flow rate of <0.5 ml/kg/hour or in infants as <1.0 ml/kg/hour. Acute-on-chronic renal failure occurs when ARF is superimposed on pre-existing renal disease, which may previously have been unrecognized. Renal failure presenting in the neonatal period requires special consideration, since newborn with congenital renal abnormalities will also suffer an apparent rapid decline in renal function with placental separation, thereby extending the differential diagnosis.

Aetiology and pathophysiology of acute renal failure

Normal renal function requires an adequate blood supply to healthy kidneys with patent urine collection and drainage systems.

For the purposes of differential diagnosis and management, there is practical merit in the classification of ARF as prerenal, intrinsic renal and postrenal.

PRERENAL ACUTE RENAL FAILURE

The causes of prerenal ARF are given in Table 50.1. Renal hypoperfusion, whatever its cause, results in prerenal ARF and, if not treated effectively, ischaemic acute tubular necrosis (ATN). True or effective hypovolaemia is detected by arterial and cardiac baroreceptors, which trigger neural and hormonal responses in an attempt to restore effective arterial blood volume, protect cardiac

Table 50.1 Causes of prerenal acute renal failure

Hypovolaemia	Vomiting
	Diarrhoea
	Gastrointestinal drainage
	Haemorrhage
	Burns
	Diuresis
	Hyperpyrexia
'Effective' hypovolaemia	Sepsis
	Cardiac failure
	Cardiopulmonary bypass surgery
	Nephrotic syndrome
	Liver failure
Vascular	Coarctation of aorta
	Renal artery stenosis[a]
Drugs	Non-steroidal anti-inflammatory drugs
	Angiotensin-converting enzyme inhibitors

[a]Bilateral or affecting a solitary kidney.

and cerebral perfusion and maintain renal perfusion and glomerular filtration. Renal compensatory mechanisms include afferent arteriolar vasodilatation as a result of the intrarenal production of vasodilator prostaglandins, kallikrein–kinins and possibly nitric oxide, and selective efferent vasoconstriction induced by angiotensin II. Non-steroidal anti-inflammatory drugs and angiotensin-converting enzyme inhibitors, which block intrarenal biosynthesis of vasodilator prostaglandins and angiotensin II, respectively, prevent effective autoregulation of renal blood flow and exacerbate prerenal ARF. They should not therefore be used in patients with or at risk of renal hypoperfusion.

INTRINSIC ACUTE RENAL FAILURE

Intrinsic ARF may result from ischaemic or nephrotoxic ATN, tubulointerstitial diseases, disorders of the renal microvasculature and glomeruli or diseases of large renal vessels (Table 50.2). ATN accounts for approximately 90% of cases of intrinsic ARF.

Ischaemic ATN is caused by renal hypoperfusion of sufficient severity to injure renal parenchymal cells, particularly tubular epithelial cells of the terminal portion of the proximal tubule and the medullary portion of the thick ascending limb of the loop of Henle. Extreme ischaemia may result in bilateral renal cortical necrosis and irreversible renal failure. The course of ischaemic ATN can be divided into three phases: during the initiation phase, the evolving ischaemic injury can be limited by restoration of the renal blood flow. The glomerular filtration rate (GFR) falls because of impaired renal blood flow and glomerular ultrafiltration pressure, disruption of the integrity of tubular epithelium with back leak of glomerular filtrate and obstruc-

tion to urine flow by intratubular cast formation. Epithelial cell injury is established during the maintenance phase and, despite correction of haemodynamic factors, GFR remains low, perhaps because of persistent intrarenal vasoconstriction and therefore medullary ischaemia, through the dysregulated release of vasoactive mediators (e.g. decreased nitric oxide, increased endothelin) from injured endothelial cells. Other putative mechanisms for the persistent reduction of GFR, include congestion of medullary blood vessels and reperfusion injury induced by reactive oxygen species and other mediators derived from leucocytes and renal parenchymal cells.

During the maintenance phase, urine output is lowest and uraemic complications arise. After a variable period of time, the recovery phase begins, during which renal function is restored by repair and regeneration of renal parenchymal cells.

Nephrotoxic ATN may be caused by a variety of exogenous drugs and poisons and also by some endogenous compounds if present in the urine in high concentrations e.g. myoglobin and uric acid. The kidney is particularly susceptible to nephrotoxic injury because of its rich blood supply and its ability to concentrate toxins and metabolize parent compounds into toxic metabolites. As with ischaemic ATN, nephrotoxins impair GFR by intrarenal vasoconstriction (e.g. cyclosporin, radiocontrast compounds, haemoglobin, myoglobin), causing direct injury to tubular epithelium (e.g. aminoglycosides, amphotericin B, cisplatin, ifosfamide) and tubular obstruction (e.g. uric acid, acyclovir).

ARF due to diseases of large renal vessels is rare in children, except in neonates. Perinatal asphyxia, hypotension and polycythaemia, complicating poorly controlled maternal diabetes, intrauterine growth retardation,

Table 50.2 Causes of intrinsic acute renal failure

Acute tubular necrosis	Ischaemic	Prerenal ARF	Treatment inadequate or delayed
	Nephrotoxic exogenous	Antimicrobials	e.g. aminoglycosides, amphotericin B
		Cyclosporin	
		Contrast agents	
		Cytotoxic agents, e.g. cisplatinum, ifosfamide	
		Heavy metals	
		Organic solvents	
	Endogenous	Myoglobin	
		Haemoglobin	
		Uric acid	
Tubulointerstitial diseases		Acute, severe bilateral pyelonephritis	
		Allergic interstitial nephritis, e.g. to antibiotics	
		Allograft rejection	
		Infiltrative disorders, e.g. sarcoid, lymphoma, leukaemia	
Diseases of the glomeruli and renal microvasculature		Acute glomerulonephritis, e.g. poststreptococcal, SLE, MCGN, anti-GBM nephritis, SBE nephritis, 'shunt' nephritis	
		Vasculitis, e.g. PAN, ANCA-positive, HSP	
		Haemolytic uraemic syndrome	
		Thrombotic thromboctypaenic purpura	
Diseases of large vessels		Renal artery occlusion	
		Renal venous thrombosis	

SLE, Systemic lupus erythematosus; MCGN, mesangiocapillary glomerulonephritis; GBM, glomerular basement membrane; SBE, subacute bacterial endocarditis; PAN, polyarteritis nodosa; ANCA, anti-neutrophil cytoplasmic antibody; HSP, Henoch–Schönlein purpura.

twin-to-twin transfusion or cyanotic congenital heart disease, predispose to renal venous thrombosis (RVT) (Mocan *et al.*, 1991). This may be unilateral or bilateral or extend into the inferior vena cava and presents with palpable unilateral or bilateral renal masses, macroscopic haematuria, thrombocytopenia and, if both kidneys are affected, renal failure. Renal arterial occlusion secondary to emboli from poorly positioned umbilical arterial catheters results in hypertension and, if bilateral or there is a solitary kidney, renal failure.

Diseases of the glomeruli and renal microvasculature account for more cases of ARF in children and adolescents. In acute glomerulonephritis (AGN), renal perfusion at the level of the glomerular capillary is decreased because of inflammatory and proliferative changes, and GFR is consequently reduced. In children, the most common cause of AGN is an antecedent streptococcal infection, although other infections have also been implicated. Following a latent period of 10–14 days, the child presents with haematuria, oliguria and oedema. There may be mild to moderate hypertension and renal insufficiency, which in some cases will progress to ARF. The diagnosis may be confirmed by serological proof of a preceding streptococcal infection, evidence of activation of the complement cascade and, if necessary, renal biopsy. Less common forms of AGN present with similar clinical findings. There may be clues to the underlying diagnosis from the history, clinical examination or specific serological tests, but renal biopsy is required for a definitive diagnosis.

Haemolytic uraemic syndrome (HUS) (Milford and Taylor, 1990; Milford *et al.*, 1990; Kleanthous *et al.*, 1990) is the most common cause of ARF in otherwise healthy children living in temperate climates. HUS is defined by microangiopathic haemolytic anaemia, thrombocytopenia and ARF. There is subendothelial swelling of glomerular capillary loops and glomerular perfusion is further impaired by partial or complete obstruction of glomerular capillaries and cortical arterioles by fibrin clots. Rare familial and sporadic forms of HUS exist, but the classical form typically follows a diarrhoeal, often bloody, prodrome due in most cases to a verotoxin-producing strain of *Escherichia coli*, commonly serotype 0157:H7. Pallor, sometimes with bruising, oliguria, oedema and hypertension follow. The peripheral blood smear shows red blood cell fragmentation and thrombocytopenia while the urinary sediment often shows red blood cells, cellular casts and proteinuria, and plasma creatinine is elevated.

POSTRENAL ACUTE RENAL FAILURE

The causes of urinary tract obstruction, which may result in ARF in children, are given in Table 50.3.

Significant obstruction causes ATN, the recovery phase of which begins when the obstruction is relieved. As one kidney has sufficient clearance to maintain body homeostasis, postrenal ARF implies infravesical obstruction, bilateral ureteric obstruction, obstruction of a solitary kidney or pre-existing renal insufficiency.

NEONATAL RENAL FAILURE

The normal newborn kidney is relatively immature and, as a consequence, more vulnerable to potential causes of ARF (Stapleton *et al.*, 1987). In addition, neonates with congenital renal anomalies may present with apparent ARF when the effects of placental separation become clear. The main causes of renal failure in the neonatal period are given in Table 50.4.

Table 50.3 Causes of postrenal acute renal failure

Congenital abnormalities	Posterior urethral valves Vesicoureteric junction obstruction[a] Pelviureteric junction obstruction[a]
Neuropathic bladder	Congenital, e.g. spina bifida, sacral agenesis Acquired, e.g. spinal trauma, transverse myelitis
Calculi[a]	Radiopaque: mixed infective cystinuria distal RTA oxalosis Radiolucent: uric acid xanthine dihydroxyadenine
Tumours	Nephroblastoma (Wilm's) tumour[a] Lower urinary tract tumours, e.g. rhabdomyosarcoma

[a]Bilateral or affecting a solitary kidney.

Table 50.4 Causes of neonatal renal failure

Reduced renal perfusion	Hypovolaemia	Birth asphyxia
	Hypotension	Perinatal blood loss
	Hypoxia	Reduced cardiac output: hypoxic damage
		congenital cardiac anomalies
		dysrhythmias
		post-cardiac surgery
		Cardiopulmonary bypass
		Extracorporeal membrane oxygenation (ECMO)
		Sepsis
		Polycythaemia
		Increased insensible water losses
		Hypoproteinaemia
		Hydrops foetalis
		Drugs: indomethacin tolazoline
Vascular		Coarctation of aorta
		Renal artery stenosis[a]
		Renal arterial occlusion[a]
		Renal venous thrombosis[a]
Toxins	Exogenous	Antimicrobials, e.g. aminoglycosides, amphotericin B
	Endogenous	Haemoglobin
		Uric acid
Congenital renal anomalies		Renal agenesis (Potter's syndrome)
		Renal dysplasia/hypoplasia
		Autosomal recessive polycystic
		Kidney disease
		Posterior urethral valves
		Vesicoureteric junction obstruction[a]
		Pelviureteric junction obstruction[a]
		Neuropathic bladder
		Tumour

[a]Bilateral or affecting a solitary kidney.

Management

The diagnosis and management of ARF should proceed simultaneously. Initial evaluation includes:

- assessment of severity of renal failure
- emergency treatment of life-threatening complications
- urgent treatment of reversible aetiological factors.

The underlying cause of the renal failure may be suggested by the clinical history or physical examination, or only revealed by specific investigation.

HISTORY

Specific inquiry should be made for causes of volume depletion, which may result in true hypovolaemia and prerenal ARF (Table 50.1) or ischaemic ATN. A history of cardiac failure, nephrotic syndrome or liver disease may be relevant. A history of bloody diarrhoea, particularly if associated with the sudden onset of pallor and bruising, suggests HUS. Severe infection, e.g. meningococcal disease, may be associated with prerenal ARF or ATN, whereas a history of preceding infection may indicate acute glomerulonephritis.

A detailed drug history, particularly for antibiotics, non-steroidal anti-inflammatory drugs and anti-cancer drugs, must be obtained. A history of rash suggests allergic interstitial nephritis, vasculitis or systemic lupus erythematosus (SLE); arthralgia or arthritis occurs in Henoch–Schönlein purpura (HSP) and SLE, whilst haemoptysis is characteristic of anti-glomerular basement membrane (GBM) disease and sinusitis of anti-neutrophil cytoplasmic antibody-positive vasculitis (Table 50.2).

For neonates a detailed account of perinatal events is mandatory (Table 50.4). A history of a poor urinary stream suggests posterior urethral valves or a neuropathic bladder and renal colic, calculi as a cause of postrenal ARF.

EXAMINATION

Physical examination is important in the assessment of severity of ARF and may also provide clues to the aetiology.

Careful assessment of intravascular fluid status is necessary to detect signs of dehydration and hypovolaemia and of circulatory overload. Signs of dehydration include decreased skin turgor, dry mucous membranes, sunken eyes and sunken fontanelle.

Hypotension implies a real or effective decrease in circulatory volume, which also results in tachycardia and poor peripheral circulation. Hypertension, in the setting of ARF, usually denotes circulatory overload due to failure of sodium and water homeostasis, or occasionally a hyperreninaemic state.

Circulatory overload also causes tachycardia and an increase in jugular venous pressure, hepatomegaly and peripheral and pulmonary oedema, which results in tachypnoea and, if severe, central cyanosis. On auscultation there are fine crepitations over the lungs and a third heart sound or gallop rhythm. However, it must be remembered that peripheral oedema may occur with true circulatory hypovolaemia in the nephrotic syndrome: in this situation the child's peripheral circulation is poor and the blood pressure often slightly elevated as a result of activation of the renin–angiotensin system. Pallor, jaundice, rashes and bruising should be sought and joints examined for signs of arthritis. Fever suggests an infective or allergic aetiology of ARF.

Abdominal examination may reveal large palpable kidneys, a distended bladder or costovertebral tenderness. If infravesical obstruction is suspected, rectal examination may identify an obstructive mass.

Abnormalities of the external genitalia may be associated with underlying renal tract malformations. The femoral pulses should be checked. Short stature and clinical signs of renal osteodystrophy suggest pre-existing renal disease. Careful neurological examination is necessary to detect consequences of ARF and occasionally clues to its cause, e.g. meningitis and cerebral involvement in HUS. Spinal and lower limb neurological abnormalities may indicate a neuropathic bladder.

MONITORING

Children with ARF require regular monitoring as outlined in Table 50.5 and, unless there is rapid reversal of ARF, transfer to a paediatric intensive care unit or specialized children's renal unit.

INVESTIGATIONS

Basic laboratory investigations essential in the initial evaluation of a child with ARF, are listed in Table 50.6

Table 50.5 Monitoring in acute renal failure

Temperature	Central Peripheral	Central–peripheral temperature monitoring is an effective means of assessing the adequacy of the circulation and renal perfusion (Aynsley-Green and Pickering, 1974)
Pulse		
Respiratory rate		
Oxygen saturation		Pulse oximetry is a sensitive means of detecting pulmonary oedema
Arterial blood pressure		Arterial line or appropriate size cuff
Central venous pressure		
ECG (continuous)		Detects abnormalities caused by hyperkalaemia, i.e. prolongation of PR interval and peaked T waves
Fluid balance	Urine flow rate Gastrointestinal losses Intravenous and oral input Weight	Measured hourly from an indwelling bladder catheter Measured at least once every 24 hours More frequently in young children

Table 50.6   Investigations

General investigations		
Biochemistry	Blood	Electrolytes, urea, creatinine, osmolality
		Calcium, phosphate, alkaline phosphatase
		Total protein, albumin
		Glucose, urate
	Urine	Sodium, urea, creatinine
		Osmolality
Blood gases		pH, standard bicarbonate, base excess
Haematology		Haemoglobin, WBC and differential, platelets
		Film
		Clotting studies
Urinalysis		Blood, protein
Microbiology	Urine	Microscopy for WBC, RBC, organisms, casts, crystals
		Culture
	Blood	Culture
Imaging		Chest X-ray
		Renal tract ultrasound examination
Specific investigations		
Biochemistry	Creatinine phosphokinase	To diagnose:
	Myoglobin in blood and urine	Myoglobinuria
Microbiology	Stool – Culture	
	CSF – Culture	
Serology/immunology		
	Anti-streptolysin O titre	
	Anti-DNAse B	Post-streptococcal
	Anti-hyaluronidase	glomerulo-nephritis
	C_3, C_4	
	Anti-nuclear antibody SLE	
	Anti-DNA antibodies	
	Anti-GBM antibodies	Anti-GBM nephritis
	Anti-neutrophil cytoplasmic antibodies	Vasculitis
Renal biopsy		
Imaging	Abdominal X-ray	Radiopaque stones
	Micturating cystourethrogram	
	Renal arteriogram	
	Radionuclide scans	
	CT scan	
	MRI	
	Left hand and wrist X-ray	Renal osteodystrophy

(General investigations). Depending on the child's condition, these may need to be initiated and monitoring, as outlined above, started before or during history taking and the physical examination. Further specific investigations, as listed in Table 50.6, may be indicated by the clinical findings or results of the general investigations.

TREATMENT

As stated previously, it may be necessary to initiate emergency treatment for the homeostatic derangements resulting from ARF, before or during history taking, examination and investigation. The sick child should be assessed according to the scheme given in Table 50.7.

Table 50.7 Critical pathway for management of acute renal failure

		Clinical assessment (see text)	Laboratory assessment (see Table 50.6)	Action
Ventilation	Inadequate ventilation	Secondary to underlying disease Convulsions (see below)	Pulse oximetry Arterial blood gases Chest X-ray	Oxygen Ventilation
	Pulmonary oedema	Cyanosis Restlessness Tachypnoea, orthopnoea Crepitations Gallop rhythm	as above	Oxygen Ventilation with positive end expiratory pressure Frusemide 5 mg/kg i.v. Dialysis/haemofiltration
Circulatory state	Dehydration/hypovolaemia	Dry mucous membranes Sunken eyes/fontanelle Tachycardia Poor peripheral circulation with central peripheral temperature gap > 6°C Hypotension or hypertension Low CVP Oliguria	Urine composition see Table 8	Restore circulation with 20 ml/kg N saline, 4.0% albumin or whole blood as appropriate. Reassess and repeat if indicated Frusemide 5 mg/kg i.v. if no increase in urine output after 2 h of normovolaemia
	Myocardial dysfunction	Tachycardia Hypotension Poor peripheral circulation Raised JVP/CVP Tachypnoea, orthopnoea Crepitations Gallop rhythm	Echocardiogram	Inotropic support with dopamine 2–10 µg/kg/min or dobutamine 2–20 µg/kg/min
	Circulatory overload	Hypertension for age[a] Tachycardia Gallop rhythm Raised JVP/CVP Hepatomegaly Dependent oedema Pulmonary oedema (see above) Ascites Pleural and pericardial effusions	Chest X-ray	Hypotensive therapy nifedipine 0.25–0.5 mg/kg sublingually labetalol 1–3 mg/kg/h i.v. sodium nitroprusside 0.5–8 µg/kg/min i-v Frusemide 5 mg/kg i-v Dialysis/haemofiltration

Table 50.7 (Continued)

	Clinical assessment (see text)	Laboratory assessment (see Table 50.6)	Action
Hyperkalaemia	Asymptomatic Cardiac dysrhythmias	Potassium > 7.0 mmol/l ECG changes: peaked T wave, prolonged PR interval	Discontinue potassium input Emergency treatment – (see Table 50.9) Dialysis
Metabolic acidosis	Tachypnoea 'Sighing' respiration	Arterial blood gases	If pH < 7.25, treat with sodium bicarbonate 2.5 mmol/kg i.v. unless there is symptomatic circulatory overload or severe hypocalcaemia (see below)
Hypocalcaemia	Tetany Convulsions	Total calcium <2.0 mmol/l	10% calcium gluconate 0.5 ml/kg/h: monitor every 4 hours Caution while phosphate is high
Sepsis	Fever Hypotension Chest X-ray	Blood, urine, CSF Culture	gentamicin: loading dose 2 mg/kg, monitor with blood levels and/or cefotaxime 50 mg/kg × 1 followed by 25 mg/kg × 2/day
Convulsions	Secondary to: hypertension, hypocalcaemia, hypernatremia or hyponatremia uraemia, hypoglycaemia or underlying disease		Prevention and correction of possible precipitating causes Diazepam 0.2 mg/kg i.v. or p.r. Phenytoin 15 mg/kg i.v. × 1 followed by 2.5–7.5 mg/kg × 2/day; monitor with blood levels

[a]Report of the Second Task Force on Blood Pressure Control in Children (1987).

Table 50.8 Urine composition in prerenal acute renal failure and intrinsic acute renal failure

	Neonates[a]		Children[b]	
	Prerenal	**Intrinsic**	**Prerenal**	**Intrinsic**
Volume (ml/kg/hour)	< 1	Variable	< 0.5	Variable
Urine sodium (mmol/l)	31 ± 19	63 ± 35	< 10	> 20
Fractional excretion of filtered sodium (%)[c]	< 2.5	≥2.5	< 1	≥ 1
Urine:plasma urea (mmol/l:mmol/l)	–	–	≥ 4:1	< 4:1
Urine osmolality (mosmol/kg)	≥ 350	< 300	≥ 1.3:1	< 1.11:1[d]

[a]Anand (1982).
[b]Millar *et al.* (1978).

[c]Fractional excretion of filtered sodium = $\dfrac{\text{urinary sodium}}{\text{plasma sodium}} \times \dfrac{\text{plasma creatinine (mmol/l)}}{\text{urine creatinine (mmol/l)}} \times 100\%.$

[d]Expressed as ratio to plasma osmolality.

MANAGEMENT OF PRERENAL ACUTE RENAL FAILURE

Prerenal ARF is, by definition, rapidly reversible after restoration of the renal blood flow and glomerular ultrafiltration pressure. The child with signs of circulatory insufficiency or severe volume depletion therefore requires urgent treatment to prevent progression to ATN (Table 50.7). Bladder catheterization to obtain a sample for urine composition (Table 50.8) (Millar *et al.*, 1978; Anand, 1982) and to monitor urine flow rate is recommended (Table 50.5). Central venous pressure monitoring may also be indicated if clinical assessment of volume status is difficult, with signs of myocardial dysfunction, or if there is no response to initial fluid replacement. In addition, specific therapy is directed to the cause of hypoperfusion.

The adequacy and effect of fluid replacement must be carefully monitored (Table 50.5) using pulse rate, respiratory rate, central–peripheral temperature difference (Aynsley-Green and Pickering, 1974), blood pressure, central venous pressure (CVP) and urine flow rate. In prerenal ARF, restoration of renal perfusion results in an increase in urine flow rate, whereas if this does not occur, it implies that prerenal ARF has progressed to ischaemic ATN. It may still, though, be possible to convert oliguric to non-oliguric ARF, which is advantageous to management and prognosis, by the use of diuretics. If frusemide 5 mg/kg b.w. i.v. produces a diuresis of >2 ml/kg/h, it may be repeated, if necessary, in a dose of 2 mg/kg at 4–6 hourly intervals. Mannitol is not recommended because it will cause volume overload unless excreted.

MANAGEMENT OF INTRINSIC ACUTE RENAL FAILURE

A child with intrinsic ARF may have life-threatening complications requiring urgent treatment at presentation (Table 50.7) – if not, management is directed to the prevention of the metabolic sequelae of intrinsic ARF, whilst its cause is identified and, if available, specific treatment given.

FLUID AND ELECTROLYTES

Salt and water balance

Intrinsic ARF impairs the ability of the kidney to excrete sodium and water and usually, therefore, results in extracellular volume overload. If there are clinical signs of hypervolaemia (see above and Table 50.7), fluid and sodium intake should be restricted to a minimum and frusemide 5 mg/kg b.w. i.v. administered: if there is a satisfactory response, frusemide 2 mg/kg b.w. i.v. may be repeated at 4–6 hourly intervals, but if the response is inadequate, dialysis or ultrafiltration will be required. If intrinsic ARF has resulted from the progression of prerenal ARF to ischaemic ATN, and there is evidence of continuing circulatory insufficiency or hypovolaemia, this must be corrected as for prerenal ARF to restore renal perfusion.

Once euvolaemia has been established, fluid and sodium balance can be maintained by matching intake with output. This is most easily achieved by giving the child an hourly volume of fluid, equal to the previous hour's urine output plus 1/24 of daily insensible losses, calculated as 300 ml/m^2 body surface area. As recovery proceeds, the fluid allowance can be calculated from a 12- or 24-hour period. If plasma sodium is within the normal range, daily sodium intake should match urinary excretion, which will increase as recovery proceeds.

Hyponatremia in intrinsic ARF is almost always due to the ingestion or administration of hypotonic fluids and usually responds to restriction of water intake and of hypotonic intravenous solutions. If there is not a satisfactory response and particularly if the child has neurological symptoms or signs, dialysis will be required.

Potassium

Potassium excretion is also impaired in intrinsic ARF and the resulting hyperkalaemia may be exacerbated by metabolic acidosis, which causes potassium efflux from cells. Oral or intravenous potassium supplements and any drugs promoting hyperkalaemia should be discontinued at diagnosis, unless the child is hypokalaemic. Dietary intake of potassium should be restricted and adequate nutrition (see below) ensured to limit catabolism and therefore cell breakdown and release of potassium. In non-oliguric ARF, frusemide will promote potassium excretion. If the potassium rises above 6.5 mmol/l or there are electrocardiographic (ECG) abnormalities due to hyperkalaemia, emergency treatment as outlined in Table 50.9 should be employed and arrangements made for urgent dialysis.

Metabolic acidosis

ARF is often complicated by metabolic acidosis because of failure to excrete the daily endogenous production (1–3 mmol/kg b.w.) of non-volatile acids. Restriction of dietary protein (see below), a calorie intake sufficient to prevent catabolism and effective treatment of infection will reduce the acid load, although sodium bicarbonate supplements (1–3 mmol/kg b.w./day) are also usually required. Refractory acidosis is an indication for dialysis.

Hyperphosphataemia

Hyperphosphataemia is common in ARF and can be severe, e.g. in catabolic patients, rhabdomyolysis and tumour lysis syndrome. Management comprises dietary phosphate restriction and the use of oral calcium carbonate as a phosphate binder, unless the plasma calcium is raised, when aluminium hydroxide should be substituted.

Table 50.9 Emergency treatment of hyperkalaemia

Agent	Dose	Comments
10% Calcium gluconate	0.5–1.0 ml/kg b.w. i.v. over 2–10 min	Use if there are ECG changes of hyperkalaemia with continuous ECG monitoring
Salbutamol	4 µg/kg b.w. i.v. in 10 ml water over 5–10 min or 2.5 mg (b.w. < 25 kg), 5.0 mg (b.w. > 25 kg) via nebulizer	Shifts potassium into cells Treatment of choice[a] Side-effect: tachycardia
8.4% Sodium bicarbonate	2.5 ml/kg b.w. i.v.	Shifts potassium into cells Avoid if there is significant circulatory overload or severe hypocalcaemia
Glucose with or without	0.5–1.0 g/kg b.w./hour i.v.	Shifts potassium into cells
soluble insulin	0.1 units/kg b.w./hour i.v.	Monitor blood sugar closely Risk of hypoglycaemia or hyperglycaemia
Ion-exchange resins	1.0 g/kg b.w., best given by enema	Use calcium/potassium exchange resin in preference to sodium/potassium exchange resins, which contribute to sodium overload Side-effect constipation

[a]Murdoch *et al.* (1991).

Hypocalcaemia

Hypocalcaemia may occur as a result of metastatic deposition of calcium phosphate, sequestration of calcium in damaged tissues or perturbation of calcium-regulating hormones. Asymptomatic hypocalcaemia should be treated by reducing plasma phosphate (see above) and, if necessary, additional calcium supplements in the form of calcium carbonate or calcium gluconate.

NUTRITION

Dietary therapy is integral to the management of ARF. Appropriate nutritional support is required to prevent catabolism and starvation ketoacidosis, while minimizing the production of nitrogenous waste and non-volatile acids. The advice of an experienced dietician is essential to provide at least 1400 kcal/m^2 body surface area per day. Initially, dietary protein should be restricted to 1 g/kg b.w. per day, but this may need to be increased in young children and in those treated by peritoneal dialysis. Very few children are able to complete the dietary prescription by mouth and the majority require nasogastric tube feeding. If enteral nutrition is not possible, parenteral nutrition should be employed to provide the necessary energy and protein requirements. The provision of adequate nutrition, particularly if the parenteral route has to be used, may precipitate the need for dialysis because of the volume of fluid required. Under no circumstances should nutrition be compromised for want of dialysis.

INFECTION

Infection is a frequent and often serious complication of ARF. Vigilance for signs of infection at the often multiple breaches of mucocutaneous barriers is essential. Redundant lines and catheters, e.g. the bladder catheter in a proven oligoanuric child, should be removed. Opinion is divided as to whether central venous dialysis catheters and temporary peritoneal catheters should be changed electively.

DRUG THERAPY

Drug therapy should be kept to a minimum and each medication prescribed should be checked as to whether a reduction in dose or frequency of dosing, or serum drug level monitoring is required in renal impairment (Wong *et al.*, 1994; British National Formularly, 1995). In the early phase of ARF, GFR should be assumed to be very low (< 10 ml/min). Thereafter, for patients not receiving dialysis, it can be calculated from plasma creatinine. Nephrotoxic drugs, e.g. aminoglycosides, amphotericin B, radiocontrast media and drugs potentiating renal injury, e.g. non-steroidal anti-inflammatory agents and angiotensin-converting enzyme inhibitors should be avoided if at all possible.

SPECIFIC TREATMENT

Once defined, some causes of intrinsic ARF require specific treatment, e.g. glomerulonephritis and vasculitis may respond to aggressive immunosuppressive therapy. Infusions of fresh plasma or plasma exchange may be useful in the management of HUS and thrombotic thrombocytopaenic purpura. Interstitial nephritis usually resolves spontaneously, particularly if it is caused by an allergic reaction to a drug, which is discontinued; however, corticosteroid therapy may accelerate recovery.

Alkaline diuresis, maintained by mannitol or frusemide, is useful in the prevention or early treatment of ARF due to myoglobinuria or haemoglobinuria and, combined with allopurinol therapy, in the management of tumour lysis syndrome.

ACUTE RENAL REPLACEMENT THERAPY

Not all children with ARF will require dialysis or haemofiltration. Absolute indications for initiating renal replacement therapy are given in Table 50.10. In addition, the underlying cause and predicted course of the renal failure need to be taken into consideration and dialysis or haemofiltration commenced before compli-

Table 50.10 Indications for acute renal replacement therapy

Extracellular volume overload	Causing pulmonary oedema and/or hypertension unresponsive to frusemide
Hyperkalaemia	Potassium > 7.0 mmol/l recorded before emergency treatment
Severe metabolic acidosis	
Uraemia	Causing symptoms or signs and/or urea > 40 mmol/l

Table 50.11 Comparison of peritoneal dialysis, intermittent haemodialysis, haemofiltration (CAVH, CVVH) and haemodiafiltration (CAVHD, CVVHD)

	Peritoneal dialysis	Intermittent haemodialysis	Haemofiltration[a] CAVH, CVVH	Haemodiafiltration CAVHD, CVVHD
Personnel	Paediatric renal nurses	Specialized paediatric dialysis nurses	Specialized paediatric intensive care unit nurses	Specialized paediatric intensive care unit nurses
Access	Intraperitoneal catheter placed percutaneously or surgically	Double lumen venous catheter placed in: internal jugular vein subclavian vein (risk of stenosis) femoral vein (risk of infection)	CAVH Arterial line: umbilical in neonates radial femoral Venous line: umbilical in neonates internal jugular vein subclavian vein femoral CVVH: as intermittent haemodialysis	As haemofiltration
Anticoagulation				
Particular indications	Neonates and small children Haemodynamically unstable patients	Following abdominal surgery or abdominal wall burns	Continuous Haemodynamically unstable patients without severe electrolyte derangement Need for TPN or blood products	Continuous Haemodynamically unstable patients with severe electrolyte derangement Need for TPN or blood products
Advantages	Easier to perform Requires less specialized personnel and equipment Less risk of dialysis disequilibrium Reduced risk of hepatitis and bleeding	Quicker and more efficient correction of biochemical derangements	Continuous controlled fluid removal better tolerated by haemodynamically unstable patients	Continuous controlled fluid removal better tolerated by haemodynamically unstable patients Continuous 'gentle' dialysis: less risk of dialysis disequilibrium
Disadvantages	Complications of catheter insertion: perforation of a viscus haemorrhage Catheter malfunction: blockage leakage Infection: peritonitis septicaemia Hypoproteinaemia Hyperglycaemia Lactic acidosis Pulmonary atelectasis Pleural effusion	Complications of vascular access: bleeding from site clotting infection damage to nearby organs Dialysis disequilibrium Excessive fluid removal causing hypotension and renal hypoperfusion resulting in delayed recovery	Complications of vascular access: see intermittent haemodialysis Clotting of filter and lines Inadequate control of uraemia Excessive fluid removal: see Intermittent haemodialysis	Complications of vascular access: see intermittent haemodialysis Clotting of filter and lines Excessive fluid removal: see Intermittent haemodialysis

[a]Nevard and Rigden (1995).

cations develop and to facilitate optimal nutrition. Historically, peritoneal dialysis has been the preferred treatment for the management of ARF in children, but continuing technical advances have made haemodialysis and haemofiltration (Nevard and Rigden, 1995) possible for all children and babies weighing more than 900 g. The chosen technique will therefore depend on the specific needs of an individual patient, the expertise of the nurses and doctors and the facilities available. The relative risks and advantages of peritoneal dialysis, intermittent haemodialysis, haemofiltration [continuous arteriovenous haemofiltration (CAVH), continuous venovenous haemofiltration (CVVH)] and haemodiafiltration [continuous arteriovenous haemodiafiltration, CAVHD, continuous venovenous haemodiafiltration (CVVHD)] are given in Table 50.11.

MANAGEMENT OF POSTRENAL ACUTE RENAL FAILURE

The management of postrenal ARF usually requires a multidisciplinary approach and collaboration between the paediatric nephrologist, urologist and radiologist. Urethral obstruction due to posterior urethral valves and functional bladder obstruction secondary to neuropathic bladder are usually treated initially by urethral catheterization. Obstruction of the ureter or at the pelviureteric junction may be relieved temporarily by an ultrasound-guided percutaneous nephrostomy pending a definitive procedure.

Recovery of renal function usually begins as soon as obstruction is relieved and is frequently accompanied by a postobstructive diuresis necessitating intravenous fluid and electrolyte replacement to prevent renal hypoperfusion and exacerbation of ATN.

Outcome and the future

Despite advances in supportive care and acute renal replacement therapy, mortality rates for patients with ARF remain between 10% (Niaudet *et al.*, 1985) and 60%. Prognosis is largely dependent on the cause of ARF and the presence of other associated medical problems, particularly multiorgan failure (July and Turney,

1990). The overall mortality in neonatal ARF varies from 14%–73% (Stapleton *et al.*, 1989). Non-oliguric ARF generally has a better prognosis.

The majority of surviving patients have good recovery of renal function in the short and longer term (Georgaki-Angelaki *et al.*, 1989). However, a small number, for example those with complete cortical necrosis, will have irreversible renal failure and others with, for example, severe HUS or HSP, having recovered initially, will have a slow progressive deterioration in renal function and eventually require renal replacement therapy.

At present, prevention and early recognition of ARF are the best means of potentially improving prognosis. The frequency of ATN can be reduced significantly by close attention to the haemodynamic status of high-risk patients. The incidence of ARF following trauma is declining as a result of prompt and effective resuscitation (July and Turney, 1990). Nephrotoxic ATN can be prevented or ameliorated by careful choice and dosing of potentially nephrotoxic drugs, e.g. pretreatment hydration, mannitol and/or saline diuresis to reduce cisplatin nephrotoxicity (Safirstein *et al.*, 1990).

In the future, increased understanding of the cellular and molecular basis of renal injury and regeneration will, hopefully, result in more effective treatment strategies and improved outcome of ARF.

CHRONIC RENAL FAILURE

Introduction

Irreversible renal failure is a continuum extending from mild renal insufficiency to end-stage renal failure, its severity being proportional to the reduction in functional renal mass (Table 50.12) (Kaufman *et al.*, 1974) For the purposes of this chapter, chronic renal failure (CRF) is defined by a glomerular filtration rate (GFR) of < 50 ml/min/1.73 m^2 surface area, i.e. to include moderate renal insufficiency, since below this level of renal function metabolic abnormalities such as acidosis and secondary hyperparathyroidism become increasingly apparent, growth may be impaired and further

Table 50.12 Renal failure

	Residual functioning (%)	Renal mass	GFR (ml/min/1.73 m^2 surface area)
Mild renal insufficiency	50–25	80–50	Asymptomatic
Moderate renal insufficiency	25–15	50–30	Metabolic abnormalities Impaired growth
Chronic renal failure	15–5	30–10	Progressive renal failure
End-stage renal failure	< 5	< 10	RRT required

progressive loss of function is likely to occur. Renal replacement therapy (RRT), either by dialysis or transplantation, is not usually necessary until the GFR falls below 10 ml/min/1.73m² surface area. The initiation of RRT defines the onset of end-stage renal failure (ESRF), and preterminal renal failure (pre-TRF) defines patients with CRF, but not yet requiring RRT.

Organization of services

Children with ESRF should be treated in specialized paediatric centres, where facilities can be concentrated and expertise developed. Because of the relatively low incidence of end-stage renal disease in children, one specialized paediatric unit per million child population has been advocated. A specialized paediatric unit must be capable of providing all modes of ESRF therapy, including automated peritoneal dialysis (APD), continuous ambulatory peritoneal dialysis (CAPD), hospital and home haemodialysis, and renal transplantation. The management of ESRF in children is complex and requires the resources of a multidisciplinary team comprising not only medical and nursing staff trained in paediatric renal medicine and surgeons experienced in paediatric urology and transplantation, but also specialist children's dietitians, social workers, psychiatrists, psychologists, teachers and play specialists. The main disadvantage to providing children's ESRF services in specialized units is that many families have to travel, sometimes considerable distances, for treatment. For some children the number of visits to the specialized centre can be reduced by co-opting the local paediatrician or nephrologist to the multidisciplinary team to share in the child's care.

Children with pre-TRF require careful conservative management in order to optimize their growth and to preserve their renal function for as long as possible which, for some, will be into adult life. They should be under the supervision of a specialized paediatric centre, but often their care can be shared with their local paediatrician.

Incidence

The incidence of ESRF in children in countries with well-established reporting registries is 3.5–11 per million adjusted population. In Europe, in recent years, the number of children commencing RRT before the age of 15 years, has been 4–6 children per million child population (pmcp), rising to 9 children pmcp or more in some countries (Loirat *et al.*, 1994).

In the UK in 1992, 106 children aged less than 15 years were accepted for renal replacement therapy, giving an incidence of 9.7 pmcp. In the same year 429 youngsters aged less than 15 years were identified

as receiving RRT, i.e. a prevalence rate of 38.8 pmcp (Report of a Working Party of the British Association for Paediatric Nephrology, 1995). The age distribution of children accepted for RRT has changed during the past two decades, with an increasing number of younger children being treated (Loirat *et al.*, 1994).

The prevalence of pre-TRF is less well defined because of differing definitions of pre-TRF, the use of different age cut-offs and the underreporting that occurs when infants or children are not referred to specialized units.

In Sweden, in the period 1978–85, the prevalence of pre-TRF, defined as a GFR of < 30 ml/min/1.73 m² surface area, in children aged 6 months to 16 years was 26.1 pmcp (Esbjorner *et al.*, 1990), while in the 1992 UK study, in units defining pre-TRF as a GFR of < 25–30 ml/min/1.73 m² surface area, the prevalence of pre-TRF in children less than 15 years old was 44.2 pmcp (Report of a Working Party of the British Association for Paediatric Nephrology, 1995).

Causes of chronic renal failure

The causes of CRF, compiled from three sources (Esbjorner *et al.*, 1990; Loirat *et al.*, 1994; Kohaut and Tejani, 1996) are summarized in Table 50.13. The primary renal diseases of 2735 children commencing RRT in Europe between 1987 and 1991 are given in column 1, and those of 3183 children transplanted in North America between January 1987 and February 1994 in column 2, while in column 3, the causes of CRF (GFR < 30 ml/min/1.73 m² surface area) in 146 Swedish children, 77 of whom required RRT during the period 1978–1985, are shown. Congenital abnormalities, which are more likely to occur in boys and in younger children, account for the largest proportion of cases in all three series and inherited conditions for a further 14–28%. CRF in over 50% of children requiring RRT, therefore, has a prenatal cause, which has important implications for antenatal diagnosis and intervention, genetic counselling and future research.

Progression of renal failure

Progressive decline in renal function is inevitable once a certain degree of renal damage has occurred, irrespective of the cause of the damage and whether or not it is still operating. The degree of renal damage may vary, but once residual GFR is less than half normal, risk for progression is high (Table 50.12). For example, male infants born with posterior urethral valves, whose plasma creatinine remains above 70 μmol/l (0.8 mg/dl equivalent to a calculated GFR of approximately 48 ml/min/1.73 m² surface area) throughout the first year of life often progress to ESRF during the first decade of life (Warsaw *et al.*, 1985).

Table 50.13 Causes of chronic renal failure

	EDTA[a] (%)	NAPRTCS[b] (%)	Sweden (pre-TRF + ESRF)[c] (%)
Congenital abnormalities	**36.0**	**42.6**	**45.9**
Aplasia/hypoplasia/dysplasia		17.0	21.0
Obstructive uropathy		16.8	17.8
Reflux nephropathy		5.7	5.0
Prune belly syndrome		3.1	2.1
Inherited conditions	**16.3**	**14.2**	**27.5**
Medullary cystic disease/nephronophthisis	4.7	2.6	11.0
Polycystic kidney disease	2.1	2.8	7.5
Hereditary nephritis with or without nerve deafness	1.5	2.2	4.1
Cystinosis	3.5	2.7	1.4
Primary oxalosis	1.6	0.8	–
Congenital nephrotic syndrome	–	3.1	1.4
Other causes	2.9	–	2.1
Glomerulonephritis	**23.6**	**19.0**	**9.6**
Focal segmental glomerulosclerosis	9.4	11.5	4.1
Other glomerulonephritis	14.2	7.5	5.5
Multisystem disease	**6.9**	**7.5**	**8.3**
Lupus erythematosus	0.7	–	2.1
Henoch–Schönlein purpura	1.7	–	2.1
Systemic immunological disease	–	4.7	–
Haemolytic uraemic syndrome	4.5	2.8	2.7
Other multisystem diseases	–	–	1.4
Miscellaneous	**8.8**	**10.9**	**8.4**
Renal vascular disease	–	2.1	3.5
Kidney tumour	0.9	0.5	0.7
Drash syndrome	–	0.5	1.4
Others	7.9	7.8	2.8
Chronic renal failure	**7.8**	**3.7**	**0.7**
Cause unknown	7.8	3.7	0.7

[a]Loirat *et al.* (1994).
[b]Kohaut and Tejani (1996).
[c]Esbjorner *et al.* (1990).

Progression of CRF is associated histologically with progressive glomerulosclerosis, interstitial fibrosis and vascular or arteriolar sclerosis. Numerous hypotheses, which are not necessarily mutually exclusive, have been proposed to explain these scarring processes. Hostetter *et al.* (1981) postulated that loss of a substantial proportion of renal function caused increased perfusion and filtration of the remaining nephrons, which although beneficial in the short term, will ultimately result in glomerulosclerosis. The damage was originally attributed to hyperfiltration, but the accompanying glomerular hypertension, which causes proteinuria, is now thought to play an important role (Johnson, 1994).

Hyperlipidaemia, which is common in CRF, has also been implicated in the pathogenesis of glomerulosclerosis and tubulointerstitial fibrosis (Moorhead *et al.*, 1982). Tubulointerstitial fibrosis, which is a better predictor of renal insufficiency than glomerulosclerosis (Risdon *et al.*, 1968), has, in animal experiments been attributed to hyperfunction of remaining tubules, nephrotoxicity of lipids, carbohydrates, iron and oxygen free radicals and a nephrotoxic effect of proteinuria. All of these pathogenetic mechanisms can stimulate tubular cells to release chemotactic factors which attract mononuclear cells capable of initiating inflammation and scarring.

The mechanisms underlying vascular sclerosis are less well studied, but clearly hypertension is a factor. Arteriolar sclerosis causes ischaemia of the remaining tubules and interstitium, which results in further scarring.

The rate of progression varies widely among primary renal diseases and is likely to be more rapid in those with already severely reduced renal function. In adults, it is also affected by age, gender and race. Hypertension and proteinuria are also important determinants. With this background it is clear that any therapeutic intervention designed to slow the progression of CRF must be tested in carefully designed prospective controlled trials, and whilst there have been many animal studies (Modi *et al.*, 1993), only two therapies – low protein diet (Klahr *et al.*, 1994) and treatment of hypertension (Alvestrand *et al.*, 1988) – have been investigated adequately in humans and only one – low protein diet – in children (Wingen *et al.*, 1991; Kist-van Holthe tot Echten *et al.*, 1993). The results and applications of these studies will be discussed later.

Clinical features

PRESENTATION

CRF in children may present in a wide variety of ways. Its onset may be silent and its progression insidious, with symptoms only developing late in its course.

ANTENATAL ULTRASOUND SCREENING

Routine antenatal ultrasound scanning has resulted in an increased detection of fetal renal tract abnormalities (Scott and Renwick, 1991), some of which will cause postnatal CRF, e.g. infantile polycystic kidney disease and obstructive uropathy due to posterior urethral valves. Such *in utero* diagnosis requires close co operation among the obstetrician, neonatologist, paediatric nephrologist and urologist to ensure appropriate management of the fetus predelivery and post-delivery and that the parents are given accurate information.

URINARY TRACT INFECTION

Investigation of the child presenting with urinary tract infection (see Chapter 49) may reveal a serious underlying renal tract abnormality or reflux nephropathy.

ENURESIS

Enuresis in very few children has an organic cause (see Chapter 64), but CRF may present in this way in a small number of children. Useful clues are a history of urinary tract infection, the presence of daytime wetting, the onset of secondary enuresis and a history of polydipsia and polyuria. Early morning urine osmolality is a very useful screening test and will often obviate the need for renal tract imaging studies.

FAILURE TO THRIVE

Chronic uraemia frequently results in anorexia, vomiting and failure to thrive, particularly in infants and young children, making assessment of renal function essential in such children. Failure to thrive, with dehydration and electrolyte disturbances, is a common presentation in children with renal tubular disorders, which are either associated with CRF, e.g. obstructive uropathy, or will progress to CRF, e.g. Fanconi's syndrome due to cystinosis.

SHORT STATURE

Poor growth velocity, short stature and pubertal delay may all be caused by and presenting symptoms of CRF (see Chapter 51).

PALLOR AND LETHARGY

Pallor, due to the normochromic–normocytic anaemia which results from chronic uraemia, and lethargy are classic symptoms of CRF, but usually do not develop until late in its course. Occasionally, a child with even less specific symptoms of ill health is found to have CRF.

HAEMATURIA

Rarely, macroscopic haematuria is the presenting symptom of a condition which will ultimately cause renal failure, e.g. Alport's syndrome or adult-type polycystic kidney disease.

NEPHROTIC SYNDROME

The outcome for children with minimal-change nephrotic syndrome is generally excellent, but for those with steroid-resistant disease the outlook is less favourable, with a significant number progressing to CRF and ESRF. Infants with congenital nephrotic syndrome also have a poor prognosis, either succumbing to infection or eventually developing CRF.

HYPERTENSION

Symptomatic hypertension is not infrequently the presenting feature of renal parenchymal scarring due, for example, to reflux nephropathy, which may also result in CRF. Assessment of renal function is therefore essential in all children with hypertension. Non-renin-dependent hypertension due to salt and water retention also occurs in children with CRF, but is less likely to be a presenting feature unless it results in cardiac failure (see below).

CONGESTIVE CARDIAC FAILURE

Congestive cardiac failure resulting from untreated hypertension and/or salt and water overload does not usually develop until late in the course of CRF, but in some children it may be the presenting symptom, requiring urgent treatment with diuretics or dialysis and occasionally ventilation.

FAILURE TO RECOVER FROM ACUTE RENAL FAILURE

Occasionally a child with acute renal failure (ARF) will make no or an incomplete recovery and be left in CRF or ESRF, e.g. as a result of rapidly progressive glomerulonephritis, or there may be a slow but progressive decline in renal function, usually heralded by hypertension and/or proteinuria, in children in whom there had apparently been a good recovery from ARF, e.g. haemolytic uraemic syndrome (Fitzpatrick *et al.*, 1991), Henoch–Schönlein purpura.

ABDOMINAL MASS

The detection of a renal mass or a palpable bladder may be the first sign of underlying CRF. Investigation, initially by renal tract ultrasound examination and assessment of renal function, will lead to the correct diagnosis.

ASYMPTOMATIC: DETECTED BY SCREENING

Very rarely, an asymptomatic child is found to be hypertensive or to have proteinuria or microscopic haematuria on routine urinalysis, which on investigation is found to be due to serious underlying renal disease. It is important to screen even the apparently healthy siblings of children with genetically determined CRF, e.g. juvenile nephronophthisis, Alport's syndrome or reflux nephropathy, whilst realizing the potentially devastating effect on the family of finding a further affected child.

Investigations

At presentation, it may not be clear, particularly if renal failure is severe, whether a child has ARF or CRF (see Chapter 51). History and examination may provide valu-

Table 50.14 Specific investigations to elucidate the underlying cause of chronic renal failure

Renal tract ultrasound
Micturating cystourethrogram
Radioisotope scans: DMSA, DTPA or MAG3
 antegrade pressure-flow studies
IVU
Urinalysis
Urine microscopy
C_3, C_4, antinuclear antibody, anti-DNA antibodies,
 anti-GBM antibodies, ANCA
Renal biopsy
White cell cystine level
Oxalate excretion
Purine excretion

able pointers to the underlying cause, but in some children this will only be revealed by specific investigations (Table 50.14). The investigations listed in Table 50.15 should be performed in all children presenting with possible CRF to assess the degree of renal impairment and the severity of any secondary metabolic derangements.

The features listed in Table 50.16 should be sought, since their presence may help to differentiate ARF from CRF.

Management of preterminal renal failure

From the child's viewpoint, the aims of conservative management of pre-TRF are to:

- feel normal, i.e. not to have uraemic symptoms such as nausea or vomiting

Table 50.15 Investigations to assess the severity of chronic renal failure

Full blood count	
Biochemistry	Blood electrolytes, urea, creatinine, calcium, phosphate, alkaline phosphatase, total protein, albumin, urate Blood pH and bicarbonate using blood gas analysis Parathyroid hormone using an intact molecule assay Urine creatinine, phosphate, protein, albumin
GFR	Of less value in severe CRF
Left-hand and wrist X-ray	For bone age and evidence of renal osteodystrophy
Chest X-ray	
ECG or echocardiogram	

Table 50.16 Features suggestive of acute and chronic renal failure

Acute renal failure	Chronic renal failure
Previously healthy	Family history of renal disease
Normal or slightly enlarged kidneys on ultrasound	Small/asymmetric kidneys, cystic kidneys, abnormal collecting systems, ureters and bladder on ultrasound
Microangiopathic haemolytic anaemia, thrombocytopenia	Normochromic, normocytic anaemia
	End-organ effects of hypertension, e.g. retinopathy
	Poor growth
	Radiological evidence of rickets or secondary hyperparathyroidism

• be normal, i.e. to be like his or her friends and have sufficient energy to take a full part in all school and social activities, or for the preschool child to achieve normal motor, social and intellectual development
• maintain normal growth

while

• preserving normal family functioning
• slowing the rate of progression to ESRF
• preparing the child and family for RRT.

For the child with moderate to severe CRF (GFR < 30 ml/min/1.73 m^2 surface area), these objectives are best met by a multidisciplinary team approach in the setting of a dedicated clinic, where ample time can be spent with each child and the family (Rees *et al.*, 1989).

The following management points need to be considered at each outpatient clinic visit.

GROWTH

The effects of CRF on growth and the management of growth retardation are discussed in Chapter 51. Growth is the most sensitive indicator of adequacy of CRF treatment. Height, weight and, for children under 2 years of age, head circumference should be measured at each visit, ideally by the same observer, using suitable equipment. Values obtained should be plotted for chronological age on appropriate centile charts and any deviation from the expected growth investigated with a view to correcting its cause, rather than simply ascribing the poor growth to CRF.

NUTRITION

Renal failure results in malnutrition and, in children, growth retardation. Nutritional therapy, if carefully applied, can ameliorate the effects of renal failure and allow improved well-being and growth; and it may also have a role in slowing the rate of decline in renal function. The services of a skilled paediatric renal dietician are invaluable in the provision of individualized nutritional therapy, without undue disruption to the family's eating pattern.

The recommended intake of nutrients for children with CRF are given in Table 50.17 (Department of Health, 1991), but the following points need to be emphasized.

(i) Prospective 3-day dietary assessments should be performed at 1–3-month intervals for analysis of nutrient intake.
(ii) Children with CRF tend to be anorexic and frequently have spontaneous energy intakes below the estimated average requirement (EAR) for age (Orejas *et al.*, 1995). Provision of adequate energy, defined as at least the EAR for age, is essential for successful nutritional therapy. To achieve this, most children require calorie supplements in the form of glucose polymers or fat emulsions, which for infants and young children may need to be added to a feed to be delivered by a nasogastric or gastrostomy tube.
(iii) In order to prevent or treat secondary hyperparathyroidism, plasma phosphate must be maintained between the mean and −2 SD for age, by restriction of dietary phosphate and the use of calcium carbonate as a phosphate binder (see below). As the major dietary sources of phosphate are dairy products, adequate phosphate restriction can usually be achieved by limiting the intake of cow's milk to less than half a pint a day and by avoiding cheese and yoghurt.
(iv) In animal models, dietary protein restriction slows the progression of renal insufficiency (Modi *et al.*, 1993). However, in patients, the use of low protein diets has proved much more problematic with, in properly controlled trials, only marginal benefit (Klahr *et al.*, 1994). In children, who have a higher protein requirement because of the demands of growth, protein restriction has been shown to be of no benefit in retarding progression of renal failure (Wingen *et al.*, 1991; Kist van Holthe tot Echten *et al.*, 1993) and in a short-term study in infants was associated with inferior growth (Uauy *et al.*, 1994). Children with CRF should therefore receive a minimum protein intake of EAR for age (Table 50.17).

Table 50.17 Recommended daily energy and nutrient intakes for children with chronic renal failure[a]

Age	Mean weight (kg)	Energy EAR (kcal)	Protein EAR (g)	RNI (g)	Sodium RNI (mmol)	Calcium RNI (mg)	Phosphorus RNI (mg)
0–3 months	5.9	115/kg	–	2.1/kg	9	525	400
4–6 months	7.7	100/kg	1.4/kg	1.6/kg	12	525	400
7–9 months	8.8	95/kg	1.3/kg	1.6/kg	14	525	400
10–12 months	9.7	95/kg	1.2/kg	1.5/kg	15	525	400
1–3 years	12.5	1230	11.7	14.5	22	350	270
4–6 years	17.8	1715	14.8	19.7	30	450	350
7–10 years	28.3	1970	22.8	28.3	52	550	450
11–14 years							
Males	43.0	2220	33.8	42.1	70	1000	775
Females	43.8	1845	33.1	41.2	70	800	625
15–18 years							
Males	64.5	2755	46.1	55.2	70	1000	775
Females	55.5	2110	37.1	45.4	70	800	625

[a]Based on UK Dietary Reference Values (Department of Health, 1991).
EAR, Estimated average requirement.
RNI, Reference nutrient intake = EAR +2SD.

If dairy proteins have been restricted as above to limit phosphate intake, and energy intake ensured to promote anabolism, further protein restriction is seldom necessary. If despite these measures, a child's blood urea remains above 20 mmol/l, a gentle step-wise protein restriction, using the child's 3-day dietary assessment as the basis for advice, should be introduced to reduce the blood urea to less than 20 mmol/l.

FLUID AND ELECTROLYTE BALANCE

At each clinic visit, the child's state of hydration should be assessed using skin turgor, mucous membrane moisture, blood pressure, jugular venous pressure and weight. Many causes of CRF in childhood are associated with excessive sodium loss, e.g. obstructive uropathy, renal dysplasia and juvenile nephronophthisis. Sodium depletion results in contraction of the extracellular fluid volume and further impairment in renal function; and is also detrimental to growth (Haycock, 1993). Sodium chloride supplements should be gradually increased until an improvement in growth is seen, without producing peripheral oedema, hypertension or hypernatraemia. Water intake is determined by the child to satisfy thirst.

Children with primary renal diseases resulting in hypertension may benefit from a reduction in sodium intake to 1–2 mmol/kg/day, but it is seldom necessary to restrict fluid until ESRF supervenes.

Most children with CRF are able to main potassium homoeostasis satisfactorily despite fluctuations in intake. If hyperkalaemia occurs, it is important to exclude catabolism and metabolic acidosis as correctable causes, as well as giving individually tailored advice based on the child's dietary assessments.

METABOLIC ACIDOSIS

Maintenance of acid–base balance is particularly important in infants and children. Persistent metabolic acidosis is associated with failure to thrive in infancy and contributes to muscle degradation, bone demineralization and hyperkalaemia. Although reducing protein intake and therefore the intake of sulphur-containing amino acids reduces endogenous acid production, sodium bicarbonate supplements in a starting dose of 2 mmol/kg/day are frequently required to correct metabolic acidosis. Treatment should be monitored and dosage adjusted according to venous blood gas determinations of pH and bicarbonate concentration.

HYPERTENSION

Hypertension may be the consequence of underlying renal pathology, e.g. reflux nephropathy or chronic glomerulonephritis, or in advanced CRF it may result from sodium and water retention. If, in the absence of circulatory volume overload, the child's systolic and/or diastolic blood pressure is repeatedly in excess of the 90th centile for age (Report of the Second Task Force on Blood Pressure Control in Children, 1987), specific hypotensive therapy should be instituted to prevent the morbidity and mortality associated with hypertension and to retard the progression of CRF. There is now convincing evidence that control of hypertension is beneficial in slowing the progression of CRF (Alvstrand *et al.*,

1988) although the hypotensive agent of choice remains controversial. At present, ACE inhibitors seem to be favoured, since they also reduce protein excretion (Gansevoort *et al.*, 1995). If there is evidence of circulatory volume overload causing or contributing to hypertension, a diuretic, usually frusemide in a dose of 1–3 mg/kg, should be commenced and sodium restricted as above. The most useful drugs in the management of hypertension in children with CRF are summarized in Table 50.18.

RENAL OSTEODYSTROPHY

Secondary hyperparathyroidism is the most prevalent form of metabolic bone disease resulting from CRF. Its treatment is controversial (Rigden, 1996a; Salusky and Goodman, 1996) but, in the author's unit, it has been shown that it is possible to prevent or, if already established, reverse secondary hyperparathyroidism over long periods, using a regimen of mild dietary phosphate restriction, as outlined above, calcium carbonate given with meals as a phosphate binder and 1α-hydroxycholecalciferol (1α-OHCC) or 1,25-dihydroxycholecalciferol (1,25-DHCC). The dose of calcium carbonate is increased until the plasma phosphate falls between the mean and -2 SD for age when, if the parathyroid hormone (PTH) level is still high, 1α-OHCC or 1,25-DHCC is introduced and increased until plasma calcium is at the upper end of the normal range. Plasma calcium and phosphate must be closely monitored to avoid hypercalcaemia and metastatic calcification. The PTH level should be checked at each clinic visit, using an intact molecule assay, and therapy adjusted accordingly. If the child is asymptomatic and the biochemical parameters are normal it is only necessary to perform an annual X-ray of the left hand and wrist to assess bone age.

INFECTION

Children with renal tract abnormalities predisposing them to recurrent urinary tract infections must have a urine sample cultured at each clinic visit. They should be maintained on low-dose prophylactic antibiotics and practise the general measures to prevent reinfection, as outlined in Chapter 49. Other bacterial infections, e.g. otitis media, should be treated promptly to reverse catabolism.

ANAEMIA

CRF is associated with a normochromic, normocytic anaemia, the pathogenesis of which includes inadequate

Table 50.18 Drugs used in the treatment of hypertension in chronic renal failure

Drug	Dose (mg/kg/day) Initial	Maximum	Number of doses/day	Action	Comments
Captopril	0.3	5	3	ACE inhibitor	May exacerbate hyperkalaemia
Enalapril	0.06	1	1	ACE inhibitor	Long-acting ACE inhibitor Drug of choice May exacerbate hyperkalaemia
Atenolol	1	2	1	Cardioselective β-blocker	Long-acting β-blocker May exacerbate hyperkalaemia
Nifedipine	0.25	0.5	3	Calcium channel blocker	Slow release preparations also available May cause sodium and water retention
Prazosin	0.05	0.4	3	α-Blocker	May cause sodium and water retention
Minoxidil	0.1	2	3	Direct vasodilator	Effective in refractory hypertension Causes sodium and water retention requiring diuretic therapy
Frusemide	0.5	15	2	Loop diuretic	Drug of choice to treat circulatory volume overload
Metolazone	0.1	1	2	Diuretic	Synergistic action with frusemide

ACE, angiotensin converting enzyme.

erythropoietin production. Recombinant human erythro-poietin (rHuEPO) is now available and widely used to treat anaemia in ESRF (Rigden *et al.*, 1990). However, the majority of children with pre-TRF can maintain satisfactory haemoglobin levels without endogenous rHuEPO therapy provided that careful attention is paid to nutrition, iron and folate supplements are given if indicated and secondary hyperparathyroidism is suppressed without the use of aluminium-containing phosphate binders.

EDUCATION AND PREPARATION

The pre-TRF clinic is the ideal environment for continuing the education and preparation of the child and family for ESRF treatment. In addition to ensuring their understanding of the rationale of pre-TRF therapy and the options available for ESRF treatment (see below), there are important practical preparations, as follows:

- Immunizations including BCG, hepatitis B and, if indicated, varicella zoster should be completed at least 3 months before RRT is anticipated to be required.
- If a child with pre-TRF is receiving an enzyme-inducing anti-epileptic drug, this should, if possible, be replaced by a non-enzyme-inducing agent such as sodium valproate or lamotrigine, to facilitate adequate immunosuppression following transplantation.
- Children with CRF associated with bladder dysfunction require very careful assessment, including urodynamic studies, to ensure that the bladder is safe prior to transplantation. Bladder augmentation surgery and/or management with clean intermittent catheterization may be necessary to achieve this.
- Children who are likely to require dialysis prior to transplantation, but who are not suitable for peritoneal dialysis, should have an arteriovenous fistula created to provide access for haemodialysis.

SOCIAL AND PSYCHOLOGICAL

The management of a child with progressive pre-TRF can be extremely stressful even to the best-adjusted families. All families should be offered practical and emotional support by an experienced social worker and some require and will benefit from referral to a child psychologist or psychiatrist.

Management of end-stage renal failure

Even with meticulous management, most children with pre-TRF eventually progress to ESRF, while other children present in ESRF. It is much more helpful to consider the treatment of ESRF as a potentially repetitive cycle (Fig. 50.1) rather than as a simple progression

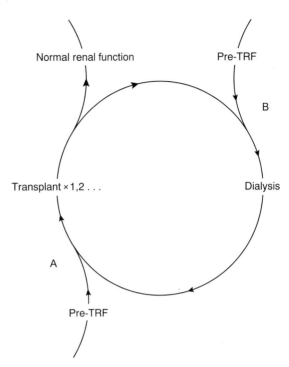

Fig. 50.1 The circular model of ESRF management.

from pre-TRF to renal transplant to cure. Children with pre-TRF may enter the cycle at point A for pre-emptive transplantation or at point B, with those presenting in ESRF for a period of dialysis prior to transplantation. The ideal exit is with normal renal function, but if this is not achieved and further treatment is appropriate, the cycle continues and the child returns to dialysis with a view to a further transplant. The author's preference is to transplant children with progressive pre-TRF just before they become symptomatic from their renal failure and require dialysis, i.e. pre-emptive transplantation (Rigden, 1996b). This is obviously easier using a live related donor, but is also possible with a well-organized cadaveric programme if the potential recipient is placed on-call for a transplant when their calculated GFR has fallen to approximately 10 ml/min/1.73 m^2 surface area.

If pre-emptive renal transplantation is not possible, indications for commencing dialysis are:

- uraemic symptoms such as lethargy, anorexia or vomiting, which interfere with daily life
- dangerous biochemical abnormalities, e.g. hyperkalaemia, unresponsive to the measures outlined above
- circulatory overload refractory to diuretic therapy
- impaired growth velocity, unresponsive to optimal conservative management. Poor growth occasionally constitutes an indication for earlier initiation of RRT, preferably by transplantation.

For children presenting in ESRF, the indications for dialysis are as in ARF.

Treatment

Successful renal transplantation is undoubtedly the treatment of choice for all children with ESRF. (Fine, 1985)

TRANSPLANTATION

Transplantation is performed using a cadaveric kidney or a kidney from a live relative over the age of consent, which for a child usually means a parent. Overall, in Europe, in the period 1987–92, 17% of children transplanted received a living related graft, although there was wide intercountry variation (Valderrabano *et al.*, 1995). In North America, live donor sources accounted for 46% of grafts performed in children and adolescents aged less than 20 years between January 1987 and February 1994 (Kohaut and Tejani, 1996).

IMMUNOSUPPRESSION

Immunosuppressive agents and regimens continue to proliferate (Welsh, 1991; Ellis, 1995), whilst the quest for immunological tolerance continues. The following general points can be made:

- The intensity of immunosuppression required is, in general, inversely related to the degree of human leucocyte antigen (HLA) matching achieved between the donor and recipient.
- Immunosuppression needs to be continued indefinitely, a fact not always appreciated by patients, particularly non-compliant teenagers.
- Cyclosporin A and FK-506 are nephrotoxic and therefore blood levels must be monitored to ensure adequate immunosuppressive effect and avoid nephrotoxicity.
- Alternate-day steroid regimens are associated with better post-transplant growth than those using daily steroids.
- The increasing use of anti-lymphocyte antibodies, particularly if monoclonal antibodies, e.g. OKT3, are also given, is associated with an increased incidence of post-transplant malignancy.

GRAFT SURVIVAL

EDTA data for children transplanted before the age of 15 years in the period 1987–92 show a 1-year graft survival for living donor grafts of 87%, falling to 80% at 3 years and, for cadaveric grafts, a 1-year survival of 76%, falling to 67% at 3 years (Valderrabano *et al.*, 1995).

Similar graft survival figures of 90% at 1 year and 74% at 5 years for live donor grafts and 76% at 1 year and 58% at 5 years for cadaveric grafts have been reported by the North American Pediatric Renal Transplantation Co-operative Study (Kohaut and Tejani, 1996).

Long-term graft survival in single-centre reports varies between 40% at 10 years (Broyer *et al.*, 1987) and 61% at 13 years (Offner *et al.*, 1988). It is thus clear that even with good graft survival a child is likely to require two or three transplants for a normal lifespan.

PATIENT SURVIVAL AND REHABILITATION

The survival of children with ESRF continues to improve: 93% of children receiving transplants in Europe between 1987 and 1992 were alive 3 years later (Valderrabano *et al.*, 1995), compared to 84% of children commencing RRT between 1977 and 1982. Long-term survival is also good following transplantation with an actuarial survival rate of 81% at 14 years reported by one centre (Offner *et al.*, 1988).

Rehabilitation following a successful renal transplant is, in general, very good (Reynolds *et al.*, 1991). However, some young adults, particularly young men, who commenced RRT during childhood still have problems (Henning *et al.*, 1988). They were concerned about their physical appearance, particularly their height, and the effect that this had on their social life and on forming lasting relationships. The challenge now is to try and ensure that the present generation of children with ESRF achieves more complete rehabilitation in adult life.

DIALYSIS

Dialysis should be seen as a complement to transplantation, which may be needed before or between transplants, but ideally not as an alternative to transplantation. When discussing dialysis options with a family, there are two basic choices: is the child to be treated by haemodialysis or peritoneal dialysis, and is the child to be dialysed at home or in hospital? There may be medical constraints to the first choice, e.g. difficult vascular access may dictate peritoneal dialysis or intraperitoneal adhesions may preclude peritoneal dialysis. The second decision depends on the family's resources. Home peritoneal dialysis, ideally using an automated machine overnight, offers advantages in terms of the child's education and psychosocial adjustment, but if continued for long periods, and particularly if the child also requires continuous nasogastric or gastrostomy tube feeding and daily injections of recombinant human growth hormone and erythropoietin, may be associated with family burnout. Home haemodialysis is now, at least in the UK, rarely undertaken (Report of a Working Party of the British Association for Paediatric Nephrology, 1995). Hospital haemodialysis relieves the family of the stresses and responsibility of performing dialysis, but as it usually needs to be carried out for 3–5 hours, depending on the child's size and residual renal function, thrice weekly, it can be very disruptive to a child's education and family life.

ACCESS

Haemodialysis requires access to the circulation, which is best provided by an arteriovenous fistula created from the radial or brachial vessels of the nondominant arm. In young children, surgically placed, double-lumen, central venous catheters may be preferable to avoid the trauma of placing dialysis needles in the fistula, although this is less of a problem since the introduction of effective local anaesthetic creams. Moreover, central venous catheters pose an infection risk and may result in stenosis or occlusion of large central veins, making further access difficult.

Peritoneal dialysis requires the placement of a soft permanent peritoneal catheter. Peritoneal catheters pose a risk of infection, either at the exit site, in the subcutaneous tunnel or within the peritoneum. They are also prone to blockage by omentum, although the modified, curled, one-cuff Tenckhoff catheter, combined with limited omentectomy, seems less prone to this complication (Alexander *et al.*, 1985).

References

Alexander, S.R., Tank, E.S. and Corneil, A.T. 1985: Five years' experience with CAPD/CCPD catheters in infants and children. In Fine, R.N., Scharer, K. and Mehls, O. (eds), *CAPD in children*. New York: Springer, 174–89.

Alvestrand, A., Guiterrez, A., Bucht, H. and Bergstrom, J. 1988: Reduction of blood pressure retards the progression of chronic renal failure in man. *Nephrology, Dialysis, Transplantation* **3**, 624–31.

Anand, S.K. 1982: Acute renal failure in the neonate. *Pediatric Clinics of North America* **29**, 791–800.

Aynsley-Green, A. and Pickering, D. 1974: Use of central and peripheral temperature measurements in care of the critically ill child. *Archives of Disease in Childhood* **49**, 477–81.

British National Formulary 1995: *British Medical Association and The Pharmaceutical Society of Great Britain*. London: Pharmaceutical Press, 29.

Broyer, M., Gagnadoux, M.F., Guest, G. *et al.* 1987: Kidney transplantation in children. Results of 383 grafts performed at Enfants Malades Hospital from 1973 to 1984. *Advances in Nephrology* **16**, 307.

Department of Health 1991: Dietary reference values for food energy and nutrients for the United Kingdom. Report on Health and Social Subjects 41. London: HMSO.

Ellis, D. 1995: Clinical use of tacrolimus (FK-506) in infants and children with renal transplants. *Pediatric Nephrology* **9**, 487–94.

Esbjorner, B., Aronson, S., Berg, U., Fodal, U. and Linne, T. 1990: Children with chronic renal failure in Sweden 1978–1985. *Pediatric Nephrology* **4**, 249–52.

Fine, R.N. 1985: Renal transplantation for children – the only realistic choice. *Kidney International* **28**, 15–7.

Fitzpatrick, M.M., Shah, V., Trompeter, R.S., Dillon, M.J. and Barratt, T.M. 1991: Long term renal outcome of childhood haemolytic uraemic syndrome. *British Medical Journal* **303**, 489–92.

Gansevoort, R.T., Sluiter, W.J., Hemmelder, M.H., Zeeuw, D. de and De Jong, P.E. 1995: Anti-proteinuric effect of blood pressure lowering agents: a meta-analysis of comparative trials. *Nephrology, Dialysis, Transplantation* **10**, 1963–74.

Georgaki-Angelaki, H.N., Steed, D.B., Chantler, C. and Haycock, G.B. 1989: Renal function following acute renal failure in childhood: a long-term follow-up study. *Kidney International* **35**, 84–9.

Haycock, G.B. 1993: The influence of sodium on growth in infancy. *Pediatric Nephrology* **7**, 871–5.

Henning, P., Tomlinson, L., Rigden, S.P.A., Haycock, G.B. and Chantler, C. 1988: Long term outcome of treatment of end stage renal failure. *Archives of Disease in Childhood* **63**, 35–40.

Hostetter, T.H., Oslon, J.L., Rennke, H.G., Venkatachalam, M.A. and Brenner, B.M. 1981: Hyperfiltration of remnant nephrons: a potentially adverse response to renal ablation. *American Journal of Physiology* **241**, F85–93.

Johnson, R.J. 1994: The glomerular response to injury: progression or resolution? *Kidney International* **45**, 1769–82.

July, U.M., Turney, J.H. 1990: Post-traumatic acute renal failure, 1956–1988. *Clinical Nephrology* **34**, 79–83.

Kaufman, J.M., DiMeola, H.J., Siegel, N.J., Lytton, B., Kashgarian, M. and Hayslett, J.P. 1974: Compensatory adaptation of structure and function following progressive renal ablation. *Kidney International* **6**, 10–17.

Kist-van Holthe tot Echten, J.E., Nauta, J., Hop, W.C.J. *et al.* 1993: Protein restriction in chronic renal failure. *Archives of Disease in Childhood* **68**, 371–5.

Klahr, S., Levey, A.S., Beck, G.J. *et al.* for the Modification of Diet in Renal Disease Study Group 1994: The effects of dietary protein restriction and blood pressure control on the progression of chronic renal failure. *New England Journal of Medicine* **330**, 877–84.

Kleanthous, H., Smith, H.R., Scotland, S.M. *et al.* 1990: Haemolytic uraemic syndromes in the British Isles, 1985–8: association with verocytotoxin producing *Escherichia coli*. Part 2: microbiological aspects. *Archives of Disease in Childhood* **65**, 722–7.

Kohaut, B.C. and Tejani, A. 1996: The 1994 Annual Report of the North American Pediatric Renal Transplant Co-operative Study. *Pediatric Nephrology* **10**, 422–34.

Loirat, C., Ehrich, J.H.H., Geerlings, W. *et al.* 1994: Report on management of renal failure in children in Europe, XXIII, 1992. *Nephrology, Dialysis, Transplantation* **11** Suppl. 1, 26–40.

Milford, D.V. and Taylor, C.M. 1990: New insights into the haemolytic uraemic syndromes. *Archives of Disease in Childhood* **65**, 713–15.

Milford, D.V., Taylor, C.M., Guttridge, B., Hall, S.M., Rowe, B. and Kleanthous, H. 1990: Haemolytic uraemic syndromes in the British Isles 1985–8: association with verocytotoxin producing *Escherichia coli*. Part 1: clinical and epidemiological aspects. *Archives of Disease in Childhood* **65**, 716–21.

Miller, T.R., Anderson, R.J., Linas, S.L. *et al.* 1978: Urinary diagnostic indices in acute renal failure: a prospective study. *Annals of Internal Medicine* **89**, 47–50.

Mocan, H., Beattie, T.J. and Murphy, A.V. 1991: Renal venous thrombosis in infancy: long term follow-up. *Pediatric Nephrology* **5**, 45–49.

Modi, K.S., O'Donnell, M.P. and Keane, W.F. 1993: Dietary interventions for progressive renal disease in experimental animal models. In El Najas, A. M., Anderson, S. and Mallick, N.P. (eds), *Prevention of progressive chronic renal failure*, vol. 1, Oxford: Oxford University Press, 117–72.

Moorhead, J.F., El Nahas, A.M., Chan, M.K. and Varghese, Z. 1982: Lipid nephrotoxicity in chronic progressive glomerular and tubulo-interstitial disease. *Lancet* **ii**, 1309–12.

Murdoch, I.A., Dos Anos, R., and Haycock, G.B. 1991: Treatment of hyperkalaemia with intravenous salbutamol. *Archives of Disease in Childhood* **66**, 527–8.

Nevard, C.H.F. and Rigden, S.P.A. 1995: Haemofiltration in paediatric practice. *Current Paediatrics* **5**, 14–16.

Niaudet, P., Maher, H. I., Gagnadoux, M.F. and Broyer, M. 1985: Outcome of children with acute renal failure. *Kidney International* **28**, S148–51.

Offner, G., Aschendorff, C., Hoyer, P.F. *et al.* 1988: End stage renal failure: 14 years experience of dialysis and transplantation. *Archives of Disease in Childhood* **63**, 120–6.

Orejas, G., Santos, F., Malaga, C., Rey, C., Cobo, A. and Simmarro M. 1995: Nutritional status of children with moderate chronic renal failure. *Pediatric Nephrology* **9**, 52–6.

Rees, L., Rigden, S.P.A., Chantler, C. and Haycock, G.B. 1989: Growth and methods of improving growth in chronic renal failure managed conservatively. In Scharer, K. (ed.), *Growth and endocrine changes in children and adolescents with chronic renal failure. Pediatric and adolescent endocrinology*, vol. 20. Basel: Karger, 15–26.

Report of a Working Party of the British Association for Paediatric Nephrology 1995: The provision of services in the United Kingdom for children and adolescents with renal disease. London: British Paediatric Association.

Report of the Second Task Force on Blood Pressure Control in Children 1987: *Pediatrics* **79**, 1–25.

Reynolds, J.M., Garralda, M.E., Postlethwaite, R.J. and Goh, D. 1991: Changes in psychosocial adjustment after renal transplantation. *Archives of Disease in Childhood* **66**, 508–13.

Rigden, S.P.A. 1996a: The treatment of renal osteodystrophy. *Pediatric Nephrology* **10**, 653–5.

Rigden, S.P.A. 1996b: Pre-emptive kidney transplantation. *Pediatric Nephrology* **10**, C44.

Rigden, S.P.A., Montini, G., Morris, M., Clark, K.G.A., Haycock, G.B., Chantler, C. and Hill, R.C. 1990: Recombinant human erythropoietin therapy in children maintained by haemodialysis. *Pediatric Nephrology* **4**, 618–22.

Risdon, R.A., Sloper, J.C. and Wardener, H.E. de 1968: Relationship between renal function and histological changes found in renal biopsy specimens from patients with persistent glomerular nephritis. *Lancet* **i**, 363–6.

Safirstein, R., Winston, J., Goldstein, M., Moel, D., Dikman, S. and Guttenplan, J. 1986: Cisplatin nephrotoxicity. *American Journal of Kidney Diseases* **8**, 356–67.

Salusky, I.B. and Goodman, W.G. 1996: The management of renal osteodystrophy. *Pediatric Nephrology* **10**, 651–3.

Scott, J.E.S. and Renwick, M. 1991: Antenatal diagnosis of congenital abnormalities of the urinary tract. *British Journal of Urology* **62**, 295–300.

Stapleton, F.B., Jones, D.P. and Green, R.S. 1987: Acute renal failure in neonates: incidence, etiology, and outcome. *Pediatric Nephrology* **1**, 314–20.

Uauy, R.D., Hogg, R.J., Brewer, E.D., Reisch, J.S., Cunningham, C. and Holliday, M.A. 1994: Dietary protein and growth in infants with chronic renal insufficiency: a report from the Southwest Pediatric Nephrology Study Group and the University of California, San Francisco. *Pediatric Nephrology* **8**, 45–50.

Valderrabano, F., Jones, E.H.P. and Mallick, N.P. 1995: Report on management of renal failure in Europe, XXIV, 1993. *Nephrology, Dialysis, Transplantation* **10** (Suppl. 5), 1–25.

Warshaw, B.L., Hyme, L.C., Trulock, T.S. and Woodard, J.R. 1985: Prognostic features in infants with obstructive uropathy due to posterior urethral valves. *Journal of Urology* **133**, 240–3.

Welsh, K.I. 1991: New strategies in immunosuppression. *Pediatric Nephrology* **5**, 622–9.

Wingen, A.M., Fabian-Bach, C. and Mehls, O. 1991: Low-protein diet in children with chronic renal failure – 1-year results. *Pediatric Nephrology* **5**, 496–500.

Wong, A.F., Bolinger, A.M. and Gambertoglio, J.G. 1994: Pharmacokinetics and drug dosing in children with decreased renal function. In: Holliday, M.A., Barratt, T.M. and Avner, E.D. (eds), *Pediatric nephrology*, 3rd ed. Baltimore, MD: Williams & Wilkins, 1305–13.

Further reading

Brady, H.R. and Singer, G.G. 1995: Acute renal failure. *Lancet* **346**, 1533–40.

Siegel, N.J., Van Why, S.K., Boydstun, I.I., Devarajan, P. and Gaudico, K.M. 1994: Acute renal failure. In: Holliday, M.A., Barratt, T.M. and Avner, E.D. (ed). *Pediatric nephrology*, 3rd ed. Baltimore, MD: Williams & Wilkins, 1176–203.

CHAPTER 51

Renal failure and growth

P.R. BETTS

Introduction
Growth in normal children
Growth measurement
Skeletal maturation
Puberty
Growth problems in infants with renal disease
Mid-childhood renal failure

Factors responsible for growth failure
Major hormonal influences on growth in chronic renal failure
Psychosocial disturbances and resulting short stature
Opportunities to improve growth in chronic renal failure
References

Introduction

The earliest recording of short stature as a recognized consequence of chronic renal insufficiency occurring during childhood was probably made by Guthrie in 1897 when he described seven children with renal failure as 'being stunted, undersized and wizened in appearance'. Sir William Gull, 25 years earlier, reported the occurrence of chronic renal failure as a cause of death in a child, commenting upon the extreme rarity of this diagnosis at that time. Growth retardation a century ago, therefore, had been linked with chronic renal failure. Later, poor appetite, osteodystrophy and delayed puberty were recognized as associated features. The possibility of preventing short stature in this condition received little attention until the 1960s, probably because no direct treatment for these children was available and death usually occurred before or during adolescence.

Rizzoni *et al.* (1985) reported that approximately 50% of adults who developed end-stage renal disease requiring dialysis or transplantation below the age of 15 years had a final height less than the third centile. Consequently, with the advent of modern treatment and long-term survival, short stature has become a major concern to parents and children alike (Reynolds *et al.*, 1995). It has been recognized for a long time that the shortest children and adults are often those whose pathology presented in the first year of life, and it is these young people who are a great challenge to the team responsible for their medical care with the aim of prevention of this growth failure.

Congenital disorders of the urinary tract and reflux nephropathy are the most common causes of renal insufficiency in infancy. These conditions frequently present to paediatric physicians and surgeons alike and it is important that the possibility of growth failure is recognized and height and weight are regularly checked during their initial management. As will be shown, a fall across the centiles in infancy may have irreversible long-term consequences for final height.

Growth in normal children

Examination of the growth pattern of a normal child demonstrates that there is a very rapid period of growth in the first few months of life and into the second year. Growth then slows down through the mid-childhood years only to accelerate again with the pubertal growth spurt (Fig. 51.1) (Tanner *et al.* 1966). The fuel for this growth is energy intake, which is divided among basal metabolic rate, physical activity and then growth. The

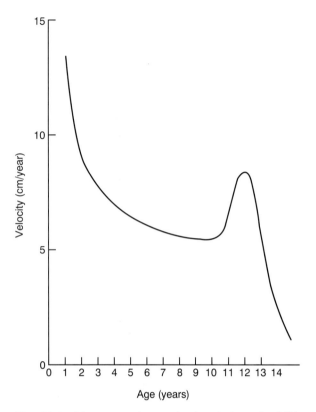

Fig. 51.1 Mean growth rate (cm/year) through childhood (adapted from Tanner *et al.*, 1966).

greatest proportion of this goes to growth in the early months of life and consequently a significant reduction in energy intake during this period, for one reason or another, may cause growth retardation and a permanent effect on later adult height (Holliday, 1975).

It should be remembered that half adult stature is reached by the age of 2 years, emphasizing the importance of growth in infancy. This period of rapid growth is traditionally stated to be mainly related to nutrition, with little hormonal input. The period of growth from infancy until the onset of the pubertal growth spurt is then described as being predominantly dependent on growth hormone. During this period growth velocity slowly reduces until the onset of puberty when there is a further rapid acceleration in response to an increase in growth hormone production and sex hormone stimulation. However, children with delayed puberty continue to exhibit a fall in velocity until, through hormonal stimulation, the physiological changes of puberty occur and growth velocity increases, albeit later.

In conclusion, therefore, the growth of the healthy child is a regular process which is carefully controlled. A child tends to grow along a set channel or trajectory which is determined by genetic constitution and modified by environmental factors. Illness or severe undernutrition may cause a fall-off in growth rate, which would

normally be counteracted after the illness by a period of increased growth velocity or catch up-growth. (Prader *et al.*, 1963). In the period of rapid growth in early life, the more prolonged the insult leading to growth retardation, the more difficult it is for catch-up growth completely to restore the child back to that preset channel and a permanent reduction in the child's growth potential may result (Widdowson and McCance, 1975).

Growth measurement

One of the hallmarks of good clinical care in chronic illness is regular and reliable measurements of height, or length according to the age of the child, and weight from birth. There is no excuse for these measurements not being available and an up-to-date growth chart being kept. Using these data, early fall-off in growth velocity or weight can easily be identified and its cause investigated and treated where appropriate. Routine measurement of all normal children should be made from birth, with height recordings at 18 months, 3 years and preschool, around 4.5 years. All children with illness should be, in addition, measured at each point of health contact up to four times per year, especially during the rapid period of growth in infancy.

LENGTH MEASUREMENTS

Length is measured up to the age of 18 months or when the child can stand. This should be measured in the supine position by two people (Doull *et al.*, 1995). Ill babies, even when in an incubator, can be measured with a Pedobaby 2 and for the larger baby the Raven Kiddimetre may be used. The equipment for measurement of height, length or weight is not expensive and should be available on all units (Child Growth Foundation, London).

HEIGHT MEASUREMENTS

Height measurements should be taken at each hospital attendance using a Harpenden Stadiometer or the cheaper Minimetre, Magnimetre or Leicester Height Measurer (Child Growth Foundation). Height may be measured from the age of 18 months or from whenever the child can stand.

The ratio of weight to height may be useful, as this is independent of age. There is a good correlation of the weight-to-height ratio and cell mass (Jones *et al*, 1982). A falling ratio is an indication for aggressive intervention.

RELIABILITY OF MEASUREMENTS

Reliable measurements may be made of length and height from birth (Doull *et al.*, 1995). The observer must

Table 51.1 Standard deviation of single length or height measurement in normal children at different ages

Age group and measurement	Standard deviation of single measurement (cm)
Newborn length	0.28
6-week length	0.42
8-month length	0.42
19–23-month height	0.55
3-year height	0.23
4–11-year height	0.23

be trained and the instrument regularly checked for its correct reading. The same observer should preferably be used for each measurement. Errors in calibration of the instrument are well recognized and avoidable (Voss *et al.*, 1990). The reproduceability decreases with different measurers. The standard deviation of a single height measurement at different ages, taken by an experienced measurer, is shown in Table 51.1. The significance of this is shown in Fig. 51.2, emphasizing how readily poor growth may be identified outside these limits.

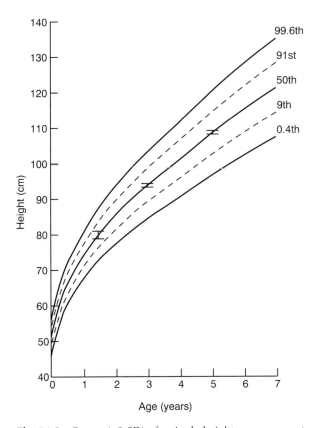

Fig. 51.2 Range (±2 SD) of a single height measurement when plotted on a centile chart in early childhood.

GROWTH CHARTS

UK cross-sectional growth charts were updated in 1994 and should now be routinely used (Fig. 51.3) (Freeman *et al.*, 1995). The previous charts of Tanner *et al.* (1966) were derived from data obtained in the 1950s and, with the secular trend in growth that has occurred in the intervening period, these charts are now outdated. The difference in absolute centiles is small; however, the new charts have an additional advantage that the different centile lines are spaced at 0.67 of a standard deviation apart and range from 99.6th centile to the 0.4th centile.

Frequent height and weight plots should be recorded to demonstrate the pattern of growth. Normal children maintain a very steady growth channel. Regular measurements will easily demonstrate a fall across the centiles indicating the need for appropriate investigation.

HEIGHT VELOCITY

Traditionally, height velocity has been calculated, but because of the error of each measurement its value has been recently questioned (Voss *et al.*, 1991). This is particularly so for any two measurements taken less than 12 months apart. Frequent plots on a growth chart are of more clinical value than assessment of growth velocity over the same period. The fastest growth velocity is in infancy.

For data collection deviation of height from the normal can be expressed for males and females as standard deviation scores (SDS) from the formula (Tanner *et al.*, 1971):

$$SDS = \frac{present\ height\ (cm) - mean\ height\ for\ age\ (cm)}{SD\ of\ height\ for\ age}.$$

Skeletal maturation

Bone age as an assessment of skeletal maturation should be examined from a radiograph of the left hand using the method of Tanner *et al.* (1975) or Greulich and Pyle (1959). In chronic renal failure there may be difficulty in interpretation of maturation because of renal osteodystrophy, osteoporosis, or both. A significant delay in bone age for chronological age demonstrates the potential capability for catch-up growth.

Puberty

Pubertal staging should be recorded using the categorization of Tanner (1962) and testicular volume assessed using an orchidometer.

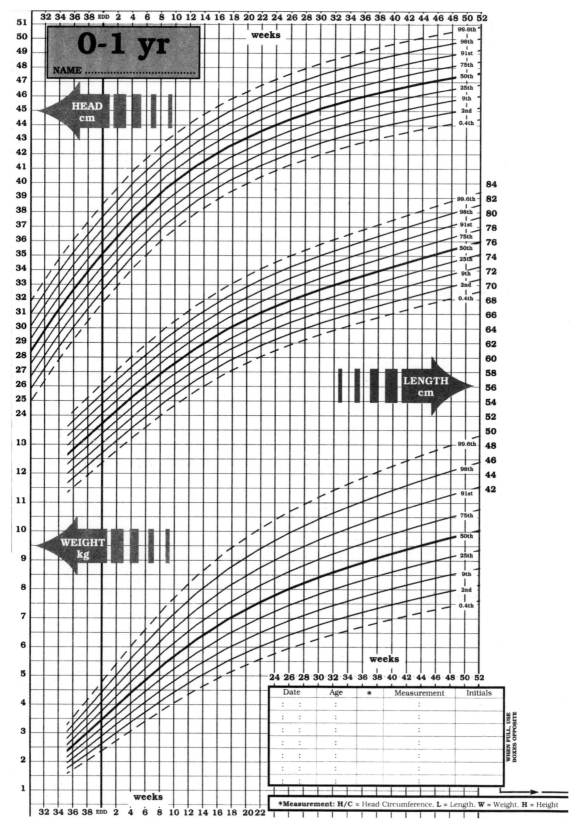

Fig. 51.3 The new UK growth charts. (Reproduced with the consent of The Child Growth Foundation, London.)

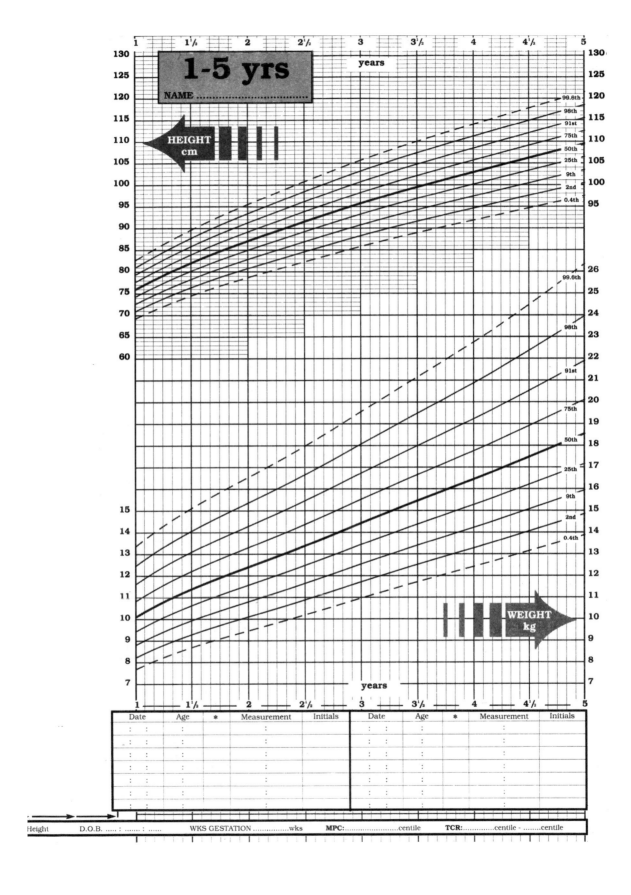

Growth problems in infants with renal disease

The pattern of growth in young people with chronic renal failure is variable and depends on the degree of impairment, the age of onset, the pattern of management and the effects of treatment itself. A significant proportion of infants with congenital renal disease are small at the time of presentation (Rees *et al.,* 1989). The typical picture of post-natal growth in chronic renal failure is shown in Fig. 51.4 (Betts and McGrath, 1974). Here it is recognized that growth failure may occur in infancy with a fall across the centiles. After this, growth is normally parallel, but below the expected centiles through the mid-childhood years, only to fall again at puberty, with the consequence of further reduction in adult height potential.

Congenital renal dysplasia and hypoplasia with or without urinary tract obstruction are the most common causes of end-stage renal disease in the first five years of life (Betts and McGrath, 1974). A gradual decline in glomerular filtration rate and tubular function occurs from birth. As 30% of poststatural growth occurs in the first 2 years of life and at the age of 2 years the child is half its adult height, any disturbance of growth in infancy will have a major effect on final height. This will be compounded if there are subsequent factors through childhood that inhibit catch-up growth.

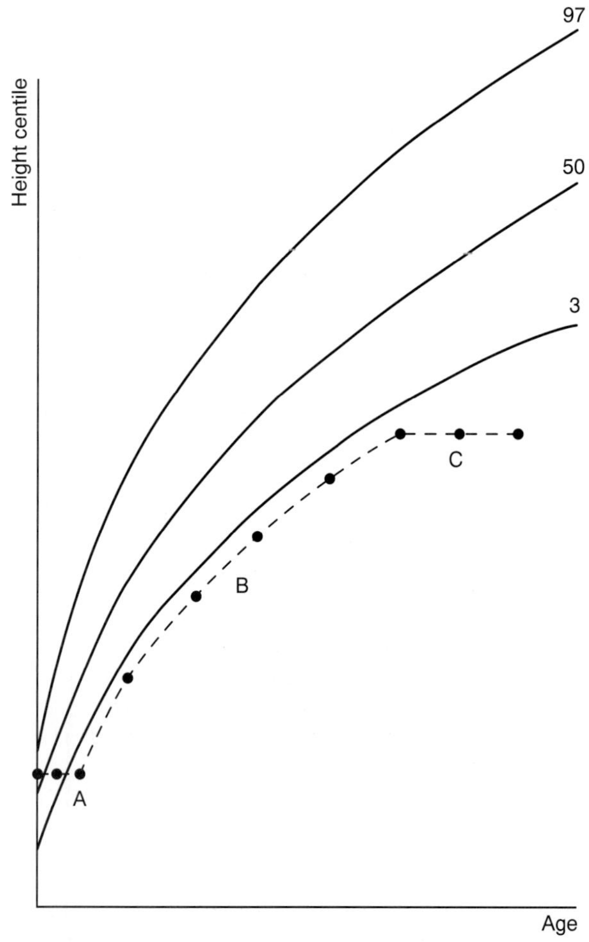

The major contributing factors to growth retardation in chronic renal failure are:

- recurrent vomiting and reduced dietary intake
- insufficient energy and protein intake
- water and electrolyte inbalance
- acidosis
- recurrent infections, especially urinary tract infections
- hyperparathyroidism and osteodystrophy.

Improved understanding of these factors has led to more effective management. It is encouraging to know that catch-up growth, even in severe renal failure, is possible, particularly in infancy (Rees *et al.*, 1989).

Mid-childhood renal failure

During the mid-childhood years, growth is usually parallel to the centiles unless renal function severely deteriorates or there is systemic illness. Treatment with growth hormone during this period has been shown to promote significant catch-up growth (Fig. 51.5) (Fine *et al.*, 1994).

GROWTH IN PUBERTY

Many young people with chronic renal insufficiency enter puberty late and two-thirds have a height below the third centile (Scharer *et al.*, 1976). Growth stops at the end of puberty and it is difficult at this stage to find ways to facilitate catch-up growth which would lead to an improvement in final adult height. The potential for significant catch-up growth diminishes the closer the patient is to full skeletal maturity.

Normally, growth velocity slows prior to the pubertal growth spurt, but remains above 3.5–4 cm/year. Boys then have an incremental gain of approximately 25 cm whilst girls grow an additional 20 cm (Buckler, 1990). In chronic renal failure growth may slow more dramatically and the pubertal spurt itself may be diminished by up to 50% of that expected (Schaefer *et al.,* 1976). The reduction in final height in these young people, therefore, is due to the reduced growth velocity in the years waiting for puberty to commence, combined with a decreased duration of the growth spurt itself.

Fig. 51.4   Schematic representation of the growth of children with renal insufficiency dating from infancy. A, B and C represent periods of growth.

FINAL ADULT HEIGHT

The consequences to growth of the factors mentioned above are demonstrated in the data from the European Dialysis and Transplant Association (Rizzoni *et al.*, 1985), which show that 50% of young people who had end-stage renal failure and were dialysed or transplanted below the age of 15 years had a reduction in adult height to below the 3rd percentile. Owing to a different pattern of pathology, boys develop renal failure earlier than girls, resulting in an earlier fall-off in growth velocity and a more stunted final height.

Factors responsible for growth failure

NUTRITION

An appropriate intake of calories and nutrients is essential for normal growth and in renal failure the frequent occurrence of anorexia interferes with this. Outside infancy there has to be a significant reduction in energy intake (Ashworth, 1978; Claris *et al.*, 1989) to less than 80% of recommended daily allowance (RDA) for growth failure to result, where RDA is defined as an

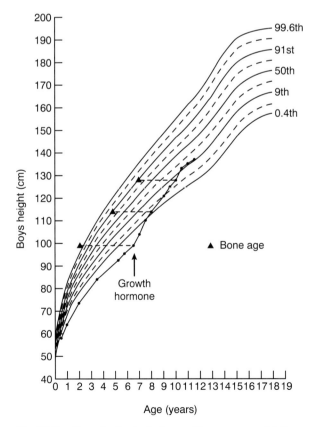

Fig. 51.5 Growth chart of a boy with severe renal failure treated with additional growth hormone therapy.

intake 'sufficient or more than sufficient for the nutritional needs of practically all healthy people in a population' (Department of Health and Social Security, 1968). The term RDA has been retained in this chapter because it has been used in previous publications. The reader should note that the terminology has now changed (Department of Health, 1991).

Intake relative to RDA needs to be tailored to individual children and those with low weight-to-height ratios may need an intake of up to 120% of RDA. As children with renal failure are small, height age rather than chronological age is used as the reference point. It also appears likely that the ratio of energy to protein intake is an important factor in the dietary management of these patients with renal failure.

Infancy appears to be the period most vulnerable to inadequate nutrition. At this time fluid balance is critical as renal tubular damage results in polyuria with large volumes of intake necessary to make up for renal loss. This high fluid intake, which is often low in calories, inhibits appropriate energy intake unless calorie supplementation is given.

Recently, more aggressive feeding methods have been recommended to promote catch-up growth in infants, with feeds being given via fine-bore nasogastric tubes or a gastrostomy (Rees *et al.*, 1988, 1989; Brocklebank and Wolfe, 1993).

Outside infancy energy intake over 80% of RDA. is usually associated with normal growth but disappointingly, higher intakes rarely promote catch-up growth (Betts and McGrath, 1974; Kleinknecht *et al.*, 1983). It has also been shown that moderate protein restriction does not impair growth so long as energy intake remains above 80% of RDA (Wingen *et al.*, 1992).

It would appear, therefore, that so long as energy intake remains near recommended levels, outside infancy nutrition does not play an important role in the growth of these children.

ELECTROLYTE–WATER IMBALANCE

Infants with congenital renal disease have reduced tubular function and as a consequence frequently exhibit polyuria leading to fluid and electrolyte imbalance. This is particularly so with obstructive uropathy and renal hypoplasia. Growth failure occurs in the animal model with salt depletion (Wassner, 1991). An increased fluid input is essential in these infants, together with appropriate electrolyte supplementation to ensure normal growth.

ACIDOSIS

Metabolic acidosis is to be expected in severe renal failure. Those children with severe acidosis due to tubular dysfunction have the poorest growth (West and Smith, 1956). Alkali in the form of supplementary bicarbonate is essential to promote normal growth.

ANAEMIA

Although anaemia is frequently mentioned as a factor that may impair growth, there have been no good studies to demonstrate that correction with erythropoietin will necessarily result in catch-up growth.

RENAL OSTEODYSTROPHY

Severe osteodystrophy with rickets used to be recognized as a regular association of renal failure and resulted in growth retardation. In this situation there was often skeletal deformity. Today, treatment with vitamin D metabolites, the monitoring and control of phosphate intake and the use of phosphate binders, should prevent osteodystrophy severe enough to cause growth retardation.

Major hormonal influences on growth in chronic renal failure

Major changes in many hormone profiles have been demonstrated in chronic renal failure. Such changes mainly reflect alterations in binding proteins and metabolic clearance. Increased levels of insulin, glucagon, parathormone, leutinizing hormone (LH) and follicular stimulating hormone have been recorded, whilst there is a decrease in erythropoetin, vitamin D, testosterone and oestrogens, together with insulin-like growth factor-1 (IGF-1) (Schaefer and Mehls, 1994). The relative importance of these changes on growth remains unclear; however, one of the most exciting areas is the possible growth accleration induced by additional growth hormone therapy (Fine *et al.*, 1994).

GROWTH HORMONE/IGF-1 AXIS

The normal growth hormone IGF-1 pathway is well described, with growth hormone itself being released by the pituitary and simulating both local and hepatic production of IGF-1. The latter is bound to circulating proteins and in particular IGF-BP3. Both growth hormone and free IGF-1 stimulate growth. Various studies have shown that in renal failure there is a physiological resistance to growth hormone with correspondingly raised plasma levels. This is probably due to abnormal hypothalamic/pituitary regulation (West and Smith, 1956).

In renal failure the bioassayable IGF-1 is low (Schwalbe *et al.*, 1977), although when measured immunologically the levels have been reported as normal. In addition circulating binding proteins are high. It is suggested that although growth hormone levels are elevated there is a reduction in receptor activity which leads to the reduction in IGF-1 and the increase in binding proteins. This leads in itself to a further lowering of free IGF-l activity. It is the increased levels of the binding protein that reduce the bioavailability of the IGFs (Mehls *et al.*, 1990).

PITUITARY GONADAL AXIS

In male adults with renal failure it is well recognized that there may be a reduction in testicular hormonal production with reduced circulating testosterone levels, reduced libido and gynaecomastia. In children the effect on gonadal function is predominantly one of delayed puberty. Detailed investigations suggest that despite normal or elevated gonadotrophin levels pulsatile release of LH from the pituitary is decreased (West and Smith, 1956), leading to a reduction in appropriate gonadal stimulation. This affects the pattern of the pubertal growth spurt as it is the activation of the hypothalamic–pituitary–gonadal axis and a transient increase in growth hormone secretion that results in the acceleration of growth during puberty. In pubertal patients with chronic renal failure, therefore, the delay in hormonal secretion, together with end-organ hyposensitivity to growth hormone, leads to a reduction in the amplitude and duration of the growth spurt.

Psychosocial disturbances and resulting short stature

Psychosocial disturbances may affect the growth of normal children. In chronic renal failure and its associated management psychological support may be needed. Growth failure in these children possibly may occur secondary to poor appetite associated with mood disurbances or an alteration in the hypothalamic–pituitary axis.

Opportunities to improve growth in chronic renal failure

Growth in children with renal insufficiency requires a team approach for its management from the paediatric surgeon, nephrologist, endocrinologist, dietician and specialist nurse.

AUXOLOGY

The early recognition of a fall-off in growth velocity is essential. All children and babies should, therefore, have regular assessment of their weight and length at each visit or admission to hospital. Height should be measured after 18 months of age or when the child can stand. These measurements must be plotted on the appropriate growth chart, from which early recognition of any growth reduction will be identified.

It should be remembered that whilst growth is likely to fall off with a glomerular filtration rate (GFR) below 25 ml/min/1.73 m^2 it may occur with any degree of renal impairment, particularly in infants.

DIETARY INTAKE

The importance of close collaborative work with a paediatric dietician with experience in renal disease cannot be overemphasized. This is particularly so in infants and toddlers. A wide variety of feeds are available, and it may be necessary to take a number of problems into consideration, e.g. fluid balance and the need for phosphate or potassium restriction.

It is essential to maximize energy intake to above 80% of RDA and to assess the level of consumed protein, although the latter makes far less contribution to growth in the presence of an adequate calorie intake. In infants it may be necessary to add calories or supplements to the diet, or to institute tube feeding to ensure sufficient intake. Following the assessment of intake, appropriate supplementation with vitamins and minerals may be necessary.

Water balance, correction of acidosis and monitoring of tubular salt loss is of vital importance. The use of phosphate binders and one hydroxylated vitamin D, combined if necessary with phosphate restriction, is usually required to manage or prevent the development of renal osteodystrophy.

In the mid-childhood period, although it is believed that poor nutrition is not such a major cause of growth retardation, it is important to assess regularly calorie and protein intake. A severe reduction may impair growth and supplementation would be necessary in these circumstances.

GROWTH PROMOTION

In recent years recombinant growth hormone has been used to stimulate an increased growth velocity during the childhood years of growth. Short normal children increase growth velocity on commencement of growth hormone therapy. Whether final height is increased is still to be determined, but certainly there is a significant increase in height by entry into puberty (McCaughey *et al.*, 1994). In chronic renal failure those children with renal disease dating from infancy have often fallen across the centiles and are short compared with their peers at school entry. There is also the expectation that they will have a later reduction in their pubertal growth spurt. Growth hormone has been seen as an opportunity to maximize growth during the prepubertal years and bring these children back to the normal height centiles before the onset of puberty (Fig. 51.5). The dose used is twice that for growth hormone-deficient children and it has been shown to be effective both before and after transplantation (Fine *et al.*, 1991, 1994). Once treatment is started it will need to continue through until final height, otherwise there is the risk of catch-down or growth arrest. As there is concern over its use around the time of renal transplantation, treatment should be started sufficiently early to maximize catch-up growth both prepubertally and pretransplant.

Possible side-effects of growth hormone treatment include glucose intolerance. This may add to the already recognized insulin resistance which may occur in renal failure, although this does not seem to be a significant clinical problem. No other significant side-effects have been identified, but renal function alters on growth hormone therapy and in normal children there is an increase in GFR (Juler *et al.*, 1989). To date there is no evidence of a deterioration in renal function of those children who have been treated.

The growth response to growth hormone treatment may be dramatic and this should be considered for all short children with chronic renal failure once other remedial causes have been excluded.

The pubertal growth spurt, as previously mentioned, may only result in half the expected height gain during this period and it is often delayed. Synthetic androgens and testosterone derivatives are used to induce puberty in normal teenage children and their short-term use in low dosage is safe and brings forward the onset of puberty without a compromise in final height (Stanhope *et al.*, 1988). Whether this will improve the situation in children with renal failure remains to be determined.

References

Ashworth, A. 1978: Energy balance and growth: experience in treating children with malnutrition. *Kidney International* **14**, 301–5.

Betts, P.R. and McGrath, G. 1974: Growth pattern and dietary intake of children with chronic renal insufficiency. *British Medical Journal* **2**, 189–93.

Brocklebank, J.T. and Wolfe, S. 1993: Dietary treatment of renal insufficiency. *Archives of Disease in Childhood* **69**, 704–8.

Buckler, J. 1990: *A longitudinal study of adolescent growth.* London: Springer.

Claris, A.A., Bianchi, M.L., Bini, P. *et al.* 1989: Growth in young children with chronic renal failure. *Pediatric Nephrology* **3**, 301–4.

Department of Health 1991: Report on Health and Social Subjects, 41. *Dietary reference values for food, energy and nutrients for the United Kingdom.* London: HMSO.

Department of Health and Social Security 1968: *Pilot study of nutrition of young children in 1963.* London: HMSO.

Doull, I.J.M., McCaughey, E.S., Bailey, B.J.R. and Betts, P.R. 1995: Reliability of infant length measurement. *Archives of Disease in Childhood* **72**, 520–1.

Fine, R.N., Kohaut, E.C., Brown, D. and Perlman, A.J. for the Genentech Cooperative Study Group 1994: Growth after recombinant human growth hormone treatment in children with chronic renal failure: report of a multicenter randomized double-blind placebo-controlled study. *Journal of Pediatrics* **124**, 374–82.

Fine, R.N., Yadin, O., Nelson, P.A. *et al.* 1991: Recombinant human growth hormone treatment of children following renal transplantation. *Pediatric Nephrology* **5**, 147–51.

Freeman, J.V., Cole, T.J., Chinn, S., Jones, P.R.M., White, E.M., and Preece, M.A. 1995: Cross sectional stature and weight reference curves for the U.K. 1990. *Archives of Disease in Childhood* **73**, 17–24.

Greulich, W.W. and Pyle, S.I. 1959: *A radiographic atlas of skeletal development of hand and wrist*, 2nd ed. California: Stanford University Press.

Gull, W., Sutton, H.G. 1872: Chronic Bright's disease with contracted kidney. *Medico-chirurgical Transactions* **LV**, 273.

Guthrie, L.G. 1897: Chronic interstitial nephritis in childhood. *Lancet* **i**, 585.

Holliday, M.A. 1975: Calorie intake and growth in uraemia. *Kidney International* **7** (Suppl.), 73–8.

Jones, R.W.A., Rigden, S.P., Barratt, T.M. and Chantler, C. 1982: The effects of chronic renal failure in infancy on growth, nutritional status and body composition. *Pediatric Research* **16**, 784–91.

Juler, H.P., Schmid, C., Zapf, J. *et al.* 1989: Effective recombinant insulin-like growth factor 1 on insulin secretion and renal function in normal human subjects. *Proceedings of the National Academy of Sciences of the USA* **86**, 2868–72.

Kleinknecht, C., Broyer, M., Huot, D., Marti, H.C. and Dartois, A.M. 1983: Growth and development of nondialyzed children with chronic renal railure. *Kidney International* **24**, S40–7.

McCaughey, E.S., Mulligan, J., Voss, L.D. and Betts, P.R. 1994: Growth and metabolic consequences of growth hormone treatment in prepubertal short normal children. *Archives of Disease in Childhood* **71**, 201–6.

Mehls, O., Tonshoff, B., Blum, W.F., Heirich, U. and Seidel, C. 1990: Growth hormone and insulin-like factor 1 in chronic renal failure – pathophysiology and rationale for growth hormone treatment. *Acta Pediatrica Scandinavia* **370** (Suppl.), 28–34.

Prader, A., Tanner, J.M. and Von Harnack, G.A. 1963: Catch-up growth following illness or starvation. *Journal of Pediatrics* **62**, 646.

Rees, L., Green, S.A., Adlard, P. *et al.* 1988: Growth and endocrine function after transplantation. *Archives of Disease in Childhood* **63**, 1326–32.

Rees, L., Rigden, S.P.A. and Ward, G.M. 1989: Chronic renal failure and growth. *Archives of Disease in Childhood* **64**, 573–7.

Reynolds, J.M., Wood, A.J., Eminson, D.M. and Postlethwaite, R.J. 1995: Short stature and chronic renal failure: what concerns children and parents? *Archives of Disease in Childhood* **73**, 36–42.

Rizzoni, G., Broyer, M., Brunner, F.P. *et al.* 1985: Combined report on regular dialysis and transplantation of children in Europe. *European Dialysis and Transplant Association* 82–8.

Schaefer, F. and Mehls, O. 1994: Endocrine, metabolic and growth disorders. In Holliday, M.A., Barratt, T.M., Avner, E.D. (eds), *Pediatric nephrology*. London: Williams & Wilkins, 1241–85.

Schaefer, F., Seidel, C., Binding, A. *et al.* 1990: Pubertal growth in chronic renal failure. *Pediatric Research* **28**, 5–10.

Scharer, K, Chantler, C., Brunner, F.P. *et al.* 1976: Combined report on regular dialysis and transplantation of children in Europe 1975. *Proceedings of the European Dialysis and Transplant Association* **13**, 3–103.

Schwalbe, S., Betts, P.R., Rayner, P.H.W. and Rudd, B. 1977: Somatomedin activity in growth disorders and chronic renal insufficiency in children. *British Medical Journal* **i**, 679–82.

Stanhope, R., Buchanan, C.R., Fenn, G.C. and Preece, M.A. 1988: Double blind placebo controlled trial of low dose oxandrolone in the treatment of boys with constitutional delay of growth and puberty. *Archives of Disease in Childhood* **63**, 501–5.

Tanner, J.M. 1962: *Growth at adolescence*. Oxford: Blackwell Scientific.

Tanner, J.M., Whitehouse, R.H., Hughes, P.C.R. and Vince, R.C. 1971: The effects of human growth hormone treatment for 1–7 years on growth of 100 children with growth hormone deficiency, low birthweight, inherited smallness, Turner syndrome and other complaints. *Archives of Disease in Childhood* **46**, 745.

Tanner, J.M., Whitehouse, R.H., Marshall, W.A., Healey, M.J.R. and Goldstein, H. 1975: *Assessment of skeletal maturity and prediction of adult height (TW2 Method)*. London: Academic Press.

Tanner, J.M., Whitehouse, R.M. and Takaishi, M. 1966: Standards from birth to maturity for height, weight, height velocity, weight velocity: British children, 1965. *Archives of Disease in Childhood* **41**, 454, 613.

Voss, L.D., Bailey, B.J.R., Cumming, K., Wilkin, T.J. and Betts, P.R. 1990: The reliability of height measurement (the Wessex Growth Study). *Archives of Disease in Childhood* **65**, 1340–4.

Voss, L.D., Wilkin, T.J., Bailey, B.J.R. and Betts, P.R. 1990: The reliability of height and height velocity in the assessment of growth (the Wessex Growth Study). *Archives of Disease in Childhood* **66**, 833–7.

Wassner, S.J. 1991: The effect of sodium repletion on growth and protein turnover in sodium-depleted rats. *Pediatric Nephrology* **5**, 501–4.

West, C.D. and Smith, W.C. 1956: An attempt to elucidate the cause of growth retardation in renal disease. *American Journal of Disease in Childhood* **91**, 460–5.

Widdowson, E.M. and McCance, R.A. 1975: A review: new thoughts on growth. *Pediatric Research* **9**, 154.

Wingen, A.-M., Fabian-Bach, C. and Mehls, O. 1992: Multicenter randomised study on the effect of a low protein diet on the progression of renal failure in childhood: one year results. *Mineral and Electrolyte Metabolism* **18**, 303–8.

CHAPTER 52

The genetics of congenital urological anomalies

J.D. ATWELL

Introduction
Chromosomal disorders
Syndrome complexes
Renal anomalies
Neoplastic disease

Congenital anomalies of the pelvicalyceal
collecting system (anomalies of the ureteric bud)
Outflow tract anomalies
Summary
References

Introduction

An understanding of the aetiology of a disease is essential if improvements in diagnosis, treatment and, more importantly, prevention are to be achieved. In genitourinary tract anomalies genetic factors probably play a more important role than environmental factors such as maternal age, birth order, season of birth, intrauterine infections, vitamin deficiencies and drugs on the developing fetus. Obstruction within the urinary tract during fetal life may cause renal dysplasia, e.g. multicystic kidney with an atretic pelviureteric junction (PUJ); however, there are many examples of genetically determined renal dysplasia. In others, when the dysplasia is associated with ectopic ureteroceles it raises the question of whether this is due to obstruction from the ureterocele or whether the genetic basis of the inheritance of double ureters and/or dysplasia affects the outcome.

The association of defects has allowed the recognition of syndrome complexes, some of which are known to have an abnormal chromosomal constitution, whilst in others the aetiology remains unknown. The next progressive stage is the identification of genes and, in years to come, gene mapping may determine the future of any individual, excluding accidents.

The following conditions will be discussed:

• chromosomal disorders
• syndrome complexes
• renal anomalies
• neoplastic disease

• congenital anomalies of the collecting system
• outflow anomalies.

Chromosomal disorders

Genitourinary tract anomalies such as horseshoe kidney, renal dysplasia, hypospadias, renal agenesis and duplications of the pelvicalyceal collecting system are commonly found associated with abnormal chromosomes. Two main factors are concerned in the causation of these defects: firstly, the chromosomal defect will affect embryogenesis and, secondly, if there is obstruction within the urinary tract this will have a secondary effect on the developing renal tract. It is possible that this may account for the different phenotypes found in concordant identical twins.

Table 52.1 lists the more common syndromes with a known chromosomal defect and the associated urological defects. Renal and genital anomalies are also found in association with many other chromosomal defects and these are listed in Table 52.2.

Syndrome complexes

A very large number of syndromes have been described but fortunately they are infrequent in surgical practice. The more common syndromes are listed in Table 52.3 with the urological defects found and, if known, the method of inheritance.

Table 52.1 Chromosome syndromes and associated congenital urinary tract anomalies

Chromosome defect	Associated urinary tract anomalies
Turner's syndrome (45 X)	Horseshoe kidney
	Duplex pelvicalyceal system
	PUJ hydronephrosis
Trisomy 21	Unilateral renal agenesis
	PUJ hydronephrosis
	Cystic disease
	Undescended testes
Trisomy 13 (47 XX or XY + 13)	Hydroureter: hydronephrosis
	Duplex pelvicalyceal system
	Polycystic kidneys
Trisomy 18 (47 XX or XY + 18)	Horseshoe kidney: fused kidneys
	Duplex pelvicalyceal system
	Unilateral agenesis
	Undescended testes
	Nephroblastoma
Klinefelter's syndrome (47 XXY)	Undescended testes
XX/XY Mosaicism	Nephroblastoma

Renal anomalies

CYSTIC DISEASE OF THE KIDNEYS

Infantile polycystic disease (Potter type I)

This is inherited as an autosomal recessive condition but it has, owing to clinicopathological findings, been subdivided into perinatal, neonatal, infantile and juvenile groups (Blyth and Ockenden, 1971). There is uniform enlargement of the kidneys, and possibly hypertension and splenomegaly. Pulmonary hypoplasia is a serious complication if there is a history of oligohydramnios. The condition is rare, with an incidence of 0.16 in 1000 live births. The affected patients usually die from renal failure within the first year of life. Renal and lower tract anomalies found in association with infantile polycystic disease include a duplex pelvicalyceal collecting system, horseshoe kidneys, hypospadias and posterior urethral valves.

Adult polycystic disease (Potter type III)

This is inherited as an autosomal dominant gene with high penetrance. The onset of symptoms of loin pain, haematuria, enlargement of the kidneys and hypertension is usually delayed until the third and fourth decades. There is an association with cystic disease of the liver, spleen, lungs, ovaries and uterus. The incidence in the general population is 1 in 4000. An α-globulin locus on the short arm of chromosome 16 has been described.

Occasionally, the adult form of polycystic disease can present in the neonatal period and there may be an association with tuberose sclerosis.

Multicystic kidney: renal dysplasia

Either the whole kidney is dysplastic or it may be segmental. In segmental renal dysplasia the distribution of the dysplasia is directly related to the abnormal opening of the ureter draining that part of the kidney (Ericsson and Ivemark, 1958). In a later study of 107 patients with dysplasia the patients were divided into three groups (Risdon, 1971a, b). In the first group there was an atretic ureter at the PUJ, whereas in the second group the dysplasia was segmental and associated with ectopic ureters, ureteroceles and vesicoureteric reflux (VUR). In the final group there was an outflow tract obstruction such as posterior urethral valves or the prune belly syndrome. There is an association of multicystic kidneys with PUJ hydronephrosis and in one review of 20 patients with a multicystic kidney (Pathak and Williams, 1964) 11 had evidence of a contralateral hydronephrosis. With the advent of prenatal diagnosis similar findings have been observed in the neonatal period.

Renal dysplasia is found in certain autosomal recessive conditions (Zellweger syndrome) and in autosomal dominant conditions (branchio-otorenal dysplasia syndrome and tuberose sclerosis).

Segmental renal dysplasia is associated with double ureters. The upper moiety is involved with ectopic ureters and ectopic ureteroceles whilst lower moiety dysplasia is associated with fetal or intrauterine reflux. A duplex pelvicalyceal collecting system is inherited as an autosomal dominant gene and therefore it is difficult to determine whether the associated dysplasia is primary or secondary.

RENAL AGENESIS

The agenesis may be unilateral or bilateral. In some patients there are remnants of the ureter on the affected side whilst in others the ureter is absent and there is a hemitrigone. Despite these clinical variations different types may occur in the same family (Crawfurd, 1980).

Bilateral renal agenesis

This condition usually arises sporadically, with an incidence of 1 in 3000 live births. The condition is recognized by the features of flattened faces, low-set ears, epicanthus and pulmonary hypoplasia. The condition is incompatible with life, the patients dying early in the neonatal period from either pulmonary hypoplasia or renal failure.

In a report of seven monozygotic twins, two were partially and two fully concordant (Crawfurd, 1980). Familial cases occur, and in another study seven of 199 siblings were affected (Carter *et al.*, 1979).

Table 52.2 Defects of individual chromosomes and associated congenital urinary tract anomalies

Chromosome defect	Associated urinary tract anomalies
Chromosome 1	Horseshoe kidney
	Renal hypoplasia
	Urethral stenosis
Chromosome 3	Polycystic kidneys
	Duplex collecting system
	Hydronephrosis
	Undescended testes
Chromosome 4	Hypospadias
	Undescended testes
	Unilateral bilateral renal agenesis
	Horseshoe kidney
	Renal dysplasia
Chromosome 5	Hypospadias
	Undescended testes
	Horseshoe kidney
	Hypoplasia
	Renal agenesis
Chromosome 6	Renal hypoplasia
Chromosome 7	Unilateral and bilateral renal agenesis
	Polycystic kidneys
	Undescended testes
	Hypospadias
	Vesico-ureteric reflux
Chromosome 8	Undescended testes
	Renal agenesis: unilateral
	Nephroblastoma
Chromosome 9	Undescended testes
	Micropenis
	Renal hypoplasia
	Renal dysplasia
Chromosome 10	Renal dysplasia: agenesis
	Renal cysts
	Undescended testes
Chromosome 11	Micropenis
	Renal agenesis
	Hypospadias
	Undescended testes
	Duplex pelvicalyceal system
	Nephroblastoma
	Renal hypoplasia: dysplasia
	Duplex pelvicalyceal system
	Renal ectopia
Chromosome 12	Micropenis
	Undescended testes
Chromosome 13	Hypospadias
	Epispadias
	Undescended testes
	Renal hypoplasia
Chromosome 14	Renal agenesis: unilateral
	Undescended testes
	Micropenis
	Hypospadias

(*Continued overleaf*)

Table 52.2 (Continued)

Chromosome defect	Associated urinary tract anomalies
Chromosome 15	Undescended testes
Chromosome 16	Undescended testes
	Micropenis
Chromosome 17	Undescended testes
	Renal hypospasia: dysplasia
	Polycystic kidneys
	Renal agenesis
	Megaureters
Chromosome 18	Micropenis
	Undescended testes
	Renal agenesis: unilateral
Chromosome 19	Hypospadias
	Multicystic kidney
	Renal ectopia
Chromosome 21	Hypospadias
	Undescended testes
	Renal agenesis: unilateral
	Duplex pelvicalyceal system
Chromosome 22	Micropenis
	Renal agenesis: unilateral

Unilateral renal agenesis

This is a more frequent finding either in isolation or associated with other urological anomalies. The author has personally treated 13 patients with VUR to a solitary kidney and six patients with PUJ hydronephrosis affecting a solitary kidney. VUR and PUJ hydronephrosis have a genetic factor in their aetiology, suggesting that a similar situation may be relevant in the aetiology of unilateral renal agenesis.

This genetic basis for unilateral renal agenesis was first suggested by Holmes (1972) and later it was argued that as unilateral renal agenesis was found in the same families as bilateral renal agenesis, the method of inheritance was by an autosomal gene of variable penetrance (Fitch, 1977; Shokeir, 1978). A subsequent investigation of first-degree relatives by ultrasonography was carried out in 41 index patients with bilateral renal agenesis and unilateral renal agenesis was found in five of 111 (Roodhooft *et al.*, 1984). The incidence in 682 normal controls was 0.3%. Such observations support a multifactorial form of inheritance.

Unilateral renal agenesis is often found in association with syndrome complexes and chromosomal disorders (Tables 52.1 and 52.2).

HORSESHOE (FUSED) KIDNEYS: RENAL ECTOPIA

There is a relationship between fused kidneys and renal ectopia, as monozygotic twins have been reported, one with a horseshoe kidney and one with crossed renal ectopia (Bridge, 1960). There is also a relationship among renal ectopia, severe grade IV VUR and renal agenesis, as the author has operated on two patients with VUR to a solitary pelvic kidney. In patients with vertebral anomalies such as spina bifida there is an increased incidence of fused kidneys and in a personal series of 96 patients with spina bifida three had a horseshoe kidney, three renal ectopia and two crossed renal ectopia.

Other examples of families with multiple renal anomalies include a mother with a right double ureter, a daughter with left renal agenesis and a son with a horseshoe kidney (Perlman *et al.*, 1976). In another family a father had adult polycystic kidneys and his son had a horseshoe kidney (George, 1981). One family has been reported with familial horseshoe kidneys, a brother and his two sisters being similarly affected.

No prospective family survey of index patients with a horseshoe kidney has been undertaken in order to elucidate the method of inheritance but the reported cases support the concept of a genetic interrelationship between congenital anomalies of the urinary tract.

Neoplastic disease

NEPHROBLASTOMATOSIS

Microscopic nodules of primitive metanephric tissue are found beneath the renal capsule in infants under 4 months of age. The disease may be diffuse or nodular

Table 52.3 Clinical syndromes and associated urological anomalies and known methods of inheritance

Syndrome	Associated urological anomaly	Method of inheritance
Prune belly	Hydronephrosis	Seen in identical twins
	Urethral stenosis	
	Undescended testes	
Meckels	Polycystic kidneys	Autosomal recessive
Tuberose sclerosis	Renal cysts	Autosomal dominant
Ehlers–Danlos	PUJ hydronephrosis	
	Polycystic kidneys	
	Hypoplastic renal artery	
Rubenstein–Taybi	Undescended testes	
	Duplex pelvicalyceal system	
	Hypospadias	
	Posterior urethral valves	
Beckwith–Wiedmann	Renal medullary dysplasia	Autosomal dominant
	Nephroblastoma	
	Renal ectopia	
	Hypospadias	
Facio-cardio-renal	Horseshoe kidney	Autosomal recessive
Silver–Russell	PUJ hydronephrosis	
	Vesico-ureteric reflux	

and in the majority of patients regression occurs with advancing age. These lesions may be a precursor of a nephroblastoma and evidence of their presence is found in up to 50% of nephroblastomas and in almost all patients with bilateral nephroblastoma (Machin and McCaughey, 1984).

NEPHROBLASTOMA

This is the second most common solid tumour of childhood, with an incidence of 1 in 10 000 live births (Cochran and Froggat, 1967). Bilateral occurrence is found in 4%. There are well-known associations with nephroblastoma which include aniridia, hemihypertrophy, horseshoe kidney, a duplex pelvicalyceal collecting system and the Wiedemann–Beckwith syndrome. The incidence of hypospadias and undescended testes is also increased.

The triad of aniridia, genitourinary tract anomalies and nephroblastoma is due to a chromosomal anomaly with deletion of part of the short arm of chromosome 11 and always includes band 11p 13 (Ricardi *et al.*, 1978; Francke *et al.*, 1978, 1979).

There are also reports of the familial nature of nephroblastoma with the occurrence in twin boys (Draper *et al.*, 1977) and in successive generations (Fitzgerald and Hardin, 1955; Strom, 1957). In a review of 58 familial cases (Knudson and Strong, 1972) tumours were found to develop at an earlier age and the incidence of bilateral tumours increased. Despite these familial examples the majority of nephroblastomas arise sporadically.

Congenital anomalies of the pelvicalyceal collecting system (anomalies of the ureter bud)

DUPLEX PELVICALYCEAL COLLECTING SYSTEM

In 1956 a family with a mother and two daughters with bifid or double ureters was reported by Girsch and Karpinski; who suggested that first-degree relatives of a patient with duplication of the upper tract should be investigated by intravenous pyelography. Two groups of workers have followed this approach in order to determine the method of inheritance of a duplex pelvicalyceal system. In the first series (Whitaker and Danks, 1966) 123 intravenous pyelograms were performed on relatives of 30 female and nine male index patients, and duplications were found in eight of 52 parents and seven of 67 siblings and one of four grandparents. In the second survey (Atwell *et al.*, 1974), 101 first-degree relatives of 30 index patients were investigated and 21 of these had bifidity of the collecting system. As there was an equal frequency of bifidity in parents and siblings the findings support the theory that a duplex collecting system is inherited as an autosomal dominant gene of variable penetrance.

Following the second survey (Atwell *et al.*, 1974), two additional observations were made. Firstly, in three families siblings were found with VUR unassociated with a bifid system (Fig. 52.1). Secondly, it was noticed that in many patients with VUR minor forms of a

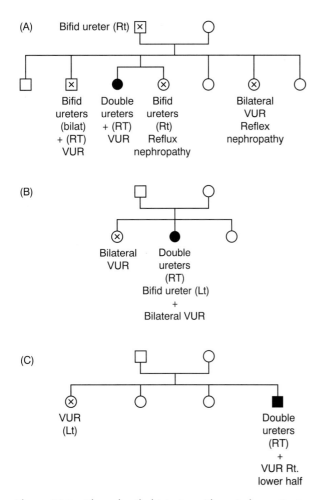

Figure 52.1   Three family histories with an index patient with double ureters with siblings with vesicoureteric reflux unassociated with double or bifid ureters.

duplex system such as a bifid renal pelvis were not reported by the radiologist. A third observation derived from the older textbooks was that urinary infection was increased 20-fold in patients with a duplex system (Campbell and Harrison, 1970). Thus, there appeared to be a relationship between VUR and a duplex collecting system.

In a survey of patients with unilateral bifid renal pelvis, or double ureters associated with VUR, contralateral VUR to the normal kidney was found in 25% (Atwell *et al.*, 1977). In these patients there was lateral ectopia of the ureteric orifice predisposing to VUR.

VESICOURETERIC REFLUX

The above observations led to a further survey in order to investigate the incidence of a duplex collecting sys-

tem in first-degree relatives of index patients with VUR (Atwell *et al.*, 1977). In 32 index patients with VUR there were seven families with familial VUR and six families with a duplex collecting system. Even in the seven families with familial VUR there were three with a duplex collecting system (Fig. 52.3).

The familial nature of VUR has been reported on numerous occasions (Tobenkin, 1964; Mulcahy *et al.*, 1970; Burger and Smith, 1971; Amar, 1972; Burger, 1972; Mebust and Forest, 1972; Bredin *et al.*, 1975; Middleton *et al.*, 1975; Vargas *et al.*, 1978; Jenkins and Noe, 1982) and in two a relationship between VUR and a duplex system was noted. These observations support the hypothesis that VUR is inherited by an autosomal dominant gene of variable penetrance.

If this hypothesis is accepted one has to consider the interrelationship among a duplex system, lateral ectopia of the ureteric orifice and VUR. There is no doubt that the main factor in preventing VUR is the length of the intramural ureter (Cass and Ireland, 1972). As previously stated, VUR was found to a contralateral normal kidney in 25% of patients with VUR and bifidity of the opposite side (Atwell *et al.*, 1977). This suggests that lateral ectopia of the ureteric orifice may be the common factor in patients with VUR, a duplex system, or both. It seems probable that both duplicity and VUR are inherited by autosomal genes of variable penetrance. However, Burger (1972) suggested that the length of the intramural ureter is determined by multiple genes with

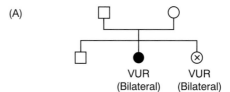

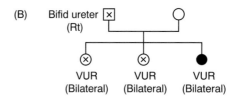

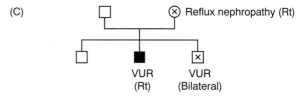

Figure 52.2   Three family histories demonstrating familial reflux.

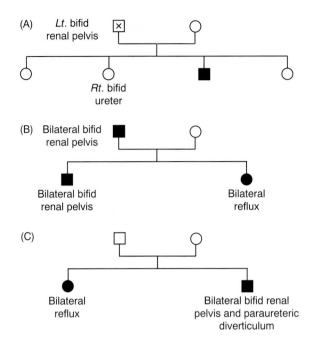

Figure 52.3 Three family histories with index patients with VUR and first degree relatives with duplex pelvicalyceal collecting systems and in family C a right paraureteric diverticulum.

a cumulative effect. This polygenic method of inheritance could explain the transmission of the trait in families, sexual and racial differences, and unilateral and bilateral VUR.

Attempts to identify a marker of the genetic susceptibility to VUR include hair and eye colour (Manley, 1981; Urrutia and Lebowitz, 1985) and HLA antigens (Sengar *et al.*, 1979; Torres *et al.*, 1980), and have not been found to be of clinical use.

PARAURETERIC DIVERTICULUM

The aetiology of a congenital paraureteric diverticulum (PUD) is unknown but its presence predisposes to the development of VUR. In the author's two surveys (Atwell *et al.*, 1974, 1977) a family was found with a relative with a PUD (Fig. 52.3). Therefore, 22 index patients with a PUD (16 male and six female) were investigated, three index patients were found to have either a bifid or double ureter (Atwell and Allen, 1980). A bifid ureter was also found in three mothers and a bifid renal pelvis in one sister. Another mother was found to have bilateral reflux nephropathy, two siblings had VUR and one brother a PUD. Another mother had a PUJ hydronephrosis and one father had adult polycystic kidneys (Fig. 52.4).

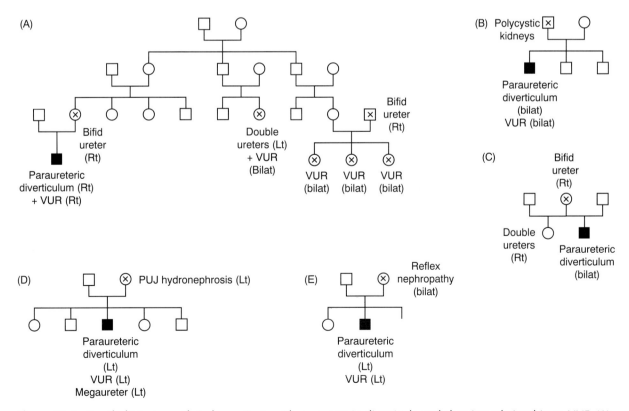

Figure 52.4 Family histories with index patients with paraureteric diverticula and showing relationship to VUR (A), polycystic kidneys (B), double and bifid ureters (C), PUJ hydronephrosis (D) and reflux nephropathy (E).

The high incidence of a duplex collecting system in index patients and their relatives suggests a direct relationship between these conditions. One possible explanation is that the PUD represents an aborted ureteric bud.

PELVIURETERIC JUNCTIONAL HYDRONEPHROSIS

Familial PUJ hydronephrosis was first reported in 1945 (Aaron and Robbins, 1948) and since then there have been six further reports (Cannon, 1954; Raffle, 1955; Jewell and Buchert, 1962; Martin and Goodwin, 1968; Simpson and German, 1970; Grosse *et al.*, 1973) and one family survey (Atwell, 1985). In the latter survey there was a marked difference in the incidence between families with one parent affected (two of six siblings affected) and those with neither parent affected (three of 33 siblings affected). These findings, together with the review (Grosse *et al.*, 1973) of the previously reported families, suggest that PUJ hydronephrosis is inherited by an autosomal dominant gene of variable penetrance. Typical family histories are shown in Fig. 52.5.

Urological conditions found in the above survey (Atwell, 1985) include VUR and double ureters with VUR to the lower pole in two index patients. Other findings included infundibular stenosis two, renal calculi one, bilateral dilatation of ureters two and reflux

nephropathy one. In addition, in nine other families not included in the survey, VUR, duplication, PUD, hypospadias, diverticulum of the posterior urethra and undescended testes were found.

The association between VUR and PUJ hydronephrosis has not often been reported (Liebowitz and Buckman, 1983; Maizels *et al.*, 1984) but is said to range between 10 and 20%. This association could be explained by a coexisting anomaly on a common ureteric bud, especially as there appears to be a relationship among VUR, duplex collecting systems, PUD and PUJ hydronephrosis (Fig. 52.6).

MEGAURETERS

The problem with megaureters is in deciding whether the dilation of the ureters is primary or secondary. Even in patients with fetal VUR the ureters are often grossly dilated (Scott and Renwick, 1988; Najmaldin *et al.*, 1990) but whether this is primary or secondary still remains unanswered.

There have been isolated reports of affected first-degree relatives of patients with megaureters (Mackay, 1945) but there are no known prospective studies of first degree relatives of index patients with mega-ureters. Therefore the precise mechanism, if any, of genetic factors involved with megaureters remains obscure at this stage and further investigation is required.

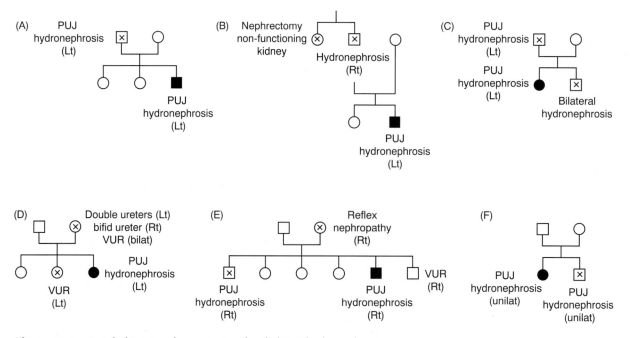

Figure 52.5   Family histories demonstrating familial PUJ hydronephrosis.

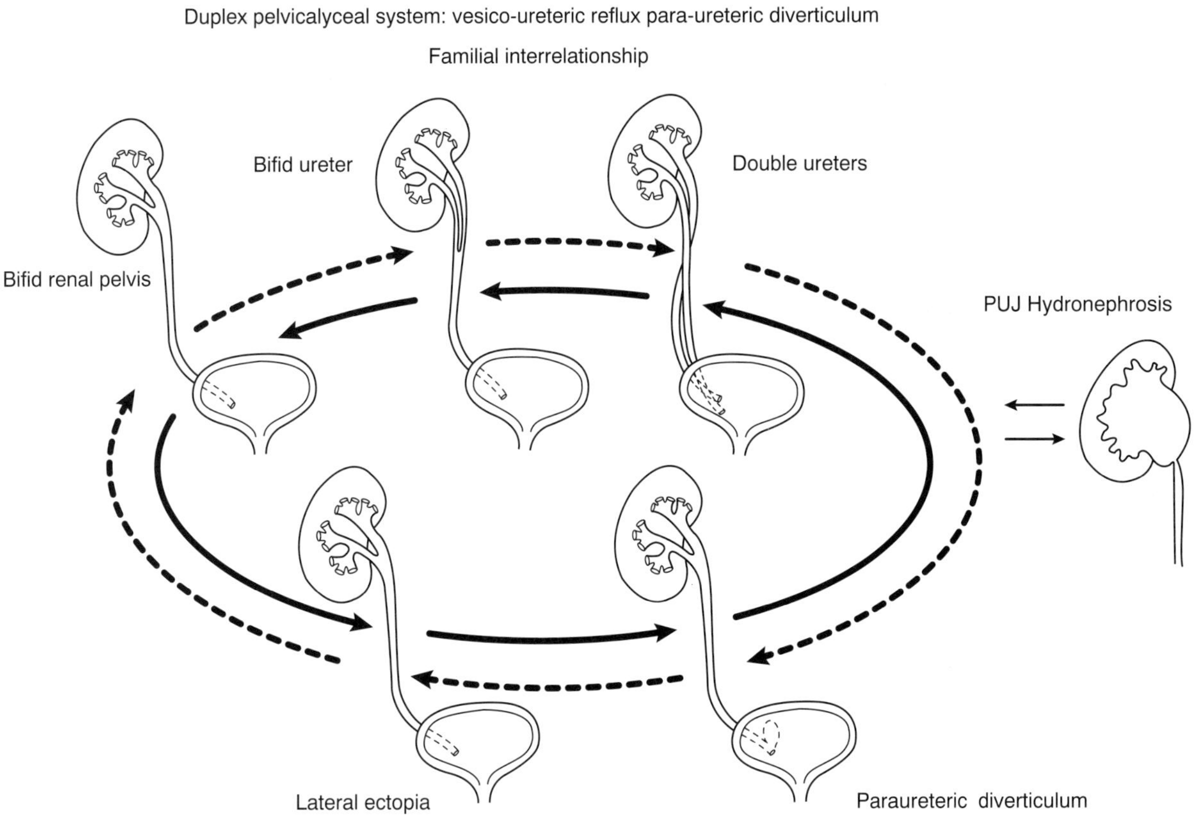

Duplex pelvicalyceal system: vesico-ureteric reflux para-ureteric diverticulum

Familial interrelationship

Figure 52.6 Familial interrelationship between duplex pelvicalyceal collecting system. Vesicoureteric reflux, paraureteric diverticulum and PUJ hydronephrosis.

ECTOPIC URETEROCELES

Ectopic ureteroceles are associated with double ureters and cystic dysplasia of the upper moiety of the affected kidney. Both of these conditions have a genetic background, although the dysplasia may be due to obstruction within the urinary tract during fetal life.

In a survey of 26 index patients with ectopic ureteroceles (Williams and Mininberg, 1979) duplicity of the contralateral side was found in 12 (47%). Of the 114 first-degree relatives investigated 12 had a duplex system, which is a 5–10-fold increase over the expected incidence. Thus the duplicity is probably due to a primary genetic effect and the dysplasia is probably secondary to obstruction.

Outflow tract anomalies

POSTERIOR URETHRAL VALVES

There is a well-known clinical association between renal dysplasia and posterior urethral valves and it is usually associated with severe VUR. In experimental animals cystic dysplasia can be caused by obstruction but the timing is important. If it occurs early, cystic dysplasia results, but if later in intrauterine life hydronephrosis occurs (Bell, 1971). In one study of renal dysplasia with ultrasonography two brothers were identified with posterior urethral valves and renal dysplasia (Al Saadi *et al.*, 1984).

BLADDER EXSTROPHY AND EPISPADIAS

The aetiology is unknown but treatment of mothers in early pregnancy with progestins led to some infants having bladder exstrophy or epispadias (Blickstein and Katz, 1991). There is a familial factor, as in a series of 66 exstrophy patients with 215 offspring there were three with exstrophy, which is well in excess of the expected incidence of 3.3 in 100 000 births (Shapiro *et al.*, 1984). Exstrophy has also been found in both of a pair of monozygotic twins (Blickstein and Katz, 1991).

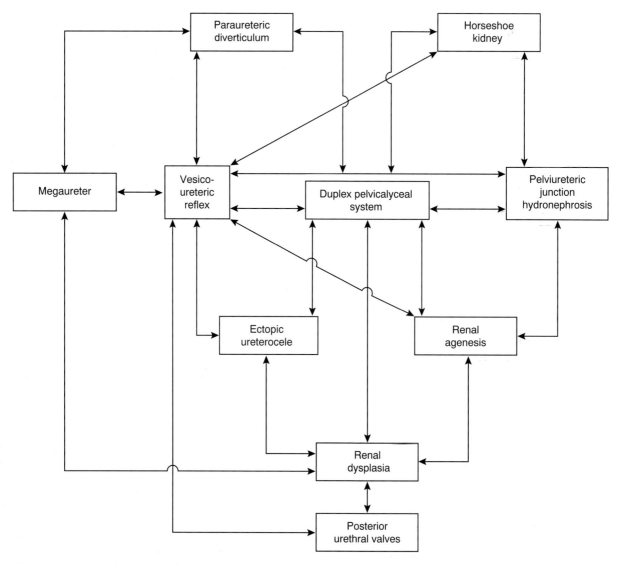

Figure 52.7 Interrelationship of common congenital anomalies of the ureteric bud and outflow tract.

Summary

In conclusion, from others' and our family studies there seems to be a direct interrelationship between the congenital anomalies affecting the ureteric bud. The duplex pelvicalyceal collecting system, VUR, paraureteric diverticulum and PUJ hydronephrosis appear to have a closer relationship than other anomalies such as megaureter, posterior urethral valves and polycystic kidneys. Renal agenesis is related as this results from an obstructed ureteric bud, e.g. multicystic kidney. There is also a relationship between renal dysplasia and PUJ hydronephrosis. The most satisfactory explanation is that the inheritance is by an autosomal dominant gene with varying degrees of penetrance. These interrelationships are shown in Fig. 52.7.

References

Aaron, G. and Robbins, M.A. 1948: Hydronephrosis due to aberrant vessels: remarkable familial incidence with report of cases. *Journal of Urology* **60**, 707–70.

Al Saadi, A.A., Yoshimoto, M., Bree, R., Farah, J., Chang, C., Sahney, S., Shokeir, M. and Bernstein J. 1984: A family study of renal dysplasia. *American Journal of Human Genetics* **36**, 119A.

Amar, A.D. 1972: Familial vesicoureteral reflux. *Journal of Urology* **108**, 969–71.

Atwell, J.D. 1985: Familial pelviureteric junction hydronephrosis and its association with a duplex pelvicalyceal system and vesicoureteric reflux: a family study. *British Journal of Urology* **57**, 365–9.

Atwell, J.D. and Allen, N.H. 1980: The interrelationship between paraureteric diverticula, vesicoureteric reflux and duplication of the pelvicalyceal collecting system: a family study. *British Journal of Urology* **52**, 269–73.

Atwell, J.D., Cook, P.L., Howell, C.J., Hyde, I. and Parker, B.C. 1974: Familial incidence of bifid and double ureters. *Archives of Disease in Childhood* **49**, 390–3.

Atwell, J.D., Cook, P.L., Strong, L. and Hyde, I. 1977: The interrelationship between vesico-ureteric reflux, trigonal abnormalities and a bifid pelvicalyceal collecting system: a family study. *British Journal of Urology* **49**, 97–107.

Bell, A.D. 1971: The effect of intrauterine urinary obstruction upon the development of the foetal kidney. *Journal of Urology* **105**, 784–9.

Blickstein, I. and Katz, Z. 1991: Possible relationship of bladder exstrophy and epispadias taken in early pregnancy. *British Journal of Urology* **68**, 105–6.

Blyth, H. and Ockenden, B.G. 1971: Polycystic disease of kidneys and liver presenting in childhood. *Journal of Medical Genetics* **8**, 257–84.

Bredin, H.C., Winchester, P., McGovern, J.H. and Degnam, M. 1975: A family study of vesicoureteral reflux. *Journal of Urology* **113**, 623–5 .

Bridge, R.A.C. 1960: Horseshoe kidneys in identical twins. *British Journal of Urology* **32**, 32–3.

Burger, R.H. 1972: A theory on the nature of transmission of congenital vesicoureteral reflux. *Journal of Urology*, **108**, 249–54.

Burger, R.H. and Smith, C. 1971: Hereditary and familial vesico-ureteric reflux. *Journal of Urology* **106**, 845–51.

Campbell, M.F. and Harrison, J.H. 1970: *Urology* 3rd ed., vol. 2. Philadelphia, PA: W.B. Saunders, 1488.

Cannon, J.F. 1954: Hereditary unilateral hydronephrosis. *Annals of Internal Medicine* **41**, 1054–60.

Carter, G.O., Evans, K. and Pescia, G. 1979: A family study of renal agenesis. *Journal of Medical Genetics* **16**, 176–88.

Cass, A.S. and Ireland, G.W. 1972: Significance of ureteral submucosal length, orifice configuration and position in vesicoureteral reflux. *Journal of Urology* **107**, 963–5.

Cochran, W. and Froggat, P. 1967: Bilateral nephroblastoma in two sisters. *Journal of Urology* **97**, 216–20.

Crawfurd, M. d'A. 1988: Renal agenesis and hypoplasia. In: *The genetics of renal tract disorders*. Oxford: Oxford University Press, 527, 529.

Draper, G.J., Heaf, M.M. and Kinnear-Wilson, L.M. 1977: Occurrence of childhood cancers among sibs and estimation of familial risks. *Journal of Medical Genetics* **14**, 81–90.

Ericsson, N.O. and Ivemark, B.I. 1958: Renal dysplasia and pyelonephritis in infants and children I–II. *Archives of Pathology* **66**, 255–69.

Fitch, N. 1977: Heterogeneity of bilateral renal agenesis. *Canadian Medical Association Journal* **116**, 381–2.

Fitzgerald, W.L. and Hardin, H.C. 1955: Bilateral Wilm's tumour in a Wilm's tumour: case report. *Journal of Urology* **73**, 468–74.

Francke, U., Holmes, L.B., Atkins, L. *et al.* 1979: Aniridia–Wilm's tumor association: evidence for specific deletion of 11p 13. *Cytogenetics Cell Genetics* **24**, 185–92.

Francke, U., Riccardi, V.M., Hitner, H.M. *et al.* 1978: Interstitial Del (11p) as a cause of the Aniridia–Wilm's tumor

association: band localization and a heritable base. *American Journal of Human Genetics* **30**, 81A.

George, C.R.P. 1981: Familial association of polycystic kidneys, horseshoe kidney and loin pain haematuria syndrome. *Journal of the Royal Society of Medicine* **77**, 77–8.

Girsh, L.S. and Karpinski, F.E., Jr. 1956: Urinary tract malformations, their familial occurrence, with special reference to double ureter, double pelvis and double kidney. *New England Journal of Medicine* **254**, 854–5.

Grosse, F.R., Kaveggia, L. and Opitz, J.M. 1973: Familial hydronephrosis. *Zentrablatt Kinder Heil Kunde* **114**, 313–22.

Holmes, L.B. 1972: Unilateral renal agenesis: common, serious, hereditary. *Paediatric Research* **6**, 419.

Jenkins, F.R. and Noe, H.N. 1982: Familial vesicoureteral reflux: a prospective study. *Journal of Urology* **128**, 774–8.

Jewell, J.H. and Buchert, W.I. 1962: Unilateral hereditary hydronephrosis: a report of four cases in three successive generations. *Journal of Urology* **88**, 129–36.

Knudson, A.G. and Strong, L.C. 1972: Mutation and cancer: a model for Wilm's tumour of the kidney. *Journal of the National Cancer Institute* **48**, 313–24.

Liebowitz, R.L. and Buckman, J.G. 1983: The coexistence of uretero-pelvic junction obtruction and reflux. *American Journal of Roentgenology* **140**, 231–8.

Machin, G.A. and McCaughey, W.T.E. 1984: A new precursor of Wilm's tumour (nephroblastoma): intralobular multifocal nephroblastosis. *Histopathology* **8**, 35–53.

Mackay, H. 1945: Congenital bilateral megaloureters with hydronephrosis. *A remarkable family history. Proceedings of the Royal Society of Medicine* **38**, 567–8.

Maizels, M., Smith, C.K. and Firut, C.F. 1984: The management of children with vesico-ureteral reflux and uretero-pelvic junction obstruction. *Journal of Urology* **131**, 722–7.

Manley, C.B. 1981: Reflux in blonde haired girls. *Society for Paediatric Urology Newsletter*, 14 October.

Martin, D.C. and Goodwin, W.E. 1968: Hereditary and familial aspects of some common urologic problems. *Urology Digest* **7**, 11–17.

Mebust, W.K. and Forest, J.D. Vesicoureteral reflux in identical twins. *Journal of Urology* **108**, 635–6.

Middleton, G.W., Howard, S.S. and Gillenwater, J.Y. 1975: Sex linked familial reflux. *Journal of Urology* **14**, 36–9.

Mulcahy, J.J., Kelalis, P.P., Stickler, G.B. and Burke, E.G. 1970: Familial vesicoureteral reflux. *Journal of Urology* **104**, 762–4.

Najmaldin, A., Burge, D.M. and Atwell, J.D. 1990: Fetal vesicoureteric reflux. *British Journal of Urology* **65**, 403–6.

Pathak, I.G. and Williams, D.I. 1964: Multicystic and cystic dysplastic kidneys. *British Journal of Urology* **36**, 318–31.

Perlman, M., Williams, J. and Orney, A. 1976: Familial ureteric bud anomalies. *Journal of Medical Genetics* **13**, 161–3.

Raffle, R.B. 1955: Familial hydronephrosis. *British Medical Journal* **1**, 580–2.

Riccardi, V.M., Sujansky, E., Smith, A.C. *et al.* 1978: Chromosomal imbalance in the Aniridia–Wilm's tumour association: 11p interstitial deletion. *Pediatrics* **61**, 604–10.

Risdon, R.A. 1971a: Renal dysplasia Part I: A clinico-pathological study of 76 cases. *Journal of Clinical Pathology* **24**, 57–65.

Risdon, R.A. 1971b: Renal dysplasia Part II: A necropsy study of 41 cases. *Journal of Clinical Pathology* **24**, 65–71.

Roodhooft, A.M., Birnholz, J.C. and Holmes, L.B. 1984: Familial nature of congenital absence and severe dysgenesis of both kidneys. *New England Journal of Medicine* **310**, 1341–5.

Scott, J.E.S. and Renwick, M. 1988: Antenatal diagnosis of congenital abnormalities in the urinary tract. *British Journal of Urology* **62**, 295–300.

Sengar, D.P.S., McLeish, W.A., Rashid, A. and Wolfish, N.M. 1978: Histocompatibility antigens in urinary tract infections and vesicoureteral reflux: a preliminary communication. *Clinical Nephrology* **10**, 166–9.

Shapiro, E., Lepor, H. and Jeffs, R.D. 1984: The inheritance of exstrophy-epispadias complex. *Journal of Urology* **132**, 308–10.

Shokeir, M.H.K. 1978: Aplasia of the Müllerian system: evidence for probable sex linked autosomal dominant inheritance. *Birth Defects Original Article Series* **14**, 147–65.

Simpson, J.L. and German, J. 1970: Familial urinary tract anomalies. *Journal of American Medical Association* **212**, 2264–5.

Strom, T. 1957: A Wilm's tumour family. *Acta Paediatrica* **46**, 601–4.

Tobenkin, M.I. 1964: Hereditary vesico-ureteric reflux. *Southern Medical Journal* **57**, 139–47.

Torres, V.E., Moore, S.B., Kurtz, S.B., Offord, K.P. and Kelasis, P.P. 1980: In search of a marker for genetic susceptibility to reflux nephropathy. *Clinical Nephrology* **14**, 217–22.

Urrutia, E.J. and Lebowitz, R.L. 1985: Relationship between hair/eye colour and primary vesicoureteral reflux in children. *Urologic Radiology* **2**, 23–4.

Vargas, A., Evans, K., Ransley, P. *et al.* 1978: A family study of vesicoureteral reflux. *Journal of Medical Genetics* **15**, 85–96.

Whitaker, J. and Danks, D.M. 1966: A study of the inheritance of duplication of the kidneys and ureters. *Journal of Urology* **95**, 176–8.

Williams, J.J. and Mininberg, D.T. 1979: *Genetics in urology,* Vol. 2. No. 1 of *Dialogues in pediatric urology.*

CHAPTER 53

Double ureters and associated anomalies

M. HOROWITZ AND M.E. MITCHELL

Embryology	**Ectopic ureters**
Duplex kidneys and ureters	**Ureteroceles**
Vesicoureteric reflux	**References**

Embryology

Urinary tract abnormalities in children often reflect abnormal development. Therefore, to understand and correct these defects a thorough understanding of genito-urinary embryology is extremely important. During embryological development the urogenital ridge produces three sets of renal organs, namely the pronephros, mesonephros and metanephros. The pronephros, which forms primitive tubules and is attached to the cloaca by a ductal system, appears in the fourth week of gestation. Late in the fourth week the pronephros is replaced by the mesonephros, which develop primitive glomeruli and tubules. The mesonephros connects to the excretory ducts of the pronephros, which are renamed the mesonephric ducts (Wolffian ducts).

During the fifth week of gestation the metanephric or ureteric buds appear at the caudal end of the mesonephric ducts near their entry into the cloaca and grow in a cephalad direction. The cephalad portion of these buds undergoes multiple divisions to form the renal pelvis, calyces and collecting tubules while the caudal portion forms the ureter. At about the same time the ureteric bud induces the formation of nephrons from the metanephric blastema. The metanephric blastema is composed of nests of primitive cells derived from the urogenital ridge. The fetal kidneys begin to contribute significant amounts to the amniotic fluid after the 16th week of gestation.

For a kidney to develop properly, a normal ureteral bud must come in contact with normal metanephric blastema and the two must interact in a normal manner (Potter, 1972). Mackie and Stephens (1975) proposed that only the midportion of the metanephric blastema could form normal mature renal tissue and this could only happen if the ureteric bud came off the mesonephric system at the correct location. A ureteric bud that comes off either proximal or distal results in the development of a dysplastic kidney. The farther away the ureteral bud arises from the normal location, the more abnormal the resulting renal segment.

By the seventh week of gestation the mesonephric duct and ureteric bud have separate orifices in the urogenital sinus. Eventually the orifice of the mesonephric duct migrates in a caudal and medial direction and that of the ureteric bud migrates in a cephalad and lateral direction. The area between these two structures is occupied by the mesoderm of the metanephric (developing ureter) duct, which will differentiate into the trigone of the bladder. In males the mesonephric ducts become the epididymis, vas deferens, seminal vesicles and ejaculatory ducts which enter the prostatic urethra. In females the mesonephric remnants include the epophoron, which is generally found in the broad ligament, and Gartner's ducts, found along the lateral wall of the uterus or in the wall of the vagina. These relationships become extremely important in understanding the pathophysiology of ureteral ectopia and duplication.

Duplex kidneys and ureters

A duplex kidney is defined as a kidney in which two pyelocalyceal systems are present and is associated with one or two ureters entering the bladder (Glassberg *et al.*, 1984). The development of two separate ureteral buds from the mesonephric duct results in complete duplication. However, early branching of the ureteric bud results in incomplete duplication, which varies from a bifid renal pelvis (where the two systems join at the ureteropelvic junction), to two ureters joining to form a single ureter just at the bladder wall. Approximately 25% of incomplete duplications join in the proximal ureter, 50% in the mid-ureter and 25% in the distal ureter (Caldamone, 1985). One ureteral orifice is the rule with incomplete duplication. With complete duplication there are two ureters and two ureteral orifices. The ureter which drains the upper pole of a complete duplication arises from a cephalad position on the mesonephric duct. However, with development, the distal upper pole ureter migrates along with the distal mesonephric duct to assume a position that is caudal and medial to the distal lower pole ureter. The lower pole ureter therefore enters the bladder lateral and cranial to the upper pole ureter. This seemingly reversed relationship of the upper and lower pole ureteral orifices in complete duplication is known as the Weigert–Mayer law (Weigert, 1877). Most duplicated systems have normal function in both segments and both ureteral orifices located in a normal location on the bladder trigone. Urinary tract anomalies, however, are present in approximately 20% of children with complete duplication. (Bissett and Strife, 1987). The greater the distance between the two ureteric buds the greater the potential for renal dysplasia. An abnormality in the location of the ureteral bud will result in an abnormal location of the ureteral orifice and usually is associated with renal dysplasia.

The incidence of incomplete duplication is about 1% and complete duplication about 0.2% (Kelalis *et al.*, 1992). In children being evaluated for urinary tract infection the incidence can be as high as 8% (Bissett and Strife, 1987). Ureteral duplication is more commonly found in female than male individuals. Unilateral duplication occurs with approximately the same frequency on the right and left sides. In a review of 230 cases, the incidence of unilateral duplication was three times more common than bilateral duplication (Nation, 1944).

Duplication is frequently accompanied by other urinary tract abnormalities. These include vesicoureteric reflux (VUR), ureteroceles, ureteral ectopia, obstruction and dysplasia, with reflux being the most common.

Ureteral triplication can occur but is a very rare anomaly, with only 75 cases published as of 1977 (Kelalis, 1985). Extending present thought, it is the result of three separate ureteric buds or a combination of two separate buds with branching. The most common abnormalities associated with triplication are contralateral duplication, ureteral ectopia, VUR and renal dysplasia. Treatment of triplication and its associated anomalies should follow the same guidelines as for duplicated systems.

The treatment of duplication and its associated anomalies must be individualized and dictated by the anatomy and function of each renal segment.

INCOMPLETE DUPLICATION OF THE URETERS

Most of the time incomplete duplication is clinically silent. The single orifice, when entering the bladder at a normal location, will not cause reflux, obstruction or incontinence. One uncommon phenomenon unique to incomplete duplication involves the reflux of urine from one of the ureteral segments to the other, also referred to as yo-yo reflux (O'Reilly *et al.*, 1984). Patients with yo-yo reflux present with either urinary tract infection, flank pain or incidental hydronephrosis. if surgery is necessary, these patients can be managed with a pyeloureterostomy or pyelopyelostomy and careful excision of the redundant ureteral segment, thus converting the bifid ureter into a bifid pelvis. The anastomosis should be between the upper pole ureter and the lower pole pelvis. If the two ureters unite close to the bladder a common sheath reimplant with excision of the distal common ureter is sometimes preferable. Yo-yo reflux is given as an argument against elective distal ureteroureterostomy.

Pelviureteric junctional (PUJ) obstruction is more common with complete duplication. The obstruction usually occurs with the lower pole renal pelvis. Patients present with the same symptoms as those with single system PUJ obstruction. With complete duplication, a customary pyeloplasty without upper pole manipulation is performed. With incomplete duplication correction requires precise knowledge of the anatomy of both systems. Anastomosis of the obstructed pelvis to the upper pole pelvis or proximal ureter will often resolve the obstruction and avoid the yo-yo reflux that could follow a standard dismembered pyeloplasty. Five children with a lower pole PUJ obstruction in incomplete duplicated systems have been reported (Joseph *et al.*, 1989). In the children with a short ureteral segment, an end-to-side pyeloureterostomy with excision of the ureter and PUJ area was performed. Those with longer ureteral segments underwent an Anderson–Hynes type pyeloplasty using the lower pole ureter for reanastomosis.

A ureter that is not associated with functioning renal tissue is referred to as a blind–ending ureter. Blind–ending ureters are associated with both complete and incomplete duplication. They are often short segments not associated with clinical findings and detected as an incidental finding on contrast studies. The longer blind–ending segments have a higher incidence of VUR and if indicated can be surgically excised.

Vesicoureteric reflux

VUR is the most common abnormality associated with ureteral duplication. The lower pole ureter has a shorter intramural tunnel and is more prone to VUR than the upper pole ureter but reflux can occur in both the upper and lower poles. When reflux occurs to both the upper and lower segments of a duplicated system, there is usually a single orifice with a short common stem. In a report on 85 duplicated ureters with reflux that required surgical treatment all ureters refluxed into the lower pole and 11 into the upper pole segment as well (Barrett *et al.*, 1975). Reflux only to the upper pole did not occur. Antenatal ultrasound will sometimes detect high-grade reflux.

The most common presentation for less severe reflux is urinary tract infection (UTI). Unfortunately, infants with UTI may not present with fever, leucocytosis or flank pain, rather simply failure to thrive. Therefore, early diagnosis of lower grades of reflux in young children can be difficult. Voiding cystourethrogram (VCUG) remains the gold standard for diagnosis of VUR (Fig. 53.1). Radionuclide cystography (RNC) can be as sensitive, with the advantage of significant reduction in radiation exposure. Grading of reflux is best accomplished with VCUG, but known VUR should be followed with periodic nuclear cystography.

Treatment of VUR in duplicated systems remains controversial. Some authors advocate surgical repair of all grades of VUR while others recommend medical surveillance and prophylactic antibiotics. Husmann and Allen (1991) compared 60 patients with grade 2 VUR into the lower pole of completely duplicated systems managed by medical surveillance with a control group who had grade 2 VUR without duplication managed by the same protocol. Resolution rate was found in 10% of the duplicated systems and 35% for the single systems over a 2-year period. However, there was no difference

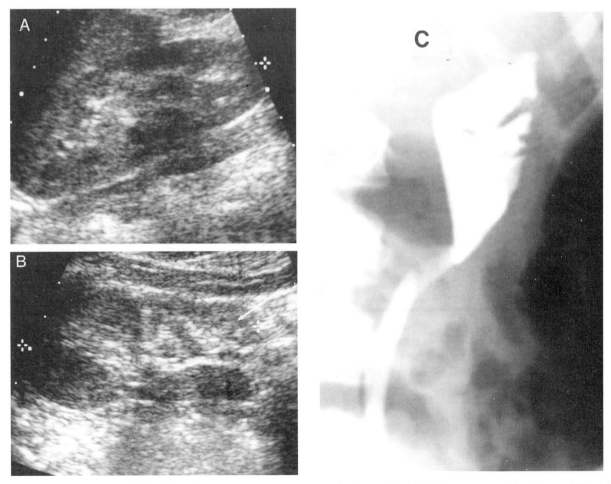

Fig. 53.1 A 10-year-old female with recurrent urinary tract infections: (A) right kidney measuring 9.7 cm; (B) left kidney measuring 6.7 cm, with lower pole scarring (white arrow); (C) VCUG shows high grade reflux to lower pole of duplicated system. (D) and (E) overleaf.

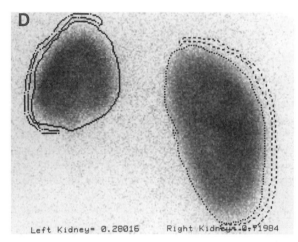

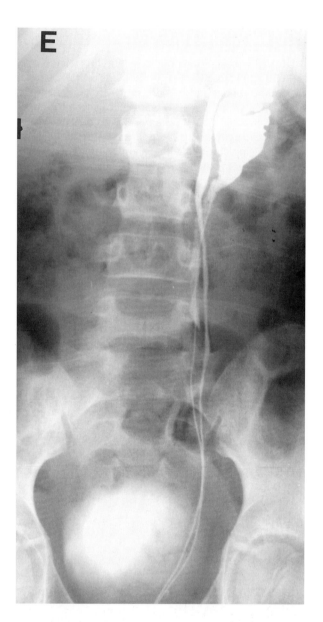

Fig. 53.1 A 10-year-old female with recurrent urinary tract infections: (D) DMSA renal scan demonstrating no function in mid- and lower portions of left kidney; (E) retrograde pyelogram showing anatomy of lower pole and small upper pole. The patient underwent left lower pole nephroureterectomy.

between the two groups with respect to incidence of breakthrough infections, progression of renal scars and findings of new scars. Earlier studies showed no resolution of VUR in duplicated systems: however, these studies were not stratified according to the grade of reflux. Patients with duplication and low-grade reflux (1–3) deserve a trial of conservative management. Surgery should be considered for progression of scars, breakthrough infection or deterioration in renal function. Patients with high-grade reflux with duplication have a very low chance of spontaneous resolution and should have surgical correction.

Prior to surgical correction of VUR an assessment of renal function in the affected segment must be made. With severe scarring and little function in the involved segment (<10% of total renal function) a partial nephrectomy and excision of the associated ureter, with care being taken not to injure the blood supply to the remaining ureter, is the treatment of choice. In children this can be achieved with an extraperitoneal approach through a single muscle-splitting flank incision. After identifying the vascular supply to both segments, the lower pole vessels should be ligated and divided. The lower pole ureteral segment can serve as a source for recurrent infection and therefore should be removed as completely as possible, without endangering the upper pole ureter. There is usually a clear demarcation between the upper and lower renal segments when function is severely reduced. In the most common case, however, the affected kidney is saved. The procedure of choice is a common sheath reimplant. Because the upper and lower ureters tend to share a common wall distally it is unwise to attempt separation of the ureters. Both are reimplanted as a unit even if only one refluxes.

Ectopic ureters

A ureter that drains into a location that is not in the normal position on the bladder trigone is known as an ectopic ureter. Ectopic ureters are more commonly seen with complete duplication but can be seen with single systems. In males the majority of ectopic ureters drain single systems, whereas more than 80% of ectopic ureters in females drain duplicated systems. About 10% of ectopic ureters are bilateral (Barrett *et al.*, 1975). In duplex systems, the ectopic ureter is associated with the upper pole segment. As noted previously, the upper pole ureter remains attached to the Wolffian duct for a longer period of time than the lower pole ureter and therefore the ectopic upper pole ureter has potential to empty into any Wolffian derivative. Hence, the male ureteral orifice can be found draining into the prostatic urethra, seminal vesicles, ejaculatory ducts or vas deferens, all proximal to the external sphincter. In the female, the most common sites of ectopic ureteral drainage are the vestibule, urethra, bladder neck, vagina, and rarely the cervix and uterus. Gartner's duct is the vestigial remains of the Wolffian duct in the female and can be absorbed into the developing Müllerian structures during embryogenesis. This explains how the ectopic ureter can drain into the Müllerian system.

Unlike boys, girls with ectopic ureters in a duplicated system can have incontinence resulting from the location of the ureteral orifice distal to the urinary sphincter (Fig. 53.2). Ureteral ectopy into the distal urethra, vestibule,

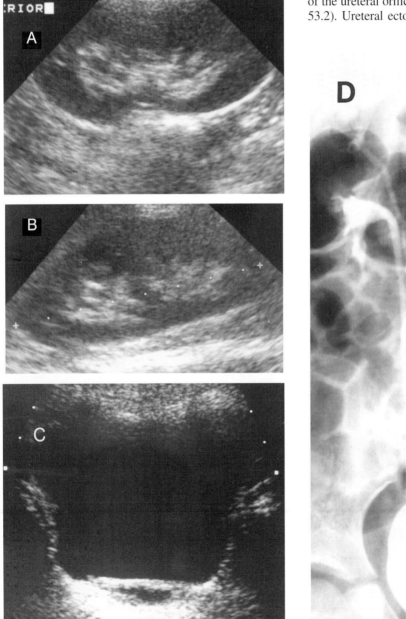

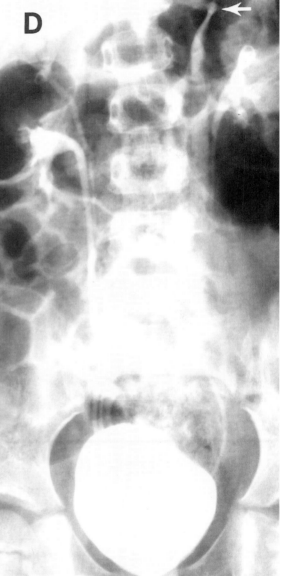

Fig. 53.2 A 4-year-old female with urinary incontinence (A) normal appearing left kidney; (B) normal appearing right kidney; (C) normal bladder without evidence of dilated or ectopic ureters; (D) intravenous urogram demonstrating bilateral duplication, drooping lily sign and left upper pole with dilated ureter (white arrow). Nuclear scan demonstrated 14% of total renal function from left upper pole and the patient underwent left proximal ureteroureterostomy with excision of the distal ureter.

vagina and cervix is manifested by incontinence. Incontinence is uncommon when the ectopic ureter enters the bladder neck or proximal urethra. More commonly, however, they present with infection from upper pole obstruction or lower pole reflux. Almost half of the females with ectopic ureters present with continuous urinary incontinence or purulent vaginal discharge. Despite being constantly wet, these children have normal voiding cycles. If, however, the ureter passes through the external sphincter, the patient may be dry and drainage of the ectopic segment occurs only when the sphincter is relaxed. The ectopic ureter in this circumstance is basically obstructed and wetting may be intermittent. Occasionally the ectopic orifice can be identified with physical examination of the vestibule, especially if the upper pole has good renal function and droplets of urine can be observed running from the ectopic orifice. The diagnosis of an ectopic ureter in girls should be suspected from history alone. The ectopic orifice of renal segments with poor renal function is often impossible to locate, even with repeat examinations and imaging studies. Ultrasound is often

the first study obtained, but it can miss a diminutive upper pole dysplastic segment. In the case of obstruction, ultrasonography may be the study of choice, demonstrating hydroureteronephrosis, thinning or dysplastic parenchyma and tortuosity of the ureter (Fig. 53.3). The excretory urogram may be more efficient and reliable but has led to missed diagnosis. With sufficient function, the upper pole can be defined and the ureter followed to its ectopic termination. Lateral and downward displacement of the lower pole system, producing the classical 'drooping lily' sign and reduction in the number of calyces may be the only indication of duplication. If the upper pole is dilated there may be increased distance from the transverse process to the medial aspect of the uppermost calyx of the lower pole system. Nuclear medicine imaging [diethylenetriaminepenta-acetic acid (DTPA) and dimercaptosuccinic acid (DMSA)] studies can help to assess the relative amount of function in the upper pole segment. A case in which magnetic resonance imaging was the only investigation that gave a definitive diagnosis has been reported (Gillatt and Feneley, 1994). A VCUG must be obtained in

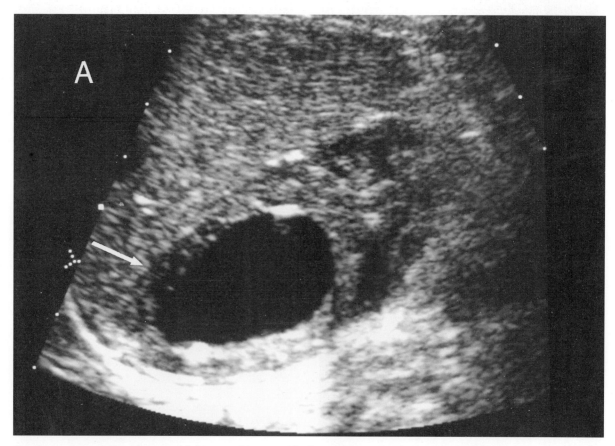

Fig. 53.3 A 6-month-old male with history of antenatal hydronephrosis: (A) ultrasound of right kidney showing moderate dilatation of upper pole collecting system and thinning of parenchyma (white arrow); (B) ultrasound of bladder showing distal ureteral dilatation (white arrow); (C) intravenous urogram showing no function in the upper pole of the right kidney, lateral and downward displacement of the lower pole system and increased distance from the transverse process to the medial aspect of the uppermost calyx (white arrow). The patient underwent right upper pole nephrectomy.

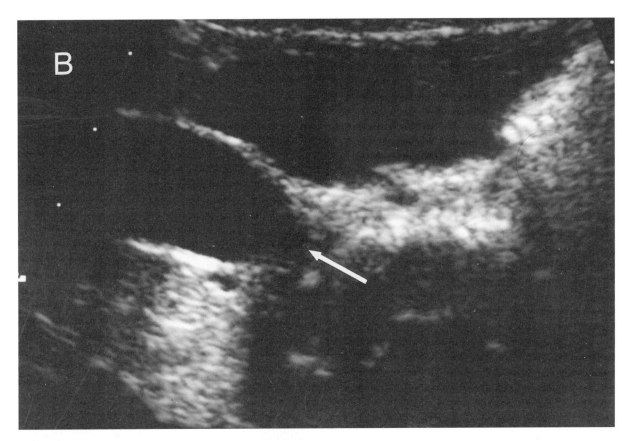

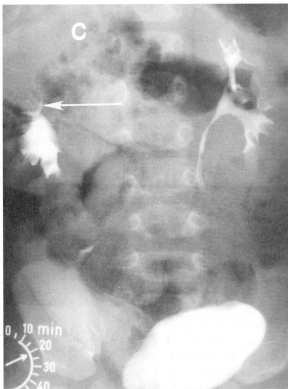

Fig. 53.3 Continued.

all patients with suspected ectopic ureters because of the high incidence of VUR to the ipsilateral lower pole. Cystourethroscopy can detect up to two-thirds of ectopic ureteral orifices (Mandell *et al.*, 1981). The authors choose to perform cystoscopy immediately before definitive surgical treatment, to avoid an additional anaesthetic.

Because the ureter terminates proximal to the external sphincter in boys, incontinence is not seen. The mode of presentation depends on the site of termination of the ureteral orifice, but UTI is the most common presenting symptom as a result of reflux, obstruction or both. A single-system ectopic ureter is usually associated with a non-visualized dysplastic kidney. Prostatitis and epididymo-orchitis occur when the ectopic ureter enters a Wolffian duct structure. When the ureter enters the bladder neck or posterior urethra, obstruction and renal dysplasia are observed and UTI often results. A cystic or boggy periprostatic mass can be felt on rectal exam when the ureter joins a seminal vesicle.

An ectopic ureter to a poorly functioning single system is managed by nephroureterectomy, with primary ureteral reimplantation being reserved for systems with good function. In a duplicated system, a poorly functioning unit should be treated by partial nephrectomy and ureterectomy, avoiding extensive dissection near the sphincter. This can be approached through a standard flank incision. There is usually a clear demarcation between the dysplastic or hydronephrotic upper segment and the normal lower segment.

After identifying and ligating the vessels to the upper pole, the upper pole is amputated transversely. All exposed lower pole calyces must be closed to prevent urinary leakage. When good function is demonstrated every effort must be made to preserve that segment. The authors favour pyeloureterostomy of the upper pole ureter to the lower pole renal pelvis for the management of a duplicated system with good function. Other options include common sheath reimplantation and, if the lower segment does not reflux, a lower ureteroureterostomy. However, the latter can result in yo-yo reflux and relative obstruction.

The last few years has seen an increase in the indications for laparoscopic surgery in adult and paediatric urology. Janetschek *et al.* (1997) recently reported on laparoscopic partial nephrectomy in 14 patients. Their experience showed that laparoscopic partial nephrectomy in children is feasible and associated with minimal blood loss, low morbidity and a low complication rate. Our last four partial nephrectomies for ureteral ectopia were performed laparoscopically. A transperitoneal approach using three ports was used in each case. The mean operating time was 118 min and there was no need for blood transfusions. There were no intraoperative complications and hospital stay was 1–3 days (mean 1.7).

Ureteroceles

Ureteroceles are defined as cystic dilatation of the distal intravesical portion of a ureter. They may drain either single systems or the upper pole of a duplicated system. The incidence of ureteroceles is approximately 1 in 500. About 10% of ureteroceles are bilateral.

Many classifications have been proposed for ureteroceles. Ericsson (1954) classified them according to the location of the ureteral orifice. Simple or orthotopic ureteroceles are entirely contained within the bladder, while ectopic ureteroceles extend into the bladder neck or urethra. Ectopic ureteroceles are commonly associated with the upper pole of a duplicated system while simple ureteroceles tend to be associated with single upper tracts. Another classification was into the following four categories:

- Stenotic: the orifice is located inside the bladder and is the presumed site of obstruction. This corresponds to the simple ureterocele of the previous classification. These account for about 40% of ureteroceles in duplicated systems.
- Sphincteric: the orifice may be normal or even patulous, but it lies in the floor of the urethra, so the ureter leading to it is obstructed by the internal sphincter mechanism. These also account for about 40% of ureteroceles in duplicated systems.

- Sphincterostenotic: a combination of the first two categories. These tend to be large and tense and cause obstruction of the bladder outlet. They account for about 5% of ureteroceles on duplicated systems.
- Cecoureterocele: the orifice is located within the bladder, but a 'caecum' or tongue of ureterocele extends submucosally into the urethra. They account for about 5% of ureteroceles on duplicated systems.

A third classification is based on grading jeopardy of the renal unit (Churchill *et al.*, 1987). Three grade exist:

- only the upper pole subtended by the ureterocele demonstrates injury
- the entire kidney ipsilateral to the ureterocele is significantly hydronephrotic or associated with high-grade reflux
- both kidneys have significant hydronephrosis and/or high-grade reflux.

The authors have found it functionally helpful to grade ureteroceles by the amount of bladder wall involved in the defect rather than the size or extension of the ureterocele into the urethra. For example, some large ureteroceles extend into the urethra but are backed by good bladder muscularis. These are not as significant as some smaller ureteroceles with large bladder wall defects. Some involve significant defects in the bladder neck. A VCUG in more significant ureterocele cases will often show a bladder diverticulum or bladder neck defect. These are the more difficult cases which will often require posterior bladder wall and sometimes bladder neck reconstruction.

In the past, the usual presentation for a child with a ureterocele was that of a urinary tract infection. The first infection usually happens within the first few months of life. Ureteroceles are being recognized more frequently in the prenatal period with the use of antenatal ultrasonography (Fig. 53.4). Other ways of presenting include a palpable mass from a dilated upper pole, distended bladder from bladder outlet obstruction, incontinence, failure to thrive, gastrointestinal symptoms and irritative voiding symptoms.

Ureteroceles in non-duplicated systems are more common in boys. The adult type is diagnosed later and is of little clinical significance but may present with pain, infection, stone or haematuria. Renal function is often normal. On an intravenous urogram (IVU), both the lumen of the ureterocele and bladder fill with contrast. However, the wall of the ureterocele is not filled with contrast and therefore is visible as a thin lucent line or halo outlining its lumen, giving it the characteristic shape of a cobra head or spring onion. Some degree of hydronephrosis and/or hydroureter can also be seen on IVU. On VCUG, the ureterocele forms a filling defect in the bladder, and with voiding the ureterocele may collapse (Fig. 53.5). The filling defect in the bladder caused by the ureterocele can also be demon-

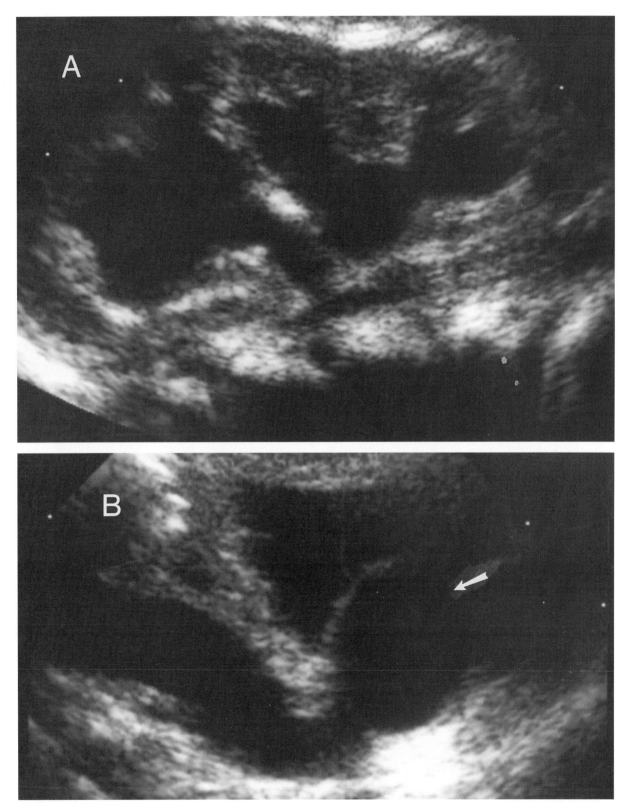

Fig. 53.4 Newborn with antenatal diagnosis of hydronephrosis: (A) ultrasound of left kidney demonstrating upper and lower pole dilatation; (B) ultrasound of bladder demonstrating ureterocele (white arrow) and distal ureteral dilatation. The patient was treated with cystoscopy and incision of the ureterocele.

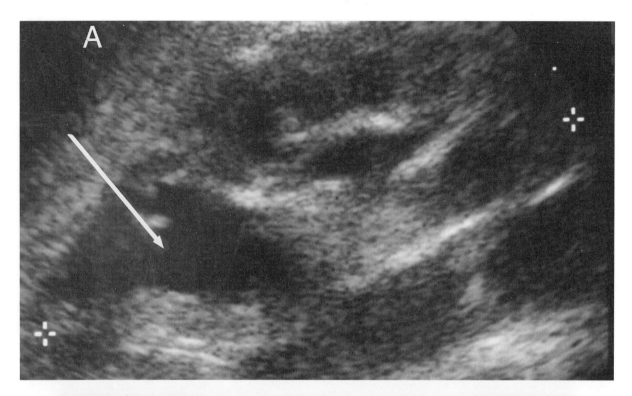

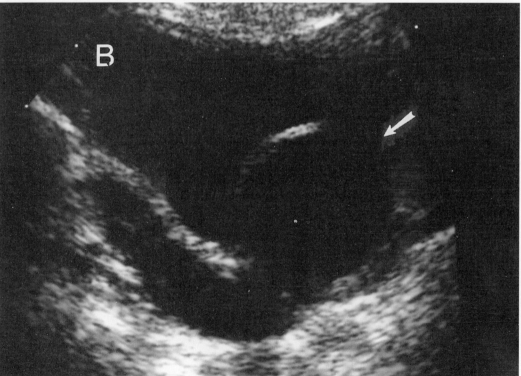

Fig. 53.5 A 5-month-old male with antenatal left hydronephrosis: (A) ultrasound of left kidney with upper pole hydronephrosis (white arrow); (B) ultrasound of bladder showing ureterocele (white arrow) and dilated distal ureter; (C) VCUG demonstrating filling defect in bladder (black arrow); (D) collapse of ureterocele with bladder filling; (E) DTPA renal scan demonstrating perfusion defect and 5% of renal function from the left upper pole. The patient underwent left upper pole nephroureterectomy.

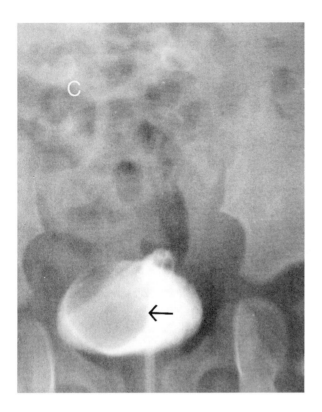

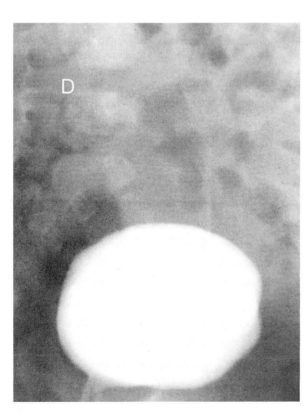

strated well on ultrasound. Management of the patient with a ureterocele involving a single ureter depends on the function of the associated renal unit and the detrusor backing behind the ureterocele. Most intravesical ureteroceles are unlikely to have a detrimental effect on the contralateral kidney or bladder neck. In such ureteroceles with good renal function and good muscular backing endoscopic incision is adequate. This can often be performed in the newborn period and relieves obstruction, resulting in recovery of renal function. Several investigators have reported reflux rates of up to 80% following incision of ureteroceles (Kelalis, 1985). A low transverse incision of the ureterocele maybe effective in preserving a flap valve mechanism (Rich *et al.*, 1985). Ureteroceles associated with a single ureter may be incised using a 3 fr. Bugbee electrode (Blyth *et al.*, 1993). The point of puncture into the ureterocele is just above its base and parallel to the floor of the bladder. Thirteen patients out of a series of 16 with single-system intravesical ureteroceles did not require a second procedure. If there is VUR following incision of a ureterocele, the patient should be managed with

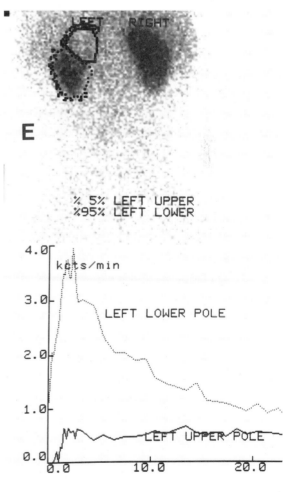

Fig. 53.5 Continued.

antibiotic prophylaxis. If the reflux persists then elective reimplant can be done in the future, when the child is older and the ureteral dilatation has had a chance to improve. If there is poor muscular support behind the ureterocele, this should be repaired at the time of reimplant to prevent later diverticulum formation and facilitate bladder emptying. Newer endoscopic equipment allows clear evaluation and safe incision of the ureterocele. Before the introduction of these instruments, the preferred management was open ureterocele excision and ureteral reimplantation. Detrusor repair and ureteral tailoring are often necessary with this approach. An extravesical ureterocele in a single system is usually associated with poorly functioning renal tissue. The approach in this case should be excision of the ureterocele with reimplantation of the ureter or a simple nephroureterectomy, depending on the renal function.

Three features of a ureterocele in a duplicated system can be seen on IVU. A mass is visible in the upper pole of the affected kidney and only 10% of these systems excrete contrast material. A radiolucent filling defect is seen in the bladder. This is seen early in the study and results from non-opacified urine in the ureterocele surrounded by opacified urine in the bladder. When the ureterocele is small, the defect lies eccentrically in the bladder on the same side of the bladder as the ureterocele and, when large, the defect is spherical. There are also changes related to obstruction and/or reflux to the lower pole of the affected side, as well as the contralateral kidney. Late in the IVU, the ureterocele may be compressed by the full bladder and not be visible. Occasionally with ureteroceles in duplicated systems there may not be any hydronephrosis or hydroureter in the upper pole, making it very difficult to diagnose by looking at the upper tracts (ureterocele disproportion) (Share and Liebowitz, 1989). Ultrasound, VCUG and scintigraphy may aid in the diagnosis of ureterocele disproportion.

Ultrasonography is often the first study that establishes the diagnosis. Findings on ultrasonography that suggest ureterocele are:

- fluid-filled mass in the upper pole of the kidney
- dilatation of the upper pole ureter
- fluid filled mass in the bladder, either occupying the entire bladder or on the same side as the fluid-filled mass in the upper pole of the kidney.

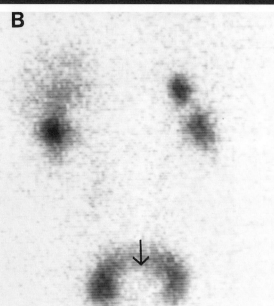

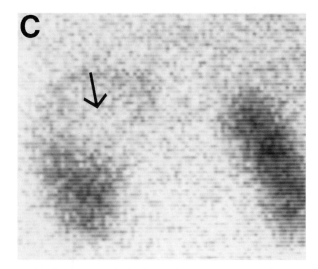

Fig. 53.6 A 9-month-old female with urinary tract infection and right upper pole hydronephrosis: (A) VCUG demonstrating filling defect in bladder (black arrow); (B) renal scan also showing filling defect in bladder (black arrow); (C) poor perfusion of left upper pole (black arrow) on renal scan.

As mentioned already hydronephrosis or hydroureter to the lower pole system and the contralateral kidney, may also be seen.

With VCUG the ureterocele is seen as a filling defect during the filling phase (Fig. 53.6). During the voiding phase there is often reflux to the ipsilateral lower pole and contralateral ureter and occasionally to the ureterocele itself. If there is poor muscle backing the ureterocele, the ureterocele can invert and resemble a diverticulum.

Surgical options in the management of the ureterocele in a duplicated system vary. The surgical approach depends on the patient's age, health, amount of function in the different renal segments and status of the lower urinary tract. The goals of treatment are to preserve as much renal function as possible, correct any bladder outlet obstruction, correct any vesicoureteral reflux and repair the detrusor defect.

The options in management are either a single procedure dealing with both the upper and lower tracts or a staged reconstruction, but the final decision is based on the amount of upper pole function. Most surgeons agree that with poor upper pole function, upper pole heminephrectomy and partial ureterectomy, which allows for decompression of the ureterocele, is the treatment of choice. If reflux is present to the lower pole or contralateral ureter, reimplant surgery can be performed at the same time or at a later date. Transvesical excision of the ureterocele can be performed at the time of ureteroneocystostomy. Patients being observed for resolution of their reflux must remain on antibiotic prophylaxis. With good upper pole function the choices are ureteropyelostomy with ureterectomy or common sheath reimplant. Again, if reflux is present, reimplantation can be performed at the time of upper tract surgery or at a later date. Transurethral incision of the ureterocele is an appropriate approach for several groups: those with questionable function who may need more time for renal recovery, sick children who cannot tolerate a major operation, patients with sepsis not responsive to conservative treatment and patients with high-grade reflux who will probably need bladder surgery at a later date.

References

Barrett, D.M., Malek, R.S. and Kelalis, P.P. 1975: Problems and solutions in surgical treatment of 100 consecutive ureteral duplications in children. *Journal of Urology* **114**, 126.

Bissett, G.S. and Strife, J.L. 1987: The duplex collecting system in girls with urinary tract infection: prevention and signifigance. *American Journal of Roentgenology* **148**, 497.

Blyth, B., Passerini-Glazel, G., Camuffo, C., Snyder, H.M. and Duckett, J.W. 1993: Endoscopic incision of ureteroceles: intravesical versus ectopic. *Journal of Urology* **149**, 556.

Caldamone, A.A. 1985: Duplication anomalies of the upper tract in infants and children. In *Urologic Clinics of North America*. Philadelphia, PA: W.B. Saunders, 75.

Churchill, B.M., Abara, E.O. and McLorie, G.A. 1987: Ureteral duplication, ectopy and ureteroceles. *Pediatric Clinics of North America* **34**, 1273.

Ericsson, N.O. 1954: Ectopic ureterocele in infants and children. *Acta Chirurgica Scandinavica* **197** (Suppl.), 8.

Gillatt, D.A. and Feneley, R.C.L. 1994: Magnetic resonance imaging in the identification of an otherwise undetectable upper pole moiety. *British Journal of Urology* **73**, 470.

Glassberg, K.I., Braren, V., Duckett, J.W. *et al.* 1984: Suggested terminology for duplex systems, ectopic ureters and ureteroceles. *Journal of Urology* **132**, 1153.

Husmann, D.A. and Allen, T.D. 1991: Resolution of vesicoureteral reflux in completely duplicated systems: fact or fiction? *Journal of Urology* **145**, 1022.

Janetschek, G., Seibold, J., Radmayr, C. and Bartsch, G. 1997: Laparoscopic heminephroureterectomy in pediatric patients. *Journal of Urology* **158**, 1928.

Joseph, D.B., Bauer, S.B. and Colodny, A.H. 1989: Lower pole ureteropelvic junction obstruction and incomplete renal duplication. *Journal of Urology* **141**, 896.

Kelalis, P.P 1985: Renal pelvis and ureter. In Kelalis, P.P., King, L.R. and Belman, A.B. (eds), *Clinical pediatric urology*, vol. 2, 2nd ed. Philadelphia, PA: W.B. Saunders, Chap. 18, 687–719.

Kelalis, P.P., King, L.R. and Belman, A.B. (eds) 1992: *Clinical pediatric urology*. Philadelphia, PA: W.B. Saunders, Chap. 15, 531.

Mackie, G, G, and Stephens, F.D. 1975: Duplex kidneys: a correlation of renal dysplasia with position of ureteral orifice. *Journal of Urology* **114**, 274.

Mandell, J., Bauer, S.B., Colodny, A.M. *et al.* 1981: Ureteral ectopia in infants and children. *Journal of Urology* **126**, 219.

Nation, E.F. 1944: Duplication of the kidney and ureter: a statistical study of two hundred thirty new cases. *Journal of Urology* **51**, 456.

O'Reilly, P.H., Shields, R.A., Testa, H.G. *et al.* 1984: Ureterouretic reflux. Pathologic entity or physiologic phenomenon? *British Journal of Urology* **56**, 159.

Potter, E.L. 1972: *Normal and abnormal development of the kidney*. Chicago, IL: Year Book Medical Publishers, 3.

Rich, M.A., Keating, M.A., Snyder, H.M. and Duckett, J.W. 1990: Low transurethral incision of single system intravesical ureteroceles in children. *Journal of Urology* **144**, 120.

Share, J.C. and Liebowitz, R.L. 1989: Ectopic ureterocele without ureteral and calyceal dilatation (ureterocele disproportion): findings on urography and sonography. *American Journal of Radiology* **152**, 567.

Weigert, C. 1877: Uber einige Bildungsfehler der Ureteren. *Virchow's Archiv (Pathol Anat)* **70**, 490.

CHAPTER 54

Vesico-ureteric reflux

J.E.S. SCOTT

Introduction	Familial ureteric reflux
Physiology	Management of ureteric reflux
Pathology	Dysfunctional voiding
Effects of reflux	Surgical management
Diagnosis	Conclusions
Fetal ureteric reflux	References

Introduction

Few topics in paediatric surgery can have prompted as many contributions to the literature as vesicoureteric reflux (VUR). From 1984 to 1994 the [mean range] (SD) number of publications appearing annually in the English language alone was 89.1 [68–106] (12.3) (source, Medline, Silver Platter). It is quite possible that a similar number was also being published in preceding decades. What more is there to write about? This author posed this question in the early 1970s but wrote at some length; he did it again in 1985 and in 1987 but hopes that something different was said on each of these occasions (Scott, 1972, 1985a, 1987a). Why is there such an abiding interest in this condition? Firstly, because it is common: it will be found in 35% of children with proven urinary tract infection (Ericsson, 1960; Rosenheim, 1963; Smellie *et al.*, 1964; Stansfeld, 1966); secondly, because the peak age incidence for the onset of urinary infection is in the first year of life, most commonly in the newborn (Smellie *et al.*, 1964; Stansfeld, 1966); and thirdly, because, despite the volume of research and writing, the condition still, with inexorable predictability, continues to be responsible for end-stage renal failure in at least 15% of adults (Markland and Kelly, 1968; Smellie *et al.*, 1980) and 30% of children (Bailey and Lynn, 1984).

Background information on the pathology and physiology of ureteric reflux may be obtained from reading Scott (1972, 1985a, 1987a) together with the books quoted in Hodson and Kincaid-Smith (1979), Bailey and Lynn (1984) and Johnston, (1984) to facilitate an understanding of what follows in this chapter the fundamentals of the condition will briefly be described.

Physiology

Urine which is secreted by the kidney is propelled into the bladder by the peristaltic activity of unstriated muscle in the wall of the ureter. This activity responds to either increased secretion rate or increased resistance to flow (i.e. by the distending bladder) by increased peristaltic contraction amplitude and frequency. Under normal conditions, having been ejected into the bladder, urine does not re-enter the ureter because the ureteric orifice in the bladder is guarded by a one-way valvular mechanism which has the following three components.

- A mucosal flap valve: this is a delicate 'flutter' valve that covers the ureteric orifice and is constructed from two layers of mucosa, one on the bladder aspect (bladder mucosa) and one on the ureteric aspect (ureteric mucosa).
- Ureteric orifice fixation: as the ureter penetrates the wall of the bladder the longitudinal muscle fibres in its wall peel off the ventral surface to join those on the dorsal surface and continue distally beneath the mucosa of the trigone beyond the orifice itself.

The fibres condense into two main bundles, one of which runs horizontally to join a similar bundle from the contralateral ureter to form the interureteric ridge, while the other runs downwards and medially to become attached to the muscle surrounding the internal urethral meatus. These bundles anchor the ureteric orifice so that it cannot displace upwards, away from the bladder neck as might otherwise tend to happen whenever there was a rise in intravesical pressure.

- The intramural tunnel: there is dispute between anatomists as to whether Waldeyer described a sheath or a space but whichever it is the ureter is only loosely attached to the detrusor muscle as it penetrates the bladder wall. Thus, as the bladder distends and its wall stretches, a greater length of the ureter becomes intramural (because the orifice cannot move as a result of uteric orifice fixation) and the intramural tunnel elongates. This increases its valvular properties just at the time when voiding is imminent and intravesical pressure is beginning to rise. This phenomenon can occasionally be seen during cystographic examinations; reflux may appear soon after contrast enters the bladder but as the bladder fills the ureter ejects the contrast and no further reflux is seen.

There is one other mechanism which is self-evident, namely ureteric peristalsis itself. Even if the apparatus protecting the orifice fails, peristalsis can continue to prevent reflux by responding in its characteristic manner to increased flow resistance. However, the response is likely to be short lived because persistently high emptying pressure will cause ureteric muscle fatigue.

Pathology

Ureteric reflux is an abnormal phenomenon and is due to a developmental abnormality of the ureteric orifice and its antireflux mechanisms. It almost certainly commences during fetal life when urine starts to be secreted at between the tenth and twelfth weeks of gestation. The incidence of fetal reflux is impossible to determine as there is at present no reliable means of detecting it; and ultrasound is inadequate. Dilatation of the fetal kidney is seen in approximately 2% of all antenatal ultrasound scans but there is no correlation between the degree of dilatation and gestational age, nor is it possible to predict whether a dilated kidney will return to normal later in pregnancy or postnatally or whether the dilatation will increase.

Effects of reflux

Two important characteristics need to be grasped in order to understand the implications of reflux.

- By itself, reflux is both asymptomatic and non-pathogenic. Thus, unless some other factor is involved there must be many individuals whose urinary tracts are affected by reflux but who are unaware of it.
- Reflux has a strong propensity to disappear spontaneously in the first few years of childhood. Estimates as to the frequency with which this happens vary from 40% to 80% by the age of 10 years.

The factors that induce pathogenicity in reflux are outflow tract obstruction and urinary tract infection.

OUTFLOW TRACT OBSTRUCTION

The male urethra has a naturally higher flow resistance than the female. Ureteric reflux in the fetus is therefore seen more commonly in males than in females and is significantly more severe. At birth, the upper urinary may be grossly dilated and tortuous and there is evidence that in some cases nephric development may be adversely affected. In the presence of an organic urethral obstruction such as posterior urethral valves a refluxing upper urinary tract is, at birth, likely to be even more dilated. There will also be serious impairment of renal development manifested by areas of cystic dysplasia together with gross dilatation and atrophy due to the back-pressure. Early end-stage renal failure is an inevitable consequence.

URINARY TRACT INFECTION

This is the most frequent manifestation of reflux and it should prompt a detailed investigation to determine whether reflux is present. The infection commences in the bladder whence bacteria are transported into the kidney in urine refluxing along the ureters. They may then be carried through the tubular orifices on the renal papillae into the tubules (intrarenal reflux) and produce areas of inflammation in the renal parenchyma which later heal and proceed to scarring. Experimental work has suggested that only certain orifices, those which are abnormally wide, permit intrarenal reflux to occur. If this is the case the process of invasion, inflammation and scarring will be initiated maximally in a solitary area of the kidney at the time of the first infection; an 'all-or-none' phenomenon. However, other observers, working in the clinical field, think that scarring occurs gradually, increasing in extent with each episode of infection, with new scars appearing at later times in the child's history. The controversy is of some importance because it influences the management of reflux and it will be discussed later in this chapter. The combination of renal parenchymal scarring and ureteric reflux is usually referred to as reflux nephropathy although, since the whole urinary tract is involved in the process, reflux uropathy might be a more sensible term. The extent to which the kidneys are affected varies from just one pole of one kidney to widespread bilateral disease. The effect of this process on a child's kidney is highly significant, although it may not become apparent until puberty. The primary disturbance produced by parenchymal scarring in the long term is interference with renal growth. This must occur at the same rate as the whole child and may do so until the pubertal growth spurt is entered. At that time the child's growth velocity increases significantly but kidneys which are extensively scarred will not grow with the same velocity. If involvement is bilateral, glomerular filtration will no longer satisfy requirement and renal failure will ensue. The effect on renal growth is particularly obvious in asymmetric or unilateral disease: the comparatively healthy kidney undergoes marked hypertrophy while the affected one may actually seem to shrink. It is evident that it is the onset of infection in the presence of reflux which triggers the process of diagnosis and the train of events which may lead to severe renal damage with its subsequent complications such as hypertension and renal failure. Once the diagnosis is made the choice is between eliminating the reflux surgically and treating the infections as and when they occur or prescribing long-term prophylactic antibacterial therapy and waiting for the reflux to resolve spontaneously. This is discussed later. However, notwithstanding the effectiveness of treatment in controlling infection and eradicating reflux it is evident that neither method has the advantage when outcome is assessed. Because reflux is seldom diagnosed until a symptomatic urinary infection has occurred, the process which culminates in reflux nephropathy has already been set in motion by the time reflux is demonstrated. What is necessary is a means of detecting reflux before the first episode of infection occurs. In turn, this means investigating the newborn and, at the moment, there are no non-invasive methods which are sufficiently reliable.

Diagnosis

REFLUX

X-ray cystography remains the standard technique for demonstrating reflux because on many occasions it is necessary to show not only whether or not reflux is present but also the degree of dilatation that it causes in the upper urinary tract and, for example, which pole of a duplex kidney it affects. In particular, it demonstrates the size and outline of the bladder, the presence or absence of diverticula and, in males, the shape and characteristics of the urethra by micturition urethrography. However, on other occasions, all that may be required is simply to reveal that reflux is or is not present. This may occur when children are under continuing supervision for reflux treated operatively or non-operatively. Furthermore, now that urinary tract disorders are being suspected in increasing numbers antenatally, it is becoming necessary to initiate the

investigations in the newborn or in the early weeks of life and thus, it is important to reduce radiation dosages to the lowest possible levels. The possibility of employing ultrasound for this purpose has been explored and although some workers have advocated this technique (Coulden *et al.*, 1990; Bergius *et al.*, 1990), others have found it unreliable (Jequier *et al.*, 1985), Rickwood *et al.*, 1992). A better method is direct radioisotope cystography, in which a solution containing a measured dose of ^{99m}Tc diethylene triamine pentacetic acid (DTPA) is injected into the bladder through a urethral catheter (Van den Abeele *et al.*, 1987; Kenda *et al.*, 1991) and images of the urinary tract are made with a gamma camera. The technique is highly sensitive in detecting reflux but the images are insufficiently detailed for anatomical analysis.

In older children, who have developed voluntary bladder control, indirect radioisotope cystography is another useful technique for supervising the progress of reflux after diagnosis by conventional cystography (Gordon *et al.*, 1990). The radioisotope is given intravenously and the renal images observed until all the radioisotope has cleared and entered the bladder. The child is then asked to empty the bladder and the kidneys immediately scanned. If reflux is present, the radioisotope will be observed again in the kidneys. The technique has the advantage of avoiding catheterization but is impractical in young infants.

RENAL SCARRING

Intravenous urography is necessary for the diagnosis of any structural defect in the upper urinary tract and is also an excellent method of detecting abnormalities in the renal parenchyma, but radioisotope imaging has been shown to be more sensitive. Since the mid-1970s, dimercaptosuccinic acid (DMSA) labelled with ^{99m}technetium has been shown to be superior to other metal chelates in demonstrating the renal parenchyma in gamma camera exposures (Enlander *et al.*, 1974; Handmaker *et al.*, 1975; MacDonald *et al.*, 1977). Sixty per cent of an administered dose concentrates in the cells of the proximal convoluted tubule (Willis *et al.*, 1977) and only 10% is excreted in the urine in the first 2 hours. It has been shown that the renal uptake of the isotope represents an accurate measurement of individual renal function (Kawamura *et al.*, 1978; Born *et al.*, 1978), and correlates well with creatinine clearance (Daly *et al.*, 1977). It is also more sensitive at detecting renal parenchymal scarring than intravenous urography (Merrick *et al.*, 1980; Verber *et al.*, 1988). Thus a DMSA scan is essential in the investigation of any child who has or may have had ureteric reflux as it demonstrates the structural integrity of the renal parenchyma and the percentage distribution of function between the two kidneys. It is of no value, however, in demonstrating obstruction to drainage.

RENAL FUNCTION

Serum creatinine is the usual method of measuring overall renal function and from this an estimate of glomerular filtration rate (GFR) in ml/min/1.73 m^2 can be made using body surface area (Counahan *et al.*, 1976), although it has been suggested that in the newborn, body weight is a more valid parameter against which to measure glomerular filtration than surface area (Coulthard and Hey, 1984). As a predictor of outcome in newborns with renal damage caused antenatally, GFR is superior to serum creatinine and the appropriate steps to measure it should be taken in such cases (Scott, 1985b). The most accurate technique for measuring GFR is by inulin clearance but this is not suitable as a routine in newborns and young children; furthermore, when renal function in the presence of VUR is under consideration, it is individual renal function that is often required. For this purpose ^{99m}Tc-labelled DTPA can be used as it provides not only an indirect measurement of glomerular filtration but, if gamma emission from the kidneys is measured by fine collimators, a time–activity curve. However, the factors that influence the shape of this curve are numerous and often misinterpreted. As with DMSA, uptake is dependent in the first instance on renal blood flow, but thereafter it is governed by the number of functioning glomeruli in the kidney. If this is reduced as a result, for example, of renal scarring, uptake will not be as high or as rapid as in the normal because less of the radioisotope is filtered from the blood each time the administered bolus passes through the kidney. Thus the time–activity curve will rise slowly and may not reach the peak achieved by a normal kidney, and a comparison between the two sides is immediately possible. It is important to note that DTPA measures glomerular filtration, but it does not measure urine transport and excretion rates and should not be used for this purpose. In the normal, mature newborn, GFR is only 25 ml/min/1.73 m^2 and it does not rise to adult values until the age of approximately 3 years. So, to attempt to measure renal excretion rates in a kidney with a low GFR using a radioisotope carrier which is filtered by the glomeruli is absurd. If there is a need to determine renal excretion and drainage rates, a carrier that is secreted by the tubules should be employed, such as ^{99m}Tc mercaptoacetyl triglyceride (MAG3). Even here, caution should be exercised because if the renal pelvis is dilated and atonic, it is customary to administer a diuretic such as furosemide in order to wash out the radioisotope, and this is supposed to distinguish an obstructed from a non-obstructed kidney. However, if there is tubular damage, the effect of the diuretic will be reduced and the radioisotope will remain in the renal pelvis even though it is not organically obstructed. Such a situation may be observed when there is advanced ureteric reflux.

Fetal ureteric reflux

What seems to have been the first observation that dilatation of the fetal upper urinary tract might be due to ureteric reflux was made by Philipson *et al.* in 1984. Subsequently, the term fetal ureteric reflux was advocated as, although none of the cases described was subjected to cystography *in utero*, the fact that reflux must have been present during intrauterine life is indisputable (Scott, 1987b). Certain features of such cases are noteworthy: (i) 80–90% are male, (ii) reflux is bilateral in 60% or more and (iii) reflux is of a high grade (MRC grade 3; Medical Research Council, 1979) in 60% or more. This type of reflux in the fetus does not include those with any form of obstructive uropathy such as posterior urethral valves. It is well known that the combination of reflux and obstruction has devastating effects on the kidney. The ominous feature of fetal ureteric reflux is that evidence of abnormalities in renal parenchymal integrity can be found at or soon after birth, before urinary infection has occurred (Anderson and Rickwood, 1991; Scott, 1993), although this is disputed by one group who claimed that renal parenchymal damage in the majority of kidneys occurs only after an episode of infection (Crabbe *et al.*, 1992). However, histological studies of nephrectomized specimens suggest that there is a strong association between hypoplastic changes in the kidney and reflux and that these changes may be present from early fetal life (Hinchcliff *et al.*, 1992). Whichever is correct it is clearly necessary to prevent infection by appreciating the need for postnatal investigation in babies who showed signs of urinary tract dilatation antenatally and, if reflux is discovered, giving them long-term antibacterial therapy. In 20–30% of the babies (Elder, 1992; Scott, 1993) reflux disappears spontaneously within the first 2 years of life but, when it does not, there is a tendency for it to deteriorate, as shown by increasing upper urinary tract dilatation. Furthermore, these children are prone to episodes of urinary infection and continuous antibacterial therapy is obligatory to prevent them. It has been suggested that if the reflux has not disappeared or shown signs of improvement by the second birthday, it should be treated surgically. Even if this operation is successful, further complications may ensue. The gross dilatation of the renal pelves caused by the reflux produces marked atony so that they have a tendency to obstruct themselves by sagging over the pelviureteric junction, and operative reconstruction of the pelviureteric junction may be required to prevent this.

Familial ureteric reflux

Possibly the first description of ureteric reflux in a family was published by Stephens *et al.* (1955) as a case report of reflux in twins. Since then the literature on the subject has expanded at a fast rate. The significant features of the phenomenon were described in a recent publication which incorporated the findings in a large series collected over 10 years (Noe, 1992). From this and other studies it appears that approximately 35% of the siblings of index cases will have reflux and of these 75% will be asymptomatic. The incidence of reflux in the offspring of mothers who have or have been treated for reflux is even higher, at 66% (Noe *et al.*, 1992). But what is the significance of this? Does familial reflux carry the same implications as symptomatic reflux? Is it justifiable to subject asymptomatic children to an invasive investigation to detect it? There is no answer to these questions because there have been no properly conducted long-term randomized prospective trials to determine what does happen to children whose reflux is discovered because one of their siblings or their mother has it. Is it advisable, for example, to administer continuous antibacterial chemotherapy to prevent urinary infection and renal scarring? It is said (Noe *et al.*, 1992) that the incidence of renal damage is lower in sibling than in index cases, but if the siblings were genuinely asymptomatic, how did any of their kidneys become damaged? Presumably, either they had occult episodes of urinary infection or the damage was due mainly to the hydrodynamic effects of the reflux.

The propensity for reflux to occur in families has now been employed as a means of identifying antenatally newborn babies who are likely to have reflux (Scott *et al.*, 1997). A group of pregnant women were screened for a history of reflux in themselves, their previous offspring or other members of their families. When the history was positive the newborn babies were subjected to cystography; reflux was present in over 20%. Early diagnosis may enable urinary infection and thus reflux nephropathy to be avoided by prescribing long-term prophylactic chemotherapy.

Management of ureteric reflux

The contentious issue has been whether to treat reflux by surgery or by non-operative measures. Again, randomized controlled trials were necessary to answer this question. The first attempt to mount such a trial was made by Scott and Stansfeld in 1968. It suggested that the outcome after 3 years for operated cases was superior to unoperated cases in terms of both kidney growth rate and incidence of urinary infection. With hindsight, it is clear that the trial contained an inadequate number of subjects for reliable results, but it did, at least, stimulate others to organize further trials, although it was nearly 15 years before their results appeared. The findings suggested that the difference between the two methods of treatment, when measured by factors such as the incidence of urinary infection, maintenance of renal function, kidney growth and scarring, was not significant. However, some researchers noted that although operated children developed bacteriuria as frequently as did unoperated children, the presence and severity of symptoms was less (Elo *et al.*, 1983). One of the difficulties in assessing the validity of the reflux trials is disagreement as to how reflux should be graded. This author has always favoured simplicity and has advocated the MRC (1979) three-grade system, but a five-grade system was chosen by the International Reflux Study Committee (IRSC) (1981). Grading reflux in children beyond the age of 3 years is of little clinical relevance because of the tendency for reflux to improve or disappear spontaneously after this age. The discovery of the reflux and decisions as to its management should nowadays have been made by that time. In a 5-year trial of surgery in children with severe reflux (Birmingham Reflux study Group, 1987), there was no significant difference between operated and non-operated cases with respect to the incidence of urinary infection, renal scarring, renal function or renal growth. Reports from the IRSC at 5 years confirmed this finding (Smellie, 1992; Smellie *et al.*, 1992; Jodal *et al.*, 1992; Weiss *et al.*, 1992). Close examination of these papers, however, revealed certain interesting features. Whenever outcome analysis segregated pyelonephritis from urinary infection as a whole, the incidence of this complication was always significantly higher in unoperated children (Hjalmas *et al.*, 1992; Jodal *et al.*, 1992; Smellie, 1992; Weis *et al.*, 1992), presumably because organisms were continuing to gain access to their kidneys via the reflux. Furthermore, although, as expected, reflux in the lower grades disappeared in 50–60% of children, particularly if it was unilateral (Tamminen-Mobius *et al.*, 1992), in the higher grades the disappearance rate was only around 25%. There were also flaws in the conduct of the trial characterized by patients being moved from one arm to the other, mostly from the medical to the surgical (Duckett *et al.*, 1992) which would inevitably affect the validity of statistical analysis. One factor taken into account by all of the contributors was the incidence, at the beginning and end of the trial, of renal scarring: it was the same in both groups and the number of new scars that appeared during the trial was also the same. In the author's view this was inevitable because there must be considerable doubt as to whether a new scar ever occurs (Scott, 1975, 1984, 1985a, 1987a). Such a hypothesis is inconvenient for those who desire clear-cut answers based on categorical data. What these workers fail to grasp is that children and their kidneys grow and that this simple fact must have a very important bearing on the radiographic and radioisotopic appearances of their kidneys. This variable which been completely ignored in the assessment of progress in children with reflux. Changes in the renal parenchyma in children included in the international reflux trial were judged on the basis of radiographic findings. There is likely to be a considerable delay following the infective event when such findings demonstrate a change. If the intravenous urogram performed a few weeks after an incident of infection in a child of, say, 6 months is normal, but when repeated at the age of 7 years reveals a renal scar, there is no proof that the scar is 'new'. It is just as likely to be caused by the infection episode which occurred at 6 months; and has become visible radiographically because the damaged area of the kidney has not grown whereas the healthy areas have. This is known as the astronomical theory: when an observer gazes at a star, the light seen was emitted from it several hundred light years previously, it is not 'new light'. This is possibly the explanation for the renal scarring noted at follow-up in a group of children, recently reported, who were managed entirely medically (Arant, 1992). With the advent of the more sensitive radioisotope test using DMSA it should be possible to prove or disprove this hypothesis.

Dysfunctional voiding

Various titles have been applied to this condition, such as uninhibited bladder, unstable bladder and bladder–sphincter dysenergia, but they all amount to the same underlying state, namely, bladder immaturity. The automatic inhibitory mechanism fails to mature so the child experiences sudden and urgent calls to void, which are overcome by energetic voluntary contraction of the external urethral sphincter assisted by the other manoeuvres (De Jonge, 1973). During these episodes, intravesical pressure will inevitably rise and potential reflux will become actual. A significant number of children with reflux do have bladder dysfunction (Van Gool *et al.*, 1992) and it is worth prescribing anticholinergic drugs such as propantheline or oxybutynin for them. Apart from helping their distressing symptoms, it will facilitate spontaneous resolution of their reflux.

Surgical management

A summary of most of the established operations for the treatment of ureteric reflux was published previously (Scott, 1972). Since then there have been two noteworthy additions to the choice of surgery, the first of which is the Cohen (1975) procedure. This involves mobilizing the ureter from within the bladder and rerouting it through a submucosal tunnel to the opposite side. Both ureters can be treated in a similar manner so that they lie on the base of the bladder like folded arms. The technique is effective in eliminating reflux but if, postoperatively, it is necessary to catheterize the ureters endoscopically for any reason, it is virtually impossible to guide a catheter through the new orifice. The second technique is the endoscopic injection of polytetrafluoroethylene (Teflon) paste submucosally under the intravesical segment of the ureter (Puri and O'Donnell, 1984; O'Donnell and Puri, 1984, 1988). This method is

undoubtedly successful in eliminating reflux in over 85% of ureters (Schulman *et al.*, 1990; Schulman and Sassine, 1992), but concern has been raised about possible complications arising from the use of Teflon. For example, granulomatous polyps have arisen at or near the injection site, probably due to introducing the substance slightly too deeply or to its leakage into surrounding tissues (Brown *et al.*, 1991). Of more significance is experimental work demonstrating migration of Teflon particles from the intravesical injection site to the brain and lungs (Rames and Aaronson, 1991; Aaronson, 1993; Aaronson *et al.*, 1993). If this occurs in human subjects to the same extent as in experimental animals, it is of serious concern. The life expectancy of the patients being treated is 60–70 years, so the long-term outcome must be speculative. Furthermore, a foreign body, albeit allegedly biologically inert, is located for many decades immediately beneath an epithelium which is notoriously unstable. The effect on the activity of the epithelium must also be speculative. Because of these concerns other materials have been investigated. One report described the use in experimental animals of a self-sealing silicone balloon. The balloon was implanted endoscopically beneath a refluxing ureteric orifice and then inflated with hydroxyethylmethyl acrylate. The technique eliminated reflux and no migration or granuloma formation was detected (Atala *et al.*, 1992). Another technique employed collagen instead of Teflon (Frey *et al.*, 1992). The antireflux success rate was reasonably good and histological examination of the collagen implants showed that they were invaded by host fibroblasts which laid down human collagen. However, the collagen was bovine in origin and now that transmission of the disease to humans has apparently occurred, the risk of introducing the agent which causes Creutzfeldt–Jakob disease must be considered.

Conclusions

Despite decades of intense study, VUR continues to be a major contributor to the incidence of chronic renal insufficiency, hypertension and end-stage renal failure. Surgical and endoscopic methods of eliminating reflux are successful and straightforward and have a low complication rate. But, with the exception of the grosser degrees of reflux, the end results, in terms of recurrent urinary infection, renal scarring and renal failure, are no better than non-operative management, although the symptoms of pyelonephritis may be relieved. It is clear that the wrong aspect of the scenario has been the source of interest. To prevent the trail of damaged kidneys that it leaves in its wake, reflux must be detected before the complications ensue, i.e. in the newborn. An effective screening method is required that can identify those babies who are at risk, because performing cystography on every newborn is absurdly unacceptable.

References

Aaronson, I.A, Rames, R., Greene, W.B. *et al.* Endoscopic treatment of reflux: migration of Teflon to lungs and brain. *European Urology* **23**, 394–9.

Aaronson, I.A. 1993: Die endoskopische Refluxkorrecktur: Einfach, aber auch sicher? *Akt Urology* **24**, 65–6.

Anderson, P.A.M. and Rickwood, A.M.K. 1991: Features of primary vesicoureteric reflux detected by prenatal sonography. *British Journal of Urology* **67**, 267–71.

Arant, B.S. 1992: Medical management of mild and moderate vesicoureteral reflux: follow-up studies of infants and young children. A preliminary report of the Southwest Pediatric Nephrology Study Group. *Journal of Urology* **148**, 1683–7.

Atala, A., Peters, C.A., Retik, A.B. and Mandell, J. 1992: Endoscopic treatment of vesicoureteral reflux with a self-detachable balloon system. *Journal of Urology* **148**, 724–7.

Bailey, R.R. and Lynn, K.L. 1984: End-stage reflux nephropathy. In Hodson, C.J., Heptinstall, R.H. and Winberg, J. (eds), *Reflux nephropathy update*. Basle: Karger, 102–10.

Bergius, A.R., Niskanen, K. and Kekomaki, M. 1990: Detection of significant vesicoureteric reflux by ultrasound in infants and children. *Zeitschrift für Kinderchirurgie* **45**, 144–5.

Birmingham Refux Study Group 1987: Prospective trial of operative versus non-operative treatment of severe vesicoureteric reflux in children: five years' observation. *British Medical Journal of Clinical Research and Education* **295**, 237–41.

Born, M.L., Grove, R.B., Jones, J.P. *et al.* 1978: Correlation of differential renal function determination by ^{99m}Tc DMSA imaging and ureteral catheterisation. *Journal of Nuclear Medicine* **19**, 721.

Brown, S., Stewart, R.J., O'Hara, M.D. and Hill, C.M. 1991: Histological changes following submucosal Teflon injection in the bladder. *Journal of Pediatric Surgery* **26**, 546–7.

Cohen, S.J. 1975: Ureterozystoneostomie: eine neue Antirefluxtechnik. *Akt Urology* **6**, 1–6.

Coulden, R.A., Hanbury, D.C. and Farman, P. 1990: Ultrasound cystography: a valuable technique. *British Journal of Radiology* **63**, 888–91.

Coulthard, M.G. and Hey, E.N. 1984: Weight as the best standard for glomerular filtration in the newborn. *Archives of Disease in Childhood* **59**, 373–5.

Counahan, R., Chantler, C., Ghazali, S., Kirkwood, B., Rose, F. and Barratt, T.M. 1976: Estimation of glomerular filtration rate from plasma creatinine concentration in children. *Archives of Disease in Childhood* **51**, 875–8.

Crabbe, D.C., Thomas, D.F., Gordon, A.C., Irving, H.C., Arthur, R.J. and Smith, S.E. 1992: The use of ^{99m}technetium-dimercaptosuccinic acid to study patterns of renal damage associated with prenatally detected vesicoureteral reflux. *Journal of Urology* **148**, 1229–31.

Daly, M.J., Jones, W.A., Rudd, T.G. and Tremaine, J.A. 1977: Differential ^{99m}Tc dimercaptosuccinic acid (DMSA) renal localisation: correlation with renal function. *Journal of Nuclear Medicine* **18**, 594–5.

De Jonge, G.A. 1973: The urge syndrome. In Kolvin, I., MacKeith, R.C. Meadow, S.R. (eds), *Bladder control and enuresis*. London: Spastics International Medical Publications, 66–9.

Duckett, J.W., Walker, R.D. and Weiss, R. 1992: Surgical results: International Reflux Study in Children – United States branch. *Journal of Urology* **148**, 1674–5.

Elder, J.S. 1992: Commentary: importance of antenatal diagnosis of vesicoureteral reflux. *Journal of Urology* **148**, 1750–4.

Elo, J., Tallgren, L.G., Alfthan, G. and Sarna, S. 1983: Character of urinary tract infections and pyelonephritic renal scarring after antireflux surgery. *Journal of Urology* **129**, 343–6.

Enlander, D., Weber, P.W. and Remedios, L.V. dos 1974: Renal cortical imaging in 35 patients: superior quality with ^{99m}Tc-DMSA. *Journal of Nuclear Medicine* **15**, 743–9.

Ericsson, N.O. 1960: Urologic viewpoints on the treatment of urinary tract infections in children. *Acta Paediatrica Scandinavica* **49**, 196–202.

Frey, P., Berger, D., Jenny, P. and Herzog, B. 1992: Subureteral collagen injection for the endoscopic treatment of vesicoureteral reflux in children. Follow up study of 97 treated ureters and histological analysis of collagen implants. *Journal of Urology* **148**, 718–23.

Gool, J.D., van, Hjalmas, K., Tamminen-Mobius, T. and Olbing, H. 1992: Historical clues to the complex of dysfunctional voiding, urinary tract infection and vesicoureteral reflux. The International Reflux Study in Children. *Journal of Urology* **148**, 1699–702.

Gordon, I., Peters, A.M. and Morony, S. 1990: Indirect radionuclide cystography: a sensitive technique for the detection of vesico-ureteral reflux. *Pediatric Nephrology* **4**, 604–6.

Handmaker, H., Young, B.W. and Lowenstein, J.M. 1975: Clinical experience with ^{99m}Tc-DMSA (dimercaptosuccinic acid), a new renal imaging agent. *Journal of Nuclear Medicine* **16**, 28–32.

Hinchliffe, S.A., Chan, Y.F., Jones, H., Chan, N., Kreczy, A. and Velzen, D., van 1992: Renal hypoplasia and postnatally acquired cortical loss in children with vesicoureteral reflux. *Pediatric Nephrology* **6**, 439–44.

Hjalmas, K., Lohr, G., Tamminen-Mobius, T., Seppanen, J., Olbing, H. and Wikstrom, S. 1992: Surgical results in the International Reflux Study in Children (Europe). *Journal of Urology* **148**, 1657–61.

Hodson, J. and Kincaid-Smith, P. (eds) 1979: *Reflux nephropathy*. New York: Masson Publishing.

International Reflux Study Committee 1981: Medical versus surgical treatment of primary vesico-ureteral reflux: a prospective international reflux study in children. *Journal of Urology* **125**, 272–83.

Jequier, S., Forbes, P.A. and Nogrady, N.P. 1985: The value of ultrasonography as a screening procedure in a first-documented urinary tract infection in children. *Journal of Ultrasound Medicine* **4**, 393–400.

Jodal, U., Koskimies, O., Hanson, E. *et al.* 1992: Infection pattern in children with vesicoureteral reflux randomly allocated to operation or long-term antibacterial prophylaxis. The International Reflux Study in Children. *Journal of Urology* **148**, 1650–2.

Johnston, J.H. (ed) 1984: *Management of vesicoureteric reflux*. Baltimore, MD: Williams & Wilkins.

Kawamura, J., Hasakawa, S., Yoshida, O., Fujita, T., Ishii, Y. and Torizuka, K. 1978: Validity of ^{99m}Tc dimercaptosuccinic acid renal uptake for an assessment of individual kidney function. *Journal of Urology* **119**, 305–9.

Kenda, R.B., Kenig, T. and Budihna, N. 1991: Detecting vesicoureteral reflux in asymptomatic siblings of children with reflux by direct radionuclide cystography. *European Journal of Pediatrics* **150**, 735–7.

MacDonald, A.F., Keyes, W.I., Mallard, J.R. and Steyn, J.H. 1977: Diagnostic value of computerised isotopic section renal scanning. *European Urology* **3**, 289–91.

Markland, G. and Kelly, W.D. 1968: Experiences with severely damaged urinary tract. *Journal of Urology* **99**, 327–36.

Medical Research Council Bacteriuria Committee 1979: Recommended terminology of urinary tract infection. *British Medical Journal* **ii**, 717–9.

Merrick, M.V., Uttley, W.S. and Wild, S.R. 1980: The detection of pyelonephritic scarring in children by radioisotope imaging. *British Journal of Radiology* **53**, 544–56.

Noe, H.N. 1992: The long-term results of prospective sibling reflux screening. *Journal of Urology* **148**, 1739–42.

Noe, H.N., Wyatt, R.J., Peeden, J.N., Jr and Rivas, M.L. 1992: The transmission of vesicoureteral reflux from parent to child. *Journal of Urology* **148**, 1869–71.

O'Donnell, B. and Puri, P. 1984: Treatment of vesicoureteric reflux by endoscopic injection of Teflon. *British Medical Journal of Clinical Research* **289**, 7–19.

O'Donnell, B. and Puri, P. 1988: Technical refinements in endoscopic correction of vesicoureteral reflux. *Journal of Urology* **140**, 1101–2.

Philipson, E.H., Wolfson, R.N. and Kedia, K.R. 1984: Fetal hydronephrosis and polyhydramnios associated with vesico-ureteric reflux. *Journal of Clinical Ultrasound* **12**, 585–7.

Puri, P. and O'Donnell, B. 1984: Correction of experimentally produced vesicoureteric reflux in the piglet by intravesical injection of Teflon. *British Medical Journal of Clinical Research* **289**, 5–7.

Rames, R.A. and Aaronson, I.A. 1991: Migration of polytef paste to the lung and brain following intravesical injection for the correction of reflux. *Pediatric Surgery International* **6**, 239–40.

Rickwood, A.M., Carty, H.M., Mc Kendrick, T. *et al.* 1992: Current imaging of childhood urinary infections: prospective survey. *British Medical Journal* **304**, 663–5.

Rosenheim, M.L. 1963: Problems of chronic pyelonephritis. *British Medical Journal* **ii**, 1433–40.

Schulman, C.C. and Sassine, A.M. 1992: Endoscopic treatment of vesicoureteral reflux. *European Journal of Pediatric Surgery* **2**, 32–4.

Schulman, C.C., Pamart, D., Hall, M., Janssen, F. and Avni, F.E. 1990: Vesicoureteral reflux in children: endoscopic treatment. *European Urology* **17**, 314–7.

Scott, J.E.S. 1987: Fetal ureteric reflux. *British Journal of Urology* **59**, 291–6.

Scott, J.E.S. 1972: A critical appraisal of the management of ureteric reflux. In Johnston, J.H., and Scholtmeijer, R.J., (eds), *Problems in paediatric urology*. Amsterdam: Excerpta Medica, 271–98.

Scott, J.E.S. 1975: The role of surgery in the management of vesicoureteric reflux. *Kidney International* **8**, S73–80.

Scott, J.E.S. 1984: Hypertension, reflux and renal scarring. In Johnston, J.H. (ed.), *Management of vesicoureteric reflux*. Baltimore, MD: Williams & Wilkins, 54–66.

Scott, J.E.S. 1985a: Vesico-ureteric reflux in children. In Whitfield, H.N. and Hendry, W.F. (eds), *Textbook of genitourinary surgery*. Edinburgh: Churchill Livingstone, 329–40.

Scott, J.E.S. 1987a: Ureteric reflux: the present position. In Hendry, W.F. (ed), *Recent advances in urology/andrology*. Edinburgh: Churchill Livingstone, 89–108.

Scott, J.E.S. 1987b: Management of congenital posterior urethral valves. *British Journal of Urology* **57**, 71–7.

Scott, J.E.S. 1993: Fetal ureteric reflux: a follow-up study. *British Journal of Urology* **71**, 481–3.

Scott, J.E.S. and Stansfeld, J.M. 1968: The treatment of vesico-ureteric reflux in children. *Archives of Disease in Childhood* **43**, 323–8.

Scott, J.E.S., Swallow, V., Coulthard, M.G., Lambert, H.J. and Lee, R.E.J. 1997: Screening of newborn babies for familial ureteric reflux. *Lancet* **350**, 396–400.

Smellie, J.M. 1980: Childhood urinary infections and their significance. In Asscher, A.W. (ed), *The management of urinary tract infection*. Oxford: Medicine Publishing, 29–38.

Smellie, J.M. 1992: Commentary: management of children with severe vesicoureteral reflux. *Journal of Urology* **148**, 1676–8.

Smellie, J.M., Hodson, C.J., Edwards, D. and Normand, I.C.S. 1964: Clinical and radiological features of urinary infection in childhood. *British Medical Journal* **ii**, 1222–6.

Smellie, J.M., Tamminen-Mobius, T., Olbing, H. *et al.* 1992: Five year study of medical or surgical treatment in children with severe reflux: radiological renal findings. The International Reflux Study in Children. *Pediatric Nephrology* **6**, 223–30.

Stansfeld, J.M. 1966: Clinical observations relating to incidence and aetiology of urinary-tract infections in children. *British Medical Journal* **i**, 631–5.

Stephens, F.D., Joske, R.A. and Simmons, R.T. 1955: Megaureter with vesico-ureteric reflux in twins. *Australian and New Zealand Journal of Surgery* **24**, 192–4.

Tamminen-Mobius, T., Brunier, E., Ebel, K.D. *et al.* 1992: Cessation of vesicoureteral reflux for 5 years in infants and children allocated to medical treatment. The International Reflux Study in Children. *Journal of Urology* **148**, 1662–6.

Van den Abeele, A.D., Treves, S.T., Lebowitz, R.L. *et al.* 1987: Vesicoureteral reflux in asymptomatic siblings of patients with known reflux: radionuclide cystography. *Pediatrics* **79**, 147–53.

Verber, I.G., Strudley, M.R. and Meller, S.T. 1988: ^{99m}Tc dimercaptosuccinic acid (DMSA) scan as first investigation of urinary tract infection. *Archives of Disease in Childhood* **63**, 1320–5.

Weiss, R., Duckett, J. and Spitzer, A. 1992: Results of a randomised clinical trial of medical versus surgical management of infants and children with grades III and IV primary vesicoureteral reflux (United States). The International Reflux Study in Children. *Journal of Urology* **148**, 1667–73.

Willis, K.W., Martinez, D.A., Hedley-White, E.T., Davis, M.A., Judy, P.F. and Treves, S. 1977: Renal localisation of ^{99m}Tc(Sn) DMSA and ^{99m}Tc(Sn) glucoheptonate in the rat by frozen section autoradiography. *Radiology Research* **69**, 475–88.

CHAPTER 55

Paraureteric diverticulum

J.D. ATWELL

Introduction	**Treatment**
Pathology	**Results**
Clinical features	**References**

Introduction

The different types of bladder diverticula found in clinical practice are shown in Table 55.1. This chapter is concerned primarily with the paraureteric diverticulum (PUD), which is of clinical importance because of its relationship to vesicoureteric reflux (VUR).

The association of vesical diverticula with outflow tract obstruction has been well documented since the early twentieth century (English, 1904). It was some years later when it became understood that some bladder diverticula were congenital in origin (Joly, 1914). The aetiology of these congenital diverticula remained obscure although the suggestion that the diverticulum represented an aborted ureteric bud was made in 1914. No evidence in support of this hypothesis was made at that time until the genetic basis and aetiology of the PUD were described by Atwell and Allen (1980) and Allen and Atwell (1980).

The relationship between a PUD and VUR was described by Hutch in 1952 but in these children the bladder was trabeculated, suggesting an obstructive cause. In retrospect this trabeculation could have been secondary to sphincter dysinergia. The presence of PUD in smooth-walled bladders (13 children) was reported by Johnston (1960), who suggested that the diverticula were examples of extreme lateral ectopia of the ureteric orifices. Meanwhile, anatomical studies of the trigone and a study of the changes occurring with growth were reported by Hutch (1961a, b).

Table 55.1 Classification of bladder diverticula

Congenital (or primary)
  Isolated bladder diverticula
  Paraureteric bladder diverticula

Acquired (or secondary)
  Obstructive/pulsion diverticula
    Secondary to posterior urethral valves or neuropathic bladder
  Unobstructive/traction diverticula
    Secondary to traction, i.e. postoperative but may also be partially pulsion.

Pathology

The paraureteric diverticulum is situated above and lateral to the ureteric orifice (Fig. 55.1). With increasing age the pulsion effect becomes more pronounced so that the diverticulum enlarges and eventually the ureteric orifice is displaced and lies within the diverticulum. This loss of the support to the intramural ureter predisposes to the development of VUR (Fig. 55.1).

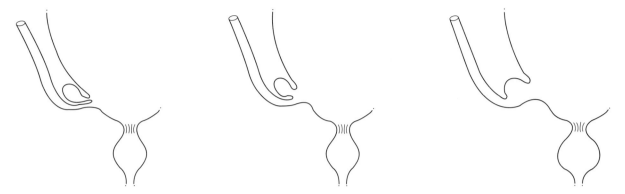

Fig. 55.1 Changes in a paraureteric diverticulum that result in the development of vesicoureteric reflux.

Clinical features

Urinary infection is the most common method of presentation but nocturnal and diurnal enuresis is seen in approximately 15%. Haematuria and abdominal pain can occur. A rare presentation in the young infant with very large PUD is acute retention, presumably due to angulation of the bladder neck.

INVESTIGATIONS

In one series of 27 patients (20 male and seven female) (Allen and Atwell, 1980) the PUD was only seen on intravenous pyelogram (IVP) in two patients. The micturating cystogram is the investigation of choice and the diverticula were seen in 21 patients of this series (Fig. 55.2). Cystoscopy confirmed the diagnosis in three patients.

The IVP is helpful, however, as upper tract dilatation and evidence of renal scars will be demonstrated which will alert the clinician to the need for further investigation.

ASSOCIATED ANOMALIES

VUR is the most common associated finding and the mechanism is seen in Fig. 55.1. Double ureters are found at a 20-fold increased frequency above that expected. Megaureters were seen in four of 27 patients (Allen and Atwell, 1980) but whether these were primary or secondary is debatable.

FAMILY HISTORY

In an investigation of the first-degree relatives of index patients with a PUD (Atwell and Allen, 1980), three mothers had varying degrees of a duplex pelvicalyceal collecting system, another mother had reflux nephropathy and another a left PUJ hydronephrosis (Fig. 55.3). One father had polycystic kidneys and another renal calculi.

In the siblings investigated one brother had a PUD, two had a duplex pelvicalyceal collecting system and two had VUR, thus in five of the 32 siblings investigated other urinary tract problems were identified, an incidence of 15.6%. Similarly, seven of the parents out of 43 had associated renal tract anomalies, an incidence of 16.6%.

As there is no gender difference in the affected relatives these results would support that the method of inheritance is by an autosomal dominant gene of variable penetrance and that there is a genetic interrelationship among PUD, VUR, the duplex pelvicalyceal collecting system and PUJ hydronephrosis (Atwell, 1985).

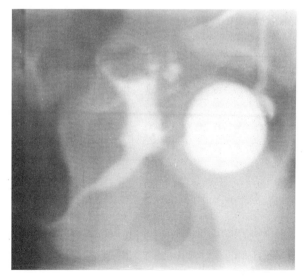

Fig. 55.2 Micturating cystogram showing a paraureteric diverticulum. Note the importance of taking oblique micturating films as the PUD may be obscured by a full bladder. (From Atwell and Allen, 1980.)

(a)
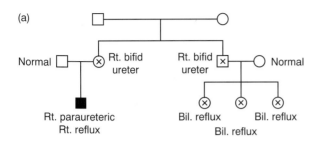

(b)
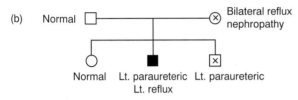

Fig. 55.3 (a) PUD and VUR in the index patient and duplication in the mother. Note the cousins with familial VUR. (b) Two brothers with PUD. Note the mother with bilateral reflux nephropathy. (From Allen and Atwell, 1980.)

Treatment

The treatment of choice is surgical excision of the PUD with reimplantation of the associated ureter. However, surgical treatment is only indicated in those patients with complications such as VUR and megaureters. If small diverticula are found, conservative treatment with continuous prophylactic chemotherapy is used with additional advice about regular micturition, avoidance of constipation and an adequate fluid intake. In some patients on such a regime VUR may occur as a complication (Allen and Atwell, 1980) due to continued enlargement of the diverticulum.

Results

The results of surgical treatment are very satisfactory. In a series of 23 operated patients (Allen and Atwell, 1980) one required reoperation because of the development of contralateral VUR and another had persistent VUR to a lower pole ureter of a duplex system which was cured by reoperation.

References

Allen, N.H. and Atwell, J.D. 1980: The paraureteric diverticulum in childhood. *British Journal of Urology* **52**, 264–8.

Atwell, J.D. 1985: Familial pelviureteric junction hydronephrosis and its association with a duplex pelvicalyceal collecting system and vesicoureteric reflux: a family study. *British Journal of Urology* **57**, 365–9.

Atwell, J.D. and Allen, N.H. 1980: The interrelationship between paraureteric diverticula, vesicoureteric reflux and duplication of the pelvicalyceal collecting system: a family study. *British Journal of Urology* **52**, 269–73.

English, J. 1904: Isolirte entzundung der blasendivertikel und perforations peritonitis. *Archives für Klinische Chirurgie* **73**, 1–67.

Hutch, J.A. 1952: Vesicoureteral reflux in the paraplegic: cause and correction. *Journal of Urology* **68**, 457–69.

Hutch, J.A. 1961a: Saccule formation at the ureterovesical junction in smooth walled bladders. *Journal of Urology* **86**, 390–9.

Hutch, J.A. 1961b: Theory of maturation of the intravesical ureter. *Journal of Urology* **86**, 534–8.

Johnston, J.H. 1960: Vesical diverticula without urinary obstruction in childhood. *Journal of Urology* **84**, 535–8.

Joly, J.S. 1914: Congenital diverticula of the bladder. *American Journal of Urology* **10**, 486–9.

CHAPTER 56

Megaureters

P.D.E. MOURIQUAND

Definition and classification	**Management of megaureters**
Pathophysiology and pathogenesis	**Conclusions**
Diagnosis	**References**

Definition and classification

A megaureter is a large ureter detected by either contrast X-rays, ultrasound scan or isotope studies. This anatomical status is the possible consequence of several different congenital abnormalities affecting the urine flow permanently or transiently. Many classifications have been reported (Kass, 1992) but, practically, two categories of megaureter may be distinguished: those which are related to an abnormal ureterovesical junction (obstructed, refluxing, or obstructed and refluxing), and those which are secondary to a dysfunctioning or obstructed lower urinary tract (neuropathic bladder or posterior urethral valve) or to a systemic disorder (prune belly syndrome). (The megaureter–megacystis syndrome, initially described by D.I. Williams, is not developed in this chapter. Its identification remains controversial. It is a rare condition where a huge bladder is associated with severe vesicoureteric reflux. It remains unclear whether this condition is a primary disorder or secondary to an occult neuropathy, although the bladder function itself seems to be preserved.)

Pathophysiology and pathogenesis

Three mechanisms can lead to the distension of the ureter: a deficient flow of urine, vesico-ureteric reflux and prune belly syndrome.

DEFICIENT FLOW OF URINE

Slow maturation of the fetal excretory system

The canalization of the ureter and the maturation of its muscular layers are slow processes which may lead to a transient dilatation of the ureters, detected by antenatal ultrasound.

The ureteral bud appears at 29th day of pregnancy and the ureteral division continues until the 22nd week of pregnancy (Gonzales, 1984). The canalization of the ureter is achieved at 9 weeks of pregnancy (or 23 mm according to Ruano-Gil et al., 1975) but the myogenesis of the ureters starts after 11 weeks, is not completed before the end of pregnancy and probably continues after birth. The elastic fibrils appear at 13–15 weeks and the longitudinal fibrils at 22 weeks. Reticulin and collagen fibrils appear during the second part of pregnancy and continue to develop after birth. Consequently, during the first few months of pregnancy a variable proportion of the total renal urine output may not flow along the urinary tract and may actually suffuse through the fetal membranes, according to the gradient of osmotic pressure existing between fetal urine and amniotic fluid. It is likely that his physiological leakage of fetal urine through the fetal membranes decreases progressively with the canalization and maturation of the excretory system.

Obstructed distal ureteric segment

A megaureter may be due to a structural obstruction of the distal segment of the ureter. The abnormal arrangement of collagen fibres at this level can cause some functional obstruction and can slow down the urine flow. Subsequent backpressure may lead to dilatation of the ureter. Obstruction does not, however, always imply high pressure because the renal output subsequently decreases and the compliance of the excretory system varies considerably with the duration and the severity of the obstruction. This explains why pressure studies usually fail to demonstrate an obstructed urinary tract, especially in equivocal situations.

Early microscopic studies (Bischof and Busch, 1961) demonstrated autonomic ganglia in the distal ureter and served to disprove the Hirschsprung-like theory postulated by Swenson. Multiple histological anomalies of the distal ureteric segment have been reported (Keating, 1993) and it is probably safe to say that no single pathological insult is responsible for the non-refluxing megaureter. Regardless of whether collagen deposition, cellular hypoplasia, muscular disarray or some other as-yet undefined injury or deficiency is involved at the microscopic level, a loss of functional continuity results.

Most studies have documented hyperplasia and hypertrophy of smooth muscle cells within the walls of the dilated proximal ureter. These presumably represent the ureter's compensatory response to distal obstruction. Urological obstruction usually occurs at the junction between two different embryological structures, i.e. between a Wolffian structure (the ureteric bud) and the urogenital sinus (bladder) (Fig. 56.1).

In other cases, the anatomical obstruction of the ureter is associated with another urological anomaly, mainly ureterocele (orthotopic or more frequently ectopic) or a duplex system.

Segmental obstruction or defect of the Wolffian tract

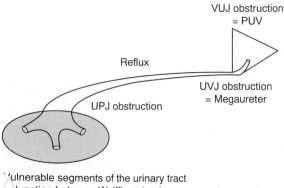

Vulnerable segments of the urinary tract
Junction between Wolffian structures
and other embryological structures

56.1   The Wolffian system.

Dysfunctioning lower urinary tract

Obstruction may be due to a dysfunctioning lower urinary tract which cannot fulfil its two major commitments: storage of urine at low pressure and regular and complete bladder emptying at physiological pressure. This is the case in the neuropathic bladder (acquired or congenital), in male children with posterior urethral valve or in female children with urethral obstruction (urethral atresia or female hypospadias).

VESICOURETERIC REFLUX

Reflux of urine into the ureter, due to a defective ureterovesical junction, can cause variable degrees of dilatation of the ureter. The defect in the ureterovesical junction may be a primary disorder or may arise secondary to bladder dysfunction (neuropathic bladder or unstable bladder) or bladder outlet obstruction (posterior urethral valve). The reflux itself can be transient or permanent and its importance can vary widely in the same patient at different times. The classification of vesicoureteric reflux in four or five grades has therefore a limited interest because it ignores these variations and in clinical practice one should distinguish reflux with and without dilatation of the upper urinary tract. The first category is usually diagnosed before birth (one-third of antenatal dilatation of the urinary tract is related to reflux), is usually found in the male population (85%) and has a resolution rate of 35% (Anderson and Rickwood, 1991). The second category is usually diagnosed after recurrent urinary tract infections in early childhood in the female population (75%) and has a resolution rate of 75%.

SYSTEMIC DISORDERS

Systemic disorders involving the ureteric wall are mainly represented by the prune belly syndrome, which consists of congenital absence or deficiency of abdominal wall musculature, cryptorchidism and anomalies of the urogenital tract. The incidence has been reported as 1 in 29 000 (Baird) to 1 in 40 000 live births (Garlinger) quoted by Greskovich and Nyberg, 1988). Thirty per cent of these patients die of renal failure or urosepsis within 2 years. Elongated, dilated and tortuous megaureters are present in 80% of the prune belly syndrome patients. The proximal ureter usually is of a more normal calibre. Although the ureteral dilatation is more marked distally the orifices usually are patent and obstruction is rare. Vesicoureteric reflux is common. Microscopically, there is a patchy distribution of muscle fibres with an increase in fibrous and collagenous tissue. Differentiation into circular or longitudinal layers is absent. Ureteric peristalsis is absent or decreased which may be due either to obstruction of nerve impulses by the collagenous and fibrous septa or to the reported marked decreases in nerve plexuses, with irregularity and degeneration of

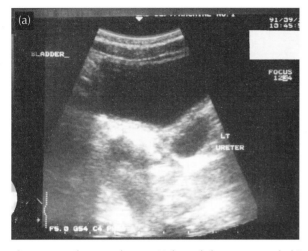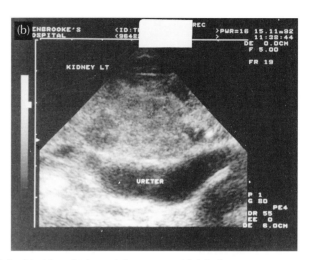

Fig. 56.2   Ultrasound scan: (a) large left ureter seen behind the bladder; (b) large left ureter and left kidney.

non-myelinated Schwann fibres. No abnormality of the ganglion cells, pelvic parasympathetic apparatus or anterior spinal nerve cells has been documented. The bladder is routinely enlarged, although trabeculation is rarely present and muscular hypertrophy is an inconsistent finding. The prostatic urethra is wide and elongated at the bladder neck, and it tapers at the level of the urogenital diaphragm (Greskovich and Nyberg, 1988).

Diagnosis

Large ureters can be picked up ultrasonically at 18–20 weeks of pregnancy. As mentioned above, some large ureters can be related to a transient event such as a slow canalization of the excretory system or a transient obstruction of the urine flow in the fetal tract (Mouriquand *et al.*, 1989). One-third of the dilated ureters picked up antenatally are related to vesicoureteric reflux. These findings are usually recorded in the male population. Investigations listed below confirm the diagnosis of a megaureter a few days after birth.

When the dilated ureter has not been detected antenatally, urinary tract infection is the most common symptom of the obstructed ureterovesical junction. Haematuria, abdominal pain and hypertension are also reported, although less common. Urinary tract infections in children should lead to paraclinical investigations which include morphological and functional studies attempting to define obstruction of the urine flow. This still raises many controversies.

MORPHOLOGICAL STUDIES

These include ultrasound scans of the urinary tract (Fig. 56.2), intravenous urography (IVU) (Fig. 56.3) and micturating cystograms (MCU) (Fig. 56.4). All three

may show the ureteric dilatation and the MCU may show the presence of vesicoureteric reflux. Distal anatomical obstruction of the ureter and vesicoureteric reflux may be concomitant.

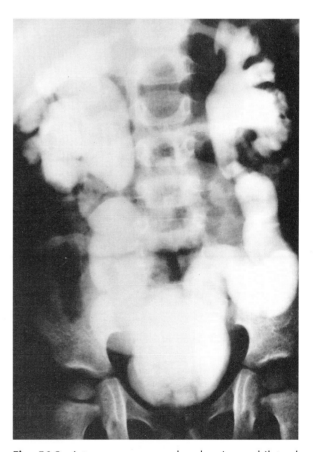

Fig. 56.3   Intravenous urography showing a bilateral megaureter.

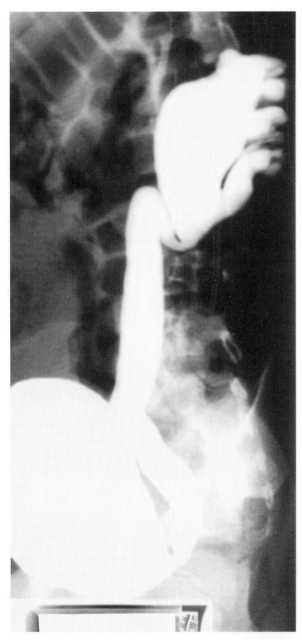

Fig. 56.4 Micturating cystogram showing reflux into the upper pole of the left kidney.

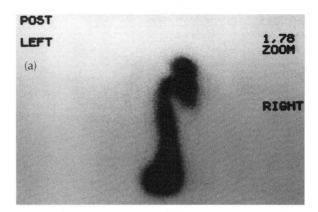

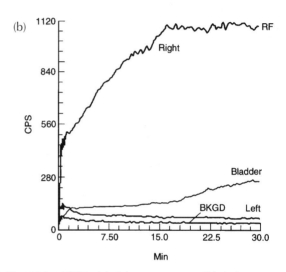

Fig. 56.5 DTPA: (a) right megaureter; (b) drainage curve of a right megaureter.

Ureteric dilatation may be permanent or evidence of a previous and transient abnormal urodynamic function. A progressive increase of the ureteric dilatation may be a reliable sign of continuous obstruction, although functional studies may be better to define this situation.

FUNCTIONAL STUDIES

These investigations include ^{99m}Tc-DTPA or ^{99m}Tc-mercapto-acetyltriglycerine (Mag 3) isotope scans (O'Reilly, 1992) with administration of diuretic (20 min before the injection of isotope) and pressure studies.

Diuretic isotope studies measure three parameters: the relative function of each kidney, the mean transit time of the isotope through the renal substance and the drainage curve of each excretory system (Fig. 56.5).

None of these three criteria has an absolute value to define obstruction and all three depend on the hydration of the patient. The renal function assessed is, by definition, relative and can be difficult to interpret, especially when the contralateral kidney is also abnormal. The relative function of the dilated tract is occasionally higher than the normal side, but this phenomenon is unclear. Some authors consider a progressive decrease of relative function as the only reliable criteria of continuous and active urine flow impairment, whereas some others also take into consideration the mean transit time and the shape of the drainage curve.

Pressure studies (Whitaker, 1979; Vela-Navarette, 1984) aim at measuring the differential pressure between the upper tract and the bladder with a constant infusion. They could be particularly useful in equivocal situations when isotope studies and morphological studies are not concordant. Whitaker stated that normal kidney pressure gradient never exceeded 15 cmH$_2$O pressure even when subjected to a fluid load of 10 ml/min; however, when an obstruction was present, the pressure regularly exceeded 22 cmH$_2$O. These pressure studies postulate that pressure is increased in obstructed systems, which is often wrong for the reasons detailed above, particularly when the system is very dilated. These studies are also quite invasive and often give false reassurance.

Management of megaureters

MEGAURETER RELATED TO LOWER TRACT DYSFUNCTION OR OBSTRUCTION

Correction of the primary disorder is required by augmentation of the bladder capacity (enterocystoplasty, gastrocystoplasty or autoaugmentation) in neuropathic bladder developing high pressure, treatment of bladder instability (anticholinergics), release of bladder outlet obstruction (posterior urethral valve), etc. Attempts to reimplant megaureters without correcting the primary disorder often lead to failures and complications. It is therefore essential to recognize any underlying bladder dysfunction before deciding upon a ureteric reimplantation.

MEGAURETER AND PRUNE BELLY SYNDROME

Children with prune belly syndrome usually require a complete assessment of their condition in a paediatric intensive care unit. This is due to the high incidence of associated anomalies (pulmonary, musculoskeletal and cardiac systems) and metabolic disorders. Controversies in the surgical management of urological anomalies exist, with urologists who favour the minimal surgical interference and urologists who prefer an aggressive surgical approach (extensive tailoring and straightening of the ureters, vesicoureteric or reimplantation, excision of the urachus with or without a reduction cystoplasty and tailoring of the bladder neck). In view of the variability of degrees of renal and urinary tract involvement with the prune belly syndrome, therapeutic options, whether medical or surgical, must be contemplated on an individual case-by-case basis (Greskovich and Nyberg, 1988). Upper tract diversion or vesicostomy may be required in patients with severe uraemia, obstruction or uncontrollable infection. Urethroscopy is recommended to exclude posterior urethral valves. Other procedures and correction of the undescended testes will not be detailed here.

MANAGEMENT OF MEGAURETERS RELATED TO AN ABNORMAL URETEROVESICAL JUNCTION

Expectative

Spontaneous improvement of ureteric dilatation is a frequent event in megaureters related to a faulty ureterovesical junction. Maturation of the obstructive or/and refluxing junction is a likely event during the first months of life. The resolution rate of antenatally diagnosed vesicoureteric reflux is around 35% (80% male), whereas it is around 75% in symptomatic reflux, usually diagnosed in female patients (75%). Resolution of obstruction alone is also common and conservative management of megaureters is recommended when renal function and dilatation of the upper tract remain stable (or improve) and when the child remains asymptomatic (Rickwood *et al.*, 1992). Antibiotic prophylaxis is recommended, especially in refluxing megaureters. Regular isotope assessments are required to follow these children.

Surgery of the ureterovesical junction

When the conservative approach fails, i.e. when symptoms recur in spite of an adequate antibiotic prophylactic cover, when renal function decreases on repeated isotope studies or when dilatation of the urinary tract increases, ureteric reimplantation is usually recommended.

The aim of the operation is to excise the distal obstructive segment of the ureter and reimplant the ureter with an antireflux mechanism. The suprahiatal reimplantation of the ureter and the transhiatal reimplantation of the ureter (Cohen's procedure or Glenn-Anderson's procedure) are the two main surgical options (Mouriquand, 1994).

Suprahiatal reimplantation of the ureter

This is the technique of choice for megaureters, although it remains a difficult procedure which has a significant complication rate.

The bladder is approached by a transverse suprapubic incision of the skin and a midline opening of the abdominal wall. The extravesical approach to the ureter is the main step of this procedure. The peritoneum covering the dome and the lateral face of the bladder should be pushed upwards, which involves the ligation of the obliterated hypogastric vessels. It is then easy to mobilize the peritoneum upwards and expose the full length of the iliac vessels. The vas deferens and its pedicle are easily located and should also be freed before the ureteric reimplantation (Fig. 56.6).

The ureter is identified passing over the iliac vessels close to their division into the external iliac and hypogastric arteries. The ureter is progressively mobilized from this point down to the bladder, preserving its blood supply and the vascularity of the bladder. There is a plethora of small vessels and nerves arising from

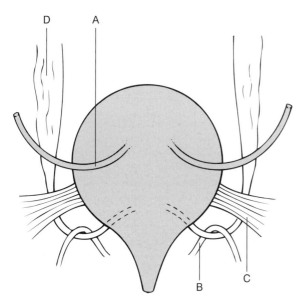

Fig. 56.6 Anatomical disposition of the distal ureters: (A) obliterated hypogastric vessels; (B) vas deferens; (C) lateral bladder vascular bundles; (D) megaureter.

the pelvic pedicles to the bladder which crosses the distal part of the extravesical ureter and these should be preserved.

In severe megaureters, the ureter is grossly dilated and kinked and its dissection should be meticulous to straighten it and maintain enough tissues around it to preserve its vascularity and innervation. The ureter is divided at its entrance into the bladder and a stay-suture facilitates its mobilization. The ureter, which normally passes under the vas deferens, should be redirected over the vas to straighten it out.

The distal segment of the ureter is usually narrowed and its excision allows urine to flow out freely (Fig. 56.7). The ureteric diameter rapidly contracts and it is then possible to decide whether the ureteric reimplantation can be achieved with or without remodelling or trimming. This decision is dictated by Paquin's law (Paquin, 1979): the length of the submucosal tunnel should represent at least five times the ureteric diameter.

If the ureter remains too large after excision of its distal end, the calibre of the ureter should be reduced either by excising a strip of ureter [Hendren's technique (Hendren, 1979) (Fig. 56.8)] or by folding the ureter [Kalicinski's technique (Kalicinski *et al.*, 1977) (Fig. 56.9)].

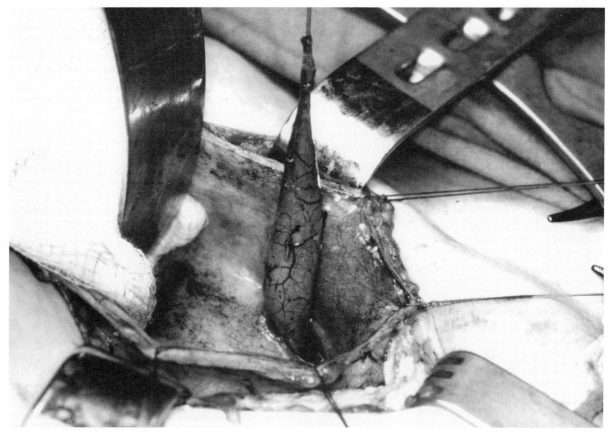

Fig. 56.7 Transvesical approach of a left megaureter. Note the narrow distal segment of the ureter.

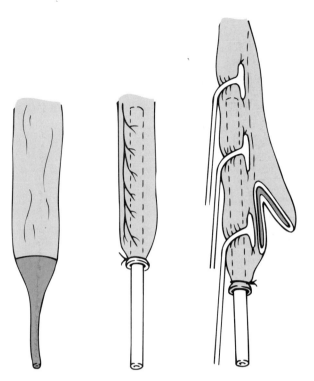

Fig. 56.8 Hendren's technique to adjust the ureteric calibre.

Excision of a strip or ureter may threaten the ureteric vascularity, whereas the ureteric infolding can create a certain degree of obstruction. Whichever technique is chosen, the length of the remodelled or the trimmed segment of ureter should not need to exceed the length of the submucosal tunnel (Fig. 56.10).

The hiatus of entrance into the bladder of the ureter should be medial and high at the top of the posterior

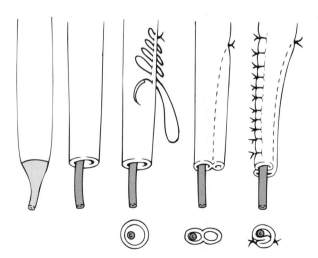

Fig. 56.9 Kalicinski's technique to adjust the ureteric calibre.

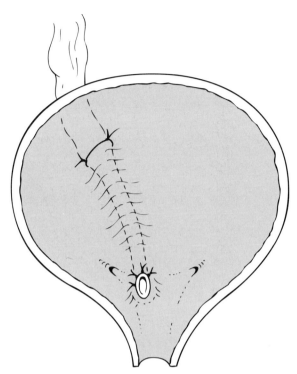

Fig 56.10 Suprahiatal reimplantation of a megaureter: the orifice of the entrance into the bladder should be medial, high and posterior. The length of the modelled segment should not exceed the length of the submucosal tunnel.

face of the bladder (Fig. 56.10). The ureter should not be constricted at this level and it is necessary to excise a disc of bladder to allow free passage of the ureter. The submucosal tunnel is fashioned as described above and should be vertical. Its distal end should be opened on the trigone. The passage of the freed ureter through the tunnel is the most difficult step of this procedure. The ureter should not be twisted or kinked, especially at the entrance into the bladder, and its pelvic course should be smooth. A few absorbable sutures are placed at its entrance into the bladder and sometimes the bladder itself is tacked down on the psoas muscle to maintain the smooth course of the ureter. The ureterovesicostomy is completed with dissolvable sutures.

Bilateral procedure may be performed. Some authors prefer to perform a transureteroureterostomy to avoid bilateral suprahiatal reimplantation. The extravesical approach of the ureter is the main step of this procedure and should be understood properly.

Transhiatal reimplantation of the ureter(s)

This is mainly represented by Cohen's procedure (Cohen, 1975), which is easier to perform than the suprahiatal reimplantation, especially in babies, although it is not always appropriate when the ureter is too large or the trigone too small. Its indications for megaureter are

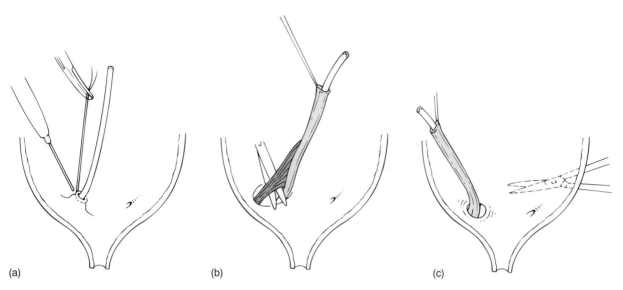

(a)   (b)   (c)

Fig. 56.11 (a) and (b) Transtrigonal dissection of the ureter (Cohen's technique); (c) construction of a submucosal tunnel (Cohen's technique).

less common because the need to reimplant megaureters in infants is much smaller than it used to be. The approach of the bladder is identical. The ureteric orifice is circumcised with diathermy and the mobilization of the distal 2 cm of ureter can be performed with diathermy alone (Fig. 56.11a) (these 2 cm will be excised later).

It is essential to enter the correct plane between the bladder and the transparietal ureter, commencing below the orifice. Sharp scissors should be avoided and Reynolds scissors make this procedure much easier. The tip of the Reynolds scissors elevates the muscle fibres that attach the ureter to the bladder musculature. These fibres are grasped with fine De Bakey forceps, coagulated and divided (Fig. 56.11b). The dissection continues progressively and circumferentially until the ureter is completely free. Coagulation of the fibres should be carried out at some distance from the ureter to avoid damaging its blood supply.

The peritoneum is visible at the end of this dissection and should be teased away from the ureter. In male patients the vas deferens may lie close to the ureter at this point and care must be taken to avoid damaging it.

In patients with ureteric duplication both ureters are dissected together and should not be separated, thus avoiding damage to their blood supply. In some the ureteric hiatus is wide and should be narrowed by one or two absorbable sutures. This is done to prevent the formation of a diverticulum. These sutures should narrow the hiatus, but still allow the free movement of the ureter and not restrict or constrict it. The sub-mucosal tunnel is then constructed (Fig. 56.11c). It is usually a horizontal tunnel, crossing the midline of the posterior surface of the bladder, just above the trigone. Its length should represent at least five times the ureteric diameter

(Paquin's rule) and, if this condition cannot be fulfilled, trimming or remodelling of the ureter and suprahiatal reimplantation should be considered.

The site of the new ureteric orifice is selected and the bladder mucosa is lifted from the underlying bladder muscles with a pair of Reynolds scissors, starting either from the hiatus or from the new ureteric orifice. Again, sharp scissors should be avoided (especially Potts scissors) and Reynolds scissors are ideal. The tunnel should be wide enough to allow easy insertion of the ureter, without constriction (Fig. 56.11c).

A similar procedure can be carried out for the opposite ureter in the case of bilateral reimplantation. The construction of the lowest tunnel which crosses the trigone can bleed a little and the lifting of the mucosa is slightly less easy (Fig. 56.12a)

A pair of artery forceps or a right-angle forceps is inserted through the tunnel, grasps the stay suture and is gently pulled to draw the ureter into place, taking care not to twist or kink it in the process.

The last 2 cm of ureter is excised (Fig. 56.12b) and the ureteric opening is spatulated with a pair of angulated Potts scissors. The 5/0 absorbable suture anchors the ureter to the bladder muscles and the ureterovesicostomy is completed with interrupted 6/0 absorbable sutures. An infant-feeding tube is inserted into the reimplanted ureter and exteriorized through the bladder wall, the rectus muscle and the skin, using the punch of a suprapubic catheter. This feeding tube is left for 2 days, or 10 days if the ureter has been remodelled. There is no consensus on the drainage of the reimplanted ureters and some authors do not leave any drain. The bladder is drained either by a transurethral catheter which will be left for 5 days or by a suprapubic catheter.

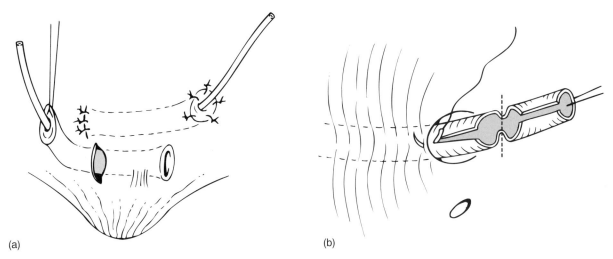

(a)   (b)

Fig. 56.12   (a) Bilateral ureteric reimplantation (Cohen's technique); (b) ureterovesicostomy of the last 2 cm.

Postoperative care

The child usually stays for 5 days in a paediatric surgical ward. The ureteric stent is removed after 2 days (or 10 days if the ureter has been remodelled). Bladder spasms are common after this surgery and a prescription of oxybutinin may be useful to reduce the patient's discomfort. A broad antibiotic cover is recommended for 10 days, followed by 3 months of antibiotic prophylactic treatment.

An ultrasound scan performed 1 month and 6 months after the procedure ensures that the dilatation improves, although complete resolution of the dilatation is uncommon. A Mag 3 scan is repeated 6 months later to detect indirect signs of reflux, persistent obstruction, a possible progression of existing scars or new scars. A micturating cystogram is certainly a more reliable method for checking the result of surgery, although it is often badly accepted by the children.

Nephroureterectomy

Nephroureterectomy is indicated when renal function is poor (<15% relative function). Two incisions are required to excise the entire system. If a ureteric stump is left *in situ* it may cause recurrent infections and therefore a total excision of the ureter is recommended.

Results of surgery

In a series of 524 megaureters (Mollard and Mouriquand, 1987), 40 underwent a nephroureterectomy straightaway, ten a nephroureterectomy after nephrostomy and 474 a ureteric reimplantation: 430 (91%) had a good anatomical result with a minimum follow-up of 6 months, while 43 (9%) were failures: 24 ureteric stenosis, 15 vesicoureteric reflux and four persistent

dilatations without stenosis and reflux (one was lost to follow-up). None of these patients underwent an isotope study.

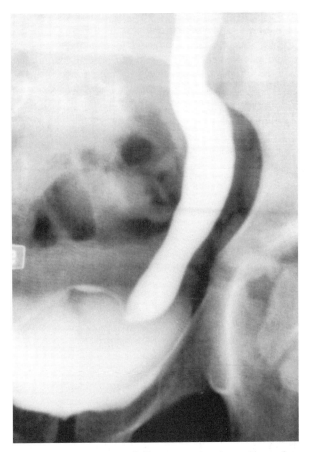

Fig. 56.13   Stenosis following reimplantation of a megaureter.

Ischaemia is a possible cause of stenosis (Fig. 56.13) and may be secondary to an excessive or inadequate trimming of the distal ureter. Other causes include a narrow entrance into the bladder, a too long submucosal tunnel or a wrongly placed tunnel. Ureteric dilatation when the bladder is full is found when the tunnel is not correctly placed (on the dome of the bladder).

Vesicoureteric reflux is due to a short submucosal tunnel or to underlying bladder dysfunction.

Conclusions

The term megaureter is somewhat inappropriate because it only reflects an anatomical status which can be secondary to many different urine flow impairments. Multiple and misleading classifications of megaureters in addition to disagreements about the definition of urinary obstruction have allowed confusion to persist. Most paediatric urologists would agree that a dilated segment of urinary tract may be the reflection of a past or present urine flow impairment of variable severity. It is therefore either an active process or a sequela of a past disorder which has been spontaneously resolved. A better knowledge of the natural history of urine flow impairment has considerably simplified the pathophysiology and the current management of megaureters, where conservative treatment appears to be a reliable option in many cases. Surgery of megaureter within limited but well-defined indications is satisfactory but has a significant complication rate even in the best paediatric urological hands (Mollard et al., 1979).

References

Anderson, P.A.M. and Rickwood, A.M.K. 1991: Features of primary vesicoureteric reflux detected by prenatal sonography. *British Journal of Urology* **67**, 267–71.

Bischof, P.F. and Busch, H.G. 1961: Origin, clinical experiences and treatment of urinary obstructions of the lower ureter in childhood. *Journal of Urology* **85**, 739.

Cohen, S.J. 1975: Ureterozystoneostomie: Eine Neue Antirefluxtechnik. *Aktuelle Urologie* **6**, 1–6.

Gonzales, J. 1984: Relation structure et fonction dans le développement de l'appareil urinaire du foetus. *Journal d'Urologie (Paris)* **91**, 108–17.

Greskovich, F.J. and Nyberg, L.M. 1988: The prune belly syndrome: a review of its etiology, defects, treatment and prognosis. *Journal of Urology* **140**, 707–12.

Hendren, W.H. 1979: Megaureter. In Ravitch, M.M., Welch, K.J., Benson, C.D., Aberdeen, E. and Randolph, J.G. (eds), *Pediatric surgery*. Chicago, IL: Year Book Medical Publishers, 1197–211.

Kalicinski, Z.H., Kanzy, J., Kotarbinska, B. and Joszt, W. 1977: Surgery of megaureters. Modification of Hendren's operation. *Journal of Pediatric Surgery* **12**, 183–8.

Kass, E.J. 1992: Megaureter. In Kelalis, P.P., King, L.R. and Belman, A.B. (eds), *Clinical pediatric urology*. Philadelphia, PA: W.B. Saunders, 782.

Keating, M.A. 1993: The non-refluxing megaureter: pathophysiology and pathogenesis. *Dialogues in Pediatric Urology* **16**, 2–4.

Mollard, P. and Mouriquand, P.D.E. 1987: Primary obstructive megaureter: technique of reimplantation, results and complications. Lecture: Gesellschaft für Kinderchirurgie der DDR XIII. Symposium: Supravesikaler Harntrakt im Kindesalter, Erfurt, Germany.

Mollard, P., Valla, V. and Sarkissian, J. 1979: Les échecs du traitement chirurgical des méga-uretères primitifs de l'enfant. *Journal d'Urologie (Paris)* **85**, 625–38.

Mouriquand, P.D.E. 1994: Surgical treatment of vesicoureteric reflux. In Carter, D.C. and Russell, R.C.G. (eds), *Rob & Smith's operative surgery*, London: Chapman & Hall.

Mouriquand, P.D.E., Mollard, P. and Ransley, P.G. 1989: Dilemmes soulevés par le diagnostic anténatal des uropathies obstructives et leurs traitements. *Pédiatrie* **44**, 357–63.

O'Reilly, P.H. 1992: Diuresis renography. Recent advances and recommended protocols. *British Journal of Urology* **69**, 113–20.

Paquin, A.J. 1979: Uretero-vesical anastomosis. *Journal of Urology* **82**, 573.

Rickwood, A.M.K., Jee, L.D., Williams, M.P.L. and Anderson, A.M. 1992: Natural history of obstructed and pseudo-obstructed megaureters detected by prenatal ultrasonography. *British Journal of Urology* **70**, 322–5.

Ruano-Gil, D., Coca-Payeras, A. and Tojedo-Mateu, A. 1975: Obstruction and normal canalization of the ureter in the human embryo. Its relation to congenital ureteric obstruction. *European Urology* **1**, 287–93.

Vela-Navarette, R. 1984: L'exploration urodynamique du haut appareil urinaire. *Annals of Urology* **18**, 81–8.

Whitaker, R.H. 1979: An evaluation of 170 diagnostic pressure flow studies of the upper urinary tract. *Journal of Urology* **121**, 602.

CHAPTER 57

Multicystic dysplastic kidney

D.C.S. GOUGH

Introduction
Embryology
Clinical features
Complications of multicystic
dysplasia
Resolution of multicystic dysplastic
kidney

The contralateral kidney in multicystic
dysplasia
Vesicoureteric reflux
Contralateral hydronephrosis
The bladder in multicystic dysplasia
Conclusions
References

Introduction

Renal dysplasia is characterized by abnormal or incomplete differentiation during development, not simple retention of fetal structure. A classification suggested by Risdon in 1975 might be simplified into: (i) hypoplasia, (ii) agenesis and (iii) multicystic dysplasia. Segmental dysplasia may affect part of the kidney or the whole of the duplex moiety.

Renal cystic disease may be developmental, genetically determined or acquired postnatally and multicystic dysplasia (MCD) is a developmental abnormality characterized by ureteric atresia, non-function of the affected kidney and multiple cysts of varying sizes.

Embryology

NORMAL RENAL DEVELOPMENT

In normal development the nephrogenic mesoderm develops as a core of tissue during the fourth week of gestation. This is divided into the cranial pronephros which disappears by the fifth week and never has excretory function. The more caudally placed mesonephros is developing at about the fifth week and mesonephric tubules enter the mesonephric or Wolffian duct, which develops in the nephrogenic mesoderm and enters the urogenital sinus by the sixth week of gestation. The mesonephros has glomerular structures which all disappear by 10 weeks, but the secretions from these may be responsible for the bulging and rupture of the cloacal membrane.

The ureteric bud branches off the mesonephric duct just before it enters the urogenital sinus and grows towards the metanephric blastema. The ureteric bud invades the loose mesenchyme of the metanephros and there is a mutually conductive interaction thought to require cell contact. The mesenchyme differentiates into epithelium. Blastema aggregates at the tips of the branching ureteric bud and forms glomeruli with proximal and distal nephron segments. These structures then connect with the branches of the ureteric epithelium to form the collecting system. By 15 weeks of gestation no further divisions in the ureteric bud are occurring. Late in this process angiogenesis occurs, leading to capillary loop formation in the glomerulus (Sukhatame, 1993).

Direct cell-to-cell contact is needed for the induction of normal renal development and agents blocking glycosylation lead to the formation of primitive ducts (Spencer and Maizels, 1987).

PATHOLOGICAL DEVELOPMENT AND CAUSATION

It has been suggested that an abnormally sited ureteric bud is responsible for inducing abnormal metanephric development (Mackie and Stevens, 1975), or further postulated that the bud itself may be abnormal, leading to developmental abnormalities (Gribetx and Leiter, 1978). Obstruction and reflux *in utero* may be associated with abnormal renal development and dysplastic lesions, but with multicystic dysplastic kidney the abnormality is an extreme one secondary to ureteric atresia and complete occlusion of the drainage system, presumably before 15 weeks' gestation. With MCD there is always non-function of the kidney. This usually affects a simplex kidney with a single ureter but may involve a duplex kidney with the upper pole being affected in every instance. The kidney is usually normally sited but MCD has been found in association with crossed ectopia and horseshoe kidney, and in the ectopic kidney.

Pathological specimens show different size cysts which may intercommunicate, islands of glomeruli and primitive tubules, primitive duct structures, frequently areas of cartilage and hypertrophic nerve trunks (Fig. 57.1). The ureter is atretic at some point.

Extreme forms of hypoplasia merging with multicystic dysplasia exist and the ureter in these patients may be rudimentary and stenotic. I can do no better than to quote Hill (1989) with regard to these lesions: 'The reader is left to classify these kidneys as he wishes'.

Clinical features

INCIDENCE

MCD is the most common form of cystic disease of the kidney in childhood. Having investigated 403 patients diagnosed prenatally with hydronephrosis, the author found 62 with multicystic dysplastic kidney. As prenatal fetal hydronephrosis complicates 1 in 600 pregnancies it is suggested that MCD complicates 1 in 4000 live births.

Four patients in the author's care have had MCD in the upper pole of a duplex system with functioning lower polar tissue, while two have had a multicystic dysplastic kidney in the pelvis.

CLINICAL PRESENTATION AND PROGNOSIS

Patients still present with an abdominal mass in the newborn period but, in the UK, most are now diagnosed prenatally and present for confirmation of diagnosis postnatally.

It is very unusual for patients to present in childhood with complications of MCD, but it needs to be considered in all patients who present with a renal mass, hypertension or chronic infection of the kidney.

MCD has been regarded as a relatively benign condition which has been the subject of removal, more for diagnostic than for therapeutic reasons. Before ultrasound or computed tomography (CT) scanning, the finding of an abdominal mass and a non-functioning kidney on intravenous urography could not be managed safely without operation, and excision was appropriate. With ultrasound and gamma camera imaging, diagnosis can be established with certainty in almost all patients, without recourse to pathological examination. Questions have recently been asked about the need for surgical removal, as the lesion seems to disappear on ultrasound (Pedicelli *et al.*, 1986).

Because MCD complications are rarely seen many authors suggest that routine removal of the kidney is not necessary. This would seem to have much merit when the current incidence of MCD is 1 in 4000 and the case reports of complications are so rare.

The safety of this approach is based on the assumptions that (i) the incidence of MCD is stable in the community; and (ii) most complications are reported.

MCD is now the most common pathological form of cystic disease encountered in childhood. The pathological literature of the nineteenth century was fully

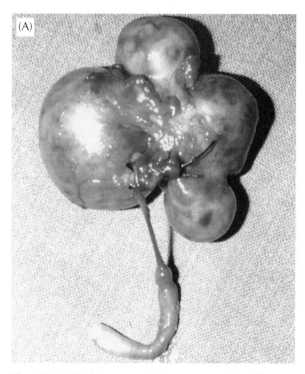

Fig. 57.1 (A) Macroscopic appearance of multicystic dysplastic kidney: partial ureteric atresia. (B) and (C) opposite.

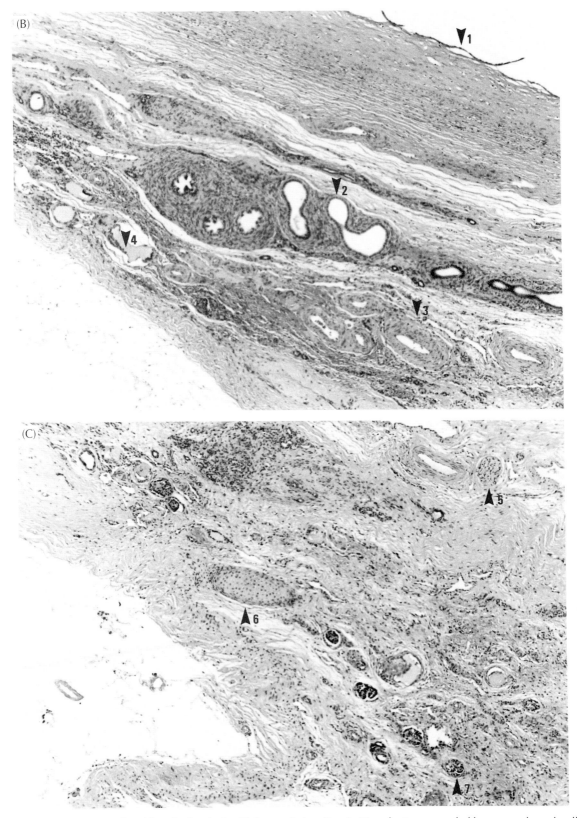

Fig. 57.1   Microscopy of multicystic dysplasia: (B) 1, cyst lining; 2, primitive ducts surrounded by mesenchymal collars; 3, thick-walled blood vessels; 4, tubule containing Tamm Horsfall protein. (C) 5, nerve trunk; 6, cartilage; 7, glomerulus.

aware of renal cystic disease in children, and a major review of renal cystic disease was undertaken in the early part of the twentieth century (Schwartz, 1926). It is noteworthy that this same author, some 9 years later, wrote of an unusual case of cystic disease in childhood, which he termed multicystic kidney, suggesting that this was a unique case (Schwartz, 1936). This casts doubt on the theory that MCD has always been a common condition.

Further evidence for the increasing incidence of developmental abnormalities of the upper urinary tract comes from a pathological study in Australia, which lends further support to the concept that MCD may be increasing in incidence during the latter part of this century (McKenna, 1974).

Not all medical complications are recorded in the literature and many case reports are turned down for publication on the basis that they offer little new insight and such situations have been recorded previously. Not all unusual events find themselves in the literature and many surgeons with great experience never write about them.

It must also be remembered that when MCD was diagnosed surgical removal was usually undertaken until quite recently and, therefore, surgery has reduced the incidence of patients retaining an MCD kidney in whom complications might have occurred.

What little we know about the incidence and pathology of this renal malformation does tends to suggest that it is relatively new, occurring more frequently in the latter half of the twentieth century, and that to base current management on past experience might not necessarily be valid.

DIAGNOSIS

Despite the apparent reliability of ultrasound in confirming the diagnosis of MCD, formal steps should be taken to confirm the diagnosis after birth (see Table 57.1). An initial ultrasound is performed, followed by upper tract imaging after 4 weeks of age with a ^{99m}technetrium dimercaptosuccinic acid (^{99m}Tc-DMSA) scan. The diagnosis is confirmed when a confident ultrasound diagnosis has been obtained and there is no function on DMSA.

Where function is present then the MCD may be the upper pole of a duplex kidney, in which case anatomical information from an intravenous urogram will be helpful in confirming the diagnosis. If it is not part of the duplex system, the diagnosis is wrong, and further investigation and exploration of the kidney may be required.

The decision to exclude vesicoureteric reflux (VUR) will be discussed later, but it is the author's practice to perform a micturating cystogram where there is any evidence of contralateral hydronephrosis or suggestion of a bladder diverticulum.

Where the patient presents with unilateral multicystic dysplasia and contralateral hydronephrosis the patient should initially have a reflux cystogram under antibiotic cover and, where reflux is present, prophylaxis and confirmation of the diagnosis of MCD kidney as shown in Table 57.2.

If the patient does not have reflux then a renogram, using ^{99m}mercaptoacetyltriglyceride (MAG3) should confirm the non-functioning nature of the multicystic dysplastic kidney and lead to functional and

Table 57.1 Confirmation of the diagnosis

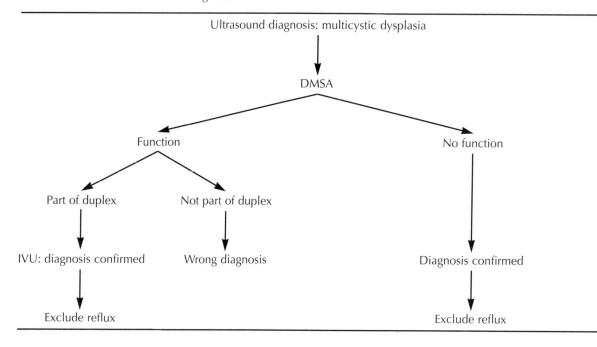

drainage information which can be attributed to the hydronephrotic kidney (Table 57.2). This may lead to further surgical treatment or observation on antibiotic prophylaxis.

Complications of multicystic dysplasia

HYPERTENSION

Systemic hypertension caused by multicystic dysplastic kidney has clearly been reported (Javadpour *et al.*, 1970; Chen *et al.*, 1985). These are classical cases in which removal of the multicystic dysplastic kidney, once identified, led to the resolution of hypertension. Further cases have been reported where removal of the kidney did not lead to a fall in blood pressure, but experience in the author's own unit has identified two further children in whom hypertension responded to nephrectomy. One patient was aged 6 months and the other 26 months.

It could be argued that routine blood pressure monitoring is now frequently undertaken in children and that the risks of missing this complication on regular follow-up would be minimal.

RENAL TUMOURS AND MULTICYSTIC DYSPLASTIC KIDNEY

Of greater concern to surgeons dealing with these patients is the risk of malignant degeneration. Renal cell carcinoma arising in a multicystic dysplastic kidney has been reported on three occasions (Barrett and Wineland, 1980; Birken *et al.*, 1985; Shiral *et al.*, 1986). These reports make it quite clear that follow-up of children with MCD needs to be lifelong before the

natural history of the condition can be understood, as one case occurred in a patient over 60 years of age.

Renal tumours in childhood are more frequently Wilms' tumours and there have been four reports of such malignant transformation arising in MCD kidneys (Uson *et al.*, 1960; Raensperger and Abouyleiman, 1968; Hartman *et al.*, 1986).

Nodular renal blastema, a histological accompaniment of Wilms' tumour has been found relatively frequently in the multicystic dysplastic kidney (Noe *et al.*, 1989). Wilms' tumourlet has been described and was again associated with nodular renal blastema (Dimmick *et al.*, 1989). Despite the fact that renal blastema elements occurred in 6.7% of the patients in this paper, a conservative approach towards MCD was advised, believing that these histological changes would not lead to the development of Wilms' tumour (Dimmick *et al.*, 1989). Support for such a conservative approach to MCD has come from flow cytometric evaluation where analysis of the DNA in patients with MCD all showed diploid results. If aneuploidy had been demonstrated it may have suggested a more definite link between dysplasia and neoplasia, although several renal malignancies have been found to have a low incidence of aneuploidy in the tumour nuclei.

Another case report of interest, regarding a patient developing a mesothelial tumour at the age of 68 years in a pre-existing MCD kidney, represents the only additional case of malignancy reported (Gutter and Hermanek, 1957).

INFECTION AND PAIN

These symptoms are impossible to assess in infants and should infection supervene in the urinary tract of a child being followed with a MCD kidney it is most likely that reflux or contralateral obstruction is the cause.

Table 57.2 Suggested diagnostic pathways for contralateral renal anomaly in MCD

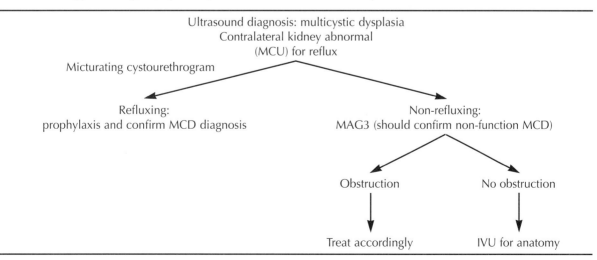

However, a literature review by Ambrose (1977) discovered 27 adults who had undergone removal of a MCD kidney for the symptoms of pain or infection. Fungal as well as bacterial infections were recorded. Despite resolution of the cystic elements in patients with MCD, these reports of complications in adult life suggest that complete resolution does not occur, despite involution of the cystic component.

Resolution of multicystic dysplastic kidney

Despite the widely held view that MCD kidney disappears there has been scant evidence that they do so. Two published series indicate that little more than one-third show progressive involution when studied over a period of years (Gordon *et al.*, 1988; Rickwood *et al.*, 1992). There has been a suggestion that the lesion completely disappears from the body in early childhood and would present later in life as renal agenesis, but childhood post-mortem studies differentiate clearly between multicystic dysplastic kidney and renal agenesis, associating the former with ureteric atresia but with a visible ureteric orifice, and the latter with absence of ureter and ureteric orifice (Barakat *et al.*, 1988).

The author's experience with MCD has been that the cystic element not infrequently resolves on ultrasound scanning, suggesting that total resolution has taken place. Unfortunately, cellular material may still exist in the renal fossa, which could conceivably cause problems later in life. The author has operated on three patients who had conservative treatment elsewhere and whose parents ultimately requested exploration of the renal fossae and excision of whatever tissue was present. Viable dysplastic renal tissue was confirmed in each case, despite negative ultrasound in all three. A CT scan was performed in one patient and was also negative, but exploration revealed cellular material in the renal fossa in the form of a shrunken, non-functioning MCD kidney (Fig. 57.2).

It would seem, therefore, that if a conservative approach to multicystic dysplasia is adopted then there is little to recommend frequent ultrasound as the cellular component of the mass shows no evidence of resolution in the long term and is unidentifiable by any conventional radiological means. Patients could not, therefore, safely be told that the lesion had disappeared from the body when ultrasound resolution has taken place.

Further confirmation about the current natural history of this condition is clearly needed before we can safely regard it as totally benign.

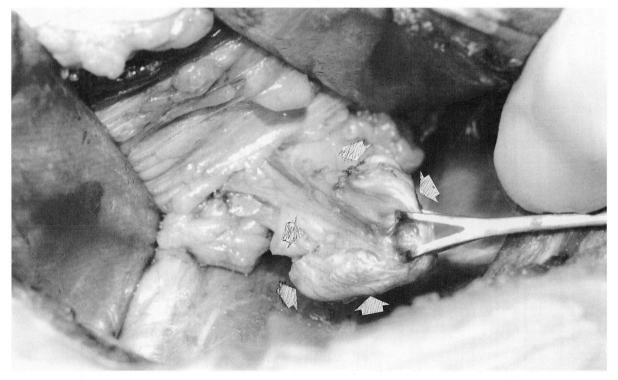

Fig. 57.2 Surgical specimen of apparently resolved multicystic dysplasia on ultrasound and CT scan. Arrows: in Babcock's forceps.

Long-term follow-up of patients with MCD is needed to answer the clinical problem as to whether significant risks to health are likely. The great difficulty here is long-term follow-up and some authors have shown that at least 10% of patients are lost to follow-up after only 3 years (Rickwood *et al.*, 1992).

The contralateral kidney in multicystic dysplasia

Previous experience led many practitioners to believe that MCD was not a benign condition. Serious renal impairment occurred in quite significant numbers of patients and several factors were associated with a poor prognosis. Bloom and Brossman (1978), noted that where the MCD kidney was large the contralateral kidney was usually normal, but where the MCD kidney was small the other kidney was abnormal.

DeKlerk *et al.* (1977) noted that if the ureter was normal in most of its length in association with MCD there was a low incidence of contralateral disease. At 1-year follow-up, 13 out of 14 patients (93%) were alive without renal disease, but one patient had died of renal failure. Where the ureter was atretic in most of its length there was a greater incidence of contralateral abnormality. More than half the patients died during the first year of life with renal failure, implying an earlier or more central defect affecting the development of the whole of the urinary tract.

With greater individual experience in MCD and more awareness of the potential problem, the contralateral kidney and its prognosis can be put into clearer perspective.

Vesicoureteric reflux

The incidence of vesicoureteric reflux has been reported to be as high as 28% in a prospective series (Flack and Bellinger, 1993), but much of this was of relatively low grade and spontaneously cured at follow-up. Despite suggesting that all patients with MCD ought to have assessment by MCU for VUR, few of the patients had complications of the reflux and by 20 months of age the majority had undergone spontaneous resolution. Only one patient came to any harm who was noted to have hydronephrosis and hydroureter on ultrasound at the initial postnatal study, and this finding of dilatation would, presumably, have led to further investigation of this patient and the discovery of the underlying cause (Flack and Bellinger, 1993).

It is not usual for patients with MCD to be screened for reflux routinely, but an incidence of VUR of 15% was found in the author's patients, and a similar study from Nottingham (Watson, personal communication) agrees with this figure.

Two patients with MCD known from prenatal diagnosis presented anuric with a combination of VUR and pelviureteric junction (PUJ) occlusion in their only functioning kidney. Both patients had been managed without antibiotic therapy and presented in the first 6 months of life. This would support the case for routine cystography and appropriate chemoprophylaxis where additional risks of infection were present in the patient's urinary tract.

Contralateral hydronephrosis

Contralateral hydronephrosis was found in 10% of the author's patients, but the majority show spontaneous resolution of this hydronephrosis with growth. PUJ obstruction does seem to be present in approximately 1.5% of patients with MCD (Williams and Kenawi, 1976). Four of the patients have had pyeloplasty. Two presented anuric, as above, and one with an acute pyelonephritis in an apparently obstructed kidney. A further patient had rapidly increasing hydronephrosis in the only functioning kidney which displayed an obstructive drainage curve on renography and was, therefore, subjected to pyeloplasty. Where the MCD involved the upper pole of a duplex kidney there was evidence of ureterocele associated with the upper pole in two patients and reflux into the lower pole ureter in a further two patients.

Overall, 6% of patients had or developed, some functional renal impairment and, therefore, the diagnosis of MCD could not be taken lightly.

The bladder in multicystic dysplasia

In the author's experience with 60 patients, three had a significant bladder diverticulum in association with non-functioning kidney and one presented with a large bladder diverticulum at the age of 1 year, leading to the finding of an atretic ureter and a partially resolved MCD kidney. Such bladder defects, which lead to diverticular formation, tend to support the abnormal ureteric bud theory.

Conclusions

The finding of MCD either prenatally or postnatally cannot be regarded lightly. At present little is known about the long-term natural history of MCD because of its relatively recent appearance, and one must be circumspect with regard to figures based on historical data suggesting that the long-term outcome will always be good. The fact that the cystic element of the multicystic kidney disappears on ultrasound should not, and cannot, be regarded as evidence of complete resolution.

Routine use of ultrasound for follow-up only until the cystic elements have disappeared would not seem logical, and follow-up needs to be lifelong in order to advance our knowledge of the natural history of this condition (Wacksman and Phipps, 1993).

The functional evaluation of the contralateral kidney, its appearance and drainage, should be established and VUR excluded. Should there be any evidence of reflux or contralateral hydronephrosis it would seem appropriate to treat the patient with prophylactic antibiotics until the reflux has ceased or the hydronephrosis resolved, with surgical treatment being reserved for those with persistent severe reflux or evidence of obstruction in the functioning system. Bladder diverticulae may be present and if these are complex removal is indicated.

The decision to remove or not to remove the multicystic dysplastic kidney remains controversial and personal, depending much on individual viewpoint and interpretation of the literature but, until clearer information from long-term natural history studies becomes available, nephrectomy remains an acceptable form of patient management (Wacksman and Phipps, 1993).

References

Ambrose, S.S. 1977: Unilateral multicystic renal disease in adults. *Birth Defects* **13**, 349–53.

Barakat, A.J., Drougas, J.G. and Barakat, R. 1988: Association of congenital abnormalities of the kidney and urinary tract with those of other organ systems in 13 775 autopsies. *Child Nephrology and Urology* **9**, 269–72.

Barrett, D.M. and Wineland, R.E. 1980: Renal cell carcinoma in multicystic dysplastic kidney. *Urology* **15**, 152–4.

Birken, G., King, D., Vane, D. and Lloyd, T. 1985: Renal cell carcinoma arising in a multicystic dysplastic kidney. *Journal of Paediatric Surgery* **20**, 619–21.

Bloom, D. and Brosman, S. 1978: The multicystic kidney. *Journal of Urology* **120**, 211–3.

Chen, Y.H., Stapleton, F.B., Roy, S. III and Noe, H.N. 1985: Neonatal hypertension from a unilateral multicystic dysplastic kidney. *Journal of Urology* **133**, 664–7.

DeKlerk, D.P., Marshall, F.F. and Jeffs, R. 1977: Multicystic dysplastic kidney. *Journal of Urology* **118**, 306–8.

Dimmick, J.E., Johnson, H.W., Coleman, G.U. and Carter, M. 1989: Wilms' tumourlet, nodular renal blastema, and multicystic renal dysplasia. *Journal of Urology* **142**, 484–5.

Flack, C.E. and Bellinger, M.F. 1993: The multicystic dysplastic kidney and contralateral vesico-ureteral reflux: protection of the solitary kidney. *Journal of Urology* **150**, 1873–4.

Gordon, A.C., Thomas, D.F.M., Arthur, R.J. and Irving, H.C. 1988: Multicystic dysplastic kidney: is nephrectomy still appropriate? *Journal of Urology* **140**, 1231–4.

Gribetz, M.E. and Leiter, E. 1978: Ectopic uterocoele, hydroureter and renal dysplasia: an embryogenic triad. *Urology* **11**, 131–3.

Gutter, W. and Hermanek, P. 1957: Maligner Tumor der Nierengegend Unter dem Bilde der Knollennierle. *Urology International* **4**, 164–6.

Hartman, G.E., Smolik, L.M. and Shochat, S.J. The dilemma of the multicystic dysplastic kidney. *American Journal of Disease in Children* **140**, 925–8.

Hill, G.S. 1989: Cystic and dysplastic disease of the kidney: developmental lesions. In Hill, G. (ed.), *Uropathology*, vol. 1. London: Churchill Livingstone, 103.

Javadpour, N., Chelouhy, E., Moncada, L. *et al.* 1970: Hypertension in a child caused by a multicystic dysplastic kidney. *Journal of Urology* **104**, 918–21.

Mackie, G.G. and Stevens, F.D. 1975: Duplex kidneys: a correlation of renal dysplasia with position of the ureteral orifice. *Journal of Urology* **114**, 274–8.

McKenna, H. 1974: A significant increase in developmental malformations of the renal tract in perinatal autopsies at Royal Women's Hospital, Brisbane. 1972–1973. *Medical Journal of Australia* **1**, 108–9.

Noe, H.N., Marshall, J.H. and Edwards, O.P. 1989: Nodular renal blastema in the multicystic kidney. *Journal of Urology* **142**, 486–8.

Pedicelli, G., Jequier, S., Bowen, A. and Bosivert, J. 1986: Multicystic dysplastic kidneys: spontaneous regression demonstrated with ultrasound. *Radiology* **160**, 23–6.

Raensperger, J. and Abouyleiman, A. 1968: Abdominal masses in children under one year of age. *Surgery* **63**, 514–21.

Rickwood, A.M.K., Anderson, P.A.M. and Williams, M.P.L. 1992: Multicystic renal dysplasia detected by prenatal ultrasonography. Natural history and results of conservative management. *British Journal of Urology* **69**, 533–40.

Risdon, R.A., Young, L.W. and Crispin, A.R. 1975: Renal hypoplasia and dysplasia: a radiological and pathological correlation. *Pediatric Radiology* **3**, 213–5.

Rubenstein, M., Meyer, R. and Bernstein, J. 1961: Congenital abnormalities of the urinary system. A postmortem survey of developmental anomalies and congenital lesions in a children's hospital. *Journal of Paediatrics* **58**, 356–66.

Schwartz, J. 1926: Polycystic disease of the kidneys. *New York State Journal of Medicine* **26**, 231–7.

Schwartz, J. 1936: An unusual unilateral multicystic kidney in an infant. *Journal of Urology* **35**, 259–63.

Shiral, M., Kitagawa, T., Nakata, H. and Urano, Y. 1986: Renal cell carcinoma originating from dysplastic kidney. *Acta Pathologica Japonica* **36**, 1263–9.

Spencer, J.R. and Maizels, M. 1987: Inhibition of protein glycosylation causes renal dysplasia in the chick-embryo. *Journal of Urology* **138**, 984–7.

Sukhatame, B.P. 1993: Renal development, challenge and opportunity. *Seminars in Nephrology* **13**, 422–6.

Uson, A.C., Del Rosario, C. and Melicow, M.M. 1960: Wilms' tumour in association with cystic renal disease: report of two cases. *Journal of Urology* **83**, 262–6.

Wacksman, J. and Phipps, L. 1993: Report of the multicystic kidney registry: preliminary findings. *Journal of Urology* **150**, 1870–2.

Williams, D.I. and Kenawi, M.M. 1976: The prognosis of pelvi-ureteric obstruction in childhood. A review of 190 cases. *European Urology* **2**, 57–63.

CHAPTER 58

Polycystic kidneys

E.R. FREEDMAN AND A.M.K. RICKWOOD

Introduction	Differential diagnosis of polycystic kidneys
Autosomal recessive polycystic kidney disease	References
Autosomal dominant polycystic kidney disease	

Introduction

Cysts occur in the kidney more commonly than in any other organ and these entities comprise a disparate group of anomalies, many of them genetically determined. Whilst the treatment of most forms of renal cystic disease is predominantly medical, an appreciation of their pathological and clinical features is helpful when evaluating an infant or child with hypertension, haematuria or renal failure. A complete classification of renal cystic disease is summarized in Table 58.1; however only a few of these conditions are relevant to paediatric surgical practice.

Polycystic kidney disease comprises two heritable forms, autosomal recessive (ARPKD) and autosomal dominant (ADPKD), which are clearly distinguishable clinically, pathologically and genetically.

Autosomal recessive polycystic kidney disease

ARPKD, often termed infantile polycystic disease, is the most common genetically determined renal cystic disease presenting during childhood. Nonetheless it is rare with an estimated birth incidence of 1 in 10 000 (Blyth and Ockenden, 1971) to 1 in 40 000 (Glassberg

and Filmer, 1992). The characteristic features are bilateral renal involvement, presentation early in childhood, a constant association with hepatic disease and an autosomal recessive mode of inheritance. As a rule, renal function deteriorates gradually and less than one-third of patients require dialysis before adult life (Broyer and Gagnadoux, 1992).

Table 58.1 Classification of renal cystic disease[a]

Genetic[b]	Autosomal dominant polycystic kidney (ADPKD)
	Autosomal recessive polycystic kidney (ARPKD)
	Cysts associated with multiple malformation syndromes
Non-genetic	Multicystic dysplasia
	Multilocular cyst
	Simple cyst (solitary or multiple)
	Parapelvic cyst
	Medullary sponge kidney (tubular ectasia)
	Acquired cystic disease (ESRD and dialysis)

[a]Adopted from Glassberg et al. (1987)
[b]Juvenile nephronophthisis: medullary cystic complex and the glomerulocystic diseases are associated with cysts only secondarily and are therefore not included in this list.

GENETICS

Inheritance is via an autosomal recessive trait and there are no reports of parents affected by the disease. As would be expected, the risk of affected siblings approximates to 1 in 4. Despite the clear genetic basis, the clinical spectrum of the disease varies widely and Blyth and Ockenden (1971) originally proposed four distant clinicopathological entities [perinatal, neonatal, infantile (with renal predominance) and juvenile (with hepatic predominance)] on the basis of possible allelic genes. Subsequent studies have shown no clear correlation between age of onset and rate of disease progression and hence this theory has largely been discarded (Kaplan *et al.*, 1989; Broyer and Gagnadoux, 1992). Nonetheless, among affected siblings, the clinical presentation and course is usually uniform (Blyth and Ockenden, 1971).

The affected chromosome has yet to be identified using known genetic markers (Broyer and Gagnadoux, 1992).

PATHOLOGY

Renal

Both kidneys are symmetrically affected and although they may be severely enlarged, up to 15 times normal size, the reniform shape is maintained. The collecting system is not obstructed, although later in the disease there may be some distortion due to compression by larger cysts. The kidneys are firm, with numerous microcysts visible beneath the capsule (Fig. 58.1; this figure also appears in colour as Plate 9). The cut surface presents a sponge or honeycomb appearance, with rounded medullary cysts and more elongated radially arranged cortical cysts (Rickwood, 1990) (Fig. 58.2; this figure also appears in colour as Plate 10). Glomerular cysts are never found. Over time, there is a tendency for larger cysts to develop along with renal parenchymal atrophy, with replacement by fibrous tissue and glomerulosclerosis (Broyer and Gagnadoux, 1992). Microdissection studies (Osathanondh and Potter, 1964) have shown that the cysts are due to segmental dilation of renal tubules

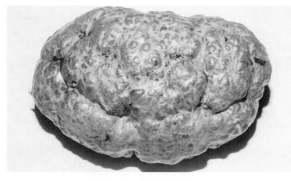

Fig. 58.1 Autopsy specimen from a neonate with ARPKD. The reniform shape is maintained and numerous microcysts are visible beneath the renal capsule.

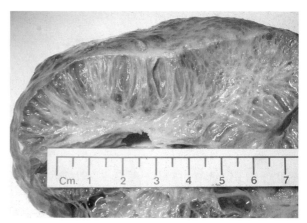

Fig. 58.2 The cut surface in ARPKD presents a spongy appearance, with the radially arranged elongated cortical cysts easily visible.

and collecting ducts and that there is no discontinuity along the entire length of any individual nephron.

Extrarenal

All patients with ARPKD have some degree of liver involvement. The extent of this varies widely from those with mild intrahepatic biliary duct ectasia (Caroli's disease) through to severe biliary fibroadenomatosis (Broyer and Gagnadoux, 1992) (congenital hepatic fibrosis or periportal fibrosis). The hepatocytes are uninvolved and liver function is normal. Macroscopically, there is an even distribution of whitish stellate spots throughout the hepatic parenchyma and which are due to periportal fibrosis. Cystic changes do not occur. Portal hypertension, with secondary hypersplenism and varices, may occur as a result of the periportal fibrosis.

CLINICAL FEATURES

The clinical features are dependent on the relative predominance of the renal or hepatic pathologies, although the majority of cases are recognized in young children presenting with renal enlargement or hypertension (Table 58.2).

Table 58.2 Clinical presentation of autosomal recessive polycystic kidney disease

Period	Primary problems
Neonatal	Respiratory failure
	Renal failure
Infantile	Systemic hypertension
	Progressive renal insufficiency
	Progressive portal hypertension
Juvenile	End-stage renal failure
	Dialysis
	Renal transplantation
	Portacaval shunt

Perinatal and neonatal

In the severely affected fetus, the disease may be suspected on prenatal ultrasonography as early as the second trimester from a combination of maternal oligohydramnios, an empty bladder and increased renal volume and echogenicity (Zerres *et al.*, 1984). It should be emphasized, however, that prenatal ultrasonography is not of value for routine screening since normal examinations at any stage in pregnancy do not exclude ARPKD (Zerres *et al.*, 1988). The massively enlarged kidneys are always easily palpable and birth may be complicated by an obstructed delivery. Ultrasound examination postnatally is diagnostic in excluding gross hydronephrosis or solid masses and in demonstrating the characteristic symmetrical renal enlargement with hyperechoism (Rickwood, 1990) due to multiple cyst interfaces. In the great majority of such cases there has been fetal oliguria leading to pulmonary hypoplasia and this, rather than the renal impairment, is the usual cause of early death. Very occasionally, the lungs are less affected and survival is possible with intensive neonatal care, including dialysis. In this circumstance, it may be necessary to perform early bilateral nephrectomy in order to relieve upward pressure on the diaphragm and thus enable the lungs to expand more fully.

With the less extreme forms, where the kidneys are not so enlarged and where renal function is less impaired, diagnosis may be delayed for months or, occasionally, for years. In these cases there is no correlation between the age at presentation and the rate of progression of renal insufficiency.

Manifestations of liver disease are never present in the neonate with ARPKD.

Infant and juvenile

In this age group, incidentally discovered bilateral renal enlargement is the most common presenting feature. Hypertension, which is not associated with elevated levels of serum renin (Kaplan *et al.*, 1989), is the first manifestation in up to one-third of patients (Gagnadoux *et al.*, 1989). Other symptoms and signs comprise recurrent abdominal pain, recurrent pyuria (with absence of haematuria or proteinuria) (Broyer and Gagnadoux, 1992) and polyuria due to loss of renal concentrating ability.

In patients where the liver disease predominates, the symptoms are consequent on the development of portal hypertension and include gastrointestinal bleeding due to oesophageal varices, thrombocytopenia due to hypersplenism, recurrent cholangitis and liver abscess. As a rule these patients do not have severe renal involvement (Broyer and Gagnadoux, 1992) and their prognosis is determined principally by the hepatic involvement.

Ultrasonography is the most useful diagnostic agent. The renal appearance is similar to that described for neonates. Larger cysts are sometimes evident, which

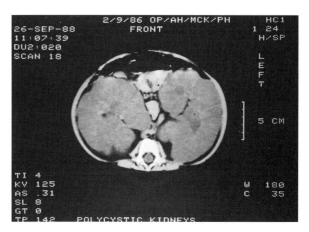

Fig. 58.3 Abdominal CT scan with contrast in a child with ARPKD demonstrating massive renomegaly and radial streaking.

can cause confusion with ADPKD. Ultrasonography may also reveal dilatation of the biliary tree, especially in the peripheral intrahepatic ducts (Gagnadoux *et al.*, 1989) biliary cysts and signs of portal hypertension. It should be emphasized that patients may have gross renal involvement with minimal hepatic changes and vice versa. Where further imaging is thought advisable, computed tomography (CT) scanning, with contrast (Fig. 58.3), has largely displaced intravenous urography, although here too the appearance is characteristic (Fig. 58.4). Liver biopsy or cholangiography is occasionally required in equivocal cases.

TREATMENT AND PROGNOSIS

Prognosis is usually determined by the degree of renal involvement. As a rule deterioration of renal function is slow and ARPKD accounts for only 2% of end-stage renal disease in children (Broyer and Gagnadoux, 1992). The probability for survival with functioning kidneys by the age of 15 years varies between 56% (Gagnadoux *et al.*, 1989) and 79% (Kaplan *et al.*, 1989). Prognosis has improved in recent years as a result of advances in medical management of renal failure and hypertension, plus surgical intervention in the form of renal transplantation and portal-systemic shunting. Some patients have undergone both procedures (McGonigle *et al.*, 1981). The number of cases surviving into the second decade and beyond is now appreciable (Broyer and Gagnadoux, 1992).

Autosomal dominant polycystic kidney disease

ADPKD is the most common form of renal cystic disease and also one of the most prevalent inherited

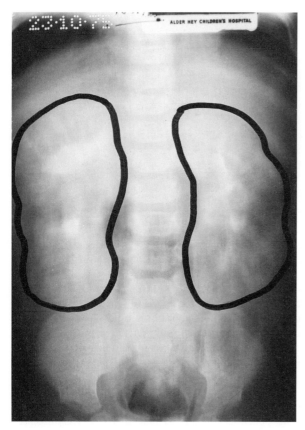

Fig. 58.4 Intravenous urogram in an infant with APRKD 2 hours after contrast injection. The characteristic massive kidneys with a 'sunburst pattern' of radially arranged cortical cysts are demonstrated.

diseases in humans, with an estimated incidence of approximately 1 in 1000 adults (Snyder, 1986). Although it accounts for approximately 10% of all patients with end-stage renal failure (Pirsen and Grunfeld, 1992), presentation during childhood is unusual.

GENETICS

Although ADPKD is well established as being inherited via an autosomal dominant trait, the expectation that any individual patient will have one parent or 50% of siblings similarly affected is often not found. This is presumably because some cases remain clinically undetected throughout their lives whilst in others the disease may occur as a result of spontaneous mutation (Pirsen and Grunfeld, 1992). While the specific defective gene, and its resultant biochemical abnormality, remains unknown, genetic linkage techniques (reverse genetics) using known flanking gene markers have enabled indirect isolation of the gene to the short arm of chromosome 16 (16P) (Reeders, 1992). In large 'informative families', where the specific allele markers

are observed to be linked to the determined gene, diagnosis is possible with an accuracy up to 95% (Zerres, 1989). In such families, prenatal diagnosis is also possible, using gene linkage studies of chorionic villi, as early as the ninth week of gestation (Waldherr *et al.*, 1989). Indirect gene testing *in utero* has many limitations and the frequency of non-linked ADPKD may be as high as 10% of all cases (Kimberling *et al.*, 1985).

PATHOLOGY

Renal

The disease is characterized by multiple spherical cysts of varying size (up to several centimetres in diameter) distributed throughout the cortex and medulla (Figs 58.5 and 58.6, these figures also appear in colour as Plates 11 and 12, respectively). In adult patients, the enlargement is almost always bilateral and symmetrical but in children it may initially be asymmetrical or, occasionally, unilateral. There are no associated urinary tract anomalies although the calyceal system is characteristically distorted by the cystic compression. Dysplastic changes, as seen in multicystic renal dysplasia (Chapter 57), are not found in ADPKD. Microdissection studies (Osathanondh and Potter, 1964) have shown that the cysts may arise from all parts of the nephron from Bowman's capsule to the collecting ducts. Histological studies of aborted fetuses from high-risk families have revealed multiple glomerular and tubular cysts as early as the first trimester (Zerres, 1989).

Extrarenal

Approximately one-third of patients with detected ADPKD have hepatic involvement, typically in the form of asymptomatic macrocysts which occasionally

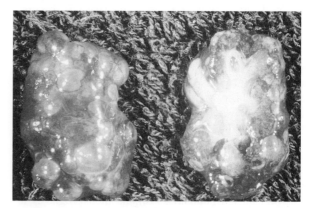

Fig. 58.5 Gross appearance of the kidneys in ADPKD, from an infant with a positive family history who died of complications of renal insufficiency. Multiple macrocysts of varying sizes are evident.

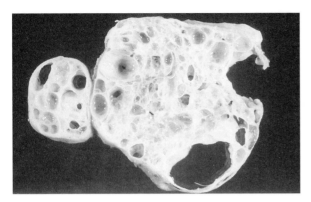

Fig. 58.6 This section of the kidney from an older individual with ADPKD demonstrates macrocysts throughout the cortex and medulla, with compression of the intervening parenchyma and collecting system.

result in massive hepatomegaly with compression symptoms. The cysts are thought to originate from biliary microhamartomas (Pirsen and Grunfeld, 1992). Unlike ARPKD, there is no periportal fibrosis and the hepatic parenchyma is well preserved. In a few cases cysts are also found in the pancreas and spleen. Intracranial aneurysms and cardiac valvular abnormalities also occur.

CLINICAL FEATURES

The peak age of presentation is around 40 years and clinical detection during childhood is comparatively rare.

Neonatal and paediatric

There are now many reports of detection of ADPKD during infancy and childhood (Kaye and Lewy, 1974; Edwards and Baldinger, 1989; Gagnadoux *et al.*, 1989; Zerres, 1989; Broyer and Gagnadoux, 1992).

Severely affected fetuses, with a positive family history and oligohydramnios, can occasionally be diagnosed prenatally, usually during the last trimester (Sedman, 1987). Early death from respiratory distress, with pulmonary hypoplasia or Potter's syndrome, should prompt a search for chromosomal and non-renal abnormalities. An association with pyloric stenosis has been described (Gagnadoux *et al.*, 1989).

Diagnosis by ultrasonography can present problems where the cystic changes are asymmetrical or unilateral, or where the cysts are small, more resembling those found in ARPKD (Broyer and Gagnadoux, 1992). The estimated sensitivity of ultrasonography during the first decade is only some 22% (Bear, 1984) and in doubtful cases imaging of older relatives is sometimes helpful.

Hypertension is the most common early manifestation of the disease in childhood and its incidence relates to the degree of renal enlargement and cyst size. The mechanism of the hypertension is unknown but is not associated with elevated levels of plasma renin (Valvo, 1985). Prompt control of blood pressure minimizes the risk of later cardiovascular complications.

Although patients with earlier clinical manifestations tend to have more rapid progression to end-stage renal failure, the course of any individual patient is difficult to predict and may vary within an affected sibship (Broyer and Gagnadoux, 1992).

Juvenile and adult

Here the clinical and radiological picture tends to be more characteristic. Recurrent loin pain and haematuria, secondary to intracystic haemorrhage or cyst distention, are the most common symptoms and become more troublesome with increasing renal enlargement, cyst size, hypertension and serum creatinine. Haemorrhage is seldom sufficient to necessitate blood transfusion. Other causes of abdominal pain in patients with ADPKD are summarized in Table 58.3. Renal cyst infections are usually ascending in origin, preceded by lower urinary tract symptoms, and are hence more common among females (Pirsen and Grunfeld, 1992). Differentiating features between renal parenchymal and cyst infections are summarized in Table 58.4. Intravenous urography or CT scans can be useful in excluding secondary obstruction from calculi or clots. Treatment of cystic infection with

Table 58.3 Aetiology of pain in autosomal dominant polycysic kidney disease

Intracystic haemorrhage and distention
Stone/clot colic
Renal parenchymal/cyst infection
Perirenal haematoma (cyst rupture)
Massive liver cyst (compression/rupture)

Table 58.4 Renal parenchymal and cyst infections in ADPKD: differentiating features

	Parenchymal	Cyst
Pyrexia	+	+
Renal pain	+	+
Blood culture	+	++
Urine culture	+	+
Pyuria	+	+
Sonograph	Anechoic	Echo complex
Antibiotic response	+	Variable

lipophobic antibiotics, i.e. aminoglycosides, penicillins and cephalospsorins (Pirsen and Grunfeld, 1992), is usually unsatisfactory owing to poor cyst penetration. The lipophilic antibiotics, i.e. trimethoprim, chloramphenicol, metronidazole and fluorinated quinolones (Bennett *et al.*, 1985) are usually more successful. Occasionally, percutaneous cyst drainage, using ultrasound or CT guidance, may be required in the acute treatment of uncontrolled sepsis. Antibiotic prophylaxis is advisable in those patients with recurrent urinary tract infections and, as a rule, urinary tract instrumentation should be avoided.

Urinary calculi occur in up to 30% of adult patients (Delaney *et al.*, 1985; Broyer and Gagnadoux, 1992), but the incidence is materially less in children. The calculi consist predominantly of uric acid, secondary to low urinary pH, hypocitraturia and stasis (Pirson and Grunfeld, 1992), and are only faintly opaque. Most can be treated initially with extracorporeal shock wave lithotripsy.

The ultrasonographic appearance in older patients is usually diagnostic, with symmetrical renal enlargement and multiple anechoic macrocysts (Fig. 58.7). There is prompt excretion on contrast studies, and while intravenous urography shows characteristic distortion of the collecting system (Fig. 58.8), CT scanning is the more sensitive imaging study (Fig. 58.9). In cyst infection, ultrasonography shows echo-complex appearances while CT scanning demonstrates irregular thickness of the cyst wall with heterogeneous contents.

Although there is a 10-fold risk of developing renal cell carcinoma in ADPKD, no such cases have been described in childhood.

Extrarenal manifestations of ADPKD are comparatively unusual. The hepatic cysts are usually asymptomatic although pain can result from compression, rupture or infection of massive cysts. The potentially

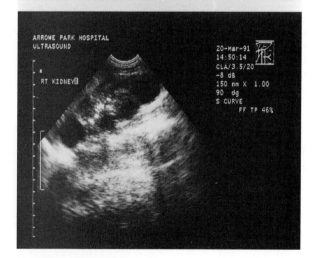

Fig. 58.7 Renal sonograph of a 10-year-old boy with ADPKD demonstrating the classical symmetrical renomegaly, with anechoic cysts of variable size in both the cortex and medulla.

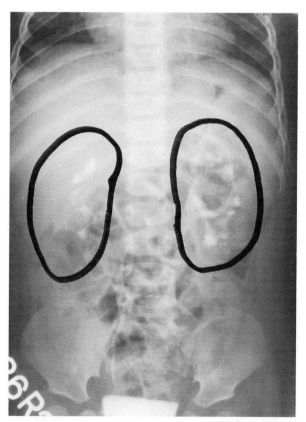

Fig. 58.8 Intravenous urogram (IVU) of a 5-year-old child with ADPKD demonstrating the early distortion of the calyces due to cyst compression and radiolucencies due to macrocysts.

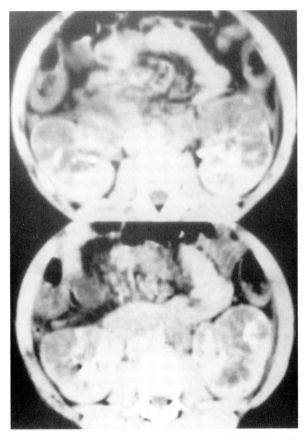

Fig. 58.9 Contrast CT scan appearance of ADPKD with symmetrical enlargement, distorted collecting system, multiple low-density cysts and areas of preserved parenchyma. High-density cysts are seen with intracystic haemorrhage.

fatal complication of intracranial Berry aneurysm is thought to occur in one-third of older patients (Lozano and Leblanc, 1992). Rupture has also been described in a few paediatric cases but the incidence and risks of rupture are not well defined because tiny aneurysms cannot be detected (Pirsen and Grunfeld, 1992). Cardiac valvular anomalies, in the form of mild mitral, tricuspid or aortic incompetence, are reported as occurring in 20% of patients (Gabow and Schrier, 1989).

SURGICAL TREATMENT

Although the treatment of ADPKD is predominantly medical, surgical intervention may be advisable for specific indications including the relief of acute or recurrent pain, and urinary tract obstruction or sepsis.

The earliest surgical treatment of ADPKD, Rovsing's operation (Walters and Braasch, 1934), took the form of open exposure and needle decompression of as many cysts as feasible. It was hoped that this would permanently relieve intrarenal pressures and prevent further pressure atrophy of the renal parenchyma. However, it proved that the cysts and pain soon recurred and that the long-term course of the disease was unaffected (Higashihara *et al.*, 1992). Nonetheless, surgical decompression of the cysts (unroofing and enucleation) does result in long-term pain relief and improved control of hypertension (Bennett *et al.*, 1987) without slowing the progression of renal insufficiency (Elzinga *et al.*, 1992). Percutaneous cyst aspiration (using ultrasound or CT guidance) is also indicated for the relief of cyst sepsis or urinary tract obstruction. Hepatic debulking in the form of partial resection and cyst fenestration has also been described in treating massive polycystic livers (Vauthey *et al.*, 1992).

PROGNOSIS

ADPKD seldom causes end-stage renal disease during childhood. Those presenting younger tend to have more rapid progression with marked renomegaly and hypertension. The probability of survival to the age of 70 years, without necessity for renal dialysis, has been estimated at 23% (Gabow *et al.*, 1992b) to 50% (Churchill *et al.*, 1984). Renal enlargement is no impediment to peritoneal dialysis. Graft survival for those undergoing renal transplantation does not differ from end-stage renal disease generally (Fitzpatrick *et al.*, 1990). Any relative offering to act as a live donor should clearly be carefully screened to exclude the disease. Indications for pretransplant nephrectomy are recurrent haematuria or renal infections.

Differential diagnosis of polycystic kidneys

There are many causes of renal cystic disease (Table 58.1) and the sonographic appearances in a fetus, neonate or infant may be inconclusive. Isotope and contrast studies are sometimes helpful. The most common cystic anomaly to be detected by prenatal ultrasonography is multicystic renal dysplasia where there is no functioning renal parenchyma (Chapter 57). Duplex system anomalies, with severe polar hydronephrosis, and multilocular, simple or parapelvic renal cysts can usually be differentiated by appropriate contrast studies and are seldom associated with appreciable renomegaly. Multiple renal cysts can be found in various multiple malformation syndromes (Table 58.5), and where the congenital anomalies involve several systems and viscera, a syndrome should be excluded. Genetic counselling, as well as sonographic monitoring of subsequent pregnancies, is advisable.

Table 58.5 Cysts associated with multiple malformation syndromes[a]

Autosomal dominant	Tuberous sclerosis
	von Hippel–Lindau syndrome
Autosomal recessive	Meckel syndrome
	Jeune's asphyxiating thoracic dystrophy
	Zellweger's cerebrohepato-renal syndrome
	Lawrence–Moon–Bardet–Biedl syndrome
	Ivemark's renohepatopancreatic dysplasia
X-linked	Orofacial digital syndrome Type I
Chromosomal disorders	Trisomy 21, 18, 13

[a]Adopted from Glassberg *et al.* (1987).

References

Bear, J.C. 1984: Age at clinical onset and at sonographic detection of adult polycystic kidney disease. *American Journal of Medical Genetics* **18**, 45–53.

Bennett, W.M., Elzinga, L., Golper, T.A. *et al.* 1987: Reduction of cyst volume for symptomatic management of autosomal dominant polycystic kidney disease. *Journal of Urology* **137**, 620–2.

Bennett, W.M., Elzinga, L., Pulliam, J.R. *et al.* Cyst fluid antibiotic concentrations in autosomal-dominant polycystic kidney disease. *American Journal of Kidney Disease* **6**, 400–4.

Blyth, H. and Ockenden, B.B. 1971: Polycystic disease of kidney and liver presenting in childhood. *Journal of Medical Genetics* **9**, 257–84.

Broyer, M. and Gagnadoux, M. 1992: Polycystic kidney disease in children. In Cameron, S., Davison, A. and Grunfeld, J. (eds), *Oxford textbook of clinical nephrology*. Oxford: Oxford University Press, 2163–71.

Churchill, D.N., Bear, J.C., Morgan, J. *et al.* 1984: Prognosis of adult onset polycystic kidney disease re-evaluated. *Kidney International* **26**, 190–3.

Delaney, V.B., Adler, S., Bruns, F.J. *et al.* 1985: Autosomal dominant polycystic kidney disease: presentation, complications, and prognosis. *American Journal of Kidney Disease* **5**, 104–11.

Edwards, O.P. and Baldinger, S. 1989: Prenatal onset of autosomal dominant polycystic kidney disease. *Urology* **34**, 265–70.

Elzinga, L., Barry, J., Torres, V. *et al.* 1992: Cyst decompression surgery for autosomal dominant polycystic kidney disease. *Journal of the American Society of Nephrology* **2**, 1219–26.

Elzinga, L., Barry, J., Torres, V. *et al.* 1992: Cyst decompression surgery for autosomal dominant polycystic kidney disease (ADPKD): long term result of renal functional and symptomatic response. *Kidney International* **37**, 247–9.

Fitzpatrick, P.M., Torres, V.E. and Charboneau, J.W. 1990: Long term outcome of renal transplantation in autosomal-dominant polycystic kidney disease. *American Journal of Kidney Disease* **15**, 535–43.

Gabow, P. and Schrier, R.W. 1989: Pathophysiology of adult polycystic kidney. *Advances in Nephrology* **18**, 19–32.

Gabow, P.A., Duley, I. and Johnson, A.M. 1992a: Clinical profiles of gross haematuria in autosomal dominant polycystic kidney disease. *American Journal of Kidney Disease* **20**, 140–3.

Gabow, P.A., Johnson, A.M., Kaehny, W.D. *et al.* 1992b: Factors affecting progression of renal disease in autosomal-dominant polycystic kidney disease. *Kidney International* **41**, 1309–11.

Gagnadoux, M.F., Habib, R., Levy, M. *et al.* 1989: Cystic renal disease in children. *Advances in Nephrology* **18**, 33–57.

Glassberg, K. and Filmer, R.B. 1992: Renal dysplasia, renal hypoplasia, and cystic disease of the kidney. In Kelalis, P., King, L. and Belman, B. (eds), *Clinical pediatric urology*. Philadelphia, PA: W.B. Saunders, 1133–84.

Glassberg, K.I., Stephens, F.D., Lebowitz, R.L. *et al.* 1987: Renal dysgenesis and cystic disease of the kidney: a report of the Committee on Terminology, Nomenclature, and Classification, Section of Urology, American Academy of Pediatrics. *Journal of Urology* **138**, 1085–8.

Higashihara, E., Nutahara, K., Minowada, S. *et al.* 1992: Percutaneous reduction of cyst volume of polycystic kidney disease: effects on renal function. *Journal of Urology* **147**, 1482–4.

Kaplan, B.S., Fay, K., Shah, V. *et al.* 1989: Autosomal recessive polycystic disease. *Pediatric Nephrology* **3**, 43–9.

Kaye, C. and Lewy, P.R. 1974: Congenital appearance of adult type (autosomal dominant) polycystic kidney disease: report of a case. *Journal of Pediatrics* **85**, 807.

Kimberling, W.J., Fain P.R., Kenyon J.B. *et al.* 1988: Linkage heterogeneity of autosomal dominant polycystic kidney disease. *New England Journal of Medicine* **52**, 313–9.

Lozano A.M. and Leblanc, R. 1992: Cerebral aneurysms and polycystic kidney disease: a critical review. *Canadian Journal of Neurological Science* **19**, 222–7.

McGonigle, R.J.S., Mowat, A.P., Bewick, M. *et al.* 1981: Congenital hepatic fibrosis and polycystic kidney disease: role of portacaval shunting and transplantation in 3 patients. *Quarterly Journal of Medicine* **199**, 269–78.

Osathanondh, V. and Potter, E.L. 1964: Pathogenesis of polycystic kidneys. Type I due to hyperplasia of interstitial portions of the collecting tubules. *Archives of Pathology* **77**, 466–73.

Pirson, Y. and Grunfeld, J. 1992: Autosomal-dominant polycystic kidney disease. In Cameron, S., Davison, A. and Grunfeld, J. (eds), *Oxford textbook of clinical nephrology*. Oxford: Oxford University Press, 2163–71.

Reeders, S. 1992: Molecular genetics of renal disorders. In Cameron, S., Davison, A. and Grunfeld, J. (eds), *Oxford textbook of clinical nephrology*. Oxford: Oxford University Press, 2155–63.

Rickwood, A.M.K. 1990: Renal cystic disease. In Lister, J. and Irving, I. (eds), *Neonatal surgery*. London: Butterworths, 685–91.

Sedman, A. 1987: Autosomal dominant polycystic kidney disease in childhood: a longitudinal study. *Kidney International* **31**, 1000–5.

Snyder, H.M. 1986: Cystic disease of the kidney, dysplasia, and agenesis. In Welch, K.J., Randolph, J.G., Ravitch, M.M., O'Neill, J.A. and Rowe, M.I. (eds), *Pediatric surgery*. Chicago, IL: Year Book Medical Publishers, 1127–34.

Valvo, E. 1985: Hypertension of polycystic kidney disease: mechanisms and haemodynamic alterations. *American Journal of Nephrology* **5**, 176–82.

Vauthey, J.N., Maddern, G.J., Kolbinger, P. *et al.* 1992: Clinical experience with adult polcystic liver disease. *British Journal of Surgery* **79**, 562–5.

Waldherr, R., Zerres, K., Gall, A. *et al.* 1989: Polycystic kidney disease in the fetus. *Lancet* **i**, 274–5.

Walters, W. and Braasch, W.F. 1934: Surgical aspects of polycystic kidney. *Surgery, Gynaecology and Obstetrics* **58**, 647–50.

Zerres, K. 1989: Cystic kidney disorders in children. In Versteegh, F.G., Ens-Dokkum, M., Ooms, E.C.M., Kuypers, J.C., Peters, P.W.J. and Velzen, D. van (eds), *First International Congress in Paediatric Pathology*. Pinjnacker: Dutch Efficiency Bureau, A1–14.

Zerres, K., Hansmann, M., Mallman, R. *et al.* 1988: Autosomal recessive polycystic kidney disease: problems of prenatal diagnosis. *Prenatal Diagnosis* **8**, 215–7.

Zerres, K., Volpel, M.C. and Weiss, H. 1984: Cystic kidneys: genetics, pathologic, anatomy, clinical picture and prenatal diagnosis. *Human Genetics* **68**, 104–35.

CHAPTER 59

Renal agenesis: ectopia and fusion

M. FISCH AND R. HOHENFELLNER

Regal agenesis   References
Ectopia and fusion

Renal agenesis

The embryological basis for renal agenesis appears to be an early insult to the developing ureteric bud which prevents normal renal organogenesis from progressing. Renal agenesis can be unilateral or bilateral, the latter being incompatible with life.

The incidence of unilateral agenesis in necropsy studies ranges between 1:600 and 1:1000 (Zollinger, 1966; Warkany, 1971) and is more often found on the left side. Males dominate in a ratio of 1.8:1(Doroshaw and Abeshouse, 1961). In the majority of patients the diagnosis is made in the second decade of life as the contralateral kidney commonly is normal. Associated anomalies occur in up to 25% of patients and involve the genitalia and the cardiovascular, gastrointestinal and skeletal systems. Investigations confirming the diagnosis include ultrasonography, excretory urography, renal function studies, computed tomography (CT) scan and magnetic resonance imaging (MRI). During cystoscopy a hemitrigone without visualization of a ureteric orifice can be found.

Bilateral renal agenesis is rare, with an incidence of 0.3 per 4000 viable births or 4 per 1000 stillborn (Potter and Craig, 1976; Kaffe et al., 1977), and males are affected more often (72% of all cases). The child shows pulmonary hypoplasia and is characteristically deformed. A prominent skinfold covers the inner canthus of each eye and the legs are often bowed and clubbed. This group of signs has been termed Potter's syndrome (Potter, 1946) and can also be found in newborns with polycystic kidney disease or urethral atresia. In 1970 Garrett et al. reported on the antenatal diagnosis of Potter's syndrome by ultrasound. Through improvements in technology and the increasing experience of investigators, today most cases of Potter's syndrome are detected antenatally by ultrasound.

Ectopia and fusion

Renal ectopia is defined as a kidney positioned outside its normal retroperitoneal location. The condition is always congenital and has to be differentiated from renal ptosis, where the renal vasculature and ureteral length are normal. Developmental arrest during renal ascent of the kidney in the embryo is responsible for the altered kidney position (pelvic, iliac or abdominal).

In crossed renal ectopia a ureter crosses the midline from the kidney on one side to the vesical orifice on the opposite side. Ninety percent of crossed ectopic kidneys are fused to the ipsilateral kidney (Kretschmer, 1925; Bagentoss, 1951). McDonald and McClellan (1957) classified crossed renal ectopic kidneys into four types: (1) crossed renal ectopia with fusion (90%), (2) crossed renal ectopia without fusion, (3) solitary crossed renal ectopia, and (4) bilateral crossed renal ectopia (Fig. 59.1a–d).

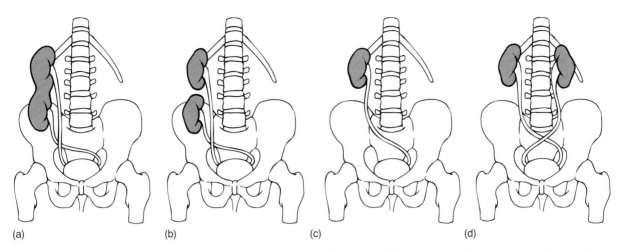

(a)   (b)   (c)   (d)

Fig. 59.1 Classification of crossed renal ectopia by McDonald and McClellan: (A) fused renal ectopia; (B) non-fused renal ectopia; (C) solitary renal ectopia; and (D) bilateral renal ectopia.

Ectopic kidneys with fusion were further classified by the nature of fusion and position. Inferior ectopia refers to a situation where the crossed ectopic kidney's upper pole adheres to the normal kidney's lower pole (two-thirds of fusions). When both kidneys are fused only at their adjacent poles in a longitudinal line this is termed a sigmoid kidney. Lump kidneys ascribes extensive fusion, L-shaped kidney means that the ectopic kidney lies transversely and disc, doughnut or pancake kidneys have variable fusions along their medial aspect.

Fusion anomalies can also be present without renal ectopia. Hence, the horseshoe kidney is the most common fusion anomaly, with fusion of the lower poles in more than 90%, the fusion site lying over the midline or asymmetrically positioned to one side (Fig. 59.2; this figure also appears in colour as Plate 13).

THORACIC KIDNEY

Thoracic renal ectopia is a very rare condition where the kidney protrudes or projects above the diaphragm. In contrast to true ectopia, in diaphragmatic hernias other abdominal viscera also occupy the chest cavity.

The embryological aetiology of the thoracic kidney is unclear. Either the kidney ascends before the diaphragmatic leaflets close normally or delayed diaphragmatic formation enhances the exaggerated renal ascent (Burke *et al.*, 1967). Because this anomaly is normally asymptomatic no therapy is required. This condition is usually diagnosed on routine chest roentgenography.

PELVIC KIDNEY

Pelvic kidney occurs when the developing metanephric blastema in the 5–7-week embryo fails to ascend normally. The incidence of this anomaly is reported to range from 1:2100 to 1:3000 births (Stevens, 1937). The pelvic kidney is served by one or more aberrant renal arteries

and veins. (Dretter *et al.*, 1971). The renal hilum is ventrally related as the kidney does not rotate until it reaches the normal lumbar position (Perlmutter *et al.*, 1986).

In up to 50% of patients the contralateral kidney is abnormal (Malek *et al.*, 1971). As in other position-associated anomalies, skeletal and genitourinary tract anomalies may coexist (Malek *et al.*, 1971; Donahoe and Hendren, 1980).

Pelvic kidneys are more susceptible than normal kidneys to calculus formation. They can also be obstructed owing to a high pelviureteric junction or anomalous blood vessels crossing the ureter. Non-obstructive dilata-

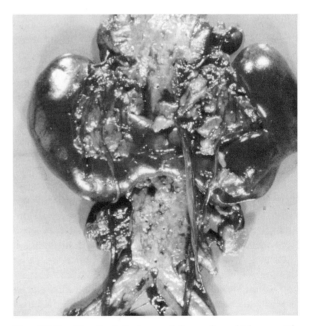

Fig. 59.2 Classical feature of horseshoe kidney with fusion of the lower poles The renal pelves are situated in front and the ureters pass anteriorly to the isthmus.

tion results from associated reflux, dysplasia or malrotation and may be difficult to differentiate from obstruction. In clinical series, ectopic kidneys are frequently symptomatic in up to 40–50% of patients (Downs *et al.*, 1973).

The correct diagnosis can be established by pelvic ultrasound. Visualization in urography may be difficult as the kidney overlies the pelvic bones.

HORSESHOE KIDNEY

Horseshoe kidneys result from an abnormal fusion of the metanephric masses in the first 2 months of fetal life. If, during this time, metanephric buds become attached to one another their normal upward migration and rotation would be blocked.

Associated anomalies occur in at least one-third of patients, including multisystem disturbances of the skeletal and cardiovascular system (Taylor *et al.*, 1987) and gastrointestinal tract, as well as genitourinary abnormalities (Boatman *et al.*, 1971). Dysplasia and neoplasia such as Wilm's tumour, angiomyolipoma, teratoma, renal cell carcinoma and transitional cell carcinoma have been reported to arise from horseshoe kidneys (Castro, 1975; Feldmann and Lome, 1982; Gray *et al.*, 1983; Schacht *et al.*, 1983; Reed *et al.*, 1984).

In 95% of cases the lower poles are fused (Fig. 59.2), whereas in only 5% of cases are the upper poles fused. The isthmus may be composed of a fibrous band but more often is composed of thick parenchymous tissue. In lower pole fusion calyces face the vertebral column and the pelves are situated in front. The ureters arch anteriorly to pass over the isthmus (Dajani, 1966).

The blood supply of the horseshoe kidney is quite variable (Graves, 1966; Boatman *et al.*, 1971): 30% have a renal blood supply that consists of one renal artery for each kidney (Bernstein *et al.*, 1986). The isthmus may be supplied by the renal arteries, aorta, inferior mesenteric, common or external iliac as well as sacral arteries, and the entire blood supply may enter through the isthmus (Berlmutter *et al.*, 1986).

At least one-third to a half of patients with horseshoe kidneys remain asymptomatic. Nevertheless, upper tract dilatation may be present in up to 80% of patients (Segura *et al.*, 1972; Odiase, 1983) (Fig. 59.3).

This upper tract dilatation may be due to pelviureteric junction stenosis which reflects the usual high insertion of the ureter into the pelvis as well as displacement by the fused isthmus. In these patients recurrent flank pain increasing after high oral fluid intake is a typical symptom. Stones as a sign of obstruction are a common finding in adults but rare in children.

During sonography the prevertebral isthmus can be visualized by an experienced investigator. The diagnosis can be established in most cases with excretory urography if both kidneys are functioning well (Fig. 59.4). The vertical line of the axis through the kidney will point towards the lumbosacral spine and there will be ureteral

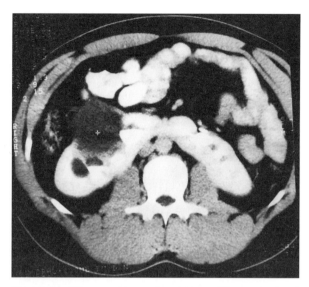

Fig. 59.3   CT scan of horseshoe kidney. Slice at the level of the isthmus. The right moiety shows dilatation.

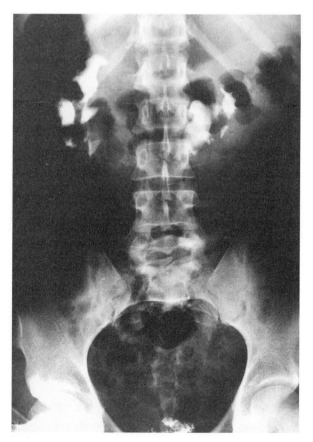

Fig. 59.4   IVP of horseshoe kidney: the vertical line of the axis through the kidneys points towards the lumbosacral spine. The pelves are anteriorally located as a sign of malrotation.

deviation by the isthmus. Radionuclide studies are helpful either to establish whether the isthmus contains functioning parenchyma (Fig. 59.5) or to show an obstruction by measuring the washout after application of frusemide. In symptomatic horseshoe kidneys with dilatation and obstruction, division of the isthmus in combination with pyeloplasty and lateropexy of the dilated part of the horseshoe kidney is the treatment of choice, and can easily be accomplished by means of a flank incision on the side of dilatation. Full preoperative investigations are required to identify the plane of separation permitting a minimum loss of functioning parenchyma.

Data evaluation by single photon emission computed tomography (SPECT) based on gamma camera renography allows three-dimensional (3D) presentation using special computer systems. The 3D picture constructed using the SPECT data clearly shows the configuration of the kidney and the portion of the isthmus presenting with the least functioning parenchyma, thereby clearly defining the optimal surgical plane (Fig. 59.6; this figure also appears in colour as Plate 14).

Between 1969 and 1991 65 patients with a horseshoe kidney were operated on at our institution, nearly half of whom (27) needed separation of the two parts of the kidney because of obstruction, either alone or in combination with a pyeloplasty.

CAKE KIDNEY (LUMBAR KIDNEY)

Complete fusion of both kidneys into a rounded, irregularly lobed mass is considered extremely rare (Fig. 59.7). Embryologically, complete fusion may be explained by abnormal course of the ureteric buds, with fusion occurring if their terminations are too close together. Alternatively, this anomaly could result from the growth of the ureteric buds into a common metanephric blastema (Parton, 1962). The vascular supply of the cake kidney is variable and is derived from the adjacent vessels. The fused kidney may remain asymptomatic and be detected at autopsy (Shiller and Wiswell, 1957). It may become infected or cause local symptoms (Glenn, 1958) and equally may be misdiagnosed as a tumour. The coexistence of cake kidney with anomalies of the cardiovascular system is well recognized (Taylor *et al.*, 1987).

CROSSED RENAL ECTOPIA

One of the rarest anomalies of the urinary tract is crossed renal ectopy. The incidence has been reported to be 1:3000 to 1:7500 autopsies and 1:5300 pyelograms (Dretschmer, 1925; Boatman *et al.*, 1972; Hendren *et al.*, 1976), with a male predominance (Cook and Stephans, 1977; Farkas and Earon, 1978; Vereb *et al.*, 1978) and affecting the right side two to three times as often as the left side (Kelalis, 1976; Vereb *et al.*, 1978). Since solitary crossed renal ectopia combines two non-related events it is extremely rare (1:1 500 000 cases) and only a few cases have been reported in the literature (Tanenbaum *et al.*, 1970; Cranidis and Terhorst, 1982; Miles *et al.*, 1985).

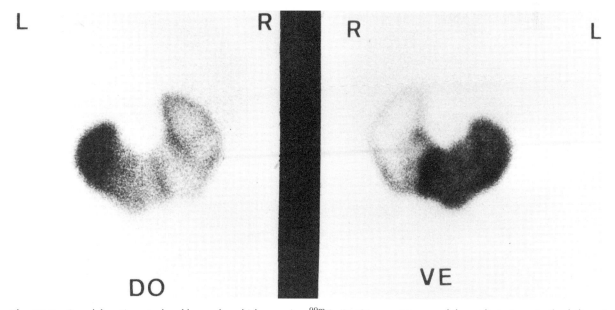

Fig. 59.5 Renal function study of horseshoe kidney using ^{99m}Tc-DMSA: persistence of the radioisotope in the left part of the horseshoe kidney 3 hours after injection. The amount of radioisotope found in the right part of the kidney is significantly lower. In the area of the isthmus there are functioning parenchyma. The mean function of the right side was calculated to be 26%, compared with 74% on the left side.

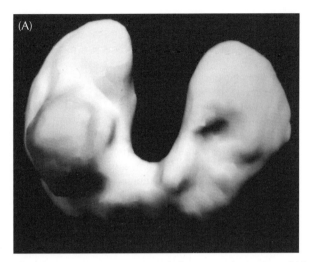
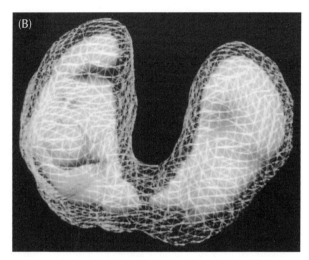

Fig. 59.6 SPECT imaging of the same horseshoe kidney: this 3D picture constructed using the SPECT data, clearly shows the configuration of the kidney. (A) For this picture the medium level of isointensity lines was used to create the surface. By illumination with light of different colours the 3D effect of the picture is achieved. (B) In this picture the medium level is transparent and only the inner level of high isointensity is solid. The portion of less function in the isthmus clearly can be identified, representing the best plane for operative separation of the kidney.

Although renal ectopia has been observed at all ages it is mostly diagnosed in patients between the ages of 21 and 30 years (McDonald and McClellan, 1957).

Theories that have been proposed to explain crossed renal ectopia are that the kidneys become attached while in the pelvis and are pulled toward one side during their ascent, that there may be abnormal vascular connections or that development of the ureteral bud may induce the development of the nephrogenic blastema of the contralateral kidney (Kelalis *et al.*, 1973; Witten *et al.*, 1977). Because of the increased frequency of skeletal abnormalities, mainly in children diagnosed with this entity, there may be a teratogenic factor affecting both systems (Kelalis *et al.*, 1973). In general, the occurrence of associated malformations is low. The most frequent are orthopaedic anomalies (4%), imperforate anus (4%), and genital and septal cardiac defects (Abeshouse and Bhisitkul, 1959; Hertz

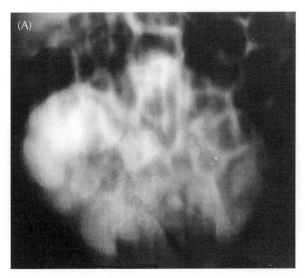
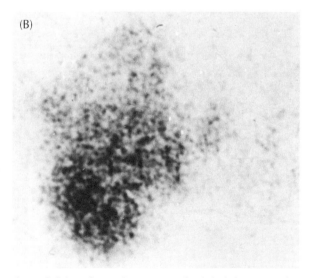

Fig. 59.7 Cake kidney: (A) IVP showing dilatation on the right and delayed visualization on the left (left part: multicystic kidney with ureteral atresia). (B) Renal function study of the same kidney showing good function of the right and impaired function of the left side.

et al., 1977; Marshall and Freeman, 1978, Kyrayiannis *et al.*, 1979). A frequently associated genitourinary anomaly is reflux with subsequent hydronephrosis, but megaureters, urethral valves, cystic dysplasia, vaginal aplasia, hypospadias and cryptorchidism have also been reported. Solitary crossed ectopic kidneys have the highest accompanying malformation rate in 40–50% (Rivard *et al.*, 1978; Miles *et al.*, 1985; Pak *et al.*, 1988).

The blood supply is abnormal to both kidneys and arteries originating from the aorta from D12 to L3–4 as well as from the common iliac arteries have been reported (Hertz *et al.*, 1977).

Many patients with crossed renal ectopy remain entirely asymptomatic. The clinical symptoms are non-specific and may or may not be related to the side of the malformation. The most common presenting clinical features are abdominal or flank pain, a palpable mass, haematuria, urinary tract infections and dysuria, and 20–30% are incidental findings (Hertz *et al.*, 1977; Marshall and Freedman, 1978; Kyrayiannis *et al.*, 1979; Perlmutter *et al.*, 1986). The urological conditions associated with crossed ectopic kidneys are hydronephrosis, reflux, renal calculi and tumours. Renal tumours in

crossed ectopic renal tissue have been reported sporadically (Langworthy and Drexler, 1942; Lee, 1949). The tumours were nephroblastoma (Berant *et al.*, 1975; Redman and Berry, 1977), mesoblastic nephroma (Williams, 1982) and renal cell carcinoma in the renal pelvis (Kyraviannis *et al.*, 1979).

Although an intravenous pyelogram (IVP) usually demonstrates crossed renal ectopy (Figs 59.8 and 59.9), additional imaging studies will be necessary if the function of the ectopic renal unit is impaired secondary to multicystic dysplasia, trauma, severe obstruction or replacement by tumour. Ultrasound confirms the absence of a renal unit on one side but also plays an important role in sorting out the differential diagnosis, establishing the aetiology of the palpable mass and planning the surgical approach. In non-functioning crossed ectopy ultrasound will demonstrate the presence of the normal and the ectopic kidney, whereas the IVP will show only a normal-sized single kidney in an essentially normal position (Rosenberg, 1984).

Placing the patient in multiple positions during the IVP has been used to shift the kidney shadows away from each other to differentiate between fused and unfused states. Ectopic pelvic kidneys have malrotated

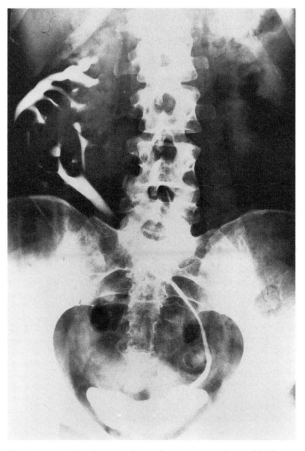

Fig. 59.8 IVP of crossed renal ectopia: L-shaped kidney.

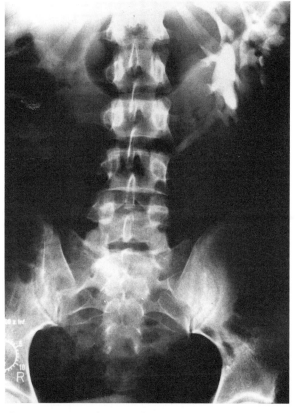

Fig. 59.9 IVP of sigmoid or S-shaped crossed renal ectopia.

renal pelves and usually some degree of dilatation which could be mistaken for pelviureteric junction obstruction. A diuretic renogram to document actual obstruction may be helpful in this clinical setting (Das and Amar, 1984). Because of the high incidence of reflux, a voiding cystogram is recommended. CT scans, MRI and antegrade or retrograde pyelography in selected cases have all been used to clarify the anomaly. Arteriography prior to surgery may be useful in demonstrating any anomalous blood supply.

Treatment of crossed renal ectopy is indicated for the complications rather than for the anomaly itself. The majority of cases do not require any surgical intervention except for complications such as hydronephrosis, stones, abscess or tumour.

References

Abeshouse, S.B. and Bhisitkul, I. 1959: Crossed renal ectopia with and without fusion. *Urology International* **9**, 63.

Bagentoss, A.H. 1951: Congenital anomalies of the kidney. *Medical Clinics of North America* **35**, 987–91.

Berant, M., Jacob, E.T. and Pevzner, S. 1975: Wilm's tumor in the crossed ectopic kidney. *Journal of Pediatric Surgery* **10**, 555.

Bernstein, J. and Gardner, K. 1986: Renal ectopic disease and renal dysplasia. In Walsh, P.C., Gittes, R. and Perlmutter, A. (ed), *Campbell's Urology*, 5th ed. Philadelphia, PA: W.B. Saunders, 1793–7.

Boatman, D.L., Cornell, S.H. and Kolln, C.P. 1971: The arterial supply of horseshoe kidneys. *American Journal of Radiology* **113**, 447.

Boatman, D.L., Culp, D.A., Jr, Culp, D.A. and Flocks, R.H. 1972: Crossed renal ectopia. *Journal of Urology* **108**, 30.

Burke, E.C., Wenzl, J.E. and Utz, D.C. 1967: The intrathoracic kidney. Report of a case. *American Journal of Diseases in Children* **113**, 487.

Castro, J.E. 1975: Complications of horseshoe kidney. *Urology* **6**, 344.

Cook, W.A. and Stephans, F.D. 1977: Fused kidneys morphologic study and theory of embryogenesis. *Birth Defects* **13**, 327.

Cranidis, A. and Terhorst, B. 1982: Crossed renal ectopia with solitary kidney. *Urological Radiology* **4**, 45.

Dajani, A. 1966: Horseshoe kidney: a review of twenty nine cases. *British Journal of Urology* **38**, 388–402.

Das, S. and Amar, A. 1984: Ureteropelvic junction obstruction with associated renal anomalies. *Journal of Urology* **131**, 872.

Donahoe, P. K. and Hendren, W.H. 1980: Pelvic kidney in infants and children. *Journal of Pediatric Surgery* **115**, 486.

Doroshow, L. and Abeshouse, B.S. 1961: Congenital unilateral solitary kidney: report of 37 cases and a review of the literature. *Urological Surgery* **11**, 219.

Downs, R.A., Lane, J.W. and Burns, E. 1973: Solitary pelvic kidney. Its clinical implications. *Urology* **1**, 51.

Dretler, S.P., Olsson, C. and Pfister, R.C. 1971: The anatomic, radiologic and clinical characteristics of the pelvic kidney:

an analysis of 86 cases. *Journal of Urology* **105**, 623–7.

Dretschmer, H.L. 1925: Unilateral fused kidney. *Surgery, Gynecology and Obstetrics* **40**, 350.

Farkas, A. and Earon, J.M. 1978: Crossed renal ectopia with crossed single ectopic ureterocele. *Journal of Urology* **119**, 836.

Feldmann, S.L. and Lome, L.G. 1982: Renal dysplasia in horseshoe kidney. *Urology* **20**, 74.

Garrett, W.G., Grunwald, G. and Robinson, D.E. 1970: Prenatal diagnosis of fetal polycystic kidney by ultrasound. *Australian and New Zealand Journal of Obstetrics and Gynaecology* **10**, 7.

Gay, B. B., Dawes, R.K. and Atkinson, G.O. 1983: Wilm's tumor in horseshoe kidneys: radiologic diagnosis. *Radiology* **146**, 693.

Glenn, J.W. 1958: Fused pelvic kidney. *Journal of Urology* **80**, 7–9.

Graves, F.T. 1969: The arterial anatomy of the congenitally abnormal kidney. *British Journal of Surgery* **56**, 533–41.

Hendren, W.H., Donahoe, P.K. and Pfister, R.L. 1976: Crossed renal ectopia in children. *Urology* **7**, 135.

Hertz, M., Rubinstein, Z.J., Shahin, N. and Melser, M. 1977: Crossed renal ectopia. Clinical and radiological findings in 22 cases. *Clinical Radiology* **28**, 339–44.

Kaffe, S., Godmilow, L., Walker, B.A. and Hirschhorn, K. 1977: Prenatal diagnosis of bilateral agenesis. *Obstetrics and Gynecology* **49**, 478.

Kelalis, P.P. 1976: Anomalies of the urinary tract. In Kelalis, P.P., King, L.R. and Belman, A.B. (eds), *Clinical pediatric urology*. Philadelphia, PA: W.B. Saunders, 475–98.

Kelalis, P.P., Malek, R.S. and Segura, J.W. 1973: Observations on renal ectopia and fusion. *Journal of Urology* **110**, 558.

Kretschmer, H.L. 1925: Unilateral fused kidney. *Surgery, Gynecology and Obstetrics* **40**, 360.

Kyrayiannis, B., Stenos, J. and Deliveliotis, A. 1979: Ectopic kidney with and without fusion. *Journal of Urology* **51**, 173–4.

Langworthy, H.T. and Drexler, L.S. 1942: Carcinoma in crossed renal ectopia. *Journal of Urology* **47**, 776.

Lee, H.P. 1949: Crossed unfused renal ectopia with tumor. *Journal of Urology* **61**, 333.

McDonald, J.H. and McClellan, D.S. 1957: Crossed renal ectopia. *American Journal of Surgery* **93**, 995–9.

Malek, R.S., Kelalis, P.P. and Burke, E.C. 1971: Ectopic kidney in children and frequency of other malformations. *Mayo Clinic Proceedings* **46**, 461.

Marshall, F.F. and Freedman, M.T. 1978: Crossed renal ectopia. *Journal of Urology* **119**, 188–91.

Miles, B.J., Moon, M.R., Belville, W.D. and Kiesling, V.J. 1985: Solitary crossed renal ectopia. *Journal of Urology* **133**, 1022–3.

Odiase, V.O.N. 1983: Horseshoe kidney. A review of 25 cases. *Journal of the Royal College of Surgeons* **28**, 41.

Pak, K., Konishi, T. and Tomoyoshi, T. 1988: Non-crossed renal ectopia with fusion associated with single ectopic ureter. *Urology* **32**, 246–9.

Parton, L.I. 1962: Renal fusion. *New Zealand Medical Journal* **61**, 506–9.

Perlmutter, A.D., Retik, A.B. and Bauer, S.B. 1986: Anomalies of the upper urinary tract. In Walsh, P.C., Gittes, R. and Perlmutter, A. (eds), *Campbell's urology*, 5th ed. Philadelphia, PA: W.B. Saunders, 1665–759.

Potter, E.L. 1946: Facial characteristics of infants with bilateral renal agenesis. *American Journal of Obstetrics and Gynecology* **51**, 885.

Potter, E.L. and Craig, J.M. 1976: *Pathology of the fetus and the infant*, 3rd ed. London: Lloyd-Luke.

Redman, J.F. and Berry, D.C. 1977: Wilm's tumor in crossed fused renal ectopia. *Journal of Pediatric Surgery* **12**, 601.

Reed, H.M. and Robinson, N.D. 1984: Horseshoe kidney with simultaneous occurrence of calculi, transitional cell and squamous cell carcinoma. *Urology* **23**, 62.

Rivard, D.J., Milner, W.A. and Garlich, W.B. 1978: Solitary crossed renal ectopia and its associated congenital anomalies. *Journal of Urology* **120**, 241.

Rosenberg, H.K. 1984: Traumatic avulsion of the vascular supply of a crossed unfused ectopic kidney: complementary roles of ultrasonography and intravenous pyelography. *Journal of Ultrasound Medicine* **3**, 89.

Schacht, M.J., Sakowica, B. and Rao, M.S. 1983: Intermittent abdominal pain in a patient with horseshoe kidney. *Journal of Urology* **130**, 749.

Segura, J.W., Kelalis, P.P. and Burke, E.C. 1972: Horseshoe kidneys in children. *Journal of Urology* **108**, 333.

Shiller, W.R. and Wiswell, O.B. 1957: A fused pelvic (cake) kidney. *Journal of Urology* **78**, 9–16.

Stevens, A.R. 1937: Pelvic single kidneys. *Journal of Urology* **37**, 610–8.

Tanenbaum, B., Silverman, N. and Weinberg, S. 1970: Solitary crossed renal ectopia. *Archives of Surgery* **101**, 616.

Taylor, D.C., Sladen, J.G. and Maxwell, T. 1987: Aortic surgery and horseshoe kidney: a challenging surgical problem. *Canadian Journal of Surgery* **30**, 431–3.

Vereb, J., Tischler, V. and Pavkovcekova, O. 1978: Differential X-ray diagnosis of renal dystopia and ectopias in children. *Pediatric Radiology* **7**, 205.

Warkany, J. 1971: *Congenital malformations*. Chicago, IL: Year Book Medical Publishers.

Williams, G.B. 1982: Mesoblastic nephroma in crossed renal ectopia. *Journal of Urology* **128**, 801–2.

Witten, D.M., Myers, E.H. and Utz, D.C. 1977: Emett's clinical urography. Philadelphia, PA: W.B. Saunders, 579–93.

Zollinger, H.V. 1966: Niere und ableitende Harnwege. In Doerr, W. and Uehlinger, E. (eds) *Spezielle pathologische Anatomie*, 3rd ed. Berlin: Springer.

CHAPTER 60

Bladder exstrophy and epispadias complex

P. MALONE

Introduction
Incidence and epidemiology
Embryology
Pathological anatomy
Classic bladder exstrophy
Cloacal exstrophy
Clinical features

Management
Investigation
Surgical treatment
Ongoing reconstructive programme
Isolated epispadias
Results
References

Introduction

Bladder exstrophy and epispadias represents a complex series of abnormalities ranging from isolated epispadias through classical bladder exstrophy to the most complex condition of cloacal exstrophy. It is a rare abnormality but its clinical significance is major because of the devastating effect of the condition on the patients and their families and the need for multiple, staged, complex operative procedures to achieve a satisfactory outcome offering a good quality of life.

The management of the exstrophy patient has undergone a number of evolutionary changes from cutaneous urinary diversion, continent diversion using uretero-sigmoidostomy to total reconstruction of the lower genitourinary tract. In 1992 the European Society of Paediatric Urology (ESPU) hosted a symposium on bladder exstrophy and a broad consensus was reached which consisted of staged reconstruction during infancy and early childhood. The management described later in this chapter will generally reflect this consensus. This move to reconstruction means that the exstrophy patient should be treated not by the 'occasional surgeon' but only by those with experience and facilities to offer a complete treatment programme from start to finish. It is only by adopting this approach that the excellent results that are possible will be achieved in most patients, an expectation to which they are certainly entitled.

Incidence and epidemiology

The reported prevalence of classic bladder exstrophy is 3.3 in 100 000 births, epispadias without exstrophy 2.4 in 100 000 and cloacal exstrophy 1 in 200 000–400 000 births (International Clearing House for Birth Defects, 1987). Classic bladder exstrophy is more common in males, with a ratio ranging from 1.5:1 to 3:1. Isolated epispadias is especially rare in females, with a male to female ratio of approximately 4:1, and the ratio for cloacal exstrophy is 1:1 (Leck *et al.*, 1968; Hendren, 1981, International Clearing House, 1987).

The aetiology of the exstrophy complex is unknown. In a number of studies no linkage has been found with maternal age, birth order, season of birth, chromosomal or genetic abnormalities or teratogens (Leck *et al.*, 1968; Ives *et al.*, 1980; Shapiro *et al.*, 1984). Blickstein and Katz (1991) reported a cluster of infants with bladder exstrophy–epispadias born to women treated with progestins in early pregnancy and suggested a causal relationship. The International Clearing House study (1987) found that high parity (≥3) increased the risk for bladder exstrophy but reduced that for epispadias. Shapiro *et al.* (1984) found nine recurrences in 2500 families, a risk of 1:275. There were 17 sets of twins and bladder exstrophy affected both in five monozygotes. Sixty-six exstrophy patients produced 215 offspring and three had exstrophy, a risk of 1:70, which is

400 times greater than in the general population. It is hoped that better genital reconstruction will improve fertility rates but parents must be counselled that the risks of recurrence are greater than previously assumed.

Embryology

The bladder develops by subdivision of the cloaca (Arey, 1974). A wedge of mesenchyme known as the cloacal or urorectal septum divides the cloaca into a dorsal rectum and a ventral bladder and urogenital sinus, a process completed by the seventh week.

The primitive bladder is continuous with the allantois, and its caudal end receives the two common stems of the paired mesonephric ducts and ureters which mark the approximate upper end of the urogenital sinus. The urogenital sinus is divided into two regions, a pelvic portion nearest the bladder and a slit-like phallic portion which extends as a solid plate into the terminal part of the genital tubercle. This whole area is covered by an entodermal–ectodermal plate, the cloacal membrane, which extends along the allantois to the body stalk. When the urorectal septum reaches the cloacal membrane, rupture follows promptly. After 8 weeks the bladder proper expands into an epithelial sac, the apex of which tapers into an elongated tube, the urachus, which is continuous with the proximal remnant of the allantoic stalk at the umbilicus. In the female the short neck connecting the bladder and the urogenital sinus elongates into the whole urethra and the urogenital sinus itself forms the shallow vestibule. In the male the counterpart of the female urethra extends from the bladder to the distal prostatic urethra, the pelvic portion of the urogenital sinus forms the rest of the prostatic and the membranous urethra while the phallic portion adds the cavernous urethra which extends through the penis.

One theory of the cause of the exstrophy–epispadias complex is early rupture of the cloacal membrane along with failure of mesoderm to invade the infraumbilical region which allows the bladder to open and evert on to the ventral abdominal wall (Arey, 1974; Ives *et al.*, 1980). If rupture of the cloacal membrane occurs very early before the urorectal septum has developed (before the fifth week) cloacal exstrophy develops (Johnston, 1913) whereas if it occurs between the fifth and seventh weeks bladder exstrophy ensues (Ives *et al.*, 1980). This theory is disputed by Marshall and Muecke (1962). They postulated an overdevelopment of the cloacal membrane, producing a wedge effect, which would hold apart the developing structures of the lower abdominal wall but leave them intrinsically normal in a diverged position. An excessive and perhaps premature split of the cloacal membrane would then be expected to extend towards the body stalk and lay open the underlying vesical primordium. It is more difficult to explain the origin of cloacal exstrophy by this hypothesis. The earlier and more extensive the split in the cloacal membrane the greater would be the tendency for the underlying structures to eventrate and this could interfere with the formation of the urorectal septum and its reaching the perineum. To derive epispadias without exstrophy it is necessary only to picture a lesser persistence or overdevelopment of the cloacal membrane.

Pathological anatomy

The anomaly of exstrophy–epispadias involves not only the urinary tract and genital system as might be expected, but also the musculoskeletal arrangements of the lower abdomen and pelvis. The deformity is sometimes so extensive as to effect the lower gastrointestinal tract, thus constituting a complex involving the urinary, genital, musculoskeletal and intestinal systems all in one continuum, i.e. cloacal exstrophy.

Classic bladder exstrophy

BLADDER AND UPPER URINARY TRACT

The urethra and bladder are open anteriorly with the bladder represented as a midline bulging mass below the umbilicus (Fig. 60.1). The exstrophied bladder changes in size as the intra-abdominal pressure varies. On the lower part of the everted mass two small elevated projections are seen, which are the ureteric orifices.

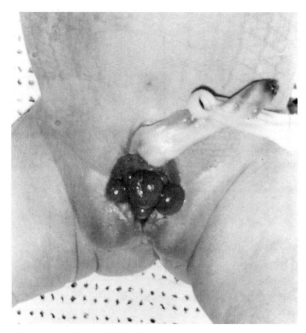

Fig. 60.1 Classical bladder exstrophy.

Occasionally, if the mucosa is oedematous, these can be difficult to identify. On each side of the lower part of the bladder there is an area of shiny skin, the paraexstrophy skin. The bladder itself can vary enormously in respect of its mucosal appearance, size, distensibility and neuromuscular function which are important when planning treatment. (Jeffs, 1986). Culp (1964) studied the histology of 23 exstrophic bladders, none of which was entirely normal. The abnormalities included: acute and chronic follicular inflammation with oedema of the submucosal layer, patchy areas of squamous metaplasia of the epithelial covering, glandular formations in the submucosal and muscular layers which bear a striking resemblance to rectal glands, cystitis cystica, marked fibrosis of the muscular layer with disorganization in the arrangement of the muscle bundles, patches of intestinal mucosa which have no connection with the intestinal tract and, finally, neoplastic change in one of the 23 bladders. This was an adenocarcinoma in a 52-year-old man. Shapiro *et al.* (1985) studied the muscarinic cholinergic receptors in exstrophy and found that the density and binding affinity of receptors were similar to control bladders. They concluded that the neurophysiological composition of the exstrophied bladder was not grossly altered. Toguri *et al.* (1978) performed gas cystometry in continent patients following bladder closure and reported normal results in 70%. However, more recent work by Hollowell *et al.* (1991) disputed these findings. They prospectively studied 36 children with exstrophy and epispadias using cystometry and cystography. Bladder function was normal only in those patients with epispadias who did not require bladder neck reconstruction, but the bladders of all of the closed exstrophies and the epispadias patients requiring bladder neck reconstruction were abnormal. The most common abnormality was detrusor instability, which was a major cause of upper tract damage. However, it seems likely that these abnormalities were not congenital but related to surgery, particularly bladder neck reconstruction.

The upper urinary tract is usually normal but horseshoe kidney, pelvic kidney, hypoplastic kidney and renal agenesis have been reported. The ureters enter the bladder with little or no obliquity and consequently following bladder closure reflux will occur in nearly 100% of cases (Jeffs, 1987).

GENITAL DEFECTS

Male

Woodhouse and Kellett (1984) studied the penis in 17 patients by cavernosograms, computed tomography (CT) scans and surgical exploration. The glans penis is wide, with a dorsal groove, and the urethra is represented by a mucosal strip on the dorsum of the short upturned penis. In most cases the corpora are normal in diameter and have a normal attachment to the inferior pubic ramus. However, the exophytic part of the penis is short, partly because so much of the corporal length is taken up in reaching the midline, but also because the total length of the corpora is reduced, producing a short penis of normal calibre. Ten corpora in six patients were rudimentary, probably because of operative damage. The neurovascular bundles are found on the dorsolateral aspect of the corpora cavernosa. Erectile deformities are also seen, which most commonly consist of a tight dorsal chordee. The chordee is due to intrinsic curves in the deep part of the corpora before they emerge from the perineum. In patients with unilateral rudimentary corpora there is deviation of nearly 90° to one side, as well as the dorsal chordee. Despite the severity of the deformity it is amenable to surgical correction with satisfactory functional results in the majority of cases. Rarely, if the penis is duplicated or severely dystrophic, sex reassignment is advised but this only occurs in every 1:50–100 cases (Jeffs, 1986). The scrotum is wide and shallow and although most testes are retractile, orchidopexy is not commonly required.

Female

Because the bladder and the abdominal wall are effectively missing, the vagina and anus are displaced forward. Indeed, in some patients, even after successful bladder reconstruction, the introitus appears to be on the lower abdomen rather than in the perineum. The clitoris is bifid and the mons pubis, labia and clitoris are divergent. The urethra and vagina are short and the vaginal orifice is frequently stenotic. The vagina and uterus are poorly supported and liable to prolapse, particularly during pregnancy and following delivery (Stanton, 1974; Dewhurst *et al.*, 1980). Septate vagina, bicornuate uterus and absent ovary have also been described (Blakaley and Mill, 1981).

MUSCULOSKELETAL DEFECTS

In all cases of exstrophy there is wide diastasis of the pubic symphysis due to lateral rotation of the iliac and innominate bones. The pubis is also rotated downwards so that the inferior pubic ramus lies horizontally when the patient is standing (Woodhouse and Kellet, 1984). This position and the normal attachment of the corpora to the inferior ramus contribute to the penile shortening. In more severe cases, such as cloacal exstrophy, there is also a lateral separation of the inferior part of the innominate bone. It has generally been believed that these deformities produce little in the way of orthopaedic abnormalities other than a waddling gait, but Thomas and Wilkinson (1989) reported two patients with dislocation of the hip prior to treatment and Blakeley and Mills (1981) also reported a similar case.

The distance between the umbilicus and anus is shortened and the bladder bulges through a triangular fascial defect limited laterally by the divergent rectus muscle and inferiorly by the open urogenital diaphragm stretched between the separated pubic bones. The tendon and the tendon sheath of the rectus muscle have a fan-like extension behind the urethra and the bladder neck that inserts into the intersymphyseal band or urogenital diaphragm. Inguinal herniae frequently occur because of a patent processus vaginalis, wide internal and external inguinal rings and lack of obliquity of the inguinal canal. Stringer *et al.* (1994) reported herniae in 86% of boys and 15% of girls undergoing staged reconstruction and in 78% of cases they were bilateral. Twenty-nine per cent of boys presented with an incarcerated hernia and there was a postoperative recurrence of 17%.

ANORECTAL DEFECTS

The perineum is broad and short and the anal canal is displaced anteriorly. The divergent levator ani and puborectalis muscles and the distorted external sphincter contribute to varying degrees of anal incontinence and rectal prolapse. Rectal prolapse virtually always disappears after closure of the bladder. Imperforate anus, anal stenosis and rectovaginal fistulae have also been reported.

Classic bladder exstrophy is rarely associated with congenital anomalies other than those discussed above, but cloacal exstrophy frequently is.

Cloacal exstrophy

The main features of classic cloacal exstrophy are an exstrophic central bowel field flanked by two hemibladders (Fig. 60.2). The central bowel field is the ileocaecal region and it has three or four orifices: the superior orifice leads from the terminal ileum and it can prolapse as the 'elephant trunk', the inferior orifice leads to a short blind-ending colonic segment, and these are flanked by the two lateral appendiceal orifices. In 90% of cases an exomphalus is present at the upper aspect of the eventrated bladder and bowel. In 30% of males the penis is absent but it is usually widely separated with two rudimentary corpora. About 20% of males have an epispadias and the testes are usually undescended. The scrotum may be absent, divided into two hemiscrota or bifid. In the female Müllerian fusion anomalies are almost always found: uterine duplication in 95%, vaginal duplication in 65% and an absent vagina in 25% (Tank and Lindenauer, 1970).

Associated anomalies occur in the majority of cases and in some series the incidence is as high as 95% (Spencer, 1965; Huruitz *et al.*, 1987; Mitchell *et al.*, 1990). They include the upper urinary tract, vertebral anomalies ranging from spina bifida to sacral agenesis, gastrointestinal anomalies such as malrotation, atresia, duplication and anatomic short bowel, central nervous system anomalies such as myelomeningocele and hydrocephalus, and cardiovascular and pulmonary anomalies including cyanotic heart disease.

Clinical features

The defect may be perfectly obvious, as in classic bladder exstrophy, but the defect of epispadias in both males and females may be less obvious on initial presentation. Classic bladder exstrophy accounts for about 50% of all cases but variations occur (Marshall and Muecke, 1962).

SUPERIOR VESICAL FISSURE

The opening in the bladder lies just below the umbilicus but the inferior portion has fused and the genitalia are usually normal. These patients have a good sphincteric mechanism so closure of the opening is usually all that is required. This is not just an example of a patent urachus, as the musculoskeletal abnormalities of exstrophy (separation of the pubic symphysis) are always present.

DUPLICATE EXSTROPHY

Sheldon *et al.* (1990) described a case of an exstrophic bladder plate with a normal-sized subjacent bladder, patulous bladder neck and associated epispadias. The author has also seen such an arrangement, which has been described as covered exstrophy and visceral sequestration by others (Cerniglia *et al.*, 1989).

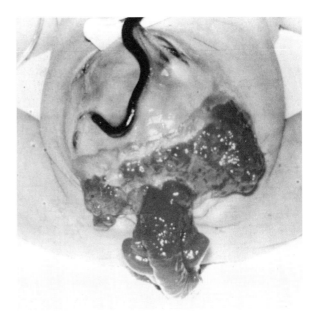

Fig. 60.2 Cloacal exstrophy.

INFERIOR VESICAL FISSURE

Marshall and Muecke (1962) suggested that an epispadias with an open bladder neck might conceivably be labelled an inferior fissure.

MALE EPISPADIAS WITHOUT EXSTROPHY

This is subdivided into glanular, penile and subsymphyseal (Jeffs, 1986). The majority of these patients are incontinent as the sphincteric mechanism is involved. The anatomical defect is similar to that seen in patients with associated bladder exstrophy and there is also symphyseal diastasis.

FEMALE EPISPADIAS WITHOUT EXSTROPHY

There are two subdivisions: bifid clitoris and subsymphyseal. The urethra is patulous and incontinent and the symphyseal area is usually abnormally widened.

CLOACAL EXSTROPHY

The cloacal exstrophy complex has been classified into two broad categories based on bladder and bowel patterns (Manzoni *et al.*, 1987). Type 1 includes the classic cloacal exstrophy patterns and comprises three subgroups: 1A, hemibladders confluent cranial to the bowel field; 1B, hemibladders on the side of the bowel; and 1C, hemibladders confluent caudal to the bowel. Type 2 includes the variants and often contains the most bizarre combination of abnormalities. In an attempt to organize such complex and unfamiliar anatomy Manzoni *et al.* (1987) constructed a grid by which the anomaly can be schematically represented.

PRENATAL DIAGNOSIS

Bladder filling and emptying can be detected from as early as 16 weeks' gestation so, in theory, exstrophy should be amenable to prenatal ultrasound diagnosis. It is disappointing, therefore, that bladder exstrophy is rarely diagnosed early in pregnancy. Cloacal exstrophy has an associated exomphalus which is commonly diagnosed prenatally, but the true extent of the condition is rarely appreciated. Shapiro *et al.* (1984) reported one patient with cloacal exstrophy where maternal α-fetoprotein levels were elevated.

Management

The aims of management are:

- to preserve renal function
- to achieve dryness with voiding or bladder emptying by clean intermittent catheterization
- to produce satisfactory abdominal wall and genital cosmesis

- to effect functional genital reconstruction to allow satisfactory sexual activity and preserve fertility in later life
- to produce an individual who can integrate normally into society.

There is no doubt that these aims are best served by functional reconstruction of the lower genitourinary tract and although urinary diversion is of historical interest in the treatment of bladder exstrophy and may still be required in the occasional patient, it will not be dealt with further in this chapter.

It is essential that the parents appreciate the nature of the abnormality so that they can understand and accept the necessity for the multiple complex operations that will be required in the future. They should have the opportunity to hold and cuddle their baby and see the exstrophy in the presence of the paediatric urologist, who can explain the nature of the anomaly to them. This frequently necessitates the transfer of mother and baby together to a specialist centre where appropriate accommodation and facilities should be made available. The introduction of urological nurse specialists has dramatically improved this aspect of care by providing liaison with the community and thus better ongoing support of the family as a whole.

Investigation

BLADDER EXSTROPHY

Initial investigations are limited to a complete clinical examination, including full blood count, blood urea, and electrolytes and creatinine estimation. The author routinely performs an ultrasound scan of the upper urinary tract and pelvis prior to bladder closure to confirm the presence of two normal kidneys and, with the recent recognition of hip dislocation, an orthopaedic consultation with an ultrasound assessment of the hip joints. Following bladder closure repeated monitoring investigations are required to assess both the continuing normal development of the upper urinary tract and the growth and capacity of the bladder, including blood testing, ultrasound scans, isotope renography and cystography.

CLOACAL EXSTROPHY

Because of the increased risk of associated anomalies meticulous assessment is required and includes clinical examination, karyotyping and imaging of the urinary, gastrointestinal and central nervous systems. These investigations should include ultrasound examination of the kidneys, abdominal X-ray to assess the gas pattern (e.g. atresia), X-rays of the spine and sacrum, chest X-ray and other more specialized investigations when indicated by the initial results. A clear picture of the exstrophy itself and other associated anomalies should be available before one embarks on treatment.

Surgical treatment

BLADDER EXSTROPHY (TABLE 60.1)

Bladder closure

There is no doubt that initial bladder closure was the consensus at the ESPU symposium in 1992. However, there was some debate on the timing of closure and this centred on whether pelvic osteotomy was used. If pelvic osteotomy is not used, closure should be performed certainly within the first 72 hours and is probably best within the first 24 hours of life. This turns the condition into an operative emergency and necessitates the separation of mother and child, and there is now a definite trend towards osteotomy and closure within the first week or 10 days.

In the past, posterior iliac osteotomies were used (Schultz, 1958; Lloy-Roberts *et al.*, 1959; Aadalen *et al.*, 1980), but recently there has been a move to anterior horizontal osteotomies of the innominate bones (Salter type). The operative technique is well described by Gibbon *et al.* (1991) who reported excellent results with their first 11 patients. Perovic *et al.* (1992a) performed anterior osteotomies through the superior pubic ramus, originally described by Frey and Cohen (1989), in 36 children, all of which were successful. Fixation of the bony pelvis or traction is usually employed following osteotomy but Allen *et al.* (1992) successfully treated six infants without any form of pelvic fixation. Anterior pelvic osteotomy may soon become routine in the initial management of all patients with bladder exstrophy, but it will be a long time before its benefits can be assessed. This approach will require the active participation and input of paediatric orthopaedic specialists.

Bladder closure is performed simultaneously with pelvic osteotomy and only very few patients are not suitable for closure (Ansell, 1979; Mollard, 1980; Osterling and Jeffs, 1987). The surgical techniques are well described by Jeffs (1986) and Ransley *et al.* (1988) and will not be dealt with in detail in this text. In 1977 Duckett advocated the use of paraexstrophy skin flaps in bladder closure but at the ESPU (1992) worry was expressed that this may cause infertility and difficulty with urethral intermittent catheterization and there was a clear trend towards abandoning their routine use (Gearhart *et al.*, 1993). The cosmetic benefits of superior translocation of the umbilical stump were also stressed and although a normal umbilicus is not produced, a satisfactory appearance is possible. The success of bladder closure has improved considerably from the 36% dehiscence reported by Williams and Savage (1966) to the 94% success rate of Oesterling and Jeffs (1987). Patients with a successful initial closure had greater bladder capacities, reduced time intervals from primary closure to bladder neck reconstruction and urinary continence. Lowe and Jeffs (1983) identified wound infection and bladder prolapse secondary to poor pelvic ring fixation and insufficient urethral and bladder neck length as the principal causes of dehiscence. Jeffs *et al.* (1982) identified the following factors in successful exstrophy closure:

Table 60.1 Staged reconstruction of classical exstrophy–epispadias

(1) Initial bladder closure combined with Salter-type osteotomy at 7–10 days
   Examination under anaesthesia at 4–6 weeks and at 6-monthly intervals to assess the bladder outlet and capacity; 6-monthly ultrasound scans of the upper tracts

(2) Repair of epispadias at 12 months following 3 months of testosterone treatment
   Sustanon 25 mg. i.m./month × 3 months

(3a) Young–Dees–Leadbetter bladder neck reconstruction
   If bladder capacity not greater than 100 ml by 4–5 years, proceed to (3b)

(3b) Young–Dees–Leadbetter with augmentation cystoplasty
   If patient remains wet or if the upper tracts deteriorate, proceed to (4)

(4) Augmentation cystoplasty (if not previously performed)
   Redo bladder neck reconstruction
   Artificial urinary sphincter or bladder neck injection
   Continent diversion
   If retention ensues, proceed to (5)

(5) Clean intermittent catheterization with or without Mitrofanoff

- bladder protection with a smooth plastic film for 7–10 days followed by closure with simultaneous osteotomy
- a heavy anterior suture for approximation of the pubic symphysis
- avoidance of infection with the use of broad-spectrum antibiotics
- effective bladder drainage with a suprapubic (not urethral) catheter and ureteric stents, again exiting suprapubically
- provision of a bladder neck and urethra of sufficient length to prevent prolapse of the anterior wall and dome of the bladder
- the use of modified Bryant's traction for 3–4 weeks. With the introduction of the Salter-type osteotomy stabilization by plaster spica (in the baby) or fixation devices in the older child are being used more commonly.

If the initial closure is unsuccessful, even if complete dehiscence occurs, reclosure can and should be attempted. Gearhart *et al.* (1993) described reclosure, for complete dehiscence in 28 cases and significant prolapse in 10, in combination with osteotomy (even if this had been previously performed). There were no cases of recurrent prolapse or dehiscence.

The aim of the initial closure is to change the exstrophy into an isolated incontinent epispadias. It is essential to ensure continued free drainage of urine from the bladder by having a loose closure of the bladder neck and urethra (20 FG). This should also minimize the risks of urinary infection secondary to vesicoureteric reflux by facilitating low-pressure bladder emptying but the use of prophylactic antibiotics as indicated. Continued upper tract surveillance with ultrasonography is advised and regular (6-monthly) examinations are carried out under anaesthesia to assess the bladder capacity.

In rare cases patients may be continent following initial bladder closure and no further bladder reconstruction will be required. Mollard *et al.* (1994) achieved this in three of 66 patients and Hollowell and Ransley (1991) in two of 86 patients. This result seems to be a fortunate accident and cannot be achieved by specific procedures.

CLOACAL EXSTROPHY

Initial surgery

A broad outline of the initial surgical treatment is indicated in Table 60.2. In selected cases the longer single-stage closure may be appropriate but in patients with severe associated anomalies staged primary closure may be more successful. Important points include the preservation of as much bowel as possible and the construction of an end colostomy rather than an ileostomy (Howell *et al.*, 1953). It has been suggested that if the

Table 60.2 The surgical treatment of cloacal exstrophy

(a) Early	
Bladder	Separate bowel from the two hemibladders
	Join bladders, converting the anomaly to 'bladder exstrophy'
	Functional closure of bladder with bilateral pelvic osteotomy
	(this may be done as a secondary procedure)
Bowel	Tubularize exstrophied bowel segment
	Preserve as much bowel length as possible
	Construct end colostomy
Genitalia	46 XY – gender reassignment to female
	Bilateral orchidectomy
	Clitoroplasty
Exomphalus	Closure with abdominal wall repair
Other	Treat all associated anomalies as required
(b) Late	
Bladder	Follow scheme as outlined for classical bladder exstrophy
Bowel	Colonic pull-through
	Faecal incontinence: permanent stoma; ACE procedure
Genitalia	Monsplasty and vaginoplasty

hemibladders are small the exstrophic ileocaecal plate can be left behind as an autoaugmentation with an end-to-end anastomosis of the ileum to the hindgut. Pelvic osteotomies are always required. The urethra is usually absent and creation of a neourethra is performed using paraexstrophy or perineal skin flaps. There is universal agreement that males with an inadequate phallus should be reassigned to female gender.

Additional procedures

Some additional operative procedures may be required during early infancy and include inguinal herniotomy and treatment of rectal prolapse. Stringer *et al.* (1994) suggest that inguinal hernia repair should be performed at the time of bladder closure as the vast majority of patients will require this procedure at some point. Rectal prolapse rarely persists following bladder closure.

Following a successful closure the infant can then be treated as normal in every way for bladder exstrophy, but those with cloacal exstrophy will need ongoing colostomy care. The continuous leakage of urine may lead to skin problems, which may be reduced by the frequent and often ingenious use of barrier creams by parents. Parents will require regular support and guidance and the importance of input from a urological nurse specialist at this stage should not be underestimated.

Ongoing reconstructive programme

BLADDER EXSTROPHY

The patient should be fitted into the planned sequence as defined in Table 60.1. The first stage in the ongoing reconstructive is the epispadias repair and the principal steps are outlined in Table 60.3. The Cantwell–Ransley repair is well described elsewhere (Ransley *et al.*, 1988), has superseded all previous forms of repair and excellent results are reported (Gearhart *et al.*, 1992; Provic *et al.*, 1992b). Gearhart and Jeffs (1989) have also demonstrated increased bladder capacity following epispadias repair, which aids subsequent bladder neck reconstruction and the achievement of continence (Peters *et al.*, 1988). Patients with isolated epispadias are managed in a similar fashion. The next operative step involves bladder neck reconstruction to produce dryness. At the ESPU (1992) there was a lack of consensus at this point. Many experts recommended the Young–Dees–Leadbetter bladder neck reconstruction in combination with ureteric reimplantation but without bladder augmentation (Dees, 1949; Leadbetter, 1964). Gearhart and Jeffs (1988) report satisfactory continence with this approach and only 12 of their 148 patients required a subsequent augmentation. More recently, Mollard *et al.* (1994) reported their results in 55 patients; 10 patients required bladder augmentation combined with a redo bladder neck reconstruction in

five, seven required an isolated redo bladder neck reconstruction and one a bladder neck suspension. However, Woodhouse *et al.* (1983) reported only 10 of 62 patients to be reliably dry following bladder neck closure and Hollowell and Ransley (1991) found that 20 of the 32 patients treated by bladder neck reconstruction alone later required an augmentation. It is difficult to reconcile these differences but many of the difficulties seemed to relate to the definition of continence. Some authors refer to a dry interval in excess of 3–4 hours, but others are more critical, demanding a continent patient who never wets. There are many sequelae of enterocystoplasty (Woodhouse, 1992a). The majority of patients with augmentation are dependent on clean intermittent catheterization to empty their bladders (Kramer, 1989; Hollowell and ransley, 1991; De Castro *et al.*, 1994), and some will require additional operative procedures such as the Mitrofanoff (1980) procedure to facilitate this (Hollowell and Ransley, 1991; Borzi *et al.*, 1992). It would seem that attempts to achieve continence by bladder neck reconstruction alone are well worthwhile but there should be a low threshold to proceed to augmentation should the patient remain incontinent or upper tract dilatation occurs. Even with this approach failure to produce continence still occurs in a minority of patients but Gearhart *et al.* (1991) have reported good results with redo Young–Dees–Leadbetter bladder neck reconstruction: 16 of 17 patients were made socially continent. Despite these advances and successes failure continues to occur, but some further procedures may help. With the technical improvements of artificial urinary sphincters their successful use is increasingly being reported in patients with bladder exstrophy–epispadias where previous surgery has failed to make them dry (Perlmutter *et al.*, 1991). Decter *et al.* (1988) report a 70% success rate with the AS 800 device in six patients, and as far back as 1983 Light and Scott reported a 90% success rate with the AS 792 device. Patients who have undergone previous urinary diversion may be suitable for undiversion or conversion to a continent diversion using the Mitrofanoff procedure (Hollowell and Ransley, 1991).

CLOACAL EXSTROPHY

Bladder reconstruction to attain continence is more difficult than in classic bladder exstrophy (Table 60.2). A limiting factor is the amount of bowel available but Mitchell *et al.* (1990) recommend the use of gastrocystoplasty. The timing and techniques of vaginal reconstruction are also controversial and perineal skin flaps or intestine may be used. Present trends favour the use of colon if sufficient length is available (Martinez-Mora *et al.*, 1992; Hitchcock and Malone, 1994). Even if vaginal reconstruction is carried out early formal revision after puberty will usually be required (Hurwitz, 1990).

Table 60.3   Cantwell–Ransley epispadias repair: essential steps

(1)	Preliminary glansplasty	Essentially the reverse of the MAGPI: it is called the IPGAM and it displaces the urethral meatus ventrally
(2)	Skin mobilization	Starts in the midline above the urethral meatus, down each side of the dorsal urethral plate, around the coronal sulcus with complete degloving of the penis
(3)	Mobilization of the urethral plate	Start on the ventral surface and preserve a pedicle from the dartos. Mobilize completely.
(4)	Mobilization of the corpora	These are freed completely with only limited dissection (1–2 cm) from the inferior pubic ramus
(5)	Mobilization of neurovascular bundles	Run laterally and ventrally
(6)	Tubularization of the urethra	Prior to this a broad strip of glans tissue is excised on each side of the glanular urethra. The urethra is closed over a 10 FG catheter and then displaced ventrally
(7)	Closure of glans	In two layers
(8)	Artificial erection	A separate injection is required for each corpus
(9)	Cavernostomy/corporal rotation	Performed at the site of maximal angulation the dorsal surface of the corpora using non-absorbable sutures
(10)	Mobilization of the preputial skin	The mucosal surface is mobilized on its vascular pedicle and brought on to the dorsal surface for skin cover
(11)	Silastic foam dressing	For 1 week
(12)	Follow up cystoscopy	At 3 months

Isolated epispadias

MALE

The penile reconstruction is best performed around 1 year of age with the aid of preoperative testosterone treatment. The Cantwell–Ransley approach is the recommended technique and excellent cosmetic and functional results can be achieved. If the patient is continent no further treatment is required but in the incontinent patient the continuing approach is similar to that employed for classical exstrophy. Some encouraging preliminary results are emerging with the use of bladder neck injection (Caoni *et al.*, 1993).

FEMALE

The correction of female epispadias was described by Hendren 1981. The cleft urethra is mobilized and tubularized throughout its length and the dilated proximal urethra is also narrowed. The thin skin above the mons is excised and the fat from the mons can be used to cover the neourethra and obliterate the space behind the pubic symphysis. The medial aspects of the clitoris are then excised, the two halves brought together and the mons closed. Hendren then describes a simultaneous Young–Dees–Leadbetter bladder neck reconstruction but in the author's experience the urethral reconstruc-

tion alone may provide an adequate increase in resistance to make the patient dry. Therefore the bladder neck reconstruction does not need to be performed simultaneously and if the patient remains incontinent it is worth trying a bladder neck injection before taking the major step of bladder neck reconstruction (Caoni *et al.*, 1993).

Results

MORTALITY

Although the exstrophy–epispadias complex is not in itself a lethal condition, deaths do occur, but largely as a result of complications of treatment. In the early twentieth century 50% of patients were dead by 10 years of age and 67% by 20 years (Woodhouse, 1991). With improvements in treatment and the advent of antibiotics mortality has fallen dramatically; Woodhouse *et al.* (1983) reported nine deaths in 101 patients, only three of which were directly attributable to the exstrophy and its management, and Connor *et al.* (1989) reported four deaths in 207 patients. Cloacal exstrophy was thought to be uniformly fatal until Rickham (1960) reported the first surgically treated survivor. Since then the reconstructive efforts have increased and with the intensive treatment of the short bowel survival rates of 80–100%

are reported (Howell *et al.*, 1983; Diamond and Jeffs, 1985; Hurwitz *et al.*, 1987). Mortality is usually a result of associated anomalies.

Malignant degeneration within the bladder is the most common cause of mortality in the classic exstrophy group. This rarely arises in the native bladder as a result of metaplasia in the bladder mucosa or the islands of intestinal mucosa seen in the exstrophic bladder (Culp, 1964; Jeffs, 1986). The tumour is usually an adenocarcinoma but rare cases of squamous cell carcinoma and rhabdomyosarcoma have been reported (Jeffs, 1986). The most common cause of a malignant tumour is following ureterosigmoidostomy and it is hoped that the declining use of this operation will reduce the number of deaths from malignant disease. Malignant change is also reported in patients with enterocystoplasty but probably to a much lesser degree; 14 neoplasms have been reported to date and the mean time to tumour development is 18 years (Woodhouse, 1992b). Life-long surveillance will be required because of this increased risk of malignant disease.

Renal failure is the other cause of mortality and a major factor in chronic morbidity, and is a direct consequence of management. Woodhouse *et al.* (1983) reported two deaths in 101 patients secondary to renal failure and Connor *et al.* (1989) reported significant renal deterioration in up to 26% of patients. In the long term the kidneys do much better with a working bladder: 25% of continent patients had renal damage compared to 50% of incontinent patients with a reconstructed bladder, but in those patients with a urinary diversion renal damage ranged from 55% to 100% (Woodhouse, 1991). Husman *et al.* (1988a) reported renal damage in 13% of 51 patients successfully reconstructed, compared to 82% with ileal conduits, 22% for non-refluxing colonic conduits and 33% for ureterosigmoidostomies.

BLADDER FUNCTION

Although good results are reported by many authors following functional reconstruction the proportion of fully continent exstrophy patients is small (Woodhouse, 1991). The results from the Hospital for Sick Children, Great Ormond Street, London, reported by Woodhouse *et al.* (1983) and updated by Woodhouse in 1991, were that completely reliable continence was only achieved in five of 21 girls and five of 41 boys. Connor *et al.* (1989) reported that for 137 patients undergoing primary anatomical reconstruction 31% eventually required urinary diversion but when the closure was performed within 72 hours of birth and followed by staged bladder neck reconstruction 'acceptable urinary continence' was achieved in 82% of patients. Jeffs (1987) claims that many patients are too young to assess complete diurnal and nocturnal continence, but a 3-hour dry interval indicates that this will eventually be achieved. Using these

criteria he claimed that patients requiring redo bladder closure had a 55% continence rate compared to 92% where the primary closure was successful. Whether these figures can be accepted as representing true continence is debatable. Ansell (1979) and Mollard *et al.* (1994) reported continence rates of 43% and 69%, respectively, but again their criteria of continence assessment were not clearly defined. Hollowell and Ransley (1991) reported on 86 patients with classic exstrophy who had undergone primary bladder closure. They classified continence as excellent with a dry interval greater than 4 hours, good greater than 3 hours, poor not greater than 2 hours with protection required, and wet patients. Only 12 with bladder reconstruction alone achieved an excellent or good result but a total of 71 patients required augmentation cystoplasty as well, some with an associated Mitrofanoff procedure. At least 55 patients in their group needed clean intermittent catheterization to empty their bladders and 80% achieved good results using this approach. At the end of the day it would seem that satisfactory dryness rather than continence can be achieved in at least 80% of patients with bladder exstrophy but long-term results of patients with augmentations, Mitrofanoff procedures or artificial urinary sphincters are as yet unknown. Life-long follow-up is required to assess renal function, bladder function and growth. Hollowell and Ransley (1991) described spontaneous bladder perforation in seven patients. Wagstaff *et al.* (1992) and Mundy and Nurse (1992) have expressed worries with respect to growth, calcium balance and skeletal mineralization in patients with cystoplasties.

It is more difficult to assess long-term bladder function in patients with isolated epispadias as large series are not available. Woodhouse (1991) stated that about half the patients have a working bladder and he had not encountered the same long-term problems as occur with classical exstrophy patients. Peters *et al.* (1988) reported satisfactory continence in 87% of patients, only one of whom required bladder augmentation. More recent work suggested that bladder neck reconstruction may produce bladder dysfunction in the isolated epispadias patient and implied that this may not be the optimum treatment (Hollowell *et al.*, 1991).

Bladder function in cloacal exstrophy is difficult to assess. Diamond and Jeffs (1985) were the first to report dry intervals of 3–4 hours in three of seven available patients, and satisfactory continence was reported by Mitchell *et al.* (1990) in 83% of 12 patients and by Ricketts *et al.* (1991) in three of 11 patients. The majority of these patients are dependent on clean intermittent catheterization and many have undergone enterocystoplasty.

BOWEL FUNCTION

In cloacal exstrophy, a significant proportion of patients have life-threatening short bowel syndrome, therefore many are malnourished and require long-term parenteral nutrition. Faecal continence has been reported in only two patients but social control with various enema programmes can be achieved in some patients following pull-through (Husmann *et al.*, 1988b; Ricketts *et al.*, 1991). The long-term effect of the antegrade continence enema (ACE) procedure has yet to be evaluated (Malone *et al.*, 1990).

SEXUAL FUNCTION

There is no doubt that the evolution of the Cantwell–Ransley repair of epispadias has produced improved cosmetic and functional results. Men appear to have normal libido but fewer casual sexual partners than would be expected in the population at large. However, they do appear to form stable partnerships with normal women and have a normal family life. Woodhouse (1991) reported that 33 of 43 patients for whom full information was available were married or lived with a partner (Woodhouse, 1991). It was also claimed that even for patients with a small penis mutually satisfactory sexual relations with female partners were the norm. It is hoped, and the expectations seem to be realistic, that with the new penile repair and its improved correction of erectile deformities, better cosmesis and function will be achieved.

In the female, although the vagina may be narrow and short, and lie horizontally, this rarely interferes with sexual function and in one series 14 out of 23 women had normal intercourse with orgasm (Woodhouse, 1991).

In cloacal exstrophy gender reassignment in all but the most unusual male will avoid the disastrous problem of the sexually inadequate male, but the future sexual potential of these gender-converted females remains uncertain.

FERTILITY

Ejaculation occurs in the majority of men but there is a high incidence of poor or absent sperm. However, it seems that patients who have an early urinary diversion have better sperm than those in whom reconstruction has been attempted (Hanna and Williams, 1972; Lattimer *et al.*, 1979). Shapiro *et al.* (1984) reviewed the literature and found reports of 18 males with exstrophy who fathered 23 children and 17 males with epispadias who fathered 23 children. In Woodhouse's series seven of the male patients have initiated one or two pregnancies from which there have been five children. A further 13 are known to be infertile, and he states that the main cause of infertility is repeated bladder and prostatic infections related to the reconstruction rather than obstruction of the vasa or ejaculatory duct systems (Woodhouse, 1991).

In the female fertility seems to be unimpaired. Shapiro *et al.* (1984) reported on 66 women with exstrophy and seven with complete epispadias who had 84 and 11 children, respectively. However obstetric difficulties are common, varying from uterine prolapse to complete procidentia (Clayton, 1945; Krisiloff *et al.*, 1978). There is no information available on fertility in the female patients with cloacal exstrophy but in patients with normal ovaries and genital tracts fertility must be possible.

SOCIAL DEVELOPMENT

In general exstrophy patients are well-motivated, well-adjusted people who are hard working and proud of their jobs, and unemployment is reported to be considerably lower than the national average (Woodhouse, 1991).

There is little doubt that with expert surgical management and continuing counselling, well-integrated individuals with satisfactory sexual and bladder function will be the end result. Parents should therefore be counselled on the major nature of the anomaly and the treatment needed, but a realistically optimistic outlook should be given. There is little long-term follow-up for patients with cloacal exstrophy.

References

Aadalen, R.J., O'Phelan, E.H., Chisholm, T.C. *et al.* 1980: Exstrophy of the bladder; long term results of bilateral posterior iliac osteotomies and two stage anatomic repair. *Clinical Orthopaedics and Related Research* **151**, 193–200.

Allen, T.D., Husmann, D.A. and Bucholz, R.W. 1992: Exstrophy of the bladder: primary closure after iliac osteotomies without external or internal fixation. *Journal of Urology* **147**, 438–40.

Ansell, J.D. 1979: Surgical treatment of exstrophy of the bladder with emphasis on neonatal primary closure: personal experience with 28 consecutive cases treated at the University of Washington Hospitals from 1962–1977: techniques and results. *Journal of Urology* **121**, 650–3.

Arey, L.B. 1974: *Developmental anatomy. A textbook and laboratory manual of embryology*, 7th ed. (revised). Philadelphia, PA: W.B. Saunders, 308–14.

Blakeley, C.R. and Mill, W.G. 1981: The obstetric and gynaecological complications of bladder exstrophy and epispadias. *British Journal of Obstetrics and Gynaecology* **88**, 167–73.

Blickstien, I. and Katz, Z. 1991: Possible relationship of bladder exstrophy and epispadias with progestins taken during pregnancy. *British Journal of Urology* **68**, 105–6.

Borzi, P.A., Bruce, J. and Gough, D.C.S. 1992: Continent cutaneous diversions in children: experience with the Mitrofanoff procedure. *British Journal of Urology* **70**, 669–763.

Caoni, P., Lais, A., De Gennaro, M. and Lapozza, N. 1993: Gluteraldehyde cross-linked bovine collagen in exstrophy/epispadias complex. *Journal of Urology* **150**, 631–3.

Cerniglia, F.R., Roth, D.R. and Gonzales, E.T.1989: Covered exstrophy and visceral sequestration in a male newborn: case report. *Journal of Urology* **141**, 903–4.

Clayton, S.G. 1945: Note of case of exstrophy of bladder with procidentia. *Journal of Obstetrics and Gynaecology of the British Empire* **52**, 177–9.

Connor, J.P., Hensle, T.W., Lattimer, J.K. and Burbige, K.A. 1989: Long-term follow up of 207 patients with bladder exstrophy: an evolution in treatment. *Journal of Urology* **142**, 793-6.

Culp, D.A. 1964: The histology of the exstrophied bladder. *Journal of Urology* **91**, 538–48.

De Castro, R., Pavanello, P., and Domini, R. 1994: Indications for bladder augmentation in the exstrophy–epispadias complex. *British Journal of Urology* **73**, 303–7.

Decter, R.M., Roth, D.R., Fishman, I.J. *et al.* 1988: Use of the AS 800 device in exstrophy and epispadias. *Journal of Urology* **140**, 1202–3.

Dees, J.E. 1949: Congenital epispadias with incontinence. *Journal of Urology* **62**, 513–22.

Dewhurst, J., Toplis, P.J. and Sheperd, J.H. 1980: Ivalon sponge hysterosacropexy for genital prolapse in patients with bladder exstrophy. *British Journal of Obstetrics and Gynaecology* **87**, 67–9.

Diamond, D.A. and Jeffs, R.D. 1985: Cloacal exstrophy: a 22-year experience. *Journal of Urology* **133**, 779–82.

Duckett, J.W. 1977: Use of paraexstrophy skin pedicle grafts for correction of exstrophy and epispadias repair. *Birth Defects* **13**, 175–9.

European Society for Paediatric Urology 1992: Third Annual Meeting, Cambridge, UK.

Frey, P. and Cohen, S.J. 1989: Anterior pelvic osteotomy. A new operative technique facilitating primary bladder exstrophy closure. *British Journal of Urology* **64**, 641–3.

Gearhart, J.P. and Jeffs, R.D. 1988: Augmentation cystoplasty in the failed exstrophy reconstruction. *Journal of Urology* **139**, 790–3.

Gearhart, J.P. and Jeffs, R.D. 1992: Bladder exstrophy: increase in capacity following epispadias repair. *Journal of Urology* **142**, 525–6.

Gearhart, J.P., Canning, D.A. and Jeffs, R.D. 1991: Failed bladder neck reconstruction: options for management. *Journal of Urology* **146**, 1082–4.

Gearhart, J.P., Leonard, M.P., Burgers, J.K. and Jeffs, R.D. 1992: The Cantwell–Ransley technique for repair of epispadias. *Journal of Urology* **148**, 851–4.

Gearhart, J.P., Peppas, D.S. and Jeffs, R.D. 1993: The failed exstrophy closure: strategy for management. *British Journal of Urology* **71**, 217–20.

Gibbon, A.J., Maffuli, N. and Fixsen, J.A. Horizontal pelvic osteotomies for bladder exstrophy – a preliminary report. *Journal of Bone and Joint Surgery* **73B**, 896–8.

Hanna, M.K. and Williams, D.I. Genital function in males with vesical exstrophy and epispadias. *British Journal of Urology* **44**, 169–74.

Hendren, W.H. 1981: Congenital female epispadias with incontinence. *Journal of Urology* **125**, 558–64.

Hitchcock, R.J.I. and Malone, P.S. 1994: Colovaginoplasty in infants and children. *British Journal of Urology* **73**, 196–9.

Hollowell, J.G. and Ransley, P.G. 1991: Surgical management of incontinence in bladder exstrophy. *British Journal of Urology* **68**, 543–8.

Hollowell, J.G., Hill, P.D., Duffy, P.G. and Ransley, P.G. 1991: Bladder function and dysfunction in exstrophy and epispadias. *Lancet* **338**, 926–8.

Howell, C., Caldamone, A., Snyder, H., Ziegler, M. and Duckett, J. 1983: Optimal management of cloacal exstrophy. *Journal of Pediatric Surgery* **18**, 365–9.

Hurwitz, R.S. 1990: Cloacal exstrophy: management of the genitalia. *Dialogues in Pediatric Urology* **13**, 5–6.

Hurwitz, R.S., Manzoni, G.M., Ransley, P.G. and Stephens, F.D. 1987: Cloacal exstrophy: a report of 34 cases. *Journal of Urology* **138**, 1060–4.

Husmann, D.A., MacLorie, G.A. and Churchill, B.M. 1988a: A comparison of renal function in the exstrophy patient treated with staged reconstruction versus urinary diversion. *Journal of Urology* **140**, 1204–6.

Husmann, D.A., MacLorie, G.A., Churchill, B.M. and Ein, S.H. 1988b: Management of the hindgut in cloacal exstrophy: terminal ileostomy versus colostomy. *Journal of Pediatric Surgery* **23**, 1107–13.

International Clearing House for Birth Defects 1987: Epidemiology of bladder exstrophy and epispadias. *Teratology* **36**, 221–7.

Ives, E., Coffey, R. and Carter, C.O. 1980: A family of bladder exstrophy. *Journal of Medical Genetics* **17**, 139–41.

Jeffs, R.D. 1986: Exstrophy of the urinary bladder. In Welch, K.J., Randolph, J.G., Ravitch, M.M., O'Neill, J.A. and Rowe, M.I. (eds), *Pediatric surgery*, 4th ed. Chicago, IL: Year Book Medical Publishers, 1216–41.

Jeffs, R.D. 1987: Exstrophy, epispadias and cloacal and urogenital sinus abnormalities. *Pediatric Clinics of North America* **34**, 1233–57.

Jeffs, R.D., Guice, S.E. and Oesch, I. 1982: The factors in successful exstrophy closure. *Journal of Urology* **127**, 974–6.

Johnston, T.B. 1913: Extraversion of the bladder complicated by the presence of intestinal openings on the surface of the extraverted area. *Journal of Anatomy* **48**, 89–106.

Kramer, S.A. 1989: Augmentation cystoplasty in patients with exstrophy–epispadias. *Journal of Pediatric Surgery* **24**, 1293–6.

Krisiloff, M., Puchner, P.J. and Tretter, W. 1978: Pregnancy in women with bladder exstrophy. *Journal of Urology* **119**, 478–9.

Lattimer, J.K., MacFarlane, M.T. and Puchor, P.J. 1979: Male exstrophy patients: a preliminary report on the reproductive capability. *Trans American Association of Genito-urinary Surgery* **70**, 42–5.

Leadbetter, G.W. 1964: Surgical correction of total urinary incontinence. *Journal of Urology* **91**, 261–6.

Leck, I., Record, R.G., McKeown, T. and Edwards, J.H. 1968: The incidence of malformations in Birmingham, England 1950–1959. *Teratology* **1**, 263–80.

Light, J.K. and Scott, F.B. 1983: Treatment of the exstrophy–epispadias complex with the AS 792 artificial urinary sphincter. *Journal of Urology* **129**, 738–40.

Lloyd-Roberts, G.C., Williams, D.I. and Braddock, G.T.F. 1959: Pelvic osteotomy in the treatment of ectopia vesicae. *Journal of Bone and Joint Surgery* **41(B)**, 754–7.

Lowe, F.C. and Jeffs, R.D. 1983: Wound dehiscence in bladder exstrophy: an examination of the etiologies and factors for initial failure and subsequent success. *Journal of Urology* **130**, 312–5.

Malone, P.S., Ransley, P.G. and Kiely, E.M. 1990: Preliminary report: the antegrade continence enema. *Lancet* **336**, 1217–8.

Manzoni, G.M., Ransley, P.G. and Hurwitz, R.S. 1987: Cloacal exstrophy and cloacal exstrophy variants: a proposed system of classification. *Journal of Urology* **138**, 1065–8.

Marshall, V.F., Muecke, E.C. 1962: Variations in exstrophy of the bladder. *Journal of Urology* **88**, 766–96.

Martinez-Mora, J., Isnard, R., Castellvi, A. and Lopez-Ortis, P. 1992: Neovagina in vaginal agenesis: surgical methods and long term results. *Journal of Pediatric Surgery* **27**, 10–4.

Mitchell, M.E., Brito, C.G. and Rink, R.C. 1990: Cloacal exstrophy reconstruction for urinary incontinence. *Journal of Urology* **144**, 554–8.

Mitrofanoff, P. 1980: Cystostomie continente trans-appendiculare dans le traitement des vessies neurologique. *Chirugica Pediatric* **21**, 297–305.

Mollard, P. 1980: Bladder reconstruction in exstrophy. *Journal of Urology* **124**, 525–9.

Mollard, P., Mouriquand, P.D.E. and Buttin, X. 1994: Urinary continence after reconstruction of classical bladder exstrophy (73 cases). *British Journal of Urology* **73**, 298–302.

Mundy, A.R. and Nurse, D.E. 1992: Calcium balance, growth and skeletal mineralisation in patients with cystoplasties. *British Journal of Urology* **69**, 257–9.

Osterling, J.E. and Jeffs, R.D. 1987: The importance of a successful initial bladder closure in the surgical management of classical bladder exstrophy: analysis of 144 patients treated at the Johns Hopkins Hospital between 1975 and 1985. *Journal of Urology* **137**, 258–62.

Perlmutter, A.D., Weinstein, M.D. and Reitelman, C. 1991: Vesical neck reconstruction in patients with epispadias–exstrophy complex. *Journal of Urology* **146**, 613–5.

Perovic, D., Brdar, R. and Scepanovic, D. 1992a: Bladder exstrophy and anterior pelvic osteotomy. *British Journal of Urology* **70**, 678–82.

Perovic, S., Scepanovic, D., Sremcevic, D. and Vukadinovic, V. 1992b: Epispadias surgery – Belgrade experience. *British Journal of Urology* **70**, 674–7.

Peters, C.A., Gearhart, J.P. and Jeffs, R.D. 1988: Epispadias and incontinence: the challenge of the small bladder. *Journal of Urology* **140**, 1199–201.

Ransley, P.G., Duffy, P.G. and Wollin, M. 1988: Bladder exstrophy closure and epispadias repair. In Spitz, L. and Nixon, H.H. (eds), *Rob and Smith's Operative surgery – paediatric surgery.* London: Butterworths, 620–32.

Ricketts, R.R., Woodard, J.R. and Zwiren, G.T. 1991: Modern treatment of cloacal exstrophy. *Journal of Pediatric Surgery* **26**, 444–50.

Rickham, P.P. 1960: Vesico-intestinal fissure. *Archives of Disease in Childhood* **35**, 97–102.

Shapiro, E., Jeffs, R.D., Gearhart, J.P. and Lepor, H. 1985: Muscarinic cholinergic receptors in bladder exstrophy: insights into surgical management. *Journal of Urology* **134**, 308–10.

Shapiro, E., Lepor, H. and Jeffs, R.D. 1984: The inheritance of the exstrophy–epispadias complex. *Journal of Urology* **132**, 308–10.

Sheldon, C.A., MacLorie, G.A., Khoury, A. and Churchill, B.M. 1990: Duplicate bladder exstrophy: a new variant of clinical and embryological significance. *Journal of Urology* **144**, 334–6.

Shultz, W.G. 1958: Plastic repair of exstrophy of bladder combined with bilateral osteotomy of ilia. *Journal of Urology* **79**, 453–8.

Spencer, R. 1965: Exstrophia splanashnica (exstrophy of the cloaca). *Surgery* **57**, 751–66.

Stanton, S.L. 1974: Gynaecologic complications of epispadias and bladder exstrophy. *American Journal of Obstetrics and Gynaecology* **119**, 749–54.

Stringer, M.D., Duffy, P.G. and Ransley, P.G. 1994: Inguinal hernias associated with bladder exstrophy. *British Journal of Urology* **73**, 308–9.

Tank, E.S. and Lindenauer, S.M. 1970: Principles of management of exstrophy of the cloaca. *American Journal of Surgery* **119**, 95–8.

Thomas, W.G. and Wilkinson, J.A. 1989: Ectopia vesicscae and congenital hip dislocation: brief report. *Journal of Bone and Joint Surgery* **72(B)**, 328–9.

Toguri, A.G., Churchill, B.M., Schillinger, J.F. and Jeffs, R.D. 1978: Gas cystometry in cases of continent bladder exstrophy. *Journal of Urology* **119**, 536.

Wagstaff, K.E., Woodhouse, C.R.J., Duffy, P.G. and Ransley, P.G. 1992: Delayed linear growth in children with enterocystoplasties. *British Journal of Urology* **69**, 314–17.

Williams, D.I. and Savage, J. 1966: Reconstruction of the exstrophied bladder. British *Journal of Surgery* **53**, 168–73.

Woodhouse, C.J.R. 1991: Exstrophy and epispadias. In *Long-term paediatric urology.* London: Blackwell Scientific, 127–50.

Woodhouse, C.J.R. and Kellett, M.J. 1984: Anatomy of the penis and its deformities in exstrophy and epispadias. *Journal of Urology* **132**, 1122–4.

Woodhouse, C.R.J. 1992a: Lower urinary tract reconstruction in young patients. *British Journal of Urology* **70**, 113–20.

Woodhouse, C.R.J. 1992b: Late malignancy in urology. *British Journal of Urology* **70**, 345–51.

Woodhouse, C.R.J., Ransley, P.G. and Williams, D.I. 1983: The patient with exstrophy in adult life. *British Journal of Urology* **55**, 632–5.

CHAPTER 61

Hypospadias

P.D.E. MOURIQUAND

Introduction
Definition
The urethral plate
Principles of hypospadias repair
A practical classification of hypospadias repair
Modern techniques
Complications

General recommendations in the
management of hypospadias
General recommendations for
hypospadias surgery
Conclusions
References

Introduction

The approach to hypospadias surgery has evolved since the mid-1980s because of a better understanding of the anatomical characteristics of this congenital anomaly. The identification and use of the urethral plate as an anatomical entity has considerably simplified this surgery, which now involves a small number of procedures using the same principles, allowing a single-stage repair in all cases.

Historically, hypospadias repair has travelled through three periods of uneven inspiration: the nineteenth century where principles of this surgery were remarkably good but technical facilities were poor (Thiersch, 1869; Duplay, 1874; Cantwell, 1895); the first two-thirds of the twentieth century where a plethora of procedures was described, often advocating multistage reconstruction, the use of inadequate tissues (hairy skin) for urethroplasty and accepting approximate results; and, finally, the current era where modern principles have been standardized (Duckett, 1986; Ransley *et al.*, 1988; Mollard *et al.*, 1991), offering better anatomical and functional results, and using some of the nineteenth-century concepts which have been resumed and revived very successfully (Thiersch–Duplay urethroplasty).

Definition

Hypospadias is classically defined as an association of three anatomical anomalies of the penis (Fig. 61.1): (1) an abnormal ventral opening of the urethral meatus which can be located at any position on the ventral

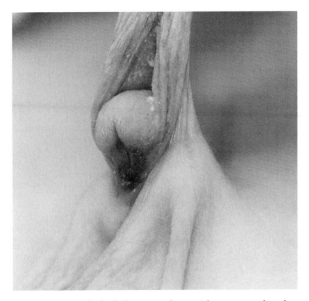

Fig. 61.1 Mid-shaft hypospadias with severe chordee and hooded foreskin.

aspect of the penis (the urethral meatus may look narrow, though exceptionally stenotic); (2) an abnormal ventral curvature of the penis (chordee); and (3) an abnormal distribution of the foreskin around the glans with the ventrally deficient hooded foreskin. The chordee and the hooded foreskin are common but not constant (Fig. 61.2).

Looking more carefully at these anomalies, hypospadias might be defined as an atresia of the ventral radius of the penis (Fig. 61.2B). The skin shaft is often poorly represented on the ventral aspect of the penis and sometimes very adherent to the underlying urethra, the ventral height of the glans is poor and the glans itself is

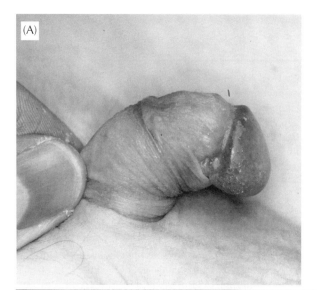

widely open. The corpus spongiosum is atretic and represents one of the major factors of the penile chordee; the frenulum artery is always missing even when the foreskin is intact, and in some rare cases the ventral aspects of the corpora cavernosum are also atretic. The aetiology of the poor development of the ventral tissues of the penis is unclear: impaired hormonal secretions or receptivity, genetic disorders or vascular anomalies have been suggested but never confirmed, although it is true that this anomaly has a higher incidence within the same family (10% incidence in first-degree relatives).

The urethral plate

The urethral plate is a strip of urethral mucosa extending from the ectopic meatus toward the glans (Fig. 61.2B). In the male embryo, the urogenital plate is the horizontal segment of the urogenital sinus, which appears at 11 weeks of pregnancy and lies under the genital tubercle. The urogenital plate is at the origin of the penile urethra but not the distal urethra (glanular urethra) which has a different embryological origin and appears later, at 4 months of pregnancy (Tuchmann-Duplessis, 1970).

Several authors have actually used the urethral plate to repair the urethra without naming it and without identifying it as an anatomical entity (Thiersch, 1869; Duplay, 1874; Mathieu, 1932; Browne, 1949; King, 1970; Devine and Horton, 1977). This concept was first used in the repair of epispadias (Ransley *et al.*, 1988) and soon after this the technique was described for use in hypospadias repair (Elder *et al.*, 1987; Hollowell *et*

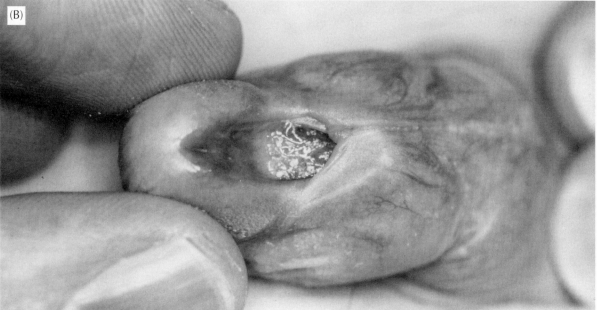

Fig 61.2 (A) Hypospadias with marked chordee and complete foreskin; (B) same patient. Note the absence of frenular artery and the wide urethral plate which will be used to reconstruct the urethra.

al., 1990). In 1991 this concept was for repair of severe posterior hypospadias (Mollard *et al.*, 1991). It became apparent that the untethering of the urethral plate was the major procedure to correct penile chordee, thus allowing reconstruction of the urethra.

Since these recent studies, it has become recognized that the urethral plate is not the cause of the chordee and is a reliable mooring plate to reconstruct the urethra.

Principles of hypospadias repair

According to the anatomical features described above, three main steps characterize hypospadias surgery: correction of the penile chordee, reconstruction of the missing urethra (urethroplasty), and fashioning of the urethral meatus (meatoplasty), the ventral aspect of the glans (glanuloplasty), the mucosal collar and the skin cover of the penile shaft.

The first step is to correct the penile chordee, which is related to four possible factors (Fig. 61.2A): (1) the abnormal distribution of the skin around the penile shaft and the tethering of the skin on to the underlying layers; (2) the tethering of the urethral plate on to the ventral surface of the corpora cavernosum; (3) the atretic corpus spongiosum which extends in a fan shape from the ectopic meatus to the glans; or (4) in rare cases, an atresia of the ventral aspect of the corpora cavernosum can be responsible for some residual chordee.

Therefore, the correction of the chordee, when it exists, implies (1) the degloving of the penis; (2) the dissection of the urethral plate which is carefully lifted off the ventral surface of the corpora cavernosum. It is remarkable to see the lengthening and the narrowing of the urethral plate as soon as it is freed from the corpora, even in posterior hypospadias. The two lateral wings of the glans are also dissected extensively at this stage (Fig. 61.3); (3) the excision of the atretic and fibrous

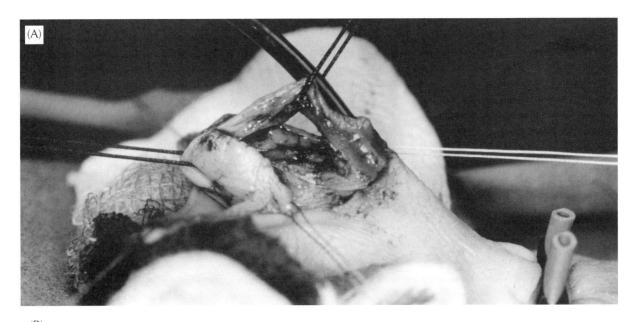

(A)

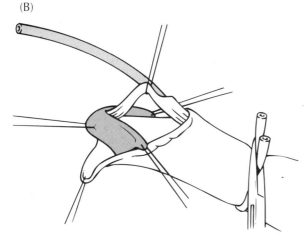

(B)

Fig. 61.3 Extensive dissection of the two wings of the glans and the urethral plate. Note the position of the tourniquet with the clip applied on the urethra: this does not damage the urethra and allows the change of urethral catheter during the procedure without removing the tourniquet.

corpous spongiosum distally to the ectopic meatus; and (4) in rare cases (less than 5%), the penis remains bent and either a dorsal plication of the tunica albuginea of the corpora (Nesbit, 1965) or a derotation of the corpora, which is a more complex procedure (Kass, 1992), can be performed.

When penile straightening is achieved it should be checked by an artificial erection test (Gittes and McLaughlin, 1974). It is then possible to perform an urethroplasty using the urethral plate, which remains attached proximally to the urethra and distally to the glans cap (Fig. 61.4). There are two options to reconstruct the missing urethra: either the urethral plate is wide enough to be rolled into a tube (Thiersch, 1869; Duplay, 1874) (Fig. 61.5) or the urethral plate is too narrow to be rolled and is then used as a mooring plate for the urethroplasty. A rectangular pediculized flap of preputial mucosa or a rectangular free graft of buccal mucosa or bladder mucosa comprise the main materials used for creating a new conduit. This rectangle of tissue is sutured to the two edges of the urethral plate creating a tube without carrying out a circular anastomosis (Fig. 61.6): this is the onlay urethroplasty (Elder *et al.*, 1987), the roof of the neourethra being the urethral plate and the floor of the neourethra being the preputial mucosa, bladder or buccal mucosa.

When the urethroplasty is completed, the meatoplasty and glanuloplasty are performed by folding the two wings of the glans over the neourethra (Fig. 61.7). A mucosal collar is brought ventrally around the corona using the excess of dorsal preputial mucosa (Firlit, 1987) (Fig. 61.8).

The skin cover (sleeve cover) uses the excess of dorsal skin which is progressively brought ventrally.

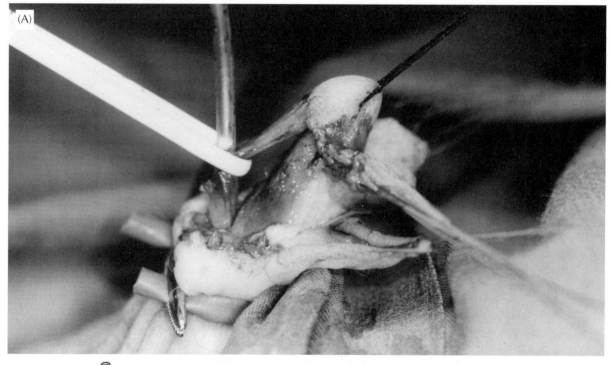

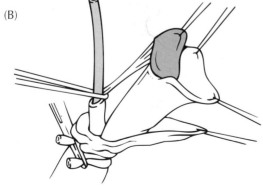

Fig. 61.4 Complete correction of the penile chordee by lifting the urethral plate off the ventral surface of the corpora. After untethering, the urethral plate remains attached by its two extremities, proximally to the urethra and distally to the glans groove.

(A)

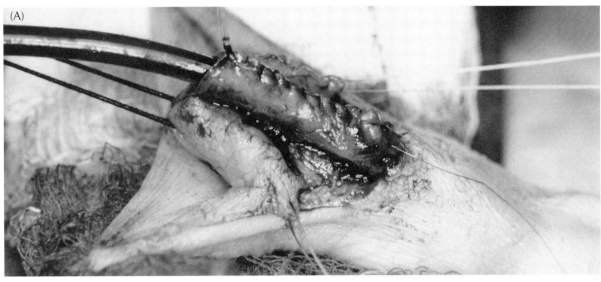

(B)

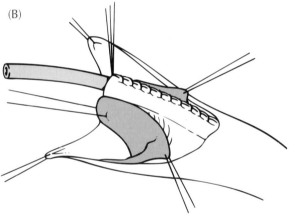

Fig. 61.5 Urethroplasty: the tubularization of the urethral plate is completed with a running suture of 7/0 PDS.

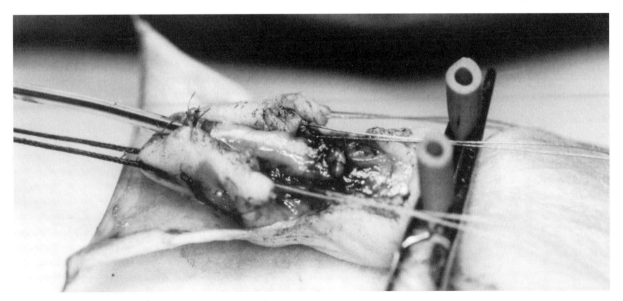

Fig. 61.6 Onlay urethroplasty with a buccal graft.

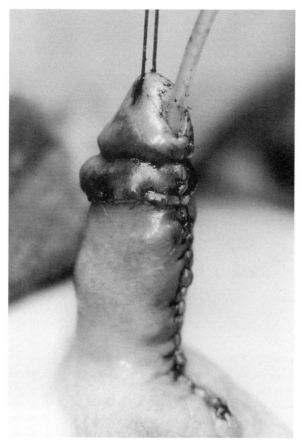

Fig. 61.7 Meatoplasty, glanuloplasty, Firlit mucosal collar and sleeve skin cover represent the third step of hypospadias reconstruction.

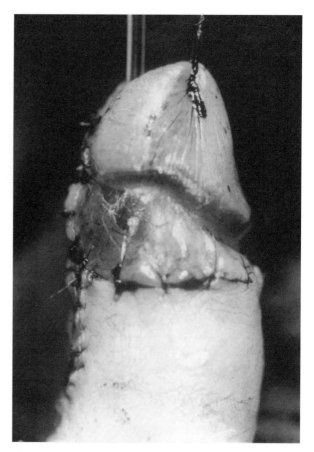

Fig. 61.8 The mucosal collar described by Firlit.

The sleeve cover gives better cosmetic results than the traditional Byars (1950) procedure (Fig. 61.9).

A practical classification of hypospadias repair

GLANULAR HYPOSPADIAS

The meatus is distal to the corona and there is usually no chordee. The most common procedure used is the MAGPI (meatoplasty advancement and glanuloplasty incorporated) (Duckett, 1981a). Other methods roll the distal urethral plate (Arap *et al.*, 1984; Zaontz, 1989; Gilpin *et al.*, 1993), while others use a flap of skin shaft (Mathieu, 1932).

PENILE HYPOSPADIAS WITHOUT CHORDEE (FIG. 61.10) (OR WITH A MINOR DEGREE OF CHORDEE)

The meatus is at any position between coronal sulcus and midshaft. When the urethral plate is wide enough to

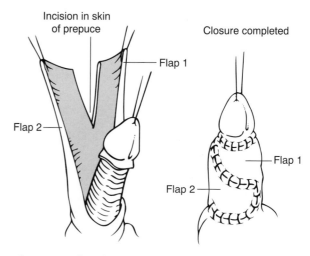

Fig. 61.9 The classical Byars procedure, which gives unsatisfactory cosmetic results because of the excess of ventral skin.

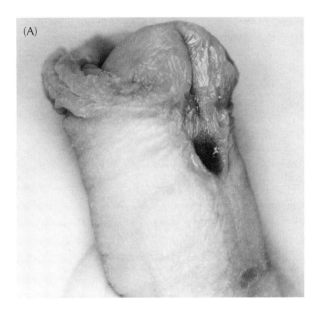

(A)

(B)

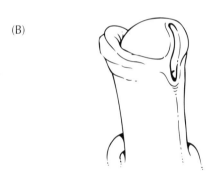

Fig. 61.10 Anterior hypospadias without chordee which will undergo a Mathieu procedure (see Figs 61.20 and 61.21).

be rolled into a tube this can be used, if not a Mathieu urethroplasty is recommended.

HYPOSPADIAS WITH CHORDEE

A three-step approach is needed in these patients with untethering and preservation of the urethral plate (Mollard *et al.*, 1991), urethroplasty, meatoplasty, glanuloplasty and skin cover.

CRIPPLE HYPOSPADIAS

A complete revision of the penis is usually required. The urethral plate, even if it scarred, can be preserved in many cases and the urethroplasty often uses an onlay buccal graft.

Modern techniques

Paediatric urologists only use single-stage procedures in hypospadias. Multistage procedures are not discussed here.

GLANULAR HYPOSPADIAS

Many techniques have been described. Surprisingly, it is often more difficult to operate on these distal hypospadias (known as 'minor') than on the posterior ones ('major').

The MAGPI operation (Fig. 61.11)

MAGPI is a popular procedure described by Duckett (1981a). It is actually not an advancement of the meatus but a reshaping of the glans which gives the illusion that the urethral meatus has been moved to the tip of the penis.

The incision line is drawn 5 mm behind the ectopic meatus and follows the cutaneomucosal junction of the prepuce. A deep vertical incision into the glanular

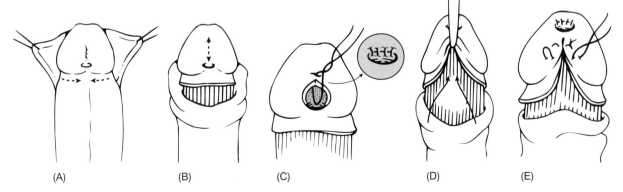

(A) (B) (C) (D) (E)

Fig. 61.11 Five main steps of the MAGPI procedure.

groove for a distance of about 1 cm opens the dorsal meatus generously. Transverse closure of the diamond-shaped defect thus created flattens out the glanular groove and allows a straight stream to emerge. The ventral lip of the urethra is fixed with a holding stitch and brought forward. This tilts the glans to a more normal conical position and allows the lateral wings of the glans to rotate to the ventrum. A sleeve approximation of the penile skin is carried out, excising all redundant tissue and leaving a circumcised appearance. The MAGPI is particularly well indicated when the glans is broad and flat (Fig. 61.12).

Other similar techniques

Other authors have slightly modified the MAGPI procedure to improve the cosmetic appearance (Arap *et al.*, 1984). This modified repair advances two flaps of lateral coronal tissue distally, approximating them in the midline, effectively lengthening the urethra. The glans is then closed over this tissue, normalizing its ventral appearance.

The idea of using the mucosa of the distal groove (Fig. 61.13) to reconstruct minor hypospadias has been described by several authors: the glans approximation procedure (GAP) (Zaontz, 1989) is possible when there is a wide glanular groove, and glanular reconstruction and preputioplasty (Gilpin *et al.*, 1993) (GRAP) relied on the same principle. Others have reconstructed the distal urethra with one cutaneous flap and one glanular flap (Barcat, 1873). In many cases of glanular or coronal hypospadias, the technique of Mathieu (1932) can be used.

PENILE HYPOSPADIAS WITHOUT CHORDEE

The Mathieu operation is the treatment of choice (Fig. 61.14). Two parallel incisions are made on either side of the urethral plate up to the tip of the glans and deep down to the corpora cavernosum. The incision line delimits a perimeatal-based skin flap which is folded over and sutured to the edges of the urethral plate. The lateral wings of the glans are generously dissected from the corpora cavernosum. The rest of the procedure follows the recommendations given above.

HYPOSPADIAS WITH CHORDEE

Preservation of the urethral plate (Fig. 61.15) (Mouriquand, 1997), with or without onlay procedures (Fig. 16.16) should be the treatment of choice.

In these cases the urethral plate is lifted off the corpora cavernosum as described previously. An onlay urethroplasty (Elder *et al.*, 1987) is done using pedicularized foreskin or buccal mucosa.

The transverse preputial island flap technique (Fig. 61.17) (Asopa *et al.*, 1971; Duckett, 1981b) can also be used for this type of hypospadias. This technique ignores the urethral plate, which is excised, and uses a tubularized pedicle flap of foreskin which is interposed between the ectopic meatus and the glans. Because there is a circular anastomosis, the risk of stricture is higher here than in the onlay procedures.

RESULTS

MAGPI

In 1992 Duckett and Snyder reported 1111 MAGPIs with 1.2% cases requiring secondary procedures. Partial ventral regression of the meatus is a complication of this procedure, which remains the most popular one for glanular hypospadias (Felfela *et al.*, 1990).

Mathieu

Distal strictures are rare (1%) and fistulae are met in 4% of cases (Mollard *et al.*, 1987). The half-moon shaped meatus is sometimes disappointing but an extensive dissection of the two wings of the glans allows a neat glanuloplasty. The overall results remain excellent.

Onlay urethroplasty

This is a relatively new procedure, so the long-term outcome is unknown. In a personal series of 84 patients, 15% have fistulae, of whom 6% required a secondary procedure (Mouriquand, 1995). No stricture has been recorded.

Transverse preputial island flap technique

The complication rate varies between 3.7% (El-Kasaby *et al.*, 1986) and 69% (Parsons and Abercombie, 1984).

Complications

These modern surgical techniques should result in a normal-looking penis with a slit-shaped apical meatus, a ventral reconstruction of the glans, normal erections and normal micturition. Complications are quite common (Mollard *et al.*, 1990) and surgical correction should be delayed until 6 months after the initial operation in order to allow recovery of the tissues.

FISTULAE (FIG. 61.18)

This complication is encountered in all urethroplasties and can be explained by three main causes: meatal strictures, infected haematomas and localized necrotic patches of the reconstructed urethra or the covering layers. Prevention of this complication starts with a proper antiseptic preparation of the penis, a broad antibiotic cover, the choice of the appropriate instruments and sutures, a moderate use of electric coagulation and an experienced operator.

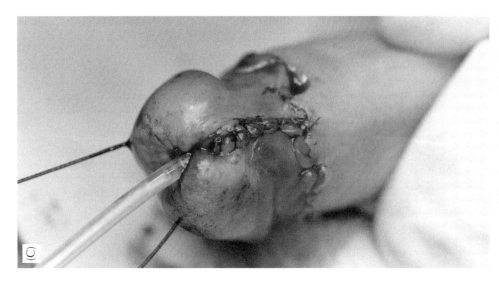

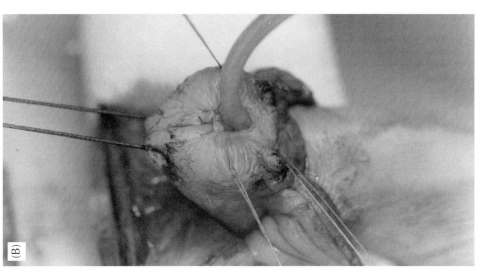

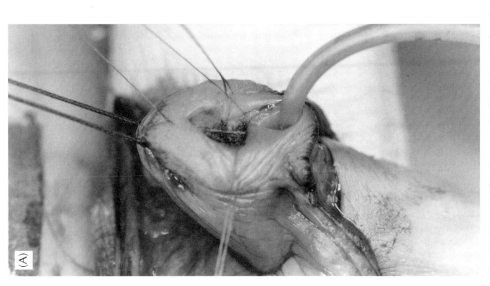

Fig. 61.12 (A) The deep vertical incision of the glans which allows the relocation of the meatus; (B) the transverse suture of the glans incision which allows the reshaping (flatening) of the glans; (C) the reconstruction of the ventral aspect of the glans.

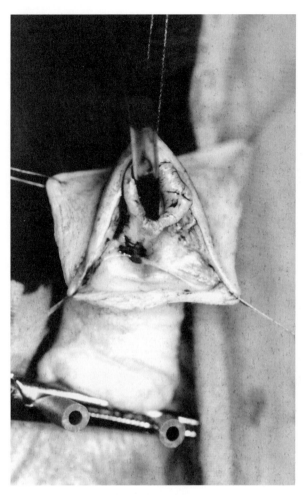

Fig. 61.13 Dissection of the distal urethral plate in a glanular hypospadias.

Some fistulae will heal spontaneously and a minimal delay of 6 months is required before deciding on a surgical closure, which can be done as a day case without drainage. The fistula is usually a tiny conduit, which can be excised and ligated at its base after dissection. Large fistulae are unusual and attest that the original urethroplasty was unsatisfactory. They require a full reconstruction of the urethra.

URETHRAL STENOSIS

This complication is rare with the modern procedures which avoid a circular anastomosis. Proximal stenoses are severe complications requiring recurrent dilatations, which are traumatic to the child and often fail to correct the stenosis. *In situ* urethrostomy followed by a urethroplasty is sometimes required. The onlay urethroplasty has made this complication extremely rare. Free grafts still have a significant rate of meatal stenosis which can be treated with a meatostomy.

MUCOSAL ECTROPION

This is due to the prolapse of a bladder mucosal graft (Mollard *et al.*, 1989) and the subsequent development of pseudopolyps requiring a resection. Recurrence and meatal stenosis are common.

Balanitis xerotica obliterans is a rare complication related to a chronic inflammation and fibrosis of the meatus and glans. Meatoplasty may be required and a short course of topical steroids may also be of value in the treatment of this condition.

URETHROCELE

Dilatation of the neourethra is usually secondary to distal stenosis either at the level of the meatus or within the glans tunnel. It can also appear when the calibration of the neourethra is inappropriate. Excision of the redun-

(A)

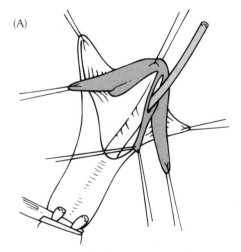

(B)

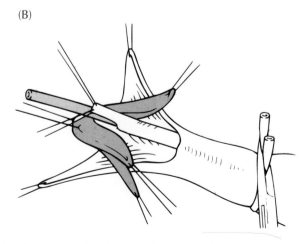

Fig. 61.14 (A) Mathieu procedure: the dissection of the skin flap is completed; (B) Mathieu procedure: the skin flap is folded over and urethroplasty can start.

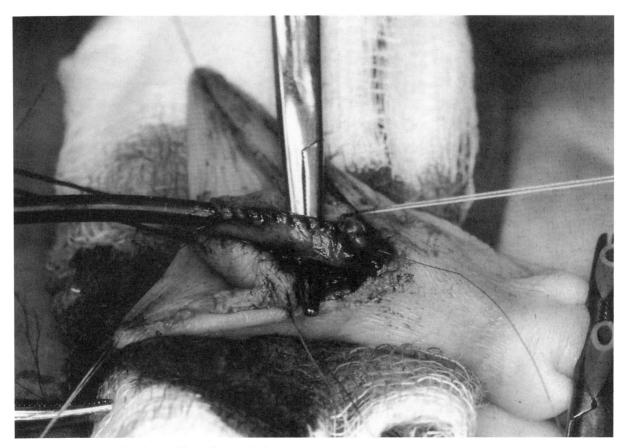

Fig. 61.15 Neo urethra formed from the urethral plate.

dant urethral tissues and treatment of the distal stenosis is required.

OTHER COMPLICATIONS

Hairy urethra should no longer be seen with modern techniques. It is due to the use of scrotal skin and requires a new urethroplasty. Urethral stones may develop in the hairy segment of the urethra.

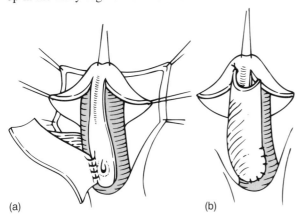

Fig. 61.16 Onlay urethroplasty with a pediculized graft of mucosal foreskin.

Meatal regression or glanular dehiscence should be avoided by adequate lateral mobilization of the glans wings and careful midline approximation of the glans. It can be corrected with a salvage Mathieu's repair.

Persistent chordee can be caused by the inexperience of the surgeon. A rigorous procedure with peroperative erection test is the only way to avoid this unacceptable complication. If the persistent chordee is minor, dorsal plication of the tunica albuginalis is a possible option, although ventral dissection is often needed.

DISASTERS: CRIPPLE HYPOSPADIAS (FIG. 61.19)

These situations are secondary to multiple surgical interventions and lead to persistent chordee, fibrous patches, scarred tissues, irregular skin and multiple fistulae partially covered by skin bridges.

Incorrect diagnosis, ignorance of the rigorous principles of this surgery and a poor follow-up are often found. Neglected chordee, missed intersexuality, traumatizing dissection, badly vascularized tissues, sutures under tension, inappropriate urine drainage and infection are the main causes of these disasters.

These cases imply a complete penile degloving and a dissection of the reconstructed urethra down to the

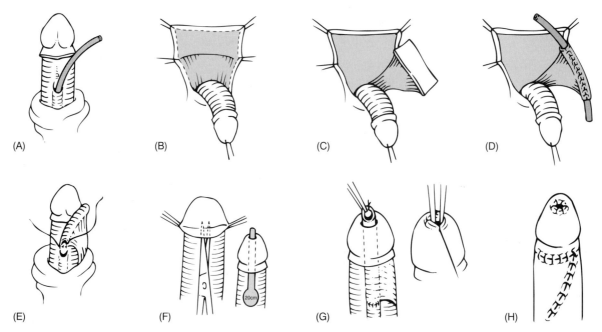

(A) (B) (C) (D)

(E) (F) (G) (H)

Fig. 61.17 The Duckett's procedure using a pediculized tube of mucosal foreskin. This procedure ignores the concept of urethral plate.

normal urethra. The most difficult step of this operation is to correct the residual chordee, which implies a complete dissection of the ventral surface of the corpora, avoiding grafts (dermal grafts or tunica vaginalis grafts) and sometimes plicating their dorsal aspect.

An onlay island flap urethroplasty is sometimes possible, although a complete excision of the reconstructed urethra is often required, leading to a free graft urethroplasty. When possible, it can be useful to keep the transglanular urethra intact to avoid further problems with the meatus.

Poor cosmetic results such as redundant ventral skin, asymmetrical foreskin or retracted meatus are badly accepted by patients and may necessitate further surgical procedures.

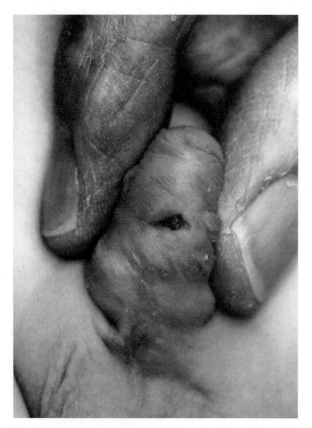

Fig. 61.18 Fistula. Most fistulae are sited laterally under the corona.

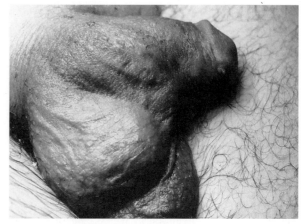

Fig. 61.19 Cripple hypospadias.

The sexual life of these patients should be normal although it often starts slightly later than usual. Erection should be normal and fertility is not affected unless the hypospadias is associated with undescended testes.

General recommendations in the management of hypospadias

The ideal age for surgery is probably between 12 and 24 months, when the penis is big enough and the psychological effects of surgery are said to be minimal.

ASSOCIATED ANOMALIES

Hypospadias associated with one or two undescended testicles or with a micropenis should have an endocrine and genetic assessment. The presence of a prostatic utricle is not uncommon in patients with hypospadias and should not require any particular treatment.

General recommendations for hypospadias surgery

MATERIAL

Magnification devices and instruments for microsurgery may be helpful to manipulate delicate tissues and small stitches (6/0 and 7/0 absorbable sutures).

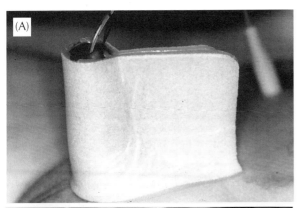

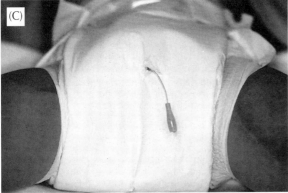

PEROPERATIVE HAEMOSTASIS

This can be achieved either by using a tourniquet or by injecting a solution of 1:100 000 of adrenaline. Electric coagulation is barely necessary during the procedure. Bipolar coagulation is said to be safer than unipolar coagulation.

URINE DRAINAGE

This depends on the surgeon's convictions and it may not be necessary to drain distal hypospadias repairs (MAGPI or Mathieu). A Ch4 or Ch6 feeding tube is left for 4 days following a Mathieu's operation and 10–12 days for onlay procedures. The extremity of the feeding tube is left open in the nappy. A suprapubic stent or a dripping stent is an alternative method of drainage.

ANTIBIOTICS

A broad cover antibiotic treatment is required perioperatively and postoperatively. An antibiotic combination of ampicillin/co-trimoxazol and aminoglycoside or cephalosporin is usually sufficient to avoid infections with *Escherichia coli*, *Klebsiella*, *Enterobacter cloacae* and *Proteus mirabilis*.

DRESSING (FIG. 61.20)

Silastic foam dressing, hydrocolloid dressing or bandage dressing can be used. The hydrocolloid dressing is very comfortable and progressively comes off without hurting the child. Repeated baths can be very helpful to remove the dressing.

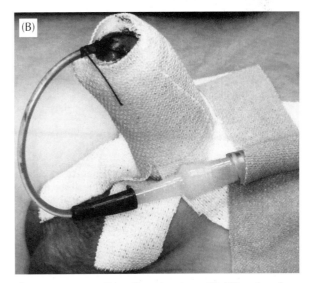

Figs 61.20 (A) Granuflex dressing; (B) Kling bandage and elstoplast; the urethral catheter is secured on the abdominal skin; (C) The double nappy system allows an efficient protection of the reconstructed penis and gives more comfort to the child.

POSTOPERATIVE CARE

The child should be confined into his cot for 2 days and regular baths can be given starting the day after surgery. Bruising and swelling of the penis may persist for 3–4 weeks.

Conclusions

Hypospadias surgery represents one of the most important activities of paediatric urology. Improvements with more simplification of procedures may be expected with urethral cell culture (Baskin *et al.*, 1993) or laser welding (Mininberg *et al.*, 1989), which may reduce the incidence of fistulae. The concept of the urethral plate has considerably simplified the surgical approach to this condition and led to better results.

References

Arap, S., Mitre, A.I. and Degoes, G.M. 1984: Modified meatal advancement and glanuloplasty repair of distal hypospadias. *Journal of Urology* **131**, 1140–2.

Asopa, H.S., Elhence, E.P., Atria, S.P. and Bansal, N.K. 1971: One stage correction of penile hypospadias using a foreskin tube. A preliminary report. *International Surgery* **55**, 435.

Barcat, J. 1873: Current concepts of treatment. In Horton, C.E. (ed.), *Plastic and reconstructive surgery of the genital area*. Boston, MA: Little, Brown, 249.

Baskin, L.S., Macarak, E.J., Duckett, J.W., Snyder, H.M. and Howard, P.S. 1993: Culture of urethral fibroblasts: cell morphology proliferation and extracellular matrix synthesis. *Journal of Urology* **150**, 1260–6.

Browne, D. 1949: An operation for hypospadias. *Proceedings of the Royal Society of Medicine* **42**, 466.

Byars, L.T. 1950: Surgical repair of hypospadias. *Surgical Clinics of North America* **30**, 1371.

Cantwell, F.V. 1895: Operative technique of episadias by transplantation of the urethra. *Annals of Surgery* **22**, 689.

Devine, C.J. and Horton, C.E. 1977: Hypospadias repair. *Journal of Urology* **118**, 188–93.

Duckett, J.W. 1981a: MAGPI (meatoplasty and glanuloplasty): a procedure for subcoronal hypospadias. *Urological Clinics of North America* **8**, 513.

Duckett, J.W. 1981b: The island flap technique for hypospadias repair. *Urological Clinics of North America* **8**, 513.

Duckett, J.W. 1986: Hypospadias. In Walsh, P.C., Gittes, R.F., Perlmutter, A.D. and Stamey, T.A. (eds), *Campbell's urology*. Philadelphia, PA: WB Saunders, 1987–9.

Duckett, J.W. and Snyder, H.M. 1992: Meatal advancement and glanuloplasty repair after 1,000 cases: avoidance of metal stenosis and regression. *Journal of Urology* **47**, 665–9.

Duplay, S. 1874: De l'hypospade périnéo-scrotal et de son traitement chirurgical. *Archives of General Medicine* **1**, 613–57.

El-Kasaby, A.W., El-Beialy, H., El-Halaby, R., Nowier, A. and Maged, A. 1986: Urethroplasty using transverse penile island flap for hypospadias. *Journal of Urology* **136**, 643–4.

Elder, J.S., Duckett, J.W. and Snyder, H.M. 1987: Onlay island flap in the repair of mid and distal hypospadias without chordee. *Journal of Urology* **138**, 376–9.

Felfela, T., Mouriquand, P.D.E. and Mollard, P. 1990: Indication de l'intervention de MAGPI dans le traitement des hypospades mineurs. *Chirurgia Pediatrica* **31**, 167–8.

Firlit, C.F. 1987: The mucosal collar in hypospadias surgery. *Journal of Urology* **137**, 80–2.

Gilpin, P., Clements, W.B.D. and Boston, V.E. 1993: GRAP repair: single stage. Reconstruction of hypospadias as an out-patient procedure. *British Journal of Urology* **71**, 226–9.

Gittes, R.F. and McLaughlin, A.P. 1974: Injection technique to induce penile erection. *Urology* **4**, 473–4.

Hollowell, J.G., Keating, M.A., Snyder, H.M. *et al.* 1990: Preservation of urethral plate in hypospadias repair. Extended applications and further experience with the onlay island flap urethroplasty. *Journal of Urology* **143**, 98–101.

Kass, E.J. 1992: Transverse dorsal plication: an alternative technique for the management of severe chordee. Poster, American Academy of Pediatrics, San Francisco.

King, L.R. 1970: Hypospadias – a one stage repair without skin graft on a new principle: chordee is sometimes produced by skin alone. *Journal of Urology* **103**, 660.

Mathieu, P. 1932: Traitement en un temps de l'hypospade balanique et juxta-balanique. *Journal de Chirurgie (Paris)* **39**, 481–4.

Mininberg, D.T., Sosa, R.E., Neidt, G. and Poe, C. 1989: Laser welding of pedicled flap skin tubes. *Journal of Urology* **142**, 623–6.

Mollard, P., Mouriquand, P.D.E. and Basset, T. 1987: Le traitement de l'hypospade. *Chirurgia Pediatrica* **28**, 197–203.

Mollard, P. Mouriquand, P.D.E. and Bringeon, G. 1989: Repair of hypospadias using a bladder mucosa graft in 76 patients. *Journal of Urology* **131**, 1140–2.

Mollard, P., Mouriquand, P.D.E. and Felfela, T. 1990: Traitement des hypospades. *Encyclopédie Médico-Chirurgicale (Paris)* **41340**, 1–17.

Mollard, P., Mouriquand, P.D.E. and Felfela, T. 1991: Application of the Onlay Island flap urethroplasty to penile hypospadias with severe chordee. *British Journal of Urology* **68**, 317–9.

Mouriquand, P.D.E. 1995: Untethering and preservation of the urethral plate in penile hypospadias with severe chordee. *British Journal of Urology* **76** (Suppl. 3), 9–22.

Nesbit, R.M. 1965: Congenital curvature of the phallus: report of three cases with description of corrective operation. *Journal of Urology* **93**, 230.

Parsons, K. and Abercombie, G.F. 1984: Transverse preputial island flap neo-urethroplasty. *British Journal of Urology* **25**, 186–8.

Ransley, P.G., Duffy, P.G. and Wollin, M. 1988: Bladder exstrophy closure and epispadias repair. In Dudley, H., Carter, D. and Russel, R.C.G. (eds), *Rob & Smith's operative surgery* London: Butterworths, 620–32.

Thiersch, C. 1869: Über die entstehungswise and operative behandlung der epispadie. *Archiv für Heitkunde* **10**, 20–5.

Tuchmann-Duplessis, H. 1970: *Embryologie – Organogenèse*. Paris: Masson, 66–87.

Zaontz, M.R. 1989: The GAP (glans approximation procedure) for glanular/coronal hypospadias. *Journal of Urology* **141**, 359–61.

CHAPTER 62

Pelviureteric junctional hydronephrosis

T.P.V.M. DE JONG AND J.D. VAN GOOL

Introduction
Pathophysiology
Clinical features
Diagnosis

Treatment of PUJ hydronephrosis
Surgical treatment PUJ obstruction
Conclusions
References

Introduction

In children, pelvicalyceal dilatation of a kidney without ureteral dilatation is commonly a result of obstruction at the level of pelviureteric junction (PUJ). Nowadays, in the western world, most cases of upper tract dilatation are detected prenatally by ultrasound. The widespread use of routine fetal sonography detects upper tract dilatation in approximately 1 in 1000 pregnancies (Flashner and King, 1992). The scenario for management of PUJ obstruction must therefore focus on two different modes of presentation: the asymptomatic neonate with prenatally detected dilatation of one or both kidneys, and symptomatic upper tract dilatation detected later in life.

Pathophysiology

At 10–12 weeks' gestation the ureteric bud and metanephros have formed a functioning kidney with a complete collecting system that starts passing urine to the bladder (Osathanodh and Potter, 1963). For successful passage of urine a patent, non-kinking PUJ that can transmit pelvic contractions to the ureter must be available for the ureter to accept and propulse a urine bolus (Koff, 1990). Since most fetuses spend an important part of intrauterine life in an upside-down position and infants are in a horizontal position most of the time, dependency of the PUJ and gravity appear to be of minor importance.

Obstruction of the PUJ and the proximal ureter can be due to intrinsic and extrinsic factors. Sometimes the cause of obstruction is identified easily, but more often a combination of factors is seen. Obstruction can be caused by a narrow ureteral segment, muscular discontinuity or severe kinking of the proximal ureter, angulation of a ureter that is inserted high in the renal pelvis, a valve-like flap covering the PUJ, a polyp in the PUJ, aberrant blood vessels and compressing fibrotic bands. The obstruction can be anatomical, the narrowed lumen of the PUJ limiting the flow, or functional, when there is no propulsion of urine from the renal pelvis into the ureter. The difference between these two mechanisms is seldom clarified at operation: is an angulated PUJ an example of a true anatomical obstruction, is it a functional problem or is it a combination of both?

Obstruction of the PUJ causes dilatation of the pelvicalyceal system and, when pressure rises too high it will eventually compromise the function of the kidney. This is the point where managing the problems with the phenomenon of PUJ obstruction arise. Many factors have to be considered in the pathogenesis. The pyelocalyceal system is a very compliant system that can show massive dilatation with low pressures that do not compromise renal function (Ransley et al., 1990). The rate of obstruction can vary immensely over a length of time. The pelvicalyceal system is not very elastic: when dilatation has occurred during a period of obstruction with high pressures, the dilatation can be permanent, even when the obstruction has long since subsided. One factor remains: a PUJ obstruction can severely damage renal function. Although it has never been proven, there seems to be a sliding scale of PUJ stenosis with, at one end, the completely obstructed afunctional multicystic dysplastic kidney and, at the other end, the completely normally functioning dilated kidney. Therefore, when a dilated upper urinary tract is seen, the aim must be to exclude obstruction.

Clinical features

THE PATIENT WITH A PUJ HYDRONEPHROSIS

Owing to fetal ultrasound, the majority of patients with a dilated collecting system of one or both kidneys are nowadays identified before any symptom arises. This brings the benefit that severe obstructions can be cured before complications have occurred, but has the disadvantage of many diagnostic studies being conducted on children with asymptomatic, non-obstructive hydronephrosis. A dilatation of more than 12 mm at fetal ultrasound around the 20th week of gestation bears a great risk for impaired function of the kidney after birth (Ransley *et al.*, 1990). Classically, a neonate with an obstructed PUJ can present with an abdominal mass, sometimes failure to thrive, and often symptoms of abdominal colic indiscernible from gastrointestinal abdominal colic. The child often presents with a urinary tract infection that in many cases is accompanied by life-threatening renal loss of sodium and water, known as pseudohypoaldosteronism (van der Heiden *et al.*, 1985). Ultrasound can often detect pus in a dilated system. Management of these children is straightforward and relatively easy in experienced hands. At any age, children and adolescents with PUJ can present with symptoms of abdominal colic, complicated urinary tract infection, spontaneous haematuria or haematuria after a relatively minor blunt abdominal trauma (Byrne *et al.*, 1985; Belman, 1991). Pathognomonic is the 'beer colic' of the adolescent who goes to a pub for the first time in his life and ends up in the local hospital with severe abdominal pains. When symptoms are clear, management will be easy. Sometimes intermittent episodes of symptoms can make detection of the origin of the pain difficult (Flotte, 1988). This can be very frustrating when an aberrant blood vessel or a polyp is the cause for the intermittent obstruction. Rarely, a kinking ureter at an aberrant lower pole artery, or a ptosis of a kidney, can produce colic in an upright position that disappears when the patient is supine. Sometimes only acute ultrasound at the moment when pain occurs can detect the source of the complaints. Colour Doppler ultrasound can probe the presence of an aberrant lower pole artery in selected cases.

Diagnosis

ULTRASOUND

Ultrasound of the urinary tract is generally the first choice. It can show the morphology of a dilated renal pelvis with signs of past or present high pressures in the collecting system. When no calyceal dilatation is apparent, obstruction is improbable and the diagnosis should be one of extrarenal enlarged renal pelvis, without the need for further investigation unless there are specific complaints. Recent publications suggest the use of Doppler ultrasound of the renal vessels as an adjunct in the detection of high pressures (Kessler *et al.*, 1993; Gottlieb *et al.*, 1989). Differences in the resistive index of the renal vessels related to obstruction have been established in acute obstruction of the upper tract. It is unreliable in children with PUJ stenosis. We have not been able to reproduce the satisfactory results as reported in the literature, especially in patients where there is doubt on the severity of obstruction. The difference between the resistive index at rest and at maximal diuresis could be of use in the future but the method has not yet been standardized. Compensatory hypertrophy of the contralateral normal kidney also indicates obstruction in the affected kidney. Again, no information on the actual rate of obstruction is obtained and the hypertrophy may be the expression of an obstruction that has long since subsided.

INTRAVENOUS UROGRAPHY

Intravenous urography (IVU) gives a morphological image of the upper urinary tract and also provides some information, although unreliable, on kidney function. The only sign of past or present obstruction on IVU comes from the pattern of the calyces: when these are sharply outlined high pressures are improbable, whereas when clubbed calyces are present high pressures can exist. Since ultrasound does not detect all duplex systems IVU still has a minor role in the imaging of PUJ obstruction.

VOIDING CYSTOURETHROGRAPHY

Voiding cystourethrography (VCUG) is mandatory in all cases of PUJ obstruction, because of the important incidence of coexisting vesicoureteral reflux in these patients (Hollowell *et al.*, 1989). Especially when a dilated ureter is visible below the level of the PUJ, vesicoureteral reflux must be suspected (Fig. 62.1). The reported incidence of reflux with PUJ stenosis varies from 8–15%.

ISOTOPE STUDIES

Isotope studies provide function-over-time information about the kidneys. A gamma camera positioned under

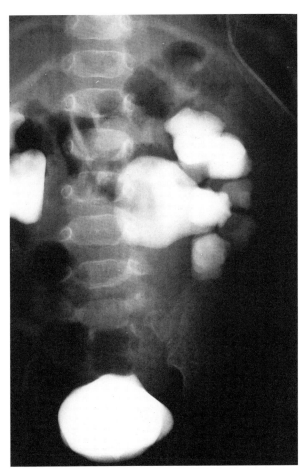

Fig. 62.1 X-ray picture, after micturition, of a voiding cystourethrogram showing reflux in both upper tracts. The left PUJ stenosis is apparent. Often it is difficult to decide whether the child needs a neoureterovescostomy, a pyeloplasty or both.

the patient registers the uptake and excretion of an intravenously administered bolus of radioactive labelled substance by the kidney parenchyma into the collecting system and from there to the bladder. Because of its high resolution and availability, ^{99m}Tc-mercaptoacetyltriglycine (MAG3) is the isotope of choice in a paediatric renography (Young, 1991). The excretion factor of ^{99m}Tc MAG3 with each renal passage is more than 80%, by glomerular filtration and active tubular excretion. The information obtained consists of the differential renal uptake of radioactivity and the evacuation time of each collecting system. The differential renal uptake is calculated from the total number of counts registered over both kidney areas in the first 2 min after intravenous injection. After 2 min, activity excreted into the collecting system can hamper the accurate measurement of differential renal uptake. In the normal situation, activity will be equally divided over both kidneys.

Decrease of differential uptake in a hydronephrotic kidney is used as an indicator for obstruction (Koff *et al.*, 1979). In patients with dilated upper tracts diuresis during the study must be standardized by maximal hydration of the patient and by the administration of a diuretic, together with the isotope bolus, or 5–10 min later. A normal kidney shows a curve with a steep rise, with maximum uptake after 2–3 min and a steep drop to zero. A kidney with a dilated upper tract will show a steep rise followed by a plateau or a gradual decline, with a sharp drop after administration of the diuretic. An obstructed kidney shows a slower increase of activity without washout after the administration of diuretic (Fig. 62.2).

Interpretation of the data provided by the isotope study is one of the cornerstones of decision making in PUJ obstructions. Since the natural history of PUJ stenosis often shows a decrease of obstruction over time, and since it is known that long-existing chronic obstruction is being observed, the information of the excretory curve of the kidney has become less important when the affected kidney shows good differential uptake. Quite a few patients are seen with unilateral obstructive PUJ stenosis, in which the obstructed kidney appears to have more function than the contralateral,

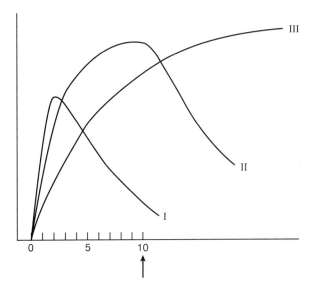

Fig. 62.2 Schematic drawing of excretion curves of ^{99m}Tc-MAG3 renography. The vertical axis shows the activity count and the horizontal axis time after injection in minutes. After 10 min, furosemide is injected. I, Normal curve; II, dilated, non-obstructed system; III, obstructed system. The differential function is calculated from the difference in uptake of activity between the two kidneys, 2 min after injection of the ^{99m}Tc-MAG3 bolus. When peak activity of both kidneys is delayed in time, this may be caused by either insufficient hydration of the patient or impaired kidney function.

normal, kidney. This phenomenon often is based on a misreading of the area of interest of the image of the gamma camera or by measuring uptake more than 2 min after injection of the bolus. It is possibly a constant factor, in some patients, owing to a compensatory mechanism of the obstructed kidney. Liver over-projection seems to be an important factor, since this phenomenon occurs more often at the right kidney. In children with bilaterally dilated upper tracts, interpretation of differential uptake is not reliable and a more aggressive approach can be justified, especially when there is a borderline serum creatinine level.

The pitfalls of isotope renography are many. The differential uptake in massively dilated kidneys with relatively thin parenchyma can give rise to faulty interpretation. Inadequate hydration of the patient can suggest insufficient uptake and obstruction of one or both kidneys. Massive dilatation of the renal pelvis can suggest obstruction due to pooling of radioactivity in the collecting system. The consequences of these pitfalls are that interpretation of isotope renography always must be done with a full understanding of the patient's history and in combination with information obtained with other imaging techniques. Furthermore, the paediatric urologist must have the experience to interpret isotope studies in situations of doubt, especially when dealing with obstruction in the neonate.

ANTEGRADE PRESSURE RECORDING

Antegrade pressure recording (Whitaker test) in PUJ stenosis (Johnston, 1969; Whitaker, 1973) is the ultimate tool to decide on obstruction when other diagnostic methods fail to provide reliable data. It can be necessary in the massively dilated upper urinary tract or in the poorly functioning kidney after a previous pyeloplasty with unremarkable amelioration of function on scintigram postoperatively. It is an invasive study with unphysiological flow rates, making its role questionable. However, it is the only study that really quantifies obstruction. Apart from cases of PUJ obstruction it can be very useful in some cases of obstructive megaureter, especially when bladder compliance is involved in the degree of obstruction. In the Whitaker test, the pressure gradient from the dilated upper urinary tract to the bladder is measured with a fixed volume load of the system. Usually, a flow rate of 4–10 ml/min, depending on age, of diluted radio-paque dye is administered. At equilibration, the pressure gradient from renal pelvis to bladder should not exceed 20 cmH$_2$O. The rather sharp cut-off point around 20 cmH$_2$O requires a meticulous recording technique with an accuracy of 1.5 cmH$_2$O. Less accurate antegrade pressure recordings are useless. This can only be achieved by a double-lumen system (double-lumen catheter or two needles) or by a microtip transducer in the renal pelvis for pressure recording. Our own technique uses a standard 5 Fr. arterial introducer set, guid-

ed percutaneously into the renal pelvis. The sheet allows easy passage of a 3 Fr. microtip transducer catheter for pressure recording, leaving enough space around the catheter to fill the system. This eliminates pump artefacts. The bladder pressure is recorded with another microtip transducer catheter. Both catheters are connected to a standard urodynamic setup. The channel that normally produces the detrusor pressure now reads the pressure difference between the renal pelvis and bladder (Fig. 62.3). When vesicoureteral reflux is present, readings should be done with both an empty and a filled bladder. Fluoroscopic control is used to avoid the trap of the low-compliant massively dilated system. In our patients the limit of 20 cmH$_2$O pressure proved to be completely justified to distinguish between operative and conservative approaches with a follow-up of 5 years and more with no mishaps in conservatively followed patients ($n = 15$).

FUTURE OF DIAGNOSIS

High-speed magnetic resonance imaging that gives accurate data on the quality of the renal parenchyma may provide valuable in the future (Cronan, 1991).

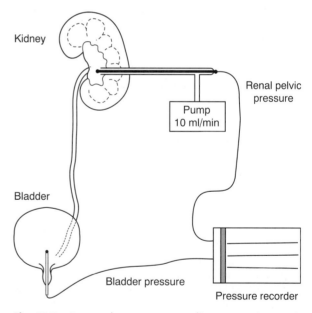

Fig. 62.3 Antegrade pressure recording set-up. An arterial introducer sheet with rubber stopcock and rectangular filling entrance is introduced into the renal pelvis. It allows passage of a 3 Fr. microtip-transducer catheter (MTC) into the renal pelvis. Filling at different flow rates is possible around the 3 Fr. catheter. Bladder pressure is recorded with a 5 Fr. MTC, with lumen, allowing recordings with both full and empty bladder. The transducers are connected to a standard urodynamic set-up. The 3 Fr. MTC can be left in place without the sheet, allowing for 24-hour pressure recording with the MTCs connected to a portable recorder.

Treatment of PUJ hydronephrosis

IN THE NEONATE

There is little doubt that any dilatation of the renal pelvis in an asymptomatic patient that has been proven to be non-obstructive should be followed conservatively. In fact, most of the prenatally discovered dilated upper tracts will resolve spontaneously (Grignon *et al.*, 1986; Homsy *et al.*, 1990). It is important to realize that, immediately after birth, a prenatally detected dilatation often seems to have resolved: the mechanical squeezing of the abdomen during birth (called the 'toothpaste phenomenon' in our department) and the change from fetal circulatory volume expansion with a high urine output to the reduced diuresis of the first postnatal days often underestimate the situation. In fact, in neonatal PU obstruction, the ultrasound 1 week after birth is more important than the very early one. The neonatal urine output is much lower than the output *in utero*, because at birth the newborn is usually volume expanded relative to his or her extrauterine needs, resulting in a negative water and sodium balance in the first few postnatal days (Shaffer and Weismann, 1992). Combined with the good compliance of the renal pelvis, the low urinary output reduces the risk of functional deterioration for the neonatal obstructed kidney in the first weeks of life (Ransley *et al.*, 1990; Elder and Duckett, 1991). Children with a persistently dilated upper urinary tract should be followed for many years, since approximately 20–25% will become obstructive later in life (Koff and Campbell, 1992).

When the child is asymptomatic in unilateral disease, it seems feasible to delay isotope study and IVU until after the first month of life, to obtain better quality pictures when tubular function of the kidney has improved.

Once obstruction has been proved, there are currently three methods for treatment, each with its own arguments supporting the chosen approach. The first supports early operative treatment of obstruction, regardless of function of the affected kidney (Hanna and Gluck, 1988; Guys *et al.*, 1988). This policy is supported by the idea that renal recovery is best when the obstruction is relieved in infancy. The second advocates watchful follow-up as long as differential uptake of the obstructed kidney is reasonable or good, regardless of the aspect of the excretory curve. In general, 35–40% uptake of the affected kidney is accepted as the lower limit (Ransley *et al.*, 1990; Cartwright *et al.*, 1991). The third advocates conservative follow-up of all obstructed kidneys, regardless of function, based on the fact that recovery in non-operated kidneys equals recovery after pyeloplasty (Koff and Campbell, 1972). Only when function deteriorates over time is pyeloplasty advised.

The second method, to operate when uptake is below 35–40%, or wait and see when uptake is more than 35–40%, appears to be the most widely accepted man-

agement at the moment. Until now it has not been possible to prove which is the best method. It is impossible to prove either that better function after surgery would not have occurred without surgery or that the outcome of conservative follow-up could not have been much better with surgery. Prospective, controlled studies are being undertaken in order to provide an answer to these questions. Recent reports on retarded growth in conservative approach of PUJ obstruction could result in a more aggressive operative approach in the future.

When obstruction is apparent, especially in combination with reflux, antibiotic prophylaxis during the first 6 months of life or until obstruction has subsided, whether by operation or not, seems to be a small price to pay in preventing complicated urinary tract infections (Daucher *et al.*, 1992). A protocol proposed by King (1993) starts with antibacterial prophylaxis at day 1, at least until reflux has been excluded, followed by ultrasound evaluation a few days after birth. When massive dilatation with unequivocal upper tract obstruction is apparent, surgical correction in the first few weeks is carried out. When isotope studies show obstruction with good function, the infant is followed monthly with ultrasound for the first 3 months, and at 3-month intervals for the first year. The isotope study is repeated at 1 year of age, or whenever ultrasound suggests increased calyectasis, whereas others, including the present authors, repeat the isotope study at a 3–6-month interval, depending on kidney function (Sheldon *et al.*, 1992). After the age of 1 year, ultrasound can be performed once every 6 months. Even when drainage improves and dilatation seems to subside, long-term follow-up is mandatory, since very late deterioration of obstructions may occur.

IN THE CHILD WITH SYMPTOMS OR COMPLICATIONS

When a child has evident abdominal complaints due to a PUJ obstruction, the obstruction must be relieved as quickly as the complaints require. Theoretically, percutaneous nephrostomy is the method of choice in acute abdominal problems. However, a percutaneous nephrostomy drain hampers secondary elective pyeloplasty owing to the oedematous, thickened renal pelvis. We prefer to perform a primary pyeloplasty, when possible, in acute presentations. Only when a child, symptomatic or asymptomatic, has a differential uptake of the obstructed kidney of less than 10% is the kidney routinely drained percutaneously, to determine whether recovery is possible or nephrectomy is indicated. When a child has a complicated urinary tract infection based on an obstructed kidney, percutaneous drainage is the therapy of first choice. In the premature and in the young infant acute drainage can be obtained by inserting an 18 G intravenous cannula, with a side-hole cut with a scalpel, into the renal pelvis under local anaesthesia.

The complicated case often presents with a unilateral pyelonephritis, sometimes accompanied by life-threatening electrolyte and acid–base disturbances, known as pseudohypoaldosteronism, despite the contralateral kidney usually being normal (van der Heiden *et al.*, 1985). Management of these children is relatively straightforward and easy in experienced hands, once the combination of infection in a dilated system with exceptionally low serum sodium and high serum potassium values has been recognized. In severe infection, ultrasound may reveal pus in the dilated system. Decompression of a severely obstructed kidney, with or without infection, can result in temporary polyuria, requiring meticulous surveillance of the fluid balance at hourly intervals. Sometimes a defect in the concentrating capacity of the operated kidney will persist. In the first 2–4 postoperative days, polyuria of the operated kidney can mimic functional problems of the contralateral normal kidney, because of maximal compensatory concentration with minimal urine output of this healthy kidney. Later in life, a diminished concentrating capacity can lead to excessive fluid intake and/or fluid overload of the urinary tract. The medical complications of fluid and electrolyte disturbances are best dealt with by experienced paediatric nephrologists.

Surgical treatment of PUJ obstruction

When operative relief of an obstructed PUJ is planned the first dilemma is to decide whether retrograde contrast studies are needed. Although retrograde studies will only very rarely alter the scheduled procedure, they can be of some use to identify ureteric obstructions at levels below the PUJ. Literature both for and against retrograde studies is available (Cockrell and Hendren, 1990; Sheldon *et al.*, 1992). A non-diverted pyeloplasty gives a relative contraindication for retrograde studies because of the possible temporary ureterovesical junction obstruction based on oedema after retrograde pyelography. Peroperative antegrade flushing of the ureter with saline or diluted contrast gives equal information on the patency of the ureter.

TREATMENT BY OPEN PYELOPLASTY

Until now open pyeloplasty has been the treatment of choice in the paediatric age group (Trendelenburg, 1890). It has a success rate nearing 100%, low morbidity and a predictable postoperative course. When pyeloplasty is planned several approaches are possible, each with its own advantages and disadvantages. The posterior approach gives good access to the PUJ and has the advantage that simultaneous bilateral pyeloplasty can be performed without the need for repositioning of the patient (Lurz, 1956; Gonzalez and Aliabadi, 1987). It

gives poor access to the renal vessels and can be cumbersome when a rotational anomaly of a poorly functioning kidney or a horseshoe kidney is missed at a preoperative examination. The posterior approach is contraindicated for a repeat pyeloplasty or if there is a large obstructed proximal segment of ureter (Sheldon *et al.*, 1992). Supracostal lumbotomy gives good access in all cases but the patient needs repositioning in bilateral pyeloplasties. Moreover, owing to the cutting of nerve fibres it often produces a temporary deformity of the abdominal wall when the child strains. This deformity always subsides after 6 months. Last, but not least, in the infant a subcostal anterior approach gives excellent extraperitoneal access to the kidney.

The dismembered Anderson–Hynes pyeloplasty (Anderson and Hynes, 1949) is the method of choice (Fig. 62.4). After incision and partial removal of the well-vascularized adventitial layer from the pelvis and proximal ureter, the lowest drainage point of the pelvis is marked and the PUJ is excised. Reduction is required only when massive dilatation of the pelvis is apparent. The ureter is spatulated until the point where adequate lumen is apparent, and anastomosed to the lowest point of the incised pelvis with 6-0 or 7-0 polyglycolic acid sutures. Running sutures give better watertight closures, whereas interrupted sutures prevent constriction of the anastomosis. To prevent calculus formation the knots should be outside the anastomosis. The safest way to make the anastomosis is to start suturing at the deepest proximal tip of the ureter, descending into the apex of the spatulation of the ureter and coming up on the plane nearest to the surgeon. This gives good visual control of the anastomosis at the deepest point going around the corner at the apex of the spatulation. After closure of the remaining pelvis the anastomosis is covered by the adventitial layer with a few approximating sutures. A soft Penrose drain or a low-pressure suction drain is placed near the anastomosis before closure.

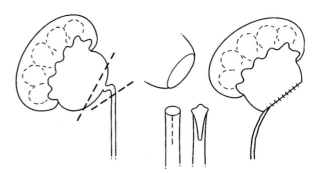

Fig. 62.4   Schematic drawing of a standard dismembered pyeloplasty. Many variations on this method are possible, such as the formation of V-flaps and spiralled flaps. The anastomosis is preferably carried out with polyglycolic acid sutures. Resection of large portions of the renal pelvis is only advised when giant hydronephrosis is present.

Stenting the anastomosis and postoperative drainage from the renal pelvis are controversial (Homsy *et al.*, 1980; Nguyen *et al.*, 1989). There is good evidence that a non-intubated, non-diverted pyeloplasty is a safe procedure. However, urinoma and secondary stenosis have been reported. Stenting the ureter with a double-J catheter combined with bladder drainage for 3 days is an elegant procedure with a short postoperative hospitalization, but it needs a second anaesthesia to remove the stent after 6 weeks unless a lengthened double-J catheter that passes outside through the wound is used. This can be removed at the outpatient clinic. Stenting has the theoretical benefit that it prevents kinking of the anastomosis immediately after the operation by fixing the dependency of the ureter. We have seen two urinomas and only one secondary obstruction in 136 diverted and stented pyeloplasties. In two premature patients of this series the small lumen of the ureter prevented safe stenting. The advantage of a diverting nephrostomy catheter is that it can be left in place, for several weeks, whenever delayed opening of the anastomosis occurs.

Several modifications of this technique are possible. One can leave the ureteric infundibulum *in situ* and create an inverted V-flap of the pelvis, anastomosing the flap to the ureter that is opened until good diameter is available. When a narrow or kinked proximal ureter needs to be bridged, a tubular flap of the pelvis can be created (Culp procedure; Culp and de Weerd, 1951). When a massively dilated collecting system exists, one can choose a ureterocalycostomy to have dependent drainage later in life. The dismembered and spatulated ureter in this procedure is anastomosed to the dilated lower pole calyx, which has been exposed by cutting a small cap off the lower pole of the kidney. In secondary obstruction after prior pyeloplasty this procedure provides an alternative method of treatment. In children with intermittent PUJ obstruction, a true kinking of the ureter on an aberrant lower pole artery is identified during operation, while the PUJ is clearly patent. In these

cases the artery can be freed from the adventitial layer and buried higher up in the pyelum with two or three sutures (Fig. 62.5). Because the urinary tract has not been opened, the postoperative hospital stay in these cases can be very short.

PYELOPLASTY IN ABNORMALLY POSITIONED AND IN DUPLEX KIDNEYS

In horseshoe kidneys infracostal lumbotomy gives good access to the PUJ and a bilateral pyeloplasty is sometimes possible through one redundant lumbotomy incision. Abnormal vasculature of the kidney is usually present and requires special care. In crossed ectopia, pancake kidney and pelvic kidney, individual access must be chosen. Sometimes a transperitoneal approach is needed. In duplex kidneys, the lower moiety is affected. In some cases pelviureterostomy from the lower moiety pelvis to the upper pole ureter is the easiest operation.

VESICOURETERIC REFLUX AND PUJ STENOSIS

In patients with high-grade reflux, the PUJ often remains a relatively narrow area that in some cases makes it difficult to decide whether obstruction is present. High-grade reflux can lead to hypertrophy of the ureteric wall and thus produce obstruction of a relatively narrow PUJ, making it difficult to decide whether relief of obstruction can be expected once the reflux has been cured. When in doubt, with a good functioning kidney, we prefer to do a reimplant first, taking care not to remove much of the ureter. This rarely saves the patient from a pyeloplasty. A combined pyeloplasty and a ureteral reimplant can be safely performed at the same time. In case of low-grade reflux, subureteric injection of Teflon, collagen or Macroplasty™ can be combined with the pycloplasty.

TREATMENT BY ENDOPYELOTOMY

Since the late 1980s many articles have been produced claiming high success rates for percutaneous antegrade or transureteral retrograde endopyelotomy (Karlin *et al.*, 1988, 1992; van Cangh *et al.*, 1989; Douenias *et al.*, 1990; Cassis *et al.*, 1991). Success rates vary from 72% to 89%, except in one series in which endopyelotomy was combined with endoscopic transpelvic retroperitoneal ureterotomy from the outside of the ureter with a reported success rate of 95%. It has yet to be proven, in paediatric PUJ obstruction, whether endopyelotomy really provides lower morbidity, less postoperative pain and equal success compared with open techniques. Disadvantages of endopyelotomy are the lower success rate, the risk of bleeding and the duration of stenting for up to 6 weeks. In the paediatric age group, resuming daily activities is of less importance than in adults.

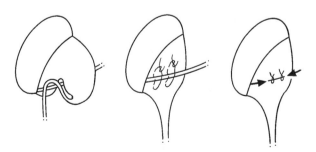

Fig. 62.5 Schematic drawing of a variation on Hellström's original operation to displace an aberrant lower pole artery causing intermittent PUJ obstruction. The artery is buried in the renal pelvis at a level above the PUJ. The renal pelvis is fixed over the artery with a 5-0 polyglycolic acid suture.

TREATMENT BY LAPAROSCOPIC PYELOPLASTY

Successful laparoscopic dismembered pyeloplasty has recently been reported. This technique may have a future, but has the disadvantage of a prolonged operating time (Kavoussi and Peters, 1993).

Conclusions

Treatment of neonates and infants with PUJ stenosis, especially when the condition is detected prenatally, still remains a challenge in paediatric urology, with dilated kidneys balancing on the edge between dilatation and obstruction. This dilemma will not be resolved until better techniques are available to recognize the kidneys at risk of deteriorating function.

References

Anderson, J.C. and Hynes, W. 1949: Retrocaval ureter: case diagnosed and treated successfully by a plastic operation. *British Journal of Urology* **21**, 209.

Belman, A.B. 1991: Ureteropelvic junction obstruction as a cause for intermittent abdominal pain in children. *Pediatrics* **88**, 1066–9.

Byrne, W.J., Arnold, W.C., Stannard, M.W. and Redman, J.F. 1985: Ureteropelvic junction obstruction presenting with recurrent abdominal pain: diagnosis by ultrasound. *Pediatrics* **76**, 934–7.

Cangh, P.J. van, Jorion, J.L., Wese, F.X. and Opsomer, R.J. 1989: Endoureteropyelotomy: percutaneous treatment of ureteropelvic junction obstruction. *Journal of Urology* **141**, 1317–21.

Cartwright, P.C., Snyder, H.M. and Duckett, J.W. 1991: The case of functional assessment of apparent PUJ obstruction. *Dialogues in Pediatric Urology* **14**, 4–5.

Cassis, A.N., Brannen, G.E., Bush, W.H., Correa, R.J. and Chambers, M. 1991: Endopyelotomy: review of results and complications. *Journal of Urology* **146**, 1492–5.

Cockrell, S.N. and Hendren, W.H. 1990: The importance of visualizing the ureter before performing a pyeloplasty. *Journal of Urology* **144**, 588–92.

Cronan, J.J. 1991: Contemporary concepts in imaging urinary tract obstruction. *Radiology Clinics of North America* **29**, 527–42.

Culp, O.S. and Weerd, J.H. de 1951: A pelvic flap operation for certain types of ureteropelvic obstruction: preliminary report. *Proceedings of the Staff of the Medical Mayo Clinics* **26**, 483.

Daucher J.N., Mandell, J. and Lebowitz, R.L. 1992: Urinary tract infection in infants in spite of prenatal diagnosis of hydronephrosis. *Pediatric Radiology* **22**, 401–4.

Douenias, R., Smith, A.D. and Brock, W.A. 1990: Advances in the percutaneous management of the ureteropelvic junction and other obstructions of the urinary tract in children. *Urology Clinics of North America* **17**, 419–28.

Elder, J.S. and Duckett, J.W. 1991: Perinatal urology. In Gillenwater, J.Y., Grayhack, J.T. and Harvards, S.S. (eds), *Adult and pediatric urology*. Chicago, IL: Year Book Medical Publishers, 1711–20.

Flashner, S.C. and King, L.R. 1992: Ureteropelvic junction. In Kelalis, P.P., King, L.R. and Belman, A.B. (eds), *Clinical pediatric urology*. Philadelphia, PA: W.B. Saunders, 693–725.

Flotte, T.R. 1988: Dietl syndrome: intermittent ureteropelvic junction obstruction as a cause of episodic abdominal pain. *Pediatrics* **82**, 792–4.

Gonzalez, R. and Aliabadi, H. 1987: Posterior lumbotomy in pediatric pyeloplasty. *Journal of Urology* **137**, 468–70.

Gottlieb, R.M., Luhmann, K. and Oates, R.P. 1989: Duplex ultrasound evaluation of normal kidneys and kidney with urinary tract obstruction. *Journal of Ultrasound Medicine* **8**, 609–11.

Grignon, A., Filion, R., Filiatrault, D. *et al.* 1986: Urinary tract dilatation *in utero*: classification and clinical applications. *Radiology* **160**, 645.

Guys, J.M., Borella, F. and Monfort, G. 1988: Ureteropelvic junction obstructions: prenatal diagnosis and neonatal surgery in 47 cases. *Journal of Pediatric Surgery* **23**, 156–8.

Hanna, M.K. and Gluck, R. 1988: Ureteropelvic junction obstruction during the first year of life. *Urology* **31**, 41–5.

Heiden, A.J. van der, Versteegh, F.G.A. and Wolff, E.D. 1985: Acute tubular dysfunction in infants with obstructive uropathy. *Acta Paediatrica Scandinavica* **74**, 584–8.

Hollowell, J.G., Altman, H.G., Snyder, H.M. and Duckett, J.W. 1989: Coexisting ureteropelvic junction obstruction and vesicoureteral reflux: diagnostic and therapeutic implications. *Journal of Urology* **142**, 490–3.

Homsy, Y.L., Serrard, J. and Dels, C. 1980: Pyeloplasty: to divert or not divert? *Urology* **16**, 577–99.

Homsy, Y.L., Saad, F., Laberge, I., Williot, P. and Pison, C. 1990: Transitional hydronephrosis of the newborn and infant. *Journal of Urology* **144**, 579–83.

Johnston, J.H. 1969: The pathogenesis of hydronephrosis in children. *British Journal of Urology* **41**, 724–34.

Karlin, G.S., Badlani, G.H. and Smith, A.D. 1988: Endopyelotomy versus open pyeloplasty: comparison in 88 patients. *Journal of Urology* **140**, 476–8.

Karlin, G.S., Badlani, G. and Smith, A.D. 1992: Percutaneous pyeloplasty (endopyelotomy) for congenital ureteropelvic junction obstruction. *Urology* **39**, 533–7.

Kavoussi, L.R. and Peters, C.A. 1993: Laparoscopic pyeloplasty. *Journal of Urology* **150**, 1891–4.

Kessler, R.M., Quevedo, H., Lankau, C.A. *et al.* 1993: Obstructive vs nonobstructive dilatation of the renal collecting system in children: distinction with duplex sonography. *American Journal of Roentgenology* **160**, 353–7.

King, L.R. 1993: Fetal hydronephrosis: what is the urologist to do? *Urology* **42**, 229–32.

Koff, S.A. 1990: Pathophysiology of ureteropelvic junction obstruction: clinical and experimental observations. *Urology Clinics of North America* **17**, 263–72.

Koff, S.A. and Campbell, K. 1992: Nonoperative management of unilateral neonatal hydronephrosis. *Journal of Urology* **148**, 525–310.

Koff, S.A., Thrall, J.H. and Keyes, J.W. Jr 1979: Diuretic radionuclide urography: a noninvasive method for evaluating nephroureteral dilatation. *Journal of Urology* **122**, 451–3.

Lurz, H. 1956: Ein muskelschonender Lumbalschnitt fur Freilegung der Nieren. *Chirurg* **27**, 125.

Nguyen, D.H., Aliabadi, H., Ercole, C.J. and Gonzalez, R. 1989: Nonintubated Anderson–Hynes repair of ureteropelvic junction obstruction in 60 patients. *Journal of Urology* **142**, 704–6.

Osathanondh, V. and Potter, E.L. 1963: Development of human kidney as shown in microdissection. *Archives of Pathology* **76**, 271.

Ransley, P.G., Dhillon, H.K., Gordon, I., Duffy, P.G., Dillon, M.J. and Barratt, T.M. 1990: The postnatal management of hydronephrosis diagnosed by prenatal ultrasound. *Journal of Urology* **144**, 584–7.

Shaffer, S.G. and Weismann, D.N. 1992: Fluid requirements in the preterm infant. *Clinical Perinatology* **19**, 233–50.

Sheldon, C.A., Duckett, J.W. and Snyder, H.M. 1992: Evolution in the management of infant pyeloplasty. *Journal of Pediatric Surgery* **27**, 501–5.

Trendelenburg, F. 1890: Uber Blasenscheidenfisteln Operationen und die Beckenhochlagerung bei Operationen in der Bauchhohle.

Whitaker, R.H. 1973: Methods of assessing obstruction in dilated ureters. *British Journal of Urology* **45**, 15–22.

Young, D.W. 1991: The use of nuclear renography and assessment of hydronephrosis. *Dialogues in Pediatric Urology* **14**, 2–3.

CHAPTER 63

Posterior urethral valves

D.F.M. THOMAS

Introduction
Incidence
Aetiology
Embryology and anatomical classification

Clinical features
Management
Conclusion
References

Introduction

Posterior urethral valves form an important condition which ultimately leads to chronic renal failure in approximately one-third of affected individuals. For paediatric urologists it is a condition that generates a significant cumulative workload because of the ongoing risk of morbidity and the need for detailed, long-term follow-up. Although since the 1970s dramatic change has been seen in the presentation and early outcome associated with the condition, as recently as 1973 Williams *et al.* reported a series of 172 cases associated with a mortality of 41% in boys under 3 months of age. With the advent of better supportive care for sick children, regional centres for paediatric nephrology and urology, and the detection of some cases by prenatal ultrasound, the mortality in infancy due to sepsis has fallen virtually to zero. Early deaths are now largely confined to neonates with pulmonary hypoplasia and lethal degrees of renal dysplasia who would previously have died without involving a paediatric urologist. During the 1970s and 1980s the introduction of specialized paediatric cystourethroscopes with rod lens optics and miniaturized working systems greatly reduced the morbidity and complications which previously resulted from urethral instrumentation and valve ablation. The use of perineal urethrostomy to gain access to the infant posterior urethra was consigned to history by the arrival of these new paediatric instruments. The 1980s saw a declining role for active upper tract intervention, e.g. ureterostomy and ureteric reimplantation, in the light of increasing evidence that it contributed little to the long-term outcome for renal function. A limited role for open surgery may now be returning in the form of augmentation cystoplasty, either with intestine or redundant megaureter, to alter the characteristics of the unstable poorly compliant 'valves' bladder, which plays an important role in some cases of later onset renal failure. A proportion of cases (around two-thirds in the author's centre) are now detected prenatally. Undoubtedly this has contributed to the reduction in early morbidity previously related to urosepsis. Can we also anticipate that prenatal detection will result in an improvement in the long-term outcome for renal function, or is this largely predetermined by events *in utero*? Detailed long-term studies would be required to provide the answer.

The purpose of this chapter is to review recent contributions to the understanding of this important condition in the context of practical management.

Incidence

Previously published estimates based on symptomatic clinically presenting cases place the incidence between 1 in 5000 and 1 in 25 000 (Atwell, 1983) live male births but these figures almost certainly underestimate the true frequency of the condition. Prenatal diagnosis has uncovered the hidden mortality of posterior urethral valves by identifying cases associated with pulmonary hypoplasia and renal dysplasia which previously resulted in death before referral to a specialist paediatric urologist or paediatric surgeon. An estimate based on the referral of 67 cases from the relatively static population of the Yorkshire region, UK (population 3.5 million), points to an incidence of around 1 in 4000 live male births. Posterior urethral valves account for approximately 20% of all obstructive uropathies presenting in the neonatal period and 10–15% of significant uropathies detected prenatally.

Aetiology

Although most cases are regarded as sporadic events, rare reports of familial cases indicate a possible genetic predisposition. The literature includes cases of both twin and non-twin affected siblings, suggesting a polygenetic mode of inheritance (Livne *et al.*, 1983). However, discordance in monozygotic twins has also been reported (Thomalla *et al.*, 1989), indicating that a random mutation may also be implicated in some cases. Regardless of the precise genetic mechanism, familial factors are sufficiently well documented to justify the postnatal ultrasound screening of male siblings (Hutton and Thomas, 1994). Posterior urethral valves are not normally associated with coexistent anomalies, other than those directly consequent on urethral obstruction *in utero*. Cases have been reported, however, in association with prune belly syndrome and Noonan's syndrome. The author's own series of 67 boys includes two with Down's syndrome but this may represent a statistical quirk rather than a previously unreported association. The association between posterior urethral valves and cryptorchidism, however, is well founded. Krueger *et al.* (1980) found an incidence of undescended testis of 12% (24 out of 207 cases) and more recently Barker *et al.* (1993) have reported an incidence of 17%. Whether this association represents a common defect of mesenchymal development or, more probably, mechanical factors interfering with testicular descent, is not known.

Embryology and anatomical classification

The embryological interactions that give rise to the posterior urethra are complex and poorly understood. It seems probable, however, that the type I form of this anomaly (see below) results from the defective interaction between the regressing wolffian ducts and the developing urogenital sinus. Embryological teaching puts the timing of these events at around the 7th week of gestation, suggesting that the obstruction is present before the fetal kidneys begin to produce significant amounts of urine at the 9th week of gestation. This concept of posterior urethral valves as a first-trimester insult to the developing urinary tract is consistent with the observation that dilatation associated with posterior urethral valves has been detected on ultrasound as early as the 12th week of gestation. It is important to acknowledge, however, that in a significant proportion of cases (approximately one-third in the author's experience) the appearances of the fetal urinary tract are entirely normal on second-trimester ultrasound and indeed may even appear normal on ultrasound performed in the latter stages of pregnancy. Such is the consistency of the anatomical findings, however, that the late onset of dilatation is more likely to reflect a mild degree of obstruction associated with an anomaly dating back to the 7th week of gestation rather than obstruction arising *de novo* in later pregnancy.

The occasional finding of a concentric constriction at a level distal to the veromontanum, characterized by Young as type III valves, may represent embryological pathology derived from the urogenital membrane. Urethral atresia, a lethal anomaly characterized by oligohydramnios and pulmonary hypoplasia, probably represents the most severe end of the spectrum of anomalies at this site. In a classic paper published in 1919, Hugh Hampton Young, one of the founding fathers of modern urology, described the anatomical appearances of posterior urethral valves at both post mortem and endoscopy. Young's paper, 'Congenital obstruction of the posterior urethra' proposed a classification (types I–III) that remained largely unchallenged for most of this century. His description of type I valves corresponds to those most commonly seen in clinical practice, i.e. a circumferentially attached membrane with valve-like cusps arising from the christi urethralis just distal to the veromontanum. According to Young, type II valves consist of folds arising from the upper aspect of the veromontanum. Their existence is now largely discounted. Valves in the third category in Young's classification, i.e. type III, were described as the concentric membrane with a central lumen sited at different levels in the posterior urethra but generally regarded as lying distal to the veromontanum. In a paper from the Hospital for Sick Children Great Ormond Street, Dewan *et al.* (1992) have questioned Young's original morphological classification, suggesting that the most of the reported variations are artefactual in origin and reflect differing degrees of damage sustained by the valve membrane during the course of catheterization or instrumentation. When the bladder has been drained suprapubically the appearance of the intact membrane when viewed from below is remarkably consistent. Dewan and his colleagues summarized the characteristics of the valve membrane as follows.

- It is attached posteriorly to the distal part of the veromontanum.
- The valve membrane has a small hole adjacent to the veromontanum.
- The membrane is attached obliquely, with the most distal attachment lying anteriorly.
- The membrane has paramedian parallel reinforcements and balloons distally to traverse the external sphincter.

Despite the uniformity of the anatomical findings, it is clear that the anomaly gives rise to widely differing degrees of obstruction and consequent upper tract damage. At one end of the spectrum severe obstruction to fetal voiding may give rise to oligohydramnios, pulmonary hypoplasia and neonatal death from pulmonary insufficiency. At the milder end of the spectrum a flimsy partially obstructing valve may give rise to little or no upper tract dilatation *in utero* and indeed may remain asymptomatic for many years in postnatal life.

URETHRAL OBSTRUCTION IN FEMALES

Posterior urethral valves are a condition confined to males and when outflow obstruction occurs in female infants it has a different embryological and urological basis. Urethral obstruction in females is exceptionally rare but when it occurs is most commonly due to occulusion of the bladder neck by a prolapsing ectopic ureterocele or some variant of the cloacal anomaly with persistence of a narrow urogenital sinus.

Clinical features

PRESENTATION

Infection represents the most common form of presentation in postnatal life. In a high-pressure obstructed urinary tract, particularly in the presence of vesicoureteric reflux (VUR), urinary infection can progress rapidly to become a life-threatening illness manifested by septicaemia and even meningitis. Until recently, it was not uncommon to be confronted with a profoundly sick and acidotic child requiring resuscitation, intensive supportive therapy and urgent decompression and drainage of the infected urinary tract. Reporting a series of 46 patients, Scott (1985) noted that 26 (57%) had presented with infection. Similarly, Egami and Smith (1982), reported urinary infection as the presenting feature in 49% of 135 boys with posterior urethral valves. Prenatal detection is changing the picture but when boys with unsuspected posterior urethral valves present clinically in postnatal life, urinary infection remains the most common form of presentation.

ABDOMINAL MASS

Abdominal masses of genitourinary origin in the neonatal period more frequently arise from the kidney (e.g. hydronephrosis, multicystic kidney) than from the bladder. However, when a hard palpable bladder is identified in a male infant the most likely explanation is posterior urethral valves. Urinary ascites is a rare presentation of posterior urethral valves and paradoxically extravasation of urine into the peritoneal cavity generally occurs from the better functioning of the two kidneys.

VOIDING SYMPTOMS

Occasionally the diagnosis comes to light following the observation, by parents or nursing staff, of a poor urinary stream or straining on voiding. In older boys it is not uncommon for posterior urethral valves to present with a voiding disorder, e.g. diurnal or nocturnal enuresis. In a multicentre review of 108 cases undertaken by Atwell (1983) on behalf of the British Association of Paediatric Surgeons, some form of voiding disorder was the presenting feature in 18 (17%) with 14 being over 5 years of age at the time of presentation. In a long-term follow-up study of 98 boys treated at the Hospital for Sick Children, Great Ormond Street, Parkhouse *et al.*, (1988) noted that 38 (39%) had been diagnosed during the 1st month of life, whilst a further 27 (28%) presented between 1 month and 1 year of age. In all, around one-third of boys in this study were destined for renal failure in either childhood or adolescence and a poor long-term outcome for renal function was significantly related to early presentation.

RESPIRATORY DISTRESS: PULMONARY HYPOPLASIA

Normal fetal lung development depends upon adequate volumes of amniotic fluid, of which fetal urine is an important constituent. Urethral obstruction of sufficient severity to result in oligohydramnios is frequently, although not invariably, associated with abnormal fetal lung development, e.g. pulmonary hypoplasia. The likelihood of pulmonary hyposplasia can be predicted on the basis of prenatal ultrasound findings. Lortat-Jacob *et al.* (1990) reported respiratory distress in 44% (eight out of 18) of their prenatally detected patients, three of whom died from pulmonary insufficiency. Reinberg *et al.* (1992) found respiratory problems in six out of nine prenatally detected cases (67%), of whom one died and the remaining five required prolonged ventilatory support. In our series of 32 prenatally detected cases fewer boys, i.e. four (13%) had respiratory problems at birth. All four died from respiratory or renal failure within the first 3 months of life. The management of these cases falls to neonatal and respiratory physicians with the urological input being limited in the first instance to suprapubic or urethral drainage in the urinary tract.

PRENATAL DETECTION

An increasing number of boys with posterior urethral valves are now being detected *in utero* as a result of obstetric ultrasound imaging. Although the definitive diagnosis is dependent on postnatal imaging, notably the micturating cystourethrogram (MCU), the following ultrasound findings point to the diagnosis of posterior urethral valves:

- male fetus
- thick-walled bladder with infrequent or incomplete emptying
- upper tract dilatation, i.e. ureters, pelves, calices
- 'bright' echogenic cortex and small kidneys: renal dysplasia
- oligohydramnios.

The main diagnostic difficulty lies in distinguishing posterior urethral valves from primary VUR in a male fetus. At the severe end of the posterior urethral valve spectrum, the ultrasound appearances may be indistinguishable from those of urethral atresia. Although it was initially thought that virtually all cases of posterior urethral valves would be potentially detectable on prenatal ultrasound, this is not proving to be the case. Although local ultrasound expertise influences the detection rate, it is becoming clear that even with state-of-the-art equipment in skilled hands, second-trimester imagining fails to detect between one-third and a half of cases, for the reason that the obstruction has not resulted in detectable upper tract dilatation at that stage. In the series of 19 prenatally detected cases reported by Dineen *et al.* (1992), in only three (16%) was the anomaly detected before 24 weeks gestation.

In a series of 31 prenatally detected cases, scanned in the second trimester, an abnormality was detected before 24 weeks in 17 cases (55%) whilst in the remaining 14 (45%) the second trimester scan was normal and it was not until later in pregnancy that dilatation became apparent on ultrasound (Hutton *et al.*, 1994). We found a close correlation between the early appearance of dilatation and poor outcome. Of the 17 cases detected before 24 weeks, four (24%) died from pulmonary and/or renal failure, six (35%) are alive but in chronic renal failure whilst only seven (41%) are alive with a normal value for plasma creatinine. In contrast, all 14 of the boys whose second trimester scans were normal and whose upper tracts only demonstrated dilatation later in pregnancy are alive and all but one (93%) have normal biochemistry.

Management

INITIAL DIAGNOSIS AND MANAGEMENT

Regardless of whether the diagnosis is suspected on the basis of prenatal ultrasound or following clinical presen-

tation in postnatal life, the starting point of diagnosis and management is invariably an ultrasound scan of the urinary tract. Ultrasound, at the bedside if necessary, should form one of the first investigations of any male infant with unexplained or overwhelming sepsis. In addition to establishing or excluding an underlying diagnosis of posterior urethral valves, ultrasound may reveal the presence of infected debris in an obstructed system, requiring drainage as well as intravenous antibiotic treatment. Ultrasound findings that characterize posterior urethral valves include hydroureteronephrosis, thick walled bladder and changes in renal cortical morphology ranging from loss of corticomedullary differentiation to gross dysplasia with cystic change. Assuming that the ultrasound findings point strongly to a diagnosis of posterior urethral valves, the next step depends on the clinical condition of the child and the presence or absence of urinary infection. In an asymptomatic child, e.g. detected prenatally, antibiotic prophylaxis is commenced and the urinary tract is not drained until a feeding tube is passed for the MCU, which is usually within 48 hours. A conventional contrast voiding cystogram remains the definitive diagnostic investigation. Typically there is an abrupt and striking transition between the dilated posterior urethra and the normal calibre anterior urethra at the level of the valve membrane below the veromontanum (Fig. 63.1). The bladder lumen is usually trabeculated, and VUR, usually high grade, is present in around 50% of cases. Once the urinary tract has been accessed via a urethral catheter or feeding tube, it is wise to leave it *in situ* until the valvular obstruction has been relieved. In some centres the lower urinary tract is visualized using contrast instilled by a suprapubic catheter, i.e. suprapubic cystogram. In the uncomplicated case the next stage consists of definitive surgical treatment, i.e. valve ablation. In the presence of infection or impaired renal function, initial management centres on the provision of adequate bladder drainage, the eradication of infection with appropriate antibiotics and appropriate medical management to correct fluid, electrolyte and acid-based disturbances. In most instances a bladder catheter, either urethral or suprapubic, will provide adequate decompression and drainage of affected urine. In those rare cases where there is an inadequate response to these measures, upper tract diversion, i.e. nephrostomy or ureterostomy, should be considered.

SURGICAL MANAGEMENT (0–5 YEARS)

Sterile urine, stable renal function (Fig. 63.2)

Valve ablation or resection is the initial and often the only form of surgical intervention now employed in many centres. The options include endoscopic resection, using the cutting loop of a miniature neonatal resectoscope, a Bugbee electrode, a fluoroscopic diathermy hook or the use of a Fogarty balloon catheter

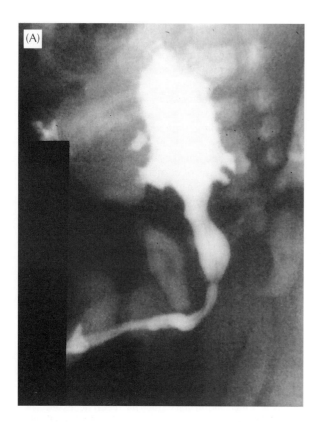

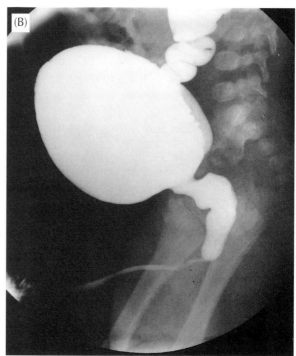

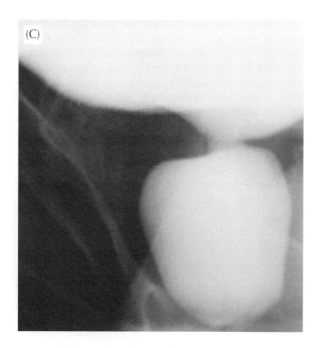

Fig. 63.1 (A) Micturating cystourethrogram showing dilatation of the posterior urethra and gross bladder trabeculation; (B) micturating cystourethrogram showing the appearances of dilatation of the posterior urethra and VUR, in this case the bladder is relatively smooth walled; (C) gross dilatation of the posterior urethra in a 9-year-old boy whose posterior urethral valve obstruction presented with voiding symptoms.

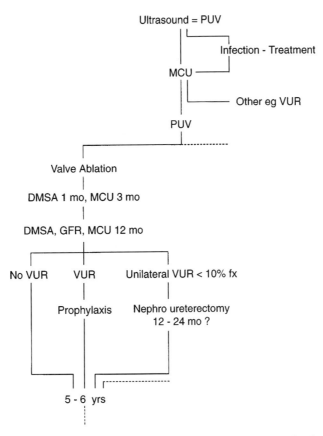

Fig. 63.2 Algorithm summarizing management of the uncomplicated case, i.e. initial valve ablation, stable renal function, freedom from significant urinary infection.

positioned in the posterior urethra and then withdrawn to disrupt the valve membrane. Many of the objections to instrumentation for the neonatal urethra have been overcome by the introduction of new neonatal resectoscopes, miniaturized down to 9 Fg. Some authors, e.g. Zaontz and Firlit (1986), have reported good results utilizing an antegrade suprapubic approach to the valve membrane. When using the neonatal resectoscope the aim is to divide rather than completely resect the valve membrane. If the view is obscured by bleeding, the procedure should be abandoned rather than risk damage to the external sphincter complex. A urethral catheter is left *in situ* for 48 hours following the procedure.

In neonates functional imaging of the upper tract is generally deferred to around 4 weeks of age to permit some maturation of function during the period of transitional nephrology.

Following presentation with acute infection in infancy or later childhood, functional imaging should also be deferred for several weeks to allow the acute pyelonephritic reaction to subside. A cystogram is performed 3 months after valve ablation to exclude the possibility of a postinstrumentation stricture, to check that there is no persisting obstruction by remnants of the valve membrane and to reassess any VUR. Even in the absence of VUR it is the authors' policy to maintain all boys with posterior urethral valves on antibiotic prophylaxis (e.g. trimethoprim 1–2 mg/kg/day during the first year of life).

Further management and the consideration of possible secondary upper tract surgery is based on re-evaluation of anatomy and function at 1 year of age, i.e.

- DMSA static isotope study: as a measure of differential renal function and to demonstrate areas of renal scarring
- MCU: to re-evaluate urethral anatomy and VUR
- estimation of GFR: plasma, urea and creatinine levels provide a crude measure of renal function, but a more reliable estimate of GFR can be generated by using the Schwartz formula, GFR = $0.55 \times L/P_{cr}$, where GFR is the glomerular filtration rate (ml/min/1.73 m^2), L is the body length (cm) and P_{cr} is the plasma creatinine (mg/dl) (Schwartz *et al.*, 1984).

Cr^{51}-EDTA and ^{99m}Tc-DTPA clearance provide the most reliable estimate of GFR but both tests involve injection of isotope and subsequent timed blood samples. In recent years, however, we have been increasingly selective in performing this investigation, on the grounds that in healthy boys with a normal plasma creatinine, the information derived from a formal clearance study rarely justifies the distress caused to the infant and his parents.

The second phase of management, i.e. from 1 to 5 years, is determined largely by the presence or absence of VUR. In the absence of VUR, antibiotic prophylaxis is discontinued but the child is seen for regular, at least annual, follow-up consisting of an ultrasound study and checks on blood pressure and plasma creatinine.

VUR can be demonstrated in 50% of cases at the time of presentation. Once outflow obstruction has been relieved, spontaneous cessation of VUR occurs in approximately 50% of refluxing units. The persistence of asymptomatic VUR is not in itself an indication for ureteric reimplantation since there is no convincing evidence that the correction of VUR is reflected in improved long-term renal function. More importantly, reimplanting wide atonic ureters into thick-walled bladders is a challenging technical exercise with a higher failure rate and greater risk of postoperative obstruction than for primary VUR. Persisting VUR following valve surgery is best treated conservatively, i.e. with antibiotic prophylaxis, usually until 3–5 years of age. If symptomatic breakthrough infections occur despite antibiotic prophylaxis, there is now a body of anecdotal evidence to suggest that circumcision is of benefit. The possible role of prophylactic circumcision in boys with posterior urethral valves has yet to be formally assessed in a randomized prospective trial.

Gross unilateral VUR with ipsilateral renal dysplasia was until recently the most frequent indication for secondary upper tract surgery. This combination of gross VUR with ipsilateral dysplasia and good preservation of function in the contralateral kidney has been likened to a protective 'pop-off' valve. Removal of the poorly functioning kidney and its refluxing ureter was undertaken to reduce the risks of infection and hypertension. Provided that these refluxing units remain asymptomatic, many paediatric urologists now prefer to leave them *in situ*, citing fears of long-term hyperfiltration damage to the remaining solitary kidney. A further argument against routine nephroureterectomy in this situation centres on the reported use of redundant refluxing megaureter for bladder augmentation, i.e. ureterocystoplasty.

EARLY MANAGEMENT (Fig. 63.3) – RENAL IMPAIRMENT AND ONGOING INFECTION

In neonates and infants with significant functional impairment and/or ongoing urinary infection, the definitive treatment of the valve membrane is of secondary importance to the need to establish reliable upper tract drainage and to eradicate infection in the renal parenchyma. In practice, these goals can sometimes only be achieved by urinary diversion. Available options include nephrostomy, ureterostomy and vesicostomy.

Nephrostomy offers short-term drainage in response to gross renal failure or profound sepsis. Unfortunately, whilst percutaneous nephrostomy has proved the technique of choice for draining hydronephroses in older children, its application in cases of posterior urethral valves, where the kidneys are often shrunken, gritty and dysplastic, has proved less successful. Open placement of nephrostomy catheters via loin incisions may be the only option.

Cutaneous ureterostomy, whilst offering effective long-term decompression of the upper tract, requires the use of drainage bags, which are difficult to manage in an active toddler and unacceptable in the long term. Whenever feasible, cutaneous vesicostomy should be performed in preference to conventional ureterostomy. The creation of a vesicostomy is technically straightforward and the stoma, which is concealed by a nappy, requires no drainage bag.

Once reliable upper tract decompression has been achieved and infection brought under control, initial management consists of careful follow-up, usually in conjunction with a paediatric nephrologist.

The degree of renal function impairment usually proves to be the factor guiding management of this group of cases in the first 5 years of life. In some the progressive onset of chronic renal failure necessitates the need for dialysis, usually continuous ambulatory peritoneal dialysis (CAPD), with a view to renal transplantation. In others, renal function stabilizes at a level at which closure of the vesicostomy or ureterostomy becomes a feasible option. The timing of valve ablation is not crucial where the urinary tract has been diverted, but it is clearly important that any underlying outflow obstruction is dealt with before closure of the diversion can be contemplated. Ideally, urodynamics should be included in the work up prior to transplantation or closure of any urinary diversion, since recent evidence suggests that poor compliance and detrusor instability shorten graft survival times and hasten the onset of renal failure in kidneys that are already compromised. In reality, however, the urodynamic findings in a defunctioned bladder are difficult to interpret. Cycling by periodically emptying and filling the bladder is not an easy option and bladder augmentation, whilst theoretically attractive is, for now, an unproven form of treatment in young boys with posterior urethral valves.

FIVE YEARS ONWARDS: MANAGEMENT OF THE 'VALVES' BLADDER

From mid-childhood onwards the threat of eventual renal failure is largely determined by two factors, i.e. pre-existing levels of renal damage, which these days tend to reflect renal dysplasia rather than postnatally acquired infective or obstructive damage, and ongoing bladder dysfunction.

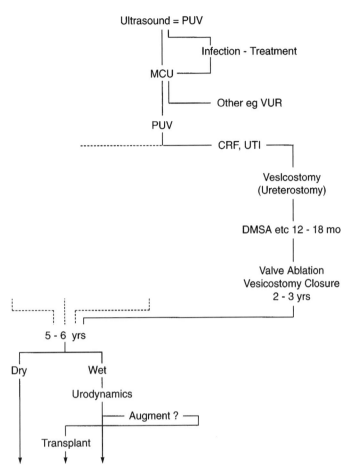

Fig. 63.3 Algorithm outlining management options for the infant with impaired renal function and/or significant symptomatic infection.

The introduction of urodynamics into paediatric urological practice has revealed the presence of ongoing bladder dysfunction throughout childhood despite the successful relief of outflow obstruction. Detrusor instability, hypocompliance and reduced functional capacity appear to pose an ongoing threat to renal function in a significant proportion of boys. In some, this bladder dysfunction may give rise to symptoms of persisting daytime incontinence, but in others bladder dysfunction poses a silent threat. Nijman *et al.* (1992) undertook urodynamic evaluation of the 'valves' bladder in 68 boys with a median follow-up of 10 years. By this time, 26 of the 68 boys had evidence of renal impairment, and 13 had already undergone renal transplantation. A combination of hyperreflexia and poor compliance was present in 22% of the boys studied and was significantly associated with a poor prognosis. Dineen *et al.* (1993) studied 51 boys with posterior urethral valves to compare their urodynamic findings with ^{51}Cr-EDTA estimations of their GFR. In 11 boys with severely reduced bladder compliance, these authors documented evidence of deteriorating GFR. Furthermore, boys with a GFR greater than 100 ml/min/1.73 m^2 had a mean bladder compliance that was significantly greater than for boys in whom GFR was equal to or less than 100 ml/min/1.73 m^2. At first sight, the solution, i.e. bladder augmentation, may appear straightforward since bladder augmentation is now a well-established form of intervention for the paediatric neuropathic bladder associated with incontinence and upper tract damage. It is important to note, however, that augmentation of the neuropathic bladder is invariably coupled with intermittent self-catheterization. Boys with posterior urethral valves, unlike the neuropathic population, have normally preserved urethral sensation, which may cause sufficient discomfort to preclude intermittent urethral catheterization. Parents may not wish a distressing urethral catheterization to be performed on an infant and older boys may refuse to submit themselves to the discomfort of catheterizing a normally innervated urethra. The use of a continent catheterizable conduit (appendicovesicostomy: Mitrofannof procedure) could circumvent this problem, but a reconstructive procedure of this overall magnitude represents a significant surgical undertaking with an appreciable risk of complications. Augmentation, using either redundant ureter (ureterocystoplasty) (Hitchcock *et al.*, 1993) or bowel (clam ileocystoplasty) is already being undertaken on a selected basis in a number of centres. Hopefully, the next 5 years will provide a clearer picture on the role of augmentation in the management of the valves bladder in later childhood and the possible benefits for renal function. In the light of current knowledge, however, it is difficult to advocate bladder augmentation other than on an exceptional basis.

PRACTICAL MANAGEMENT: 5 YEARS AND UPWARDS

Continent with stable renal function

Follow-up is maintained as before, i.e. regular annual or biannual ultrasound, blood pressure and plasma creatinine. Follow-up should be maintained through puberty since, although the majority of boys in this group do well, a small proportion progress to renal failure when their renal reserve is overcome by the increased metabolic demands of puberty. The development of proteinuria may herald this process by a number of years.

In the authors' centre boys who are dry and have stable renal function are not routinely investigated with urodynamics since it is unlikely that the findings would be translated into any form of active intervention. It is recognized, however, that this is not a universal view.

Diurnal incontinence and deteriorating renal function

In the past, incontinence was a relatively common complication of treatment – usually attributable to damage sustained by the striated sphincter during instrumentation and valve ablation. With modern miniaturised instruments in skilled hands, however, the risk to the sphincter complex is minimal and in most instances incontinence is related to detrusor instability and poor compliance. Deteriorating tubular function and high obligatory urine output also contribute to incontinence (particularly at night) and high resting intravesical pressures. In the light of urodynamic findings treatment consists of oxybutinin 2.5–5 mg three times daily combined with a regular voiding regimen if there is evidence of incomplete emptying. In the author's experience it is rare for diurnal enuresis to be of sufficient severity to represent an indication for bladder augmentation in its own right. When combined with evidence of upper tract dilatation and deteriorating renal function, augmentation may prove to be a justifiable option.

Renal transplantation

Ultimately, 15–20% of boys with posterior urethral valves come to renal transplantation and it has been shown that graft survival is significantly reduced (Cairns *et al.* 1991) by the presence of hostile bladder dynamics, i.e. hypocompliance, detrusor instability, etc. Careful urodynamic evaluation should be performed before transplantation and, if necessary, augmentation with or without appendicovesicostomy considered to render the bladder safe before transplantation.

Conclusion

Posterior urethral valves are an important condition that poses challenges to the paediatric urologists from the prenatal period throughout childhood and into adolescence. Careful follow-up, ideally shared with a paediatric nephrologist, is essential to maximize the prognosis for renal function. Further work is needed to identify the benefits, if any, of prenatal detection and to define the role of bladder augmentation in the management of the valves bladder.

References

Atwell, J.D. 1983: Posterior urethral valves in the British Isles: a multicenter BAPS review. *Journal of Pediatric Surgery* **18**, 70–4.

Barker, A.P., McMullin, N.D. and King, P.A. 1993: Posterior urethral valves and testicular maldescent: an under-reported association? *Pediatric Surgery International* **8**, 51–3.

Cairns, H.S., Leaker, B., Woodhouse, C.R. Rudge, C.J. and Neild, H.R. 1991: Renal transplantation into abnormal lower urinary tract. *Lancet* **338**, 1376–9.

Dewan, P.A., Zappala, S.M., Ransley, O.G. and Duffy, P.G. 1992: Endoscopic reappraisal of the morphology of congenital obstruction of the posterior urethra. *British Journal of Urology* **70**, 439–44.

Dineen, M.D., Dhillon, H.K., Ward, H.C., Dufy, P.G. and Ransley, P.G. 1992: Antenatal diagnosis of posterior urethral valves. *British Journal of Urology* **3**, 364–9.

Dineen, M.D., Duffy, P.G., Godley, M.L. and Ransley, P.G. 1993: Renal and vesical function in boys with posterior urethral valves. Data presented to the British Association of Urological Surgeons, Annual Meeting, Harrogate, UK.

Egami, K. and Smith, E.D. 1982: A study of the sequelae of posterior urethral valves. *Journal of Urology* **127**, 84–7.

Hitchcock, R.J.J., Duffy, P.G. and Malone, P.S. 1993: Ureterocystoplasy: the bladder augmentation of choice. Data presented to the British Association of Urological Surgeons, Annual Meeting, Harrogate, UK.

Hutton, K.A.R. and Thomas, D.F.M. 1994: Prenatal diagnosis of posterior urethral valves in siblings. *British Journal of Urology* **73**, 718–19.

Hutton, K.A.R., Thomas, D.F.M., Arthur, R.J., Irving, H.C. and Smith, S.E.W. 1994: *Journal of Urology* **152**, 698–701.

Krueger, R.P., Hardy, B.E. and Churchill, B.M. 1980: Cryptorchidism in boys with posterior urethral valves. *Journal of Urology* **124**, 101–2.

Livne, P.M., Delaune, I. and Gonzales, E.J. 1983: Genetic etiology of posterior urethral valves. *Journal of Urology* **130**, 781–4.

Lortat-Jacob, S., Fekete, C.N., Dumez, Y., Muller, F., Aubry, M.C. and Aubry, J.P. 1990: Diagnostic ante-natal et prise en charge neo-natale des valves de l'uretre posterieur: a propos de 33 observations. *Acrta Urol Belg* **58**, 29–37.

Nijman, R.J., Scholtmeijer, R.J., Groenewegen, A.A. 1992: Urodynamic studies in boys treated for posterior urethral valves. Data presented to the European Society of Paediatric Urology, Third Annual Meeting, Cambridge, UK.

Parkhouse, H.F., Barratt, T.M., Dillon, M.H., *et al.* 1988: Long-term outcome of boys with posterior urethral valves. *British Journal of Urology* **62**, 59–62.

Reinberg, Y., de Castano, I. and Gonzalez, R. 1992: Prognosis for patients with prenatally diagnosed posterior urethral valves. *Journal of Urology* **148**, 125–6.

Schwartz, G.J. Feld, L.G. and Langford, D.J. 1984: A simple estimate of glomerular filtration rate in full-term infants during the first year of life. *Journal of Pediatrics* **104**, 849–54.

Scott, J.E. 1985: Management of congenital posterior urethral valves. *British Journal of Urology* **57**, 71–7.

Thomalla, J.V., Mitchell, M.E. and Garett, R.A. 1989: Posterior urethral valves in siblings. *Urology* **33**, 291–4.

Williams, D.I., Whitaker, R.H., Barratt, T.M. and Keeton, J.E. 1973: Urethral valves. *British Journal of Urology* **45**, 200–10.

Young, H.H., Frontz, W.A. and Baldwin, I.C. 1919: Congenital obstruction of the posterior urethra. *Journal of Urology* **3**, 289–365.

Zaontz, M.R. and Firlit, C.F. 1986: Percutaneous antegrade ablation of posterior urethral valves in infants with small caliber urethras: an alternative to urinary diversions. *Journal of Urology* **136**, 247–8.

CHAPTER 64

Nocturnal enuresis

R. MEADOW

Introduction
Prevalence
Aetiology
Organic factors
Management

Assessment
Investigations
Treatment
References

Introduction

The term enuresis is derived from the Greek word *enourein,* to micturate. The term is applied to inappropriate voiding of urine at an age when control of micturition is to be expected. The age at which individual children achieve this developmental skill varies. Most children, providing they have convenient clothing and the help of a sympathetic adult, are dry by day by the age of 2.5 years. Most children achieve daytime dryness ahead of night dryness, but nevertheless by the age of 3.5 years 75% of children are dry by day and night (DeJonge, 1973). The remainder gradually acquire dryness. It is the substantial number of children with nocturnal enuresis who, either occasionally or regularly, wet their bed whilst asleep at night who are a world-wide cause of parental exasperation, childhood tears and, at times, doctor insecurity.

Prevalence

The prevalence varies in different countries and it is notable that most of the surveys come from the developed countries, particularly those which have, at least for part of the year, a cold climate (where the inconvenience of wet beds is that much greater). The prevalence in the USA and Australia seems to be slightly higher than in western Europe and Scandinavia. For western countries it can be said that at the age of 5 years, between 10% and 15% of children wet their beds at least once a month. Most of these will be wetting their beds several times a week. By the age of 10 the figure is just over 5% and by 15 years 1% (Essen and Peckham, 1967). The prevalence in young adults is uncertain. Studies of recruits to the armed services suggest that up to 1% of that group may have nocturnal enuresis.

Boys achieve dryness slightly later than girls, which is one reason why most studies of young children show that nocturnal enuresis is twice as common in boys as in girls. After the age of 11, the gender incidence is more equal and, if anything, weighted towards girls. For research purposes it is unwise to use the term nocturnal enuresis for boys under the age of 6, or girls under the age of 5 years, because below those ages the wetting can be considered part of the normal distribution curve for the development of night-time dryness (Verhault *et al.*, 1985).

The spontaneous remission rate improves with age. One study of untreated children showed that the annual spontaneous cure rate between the ages of 10 and 19 was 16%, compared with a 14% rate between the ages of 5 and 9 years (Forsythe and Redmond, 1974).

It is usually said that 10% of children with nocturnal enuresis also have diurnal enuresis (daytime wetting). However, in practice marked diurnal enuresis, which is nearly always an urge-incontinence dribbling of urine, in a school-age child is a much more troublesome symptom than bedwetting and tends to be an earlier cause of referral to the doctor. Therefore, if one limits assessment to those children who are referred because of bedwetting, considerably less than 10% have significant daytime wetting.

Some authorities still classify nocturnal enuresis as primary or secondary. Secondary enuresis is reserved for children who have had at least 1 year reliably dry in the past. Such children form a minority. Much more common are children who have never been reliably dry. Even though some people apply the term primary nocturnal enuresis to these cases, nearly all children over the age of 6 years will be found to have had at least one or two nights dry in the past. Thus it is rare to encounter a child of school age who has never had a single night dry. Therefore, the term intermittent enuresis is preferable.

Aetiology

Enuresis is a symptom and its origins are multiple. It is more common in first-born children and in the lower socioeconomic classes.

GENETIC FACTORS

Family studies show that enuresis occurs frequently in other members of the family. There is a greater frequency of enuresis in both of identical twins than in both of non-identical twins (Bakwin, 1971). It is common to find that the child with bedwetting has another first-degree relative with bedwetting. About three-quarters of boys, and half of the girls who wet their beds have at least one parent who themselves had nocturnal enuresis as a child (Dorfmuller, 1974).

STRESS

Stress is an important cause of enuresis and operates at different stages. If it occurs during the sensitive learning period for developing night-time bladder control (2.5–4 years) it tends to interfere with the development of the normal skill, and even though dryness may be achieved, it is not as secure as it would otherwise have been. It has been shown that the chance of enuresis is related to both the severity of the stress and the number of stressful events that occur in the third and fourth years. Thus the arrival of a new sibling, move of home, parental separation, prolonged hospitalization or other unpleasant experience may each affect the acquisition of dryness (Douglas, 1973; Jarvelin *et al.*, 1990). The optimal period for achieving bladder control passes, and though the stress may have disappeared the symptom of enuresis persists. Moreover, if enuresis persists

long enough then it generates additional anxiety within the family, so making it a difficult environment in which to achieve dryness. The symptom has persisted although the cause has changed.

It is also apparent that a child who has been dry may relapse into wetting as a result of a sudden stress, whether it be feverish illness, loss of a parent or admission to hospital.

Although children with learning difficulties and those with mental illness have an increased tendency to wet their beds, it is important to stress that most children who present with bedwetting do not have mental illness, they have neither learning difficulties nor significant behaviour disturbance. The minority of children whose nocturnal enuresis is combined with daytime enuresis have a greater frequency of behaviour disturbance and antisocial behaviour, with soiling being more common in boys and neurotic disorders in girls (Berg *et al.*, 1977).

BLADDER FUNCTION

Most, but not all, studies show that children with nocturnal enuresis have a smaller functional bladder capacity (Starfield, 1967; Esperanca and Gerrard, 1969). Thus, as a group, they tend to micturate more frequently by day than non-wetters. The minority who also have diurnal enuresis tend to have considerably urgency of micturition and, on urodynamic investigation, features of an unstable bladder (Whiteside and Arnold, 1975).

One of the most common reasons proposed by parents of a wetting child is that the child sleeps particularly deeply. However, there have been many careful sleep studies of children who wet, comparing them with those who do not, together with assessments of their rousability. Most of these do not show a significant difference between wetters and non-wetters.

Organic factors

URINARY TRACT INFECTION

Urine infection predisposes to nocturnal enuresis, as well as to diurnal enuresis. Many children with recent onset of urine infection present with enuresis, and the many schoolgirls with covert bacteruria have, as a group, a higher incidence of nocturnal enuresis. It is generally considered that the bacteruria irritates the bladder and predisposes to enuresis, but it can also be suggested that the wet perineum of a child with enuresis predisposes to ascending infection. It is noteworthy that the association between urine infection and enuresis is much stronger for girls than for boys (Stansfield, 1973). Although there is an important association between urine infection and nocturnal enuresis, it is nothing like so strong as that with diurnal enuresis, where up to 50% of girls with daytime wetting are found to have significant bacteruria (Berg *et al.*, 1977).

POLYURIA

If a child has been previously healthy and then develops a condition that causes excessive urine output, nocturnal enuresis may occur. Thus diabetes mellitus, diabetes insipidus or renal insufficiency may all cause the child to wet the bed. Nevertheless, it is extraordinarily rare for a child who presents because of bedwetting to have one of these conditions, not just because they are rare, but rather that they present with more dramatic illness symptoms that cause the parents to consult the doctor for other reasons.

There has been considerable interest in the finding that a selected group of older children and adolescents with nocturnal enuresis appeared to have significantly lower levels of nocturnal vasopressin activity (Rittig *et al.*, 1989). They did not show the usual raised level of antidiuretic hormone at night, compared with the daytime, and therefore did not reduce urine output at night in the usual way. The original studies were performed carefully but have not been replicated in other groups of younger children and therefore it is difficult to assess the relevance of the original finding. It is all the more difficult to understand because of several previous studies that have shown that young children who wet their beds do not have an increased output of urine compared with those who do not wet their beds (Vulliamy, 1956; Troup and Hodgson, 1971).

Neither major nor minor anatomical abnormalities of the urinary tract are of importance. If someone has an ectopic ureter they do not present with an occasional, or even frequent, wet bed; instead, they have an awkward dribble or dampness all the time. Similarly, although vesicoureteric reflux and bladder diverticulum may predispose to urinary tract infection, which in turn increases the chance of nocturnal enuresis, in themselves these bladder abnormalities do not cause bedwetting. There are many reports suggesting that minor genitourinary abnormalities, ranging from phimosis and long foreskin to specific findings on cystourethrogram and endoscopy, are a reason for nocturnal enuresis, but the wide variety of minor abnormalities reported and the discrepancy between the different surveys lead to the conclusion that none is of aetiological importance.

Management

Children with nocturnal enuresis will be managed by many different people with varied levels of skill and experience.

Most parents will seek advice from general practitioners or other primary care doctors. If the child is under the age of 5 years it is likely that, after an initial quick check of the child's general health, the parent will be reassured and given some general advice about ways of encouraging the child to become dry.

Hospital specialists, whether they be surgeons or physicians, are likely to be referred children over the age of 5 years who are still wetting their beds. In some areas a primary care doctor will be making the referral to a specific clinic, run by a paediatrician or a clinical psychologist, primarily for children with wetting problems. However, since there are few of these, most children will be referred to hospital outpatient clinics run by paediatricians, paediatric surgeons, urologists or nephrologists. It is probable that the latter groups see their role as merely excluding organic disease rather than embarking on a management regime to help the child become dry.

Assessment

A full history and examination is essential. Even though the doctor knows that an organic cause for the bedwetting is extremely unlikely, it is common for either the parents or the child to believe that there is an illness or abnormality responsible for the wetting. Moreover, the history taking provides an opportunity to reassure the child and parents about certain issues and to set the scene for successful management.

It is important to establish whether the child has ever been dry at night. Most children over the age of 5, presenting with nocturnal enuresis, will have had several nights completely dry and many will have had several consecutive nights dry. That proves to both the doctor and the family that dryness is possible and there is no permanent leak in the plumbing.

Information should be sought about night-wear: if the child is still being clad in pads and nappies at night, he or she is highly unlikely to stop wetting, and sometimes the advice to remove nappies is followed by immediate dryness.

The pattern of micturition needs to be checked. If the child passes a good stream of urine and micturates about as often as his or her school-mates, he or she is likely to be as healthy as them. Mild frequency by day is common, partly because of the tendency for bedwetters to have a smaller functional bladder capacity. A minority will have marked urgency with mild urge incontinence causing dampness of their pants, but these cases are easily differentiated from the very rare dribbling of an ectopic ureter or obstructed urethra.

It is helpful to seek information about familial or developmental factors contributing to bedwetting because it can help the child and parent to understand more about its origins and to feel less guilty about it.

The main purpose of the physical examination is to reassure rather than to expect to find an abnormality. A quick check should be made to ensure that the child's height and weight are appropriate for their age. It is logical to examine the abdomen and genitalia carefully and also to examine for any external signs, naevi, lipoma or tuft of hair, that might indicate spina bifida occulta. However, if spina bifida occulta was associated with sacral nerve impairment and bladder dysfunction, it would not present with bedwetting, but rather with continued dribbling and incontinence. The most relevant neurological test in relation to bladder function is to check the ankle jerks (innovation S1–2). When examining the perineum it is worth bearing in mind that many children who are being sexually abused develop bedwetting (some suggest as a deterrent to the abuser). The examination should include observation of the anus during gentle traction on the buttocks to see if there is any sign of a gaping anus. During the taking of the history and the examination of the child, the opportunity should be taken to allow the child and parents to voice their worries and concerns about the symptoms and for the doctor to establish the problems that enuresis is causing for the child and family.

Investigations

Assuming that the history is unremarkable and the child appears healthy, investigations should be limited.

Examination of a fresh urine sample is mandatory, but only requires dipstix testing for glucose, blood and albumin, together with a reliable test for urine infection (either microscopy by an experienced person, or a colony count culture).

Spinal X-ray is not needed unless there are definite neurological symptoms or signs. Renal tract ultrasound or intravenous urogram is not required. If the child has had a recent urine infection, or is found to have bacteriuria, then the routine tests customary in that unit (e.g. straight abdominal X-ray and ultrasound) would be carried out, because of the bacteriuria not because of the enuresis. Other more invasive tests such as voiding cystourethrogram or cystoscopy have no place in the investigation of the usual child with bedwetting.

Treatment

GENERAL

Both the child and family need a doctor who will show concern and involvement, and provide adequate time to listen and explain. Nocturnal enuresis is one of the few conditions for which one can promise cure, but it is necessary to explain that a condition that has been present for several years may take several months to resolve completely.

There are many possible therapeutic approaches and they need to be tailored to fit the preconceptions of the family and their lifestyle. It is important to involve the child directly in any management regime and to give the child as much responsibility as is appropriate to their age.

The parents' attitude is important. Often they are exasperated or angry, but they need to be counselled about the misuse of rewards or punishments. Skills may be acquired more surely under a little stress but, when there is much stress, it is difficult to acquire new skills. Therefore rewards or punishments must be used with caution. The child must want to be dry and should know that the parents and doctor want him to be dry, but too much attention, perhaps caused by extravagant bribes on the one hand or fear of punishment on the other, can create too much tension and make dryness difficult to achieve.

Parents often ask about the need to restrict fluids. Usually they have tried it before seeking help from the doctor and found that it does not prevent the bedwetting.

Normal drinking should be allowed and the child can be cautioned to avoid excessive drinking in the evening. The suggestion that bedwetting children should avoid drinks containing caffeine at night (e.g. coffee, tea or cola) is based on the diuretic activity of caffeine. Some parents report that children are more likely to wet the bed if they have had an excess of these drinks, similarly to the way in which a few adults will wet the bed after heavy ingestion of alcohol.

Many people lift or awaken their child at about 11 pm before they go to bed themselves. They persuade the half-asleep child to micturate, and that reduces the subsequent degree of wetting. The manoeuvre does not train children to stop wetting, but it may help with the laundry and there is no harm in it unless it is interfering with one of the more specific therapies detailed below.

Record keeping is essential and the child must play a full role in keeping a diary or record card of wetting events. The record card should be brought to the doctor or therapist at every visit so that progress can be monitored accurately. It is very easy for families, depressed by the continuation of bedwetting and the daily mountain of sodden, smelly bedding, to feel that there has been no improvement in the wetting, whereas a study of the records may show that since treatment started there have already been 15% more dry nights.

There is a considerable cure rate as a result of initial assessment, examination and the first 2 weeks of record keeping. In research trials some people call this the placebo effect, whereas others call it good doctoring. Bearing in mind this cure rate from general measures and also the spontaneous cure rate without treatment, one has to be rigorous in assessing the many reports of different medical and surgical treatments for nocturnal enuresis. Unless those studies are performed carefully with a preceding observation period, careful allocation of patients into similar groups and placebo control of any therapeutic procedure, it is very difficult to know whether the demonstrable improvement is the result of the new treatment or merely the general placebo effect combined with the spontaneous cure inherent in the natural history of nocturnal enuresis (Butler, 1991).

DRUGS

Through the centuries many different drugs have been used for children with nocturnal enuresis. Most of them have not been subjected to properly conducted controlled trials, without which therapeutic reliability is unsure (Blackwell and Currah, 1973). Bearing in mind that there are only two groups of drugs that have been shown to be beneficial in the course of properly conducted clinical trials, and that even these are of limited benefit, the conclusion must be that drugs are greatly overused for children who wet their beds. They are overused because they are easy to prescribe, and less time-consuming than conditioning and other behavioural therapies.

The two groups of drugs shown to be of some benefit are tricyclic antidepressants and antidiuretics.

Triclyclic antidepressants

The two drugs that have been used most are imipramine and amitriptyline. Benefit occurs in up to 50% of children and, if it is going to occur, is seen within the first 10 days of treatment. Tricyclic antidepressants seem to be more effective for girls and for those with severe enuresis (Blackwell and Currah, 1973). Unfortunately, half the children receiving these drugs do not benefit and, of those who do benefit, only a small proportion remain dry when the drug therapy stops. Therefore it is easier to make out a case for these drugs being used for short-term treatment to help a child through a difficult time, or for a holiday or visit to someone else's home, than to suggest them as long-term treatment (Meadow, 1974).

If imipramine is being used, it can be prescribed initially in a dose of 25 mg to be taken at night (or if the child wets before midnight the drug is best given at about 6 pm) (Alderton, 1970). The dose can be increased at 2-weekly intervals by 25 mg up to a maximum of 75 mg each night. In some children mood disturbance and dry mouth prevent using the larger dose. The mode of action of the tricyclic antidepressants for enuresis is unsure. They are complex drugs which, in addition to antidepressant activity and anticholinergic activity, have a local anaesthetic activity on the bladder, as well as other central affects including altering sleep patterns. The benefit seems to come from a combination of these rather than any one specific activity. The drugs

should be used with care because of the well-known toxic effects in large doses (cardiac arrhythmia and death) if a younger member of the family accidentally ingests them.

Antidiuretics

Desmopressin acetate (DDAVP) given in the evening enables about a third of children to become dry (Birkasova *et al.*, 1978). It can be given as a tablet in a dose of 200–400 μg at bedtime. Children who will not swallow tablets can use the metered dose aerosol nasal spray, for which the equivalent dose is 20–40 μg (two to four squirts) of desmopressin (Meadow and Evans, 1989; Evans and Meadow, 1992). It is recommended only for children over the age of 5 years. Since desmopressin suppresses the excretion of water, binge drinking should be avoided. In addition to the children becoming dry whilst using it, many others have a lesser degree of wetting as a result of passing less urine during the night. Unfortunately, once the drug is stopped most of the children relapse, thus, in terms of long-term cure, the results are as disappointing as for the tricyclic antidepressants, the long-term cure rate being only slightly higher than the spontaneous remission rate without treatment (Evans and Meadow, 1992). Desmospray supresses the excretion of water and therefore should be used with caution if there is any reason to suspect fluid overload. If it produces benefit, it is reasonable to continue the treatment for 3 months before having a period without the drug. Repeated courses of Desmospray do not seem to be associated with long-term problems for children. However, it is a much more expensive drug than the tricyclic antidepressants.

Other drugs are widely used and come in and out of favour according to fashion. When using them it is important to bear in mind that only the tricyclic antidepressants and DDAVP have been shown to be of definite therapeutic benefit in controlled clinical trials, whereas the apparent benefit from other drugs is likely to be coming from the placebo effect plus spontaneous cure rate. Therefore it is wrong to use alternative drugs which are potentially dangerous for the child. Other anticholinergic drugs have been widely used and since the mid-1980s oxybutynin has been favoured. Despite widespread use, there are relatively few published studies, most of which do not fulfil the criteria for proper evaluation (Bradbury and Meadow, 1994). The one properly conducted clinical trial, using a double-blind placebo-controlled method for children with nocturnal enuresis who were otherwise normal, failed to show that oxybutynin in a dose of 10 mg at night was more effective than placebo (Lovering *et al.*, 1988). As with other anticholinergic drugs, minor side-effects including dry mouth, constipation, blurred vision, facial flushing, nausea and abdominal discomfort are common.

CONDITIONING THERAPY

The two main alternatives are enuresis alarms and dry-bed training. In most countries there has been much more experience with enuresis alarms.

Enuresis alarms

The system is arranged so that the wetting event completes an electrical circuit which sounds an alarm and awakens the child. The child is instructed to try and wake up as soon as the alarm sounds, i.e. 'to beat the alarm'. At first, the child awakens in a soaked bed, but after a few weeks is awakening with only a tiny damp patch. With continued use the child either learns to awaken before the wetting event or, more commonly, sleeps through without the need to micturate at night (Forsythe and Butler, 1989).

There are two main sorts of alarm. The 'pad and bell' involves the child sleeping on a detector mat, in the form of mesh, foil or printed circuit on plastic mat, with leads passing to an alarm box placed just out of reach of the sleeping child (Figs 64.1 and 64.2). When the child

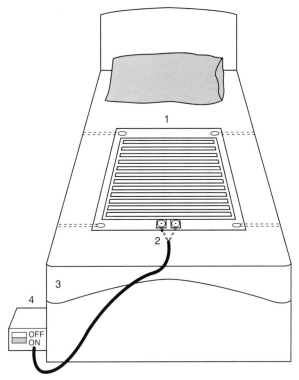

Fig. 64.2 The detector mat (1) is attached firmly to the bed mattress. The lead (2) connects the mat to the alarm box (4), which is placed out of reach of the child.

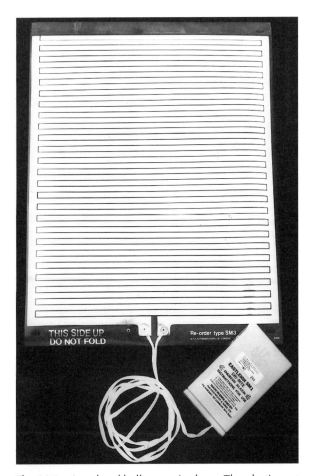

Fig. 64.1 A pad and bell enuresis alarm. The plastic mat incorporates a printed circuit.

wets and the alarm sounds, he or she has to get out of bed to turn the alarm off, go to the toilet, empty the bladder and then return to bed, setting up the system again. The body-worn alarm (Fig. 64.3) involves a wet detector strip or system by the child's perineum so that the first wetting completes the electrical circuit. The alarm itself is attached to the child's shoulder or wrist. Alarms are awkward to use, and it is difficult for young children to wake up in the middle of the night to an alarm and to sort out what is happening. However, providing there is satisfactory motivation and appropriate help from the parents, most children over the age of 7 years will use the alarm effectively. They will need to use it for a minimum of 2 months and usually for about 4 months before becoming reliably dry. Once they have been reliably dry for a month, the subsequent relapse rate is in the 10–15% range. In the event of relapse a subsequent short course of the alarm usually produces permanent cure. Families using the alarm need regular help with the problems that occur and an experienced therapist who can help them with those problems. The cure rates are much lower if the family is merely given an alarm and sent away without frequent follow-up appointments and continued support. For the minority of children who relapse after successfully becoming dry, it can be helpful to use the technique of overlearn-

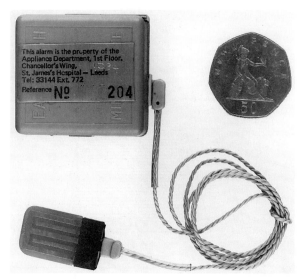

Fig. 64.3 A body-worn alarm. The sensor strip (at the bottom) is inserted either into a pouch in the pants, for a boy, or into a self-adhesive tampon pad pressed against the perineum for a girl. The mini alarm is put in the pyjama pocket or pinned to the jacket or shirt shoulder.

ing when using the alarm again, with the child being asked to drink excess fluid in the evening so as to make wetting events more likely (Morgan, 1978). The relapse rate is then lower. The alarm is more difficult to use for children with behaviour disturbance or learning difficulties, or those in very poor social circumstances, but even for those patients therapists can achieve good results providing that there is a modicum of support within the home. Children with severe wetting and those with family and behavioural problems have been shown to use the alarm more effectively if they are given desmopressin during the first 4 weeks of treatment, possibly because the degree of wetting is lessened, providing early encouragement and making it easier for the family to cope with the management regime (Bradbury and Meadow, 1995). There are several useful guides to the effective use of enuresis alarms (Meadow, 1977). The pad and bell and the body-worn alarms are of similar efficacy. Some older children prefer the body-worn alarm because it is discrete. However, many younger children cannot resist the temptation to switch off the body-worn alarm before it has sounded, and they can do that less easily when using the pad and bell with the alarm bell out of reach from their bed. With enthusiastic management up to 75% of children over the age of 7 years can be expected to become reliably dry using an enuresis alarm.

Dry-bed training

Dry-bed training developed in the USA from methods that had been used for treating adults with severe learning difficulties to become dry by day. In a modified form it can be used very successfully for healthy children with nocturnal enuresis (Azrin and Thienes, 1978). It relies on teaching the child to awaken quickly from sleep, to practise holding on to urine and inhibiting micturition, and involves imprinting on the child that the consequences of a wet bed lead to annoyingly massive toileting procedures. It is in many ways a mildly punitive regime and certainly one that can exasperate the child and the parents. Those skilled with the method may cure the child more quickly than is usual for treatment with enuresis alarms (Azrin and Beasabel-Azrin, 1979). The main limitation is the availability of experienced therapists, usually clinical psychologists or child psychiatrists, and the fact that it requires a highly motivated and compliant child and family. At its best it is a most effective treatment that may be used for some children as young as 4 years (Griffiths *et al.,* 1982).

OTHER TREATMENTS

It is inevitable that for such a common and distressing condition a wide variety of other treatments has been used. Hypnosis has been reported to help some children, but the success rate does not seem to be as high as for conditioning therapy (Olness, 1975). In some countries minor forms of surgery have been used, ranging from circumcision to urethral procedures. None has stood the test of time nor been shown to be helpful in a properly conducted trial. Specific diets, including non-allergenic ones, have been used but there is a lack of evidence relating to their efficacy. Psychotherapy and physiotherapy, involving exercises for perineal muscles and retention training, have also been used but in an uncontrolled way, and they do not appear to be anywhere near as successful as either conditioning therapy or dry-bed training.

References

Alderton, H.R. 1970: Imipramine in childhood enuresis: further studies on the relationships of time of administration to effect. *Canadian Medical Association Journal* **102**, 1179.

Azrin, N.H. and Besabel-Azrin, V. 1979: *Bedwetting eliminated through training.* New York: Simon & Schuster.

Azrin, N.H. and Thienes, P.M. 1978: Rapid elimination of enuresis by intensive learning without a conditioning apparatus. *Behaviour Therapy* **9**, 342–54.

Bakwin, H. 1971: Enuresis in twins. *American Journal of Disease in Children* **121**, 222–5.

Berg, I., Fielding, D. and Meadow, R. 1977: Psychiatric disturbance, urgency and bacteriuria in children with day and night wetting. *Archives of Disease in Childhood* **52**, 651–7.

Birkasova, M., Birkas, O., Flynn, M.J and Cort, J.H. 1978: Desmopressin in the management of nocturnal enuresis in children: a double-blind study. *Pediatrics* **62**, 970–4.

Blackwell, B. and Currah, J. 1973: The psychopharmacology of nocturnal enuresis. In Kolvin I., MacKeith, R.C. and Meadow, S.R. (eds), *Bladder control and enuresis (Clinics in Developmental Medicine* 48/49). Philadelphia, PA: Lippincott, 231.

Bradbury, M. and Meadow, R. 1994: Oxybutynin in nocturnal enuresis. *Contemporary Pharmacotherapy* **5**, 203–7.

Bradbury, M.G. and Meadow, S.R. 1995: Combined treatment with enuresis alarm and Desmopressin for nocturnal enuresis. *Acta Pediatrica* **84**, 1014–8.

Butler, R.J. 1991: Establishment of working definitions in nocturnal enuresis. *Archives of Disease in Childhood* **66**, 267–71.

Dejonge, G.A. 1973: Epidemiology of enuresis: a survey of literature. In Kolvin, I., MacKeith, R.C. and Meadow, S.R. (eds), *Bladder control and enuresis (Clinics in Developmental Medicine* 48/49). Philadelphia, PA: Lippincott, 39.

Dorfmuller, M. 1974: Enuresis. Zur Frage der Hereditaren Disposition. *Medizinische Klinik* **69**, 637–40.

Douglas, J.W.B. 1973; Early distributing events and later enuresis. In Kolvin, I., MacKeith, R.C. and Meadow, S.R. (eds), *Bladder control and enuresis (Clinics in Developmental Medicine* 48/49). Philadelphia, PA: Lippincott, 109.

Esperanca, M. and Gerrard, J.W. 1969: Nocturnal enuresis: studies in bladder function in normal children and enuretics. *Canadian Medical Association Journal* **101**, 324.

Essen, J. and Peckham, C. 1976: Nocturnal enuresis in childhood. *Developmental Medicine and Child Neurology* **18**, 577–89.

Evans, J. H.C and Meadow, S.R. 1992: Desmopressin for bed wetting: length of treatment, vasopressin secretion, and response. *Archives of Disease in Childhood* **67**, 184–8.

Fordham, K.E. and Meadow, S.R. 1989: Controlled trial of standard pad and bell alarm against mini alarm for nocturnal enuresis. *Archives of Disease in Childhood* **64**, 651–6.

Forsythe, W.I. and Butler, R.J. 1989: Fifty years of enuretic alarms. *Archives of Disease in Childhood* **64**, 879–85.

Forsythe, W.I. and Redmond, A. 1974: Enuresis and spontaneous cure rate. *Archives of Disease in Childhood* **49**, 259–63.

Griffiths, P., Meidrum, C. and McWilliam, R. 1982: Dry bed training in the treatment of nocturnal enuresis in childhood: a research report. *Journal of Child Psychology and Psychiatry* **23**, 485–95.

Jarvelin, M.R., Moilanen, I., Vikevainen-Tervonen, I. and Huttunen, N.P. 1990: Life changes and protective capacities in enuretic and non-enuretic children. *Journal of Child Psychology and Psychiatry* **31**, 763–74.

Lovering, J.S., Tallett, S.E. and McKendry, J.B.J. 1988: Oxybutynin efficacy in the treatment of primary enuresis. *Pediatrics* **82**, 104–6.

Meadow, R. 1977: How to use buzzer alarms to cure bedwetting. *British Medical Journal* **ii**, 1073–5.

Meadow, S.R. 1974: Drugs for bed-wetting. *Archives of Disease in Childhood* **49**, 257.

Meadow, S.R. and Evans, J.H.C. 1989: Desmopressin for enuresis. *British Medical Journal* **298**, 1596–7.

Morgan, R.T.T. 1978: Relapse and therapeutic response in the conditioning treatment of enuresis: a review of recent findings on intermittent reinforcement, overlearning and stimulus intensity. *Behaviour Research and Therapy* **16**, 273–9.

Olness, K. 1975: The use of self-hyponosis in the treatment of childhood nocturnal enuresis: a report on 40 patients. *Clinical Paediatrics* **14**, 273–9.

Rittig, S., Knudsen, U.B., Norgaard, J.P. *et al.* 1989: Abnormal diurnal rhythm of plasma vasopressin and urinary output in patients with enuresis. *American Journal of Physiology* **256**, 664–71.

Stansfield, J.M. 1973: Enuresis and urinary tract infection. In Kolvin, I., MacKeith, R.C. and Meadow, S.R. (eds), *Bladder control and enuresis (Clinics in Developmental Medicine* 48/49). Philadelphia, PA: Lippincott, P 102.

Starfield, B. 1967: Functional bladder capacity in enuretic and non-enuretic children. *Journal of Pediatrics* **70**, 777.

Troup, C.W. and Hodgson, N.B. 1971: Nocturnal functional bladder capacity in enuretic children. *Journal of Urology* **105**, 129–32.

Verhulst, F.C., Van Der Lee, J.H., Akkerhuis, G.W., Sanders-Woudstra, J.A., Timmer, F.C. and Donkhorst, I.D. 1985: The prevalence of nocturnal enuresis: do DSM III criteria need to be changed? A brief research report. *Journal of Child Psychology and Psychiatry* **26**, 989–93.

Vulliamy, D. 1956: The day and night output of urine in enuresis. *Archives of Disease in Childhood* **31**, 439–43.

Whiteside, C.G. and Arnold, E.P. 1975: Persistent primary enuresis: a urodynamic assessment. *British Medical Journal* **i**, 364.

CHAPTER 65

Urinary and faecal incontinence

J.P. ROBERTS AND P. MALONE

Introduction
Causes of urinary and faecal incontinence
Clinical features

Management of incontinence
Results
References

Introduction

Wetting and soiling comprise an often neglected but serious cause of problems during childhood. Children taunted for being wet and smelly can grow into withdrawn and isolated adolescents and adults. When an adult is seen with either urinary or faecal leakage the diagnosis of incontinence is automatic. The situation is much more complex in paediatric practice as only a small proportion of wetting or soiling children will be truly incontinent, and it is important not to investigate or treat inappropriately. Many wetting or soiling children will be enuretic or encopretic and in the majority spontaneous improvement is to be expected. All that is required in many instances is an explanation of the condition and reassurance (Novello and Novello, 1987; Scharf *et al.*, 1987; Jarvelin *et al.*, 1988). However, this approach can cause its own problems as there is a tendency to label all children with wetting and soiling as being enuretic and encopretic, and thus fail to recognize true incontinence. The art is to recognize the incontinent patient so that appropriate investigations and treatment can be instituted without undue delay.

When a wetting or soiling child is first seen it is essential that the diagnosis of incontinence is actively excluded. This can be done in the majority of patients with a proper history and examination, and a knowledge of the conditions that cause incontinence, particularly those that are easily missed. If incontinence is not actively sought it will continue to be misdiagnosed.

Causes of urinary and faecal incontinence

Urinary and faecal dysfunction commonly coexist and it is important that both systems are assessed and treated simultaneously (see Tables 65.1–65.3). Chronic constipation, for example, not only is the most common cause of faecal incontinence but may also cause secondary urinary incontinence. The major causes of incontinence are due to dysfunctional emptying, neuropathic and structural abnormalities. Neuropathic incontinence can affect the urinary and gastrointestinal tracts to a varying extent and structural anomalies of one system may affect the other. It is becoming increasingly clear that anorectal

Table 65.1 Causes of isolated urinary incontinence

Structural	Duplex with ectopic ureter
	Exstrophy–epispadias complex
	Posterior urethral valves
	Miscellaneous bladder outlet obstruction
	Urethral duplication
	Vesical fistula
	Small fibrotic bladder (surgery, radiotherapy)
	Labial adhesions
Dysfunctional	Idiopathic detrusor instability
	Urge syndrome

Table 65.2 Causes of isolated faecal incontinence

Structural	Anorectal malformations
	Anal stenosis
	Sphincter trauma
Dysfunctional	Hirschsprung's disease
	Neuronal intestinal dysplasia
	Segmental colonic dilatation
	Chronic constipation with overflow
	Chronic diarrhoea

Table 65.3 Causes of combined urinary and faecal incontinence

Neuropathic	Spina bifida
	Spinal dysraphism
	Sacral agenesis
	Spinal tumours
	Transverse myelitis
	Spinal cord ischaemia
	Sacrococcygeal teratoma (Malone *et al.*, 1990b)
	Trauma
	Occult neuropathic bladder
	Generalized neurological conditions
Structural	Anorectal malformations
	Cloacal anomalies
	Cloacal exstrophy
Dysfunctional	Chronic constipation

malformations are commonly associated with abnormal bladder function, probably due to spinal dysraphism, but the effects of the surgical procedures need further investigation (Karrer *et al.*, 1988; Sheldon *et al.*, 1991).

Clinical features

A thorough history and examination is all that is required in most cases to differentiate enuresis or encopresis from true incontinence.

HISTORY

A detailed micturition history is essential. This should include details of frequency, urgency, urge incontinence, urine volumes, hesitancy, quality of stream, continuous or intermittent stream, terminal dribbling and the duration the patient can stay dry. It is also important to establish the duration of the wetting problem, as a patient who has never been reliably dry in the upright position probably has true incontinence secondary to a duplex upper tract with an ectopic ureter or sphincter

weakness. This history would direct the subsequent examination and choice of investigations. Frequency, urgency and urge incontinence is suggestive of dysfunctional voiding as occurs with idiopathic detrusor instability, neuropathic bladder or the urge syndrome (Van Gool and De Jonge, 1989). A history of a weak stream raises the possibility of bladder outflow obstruction, e.g. posterior urethral valves. An intermittent stream or staccato voiding is suggestive of a functional outflow obstruction, detrusor sphincter dyssynergia. An accurate assessment of the quantity, type and timing of fluid intake is also important. It is now clear that blackcurrant- and caffeine-containing drinks such as cola, tea and coffee can provoke detrusor instability in susceptible patients. A change in drinking habits is always worth trying before embarking on invasive and expensive investigations or prescribing drug therapy. In many cases there is a dramatic improvement in symptoms and nothing more needs doing.

The severity of wetting should also be assessed by exploring the number of changes of clothing per day or the use of pads or other incontinence aids. The effects of wetting on the child's development are also important. Emotional or behavioural problems may also be present but it can be very difficult to distinguish between those causing the wetting and those that are secondary to it. The involvement of an interested psychologist in these patients may be valuable. A detailed family history should also be taken.

When assessing the soiling patient chronic constipation must always be excluded. A history of infrequent and difficult passage of large hard stools and constant soiling with liquid or soft stool is classical in overflow incontinence. The call to stool and the sensation of rectal fullness is often lost with neuropathic incontinence, but may also be absent in chronic constipation with megarectum. Urge faecal incontinence may occur with voluntary muscle weakness (solid stool) or with proctitis (often liquid stool). Voluntary muscle weakness is also suggested by stress incontinence, leakage between episodes of normal defecation indicates low resting pressure usually due to internal sphincter dysfunction. The degree of incontinence is estimated by the frequency and amount of leakage, and the type of contents leaked.

EXAMINATION

The examination is similar for patients with wetting or soiling, and begins by assessing the gait as the child walks into the consultation room. An abnormal gait is suggestive of a neuropathic aetiology. The abdomen is palpated for a full bladder and for faecal masses. If possible it is useful to observe the urinary stream and re-examine the abdomen to see whether bladder emptying is complete. The spine should be inspected for cutaneous stigmata of dysraphism. The entire spine is palpated and this must include palpation of the coccyx.

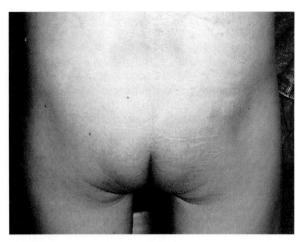

Fig. 65.1 Appearance of sacral agenesis (note the loss of the normal intergluteal cleft).

This is the best means of diagnosing sacral agenesis as the intergluteal cleft is short and the buttocks are flattened (Fig. 65.1).

Inspection of the perineum and introitus is necessary to exclude labial adhesions which may cause post-micturition dribbling, and to assess the position of the anus. A bifid clitoris with diastasis of the pubic symphysis is typical of female epispadias (Fig. 65.2). The presence of a urogenital sinus is suggested by a single urogenital orifice. In the male the presence of phimosis or a meatal stenosis must be excluded. Perineal sensation and the anocutaneous reflex are assessed and a rectal examination may be carried out to assess rectal loading and the resting sphincter tone.

A full neurological examination of the lower limbs should be performed in all patients.

Management of incontinence

INVESTIGATION OF URINARY INCONTINENCE (TABLE 65.4)

Urinalysis is mandatory in all cases of wetting to exclude infection, but if polyuria is suspected analysis should include protein, glucose and osmolality estimation. In occasional cases a 24-hour collection before and after water deprivation may be required. In isolated nocturnal enuresis further investigations are rarely indicated but with daytime wetting further studies are frequently required, and the studies chosen should be individually selected.

Spinal X-rays are advisable if the history and/or examination suggest dysfunctional voiding or a neuropathic bladder. Anteroposterior and lateral views of the lumbosacral spine are initially performed but more extensive imaging may be indicated depending on the

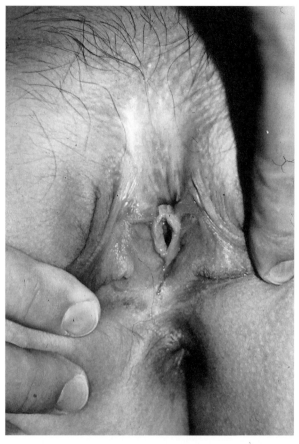

Fig. 65.2 Typical appearance in female epispadias with split clitoris and diastasis of the pubic symphysis.

findings of these and other investigations. These include magnetic resonance imaging (MRI), computed tomography (CT) scans and CT myelography and, if these are abnormal or inconclusive lower limb electromyographic studies may be helpful. The involvement of a neurologist or neurosurgeon is recommended at this stage.

Ultrasonography is the first choice for imaging the urinary tract. It can diagnose abnormalities such as

Table 65.4 Investigation of urinary incontinence

- Urinalysis
- Spinal imaging
- Ultrasonography
- Videourodynamics
- Intravenous urography
- Cystography
- Isotope renography
- Patent Sky Blue dye test
- Cystoscopy/vaginoscopy
- EMG studies

duplication with ectopic ureter, thick-walled bladder associated with posterior urethral valves or a neuropathic bladder. The value of the ultrasound is greatly enhanced by performing pre- and postmicturition bladder views with a simultaneous assessment of the free flow rate. A poor flow rate with incomplete emptying raises the suspicion of detrusor sphincter dyssynergia or of a bladder outflow obstruction. Further investigations are selected dependent on the findings.

In the majority of patients no further studies are required, and if the clinical diagnosis is suggestive of detrusor instability a trial of anticholinergic therapy (oxybutynin) is justified, with further investigations reserved for those patients who do not respond.

Videourodynamics are the next step. They are indicated for all patients with a suspected neuropathic bladder, all incontinent patients with posterior urethral valves, all patients with suspected detrusor sphincter dyssynergia and patients with detrusor instability who do not respond to oxybutynin. Occasionally urodynamics are indicated in patients with enuresis that does not resolve spontaneously, particularly if emotional problems are developing. Weerasinghe and Malone (1993) demonstrated their value in these circumstances, but they are invasive studies and approximately 30% of patients needed suprapubic lines, inserted under general anaesthesia. It is only by using urodynamic studies that conservative treatment can logically be chosen for patients with neuropathic bladders or that appropriate surgery can be planned. Videourodynamics are also invaluable in the postoperative assessment of patients undergoing bladder reconstruction. It is not in the scope of this chapter to describe the detailed urodynamic features of these conditions but many excellent references are available (Rickwood *et al.*, 1982; Mundy *et al.*, 1985). Ambulatory urodynamics are now growing in popularity and there seems to be little doubt that they will replace the standard studies in the majority of patients (Passerini-Glazel *et al.*, 1992).

As urodynamic studies provide so much more additional information, micturating cystourethrography is rarely indicated except where an ultrasound scan demonstrates a thick-walled bladder, and posterior urethral valves are the most likely diagnosis.

Intravenous urography (IVU) should be performed when duplication with an ectopic ureter is suspected. This will usually confirm the diagnosis, but in rare circumstances, with a classical history, the IVU will be normal and further investigations will be needed.

Patent Sky Blue can be instilled into the bladder and a pad is then placed over the perineum. This is inspected every 15 min until the pad becomes wet: if it is clear urine then there is no doubt that one is dealing with an ectopic ureter. Great care is needed when the catheter used to instil the dye is removed, to avoid staining the perineum and causing a false result. If the diagnosis is

duplex incontinence but ultrasound and IVU cannot identify the side, contrast-enhanced CT scanning or MRI is needed. A classical history of duplex incontinence, where a single kidney is seen on imaging, requires further investigation as the likely diagnosis is a simplex dysplastic ectopic kidney and ureter. Isotope renography, CT and MRI may all have a role to play here.

Isotope renography should be performed to assess the renal function, particularly in duplex kidneys when an upper moiety heminephroureterectomy is considered and in all cases of neuropathic bladder and bladder outflow obstruction to look for scarring. Excretory renography may also help in assessing upper tract obstruction and is particularly useful in studying postoperative results.

Cystoscopy is essential for all patients who remain incontinent following reconstructive surgery but is not so valuable in other wet patients. If a cystoscopy is performed the bladder capacity should be measured and compared to the functional capacity assessed at urodynamics. In cases of duplex the site of the ectopic ureteric orifice may be identified, but these can be very difficult to find and this should not influence either the diagnosis or the treatment.

INVESTIGATION OF FAECAL INCONTINENCE

The search for spinal cord pathology applies equally to children presenting with faecal incontinence as to those with urinary incontinence (see Table 65.5).

Anal manometry gives objectivity to information which may be gained from simple rectal examination. There are many reports correlating incontinence following anorectal surgery with resting sphincter pressures below 20 cmH$_2$O (Arhan *et al.*, 1976; Nagasaki *et al.*, 1983; Iwai *et al.*, 1988). There is, however, considerable overlap of sphincteric pressures between incontinent and normal subjects. Calculation of a pressure gradient from rectum to anus may be a more reliable indicator of faecal incontinence than sphincter pressures (Rasmussen *et al.*, 1992). Anal manometry is difficult to perform in patients too young to co-operate. This led Shandling and Gilmore (1987a) to develop the

Table 65.5 Investigations of faecal incontinence

- Spinal imaging
- Anorectal manometry
- Transanal ultrasound
- Contrast enema
- Rectal biopsy
- Endoscopy
- MRI/CT
- EMG studies

measurement of anal sphincter force (the force required to extract a balloon from the rectum), which is greater than 500 g in normal subjects of all ages.

Ambulatory anorectal manometry can provide more information. Persistence of high-amplitude colonic manometric waves may be seen in the neorectum following pull-through and is associated with incontinence, probably due to a compromised sphincter (Roberts and Williams, 1992).

Transanal ultrasound may provide further anatomical information of the external sphincter mechanism (Law and Bartram, 1989; Law *et al.*, 1991).

Vector anal manometry provides circumferential anal pressure profiles and a three-dimensional pressure diagram of the sphincter can be constructed (Perry *et al.*, 1990). These studies should have replaced electromyographic sphincter mapping.

Magnetic resonance imaging is a useful method of determining the position of the bowel, following pull-through, in relation to the sphincter complex and puborectalis in incontinent patients being considered for further surgery (Grier *et al.*, 1992).

Rectal biopsy should be considered in any child with symptoms of constipation predating toilet training, to exclude Hirschsprung's disease.

Contrast enema is not routinely indicated in the investigation of faecal incontinence but may be helpful in cases of overflow incontinence following surgery where isolated segmental colonic dilatation may occur (Pena and El Behery, 1993).

Endoscopy is of limited value but may detect proctitis or inflammatory bowel disease.

The importance of sphincter function in the maintenance of continence has probably been over-emphasized; equally important factors demonstrated in the adult include reduced compliance of the rectum and the absence of anorectal sensation, but these are difficult to assess objectively (Wakeman and Allen-Mersh, 1989; Sun *et al.*, 1990).

TREATMENT

It is essential to consider the management of the urinary tract and bowel simultaneously. However, for simplicity of presentation they will be presented separately here.

Urinary incontinence

The management of isolated urinary incontinence is individualized for each patient depending on the underlying cause (see Table 65.6). Patients with duplex upper tracts and an ectopic ureter usually have a dysplastic upper moiety (Mackie and Stephens, 1975) and can be made dry by a simple upper moiety heminephroureterectomy. In the rare patient with a functioning moiety a pyelopyelostomy or a ureteroureterostomy is indicated. If a

patient has an ectopic single dysplastic kidney a simple nephrectomy will produce continence. Incontinence secondary to posterior urethral valves will frequently be cured by valve ablation alone. Some patients will continue to wet and these will need further investigation and treatment of their underlying detrusor abnormality. These techniques are similar to those used in the management of the neuropathic bladder, which will be discussed in detail below. The management of other forms of bladder outlet obstruction may require dilatation of a urethral stricture or a meatal stenosis. Vesical fistulae can be closed and urethral duplications can be excised. A simple separation of labial adhesions may be all that is required in some girls who suffer postmicturition dribbling.

The management of detrusor instability or the wide variety of dysfunctional voiding states, e.g. the urge syndrome (Van Gool and De Jonge, 1989) is much more difficult and demanding. The history should give a clue to the underlying condition. Modification of the type and timing of fluid intake is helpful. In many patients just stopping cola, blackcurrant juice or caffeine-containing drinks will make the patient dry. A regular voiding habit is vital and initially 2-hourly micturition is advisable, along with double voiding if there is evidence of incomplete bladder emptying. If there is a convincing history of detrusor instability and pre- or postmicturition bladder ultrasound and a free flow rate excludes incomplete emptying or outlet obstruction, a trial of oxybutynin is worthwhile, starting at 2.5 mg twice daily, building to a maximum dose of 5 mg four times a day (Robinson and Castleden, 1994). If this approach is not successful videourodynamic studies are indicated (Weerasinghe and Malone, 1993). If the clinical diagnosis of detrusor instability is confirmed a further more concerted use of oxybutynin or other anticholinergics is worth trying. However, the response to these agents can be disappointing (Brading and Turner, 1994). In refractory cases intravesical oxybutynin should be considered. It is more effective but requires intermittent catheterization (Madersbacher and Jilg, 1991). It is important to treat all urinary infections, even asymptomatic bacteriuria, at the same time. Failure to make the patient dry with this regime is not uncommon and this led Van Gool and De Jong (1989) to introduce a programme of 'cognitive bladder retraining', for which success rates in the order of 70% are reported. This programme employs biofeedback and psychotherapy to teach the children how and when to void. The main problems with this system are the large number of personnel required and the cost. However, the authors have found that by using the urodynamic studies to educate both the patients and their parents about the bladder problems and the need for a specific treatment, similar results can be achieved. It is probably the interest and input that are important, rather than the exact management regime used. Even with this intensive approach some 30% of patients will continue

Table 65.6   Treatment options for urinary incontinence

Pharmaceutical	Oxybutinin: detrusor inhibition Ephedrine: increase outlet pressure Phenoxybenzamine
Collection devices	Urinary catheters/appliances Incontinence pads
Biofeedback/toilet training	
Intermittent bladder emptying	Bladder expression Clean intermittent catheterization (CIC) Mitrofanoff principle
Urinary diversion	Ileal conduit urostomy Colonic conduit Ureterosigmoidostomy Vesicostomy, ureterostomy
Continent reservoirs	Kock pouch Caecoileal (Indiana)
Bladder augmentation[a]	Ileocystoplasty Ileocaecocystoplasty Colocystoplasty Gastrocystoplasty Ureterocystoplasty
Bladder substitution	Colon/ileocaecal
Increase bladder outlet resistance[a]	Bladder neck reconstruction Young–Dees–Leadbetter Urethral lengthening (Kropp or Pippi-Salle procedure) Artificial sphincter Muscle transplantation Submucosal injection (Teflon, collagen)
Spinal surgery	Release cord tethering Decompressive duroplasty Division of filum terminale
Implantable neuroprosthesis	Pudendal nerve stimulation
Transcutaneous electrical nerve stimulation (TENS)	

[a]Except with artificial sphincters these procedures are usually combined with a method of emptying the bladder such as CIC via the urethra or a Mitrofanoff (cutaneous appendicovesicostomy).

to wet and the difficulty is how to treat these. In refractory cases it is also worthwhile reviewing all the imaging, as occasionally a structural anomaly such as an ectopic ureter may have been missed. If incomplete bladder emptying is present clean intermittent catheterization should be considered and will also provide the facility to give intravesical oxybutynin. Transcutaneous electrical nerve stimulation (TENS) has also been shown to be of help in treating instability but it is a technique not widely employed as it is cumbersome and

does not produce a long-lasting effect (McGuire *et al.*, 1983; Read *et al.*, 1985; Fossberg *et al.*, 1990).

If stress incontinence is a feature of the history, pelvic floor exercises, ephedrine hydrochloride (15 mg, three times a day) or injection of the bladder neck with either macroplastique or collagen is worth considering (Caoni *et al.*, 1993; Buckley *et al.*, 1993).

A small, but very difficult, group of patients will continue to wet despite all treatment and these pose a major challenge to the urologist. Should this group undergo bladder reconstructive surgery for a condition that is possibly, though not definitely, self-limiting or should they continue to wet throughout childhood until it is clear that spontaneous resolution will not occur? There is no one correct answer but the authors believe that reconstruction should only be considered if normal development is being interfered with. If reconstructive surgery is being performed clam ileocystoplasty is an effective procedure, but a significant number of patients will require intermittent catheterization to empty their bladders (Mundy and Stephenson, 1985). These patients may well require psychological assessment and support, and the help of trained incontinence advisors is invaluable.

Although complex in one way, the management of the neuropathic or other abnormal bladders is easier, as spontaneous improvement will not occur. The management of bladder exstrophy is considered in detail in Chapter 60, and in this chapter we will concentrate on the neuropathic bladder, using it as the template to explain the basic principles used in all lower-tract reconstructive surgery. The first aim is to prevent renal damage and preserve normal renal function and, if this can be safely achieved, to make the patient dry. This usually involves a compromise and there is little doubt that in many cases making a patient dry puts the kidneys at risk unless a strict postoperative regime is adhered to.

The bladder should be able to store an adequate volume of urine at low pressure and empty completely on voiding. The sphincters should be able to exert a variable resistance to maintain continence during storage and allow free unobstructed voiding. In the neuropathic bladder a number of different abnormalities exist and treatment needs to be individualized. Urodynamics are essential if logical treatment is to be selected.

The acontractile bladder accounts for about 9% of neuropathic bladders in children. When this is associated with a fixed urethral resistance, chronic retention will ensue until the intravesical pressure exceeds urethral resistance when overflow incontinence will occur. If the storage pressure exceeds ureteric pressure upper tract dilatation will occur and renal damage will certainly follow. Complete bladder emptying is all that is required here to protect the kidneys and make the patient dry and a number of approaches are available. Clean intermittent catheterization was introduced by Lapides *et al.* (1972) and is the cornerstone in achieving bladder emptying. Long-term results are very encouraging (Perez-Marrero *et al.*, 1982; Wyndade and Maes, 1990) and in many patients it is all that is required. There is no longer a routine place for manual expression or indwelling catheter drainage. However, in 1993 Barnes *et al.* reported excellent results in adult spinal injury patients using an indwelling catheter with intermittent clamping and drainage and this may be worth considering in individual cases. A significant number of patients with acontractile bladders have lower motor neurone lesions and will have associated sphincter weakness incontinence (Rickwood *et al.*, 1982; Mundy *et al.*, 1985). If the sphincter weakness is borderline the use of an α-sympathomimetic such as ephedrine hydrochloride (15 mg, three times a day) is worth trying and in a small number of patients may make them dry. In males with sphincter weakness incontinence a penile appliance with a leg bag may work well but this management is now less acceptable to patients with the advent of newer techniques. Penile clamps no longer have a place in modern practice because of the high rates of erosion but in the female urethral plugs may be useful in the management of sphincter weakness incontinence (Nielson *et al.*, 1990); however complications such as migration of the device have been reported and long-term follow up is not available (Boemers *et al.*, 1993).

The only remaining approach is surgery and a wide variety of procedures are available. A variable urethral resistance can only be achieved with the artificial urinary sphincter (AUS). All other techniques produce a fixed outlet resistance and thus the need for intermittent catheterization. Even when artificial sphincters are used, around 60% of patients with congenital neuropathic bladders will need to catheterize postoperatively (Nurse *et al.*, 1993). This surely must raise doubts about the value of sphincters in this group. Continence rates of 75–90% are claimed in the short term (Gonzalez *et al.*, 1989; Barrett and Parulkar, 1989; Bosco *et al.*, 1991; Montague, 1992), although these may fall with long-term follow-up (Bosco *et al.*, 1991). Complications of the AUS are common; device failure in 7–20%, cuff erosion in 7% and infection in 1–2% (Gonzalez *et al.*, 1989; Barrett and Parulkar, 1989; Montague, 1992). Cuff erosion is reduced by using lower pressure cuffs (< 80 cmH$_2$O) and reoperation rates are falling with the newer devices and more experience (Bosco *et al.*, 1991). Erosion is much more common in girls and some practitioners would now advocate reserving their use for males only (Rickwood, personal communication). Considering the high complication rates and the need for intermittent catheterization in such a large number of patients, the authors see little benefit in the use of AUS and would advocate procedures to provide a fixed increase in outlet resistance with emptying performed by clean intermittent catheterization (CIC). Complication rates are reported to be lower for these bladder outlet procedures (Sidi *et al.*, 1987).

The simplest way of increasing bladder outlet resistance is by the injection of inert substances into the bladder neck, Teflon, collagen and macroplastique (Wan *et al.*, 1992; Caoni *et al.*, 1993; Buckley *et al.*, 1993). Teflon may produce a marked inflammatory response with fibrosis, make subsequent surgery very difficult and is probably best avoided, but the other substances may well have a role to play.

Surgical suspension of the bladder neck is another approach and may entail the Marshall–Marchetti, colposuspension and a variety of other sling procedures. Freedman *et al.* (1993) reported excellent results with colposuspension and clam ileocystoplasty in spina bifida girls. The bladder neck can be reconstructed using the Young–Dees–Leadbetter technique (Leadbetter, 1964) or a modification of this procedure (Jones *et al.*, 1993) and the urethra can be lengthened using the Kropp procedure (Kropp and Angwafo, 1986; Nill *et al.*, 1990). Dryness can be achieved in 80–90% of patients but reoperation may be required in 20–40% of cases (Mollard *et al.*, 1990; Jones *et al.*, 1993). Finally, the bladder neck or urethra can be closed off and access for emptying is then established via a continent abdominal stoma. There are two broad categories of continent stoma; one of which employs a hydraulic valve mechanism originally described by Benchekroun *et al.* (1987), but long-term problems with stomal stenosis do occur (Quinlan *et al.*, 1991), while the other uses the Mitrofanoff principle first described in 1980, where the appendix was reimplanted into the bladder to produce a continent catheterizable channel. The technique has been developed further and other tubular structures used include the ureter, fallopian tube, tapered small bowel or a tubularized detrusor tube (Woodhouse and Gordon, 1994). Continence rates of 94% are reported using the Mitrofanoff (Dykes *et al.*, 1991; Woodhouse and Gordon, 1994).

It is now well recognized that when the outlet resistance is increased an acontractile bladder can become contractile and produce upper tract damage (Churchill *et al.*, 1987; Murray *et al.*, 1988). Simultaneous bladder augmentation should always be considered when an outlet procedure is performed.

Contractile bladders (sufficient detrusor activity to give a useful degree of bladder emptying) account for about 31% of congenital neuropathic bladders and demand separate consideration. Free and complete emptying may be prevented by detrusor sphincter dyssynergia. The use of α-antagonists such as phenoxybenzamine may occasionally help and allow complete bladder emptying, thus preventing upper tract deterioration and producing continence (Rickwood, 1984). In males, when there is a competent bladder neck an external sphincterotomy should also be considered.

Sixty per cent of congenital neuropathic bladders are of the intermediate type. There are variable degrees of detrusor hyperreflexia, reduced compliance, sphincter weakness and detrusor sphincter dyssynergia. Videourodynamics are vital in selecting the correct treatment option. With the selective use of CIC and adjuvant drug therapy with oxybutynin and/or ephedrine, 75–90% of patients can be made dry (Mulcahy and James, 1979; Borzyskowski *et al.*, 1982; Wyndaele and Maes, 1990). If conservative treatment fails surgery is the only other option. The bladder outlet procedures just discussed all

have a place in treatment and the correct operation must be chosen for the right patient. One of the principal objectives is to produce a low-pressure reservoir of sufficient capacity. This usually involves some form of bladder augmentation.

The least invasive form of bladder augmentation is autoaugmentation (Malone *et al.*, 1994). It involves excising the detrusor of the dome of the bladder and allowing the mucosa to expand as a giant diverticulum. However, the results are very variable and unpredictable and the procedure does not have a routine role to play. The clam ileocystoplasty remains the most common procedure to augment the bladder. Many modifications have been made with the use of colon or stomach (Dykes and Ransley, 1992). If the bladder is particularly diseased a 'clam' procedure may not be sufficient and a substitution cystoplasty will be required. Intestinal segments used include the caecum or pouches made from any part of the colon, small bowel or stomach. In girls there is a place for total cystectomy because of problems experienced with painful bladder spasm during sexual arousal in later life (Woodhouse, 1992). There are many disadvantages with enterocystoplasty, including mucus production which causes catheter blockage, infection and stone formation, absorption of urea and electrolytes which can cause serious metabolic problems when renal function is compromised, inhibition of normal growth and metabolic bone disease, increased acid production with ulceration and haematuria when the stomach is used, spontaneous perforation of the augmented bladder and, finally, though perhaps most importantly, the risk of subsequent malignancy (Woodhouse, 1992; Mundy and Nurse, 1992; Wagstaff *et al.*, 1992). Because of this long list of serious complications every effort is being made to avoid the use of enterocystoplasty whenever possible. Recently, there has been a revival in the use of megaureters to augment bladders and in the appropriate case excellent results are achievable (Eckstein and Martin, 1973; Churchill *et al.*, 1993; Hitchcock *et al.*, 1994). An exciting new concept is the use of intestinal segments stripped of their mucosal lining, used to cover the autoaugmentation and, for the future, the use of cultured urothelium to line augmentations (Dewan and Byard, 1993; Atala *et al.*, 1993). Standard urinary diversion is no longer routinely practised, although it still has an important role to play in the occasional patient. However, continent diversion has grown in popularity in recent years and a large number of different operative procedures are described: the ileal, reservoir–Kock pouch (Kock *et al.*, 1982), caecoileal, Indiana pouch (Rowland *et al.*, 1987) and the Mainz reservoir (Thuroff *et al.*, 1986), to name a few. Complications are more frequent than with simple diversion but continence rates in the order of 90% are reported.

The widespread use of these reconstructive techniques has undoubtedly improved the quality of life and increased the independence of these patients, but con-

Table 65.7 Treatment options of faecal incontinence

Pharmaceutical	Stimulant laxatives/suppositories
Biofeedback/toilet training	
Physical colonic emptying	Manual evacuation Continence enema (per-anal) Antegrade colonic enema (ACE)
Faecal diversion	Colostomy Kock ileal pouch
Pelvic floor/sphincter procedures	Repeat pull-through Levatorplasty Gracilis sling Stimulated gracilis sling Artificial sphincter
Colonic	Repeat pull-through Segmental colonic resection
Implantable neuroprothesis	Pudendal nerve stimulation
Transcutaneous electrical nerve stimulation (TENS)	

tinued support and follow-up are mandatory. The part played by urological nurse specialists is vital here and the long-term results still need to be assessed.

Faecal incontinence

The various treatment modalities are summarized in Table 65.7. Careful individual assessment of the degree and underlying causes of incontinence, motivation and consideration of the physical limitations of the patient are essential if successful intervention is to be achieved.

Manual evacuation with or without laxatives is a common technique in the long term in patients with spina bifida; however, many will continue to soil to some degree with this treatment and it usually requires reliance on other people to achieve.

Biofeedback has been described in the management of incontinence with spina bifida or following correction of anorectal anomalies (Rintala *et al.*, 1988; Gil-Vernet *et al.*, 1992; Iwai *et al.*, 1993). It is already established as a useful therapy in encopretic children (Benning *et al.*, 1993). In spina bifida eight out of 10 patients became clean with biofeedback but the importance of selection, particularly regarding patient motivation was stressed by Gil-Vernet *et al.* (1992). Loening-Bauke *et al.* (1988), conversely, found no differences in outcome between spina bifida children having conventional treatment alone or in combination

with biofeedback. In addition biofeedback did not improve anal sensation or squeeze pressure.

Biofeedback benefited 80% of selected patients following surgery for anorectal anomalies (Rintala *et al.*, 1988). An adequate anal resting pressure, ability to contract the sphincter voluntarily and some anorectal sensation appear to be prerequisites for biofeedback in this situation (Rintala *et al.*, 1988; Iwai *et al.*, 1993).

Although recognized for some years, the use of enemas to maintain cleanness was not popularized until the description, by Shandling and Gilmour (1987b), of a balloon catheter to facilitate instillation and retention of the enema. They used saline enemas (20 ml/kg) by this method in 112 children with spina bifida and claimed a 100% success rate of cleanness. Although complications of the technique are few, the compliance rate may drop to only 50% after 30 months (Liptak and Revell, 1992). Despite modifications to the apparatus to increase the ability to be used independently, many spina bifida patients are not physically capable of using the technique without assistance.

A progression of the enema technique described by Malone *et al.* (1990a) was to provide a catheterizable colonic stoma to enable antegrade continence enemas (ACE). This has the disadvantage of requiring operation, but the siting of the stoma enables much easier catheterization than by the rectal route for many patients. A reversed appendicocaecostomy was originally described, but subsequently an orthotopic appendicoscaecostomy technique has been employed (Squire *et al.*, 1993). A non-refluxing implantation is necessary. In the absence of an appendix a tubularized caecal flap may be used and reported results are good. ACE has been reported to result in total cleanness in 19 of 24 patients with up to 31 months follow-up (Squire *et al.*, 1993). Problems with the stoma occur in about 25% but rarely require revision. It may take several weeks to adjust the enema fluid and frequency of washouts required to achieve optimum results. In general, washouts are commenced with 60 ml of phosphate enema diluted in an equal quantity of saline. This is followed by saline washout to complete irrigation which may require up to 1000 ml. Arachis oil may be used to soften hard stool. Dizziness and nausea may be experienced with rapid instillation of enema or saline. Abdominal colic may also occur, which sometimes responds to mebeverine. Care must be taken with administration of phosphate enemas as their retention may lead to severe metabolic problems (Hunter *et al.*, 1993).

In the presence of incontinence following anorectal surgery a further pull-through should be considered only if the colon is demonstrated to be outside the sphincteric complex. Unless reasonable sphincteric muscle and a normal sacrum are present, patients are likely to remain incontinent.

Various operative procedures on the pelvic floor have been reported for the treatment of faecal incontinence. Puri and Nixon (1976) described the levatorplasty, which combines a posterior plication of the levator with a mobilization of the anterior part of the muscle complex to augment the puborectalis sling. Long-term follow-up (up to 10 years) of 24 patients has shown that 75% became socially clean (Nixon, 1984). It is difficult to know how many of these would have become socially clean with increasing age without treatment, and the procedure has not become widely established.

The gracilis sling, mobilizing the gracilis muscle from the leg and encircling the subcutaneous bowel, was originally reported by Pickrell *et al.* (1952). It has subsequently undergone various modifications of the configuration of the muscle and its fixation (Holle *et al.*, 1975), or the use of both gracilis muscles (Hartl, 1972). Long-term results have been conflicting: satisfactory continence has been reported in 80–100% (Holscheider and Hecker, 1984; Sonnino *et al.*, 1991), but Konsten *et al.* (1992) found none of their 10 patients to be helped by graciloplasty. The main long-term problems with graciloplasty are atrophy of the muscle, more likely if innervation is abnormal (i.e. many cases of spina bifida), muscle fibrosis causing stenosis and loosening of the sling resulting in late failure. Early fibrosis of the muscle may occur owing to devascularization, which can be overcome by delayed transposition after ligating the distal two or three pedicles of blood supply *in situ*. A recent development is the use of the stimulated graciloplasty

(Cavina *et al.*, 1990; Williams *et al.*, 1991), in which the transposed gracilis muscle is stimulated electrically by an implantable device. There is histological evidence that long-term stimulation of the muscle converts it from predominantly fast-twitch type II skeletal muscle fibres to type I fibres capable of prolonged contractions. The long-term outcome of the technique is unknown.

Artificial urinary sphincters have been inserted around the anal canal in adults with faecal incontinence (Christiansen and Lorentzen, 1989). The use has not been reported in children and there must be grave concerns of the long-term risk of infection and sphincter failure.

Combined urinary and faecal incontinence

Bladder neck reconstruction with or without Mitrofanoff stoma has been simultaneously combined with formation of an ACE stoma in nine patients with urinary and faecal incontinence (Roberts and Malone, 1994). It was possible to split the appendix for both stomas in one case, while in the others the ACE stoma was fashioned from a caecal flap. Short-term review shows no additional morbidity from combining procedures and the outcome was the same as that expected from each individual procedure. It must be stressed, however, that patient selection is of vital importance in the success of this type of reconstruction. Sufficient motivation and manipulative skills are essential to

Table 65.8 Classification of results of surgery for incontinence[a]

(1) **Excellent**	Dry day and night
	Catheter/void > 4 h
	No restrictions on fluid intake or activity
(2) **Good**	Dry day
	Some nightime wetting
	Catheter/void > 3 h
	Minor restriction activity or fluid intake
(3) **Poor**	Dry intervals not > 2 h
	Protection required
(4) **Wet**	Continuous leaking

Scoring system for the assessment of faecal incontinence[b]

Incontinence to:	Frequency:
0 = none	0 = never
1 = flatus/mucus	1 = occasionally
2 = diarrhoea	2 = weekly
3 = solid stool	3 = daily

Score from 0 (normal continence) to 6 (severe total incontinence).

[a]Modified from Hollwell and Ransley (1991).
[b]Pescatori *et al.* (1992).

achieve satisfactory outcome. Patients and their families require many hours of instruction and encouragement, and a nurse specialist dedicated to managing such patients is invaluable in this respect.

In a few highly selected cases of spina bifida with intact motor fibres in the sacral and pudendal nerves, neuroprosthetic implants may be used. This approach may result in dramatic improvement in both bladder and bowel continence, but experience of the technique remains limited (Schmidt *et al.*, 1990). There have also been reports of successful treatment of urinary urge incontinence (McGuire *et al.*, 1983) and faecal incontinence, secondary to imperforate anus (Kirsch *et al.*, 1993), utilizing TENS.

Results

Comparison of results of treatment of urinary and faecal incontinence has undoubtedly been hampered by the lack of standardised objective assessment of the degree of incontinence. Patient conception of a good result does not always correspond to that of the surgeon. From the urinary point of view a result is only satisfactory if there is dryness between bladder emptying, and if the periods between bladder emptying are of acceptable duration. Most contention relates to what constitutes an acceptable minimum period between bladder emptying. A reasonable classification of results in continence surgery has been described by Hollowell and Ransley (1991) (Table 65.8).

With faecal incontinence many scoring systems have been described. Most concentrate on the degree and frequency of soiling and the relation of this to the type of stool. Some incorporate some assessment of sphincter function, although voluntary contraction during manometry does not appear to correlate with postoperative symptoms in adults (Keighley and Fielding, 1983; Womack *et al.*, 1988). These scoring systems have been well reviewed, and a new clinically orientated system has been suggested by Pescatori *et al.* (1992) (Table 65.8).

References

Anagnostopoulos, D., Mavromihalis, J., Markantonatos, A. and Lappas, E. 1989: Constipation: a cause of enuresis. *Pediatric Surgery International* **4**, 171–4.

Arhan, P., Faverdin, C., Devroede, Dubois, F., Coupris, L. and Pellerin, D. 1976: Manometric assessment of continence after surgery for imperforate anus. *Journal of Pediatric Surgery* **11**, 157–66.

Atala, A., Freeman, M.R. and Vacanti, J.P. 1993: Human bladder muscle and urothelial formation *in vivo* following attachment to biodegradable polymer scaffolds [Abstract]. Lisbon: European Society of Paediatric Urology, 55.

Barnes, D.G., Shaw, P.J.R., Timoney, A.G. and Tsokos, N. 1993: Management of the neuropathic bladder by suprapubic catheterisation. *British Journal of Urology* **72**, 169–172.

Barrett, D.M. and Parulkar, B.G. 1989: The artificial sphincter (AS800). Experience in children and young adults. *Urologic Clinics of North America* **16**, 119–32.

Benchekroun, A., Marzouk, M., Hachimi, M. *et al.* 1987: Urostomie continente. Poche ileale et valve de Benchekroun. *Acta Urologica Belgica* **55**, 522–7.

Benninga, M.S., Buller, H.A. and Taminiau, J.A. 1993: Biofeedback training in chronic constipation. *Archives of Disease in Childhood* **68**, 126–9.

Boemers, T.M., Van Gool, J.D. and De Jonge, T.P. 1993: Displacement of incontinence device into the bladder. *British Journal of Urology* **72**, 985.

Borzyskowski, M., Mundy, A.R., Neville, B.G., Park, L., Kinder, C.H., Chantler, J.C. and Haycock, G.B. 1982: Neuropathic vesicourethral dysfunction in children. A trial comparing clean intermittent catheterisation with manual expression combined with drug treatment. *British Journal of Surgery* **54**, 641–4.

Bosco, P.J., Bauser, S.B., Colodny, A.H., Mandell, J. and Retik, A.B. 1991: The long-term results of artificial sphincters in children. *Journal of Urology* **146**, 396–9.

Brading, A.F. and Turner, W.H. 1994: The unstable bladder: towards a common mechanism. *British Journal of Urology* **73**, 3–8.

Bramble, F.J. 1982: The treatment of adult enuresis and urge incontinence by enterocystoplasty. *British Journal of Urology* **54**, 693–6.

Buckley, J.P., Lingam, K. and Meddings, R. 1993: Injectable silicone macroparticles for female urinary incontinence [Abstract]. *British Association of Urological Surgeons* 92.

Caoni, P., Lais, A., De Gennaro, M. and Lapozza, N. 1993: Gluteraldehyde cross-linked bovine collagen in exstrophylepispadias complex. *Journal of Urology* **150**, 631–3.

Cavina, E., Seccia, M., Evangelista, G., Chiarugi, M., Bucciante, P., Torora, A. and Chirico, A. 1990: Perineal colostomy and electrically stimulated gracilis neosphincter after abdominoperineal resection of the colon and anorectum. A surgical experience and follow-up study in 47 cases. *International Journal of Colorectal Disease* **5**, 6–11.

Christiansen, J. and Lorentzen, M. 1989: Implantation of artificial sphincter for anal incontinence, report of 5 cases. *Diseases of Colon and Rectum* **32**, 432–6.

Churchill, B.M., Aliabadi, H., Landau, E.H., McLorie, G.A., Steckler, R.E., McKenna, P.H. and Khoury, A.E. 1993: Ureteral bladder augmentation. *Journal of Urology* **150**, 716–20.

Churchill, B.M., Gilmour, R.F., Khoury, A.D. and McLorie, G.A. 1987: Biological response of bladders rendered continent by insertion of artificial sphincter. *Journal of Urology* **138**, 1116–19.

Dewan, P.A. and Byard, R.W. 1993: Autoaugmentation gastrocystoplasty in a sheep model. *British Journal of Urology* **72**, 56–9.

Dykes, E.H. and Ransley, P.G. 1992: Gastrocystoplasty in children. *British Journal of Urology* **69**, 91–5.

Dykes, E.H., Duffy, P.G. and Ransley, P.G. 1991: The use of the Mitrofanoff principle in achieving clean intermittent catheterisation and urinary continence in children. *Journal of Pediatric Surgery* **26**, 535–8.

Eckstein, H.B. and Martin, M.R. 1973: Uretero-cystoplastik. *Actuelle Urologie* **4**, 255–7.

Fossberg, E. Serensen, S. and Ruutu, M. 1990: Maximal electrical stimulation in the treatment of unstable detrusor and urge incontinence. *European Urology* **18**, 120–3.

Freedman, E.R., Singh, G., Rickwood, A.M. and Thomas, D.G. 1993: Bladder neck suspension plus augmentation cystoplasty for neuropathic incontinence in females [Abstract]. *British Association of Urological Surgeons, Harrogate* 92.

Gil-Vernet, J.M., Marhuenda, C., Sanchis, L. and Boix-Ochoa, J. 1992: Biofeedback in spina bifida. *Pediatric Surgery International* **7**, 30–3.

Gonzalez, R., Nguyen, D.H., Koleilat, N. and Sidi, A.A. 1989: Compatibility of enterocystoplasty and the artificial urinary sphincter. *Journal of Urology* **142**, 502–4.

Grier, D., Duncan, A., Goddard, P. 1992: Magnetic resonance imaging following surgery for anorectal anomalies. *British Journal of Radiology* **65** (Suppl.), 43.

Hartl, H. 1972: A modified technique of gracilis plastic. *Paediatrie und Paedologie* (Suppl.) 2, 99–107.

Hitchcock, R.J., Duffy, P.G. and Malone, P.S. 1994: Uretero-cystoplasty: the bladder augmentation of choice. *British Journal of Urology* **73**, 575–9.

Holle, J., Freilinger, G., Mamoli, B., Spengle, H.P., Braun, S. and Krenn, R. 1975: Neue wege zur chirurgischen rekonstruktion der analen sphinctermuskulatur. *Weiner Medizinische Wochenschrift* **125**, 735–43.

Hollowell, J.G. and Ransley, P.G. 1991: Surgical management of incontinence in bladder exstrophy. *British Journal of Urology* **68**, 543–8.

Holschneider, A.M. and Hecker, W.Ch. 1984: Smooth muscle reverse plasty. A new method to treat anorectal incontinence in infants with high anal and rectal atresia. Results after gracilis plasty and free muscle transplantation. In Rickham, P.P., Hecker, W. and Prevot, J (eds), *Progress in pediatric surgery*, vol. 17. Baltimore, MD: Urban & Schwarzenberg, 131–46.

Hunter, M.F., Ashton, M.R., Roberts, J.P., Griffiths, D.M., Ilangoven, P. and Walker, V. 1993: Hyperphosphataemia following enemas in childhood: prevention and treatment. *Archives of Disease in Childhood* **68**, 233–4.

Iwai, N., Nagashima, M., Shimotake, T. and Iwata, G. 1993: Biofeedback therapy for fecal incontinence after surgery for anorectal malformations: preliminary results. *Journal of Pediatric Surgery* 863–6.

Iwai, N., Yanagihara, J., Tokiwa, K., Deguchi, E. and Takahashi, T. 1988: Voluntary anal continence after surgery for anorectal malformations. *Journal of Pediatric Surgery* **23**, 393–7.

Jarvelin, M.R., Vikevainen-Torronen, L. and Moilanen, I. 1988: Enuresis in seven year old children. *Acta Paediatrica Scandanavia* **77**, 148–53.

Jones, J.A., Mitchell, M.E. and Rink, R.C. 1993: Improved results using a modification of the Young-Dees–Leadbetter bladder neck repair. *British Journal of Urology* **71**, 555–61.

Karrer, F.M., Flannery, A.M., Nelson, M.D., McLone, D.G. and Raffensperger, J.G. 1988: Anorectal malformations: evaluation of associated spinal dysraphic syndromes. *Journal of Pediatric Surgery* **23**, 45–8.

Keighley, M.R. and Fielding, W.L. 1983: Management of faecal incontinence and result of surgical treatment. *British Journal of Surgery* **70**, 463–8.

Kirsch, S.E., Shandling, B., Watson, S.L., Gilmour, R.F. and Pape, K.E. 1993: Continence following electrical stimulation and EMG biofeedback in a teenager with imperforate anus. *Journal of Pediatric Surgery* **28**, 1408–10.

Kock, N.G., Nilson, A.E., Nilsson, L.O., Norlen, L.J. and Philipson, B.M. 1982: Urinary diversion via a continent ileal reservoir: clinical results in 12 patients. *Journal of Urology* **128**, 469–75.

Konsten, J., Heineman, E. and Baeten, C.G. 1992: Letter. *Journal of Pediatric Surgery* **27**, 695–6.

Kropp, K.A., Angwafo, F.F. 1986: Urethral lengthening and reimplantation for neurogenic incontinence in children. *Journal of Urology* **135**, 533–6.

Lapides, J., Diokno, A.C., Silber, S.J. and Lowe, B.S. 1972: Clean intermittent self-catheterization in the treatment of urinary tract disease. *Journal of Urology* **107**, 458–61.

Law, P.J. and Bartram, C.I. 1989: Anal endosonography-technique and normal anatomy. *Gastrointestinal Radiology* **14**, 349–53.

Law, P.J., Kamm, M.A. and Bartram, C.I. 1991: Anal endosonography in the investigation of faecal incontinence. *British Journal of Surgery* **78**, 312–14.

Leadbetter, G.W. 1964: Surgical correction of total urinary incontinence in children. *Journal of Urology* **91**, 261–6.

Lewis, D.K., Morgan, J.R., Weston, P.M. and Stephenson, T.P. 1990: The 'clam': indications and complications. *British Journal of Urology* **65**, 488–91.

Liptak, G.S. and Revell, G.M. 1992: Management of bowel dysfunction in children with spinal cord disease or injury by means of the enema continence catheter. *Journal of Pediatrics* **120**, 190–4.

Loening-Bauke, V., Desch, L. and Wolraich, M. 1988: Biofeedback training for patients with myelomeningocele and fecal incontinence. *Developmental Medicine and Child Neurology* **30**, 781–90.

Mackie, G.G. and Stephens, F.D. 1975: Duplex kidneys: a correlation of renal dysplasia with position of ureteral orifice. *Journal of Urology* **114**, 274–80.

Madersbacher, H. and Jilg, G. 1991: Control of detrusor hyperreflexia by the intravesical instillation of oxybutynin hydrochloride. *Paraplegia* **29**, 84–90.

Malone, P.R., Gordon, E.M. and Duffy, P.G. 1994: Autocystoplasty. Unpublished data.

Malone, P.S., Ransley, P.G. and Kiely, E.M. 1990: Preliminary report: the antegrade continence enema. *Lancet* **336**, 1217–18.

Malone, P.S., Spitz, L., Kiely, E.M., Brereton, R.J., Duffy, P.G. and Ransley, P.G. 1990: The functional sequelae of sacrococcygeal teratoma. *Journal of Pediatric Surgery* **25**, 679–80.

McGuire, E.J. Shi-Chun, Z., Horwinski, E.R. and Lytton, B. 1983: Treatment of motor and sensory detrusor instability by electrical stimulation. *Journal of Urology* **129**, 78–9.

McGuire, E.J., Shi-Chun, Z., Horwinski, E.R. and Lytton, B. 1983: Treatment of motor and sensory detrusor instability by electrical stimulation. *Journal of Urology* **129**, 78–9.

Mitrofanoff, P. 1980: Cystostomie continente trans-appendiculaire dans le traitement des vessies neurologiques. *Chirugica Paediatica* **21**, 297–305.

Mollard, P., Mouriquand, P. and Joubert, P. 1990: Urethral lengthening for neurogenic urinary incontinence (Kropp's procedure): results of 16 cases. *Journal of Urology* **143**, 95–97.

Montague, D.K. 1992: The artificial urinary sphincter (A5800); experience in 166 consecutive patients. *Journal of Urology* **147**, 380–2.

Mulcahy, J.J. and James, H.E. 1979: Management of neurogenic bladder in infancy and childhood. *Urology* **13**, 235–40.

Mundy, A.R. and Nurse, D.E. 1992: Calcium balance, growth and skeletal mineralization in patients with cystoplasties. *British Journal of Urology* **69**, 257–9.

Mundy, A.R. and Stephenson, T.P. 1985: 'Clam' ileocystoplasty for the treatment of refractory urge incontinence. *British Journal of Urology* **57**, 641–6.

Mundy, A.R., Shah, P.J.R., Borzyskowski, M. and Saxton, H.M. 1985: Sphincter behaviour in myelomeningocele. *British Journal of Urology* **57**, 647–51.

Murray, K.H.A., Nurse, D.E. and Mundy, A.R. 1988: Detrusor behaviour following implantation of the Brantley Scott artificial urinary sphincter for neuropathic incontinence. *British Journal of Urology* **61**, 122–8.

Nagasaki, A., Ikeda, K., Hayashida, Y., Sumitomo, and Sameshima, S. 1983: Assessment of bowel control with anorectal manometry after surgery for anorectal malformation. *Japanese Journal of Surgery* **14**, 229–34.

Nielson, K.K., Kromann-Andersen, B. and Jacobsen, H. The urethral plug: a new treatment modality for genuine urinary stress incontinence in women. *Journal of Urology* **144**, 1199–202.

Nill, T.G., Peller, P.A. and Kropp, K.A. 1990: Management of urinary incontinence by bladder tube urethral lengthening and submucosal reimplantation. *Journal of Urology* **144**, 559–61.

Nixon, H.H. 1984: Possibilities and results of management of bowel incontinence in children. In Rickham, P.P., Hecker, W. and Prevot, J. (eds), *Progress in pediatric surgery*, vol. 17. Baltimore, MD: Urban & Schwarzenberg, 105–114.

Novello, A.C. and Novello, J.R. 1987: Enuresis. *Pediatric Clinics of North America* **34**, 719–33.

Nurse, D.E., Britton, J.P. and Mundy, A.R. 1993: Relative indication for orthotopic lower urinary tract reconstruction, continent urinary diversion and conduit urinary diversion. *British Journal of Urology* **71**, 562–5.

Passerini-Glazel, G., Cisternino, A., Artibani, W. and Pagano, F. 1992: Ambulatory urodynamics: preliminary experience with vesico-urethral holter in children. *Scandanavian Journal of Urology and Nephrology* **141** (Suppl.), 87–92.

Pena, A. and El Behery, M. 1993: Megasigmoid: a source of pseudoincontinence in children with repaired anorectal malformations. *Journal of Pediatric Surgery* **28**, 199–203.

Perez-Marrero, R., Dimmock, W., Churchill, B.M. and Hardy, B.E. 1982: Clean intermittent catheterization in myelomeningocele children less than 3 years old. *Journal of Urology* **128**, 779–81.

Perry, R.E., Blatchford, G.J., Christensen, M.A., Thorson, A.G. and Attwood, E.A. 1990: Manometric diagnosis of anal sphincter injuries. *American Journal of Surgery* **159**, 112–17.

Pescatori, M., Anastasio, G., Bottini, C. and Mentasti, A. 1992: New grading and scoring for anal incontinence, evaluation of 335 patients. *Diseases of Colon and Rectum* **35**, 482–7.

Pickrell, K.L., Broadbent, T.R., Masters, F.W. and Metzger, J.D. 1952: Construction of a rectal sphincter in restoration of anal continence by transplanting the gracilis muscle. *Annals of Surgery* **135**, 853–62.

Puri, P. and Nixon, H.H. 1976: Levatorplasty: a secondary operation for fecal incontinence following primary operation for anorectal agenesis. *Journal of Pediatric Surgery* **11**, 77–82.

Quinlan, D.M., Leonard, M.P., Brendler, C.B., Gearhart, J.P. and Jeffs, R.D. 1991: Use of the Benchekroun hydraulic valve as a catheterizable continence mechanism. *Journal of Urology* **145**, 1151–5.

Rasmussen, O.O., Sorensen, M., Tetzschner, T. and Christiansen, J. 1992: Anorectal pressure gradient in patients with anal incontinence. *Diseases of Colon and Rectum* **35**, 8–11.

Read, D.J., James, E.D. and Shaldon, C. 1985: The effect of spinal cord stimulation on idiopathic detrusor instability and incontinence: a case report. *Journal of Neurosurgery and Psychiatry* **48**, 832–4.

Rickwood, A.M.K. 1984: The neuropathic bladder in children. In Mundy, A.R., Stephenson, T.P. and Wein, A.J. (eds), *Urodynamics principles, practice and application.* Edinburgh: Churchill Livingstone, 326–47.

Rickwood, A.M.K., Thomas, D.G., Philp, N.G. and Spicer, R.D. 1982: Assessment of congenital neurovesical dysfunction by combined urodynamic and radiological studies. *British Journal of Urology* **54**, 512–18.

Rintala, R., Lindahl, H. and Louhimo, I. 1988: Biofeedback conditioning for fecal incontinence in anorectal malformations. *Pediatric Surgery International* **3**, 418–21.

Roberts, J.P. and Malone, P.S. 1995: Treatment of neuropathic urinary and faecal incontinence with synchronous combined bladder reconstruction and ACE procedure. *British Journal of Urology* **75**, 386–9.

Roberts, J.P. and Williams, N.S. 1992: The role and technique of ambulatory anal manometry. In Henry, M.M. (ed.), *Baillière's clinical gastroenterology: anorectal disorders.* London: Baillière Tindall, 163–78.

Robinson, T.G. and Castleden, C.M. 1994: Drugs in focus 11. Oxybutinin hydrochloride. *Prescribers Journal* **34**, 27–30.

Rowland, R.G., Mitchell, M.E., Bihrle, R., Kahnoski, R.J. and Piser, J.E. 1987: Indiana continent urinary reservoir. *Journal of Urology* **137**, 1136–9.

Scharf, M.B., Pravda, M.F. and Jennings, S.W. 1987: Childhood enuresis. A comprehensive treatment program. *Psychiatric Clinics of North America* **10**, 655–66.

Schmidt, R.A., Kogan, B.A. and Tanagho, E.A. 1990: Neuroprostheses in the management of incontinence in myelomeningocele patients. *Journal of Urology* **143**, 779–82.

Shandling, B. and Gilmour, R.F. 1987a: The anal sphincter force in health and disease. *Journal of Pediatric Surgery* **22**, 754–7.

Shandling, B.and Gilmour, R.F. 1987b: The enema continence catheter in spina bifida: successful bowel management. *Journal of Pediatric Surgery* **22**, 271–3.

Sheldon, C., Cormier, M., Crone, K. and Wacksman, J. 1991: Occult neurovesical dysfunction in children with imperforate anus and its variants. *Journal of Pediatric Surgery* **26**, 49–54.

Sidi, A.A., Reinberg, Y. and Gonzalez, R. 1987: Comparison of artificial sphincter implantation and bladder neck reconstruction in patients with neurogenic urinary incontinence. *Journal of Urology* **138**, 1120–2.

Sonnino, R.D., Reiberg, O., Bensoussan, A.L., Laberge, J.M. and Blanchard, H. 1991: Gracilis muscle transposition for anal incontinence in children: long-term follow up. *Journal of Pediatric Surgery* **26**, 1219–23.

Squire, R., Kiely, E.M., Carr, B., Ransley, P.G. and Duffy, P.G. 1993: The clinical application of the Malone antegrade colonic enema. *Journal of Pediatric Surgery* **28**, 1012–15.

Sun, W.M., Read, N.W. and Miner, P.B. 1990: Relation between rectal sensation and anal function in normal subjects and patients with faecal incontinence. *Gut* **31**, 1056–61.

Thuroff, J.W., Alken, P., Reidmuller, H., Engelman, U., Jacobi, G.H. and Hohenfellner, R. 1986: The Mainz pouch (mixed augmentation ileum and cecum) for bladder augmentation and continent diversion. *Journal of Urology* **36**, 17–26.

Van Gool, J.D. and De Jonge, G.A. 1989: Urge syndrome and urge incontinence. *Archives of Disease in Childhood* **64**, 1629–34.

Wagstaff, K.E., Woodhouse, C.R., Duffy, P.G. and Ransley, P.G. 1992: Delayed linear growth in children with enterocystoplasties. *British Journal of Urology* **69**, 314–17.

Wakeman, R. and Allen-Mersh, T.G. 1989: Puborectalis and external anal sphincter paralysis with preservation of fecal continence. *Diseases of Colon and Rectum* **32**, 980–1.

Wan, J., McGuire, E.J., Bloom, D.A., Ritchey, M.L. 1992: The treatment of urinary incontinence in children using glutaraldehyde cross-linked collagen. *Journal of Urology* **148**, 127–30.

Weerasinghe, N. and Malone, P.S. 1993: The value of videourodynamics in the investigation of neurologically normal children who wet. *British Journal of Urology* **71**, 539–42.

Williams, N.S., Patel, J., George, B.D., Hallan, R.I. and Watkins, E.S. 1991: Development of electrically stimulated neoanal sphincter. *Lancet* **338**, 1166–9.

Womack, N.R., Morrison, J.F. and Williams, N.S. 1988: Prospective study of the effects of postanal repair in neurogenic fecal incontinence. *British Journal of Surgery* **75**, 48–52.

Woodhouse, C.R. 1992: Reconstruction of the lower urinary tract for neurogenic bladder: lessons from the adolescent age group. *British Journal of Urology* **69**, 589–93.

Woodhouse, C.R.J. and Gordon, E.M. 1994: The Mitrofanoff principle for urethral failure. *British Journal of Urology* **73**, 55–60.

Wyndaele, J.J. and Maes, D. 1990: Clean intermittent self-catheterisation: a 12-year follow up. *Journal of Urology* **143**, 906–8.

CHAPTER 66

Urolithiasis in children

F.M.J. QUINN AND W.G. VAN'T HOFF

Introduction
Investigation of children with
renal calculi
Management of renal calculi
Calculi secondary to stasis and
infection
Metabolic causes of renal calculi

Endemic bladder stone disease
Recurrent stones
Surgical management
Summary
References
Further reading

Introduction

In western countries the incidence of urinary tract calculi in children is low, varying between 1 in 1000 and 1 in 8000 paediatric admissions per year. In developing countries, particularly in the Middle East and Asia where stones are endemic, they are amongst the most common problems in paediatric urology. These tend to be urate in formation and they tend to occur in the lower urinary tract. In developed countries, however, the calculi tend to form in the upper tracts and are caused either by metabolic disorders or by anatomical abnormalities associated with urinary stasis. Most of the latter are triple phosphate stones associated with infection and have a peak incidence around 4 years of age, whereas metabolic stones can occur at any age. The presentation of calculus disease in children regardless of the aetiology, is similar to that in adults. In older children, the symptoms and signs include colicky flank pain, nausea and vomiting, haematuria, dysuria and infection. In the younger child the symptoms may be confusing, particularly in those with known congenital abnormalities of the urinary tract. Therefore stone disease must be considered as a possible aetiology of any acute illness in such a child.

Investigation of children with renal calculi

All children who develop renal calculi should have extensive investigation to determine the cause and also the effect on their renal function. This requires close liaison between the clinician, radiologist and biochemist and should ideally be performed in a centre with experience of paediatric calculi. If a calculus has been passed or is removed surgically it should be analysed to determine its composition (Table 66.1).

Table 66.1 Causes of calculi and their chemical analysis

Disorder	Composition of calculus
Infection	Magnesium ammonium phosphate
Idiopathic/hyperoxaluria	Calcium oxalate
Hypercalciuria/idiopathic	Calcium phosphate
Gout/Lesch–Nyhan/leukaemia	Urate
Cystinuria	Cystine

If no calculus is available, the following tests should help to determine the cause:

- early morning urine for pH, microscopy (cystine crystals), culture and calcium/creatinine ratio, and quantitative amino acid chromatography (cystinuria)
- 24-hour urine (with acid preservative) for oxalate, glycolate and creatinine (hyperoxaluria)
- 24-hour urine for purine metabolites (urate, dihydroxyadenine and xanthine)
- blood biochemistry, including calcium, bicarbonate, creatinine and urate
- plain abdominal X-ray to view the kidneys, ureters and bladder. Most stones are radiopaque, the exceptions being those composed of urate or other purine metabolites
- ultrasound of the kidneys to demonstrate renal calculi including radiolucent stones (Fig. 66.1) and the presence of associated urinary tract obstruction
- intravenous urography may be helpful during an episode of renal colic
- micturating cystourethrogram after stone clearance in children less than 3 years old for abnormalities which may predispose to stones or their recurrence,

e.g. vesicoureteric reflux (VUR) or urethral abnormalities
- DMSA or DTPA renogram to give baseline relative renal function, especially before treatment with percutaneous nephrolithotomy (PCNL) or extracorporeal shock-wave lithotripsy (ESWL) (this is discussed in more detail later in this chapter).

Management of renal calculi

The treatment of renal calculi can be divided into general and specific management, some of which is medical and some surgical (or interventional). Specific measures are described in the following sections on infective and metabolic stones. General measures are very important and can be listed as follows:

- High fluid intake: children with renal stones should aim to have for a fluid intake of approximately 150% of their normal daily requirement (more in hot weather and during fever). A significant part of this (e.g. 30%) should be taken during the night (Pak *et al.*, 1980; Fine *et al.*, 1995).

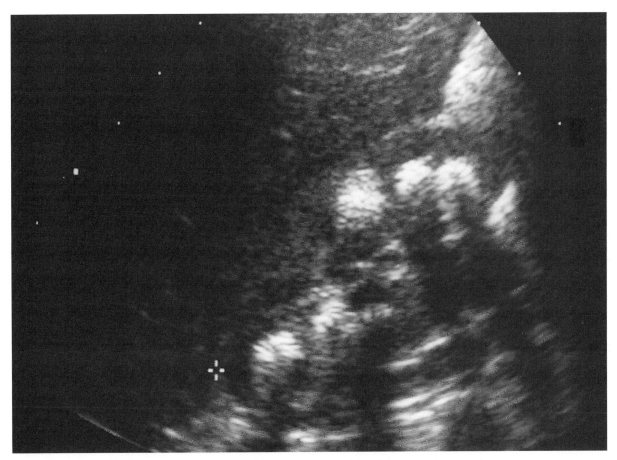

Fig. 66.1   Renal ultrasound scan showing multiple calculi in a child with hyperoxaluria.

- Avoidance of dehydration: minor illnesses such as upper respiratory infections or gastroenteritis can lead to a reduced oral intake or excessive fluid losses. Children with calculi need more aggressive fluid therapy, e.g. by nasogastric tube or intravenous infusion. Children undergoing surgery or receiving a general anaesthetic should have an intravenous infusion to cover the fasting period.
- Avoidance of urinary tract infection: prophylactic antibiotics may be required in children with recurrent calculi (Androulakakis *et al.*, 1982; Diamond *et al.*, 1994).

Calculi secondary to stasis and infection

The formation of calculi is one of the main complications of urinary tract infections and urinary stasis in children. Children with anomalies such as neuropathic bladder (congenital or acquired), obstructive lesions such as posterior urethral valves or pelviureteric junc-tion obstruction, bladder exstrophy (Fig. 66.2), prune belly syndrome and VUR may have dilated segments of the urinary tract with diminished peristalsis and stasis predisposing to urinary infection and stone formation. The high incidence of *Proteus miribalis* infection is common to all series of paediatric urolithiasis in the UK (Androulakalis *et al.*, 1982; Diamond *et al.*, 1994).

Proteus has urease activity, which degrades urea to form ammonia, producing alkaline urine (pH > 7.5), enabling calcium, magnesium and ammonium phosphate (struvite) and calcium carbonate to precipitate (i.e. triple phosphate stones). Under these circumstances stone formation may be rapid, leading to staghorn calculi. Other urease-producing organisms include: *Klebsiella*, *Pseudomonas*, and *Staphylococcus* species, *Escherichia coli* and *Serratia*.

Intravesical foreign bodies may serve as a nidus for calculus formation. Phosphate encrustation is frequently seen in patients with chronic indwelling catheters and calculi can form around unabsorbable suture material, surgical clips or foreign bodies introduced during self-catheterization. These calculi are also frequently seen in augmentation enterocystoplasties, especially if there is

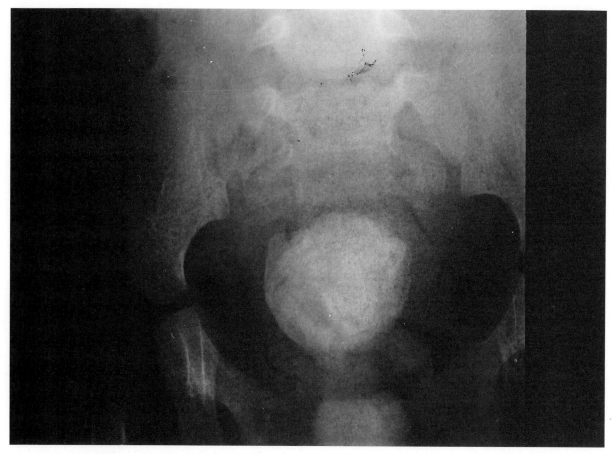

Fig. 66.2 Plain abdominal radiograph showing a large bladder calculus in a child with a repaired bladder exstrophy.

excess mucus production. The risk of stone formation may be related to the production of mucus by the enteric segment or may be due to poor self-catheterization technique leaving behind residual mucus in stagnant urine. Intravesical foreign body calculi are usually associated with infected, foulsmelling urine and must be removed surgically and intact if possible, lest a nidus for further stone formation be left behind. Calculi in augmented bladders are therefore not as amenable to transurethral lithopaxy as calculi that form in a normal bladder. In these patients adequate hydration, frequent catheterization and occasionally antibiotic prophylaxis can decrease the risk of stasis and further formation.

Xanthogranulomatous pyelonephritis is a chronic inflammatory disease of unknown origin usually found in the adult female population, but increasingly reported in children. These patients present with fever, leucocytosis, severe anaemia and a raised erythrocyte sedimentation rate (ESR). In a recent review of 28 paediatric cases, 22 had multiple renal calculi in a nonfunctioning kidney. In 75% of these the calculi were staghorn. Nephrectomy was curative in all cases (Quinn and Guiney, 1998).

Metabolic causes of renal calculi

HYPERCALCAEMIA AND HYPERCALCIURIA

Hypercalcaemia in children may lead to nephrocalcinosis and/or urolithiasis and will usually be associated with hypercalciuria. Hypercalcaemia in children may be idiopathic (e.g. in Williams–Beuren syndrome) or may be secondary to prolonged immobilization (e.g. in patients with severe motor disability) or vitamin D intoxication. Hypothyroidism is also associated with hypercalcaemia. Some other causes of hypercalcaemia more often seen in adult practice (e.g. hyperparathyroidism and sarcoidosis) are very rare in children.

Hypercalciuria, defined as a urinary calcium: creatinine ratio > 0.74 mmol/mmol in a second morning urine sample, can present with haematuria, recurrent abdominal pain, nephrocalcinosis or symptoms of urolithiasis (Ghazali and Barratt, 1974). Increased gastrointestinal calcium absorption or increased bone turnover may be the cause. In addition, hypercalciuria is seen in a variety of renal tubular disorders including renal tubular acidosis (classically distal RTA, but also in some forms of generalized proximal tubular dysfunction, e.g. renal Fanconi syndrome), in Bartter's syndrome and in Dent's disease. Commonly, however, no cause is found and the child is said to have idiopathic hypercalciuria. Treatment is directed towards the underlying cause in addition to a high fluid intake. Thiazide diuretics which reduce urinary calcium excretion are sometimes prescribed.

HYPEROXALURIA

Oxalate is derived partly from the diet but mainly from the hepatic metabolism of glyoxalate and ascorbate. It is a metabolic end-product, excreted via the kidneys and is relatively insoluble so that hyperoxaluria can lead to nephrocalcinosis or calculus formation (Fig. 66.3). Patients with chronic diarrhoea (e.g. due to enteropathy) have a reduced calcium absorption and, as a secondary phenomenon, absorb increased amounts of oxalate leading to enteric hyperoxaluria.

There are two rare, autosomal recessive disorders of oxalate metabolism which lead to primary hyperoxaluria (PH). The more common of these, primary hyperoxaluria type 1 (PH1), is due to a deficiency of hepatic peroxisomal alanine-glyoxalate transferase (AGT) and leads to increased urinary excretion of glycolic acid in addition to oxalate (see Cochat and Watts, 1995, for a review). Patients usually present in childhood with symptoms of renal calculi and, without treatment, develop progressive renal failure. Since the kidney is the only source of oxalate excretion, renal failure leads to a systemic accumulation of oxalate (systemic oxalosis) which manifests as osteopathy, cardiomyopathy and arterial lesions causing gangrene. Rarely, PH1 presents in infants with nephrocalcinosis and complications of systemic oxalosis but not with calculi. Primary hyperoxaluria type 2 is rarer and is due to a deficiency of D-glycerate dehydrogenase and glyoxylate reductase. It is characterised biochemically by elevated urinary L-glycerate and oxalate excretion, and clinically by calculus formation.

Primary hyperoxaluria can be diagnosed by chemical analysis of a calculus and by measurement of urinary oxalate and glycolate excretion, preferably in a 24-hour urine collection stored in a bottle with acid preservative. Patients with renal failure may have a reduced oxalate excretion and a plasma oxalate is useful but requires specialist handling. A liver biopsy can be used to determine the AGT activity. Specific treatment involves administering agents that inhibit oxalate crystallization (e.g. phosphate or citrate) and offering a trial of pyridoxine (which is a cofactor for AGT) in patients whose liver biopsy demonstrates some residual AGT catalytic activity. Most patients, however, will progress into renal failure and it is very important to consider further treatment before they require dialysis. Both peritoneal dialysis and haemodialysis are inefficient methods of clearing plasma oxalate, which therefore progressively accumulates. Renal transplantation alone does not cure the metabolic defect and the systemic oxalate load damages the graft, thereby dramatically reducing graft survival. Liver transplantation will cure the metabolic defect and is a feasible option for patients who are not yet in renal failure, e.g. glomerular filtration rate (GFR) > 40–50 ml/min/1.73 m^2. Patients in renal failure (GFR < 40 ml/min/1.73 m^2) should be considered for combined liver and kidney transplantation, which has been highly successful in this disorder.

CYSTINURIA

Cystinuria is a relatively common inherited disorder, with a prevalence of between 1 in 2000 and 1 in 15 000. It accounts for approximately 7% of childhood cases of calculi (see Rose, 1992, for a review). The disorder is due to defective transport of cystine and dibasic amino acids (arginine, ornithine and lysine) in the epithelia of the renal tubule and small intestine. Defective transport in the renal tubule leads to high concentrations of urinary cystine which, because of its low solubility, predisposes to the formation of cystine calculi causing obstruction, infection and renal failure. Individuals with cystinuria can be divided into three types according to differences in intestinal amino acid transport, response to an oral cystine load and urinary excretion of lysine.

Patients usually present in adolescence or early adulthood but symptoms can occur in children. Renal colic and infection are common presentations and plain X-ray or ultrasound will demonstrate radiopaque calculi. Urine microscopy may reveal hexagonal cystine crystals (which are diagnostic) but formal confirmation requires quantitative urine amino acid analysis. Patients should take a fluid intake large enough to lower the urinary cystine concentration to less than 1 mmol/l, a concentration below which cystine crystalluria is less likely to occur. Alkalinization of the urine is theoretically helpful, preferably with potassium bicarbonate or citrate since increased sodium intake promotes cystine excretion. Rarely, pharmacological treatment is used. D-penicillamine undergoes disulphide exchange with cystine, forming penicillamine–cysteine, which is much more soluble. However, some patients on penicillamine develop skin rashes and proteinuria. Captopril has also been used in the treatment of cystinuria.

OTHER CAUSES OF METABOLIC STONE DISEASE

Hyperuricaemia with consequent hyperuricosuria can occur in gout, in children with disorders of purine metabolism (e.g. Lesch–Nyhan syndrome) and as a complication of malignancies (e.g. lymphoma and

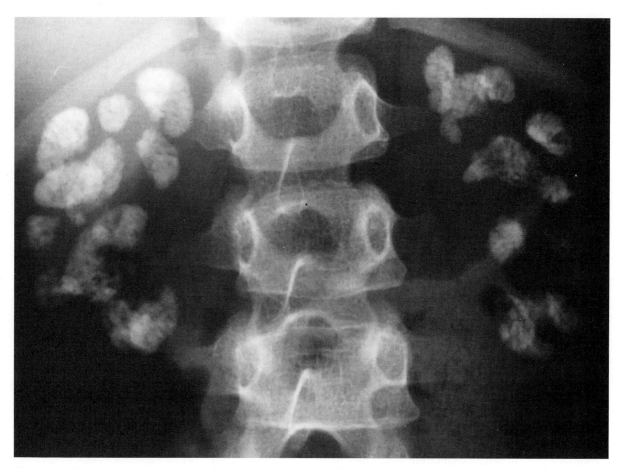

Fig. 66.3 Plan abdominal radiograph showing multiple renal calculi in a child with hyperoxaluria.

leukaemia) (Rose, 1992). Allopurinol is very effective in reducing uric acid production and thus preventing stone formation in these patients. Dihydroxyadenine or xanthine stones occur in two other disorders of purine metabolism. All of these stones are radiolucent and therefore not visible on plain X-ray. The diagnosis may be suspected by the demonstration of stones on ultrasound or of a filling defect on intravenous urography. Confirmation of the diagnosis may involve stone analysis and specialized assays of plasma and urine purine metabolites.

Endemic bladder stone disease

Bladder stones in industrialized countries are almost always related to infection underlying anatomic or functional abnormalities of the bladder and are occasionally due to an underlying metabolic cause of stone formation. Endemic stone formation has been a major health problem in many areas of the developing world, especially in the Middle East, Asia and Africa. Calculi were also widespread in the UK before the industrial revolution. Endemic stones are usually composed of calcium oxalate, calcium phosphate, ammonia and urate. They frequently occur in boys in the first decade of life and tend not to recur after removal. The cause of these stones varies from country to country and even between regions within a country. They are not associated with bladder outlet obstruction or neurovesical dysfunction. Diet and feeding patterns, infection, infestation and dehydration have all been implicated. Diets high in oxalate precursors and oxalate appear to be a major factor in calcium oxalate crystalluria and stones. Phosphate supplementation appears to prevent the stone formation.

Recurrent stones

Factors implicated in stone recurrence are incomplete removal at the initial procedure, recurrent or persistent urinary tract infection and failure to deal with the underlying metabolic or anatomic abnormality. Even if a patient has had all the stones removed recurrent calculi occur in 7–14% of patients per year (Fine *et al.*). However, using a variety of specific medical treatments for metabolic derangements, new stone formation or growth can be controlled in many of these patients irrespective of whether or not residual stone fragments are present. Persistent infection after stone removal is associated with recurrence rates up to 50% within 1 year and 100% at 2 years. Moreover, the risk of recurrence increases in proportion to the duration of post-operative infection. Prompt eradication of urinary infection in the immediate postoperative period is therefore the most crucial factor in preventing new recurrences. As most

recurrences occur between 12 and 24 months after the initial surgery, aggressive medical treatment in the first few months after surgery and long-term antibiotic prophylaxis constitute the most efficient measures for preventing stone recurrence. In some patients the recurrent calculi occur many years after surgery, so long-term follow-up is indicated (Androulakakis *et al.*, 1982).

Surgical management

The indications for removal of stones in children are similar to those in adults. They must be symptomatic, causing obstruction or acting as a source of infection. Until 15 years ago almost all stones in the paediatric age group as well as in adults required an open surgical approach for removal. The development of various minimally invasive techniques over this period of time has reduced the incidence of open surgery in most adult practices to around 5% of cases.

EXTRACORPOREAL SHOCK WAVE LITHOTRIPSY

Shock waves are generated by one of four systems: spark-gap, piezoelectric, electromagnetic and explosive pellet. The procedure is usually performed under general anaesthesia in children and the stone is localized using fluoroscopy, ultrasound or plain X-ray film. Because stones in children are rare, there are no large series comparing any of the above methods as there are in adults. Stone-free rates vary from 60–90% for renal stones to around 90% for ureteric stones. Interpretation of such results is complicated by variable definitions of success used by different authors. Success rates fall well below these figures when treating hard stones, e.g. cystine stones, calcium oxalate monohydrate and calcium hydrogen phosphate stones. Stones in kidneys with poor drainage do not respond well to ESWL because the fragments fail to be expelled from the system and ancillary procedures such as ureteric stents or nephrostomy tubes are occasionally necessary both before and after treatment. These stones should no longer be referred for lithotripsy but should be treated by one of the other modalities mentioned below. ESWL has now been shown to be most appropriate for children with small simple stones (<20 mm). When used to treat stones more than 25 mm or a large stone burden the resulting large fragments can block the ureter below (Stienstrasse). ESWL may have a useful adjuvent role in treating patients with residual stones after initial open surgery or PCNL.

Complications are rare and are most commonly related to the skin overlying the kidney, i.e. ecchymoses and bruising (Kramolowsky *et al.*, 1987). Subcapsular haematomas and intraparenchymal haemorrhage have been demonstrated. These cause mild haematuria that can persist for up to 24 hours after treatment. In adult animal studies ESWL generates similar parenchymal damage which does not appear to be of long-term significance, whereas in young animals the morphological changes are more substantial and can be permanent. These studies also show that these morphological changes are dose dependent and transient, and long-term damage only occurs when the shock wave dose is vastly exceeded. In children there are some data showing immediate but temporary reduction in function on DTPA renography following treatment (Corbally *et al.*, 1991). This should be borne in mind when treating a child with a solitary kidney or with an asymptomatic stone. An increased risk of hypertension in patients treated with ESWL has been reported, but these reports were not adequately controlled and further study is necessary. Haemoptysis following lung contusions, especially in those with spinal deformities, has been reported; however the use of lung shields has decreased the incidence of this problem (Kroovand *et al.*, 1987). There are no long-term studies that can answer the question of safety of lithotripsy in children.

PERCUTANEOUS NEPHROLITHOTOMY

Despite the high success rates of ESWL in both adults and children there are certain situations (e.g. associated urinary obstruction or anatomic abnormality) when ESWL cannot be employed. In addition, if a previous treatment with ESWL has failed or has achieved incomplete clearance, an alternative approach is needed. Advances in fluoroscopic techniques allow percutaneous puncture of the renal pelvis and subsequent dilatation of a small nephrostomy tract. This enables insertion of endoscopic instruments to inspect the collecting system and to grasp or disintegrate calculi. Initial experience with PCNL was encouraging, but it was only recommended in children over 8 years old because of the relatively large size of the endourological equipment (Hulbert *et al.*, 1985). PCNL can now be performed in children at 18 months with no increase in complication rates (Mor *et al.*, 1998). This is a significant advance as many children with stones in Europe are less than 5 years old. The initial concern that significant renal damage could occur following PCNL owing to the establishment of a wide tract through the renal parenchyma has not been borne out as several studies have shown minimal scar formation and insignificant loss of renal function. PCNL now compares well with open surgery and is established either as the only therapy or in combination with other procedures such as endoscopic pyelolysis or balloon dilatation of the pelvi-ureteric junction if obstruction is present. If these treatment strategies are successful in the long term, subsequent open surgery may be avoided. PCNL can also be a used to deal with retained stones and fragments following ESWL and open surgery. There seems little doubt now that the correct management of large staghorn calculi should consist of an initial PCNL or, rarely, open surgery followed by ESWL to remove any retained fragments in the calyces (Fig. 66.4).

URETEROSCOPY

In the early 1980s ureteroscopy was considered dangerous because of the size mismatch of the instruments and it was recommended that the procedure should not be used in children under 5 years old (Shroff and Watson, 1995). However, with the introduction of miniaturized ureteroscopes it is now feasible for the experienced

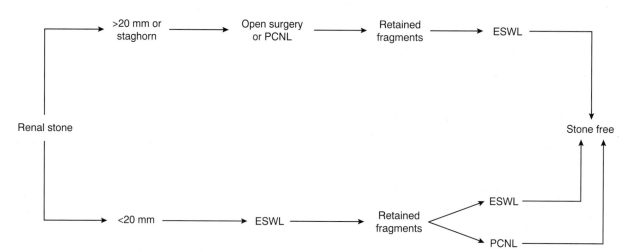

Fig. 66.4   Suggested algorithm for treatment of renal calculi. The treatment of an individual patient depends on many factors, e.g. the size, shape and number of calculi and the age of the patient. Bilateral renal and ureteric calculi will also need an individualized approach.

ureteroscopist to undertake this procedure safely in children with ureteric stones. With these smaller scopes dilatation of the ureteric orifices is now seldom required and there have been no reported new cases of VUR after these procedures. Ureteroscopy has also been combined with intracorporeal lithotripsy procedures, e.g. laser, pneumatic or ultrasonic lithotripsy, to break up ureteric stones. One of the authors has successfully removed a 20 mm lower ureteric stone using the Lithoclast through a 7.5 F flexible ureteroscope in a 2-year-old child.

Summary

ESWL, PCNL and ureteroscopy have changed the concept of surgical management of urinary tract calculi in recent years and the role of these modalities is still evolving. However, these methods require specific expertise which can only be acquired in specialist centres treating large numbers of stones. Despite the possibility that these techniques may eventually replace open renal stone surgery, the frequency of underlying urological abnormalities indicates that there is still a role for open renal surgery with simultaneous correction of the anomaly. Open surgery should also be considered when calculi are multiple and widely spread throughout the urinary tract (MacDonald *et al.*, 1988; Losty *et al.*, 1993; Pelzer *et al.*, 1994) (Fig. 66.5).

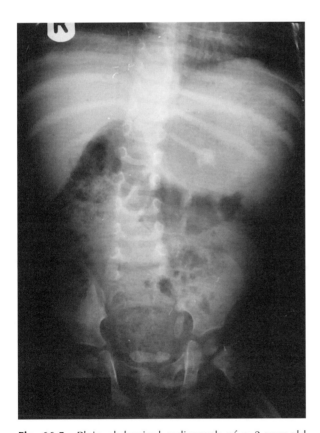

Fig. 66.5 Plain abdominal radiograph of a 2-year-old child with muliple urinary tract calculi. These were removed by a combination of pyelolithotomy and endoscopic cystolithotomy.

References

Androulakakis, P.A., Barratt, T.M., Ransley, P.G. and Williams, D.I. 1982: Urinary calculi in children. A 5–15 year follow-up with particular reference to recurrent and residual stones. *British Journal of Urology* **54**, 176–80.

Cochat, P. and Watts, R.W.E. 1995: Primary hyperoxaluria. *Neph Dial Transplant* **10**, Suppl. 8.

Corbally, M.T., Ryan, J., Fitzpatrick, J. and O'Donnell, B. 1991: Renal function following extracorporeal shock wave lithotripsy in children. *Journal of Pediatric Surgery* **26**, 539–40.

Diamond, D.A., Rickwood, A.M.K., Lee, P. and Johnston, J.H. 1994: Infection stones in children: a twenty-seven year review. *Urology* **43**, 525–7.

Fine, J.K., Pak, C.Y.C. and Preminger, G.M. 1995: Effect of medical management and residual fragments on recurrent stone formation following shock wave lithotripsy. *Journal of Urology* **153**, 27–33.

Ghazali, S. and Barratt, T.M. 1974: Urinary excretion of calcium and magnesium in children. *Archives of Disease in Childhood* **49**, 97–101

Hulbert, J.C., Reddy, P.K., Gonzalez, R. *et al.* 1985: Percutaneous nephrolithotomy: an alternative approach to the management of pediatric calculus disease. *Pediatrics* **76**, 610–12.

Kramolowsky, E.V., Willoughby, B.L. and Loening, S.A. 1987: Extracorporeal shock wave lithotripsy in childhood. *Journal of Urology* **137**, 939–41.

Kroovand, R.L., Harrison, L.H. and McCullough, D.L. 1987: Extracorporeal shockwave lithotripsy in childhood. *Journal of Urology* **138**, 1106–8.

Losty, P., Surana, R.J. and O'Donnell, B. 1993: Limitations of extracorporeal shock wave lithotripsy for urinary tract calculi in young children. *Journal of Pediatric Surgery* **28**, 1037–9.

MacDonald, I. and Azmy, A.F. 1988: Recurrent and residual renal calculi in children. *British Journal of Urology* **61**, 395–8.

Mor, Y., Elmasry, Y.E.T., Kellet, M.J. and Duffy, P.G. 1998: The role of percutaneous nephrolithotomy in the management of pediatric renal calculi (in press).

Pak, C.Y.C., Sakhaee, K., Crowther, C. and Brinkley, L. 1980: Evidence justifying a high fluid intake in treatment of nephrolithiasis. *Annals of Internal Medicine* **93**, 36–9.

Pelzer, J.O., Leumann, E. and Schwobel, M.G. 1994: The role of surgery and lithotripsy in childhood urolithiasis. *European Journal of Pediatric Surgery* **4**, 196–8.

Quinn, F.M.J. and Guiney, E.J. 1998: Xanthogranulomatous pyelonephritis in childhood (in press).

Rose, G.A. 1992: The medical management of renal stone disease. In Cameron, S., Davison, A.M., Grunfeld, J.-P., Kerr, D. and Ritz, E. (eds.) *Oxford textbook of clinical nephrology*. Oxford: Oxford University Press, Chap. 14.5, 1845–69.

Shroff, S. and Watson, G.M. 1995: Experience with ureteroscopy in children. *British Journal of Urology* **75**, 395–400.

Further reading

Levin, R.K. and Hensle, T.W. 1990: Pediatric urolithiasis. In Ashcraft, K.W. (ed.), *Pediatric urology*. Philadelphia, PA: W.B. Saunders, 461–88.

Smith, L.H. and Segura, J.W. 1992: Urolithiasis. In Kelalis and King (eds), *Pediatric urology*, 3rd ed. Philadelphia, PA: W.B. Saunders, 1327–52.

PART V

Trauma

CHAPTER 67

Reception and resuscitation of trauma patients

R.A. SLEET

Introduction	Safe transfer to the next stage
Primary assessment and resuscitation	of patient care
Secondary assessment	References

Introduction

Trauma is the leading cause of death in childhood, with almost seven children in every 100 000 of the population being killed per year (Office of Population Census and Survey, 1991). The majority of deaths result from blunt injury following falls and motor vehicle accidents. Penetrating injury is rare before the age of 10 years and still remains uncommon in the UK. The majority of seriously injured children are treated in accident and emergency departments of district general hospitals rather than in specialized paediatric accident units. The basic principles of trauma management are similar to those adopted for adult patients, but special requirements are necessary for the management of the injured infant or child (Skinner *et al.,* 1991).

Successful management is dependent on an organized system which co-ordinates prehospital ambulance care with that of the receiving accident unit. Ambulance paramedic personnel trained to national standards in trauma care and working with all necessary resuscitation aids, observing and documenting patient progress during transfer, have the responsibility for alerting the receiving trauma team of the imminent arrival of the injured casualty, using a protected telephone or radio link. This allows for the rapid assembly of the receiving team and for the delegation of specific tasks in patient care.

The resuscitation room of the accident department should be adjacent to the ambulance arrival bay, allowing for rapid transfer of the casualty. The room should be fully equipped for the resuscitation of children of all ages. There should be adequate additional heating units to improve the ambient temperature where necessary to prevent hypothermia in the small child. Nomograms or Broselow tape should be available to allow for the calculation of the child's weight from measured length to aid the estimation of drug dosage and fluid replacement (Oakley, 1988).

The receiving trauma team should be a balanced unit of medical and nursing personnel led by an experienced physician or surgeon aware of the special needs of the injured child.

The medical team leader has the responsibility of co-ordinating all aspects of the patient's care whilst in the resuscitation facility. This includes the primary assessment of the patient for life-threatening injuries, and directing and completing the resuscitation procedures before undertaking a secondary survey to assess for potentially life-threatening and other injuries. The leader is responsible for obtaining necessary paediatric and other specialist opinion and co-ordinating investigations and the safe transfer of the patient to the next stage of hospital care, whether in the receiving hospital or in a regional centre. The team should have the support of an experienced paediatric anaesthetist responsible for airway care, ventilation and the insertion of monitoring lines as needed. A third doctor is required to insert intravenous lines, obtain blood samples and manage other problems as directed by the team leader.

Co-ordinating nursing activity is the responsibility of the senior nurse, who will delegate support to the anaesthetist and other medical members of the team, and delegate responsibility for the recording of all data related to the patient's treatment and progress on to a suitable trauma form, which can later be used to evaluate the care given. Prehospital data regarding pulse and respiratory rate, blood pressure and Glasgow Coma Score (GCS) should be recorded on the form.

The trauma team caring for the child should have rapid access to all necessary diagnostic facilities, early paediatric and other specialist opinion and an agreed system of rapid access to emergency theatres. It is important that all members of the trauma team should be knowledgeable of their role in the management of the injured child and competent in the use of resuscitation equipment, and while awaiting the arrival of the patient should be briefed of their tasks in the management of the patient. Successful outcome depends on effective teamwork, adequate equipment and a system of management that allows for rapid assessment and resuscitation.

By virtue of size, infants and small children are vulnerable to multiple injury, particularly affecting the thorax and abdomen, which has the potential for rapid deterioration and the development of life-threatening complications. Anatomical variations from the adult may lead to problems of airway control and venous access and the greater body surface area in infants carries the risk of hypothermia. Injured children are frightened and in pain, and require reassurance during management from a parent or in their absence, from a delegated member of the nursing staff.

Successful outcome is dependent on a system of trauma management that allows for rapid assessment, identification of life-threatening injuries and appropriate resuscitation. The system employed in the UK since 1988 is that of the American College of Surgeons. Advanced trauma life support (ATLS) (Committee on Trauma, 1993), provides guidelines on patient management, highlighting the specialist needs of the paediatric casualty. It has been widely adopted by hospitals throughout the UK and a paediatric advanced life support (PALS) course is now available. Relevant aspects of the system have been incorporated into the National Health Service Training Directorate's (1993) ambulance paramedic training programme, and by the Royal College of Nursing into nursing practice. A trauma system has been introduced by the Royal College of Surgeons (1993–4) for doctors and others working in the prehospital situation. ATLS categorizes priorities of care into:

- primary assessment and resuscitation
- secondary assessment and necessary emergency treatment
- safe transfer to the next stage of patient care.

Primary assessment and resuscitation

These are carried out simultaneously. The team leader rapidly assesses the child for life-threatening injuries whilst the anaesthetist is managing the airway and intravenous access is obtained by the third member of the team. Regular recording of pulse and respiratory rate, blood pressure, GCS and patient temperature should be initiated. If more than one casualty is involved the team may have to split until reinforced. Under these circumstances airway management takes priority over breathing problems which, in turn, are corrected before circulatory problems are addressed.

AIRWAY MANAGEMENT

Ambulance paramedic personnel will have ensured a patent airway, inserted an oropharyngeal airway and administered oxygen in the prehospital phase of management of the child. Annual evaluation of ambulance paramedic skills, however, reveals that intubation of infants and small children is relatively uncommon (NHS Training Directorate Audit, 1992).

On arrival, the airway should be checked and the oropharynx aspirated of blood and mucus. Where clinically indicated, an oropharyngeal tube of the correct size for the child should be inserted. There are resuscitation charts are available which relate the age of the child to the size of the tube (Skinner *et al.*, 1991). In the teenage child the insertion process is the same as for an adult, with the tube being inserted with the concavity towards the palate and then rotated through 180° to lie over the tongue. In the infant and small child this technique may damage the soft palate and it is recommended that the oropharyngeal tube should be inserted directly over the tongue using a tongue depressor or the laryngoscope blade. All injured children require supplemental oxygen at high flow rate, administered through a tight-fitting facemask with a reservoir. Some children will not tolerate a face mask and nasal tongs can be used.

Endotracheal intubation is necessary in unconscious children with head injuries who are unable to protect their airway. In the infant the relatively small oral cavity and the large tongue and soft tissues make visualization of the vocal cords difficult particularly as they are placed at a higher level than in the adult; i.e. C3 as opposed to C5. In the infant and preschool child a straight-bladed laryngoscope is helpful and an uncuffed tube mandatory in order to prevent pressure necrosis. The tube should be placed just below the vocal cords to prevent intubation of the right main bronchus. On ventilation a slight air leak is necessary and in the absence of such a leak a smaller tube should be selected. In the schoolchild a cuffed tube of suitable size is recommended. Following intubation the stomach should be decompressed by the passage of a nasogastric tube in the absence of evidence of a basal skull fracture or an orogastric tube in the presence of such an injury. This is to prevent the inadvertent passage of the tube through a fractured cribiform plate into the cranial cavity. Children often swallow large quantities of air when frightened or in pain, which splints the left hemidiaphragm, impairing ventilation, and carries the risk of regurgitation and aspiration.

Severe facial injury may make oral endotracheal intubation impossible. Under these circumstances surgical cricothyroidotomy should be considered. This requires a surgeon experienced in the technique. An alternative simple effective method is needle cricothyroidotomy using a 14-gauge cannula (Committee on Trauma, 1993). The cricothyroid membrane is identified by running the examining finger down the midline from the chin to the thyroid notch and then down until the first space i.e. the cricothyroid membrane, is palpated. The needle is inserted through the skin and membrane, and the entrance into the trachea is confirmed by the aspiration of air. The needle is withdrawn and the cannula advanced. This will provide an effective temporary airway, which allows for jet insufflation until formal cricothyroidotomy can be performed.

It is essential that the cervical spine is immobilized during airway management, especially if the patient is unconscious or signs of cervical injury are present. A semirigid collar will have been applied by the ambulance service and this should be retained and supplemented with sandbags on either side of the neck and taping the head to the examination trolley. This can be a potentially upsetting experience for the conscious child and reassurance is necessary. There will be occasions where the child will resist the application of sandbags and tape. This may be due to hypoxia, hypotension, pain from tight dressings or splints and, on occasion, a full bladder. These problems should be addressed and corrected.

Adequate oxygenation should be confirmed by the application of pulse oximetry. Ventilation, if necessary, should be at a rate of 40 breaths per minute for infants, reducing to 20 breaths per minute for the older child. Paediatric bag-valve mask devices limit the pressure that can be applied, thus reducing the risk of damage to the immature lungs.

BREATHING

Blunt trauma to the chest is common in children and often requires immediate intervention to establish adequate ventilation. Mobility of the mediastinal structures makes the child more sensitive to tension pneumothorax and the effects of flail segments. The pliable chest wall increases the frequency of lung contusion and direct intrapulmonary haemorrhage, usually without overlying rib fractures. Rib fractures in young chil-

dren imply massive energy transfer, associated underlying severe organ injury and a poor prognosis. Primary assessment identifies life-threatening tension pneumothorax, haemothorax and massive lung contusion. Penetrating thoracic injury is rare in children under the age of 10 years but in the older child life-threatening open pneumothorax and cardiac tamponade require early recognition and treatment. The mechanisms of injury described by ambulance personnel and accompanying relatives, and the clinical symptoms and signs aid the early recognition of life-threatening problems.

Tension pneumothorax requires rapid recognition and chest drain decompression. Diagnosis is made on clinical suspicion from external injury patterns and clinical signs. Chest X-ray films delay management and are contraindicated. A 14-gauge cannula over a needle should be inserted over the third rib into the second intercostal space at the mid-clavicular line on the suspected side of the pneumothorax. The aspiration or audible release of air confirms the diagnosis. The cannula should be left in position until the tension pneumothorax is relieved by the insertion of a chest drain. The drain should be inserted at the level of the fourth intercostal space on the affected side after infiltration of the skin and intercostal muscles with local anaesthetic. A skin incision is made down on to the fifth rib and the intercostal muscles are dissected bluntly until the pleural cavity is entered. The closed forceps are then opened and withdrawn. The chest drain without trocar is inserted towards the apex of the lung. The drain is connected to an underwater sealed system and secured as the wound is sutured. Clinical examination will confirm the re-expansion of the lung and the position of the drain can be checked by chest X-ray during the secondary assessment of the patient. A continuing air leak raises the suspicion of a bronchial injury and a second chest drain may be necessary to prevent the recurrence of a tension pneumothorax. Bronchial injuries are often associated with subcutaneous emphysema, which will be evident on clinical examination.

Penetrating injuries may be associated with an open pneumothorax. The wound needs to be closed with an airtight dressing to ensure effective ventilation but the closure of the wound may lead to a tension pneumothorax. It is recommended that the wound be closed initially with a dressing sealed on three sides only, allowing the egress of air during inspiration, and closed on the fourth side to seal the wound only when a chest drain has been inserted through a separate incision.

Massive haemothorax is suspected from impaired respiratory movements on the injured side of the chest, reduced breath sounds and dullness to percussion. Prior to the insertion of a chest drain, intravenous access with a wide-bore cannula at one or more sites should be obtained and fluid replacement commenced.

Stab wounds to the chest, particularly inside the nipple line anteriorly or inside the scapular line posteriorly, have the potential for heart and large vessel injury and possible cardiac tamponade. Cardiac tamponade should be suspected in penetrating injuries when there is evidence of hypovolaemic shock, diminished heart sounds and increased cardiac dullness to percussion. Distended neck veins may not be evident, owing to the degree of hypovolaemia. Pericardiocentesis can be life saving. A 14-gauge cannula with an electrocardiogram (ECG) lead attached is advanced into the pericardial sac using the infrasternal approach. The needle, with a two-way tap and 50 ml syringe attached, is inserted to the left of the xiphisternum and advanced aiming towards the tip of the left scapula. The syringe is aspirated during the needle advancement and the ECG monitored to detect myocardial irritation. Entry into the pericardium is confirmed by the aspiration of blood without evidence of injury on the ECG monitor. The amount of blood aspirated will be small and often straw coloured, but will produce a clinical improvement out of proportion to the quantity aspirated. The beneficial effect is often short lived and arrangements should be made for rapid formal thoracotomy.

ECG monitoring should be initiated during the primary assessment of the chest and evidence of cardiac contusion noted. Life-threatening arrhythmias secondary to cardiac contusion are rare. External chest compression is ineffective in cardiac arrest situations secondary to major thoracic injury, and emergency thoracotomy and internal cardiac massage after cross-clamping of the descending aorta may be necessary.

CIRCULATION

Signs of early blood loss in infants and children can be very subtle and difficult to detect. External bleeding may be obvious and ambulance paramedics will have estimated external blood loss and applied appropriate pressure dressings. As in adults, children can lose significant amounts of blood into the thoracic and peritoneal cavities, the retroperitoneal space and at the site of long bone fractures, and in young infants occasionally into the cranial cavity.

Skin pallor, restlessness and tachycardia are the warning signs of incipient hypovolaemic shock, which requires aggressive treatment. Evidence of hypotension or inadequate organ perfusion requires urgent surgical evaluation. Hypotension in the child is indicative of severe blood loss and inadequate resuscitation. Infants and small children have a greater blood volume than do older children, and have different parameters for fluid replacement.

Shock can be classified for infants and preschool children as early, prehypotensive and hypotensive, representing a blood loss of < 25%, 25–45% and > 45%, respectively. Early shock is characterized by an irritable child with a cool clammy skin, tachycardia and reduced pulse volume; prehypotensive shock by a lethargic child

Table 67.1 Average paediatric values

Age (years)	Pulse rate (beats/min)	Respiratory rate (breaths/min)	Systolic BP (mmHg)
<1	160	40	80
1–5	130	30	90
5–12	100	20	100

Blood pressure (BP) = 80 + (age × 2).

with a reduced pain response, a cool clammy skin, extended capillary refill time and a marked tachycardia; and hypotensive shock by a child with a grossly impaired conscious level, marked tachycardia and respiratory rate, and a low systolic blood pressure. In order to classify the degree of shock the normal values for pulse, respiratory rate and blood pressure must be available (Table 67.1).

The older child and teenager has blood reserves similar to adults on a volume-to-weight basis. Therefore assessment of hypovolaemic shock follows adult guidelines classifying blood loss into four classes. Class 1 covers up to 15% blood volume loss. There may be few signs suggestive of blood loss, apart from skin pallor and a slight tachycardia. Class 2 covers up to 30% of blood loss. The skin is pale and clammy and there may be a degree of anxiety and irritability, with a tachycardia of 100 beats/min, a slight increase in respiratory rate, no change in systolic blood pressure but a decrease in pulse pressure. Class 3 represents 40% blood loss, which can be as much as 2 litres in the teenage child. Signs of inadequate perfusion are evident, with a pale clammy skin, clouding of conscious level, tachycardia, tachyopnea and a fall in blood pressure. Class 4 represents a blood loss in excess of 40% and severe uncompensated shock, with a marked increase in pulse and respiratory rate, clouding of consciousness and a rapidly deteriorating blood pressure. Successful management of blood loss requires early recognition of the signs, and aggressive fluid replacement with warmed crystalloid or colloid solutions and blood.

Resuscitation should have started in the prehospital situation with the insertion of intravenous lines and crystalloid fluid infusion. However, venous access in the small child may be difficult owing to subcutaneous fat, environmental chilling and hypovolaemia. On arrival at the hospital, the establishment of two intravenous lines with large-bore cannulae suitable for the age of the child is essential. Central venous pressure monitoring lines are unsuitable for resuscitation purposes. If there is difficulty in visualizing or palpating suitable vessels, venous cutdown should be considered using the long saphenous vein at the ankle or the antecubital vein at the elbow. If venous cannulation is difficult in the young child intraosseous infusion should be the method of choice (Fiser, 1990). This technique requires the insertion of an intraosseous transfusion needle into the bone marrow of an uninjured tibia just below the tibial tubercle or the lower end of the femur. This is a simple and rapid technique and allows for adequate resuscitation flow rates. The infusion should be stopped as soon as venous access can be achieved.

Fluid replacement for infants and small children requires the infusion of 20 ml/kg of crystalloid as Hartman's or Ringer's lactate solution. The fluid should be administered using an adult drip set to ensure rapid volume replacement. A second bolus of fluid should be given if there is little improvement. If the child's condition stabilizes observation is continued and a surgical opinion obtained. A failure to respond to the initial fluid therapy requires the infusion of blood. O-negative or type-specific blood can be used, infusing 20 ml/kg of whole blood or 10 ml/kg of packed cells. Surgical opinion is essential and an urgent operation may be required.

In the older child blood loss is estimated and classified, and appropriate volume replacement initiated. Class 3 and 4 haemorrhage will require surgical evaluation and operative intervention, whereas lesser blood loss will usually require continuing observation and surgical review.

Neurogenic shock should be suspected when there is evidence of spinal cord injury and a low blood pressure in association with bradyrhythmia. Initial treatment includes elevation of the lower limbs, fluid replacement and intravenous atropine (20 µg/kg).

Cardiogenic shock in trauma is the result of tension pneumothorax, pericardial tamponade and severe hypovolaemia. Successful resuscitation depends on the early recognition and treatment of the underlying cause.

Following completion of the primary assessment and the resuscitation of the child it is usual to assess for neurological dysfunction. An assessment of the level of consciousness is made and recorded as alert, responding to verbal stimuli, pain only or unresponsive. Pupillary size and reaction are noted, as are limb movements. The GCS chart is reviewed and the score noted. The GCS will have been recorded on the ambulance record before arrival in the resuscitation room and transcribed to the trauma chart and the observations continued during resuscitation. It is necessary to use charts modified for the verbal response for children under the age of 2 years, and for children between 2 and 5 years, after which adult observation charts are used. The total score is related to the age of the patient (Table 67.2).

Table 67.2 Paediatric Glasgow Coma Score

Age (years)	Normal aggregate score
<1	12
1–2	13
>2	14

Secondary assessment

Secondary assessment is a top-to-toe examination, which requires total exposure of the child. The high ratio of body surface area to body mass makes the child vulnerable to heat loss and hypothermia. Every effort should be made to prevent chilling by the use of room heaters and adequate covering of the child after examination. Without total exposure external injuries and other clinical signs which direct attention to any underlying injuries will be missed and assessment will be incomplete. The secondary assessment requires examination of the posterior surface of the head, trunk and limbs, and a log-rolling technique is necessary to avoid complicating spinal injury.

Before starting the assessment there is an opportunity to order essential X-rays which, in the resuscitation room, are limited to lateral cervical spine, chest and pelvic films. Providing the patient is stable any subsequent X-rays can be undertaken in the radiology department during transfer to the theatre or wards. Essential treatment should not be delayed by unnecessary radiology. Blood samples, including arterial gas anaylsis, can be taken at this time.

It is usual to start the secondary assessment with the examination of the head. Serious head injuries in children usually result in diffuse axonal injury rather than mass lesions. Children with such injuries are prone to vomiting and fits. It may be necessary to control fits with intravenous or rectal diazepam (0.25 mg/kg) and to prevent further episodes by the infusion of phenytoin (15–20 mg/kg) administered at the rate of 1 ml/kg/min. It may be necessary to paralyse, intubate and ventilate the child during the primary assessment if there is evidence of clinical deterioration. Prompt attention to the airway, ventilation and correction of hypovolaemic shock prevents secondary brain swelling and improves survival. If there are clinical indications for computed tomography (CT) scanning and intracranial pressure monitoring, arrangements should be made for transfer to the appropriate neurosurgical facility. Secondary assessment should be completed before transfer. Life threatening thoracic and abdominal injuries may require urgent treatment and therefore an operation priority is essential.

The neck should be examined for soft tissue and tracheal injuries. This will require the removal of the semirigid collar and manual immobilization of the neck. Care must be taken during immobilization not to cover the child's ears with the immobilizing hands so that reassurance can be continued. The lateral cervical spine X-ray should be available at this stage. Because of anatomical differences, including pseudoluxation, in many young children interpretation of the film requires experience. If a radiological opinion is not available at this stage immobilization of the neck should be maintained.

Blunt injury to the chest is common in children and re-evaluation of the thorax is necessary. The chest film will confirm the successful re-expansion of the lung and the correct placement of the chest drain. Rib fractures, lung contusion, mediastinal abnormalities and injury to the diaphragm will be evident.

Abdominal injuries are commonly the result of blunt rather than penetrating trauma. Penetrating injury with evidence of hypovolaemic shock must be regarded as a life-threatening condition meriting urgent surgical opinion and operative intervention. In blunt injury, assessment of the conscious child requires warm hands and gentle palpation if subtle signs are to be elicited. Prior to this examination the stomach should have been decompressed with a gastric tube. Peritoneal lavage can be valuable in assessing the haemodynamically unstable child but should be performed by the surgeon undertaking eventual treatment of the patient. CT scanning and ultrasound examination are of value in eliciting evidence of liver, spleen, renal and bladder injury but should only be undertaken on a stable patient.

The limbs should be examined and wounds noted. This will require the removal of the primary dressing applied by the paramedic. It is helpful if good quality polaroid photographs can be taken at this stage. The dressings can then be reapplied and left until definitive treatment in theatre, thus reducing the risk of infection from multiple examinations. Deformity and swelling of limbs indicative of fracture require appropriate splintage and radiological examination, and an orthopaedic opinion is sought. Orthopaedic injuries are seldom life threatening and their investigation should not delay the treatment of urgent conditions discussed previously. Limb sensation and circulation should be noted, and vascular compromise which cannot be corrected by gentle realignment necessitates further investigation and a surgical opinion.

Log rolling of the patient will allow access for examination of the spine and the posterior surface of the trunk, as well as perineal examination. At this stage, in the absence of evidence of urethral injury, a catheter should be inserted and urine output measured, providing an assessment of the adequacy of fluid replacement (1 ml/kg/h). If urethral injury is suspected a suprapubic catheter provides an alternative method of bladder drainage.

On completion of the secondary survey previous medical and drug history, tetanus status and past history of allergies to medication and adhesives should be obtained from accompanying relatives or telephone communication with the family practitioner. With this knowledge tetanus toxoid injection can be administered if indicated, and necessary antibiotic therapy in the case of compound fractures, and analgesic medication given. Analgesia may have been necessary earlier during primary or secondary assessment and should be given intravenously using morphine 25 µg/kg titrated slowly against the patient's needs. Further doses should be titrated slowly, giving 10 µg/kg. Narcotic analgesics should not be given to patients with severe head injuries.

Safe transfer to the next stage of patient care

Once resuscitation has been completed, injuries identified and emergency treatment administered, priorities of subsequent management have to be identified in consultation with the appropriate surgical specialist. The child's parents should be informed of the extent of the injuries and the treatment discussed. All documentation should be completed and arrangements made with the receiving theatre, intensive care unit or regional centre for the transfer of the patient. Prior to transfer, the endotracheal tube, chest drain, intravenous lines, splints and dressings need to be checked and secured. X-rays and the results of investigations are attached to the patient's notes and the patient is transferred with the necessary trained staff and monitoring equipment to the next stage of care.

A copy of the trauma chart should be retained for subsequent evaluation of the care administered to the patient. Strengths and weaknesses in the management of the child need to be addressed and deficiencies of training, organization or equipment identified and corrected as part of a quality assurance programme. Audit of standards of paediatric trauma care should be routine practice (Committee on Trauma, 1989). Data should also be submitted to the UK Major Trauma Outcome Study as part of a national survey of trauma management for all ages using the TRISS methodology (plotting revised trauma score against injury severity score), which determines the potential for survival and thus compares the hospital's performance with those of a similar case mix (Boyd *et al.*, 1987). This is essential if the government's target under the 'Health of the Nation' is to reduce paediatric death from 6.7 per 100 000 in 1990 to no more than 4.5 per 100 000 in 2005 (Department of Health, 1992).

References

Boyd, C., Tolson, M. and Copes, W. 1987: Evaluating trauma care: the TRISS method. *Journal of Trauma* **27**, 370–80.

Committee on Trauma 1989: *Resources for optimal care of the injured patient*, vol. 12. American College of Surgeons, **12**, 51.

Committee on Trauma 1993: *Advanced trauma life support – instructor's manual*, 5th ed. American College of Surgeons.

NHS Training Directorate Audit, Paramedic Services 1992: *Health of the nation: accidents*. London: HMSO, 19.

Fiser, D.H. 1990: Intraosseous transfusions. *New England Journal of Medicine* **322**, 1579–81.

National Health Service Training Directorate 1991: *Ambulance paramedic training – audit report* 7.

National Health Service Training Directorate 1993: *Ambulance service paramedic training manual*, 3rd ed.

Oakley, P.A. 1988: A paediatric resuscitation chart. *British Medical Journal* **297**, 817–9.

Office of Population Census and Survey 1991: *Mortality Statistics*, Series DH 2, vol. 18, 104–5.

Royal College of Surgeons of England 1993/94: *Training prospectus*, Pre Hospital Life Support Course. 14.

Skinner, D., Driscoll, P. and Earlham, R. (eds) 1991: *ABC of major trauma*. London: BMJ Publishing, 73–82.

CHAPTER 68

Regional trauma units for children

J.A. HALLER, JR

Introduction
Emergency medical service system

Comprehensive paediatric emergency service
References

Introduction

Experience in the management of severely injured soldiers during World War II (1940–1945) clearly indicated the need for special trauma units for the resuscitation and subsequent management of severely injured patients (Trunkey, 1983). During and following this conflict the concept of the 'golden hour' evolved, emphasizing the importance of moving the patient rapidly to an appropriate treatment centre with the initiation of aggressive resuscitation within the first 60 min (Haller, 1978). This necessitated a means of rapid transport from the site of injury and the introduction of helicopters for such transport became routine. The body of knowledge of the pathophysiology of trauma and shock which evolved from this battlefield experience was embodied in the advanced trauma life support (ATLS) course of the American College of Surgeons in the 1950s (Haller, 1973).

With this recognition of the importance of focused trauma care in regional sites, the birth of trauma centres occurred, especially in the USA, but also in other western European countries (Accidental death and disability, 1966). Countries organized their transport and prehospital care differently: some used trauma physicians in the field (Germany and Austria) and others trained a new cadre of prehospital professionals, the emergency medical technicians and paramedics (Trunkey, 1983). Not until the 1970s did it become obvious that children should be included in a comprehensive

emergency medical system for the care of their life-threatening injuries, just as for adults (Haller, 1983). Since there is considerable overlap in the basic principles of trauma resuscitation and the management of shock between children and adults, most children's regional trauma programmes developed as a part of an overall emergency medical system. This sharing of trauma facilities made it possible to utilize the special expertise of a small number of paediatric surgeons who had trauma experience and to incorporate their skills into the broader concept of comprehensive regional trauma centres for adults and children (Harris, 1989).

Preliminary data derived from early regional trauma centres for children helped to identify some of the special needs of children and teenagers. Specifically, young children are not just less mature and smaller adults, but have special responses and different patterns of injury. Trauma is the number one killer in the paediatric age group (Haller, 1983). Not only was trauma found to be responsible for most of the deaths between the ages of 1 and 14 years, but injuries from automobile crashes, falls and burns from house fires were responsible for 50% of the overall mortality in children (Fig. 68.1) (Gratz, 1979).

Most children's injuries result from blunt forces such as crushing, compressing or decelerating from impact with a motor vehicle which is the most common vector for serious injuries in children, (Fig. 68.2). School-age children are usually injured as pedestrians or on bicycles. In addition, falls from buildings, walls and trees

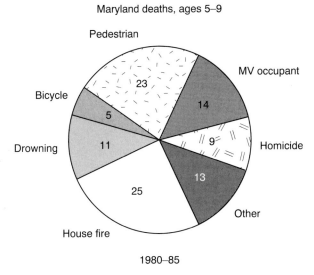

Maryland deaths, ages 5–9

1980–85

Fig. 68.1 Maryland deaths, ages 5–9 years.

are a frequent cause of blunt injury. Clearly, most of the life-threatening injuries in children result from blunt forces and are most often associated with motor vehicle crashes.

Children and adults respond differently to the same severity of trauma. The ABC of trauma management (airway, breathing and circulation) is a basic ingredient in the management of any patient, but there are important differences in children. Extensive information regarding the special response of children to life-threatening injuries was published in the 1970s from regional paediatric trauma centres, notably from the Hospital for Sick Children in Toronto, the Boston Floating Children's Hospital, the Detroit Children's Hospital and the Johns Hopkins Children's Center in Baltimore (Haller *et al.*, 1983). Some of these regional trauma centres were in independent children's hospitals while others were components of a larger university hospital environment. The most important principle derived from this experience was that a regional system of trauma management for children must be a part of an overall comprehensive emergency medical service (EMS) system.

Emergency medical service system

Such an EMS-C (children's system) should include the following eight components.

COMMUNICATION SYSTEM

Two-way radio communication with the emergency medical technicians at the scene of an emergency not only allows for communication with and advice from the physician but also identifies the presence or absence of medical specialists in nearby hospitals and determines the destination of the individual patient, whether a child or an adult.

TRANSPORT SYSTEM

A transport system is an integral part of the regional trauma centre concept. The support components of the system include police helicopter on a radio-controlled basis, initiated through an emergency medical relay centre which functions as a communication link for the system. Transportation is arranged through a relay centre for each case and the appropriate specialty facility to which the patient should be taken is determined.

FIRST RESPONDER AT THE TRAUMA SITE

The emergency medical technicians must receive specialized training in the care of newborn infants and children from medical specialists such as neonatologists, paediatric surgeons and anaesthesiologists. They are then qualified to begin i.v. treatment of small infants

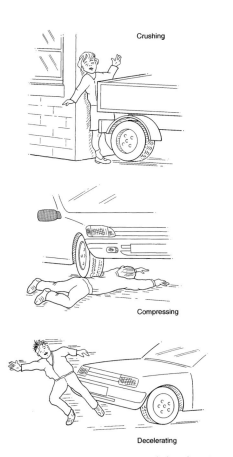

Crushing

Compressing

Decelerating

Fig. 68.2 Crushing, compressing and decelerating.

and to intubate babies and young children if this is indicated. Their training must be a part of the ongoing training programme for emergency medical personnel within the regional system.

PAEDIATRIC TRAUMA CENTRE

A resuscitation unit is a basic component of a regional paediatric trauma system. After communication from the scene of the life-threatening injury, a child is brought by appropriate transportation to the emergency room. The child is met by a team of paediatric resuscitation and paediatric surgery specialists who are trained in the initial management of life-threatening injuries.

The child should be managed in a resuscitation unit designed specifically for children, with miniature intubation equipment, including tracheostomy tubes and other specialized equipment such as central venous pressure lines for children. The captain of the trauma resuscitation team should be either a senior resident in paediatric surgery or a staff paediatric surgeon working closely with well-trained paediatric emergency medicine staff. Key paediatric surgical specialists, such as a paediatric neurosurgeons and paediatric orthopedic surgeons must be available on call within minutes. X-ray equipment must be immediately available in the unit for both the initial diagnostic studies and subsequent special films. It is important to emphasize that all children with major injuries are resuscitated by paediatricians and paediatric surgeons, all of whom are part of the paediatric trauma team. After emergency stabilization, appropriate diagnostic tests and specialty consultations, a child may go directly to the operating room or be admitted to a paediatric intensive care unit (Beaver *et al.*, 1987).

PAEDIATRIC INTENSIVE CARE UNIT

Paediatric intensive care units should also be regionally centralized. All of the patient stations should be equipped with multiple channel monitoring equipment and ventilators and staffed for the immediate detection of cardiopulmonary arrest, for resuscitation and for continuing post-trauma management. Other equipment may include a mass spectrometer, cardiac output computers, blood gas analysers, ionized calcium analysers and gamma cameras for the determination of cardiac output and similar clinical research studies. A small dedicated onsite blood gas laboratory should provide immediate blood gas determination.

Three important additional facilities complete the total concept of a regional centre for the care of major trauma in children: (i) an intermediate care unit under the direction of paediatric neurologists; (ii) a paediatric subacute rehabilitation unit under the direction of a paediatric physical medical consultant; and (iii) an intermediate and long-term facility for children with chronic rehabilitation and nursing needs.

NEUROLOGY–NEUROSURGERY INTERMEDIATE CARE UNIT

Neurology–neurosurgery intermediate care unit for paediatric trauma is directed by a paediatric neurosurgeon and a paediatric neurologist, who both have special interests in the care of the child with head injuries. This is a direct continuation of the intensive care of children with severe brain injuries including continued monitoring of their neurological recovery when they no longer require constant monitoring and the use of intracranial pressure measurements. Within this unit, paediatric rehabilitation begins and the interplay with the paediatric physical medical consultant becomes an increasingly important component of patient management. Preliminary evidence from personal experience strongly suggests that children with major head injuries producing coma lasting longer that 24 hours have a greatly improved recovery rate over that reported in the literature (Mahoney *et al.*, 1983). These data suggest that only 12% of the surviving children have a residual intellectual or motor impairment and 88% of the survivors over 2 years of age have good recovery without major motor or intellectual deficits that can be measured. It remains to be seen whether these preliminary data will reflect continuing trends but certainly they are encouraging.

PAEDIATRIC TRAUMA REHABILITATION UNIT

This is designed to allow for inpatient care and parent participation in ongoing subacute and intermediate rehabilitation programmes and evaluation. This provides not only for better day-to-day patient care but also an opportunity for studying the emotional and physical responses to rehabilitation and for designing new protocols for early rehabilitation.

PAEDIATRIC TRAUMA LONG-TERM REHABILITATION AND MANAGEMENT UNIT

This is another important component of an integrated programme. It must be committed to intermediate and long-term management of children with residual neurological and physical problems following major injuries. Supervision by a full-time paediatrician is required.

Within such a paediatric trauma system (Fig. 68.3), the resuscitation should be performed by the paediatric surgical trauma team. This team consists of a senior paediatric surgical resident (postgraduate year 6–7), paediatric intensivist, general surgical resident (postgraduate year 4) and a paediatric intern (postgraduate year 1).

Diagnostic studies must be obtained in the emergency room and the adjacent computerized tomography area. Patients can then be transferred to the operating room, paediatric intensive care unit or paediatric

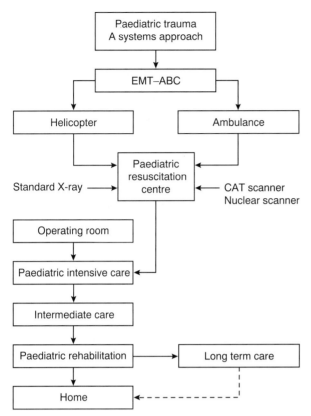

Fig. 68.3 Components of regional trauma system for children, emphasizing the sequential use of integrated facilities and personnel.

surgical ward for definitive care. A trauma registry (Tepas *et al.*, 1989) is used to record prospectively the demographic data, mechanism of injury, system injured, types of injuries, vital signs, trauma scores including Glasgow Coma Scores and patient outcome.

From the experience accumulated from a number of regional trauma centres for children, several unique aspects of trauma in children have been documented. The increased incidence of head injury in children with blunt trauma and the associated morbidity and mortality with the central nervous system required a more aggressive approach. The management of brain injury must include intracranial monitoring to facilitate the control of cerebral oedema. Computed tomography (CT) in the immediate postinjury period and sequential scanning are invaluable in following the clinical course of these children.

CT scanning plays a major role in assessing blunt abdominal injury. It has become the method of choice in those children who have altered neurological status and whose physical examination is unreliable. It is obviously necessary to locate the radiological facility close to the main trauma room to permit this early evaluation.

The multidisciplinary approach to the management of the injured children is co-ordinated through the general paediatric surgeon, who consults with neurosurgeons, orthopaedic surgeons, anaesthesiologists and intensivists. For the child to be managed non-operatively (Fig. 68.4) a team consisting of surgeons and paediatric intensivists is necessary and constant monitoring of the child is required in a paediatric intensive care unit (Douglas and Simpson, 1971). Extensive experience has indicated that an approach using a comprehensive system of prehospital support, transport, hospital resuscitation and rehabilitation will offer the injured child the best chance for long-term survival with minimal morbidity (Haller, 1989).

Comprehensive paediatric emergency service

In a further extension of this concept of trauma units for children, paediatric surgeons and general surgeons involved in trauma care have offered leadership to expand the EMS system for children to include life-threatening illness. Comprehensive paediatric emergency services should be integrated into an overall emergency care system, but must be organized regionally to address the special needs of children with life-threatening injuries and illness (Seidel, 1989). This EMS system will allow the natural overlap of many emergency services, such as obstetrics, prenatal, adolescent and young adult programmes, all of which will be strengthened by such integration (Seidel, 1986). The one non-negotiable principle must be that any emergency medical system that includes children must use

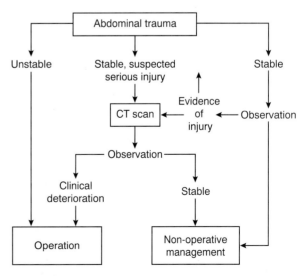

Fig. 68.4 Abdominal trauma.

the best and most experienced paediatric specialists available in the area. The exact location of the regional paediatric emergency care facility (i.e. in a self-standing children's hospital vs the children's component of a general hospital) is not as important as the total commitment of that institution and its medical personnel to the optimal care of acutely ill and severely injured children.

It has been shown that regional trauma centres not only improve the outcome of resuscitation and life-threatening injuries, but also, through this focused attention, result in better systems of transportation from the scene of the injury to the appropriate centre (Mayer *et al.*, 1980).

Surgeons and paediatricians must work closely together in the organization and implementation of emergency medical services for treating life-threatening injuries and illness. The use of an organizational framework, based on a regional trauma unit concept, but expanded to include illness, will result in improved teamwork and more efficient management of children with life-threatening conditions (Seidel *et al.*, 1984). The basic principles of rapid, careful evaluation and sequential correction of altered physiology remain the backbone of successful therapy in children with life-threatening conditions. The unique metabolic demands and miniature anatomical relationships, especially of a small child, present the emergency paediatrician and paediatric surgeon with a special challenge and a great responsibility. The organization of regional emergency medical services for children permits the highest quality management of children with life-threatening injuries and illness (Durch and Lohr, 1983).

References

Accidental death and disability: the neglected disease of modern society 1966: Washington, DC: National Academy of Science Publication.

Beaver, B., Fal, A., Fishman, E. *et al.* 1987: The efficacy of computed tomography in evaluating abdominal injuries in children with major head trauma. *Journal of Paediatric Surgery* **22**, 19–23.

Douglas, G.J. and Simpson, J.S. 1971: The conservative management of splenic trauma. *Journal of Paediatric Surgery* **6**, 565–70.

Durch, J.S., and Lohr, N.H. (eds) 1983: Institute of Medicine: *Emergency medical services for children.* Washington, DC: National Academy Press.

Gratz, R.R. 1979: Accidental injury in childhood: a literature review on paediatric trauma. *Journal of Trauma* **19**, 551–55.

Hailer, J.A., Shorter, N., Miller, D., Colombani, P., Hall, J. and Buck, J. 1983: Organization and function of a regional paediatric trauma center: does a system of management improve outcome? *Journal of Trauma* **23**, 691–6.

Haller, J.A. (ed.) 1989: *Emergency medical services for children.* Report of the 97th Ross Conference on Paediatric Research. Columbus, OH: Ross Laboratories, 22–30.

Haller, J.A. 1978: An overview of paediatric trauma. In Touloukian, J. (ed.) *Paediatric trauma.* New York: Wiley, 3.

Haller, J.A. 1983: Paediatric trauma, the no. 1 killer of children. *Journal of the American Medical Association* **249**, 47.

Haller, J.A., Jr 1973: Newer concepts in emergency care of children with major injuries. *Maryland State Medical Journal* **22**, 65–70.

Harris, B.H. 1989: Creating paediatric trauma systems. *Journal of Paediatric Surgery* **24**, 149–52.

Mahoney, W.J., D'Souza, B.J., Haller, J.A., Rogers, M.C., Epstein, M.H. and Freeman, J.M. (1983) Long term outcome of children with severe head trauma and prolonged coma. *Paediatrics* **71**, 756–62.

Mayer, T. Matlak, M., Johnson, D. *et al.*, 1980: The modified injury severity scale in paediatric multiple trauma patients. *Journal of Paediatric Surgery* **15**, 719–26.

Seidel, J.S. 1986: A needs assessment of paediatric advanced life support and emergency medical services for the paediatric patient: state of the art. *Circulation* **74** (Suppl. IV), 129–33.

Seidel, J.S. 1989: EMS-C in urban and rural areas: the California experience. In Haller, J.A. (ed.) 1989: *Emergency medical services for children.* Report of the 97th Ross Conference on Paediatric Research. Columbus, OH: Ross Laboratories, 22–30.

Seidel, J.S., Hornbein, M., Yoshiyama, K. *et al.* 1984: Emergency medical services and the paediatric patient: are the needs being met? *Paediatrics* **73**, 769–72.

Tepas, J.J., Ramenofsky, M.L., Barlow, B. *et al.* 1989: National Paediatric Trauma Registry. *Journal of Paediatric Surgery* **24**, 156–8.

Trunkey, D.D. 1983: Trauma. *Scientific American* **249**, 28–35.

CHAPTER 69

Head injuries

D. LANG

Introduction	Radiology
Epidemiology	Management of head-injured patients
Pathophysiology of head injury	Specific complications of head injury
Mechanisms of injury and patterns	Results
of recovery	References

Introduction

Management, morbidity and mortality due to acute traumatic brain damage have significantly reduced since the 1960s, reflecting increasing neurosurgical involvement in the management of mild, moderate and severe head injury, the introduction of head injury management protocols, increased emphasis on neurosurgical intensive care and guidelines for the non-specialist in the care of the head-injured patient (Committee on Trauma, 1985; Royal College of Surgeons, 1986; Teasdale et al., 1990; Report of a Working Party, 1991; Miller et al., 1991a).

Central to the management of the head-injured patient has been the emphasis placed on establishing a stable, optimal milieu for the brain to promote recovery. The need to avoid secondary insults such as hypotension and hypoxia has been underlined by neurosurgeons and, more recently, the use of brain protectants is being reviewed in the experimental and clinical setting (Eisenberg et al., 1983; Miller et al., 1978; Gildenberg and Mekela, 1985; Marmarou et al., 1991).

Epidemiology

Acute head injury remains one of the most important causes of morbidity and mortality in children (< 15 years old). In the USA 10 children in 100 000 die per annum as a result of an acute head injury (Annegers et

al., 1980). One child in 10 is reported to sustain a head injury with loss of consciousness (Melchior, 1961). The overall incidence of paediatric head injury ranges from 180 to 295 per 100 000 (Klauber et al., 1981; Annegers, 1983). Head injury in infancy (< 2 years old) represents some 31% of all head-injured children (Choux et al., 1990).

In developed countries a road traffic accident (RTA) is responsible for 22% of fatal head injuries in children aged from 5–14 years. Falls and assaults are a frequent cause of injury, whilst injuries during sport and leisure are less common. Tables 69.1 and 69.2 illustrate the causes of head injury in children of different ages. Non-accidental injury is estimated to represent some 10% of all traumatic injuries in children under 5 years of age. Some 25–40% of abused children suffer a head injury

Table 69.1 Causes of head injury in children

	Falls (%)	RTA (%)
Hendrick et al. (1964)	53	32
Craft et al. (1972)	47	33
Boulis et al. (1978)	93	5.5
Annegers (1983)	55	32
Di Rocco and Velardi (1986)	59	31
Choux (1986)	71	22

RTA, Road traffic accident.

Table 69.2 Causes of head injury in different age groups

Age (months)	Percentage	Cause	Percentage
0–2	4	Falls	79
2–6	17	RTA	8
6–12	31	NAI	2
12–18	22	Other	11
18–24	26		

RTA, road traffic accident; NAI, non-accidental injury.

and half of these survivors suffer permanent neurological and intellectual impairment. Non-accidental injury usually results in subdural haematomas, skull fractures and intracerebral haematomas (McClelland *et al.*, 1980).

Pathophysiology of head injury

ARE CHILDREN DIFFERENT FROM ADULTS?

Anatomical, physiological and developmental differences in children account for the biological differences and consequences of trauma. Infants (<2 years old) have a high incidence of haematomas (subgaleal, subperiosteal and extradural), even in the absence of a skull fracture, because of the high vascularity of the vault of the skull and the dura. The brain is generally better protected because the unfused sutures and open fontanelles increase the flexibility of the vault which is therefore more easily deformed by external forces. The anterior and middle cranial fossa floors are smooth and the brain can glide with little opposing resistance. The subarachnoid space is small and the growing brain closely applied to the dura.

The biomechanical properties of the growing brain have not been extensively studied, but pressure–volume relationships can be represented by an exponential curve as in adults (Shapiro *et al.*, 1980) (Fig. 69.1). In children the slope of the curve depends on the volume of the neuraxis. Thus an infant has less ability to buffer equal increments of volume.

CEREBRAL CIRCULATION

Cerebral blood flow (CBF) is relatively low in immature animals. Blood flow rates then increase and subsequently decrease some weeks after birth to levels comparable with those of mature animals. There is uncertainty about autoregulation and CO_2 reactivity and CBF may passively follow mean systemic arterial blood pressure. The immature brain tolerates hypoxia better than an adult brain, and this may reflect the lower metabolic requirement of the immature brain.

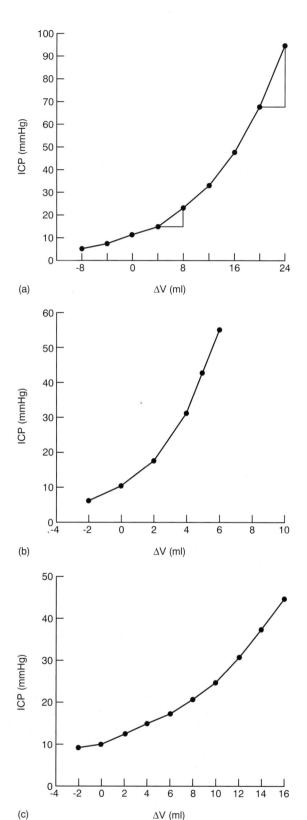

Fig. 69.1 Pressure–volume curve: (a) normal adult; (b) infant; (c) adolescent.

CEREBRAL PERFUSION PRESSURE AND INTRACRANIAL PRESSURE

Cerebral perfusion pressure (CPP)
= mean arterial blood pressure (mABP)
−intracranial pressure (ICP).

In adults a CPP of at least 50 mmHg is required to maintain adequate cerebral perfusion. CPP in normal children may not reach 50 mmHg and the levels of CPP tolerated by infants and immature animals have not been studied.

Mechanisms of injury and patterns of recovery

Sparing of function after injury may depend on the degree of commitment of the neural tissue at the time of the injury. Whilst immaturity may confer some advantages in recovery after focal brain damage there is evidence that the immature brain is susceptible to diffuse damage. This means that in young children residual neuropsychological deficits may be more severe than those observed in older children or adolescents (Brink *et al.*, 1970). Prior to attainment of language aphasia will not occur with extensive hemisphere damage. After the age of 10 years aphasia may be permanent because of the functional commitment of the left hemisphere with the onset of puberty.

FRACTURES OF THE SKULL

Injury to the head may cause superficial damage to the scalp or skull vault. Skull lesions occur more commonly in paediatric patients and it is advisable for all head-injured children to have skull X-rays (anterior–posterior, lateral and Towne's views). Fractures occur in 25% of head-injured children and 40% of infants after an acute head injury (Choux, 1986). They are classified as linear, depressed, growing or basal. Suture diastasis is commonly seen and fractures often extend between sutures. Depressed fractures in children are associated with a dural tear and/or cortical injury in some 30–40% of cases. Surgical elevation is the most suitable form of treatment, except for 'ping-pong ball' fractures which may elevate spontaneously. Fractures adjacent to venous sinuses may be treated conservatively. Late epilepsy is reported to occur in 20% of children with a depressed fracture (Jennett, 1974). An aggressive surgical approach, with routine elevation of all depressed fractures, has been reported to reduce this to 1.2% (Choux and Genitori, 1985). A growing fracture occurs in 1–15% of fractures, usually in infants. The fracture is associated with a dural tear and/or underlying brain injury. Cerebrospinal fluid (CSF) pulsations lead to pro-gressive enlargement of the fracture and a cranial defect. This may involve the roof of the orbit or anterior cranial fossa floor resulting in a traumatic encephalocoele (Choux *et al.*, 1990). Orbital roof fractures have a high incidence of dural tear and should routinely be explored. (Penfold *et al.*, 1992) Growing fractures require a dural repair and cranioplasty. Compound fractures in children are less common than in adults and basal fractures are rare; in children a CSF leak occurs in only 0.5% (Choux *et al.*, 1990).

EXTRACRANIAL HAEMATOMAS

Infants and young children may develop extensive sub-cutaneous or subgaleal haematomas. This may lead to anaemia. A cephalhaematoma is due to bleeding between the periosteum and the bone and occurs in 0.5–2% of neonates delivered by primaparous mothers. In 10% of babies this will calcify and require surgical excision. The vast majority of extracranial haematomas can be treated conservatively.

INTRACRANIAL LESIONS

Injury to the brain

Perhaps the most useful method of classifying brain damage is to consider focal and diffuse brain damage (Adams and Graham, 1984). This classification is equally applicable to adults and children. Focal damage includes contusions, haematomas and abnormalities resulting from raised ICP. Diffuse brain damage includes diffuse axonal injury, diffuse brain swelling, hypoxic brain damage and diffuse vascular injury. All of the examples of diffuse brain damage have been produced by in subhuman primates using the Penn I and Penn II inertial acceleration devices (Gennarelli *et al.*, 1982).

Focal brain damage

Contusions

Contusions tend to occur in the frontal and temporal lobes where the brain may be injured by bony protuberances on the skull base. Superficial contusions are confined to the gyri, whereas more extensive contusions involve the subcortical and deep white matter. In the presence of a skull fracture contusions tend to be more severe. In the absence of coexistent axonal injury and secondary complications patients with severe contusions may have a favourable outcome. By and large, because of the smooth contours of the anterior and middle cranial fossa floors contusions may be less frequent in infants and young children. Contusions are reported in 16% of children, compared with 33% of adults with head injuries (Zimmerman and Bilaniuk, 1981).

Haematomas

Intracranial haematomas occur in 3% of all head-injured patients admitted to hospital and in 40% of unconscious victims of a head injury.

An extradural haematoma (EDH) is a complication of a skull fracture with separation of the dura from the inner table and most commonly results from middle meningeal arterial haemorrhage or bleeding from a venous sinus. In children the source of bleeding may be the bone edges or the richly vascularized dura. Two per cent of head-injured children develop an EDH (Choux *et al.*, 1990). In adults the clot often occurs after a mild head injury and early removal results in a neurologically intact patient (Miller *et al.*, 1992b). In children 70–75% have a skull fracture (Choux *et al.*, 1990). The haematoma may be extensive. Twelve per cent of children have a normal conscious level, 20% are drowsy or confused, 45% have a lucid interval and 23% are in coma. Anaemia commonly occurs in infants (Choux *et al.*, 1990). Delayed presentation and late deterioration are common because of the exceptional tolerance of children for this lesion.

Craniotomy and evacuation is the treatment of choice. Small haematomas in children with a normal level of consciousness may be managed conservatively, in a neurosurgical unit (NSU), with serial assessments of conscious level and repeat computed tomography (CT) scanning. The reported mortality rate varies from 9% to 17%. In patients without associated brain damage mortality and morbidity should approach 0% and the poor results reflect delayed diagnosis, rigid CT scanning policies and delayed referral to a NSU.

Subdural haematomas (SDH) occur when bridging cortical veins are torn, or there is laceration of the brain surface, a torn venous sinus or a dural laceration. They are the most common post-traumatic haematomas in children, occurring in 4–12% of all head-injured children (Ingraham and Matson, 1944; Hendrick *et al.*, 1964; Choux *et al.*, 1990). They are more common in the first 6 months of life and most are due to a fall. A high incidence of SDH (58%) has been reported in children with non-accidental injury. Birth trauma (breech delivery) may cause an acute SDH in a neonate. Following injury the patient may be in coma and signs of brainstem compression rapidly develop. In infants and neonates the presentation is less dramatic. The conscious level is usually impaired and pallor, irritability and a tense fontanelle are apparent. There may be focal neurological signs and epilepsy occurs in 50–70% of cases. Management involves craniotomy and evacuation. Reported mortality is 17–20% but in the context of the older child with a severe head injury mortality is considerably higher (Gutierrez and Raimondi, 1975; Choux and Lena, 1984; Marshall *et al.*, 1991b).

Chronic subdural haematomas may occur and often present with macrocrania (30%), seizures (50%), vomiting (51%), weight loss, anaemia and fever. Subdural

taps via the anterior fontanelle or burr holes may be sufficient to treat the collection. A subduroperitoneal shunt may be required and in refractory cases where there is a chronic membrane a craniotomy may be required to drain the subdural (which may be compartmentalized) and excise the membrane.

Intracerebral haematomas (ICH) may occur after a penetrating injury or in association with a contusion. They are associated with raised ICP, a focal neurological deficit and an increased incidence of severely brain-damaged patients (Teasdale *et al.*, 1982). Intracerebral clots occur in 3% of paediatric head injuries, while in adults ICH are diagnosed in 10% of patients. It is relatively unusual in paediatric practice for the clot to be large enough to merit craniotomy and evacuation.

Raised intracranial pressure

An increase in the volume of the skull contents leads to an increase in ICP. The intracranial constituents by

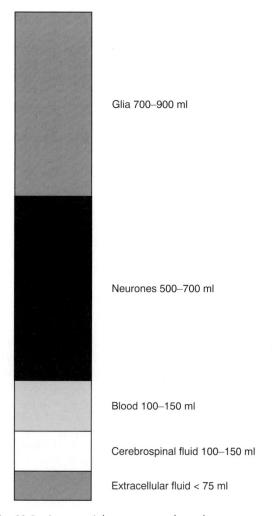

Fig. 69.2   Intracranial components by volume.

volume are shown in Fig. 69.2 and the relationship between pressure and volume is illustrated in Fig. 69.1. A rise in ICP is initially deferred by compensatory loss of CSF into the lumbar thecal sac or a reduction in cerebral blood volume (CBV). The slope of the pressure–volume curve depends on the rate of volume change. Eventually, brain tissue is compressed, brain shifts and intracranial herniation occur and CBF falls, resulting in global cerebral ischaemia. In the context of an acute head injury raised ICP results from an expanding intracranial haematoma, brain swelling or cerebral oedema (focal or generalized).

The ICP normally ranges between 0 and 10 mmHg in children and adolescents. Raised ICP in head-injured patients is associated with increased mortality. Patients in whom ICP ranges from 0 to 20 mmHg have a mortality of 23%. If the ICP rises above 60 mmHg mortality is 100% (Marmarou *et al.*, 1991). An expanding intracranial lesion produces a well-recognized sequence of events, which is summarized in Table 69.3.

At post mortem, pressure necrosis in the parahippocampal gyri is the cardinal pathological sign of raised ICP in life (Adams and Graham, 1976). In practice, aggressive management of raised ICP has resulted in improved patient outcome without any increase in severely disabled or vegetative survivors. Selective ICP monitoring, guided by CT appearances, assessment of the buffering capacity of the neural axis, ICP pulse wave analysis and appropriate use of CSF drainage, hyperventilation, propofol and barbiturates, mannitol and frusemide, may avoid refractory intracranial hypertension and prevent secondary global cerebral ischaemia in children (Marmarou, 1987; Dearden and Miller, 1989).

Diffuse brain damage

The proportion of high-velocity injuries has led to an increasing appreciation of the clinical consequences, severity and pathogenesis of closed diffuse brain damage.

Diffuse axonal injury

Pathologically, the syndrome of diffuse axonal injury (DAI) includes a focal lesion in the corpus callosum, a focal lesion in the dorsolateral brainstem and evidence of diffuse injury to axons. Lesions in the corpus callosum and brainstem can be detected macroscopically in the fixed brain. In young children brainstem and corpus callosum lesions are less common than subcortical white matter lesions. Histological evidence of axonal injury must be present if the diagnosis is to be established. If survival is short (i.e. days) there are axon retraction bulbs throughout the white matter of the hemispheres, cerebellum and brainstem. If the patient survives for weeks microglial clusters can be identified. Patients who remain vegetative for months exhibit long tract degeneration throughout the hemispheres, brainstem and spinal cord. However, DAI cannot be diagnosed in patients with short survival times (48 hours). Patients with DAI have been shown to have a lower incidence of skull fracture, contusions, haematomas and raised ICP but the frequency of hypoxic brain damage and brain swelling is similar to that in patients without DAI (Adams *et al.*, 1980a).

In subhuman primates it has proved possible to quantify axonal injury using a grading system (Gennarelli, 1983). Animals with only retraction bulbs or microglial stars were classified as grade 1. Animals with corpus callosum lesions were grade 2 and those with brainstem lesions grade 3. Pilz (1983) has suggested that differing degrees of axonal injury occur in humans, and Povlishock *et al.* (1983) has found axon retraction bulbs in cats after minor head injury and also identified axon swellings without axon disruption.

Whilst patients with grade 3 axonal injury probably remain severely disabled or vegetative, those with less severe axonal injury have persisting intellectual or cognitive problems.

Hypoxic brain damage

Hypoxic brain damage is found in 43% of patients, (Adams *et al.*, 1980b), usually in the arterial boundary zones, but also diffusely distributed throughout the brain. Patients with documented hypoxia, hypotension and raised ICP are more likely to develop hypoxic brain damage, which probably results from an inadequate CPP.

Table 69.3 Raised intracranial pressure: brain shifts and clinical consequences

Brain shift	Consequence
Subfalcine shift	Possible ipsilateral anterior cerebral artery occlusion
Tentorial herniation	Deterioration in level of consciousness Limb weakness on the same side as lesion Dilation of pupil: no reaction to light
Tonsillar herniation	Brainstem compression Deterioration in level of consciousness Respiratory and cardiovascular irregularities

Diffuse brain swelling

This type of diffuse damage is reported to occur more commonly in children and has been emphasized in patients with trivial injuries (Bruce *et al.*, 1981) who may be at risk from delayed deterioration. It is likely that brain swelling initially occurs because of changes in cerebral blood volume but later vasogenic oedema may supervene. Early seizures and enhanced small vessel permeability may contribute to this sort of brain swelling, which may also follow diffuse hypoxic brain damage. The diagnosis is made on a CT scan which shows obliteration of the third ventricle, basal cisterns or both. Delayed deterioration is more frequent in patients who are in coma for more than 1 hour and in those who sustain a hypotensive insult (Lang *et al.*, 1994). Children who are in coma for less than 1 hour and those who are not systemically shocked rarely deteriorate and in these patients a full recovery may be anticipated. All patients with diffuse brain swelling should be managed in a NSU. If refractory intracranial hypertension persists despite intensive medical management a small selected group of patients may require a cranial expansion procedure.

Diffuse vascular injury

Tomlinson (1970) has reviewed the importance of this type of brain damage, thought to be the result of severe shearing injury and incompatible with survival. This form of brain damage tends to occur in victims of road traffic accidents.

Radiology

CT SCAN CLASSIFICATION

Table 69.3 depicts the diagnostic categories used for adult patients by the Traumatic Coma Data Bank (Marshall *et al.*, 1991a), and this can be used to classify patterns of CT brain damage in children. Included in this classification are:

(1) mass lesions (intracerebral or extracerebral, high density, 15 cm^3 or greater)
(2) bilateral diffuse swelling (compressed or obliterated cisterns)
(3) diffuse brain swelling with shift (>3 mm)
(4) diffuse axonal injury, small parenchymal or intraventricular haemorrhages (<15 cm^3) without swelling or shift (>3 mm) or a mass lesion
(5) other abnormality
(6) normal CT scan.

This method of classifying CT scans has been shown to be reliable across different personnel and the overall outcome relates to the findings on the CT scan.

Management of head-injured patients

The immediate priorities are control of the airway, maintenance of normal arterial blood gases and maintenance of normal systemic blood pressure. This includes the recognition and first-aid management of extracranial injuries to avoid hypoxia and hypotension.

In severe head injury some 32% of patients have a long bone or pelvic fracture, 22% a maxillofacial injury, 23% a major chest injury, 7% abdominal trauma and 2% had a spinal injury (Miller *et al.*, 1978). The increased morbidity and mortality in hypoxic and hypotensive patients has been clearly established. Hypotension results in poor cerebral perfusion which, in turn, causes microvascular damage and ultimately ischaemic cell death. This can be compounded by hypoxia which, in turn, results in membrane disruption and anoxic cell death due to altered metabolism.

Subsequent treatment of a head-injured patient depends on the nature and severity of the head injury and whether or not there are related extracranial injuries requiring definitive management.

ADMISSION TO HOSPITAL

Some 80% of head-injured patients have a mild head injury. These patients have either not been unconscious or have regained consciousness within 5 min. Most children who have sustained such an injury can be discharged to the care of a responsible adult provided clear instructions are given about the changes to look for and how to respond should they occur. These children should be alert and have no abnormal neurological signs. A skull fracture must be excluded on skull X-rays. Children are more difficult to assess than adults and the threshold for admission should be lower. Clinical common sense must always be used and it may be prudent to admit children with a coexisting medical problem such as a coagulopathy.

Any patient with an altered conscious level, i.e. Glasgow Coma Scale (GCS) < 15, a skull fracture, a CSF leak, epilepsy or abnormal neurological signs should be admitted to hospital. In the UK patients are usually admitted to orthopaedic or paediatric surgical wards for assessment and continued observation.

Observation includes the initial assessment and continuing assessment of respiratory function, blood pressure, conscious level and neurological signs.

EFFECT OF INJURY ON CONSCIOUS LEVEL

The simplest method available to assess conscious level is the GCS (Teasdale and Jennett, 1974). Three features are independently observed: eye opening, verbal response and motor response. A modification of the

Table 69.4 Glasgow Coma Scale: adults and children

Function	Adults	Infants and children	Score
Eye opening	Spontaneous	Spontaneous	4
	To command	To sound	3
	To pain	To pain	2
	None	None	1
Verbalization	Orientated	Appropriate for age Fixes and follows Social smile	5
	Disorientated	Cries but consolable	4
	Inappropriate	Persistently irritable	3
	Incomprehensible	Restless, lethargic	2
	None	None	1
Motor	Obeys commands	Spontaneous	6
	Localizes pain	Same	5
	Withdraws	Same	4
	Reflex reflexion	Same	3
	Reflex extension	Same	2
	None	Same	1
Total score			15

system is used in children, (Table 69.4). Using this system a baseline score is recorded, which reflects the severity of the impact. Subsequent scores are then recorded so that the patient's progress can be determined. Later recordings reflect recovery from the initial effects of the head injury and the effects of secondary brain damage.

GUIDELINES FOR CT SCANNING

After a head injury the CT appearances allow classification of head injury based on the pathophysiological disturbances described above. This facilitates management decisions but, more importantly, the CT appearances in patients with a severe head injury are an independent predictor of outcome.

GUIDELINES FOR TRANSFER TO A REGIONAL NEUROSURGICAL UNIT

A small proportion (3–5%) of head-injured patients are transferred to a regional NSU (Jennett and MacMillan, 1981) usually because of a deterioration in conscious level, the presence of abnormal neurological signs, the detection of recognized risk factors for developing intracranial haematomas or because specific complications of head injury requiring neurosurgical intervention are diagnosed. Whilst the transfer of comatose children for neurosurgical management is generally accepted, the transfer of less severely head-injured children, for neurosurgical assessment, is also appropriate

if morbidity and mortality from head injury is to be reduced (Klauber *et al.*, 1989). Because patients with minor and moderate head injuries are more likely to have extracranial injuries they should have access to a regional trauma service (Miller *et al.*, 1992a).

What happens in the NSU

The principal remit of a neurosurgical service is intensive management of the head-injured patient. Operative intervention would include evacuation of intracranial haematomas, removal of contusions causing mass effect and ICP monitoring. Indications for pressure monitoring include:

- diffuse head injury, patient in coma (GCS < 8)
- diffuse head injury, altered conscious level
- CT scan showing raised ICP
- patient intubated, paralysed and ventilated
- focal brain damage, occult intracranial mass lesion
- postoperatively after removal of all intradural lesions
- postoperatively after EDH, patient in coma preoperatively.

Other responsibilities of the NSU include non-operative management of occult intracranial traumatic mass lesions and treatment of specific complications of head injury. The intensive care of the mild, moderately severe or severe head injury in the context of severe polytrauma must constitute one of the most important responsibilities of the neurosurgeon. This is all the more crucial given the evidence that intensive treatment of head-injured patients does not increase the proportion of severely disabled or vegetative survivors (Becker *et al.*, 1977; Bowers and Marshall, 1980; Miller *et al.*, 1981; Marshall *et al.*, 1983).

Specific complications of head injury

SCALP INJURIES

Some 20% of the cardiac output is to the head and neck. Substantial blood loss from the scalp may occur over a very short period, particularly in the infant and small child. Most scalp wounds can be simply closed after haemostasis and debridement. A tetanus booster should be given to a child older than 10 years if the wound is contaminated. Where there has been tissue loss, hair bearing scalp is mobilized with a blood supply and used in the repair. Most wounds can be dealt with using an advancement flap, but transposition and rotation flaps may be required. Large defects need pedicled, cutaneous or myocutaneous flaps. Tissue expansion may be required. Complex flaps require collaboration between the neurosurgeon and plastic surgeon.

DEPRESSED SKULL FRACTURES

Approximately 50% of depressed fractures occur in children (Millett and Jennett, 1968; Braakman, 1972; Jennett *et al.*, 1979). Non-compound depressed fractures are elevated if there is a cosmetic deformity or neurological deficit. Compound fractures, unless located over a major venous sinus, are usually elevated, any associated dural tear is repaired and the bone fragments are cleaned and replaced unless heavily contaminated. Complications of a depressed fracture include an intracranial haematoma, intracranial infection (meningitis or an intracerebral abscess), epilepsy (30% if the dura is torn) and associated cortical contusion or laceration. A neurological deficit is seen in some 10% of children (Steinbok *et al.*, 1987). The ping-pong fracture may be seen in the neonate and management is controversial. Operation is usually advised when there is a neurological deficit, evidence of raised ICP or CSF deep to the galea, or when conservative treatment has failed (Loeser *et al.*, 1976).

CSF LEAKS

Skull base fractures occur in 5% of head-injured children (Einhorn and Mizrahi, 1978). Anterior fossa fractures, with CSF rhinorrhoea, are more common than a fracture of the petrous pyramid. Conscious patients should be nursed head-up to reduce the intracranial CSF pressure. Prophylactic antibiotics are not given routinely because there is no clear evidence supporting their use (Klastersky *et al.*, 1976).

Spontaneous cessation of the leak may occur but CSF rhinorrhoea persisting for more than 2 weeks should be surgically repaired. CSF otorrhoea usually stops spontaneously. The decision on surgical repair should be deferred for at least 3 weeks.

The spontaneous settling of a CSF leak does not protect the patient from subsequent meningitis and early investigation should be carried out in patients with CSF rhinorrhoea to localize the fistula. This is best done by scanning the anterior cranial fossa using 2 mm CT scans windowed on a bone algorithm. Examinations with intrathecal contrast may be required but are only of value in patients with an active CSF leak.

Once the fistula has been identified operative repair is undertaken. Postoperative CSF leaks may occur, but this risk has to be balanced against the risk of meningitis (Eljamel and Foy, 1990).

TRAUMATIC AEROCOELE

Air may enter the skull after basal fractures and is usually readily visible on 'brow up' lateral views. The air may be subarachnoid, subdural, intraventricular or intracerebral. Urgent decompression may be required if the aerocoele is responsible for a clinical deterioration but usually a deferred dural repair is required after the patient has recovered from the acute effects of the head injury.

CRANIOFACIAL REPAIR

Complex disruption of the craniofacial skeleton with associated cerebral and ophthalmological problems may occur after a severe craniofacial injury. Effective management depends on accurate assessment of the primary brain damage, safe initial care, early transfer to a neurosurgical unit and early (<48 hours) single stage craniofacial repair in selected patients. Close co-operation among neurosurgeons, maxillofacial surgeons and ophthalmologists is required. CT in axial and coronal planes with bone algorithms is essential to visualize fractures of the anterior cranial fossa, orbits, skull base and facial skeleton.

Craniofacial repair involves a bifrontal craniotomy and total subperiosteal exposure of the upper and midfacial skeleton. A superior orbitotomy may be required to improve access to the anterior cranial fossa floor and reduce brain retraction. Retraction is also minimized by the use of routine intraoperative spinal drainage. The operation is tailored to the individual patient but routinely involves reconstruction of the anterior cranial fossa, a dural repair, orbital reconstruction, decompression of the optic nerves and reconstruction of the upper facial width and projection (preceded by reduction and immobilization of the zygoma) followed by reconstruction of the nasoethmoidal complex, midface and mandible. Autogenous bone (split or full-thickness calvarium in infants and young children) and rigid fixation are used to achieve an accurate and three-dimensional repair. This allows continued growth with a good functional and cosmetic result.

GROWING SKULL FRACTURES

These lesions are usually seen in infants less than 1 year old and rarely seen after the age of 3 years. Surgical repair may be complex. The dural edges tend to retract beneath the limits of the bone defect. There may be an underlying cyst to fenestrate. The dura must be repaired: in the older child cranioplasty (partial-thickness calvarium) is required while in the younger child calvarial reconstruction may be deferred with the expectancy that the defect will close spontaneously.

TRAUMATIC ANEURYSMS

These are rare but an estimated 20% of the total reported occurred in children (Fox, 1983). A traumatic aneurysm may present with haemorrhage, (delayed) epistaxis or a cranial nerve palsy. Angiography is required and clipping or excision and reconstruction are recommended.

CAROTICOCAVERNOUS FISTULA

These complicate fractures of the sphenoid and the aneurysm or dissection then produces a cavernous sinus syndrome. Endovascular treatment is preferred, with direct surgical repair usually being reserved for failed endovascular treatment.

Results

There are a number of predictors of outcome after a severe head injury, including the postresuscitation GCS, pupillary responses, age, ICP and intracranial diagnosis (CT scan) (Marmarou *et al.*, 1991; Marshall *et al.*, 1991a). After a severe head injury overall mortality in children at 6 months is 6% in patients looked after in NSUs, which are experienced and committed to the care of head-injured children. Severe disability or persistent vegetative state is rare (1–2%) in children (Bruce *et al.*, 1978; Berger *et al.*, 1985; Walker *et al.*, 1985). A good recovery or moderate disability has been reported in 90% of children in coma for 3 months or less (Brink *et al.*, 1970, 1980; Bruce *et al.*, 1978). Of 120 infants rendered comatose after a head injury, Hoffman and Taecholan (186) reported that 84 were neurologically intact, two were mentally retarded, eight had neurological and intellectual deficits, four had neurological deficits, seven had epilepsy and six developed hydrocephalus. The most common sequel to a severe head injury is ataxia and spasticity (Bruce *et al.*,

1978). After prolonged coma, intellectual deficits, instability, hyperkinesia and aggressive behaviour occur, and are more severe in young children (Levin *et al.*, 1983).

POST-TRAUMATIC EPILEPSY

One to five per cent of head-injured children develop epilepsy, compared with 8–15% of adult patients (Hendrick and Harris, 1968; Hauser, 1983). Early epilepsy occurs in 2–5% of children. Late epilepsy tends to occur when children have been in prolonged coma, after a depressed fracture or in association with an intracranial haematoma. The incidence of epilepsy in this group is 12%.

TRANSFER FROM THE NSU

In the UK, once there is no further need for acute neurosurgical observation or intervention it is standard practice to discharge the patient to a district hospital paediatric unit for continuing care. This usually involves respiratory care, nutritional support and aggressive treatment of any residual extracranial problems. Ideally, the patient should then commence rehabilitation.

REHABILITATION OF THE HEAD-INJURED CHILD

Multiple disabilities are frequent and include cognitive problems, due to amnesia or deterioration in IQ, behavioural difficulties, communication problems, physical disabilities and impairment of the special senses, including vision and hearing. Control of epilepsy may be difficult and anticonvulsants may aggravate existing cognitive problems. Effective rehabilitation includes social reintegration of the child, resumption of education and assistance with physical requirements to ensure mobility.

References

Adams, J.H. and Graham, D.I. 1976: The relationship between ventricular fluid pressure and the neuropathology of raised intracranial pressure. *Neuropathology and Applied Neurobiology* **2**, 323–32.

Adams, J.H. and Graham, D.I. 1984: Diffuse brain damage in non missile head injury. In Anthony, P.P. and MacSween, R.M.N. (eds), *Recent advances in histopathology*, vol. 12. Edinburgh: Churchill Livingstone.

Adams, J.H., Graham, D.I., Murray, L.S. and Scott, G. 1980a: Diffuse axonal injury due to non missile head injury in humans: an analysis of 45 cases. *Annals of Neurology* **12**, 557–63.

Adams, J.H., Graham, D.I., Scott, G., Parker, L.S. and Doyle, D. 1980b: Brain damage in fatal non missile head injury: observations in man and subhuman primates. *Journal of Clinical Pathology* **33**, 1132–45.

Annegers, J.F. 1983: The epidemiology of head trauma in children. In Shapiro, K. (ed.), *Paediatric head trauma.* New York: Futura, 1–10.

Annegers, J.F., Grabow, J.D., Kurland, L.T. and Laws, E.R. 1980: The incidence, causes and secular trends of head trauma in Olmsted County, Minnesota, 1935–1974. *Neurology* **30**, 912–19.

Becker, D.P., Miller, J.D., Ward, J.D., Greenberg, R.P., Young, H.F. and Sakalas, R. 1977: The outcome from severe head injury with early diagnosis and intensive management. *Journal of Neurosurgery* **47**, 491–502.

Berger, D.P., Pitts, L.H., Lovely, M., Edwards, M.S.B. and Bartkowski, H.M. 1985: Outcome form severe head injury in children and adolescents. *Journal of Neurosurgery* **62**, 194–9.

Bowers, S.A. and Marshall, L.F. 1980: Outcome in 200 consecutive cases of severe head injury treated in San Diego County: a prospective analysis. *Neurosurgery* **6**, 237–42.

Boulis, Z.F., Dick, R. and Barnes, N.R. 1978: Head injuries in children – aetiology, symptoms, physical findings and X-ray wastage. *Journal of Radiology* **51**, 851–4.

Braakman, R. 1972: Depressed skull fracture: data, treatment and follow up in 225 consecutive cases. *Journal of Neurology, Neurosurgery and Psychiatry* **35**, 395–402.

Brink, J.D., Garrett, A.L., Hale, W.R., Woo-Sam, J. and Nickel, V.L. 1970: Recovery of motor and intellectual function in children sustaining severe head injuries. *Developmental Medicine and Child Neurology* **12**, 565–71.

Brink, J.D., Imbus, C. and Woo-Sam, J. 1980: Physical recovery after severe closed head trauma in children and adolescents. *Journal of Pediatrics* **97**, 721–7.

Bruce, D.A., Alavi, A., Bilanuik, L.T., Kolinskas, C., Obrist, W. and Uzzell, B. 1981: Diffuse cerebral swelling following head injuries in children: the syndrome of 'malignant brain oedema'. *Journal of Neurosurgery* **54**, 170–8.

Bruce, D.A., Schut, L., Bruno, J., Wood, J. and Sutton, L. 1978: Outcome following severe head injuries in children. *Journal of Neurosurgery* **48**, 679–88.

Choux, M. and Lena, G. 1984: Les epanchements sous duraux du nourrisson. In David, M. and Floret, D. (eds), *Pediatrie.* Villeurbanne: SIMEP, 445–51.

Choux, M. 1986: Incidence, diagnosis and management of skull fractures in infants. In Raimondi, A.J., Choux, M. and Di Rocco, C. (eds), *Principles of paediatric neurosurgery: head injuries in newborn and infant,* New York: Springer, 163–82.

Choux, M. and Genitori, L. 1985: Depressed skull fractures in children. *Journal of Paediatric Neuroscience* **1**, 157–67.

Choux, M., Lena, G., Genitori, L., Empime, E. and Dechambenois, G. 1990: Paediatric head injuries. In Vinken, P.J., Bruyn, G.W. and Klawans, H.L. (eds), *Handbook of clinical neurology*, vol. 13 (57). Amsterdam: Elsevier, 327–44.

Committee on Trauma 1985: *Advanced trauma life support.* Chicago, IL: American College of Surgeons.

Craft, A.H., Shaw, D.A. and Cartlidge, N.E. 1972: Head injuries in children. *British Medical Journal* **834**, 200–3.

Dearden, N.M. and Miller, J.D. 1989: Paired comparison of hypnotic and osmotic therapy in the reduction of intracranial hypertension after severe head injury. In Hoff, J.T. and Betz, A.L. (eds), *ICP*, vol. VII. Berlin: Springer, 474–81.

DiRocco, C. and Verladi, F. 1986: Epidemiology and etiology of craniocerebral trauma in the first two years of life. In Raimondi, A.J., Choux, M. and DiRocco, C. (eds), *Principles in paediatric neurosurgery: head injuries in the newborn and infant.* New York: Springer, 927–34.

Einhorn, A. and Mizrahi, E.M. 1978: Basilar skull fractures in children. The incidence of CNS infection and the use of antibiotics. *American Journal of Disease in Children* **132**, 1121.

Eisenberg, H.M., Cayard, C. and Papanicolaou, F.F. 1983: The effects of three potentially preventable complications on outcome after severe closed head injury. In Ishal, S., Nagai, H. and Brock, M. (eds), *Intracranial pressure V.* Tokyo: Springer, 549–53.

Eljamel, M.S. and Foy, P.M. 1990: Acute traumatic CSF fistula: the risk of intracranial infection. *British Journal of Neurosurgery* **4**, 381–6.

Fox, J.L. 1983: Traumatic intracranial aneurysms. In Fox, J.L. (ed.), *Intracranial aneurysms.* New York: Springer, 1453–63.

Gennarelli, T. 1983: Head injury in man and experimental animals – clinical aspects. *Neurochirurgie* **32**, 1–13.

Gennarelli, T., Thibault, L.E. and Adams, J.H. 1982: Diffuse axonal injury and traumatic coma in the primate. *Annals of Neurology* **12**, 564–74.

Gildenberg, P.L. and Mekela, M.E. 1985: The effect of early intubation and ventilation following head trauma. In Dacey, R.G., Winn, R.R. *et al.* (eds), *Trauma of the central nervous system.* New York: Raven Press.

Gutierrez, F.A. and Raimondi, A.J. 1975: Acute subdural hematoma in infancy and childhood. *Child's Brain* **1**, 269–90.

Hauser, W.A. 1983: Post traumatic epilepsy in children. In Shapiro, K. (ed.), *Pediatric head trauma.* New York: Futura, 241–69.

Hendrick, E.B. and Harris, L. 1968: Post traumatic epilepsy in children. *Journal of Trauma* **8**, 547–55.

Hendrick, E.B., Harwood-Nash, D.C. and Hudson, A.R. 1964: Head injuries in children: a survey of 4465 consecutive cases at the hospital for sick children, Toronto. *Clinical Neurosurgery* **11**, 46–65.

Hoffman, H. and Taecholan, C. Outcome of craniocerebral trauma in infants In Raimondi, A.J., Choux, M. and Di Rocca, C. (eds), *Head injuries in the newborn and infant.* New York: Springer, 257–62.

Ingraham, F.D. and Matson, D.D. 1944: Subdural haematoma in infancy. *Journal of Pediatrics* **24**, 3–37.

Jennett, B. 1974: Epilepsy after non missile depressed fracture. *Journal of Neurosurgery* **41**, 208–15.

Jennett, B. and MacMillan, R. 1981: Epidemiology of head injury. *British Medical Journal* **282**, 101–4.

Jennett, B., Miller, J.D. and Braakman, R. 1979: Epilepsy after non missile depressed fracture. *Journal of Neurosurgery* **41**, 208.

Klastersky, J., Sadeghi, M. and Brihaye, J. 1976: Antimicrobial prophylaxis in patients with rhinorrhoea or otorrhoea: a double blind study. *Surgical Neurology* **6**, 111–14.

Klauber, M.R., Barrett-Connor, E., Marshall, L.F. and Bowers, S.A. 1981: The epidemiology of head injury. *American Journal of Epidemiology* **113**, 500–9.

Klauber, M.R., Marshall, L.F., Luerssen, T.G. *et al.* 1989: Determinants of head injury mortality: importance of the low risk patient. *Neurosurgery* **24**, 31–6.

Lang, D.A., Macpherson, P., Lawrence, A. and Teasdale, G.M. 1994: Diffuse brain swelling after head injury – more often malignant in children than adults. *Journal of Neurosurgery* **80**, 675–80.

Levin, H.S., Eisenberg, H.M. and Miner, M.E. 1983: Neuropsychological findings in head injured children. In Shapiro, K. (ed.) *Pediatric head trauma.* New York: Futura, 241–69.

Loeser, J.D., Kilburn, H.L. and Jolley, T. 1976: Management of depressed skull fracture in the newborn. *Journal of Neurosurgery* **44**, 62.

Marmarou, A.D. 1987: Contribution of CSF and vascular factors to elevation of ICP in severely head injured patients. *Journal of Neurosurgery* **66**, 883–90.

Marmarou, A.M., Anderson, R.L., Ward, J.D. *et al.* 1991: Impact of ICP instability and hypotension on outcome in patients with severe head injury. *Journal of Neurosurgery* **75**, 559–66.

Marshall, L.F., Becker, D.P., Bowers, S.A. *et al.* 1983: The National Traumatic Coma Data Bank Part 1. Design, purpose, goals and results. *Journal of Neurosurgery* **59**, 276–84.

Marshall, L.F., Eisenberg, H.M., Jane, J.A. *et al.* 1991a: A new classification of head injury based on computerised tomography. *Journal of Neurosurgery* **75**, 14–20.

Marshall, L.F., Gautille, T. and Klauber, M.R. 1991b: The outcome of severe closed head injury. *Journal of Neurosurgery* **75** (Suppl.) 28–36.

McClelland, C.Q., Rekate, H., Kaufman, B. and Persse, L. 1980: Cerebral injury in child abuse: a changing profile. *Child's Brain* **7**, 225–35.

Melchior, J.C. 1961: The incidence of head injuries in children. *Acta Paediatrica* **50**, 47.

Miller, J.D. and Jennett, B. 1968: Complications after depressed skull fracture. *Lancet* **ii**, 991.

Miller, J.D., Butterworth, J.F., Gudeman, S.K. *et al.* 1981: Further experience in the management of severe head injury. *Journal of Neurosurgery* **54**, 289–99.

Miller, J.D., Jones, P.A., Dearden, N.M. and Tocher, J.L. 1992a: Progress in the management of head injury. *British Journal of Surgery* **79**, 60–4.

Miller, J.D., Narayan, R., Sweet, R.C. and Becker, D.P. 1978: Early insults to the injured brain. *Journal of the American Medical Association* **240**, 439–42.

Miller, J.D., Tochler, J.L. and Jones, P.A. 1992b: Extradural haematoma – earlier detection, better results. *Brain Injury* **2**, 83–6.

Penfold, C.N., Lang, D.A. and Evans, B.T. 1992: The management of orbital roof fractures. *British Journal of Oral and Maxillofacial Surgery* **30**, 97–103.

Pilz, P. 1983: The significance of nerve fibre tearing in brain trauma. *Acta Neurochirgica* **32**, 119–23.

Povlishock, J.T., Becker, D.P., Cheng, C.L.Y. and Vaughan, G.W. 1983: Axonal change in minor head injury. *Journal of Neuropathology and Experimental Neurology* **42**, 225–42.

Report of a Working Party of the British Paediatric Association and British Association of Paediatric Surgeons Joint Standing Committee on Childhood Accidents 1991: *Guidelines on the management of head injuries in childhood.* London: British Paediatric Association.

Royal College of Surgeons of England 1986: *Report of the Working Party on Head Injuries.*

Shapiro, K., Marmarou, A.D. and Shulman, K. 1980: Characterisation of clinical CSF dynamics and neural axis compliance using the pressure volume index. *Annals of Neurology* **7**, 508–14.

Steinbok, P., Flodmark, O., Martens, D. and German, F.T. 1987: Management of simple depressed skull fractures in children. *Journal of Neurosurgery* **66**, 506–10.

Teasdale, G. and Jennett, B. 1974: Assessment of coma and impaired consciousness. *Lancet* **ii**, 81–4.

Teasdale, G.M., Galbraith, S. and Murray, L. 1982: Management of traumatic intracranial haematoma. *British Medical Journal* **285**, 1695–7.

Teasdale, G.M., Murray, G., Anderson, E. *et al.*, 1990: Risks of acute traumatic intracranial haematoma in children and adults: implications for managing head injuries. *British Medical Journal* **300**, 363–7.

Tomlinson, B.E. 1970: Brainstem lesions after head injury In: Sewitt, S. and Stoner, H.B. (eds), *The pathology of trauma*, vol. 4. Royal College of Pathologists. *Journal of Clinical Pathology* **23** (Suppl.) 178–86.

Walker, M.L., Mayer, T.A., Storrs, B.B. and Hylton, P.D. 1985: Pediatric head injury: factors which influence outcome. In Chapman, P.H. (ed.), *Concepts in pediatric neurosurgery.* Basel: Karger, 84–97.

Zimmerman, R.A. and Bilaniuk, L.T. 1981: Computed tomography in pediatric head trauma. *Journal of Neuroradiology* **8**, 257–71.

CHAPTER 70

Thoracic injuries

S.W. BEASLEY

Introduction	**Traumatic asphyxia**
Severe respiratory distress	**Pulmonary contusion**
Pericardial tamponade	**Aortic injuries**
Flail chest	**Oesophageal injuries**
Open pneumothorax	**Further reading**

Introduction

Thoracic injuries in children usually occur in association with multiple injuries of other organs. The ribcage of the child is elastic and pliable, which means that although fractures of the ribs are not often seen, compression injuries of the lungs and upper abdominal organs are common.

A significant thoracic injury should be suspected in any child who presents following multisystem trauma with symptoms of respiratory difficulty or evidence of blood loss. The first priority is to exclude upper airway obstruction by inspecting the mouth and pharynx for secretions, blood and vomitus. It should be checked that the tongue is not obstructing the oropharynx. Early life-threatening complications of thoracic trauma, while not common, must be recognized and treated promptly (Table 70.1).

Table 70.1 Early life-threatening complications

- Tension pneumothorax
- Major haemothorax
- Open pneumothorax
- Cardiac tamponade
- Flail chest

The most common intrathoracic injury is pulmonary contusion. In the presence of multiple injuries, contusion of the lung and traumatic rupture of the diaphragm may not be recognized unless a chest X-ray is taken as a routine. Pneumothorax, with or without haemothorax, can be a complication of pulmonary contusion.

Severe respiratory distress

There are a number of causes of sudden severe respiratory distress following major trauma. Compression of the chest may tear a major airway and cause leakage of air into the mediastinum or pleural cavity. Fractured ribs may also lacerate the lung and cause a tension pneumothorax. Air moves into the pleural space with each inspiration and remains there during expiration (Fig. 70.1). As the volume of air increases, there is a corresponding rise in pressure (tension) and the ipsilateral lung collapses. In addition, increasing tension causes a shift of the mediastinum to the contralateral side, with compression of the contralateral lung. Mediastinal shift also interferes with venous return to the heart. If unrecognized and left untreated, ventilation of the lungs becomes inadequate and cardiac output decreases.

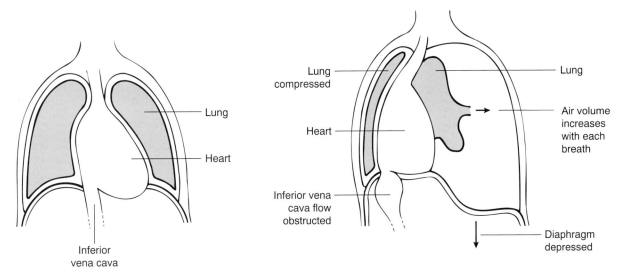

Fig. 70.1 Effect of tension pneumothorax on ventilation and venous return.

TENSION PNEUMOTHORAX

Tension pneumothorax must always be considered where there has been a major thoracic injury or fractured ribs in a child who develops rapidly progressing respiratory distress (Fig. 70.2). The chest wall moves little on the side of the pneumothorax. There is a decrease in ipsilateral breath-sounds and hyperresonance on percussion. The tracheal deviation to the contralateral side is a manifestation of mediastinal shift. In left-sided lesions, the heart-sounds become audible more easily in the right chest. As venous return is impeded by increased intrathoracic pressure, the neck veins become distended. The diagnosis is confirmed on chest X-ray, but in an emergency a 14- or 16-gauge needle should be inserted through the fourth intercostal space at the anterior axillary line of the side in which the tension pneumothorax is suspected. A chest-tube connected to an underwater drain is inserted subsequently. These manoeuvres may be life-saving. The child should be given high-flow oxygen.

HAEMOTHORAX

Laceration of an intercostal artery during rib fracture may cause major blood loss into the thorax (haemothorax). The clinical signs are similar to those seen in tension pneumothorax except that there is evidence of hypovolaemic shock, the neck veins are flat and the ipsilateral chest is dull on percussion, rather than hyper resonant.

Management involves fluid and blood resuscitation, administration of oxygen and insertion of a chest-drain to evacuate the haemothorax. Thoracotomy may be required if major intrathoracic bleeding continues, but this is uncommon.

Pericardial tamponade

Pericardial tamponade is caused when the heart is compressed between the anterior chest wall and the vertebral column, such as in crush injuries and motor vehicle accidents. There is contusion of the myocardium, with bleeding into the pericardial sac. Tamponade may also occur from penetrating wounds, e.g. stab wounds, but in most civilized areas these are uncommon in young children.

Blood in the pericardial space prevents effective contraction and refilling of the chambers of the heart, producing systemic hypotension with poor cardiac output. The child presents with increasing respiratory distress, hypotension and distended neck veins. The pulse pressure is narrow, and the pulse volume decreases with inspiration – the 'pulsus paradoxus'. The heart sounds are muffled and difficult to hear, and sometimes a pericardial friction rub is audible. Perhaps the most obvious features are the grossly distended neck veins in the presence of severe pallor and shock.

Although cardiac tamponade is anticipated after penetrating chest trauma, the diagnosis must always be considered in children after blunt trauma, when a child becomes hypotensive without an obvious source of major blood loss.

Insertion of a needle just below the xiphisternum, directed towards the left shoulder at an angle of 45° to the skin, is both diagnostic and therapeutic. There is an immediate and dramatic improvement in the child's condition. As blood is aspirated from the pericardium, the temporary relief so achieved allows a left anterolateral thoracotomy to open the pericardium and repair the underlying injury.

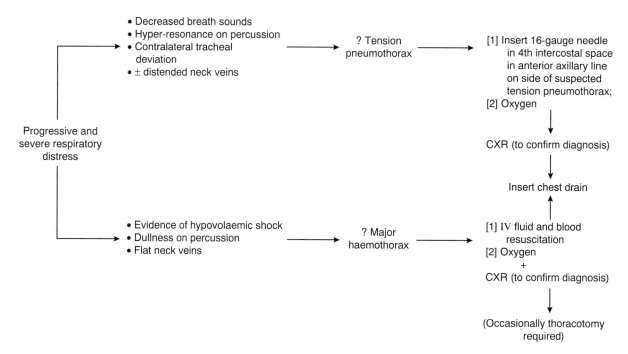

Fig. 70.2   Progressive and severe respiratory distress after thoracic trauma.

Flail chest

Flail chest is uncommon in young children because the elasticity of the thorax means that multiple fractures of the ribs occur rarely. Flail chest is more likely to be seen in the older child with multiple rib fractures. The chest wall moves asymmetrically and the flail segment moves paradoxically with respiration. It should be assumed that there is pulmonary contusion associated with flail chest. The flail segment may cause a significant haemothorax with mediastinal shift to the contralateral side. When the flail area is large enough to cause respiratory embarrassment, internal splinting by positive pressure ventilation is required. External compression or splinting is not appropriate in children.

Open pneumothorax

Although very rare in children, it is easily recognized when there is an open wound through which air and blood bubble during ventilation. The defect should be covered with an air-tight dressing, e.g. Tegaderm or Opsite, to prevent further air movement. A chest tube is inserted to allow re-expansion of the lung.

Traumatic asphyxia

Severe compression of the chest may compromise venous return through the large veins of the thoracic inlet and cause high venous pressures in the head,

neck and upper extremities. This leads to rupture of small capillaries, giving a petechial rash in the skin and subconjunctival haemorrhages. This type of injury is seen when a child has been run over at low velocity or trapped by a heavy object across the chest.

The face, neck and, to a lesser extent, the shoulders and arms, are covered with numerous red spots. The cutaneous petechiae resolve after 3 or 4 days, but the conjunctival haemorrhages may last for several weeks. When features of traumatic asphyxia are apparent, the child should be carefully observed for evidence of pulmonary contusion and other major injuries of the chest and abdomen.

Pulmonary contusion

Pulmonary contusion is the most common parenchymal injury caused by blunt trauma to the chest. There is interstitial haemorrhage into the parenchyma of the lung, with alveolar collapse. Blood and plasma extravasate into the alveoli. These changes cause a decrease in pulmonary compliance, with a concomitant increase in the work of breathing. In more severe cases, there is shunting and systemic hypoxia. The plain radiological features range from a poorly-defined infiltrate to extensive opacity.

Moderate or severe pulmonary contusion is treated by increasing the alveolar pressure with positive end expiratory pressure or continuous positive airway pressure. Its effect on ventilation peaks between 24 and 72 hours of the injury but, in severe cases, may take several weeks to resolve completely.

Aortic injuries

Thoracic aortic injuries occur after rapid deceleration and with crush injuries. They usually occur in association with other major injuries, particularly of the heart. There may be fractures of the first rib, clavicle and sternum, and plain radiology may reveal a widened mediastinum. When suspected, aortography and computer tomography (CT) imaging will confirm the diagnosis. Aortic injuries require surgical repair, and in the case of blunt trauma injuries to the ascending aorta, this is done under cardiopulmonary bypass.

Oesophageal injuries

Iatrogenic injuries to the oesophagus are seen following oesophagoscopy, particularly after oesophageal dilatation. Oesophageal perforation may also result from foreign body impaction, either by direct penetration by a sharp object or by gradual erosion of the oesophageal wall by an unrecognized object which has been stuck in the oesophagus for a long period. In iatrogenic injuries, the procedure that caused the injury is ceased immediately, oral feeds are withheld and intravenous antibiotics (e.g. cephalosporin and metronidazole) are commenced. Operative repair is reserved for those in whom an extensive laceration has occurred, or where there is established or likely mediastinal sepsis.

Further reading

Nakayama, D.K., Ramerofsky, M.L. and Rowe, M.I. 1989: Chest injuries in childhood. *Annals of Surgery* **210**, 770–5.

Peclet, M.H., Newman, K.D., Eichelberger, M.R., Gotschall, G.S., Garcia, V.F. and Bowman, L.M. 1990: Thoracic trauma in children: an indicator of increased mortality. *Journal of Pediatric Surgery* **25**, 961–6.

Scherer, L.R. 1997: Thoracic trauma. In Oldham, K.T., Colombani, P.M. and Foglia, R.P. (eds), *Surgery of infants and children: scientific principles and practice.* Lippincott–Raven, Philadelphia, PA, 455–61.

CHAPTER 71

Blunt trauma to the abdomen

R.A. BROWN

Introduction   Sequelae and outcome
Management   References
Specific visceral injuries

Introduction

Paediatric trauma is the major cause of childhood morbidity (Haller, 1983; Zorludemir *et al.*, 1988), and blunt trauma accounts for up to 80% of multiple paediatric injuries. Increasingly, recognition is being given to the differences that exist between children and adults, in their response to trauma as well as its sequelae. Dedicated paediatric trauma units and a modified paediatric trauma score (PTS) further emphasize its unique nature, and management protocols have evolved specifically for the paediatric trauma victim (Eichelberger and Randolph, 1985; Jaffe and Wesson, 1991). Boys are more prone to trauma than girls (2:1), and the 5–14-year-old group is particularly at risk. The abdomen is vulnerable to blunt trauma, being protruberant and thin-walled; the victim's short stature brings it closer to the site of impact. Rapid assessment of all the injuries and appropriate immediate treatment must be the aim of all those who are involved in paediatric trauma care.

CHILDREN VERSUS ADULTS

Physical size is markedly reduced with a high body surface-to-mass ratio, which is maximum at birth. The total blood volume is deceptively small, despite being proportionally higher in terms of body weight than in adults (7–8% vs 5–6%). Compensated blood loss is initially well tolerated, which may mask large volume losses, with the systemic blood pressure only falling after a loss of 25% of the circulating blood volume. With ongoing losses, however, sudden decompensation often follows. The possibility of underlying congenital abnormality must be taken into account as they may present with complications after minor trauma (e.g. 23% congenital renal abnormalities compared to 2% in the general population) (Murphy, 1990). Even if conscious, children are unable to explain or localize their symptoms, placing further responsibility on the attending physician.

The PTS, which includes factors specifically designed for paediatric trauma victims (e.g. size and airway), shows a significant correlation to final morbidity and mortality (Tepas *et al.*, 1988) (see Table 71.1).

AETIOLOGY

Up to 90% of trauma admissions and 90% of trauma deaths in children are due to blunt trauma (Templeton, 1993). The motor vehicle is responsible for up to 80% of victims in developing countries (Cywes *et al.*, 1990b). In developed countries, falls are the other major cause, constituting 35–45% (Eichelberger *et al.*, 1988), reflecting the child's inquisitive and at times irrational behaviour. Bumps, assaults, bicycle handlebars and sports injuries are other causes. One important group of victims of blunt trauma, constituting up to 5%, is those suffering child abuse. This cause should not be overlooked because of the proffered plausible story, and an unlikely explanation of new wounds, together with those in various stages of

Table 71.1 Paediatric trauma score

Component	+2	+1	−1
Weight (kg)	> 20	10–20	< 10
Airway patency	Normal	Maintained	Unmaintained
Systolic blood pressure (mmHg)	> 90	90–50	< 50
Neurologic status	Awake	Obtunded	Comatose
Open wound	None	Minor	Major/penetrating
Skeletal trauma	None	Closed	Open/multiple
Total (maximum 12)	> 6 Reasonable prognosis		
	< 6 ↑ injury severity/potential for mortality increases		

From Tepas *et al.* (1987).

healing, is suspicious and requires assessment and investigation by appropriately trained staff (see Chapter 74, Non-accidental injury: physical abuse).

Management

ASSESSMENT

Because of initial cardiovascular compensation for blood loss the severity of the underlying injury may be masked. The most common causes of post-traumatic shock other than intra-abdominal haemorrhage include multiple long bone and pelvic fractures, and cardiogenic shock caused by a tension pneumothorax or myocardial contusion. Even without external evidence there may be intra-abdominal visceral injury, and this must be evaluated as a potential source of blood loss. Intra-abdominal organs are particularly susceptible to trauma in the toddler and young child because the abdominal wall is thin and protruberant, the viscera are relatively large and the retroperitoneal and anterior abdominal wall fat are not as well developed. Pain, apprehension and fear which inevitably accompany a child trauma victim may make examination difficult, and the administration of an analgesic may be necessary prior to performing an objective examination. Finally, children swallow large volumes of air after an injury, resulting in acute gastric dilatation. A nasogastric tube should always be passed to deflate the stomach and so facilitate abdominal assessment (Table 71.2).

Table 71.2 Initial assessment

- Airway
- Intravenous access
- Nasogastric tube
- Urinary catheter
- Analgesia
- Maintain warmth

INITIAL MANAGEMENT AND RESUSCITATION

A systematic approach will improve the management of all paediatric trauma victims (Jaffe and Wesson, 1991). This includes a primary survey along with resuscitation, a secondary survey and appropriate investigation of selected organs with subsequent definitive treatment.

PRIMARY SURVEY AND RESUSCITATION

The first priority is to establish airway patency and adequate oxygenation. An oral airway, oxygen mask and self-inflating AMBU bag, or endotracheal intubation and mechanical ventilation are steps to ensure this. Nasogastric tube decompression of stomach may improve ventilation, and an intercostal chest drain should be inserted if a lung injury is suspected in the ventilated patient.

Restoration and maintenance of circulation is the next priority, and is covered in Chapters 14 and 15. Fluid management is summarized in Fig. 71.1. Inadequate circulation will manifest itself by tachycardia, poor peripheral tissue perfusion and hypotension, and resuscitation should aim to prevent this. A drop in systolic blood pressure is the easiest and most accurate guide for assessing blood loss and a systolic blood pressure of less than 80 mmHg in children under 5 years and less than 90 mmHg in children over 5 years old is evidence of hypovolaemia.

Intravenous access is vital, but may be problematical in a small hypotensive infant with collapsed peripheral veins. If a suitable peripheral site cannot be found, an open cutdown over one of the larger veins, e.g. long saphenous or brachiocephalic, with insertion of a cannula under direct vision, or alternatively a push-in into one of the large veins of the neck (internal jugular or subclavian) or groin (femoral), should be considered. Although not regularly used at our institution, intraosseous infusion is a reliable method for initial resuscitation, most useful in children under 6 years of age, and the technique is simple (Fiser, 1990) without

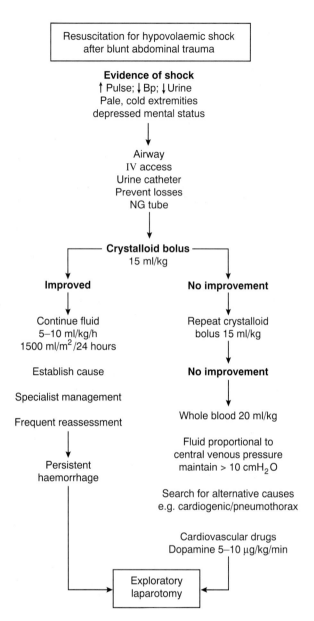

Fig. 71.1   Resuscitation regime.

major sequelae and capable of delivering up to 100 ml/h. A protocol for emergency intravenous access using a sequence of measures, i.e. peripheral line, cutdown and intraosseus infusion, has been shown to be more effective than a non-structured approach (Kanter *et al.*, 1986). Urinary output is an easy measure of confirming adequate fluid resuscitation, and a urine output of >1–2 ml/kg per hour is proof; this is best measured by insertion of a small urinary catheter early on, removed once the patient is stable.

A primary survey is conducted of other systems, including the central nervous system which is scored on the modified Glasgow coma scale (Teasdale and Jennett, 1974), examination of the neck, the chest, the back and the limbs, and appropriate emergency first-aid management is carried out where required.

SECONDARY SURVEY

This is a systematic physical examination of all body systems. Once completed, the abdomen can be scrutinized for external evidence of trauma, e.g. bruises or abrasions. Palpation may elicit areas of tenderness, and bowel sounds should be auscultated for, even though they may persist with localized injury. A rectal examination will exclude perineal injury, and macroscopic haematuria suggests renal tract damage.

Urgent laparotomy is indicated in children with evidence of massive or ongoing blood loss (> 40 ml/kg) or those with frank peritonitis. For the remainder, special investigations may be required at this stage to delineate the pathology and aid in the decision making.

ANALGESIA

No paediatric trauma victim should suffer further unnecessary pain. Tilidine hydrochloride (Valoron) drops (one per year of age) can be given sublingually and have been used at our institution, or paracetamol (20 mg/kg) orally. Alternatively, an initial bolus dose of 0.05 mg/kg followed by a continuous intravenous infusion of morphine sulphate (0.2 mg/kg in 20 ml 5% dextrose at 1–3 ml/h) is effective. Systemic response to infection, blood loss and signs of peritonitis will not be masked by providing adequate analgesia, and its action will rapidly cease on withdrawal.

INVESTIGATIONS

These play a vital role in the overall management of the blunt trauma victim, particularly with the advent of increasingly conservative management. Investigations should never be performed or interpreted in isolation, as they do not supersede the importance of careful and repeated clinical assessment of the child. They should be requested only if the information obtained will alter further management and surgical decision making (Eichelberger and Randolph, 1985). The time delay and the expense involved in special investigations may outweigh their benefit.

Routine investigations

- Conventional radiology: chest and abdominal radiographs are essential primary investigations, which can identify both visceral and pleural abnormalities as well as showing any associated skeletal injury.
- Blood investigations: these include an estimation of haemoglobin level, white cell count, mean corpuscular volume, platelet count, arterial blood gases, serum electrolytes, urea and creatinine, and amylase.

- Urine investigations/intravenous pyelogram (IVP); haematuria: see kidney and bladder sections for more details.

Immediate laparotomy without further special investigations

- Haemodynamically unstable, or failure to maintain blood pressure despite blood transfusion >40 ml/kg.
- Overt peritonitis.
- Injuries requiring surgical repair, i.e. hollow viscus rupture or diaphragm rupture.

Diagnostic peritoneal lavage (DPL)

This is a simple, low-cost investigation, which has a low complication rate (1%) with a reported accuracy of 96–98% if performed correctly (Feliciano, 1991). The bladder is emptied with gentle catheterization first. A vertical infraumbilical incision is made under local anaesthesia and a catheter inserted into the peritoneal cavity under direct vision. Normal saline (10 ml/kg) is rapidly infused, and then the infusate is drained and sent for laboratory assessment. A positive test is defined as >100 000 red blood cells (RBC)/ml, >500 white blood cells (WBC)/mm^3, bacteria or vegetable matter on microscopy, or raised bile or amylase levels. If the presence of blood alone is taken as positive, it will result in an unacceptably high incidence of unnecessary laparotomy in 34–67% (Fischer *et al.*, 1978; Fabian *et al.*, 1986). DPL lacks organ specifity, may fail to detect diaphragmatic and retroperitoneal visceral injury and may make interpretation of further abdominal examinations difficult because of tenderness at the trochar site. As stated by Trunkey and Federle (1986), 'it is extremely sensitive, perhaps too sensitive, in detection of intraperitoneal haemorrhage' which *per se* is not an indication for surgery in a child. For these reasons, DPL is not routinely used in the assessment of our blunt trauma victims, although it may be particularly useful in the unconscious patient, or where serial examinations are impossible (e.g. during long neurosurgical or orthopaedic operations). The results must be interpreted together with the physical status of the patient, and should be but one factor in the decision whether to proceed to exploratory surgery (Drost *et al.*, 1991).

Ultrasound

This is a non-invasive, relatively low-cost but highly operator-dependent modality with a reported 84% sensitivity and 88% specificity (Feliciano, 1991). There is, however, a 20–25% incidence of failure to detect splenic or liver injuries (Gruessner *et al.*, 1989). In a distressed unsedated child with a tender gas-filled abdomen, examination and interpretation may be difficult. It serves as a useful screening measure at initial assessment but is best suited for follow-up studies.

Computed tomography (CT)

This imaging modality may not be available in all centres. Even when present, the examination is time consuming, taking 20–40 min to perform, with a delay of 2.5–3.0 hours from ordering to completion. It is, however, non-invasive unless contrast is used and accurately localizes the injured solid viscus in 92–98% of cases (Feliciano, 1991). Its use is of particular benefit in the patient when examination is difficult (e.g. the unconscious patient where extended operation time is anticipated) and in the patient with multiple injuries if haematuria and a renal injury is suspected and functional assessment of the kidneys is essential. Simultaneous intravenous injection of contrast material can assess the anatomy and function of the involved viscus. An incidental finding is the visual demonstration of post-traumatic shock, or an anatomical snapshot in time (Kirks *et al.*, 1992), where despite clinical stability after resuscitation, there is evidence on dynamic scan of a hypoperfusion complex, more common in young patients, which is a marker of severe injury with a high incidence (85%) of fatal outcome (Sivit *et al.*, 1992).

Provided the facility is available and the patient is haemodynamically stable, CT is the primary mode of evaluating blunt abdominal trauma in children, as it surveys the entire abdominal cavity, as well as detecting extra-abdominal injuries, particularly thoracic and musculoskeletal. Clinical signs (e.g. haematuria, tenderness, abrasions or pelvic fractures) and mechanism of trauma (e.g. assault or lap belt injury) in a patient with a low PTS (Table 71.1) have been shown to correlate accurately with an increased risk of abdominal injury and more than 50% of these children will have a significant abdominal injury on CT scan (Taylor *et al.*, 1991). It is less accurate in detecting bowel injuries (Fischer *et al.*, 1988; Bulas *et al.*, 1989) and may be oversensitive in detecting intraperitoneal haemorrhage (Trunkey and Federle, 1986), but it is almost 100% accurate in distinguishing a surgical from a non-surgical abdomen.

Scintiscan

This technique requires a gamma camera, radioactive isotope material, an experienced radiographer and a radiologist, and is often unavailable in the emergency setting. A technetium-labelled sulphur colloid scan has been shown at our hospital to be more sensitive in detection of liver and spleen injuries than CT (Bass *et al.*, 1990), although it fails to assess any adjacent visceral or extra-abdominal injuries.

Arteriography

Arteriography is now rarely indicated as an investigation modality. The major indication for angiography was previously to evaluate the renal artery of a kidney showing absent dye excretion on IVP. The usage of dynamic CT scans has reduced its indications. Interventional radiologic techniques for identifying the source and control of pelvic bleeding with embolization are now accepted practice.

Laparoscopy

With the recent increasing safe application of laparoscopic surgery (complication rate 3% and mortality 8/100 000) (Paterson Brown, 1991) this new technique has a role to play inimproving diagnosis. Removal of excess intraperitoneal blood is easily achieved, as is excellent exposure with good localization of any visceral injury, and the injured viscus can even be repaired via the laparoscope (Lobe and Schropp, 1993).

Missed injuries are the major concern in blunt abdominal trauma, particularly as clinical examination may fail to disclose any evidence of underlying serious visceral damage. The sequelae are exacerbated by the increasing application of non-operative management. The safest approach is to suspect an injury, and to follow-up with careful initial and then repeated physical examinations, preferably by the same attending doctor, complemented by appropriate and available diagnostic modalities. These investigations should aim to detect injuries rather than avoid operations and to expedite prompt treatment. A laparotomy is indicated in a child requiring a persistently high fluid volume to maintain the circulation, if there is evidence of toxaemia, i.e. increasing pulse rate, decreasing blood pressure and urine output, and a rising temperature, or if there are deteriorating local signs. A tertiary survey by an independent observer has been proposed for those not requiring surgical intervention, which may reveal up to a further 10% of injuries by thorough re-examination (Enderson and Maull, 1991).

Specific visceral injuries

The relative incidence of specific visceral injuries at our institution over an 11-year period is shown in Table 71.3 (Cywes *et al.*, 1990a). Despite the 732 visceral injuries in 587 patients, the laparotomy rate was only 11%, including those constituting mandatory surgery (e.g. bowel, bladder or diaphragm injury). This underlines the success of a conservative management regimen, which can be adopted in the paediatric age group as outlined in Fig. 71.2. The emphasis is placed on resuscitation, identification of the involved viscus by appropriate special investigations, and then non-surgical management unless resuscitation cannot be completed or maintained, or there are mandatory surgery visceral injuries. The advantages of non-operative management include the avoidance of anaesthetic complication, intra-abdominal sepsis, postoperative pain and

Table 71.3 Incidence of specific visceral injuries (587 children, 732 organs)

Organ	*n*	Percentage
Kidney	333	57
Liver	228	39
Spleen	96	16
Pancreas	40	7
Bowel	26	4.5
Bladder	5	0.8
Diaphragm	4	0.7

complications, as well as a decrease in the length of hospital stay and overall expense. Certain mechanisms of injury are associated with recognized patterns of visceral damage (Table 71.4).

(I) INJURY

There is a higher incidence of renal injuries after blunt trauma in the child than in the adult. Anatomical reasons play a role in this because the kidney in a child is proportionately larger and more mobile, there is less protection from a thin abdominal wall and decreased retroperitoneal fat, fetal lobulations may initiate cleavage plains, and an underlying hydronephrosis may be present. Although the victims may be asymptomatic, the nature and severity of the trauma, together with local flank tenderness or a mass point to renal injury. The efficacy of non-operative management in blunt renal trauma is now well established (Bass *et al.*, 1991; Baumann *et al.*, 1992; McAnish, 1992). In our series, only 14 out of 91 (15.3%) required surgical intervention, and of the remaining 77 only five (6.5%) developed complications (Bass *et al.*, 1991). Initial presentation with asymptomatic microscopic haematuria does not correlate with renal injury (Taylor *et al.*, 1991) and 1–3+ microscopic haematuria on testing will only identify ± 10% of minor degrees of injury on IVP. In the case of hypovolaemia or renal artery occlusion, haematuria may be absent. The IVP is the quickest, most available and cost-effective means of investigating suspected blunt renal trauma and is used in our unit. If there is macroscopic haematuria, or 4+ microscopic haematuria together with loin tenderness, the diagnostic yield may be as high as 42%, embracing all those requiring surgery. The IVP can also classify the injury, as described by Sargent and Marquard (1950); i.e. grade intrarenal contusion; grade II, parenchymal lacerations involving the renal capsule and/or the collecting system; grade III, shattered kidney or transection with nonfunction of either pole; or grade IV, injuries to the vascular pedicle.

CT, if available, has advantages over the IVP since the renal injury as well as adjacent abdominal viscera can be assessed, and simultaneous administration of contrast

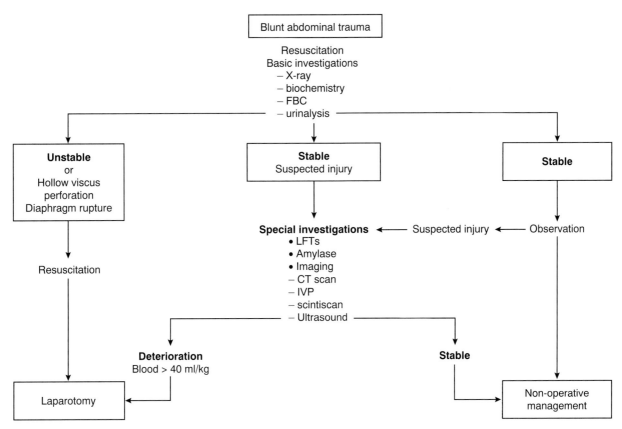

Fig. 71.2   Management protocol for blunt abdominal trauma.

demonstrates both the function of the affected as well as the contralateral kidney. The majority of injuries are grade I or II, which do not require surgical intervention and will heal on broad-spectrum antibiotics and bed rest until the haematuria clears. Grade III injuries may result in a higher complication rate, but the surgical manage-

ment in most cases consists of total nephrectomy (Guice *et al.*, 1983; Bass *et al.*, 1991) and therefore patients who remain stable after initial resuscitation are best served by non-operative management (Baumann *et al.*, 1992). Fortunately, Grade IV (renal pedicle) injuries are uncommon in children, constituting 0–5% (Karp

Table 71.4   Association with blunt abdominal trauma

Association	Organ	Features
Minor trauma	Kidney	Underlying congenital abnormality
Blunt trauma	Significant intra-abdominal injury	Incidence 30%
Head injury/neurologic impairment	Multiple abdominal viscera	Incidence 16.7% if GCS[a] < 8; 4.6% if GCS > 8
Lap belt	Intestinal injury Hyperflexion lumbar spine	Ecchymoses anterior abdominal wall Lumbar spine X-ray abnormal
Bicycle handle bar	Pancreas	
Pelvic fracture	Genitourinary	80% if multiple fractured pelvis 11% if simple fractured pelvis
Child abuse	Multiple: duodenum pancreas, kidney, bowel, liver, spleen	Higher fatal outcome. Be alert to possibility

[a]GCS: Glasgow Coma Scale (Teasdale and Jennett, 1974).

et al., 1986). Renal salvage by early vascular repair is desirable, but few (5%) truly successful revascularizations after blunt trauma have been reported (Clark *et al.*, 1981), and therefore should probably only be attempted in a patient without associated major injuries and where the kidney has been shown to be intact on preoperative scanning. Adequate proximal control of the renal artery and vein should be obtained before exploring the kidney. Warning signs for the need for surgery include major parenchymal laceration with urinary extravasation and >20% non-viable parenchyma (McAnish, 1992), or recurrent severe haematuria after >72 h observation.

Follow-up of patients should include a [99]technetium dimercaptosuccinic acid (DMSA) scan at 8 weeks to confirm resolution without scarring and a blood pressure check at 1 year to exclude the late development of hypertension. A study 1 year after conservative management showed normally functioning kidneys and one mild hypertensive out of 26 patients (Baumann *et al.*, 1992) thus supporting an initial non-operative approach. One late complication that has been reported is massive haematuria secondary to a pseudoaneurysm of an intrarenal branch of the renal artery (Teigen *et al.*, 1992). This can be diagnosed and successfully treated by embolization.

(II) HEPATOBILIARY

Haemorrhage from the liver, rather than the spleen, is the most common cause of death attributable to abdominal injury. The introduction of conservative management in the 90–95% of children who do not present with massive blood loss has been shown to be successful in 76–92% (Oldham *et al.*, 1986; Cywes *et al.*, 1991), although there is a 4–8% incidence of late complications. Liver haematomas, the most common form of liver injury after blunt trauma, expand, undergo liquefaction and are reabsorbed, as confirmed by serial ultrasound examinations.

Urgent laparotomy is indicated if there is massive bleeding (>40 ml/kg). In the remainder, the diagnosis of liver injury can be confirmed by an increase in liver enzymes [serum glutamic pyruvic transaminase (SGPT) or serum glutamic oxaloacetic transaminase (SGOT; Oldham *et al.*, 1986], CT scan or [99]technetium isotope scan (Bass *et al.*, 1990). In the conservatively managed group 21–40% require blood transfusion (Oldham *et al.*, 1986; Cywes *et al.*, 1991). Bleeding usually ceases within 72 hours. The patient can then be returned from the intensive care unit to the ward, where bedrest is advised for a further 4–7 days.

At laparotomy in the unstable group, a subcostal chevron incision is made, with a vertical xiphisternal extension if necessary. Autotransfusion of blood aspirated from the peritoneal cavity has major advantages and has been successfully used in children (Wesson *et*

al., 1980). If no significant active bleeding is present, the liver should be left alone and drained with closed suction drainage. Where there is active bleeding, suture ligation of identified bleeding points, application of local haemostatic agents (e.g. tissue glue, gelfoam or Surgicell), mattress suture hepatorraphy, local or segmental resections of devitalised parenchyma and omental packing may be employed. If these measures are unsuccessful, two techniques can temporarily halt the blood loss while the anaesthetist corrects the hypovolaemia and replaces clotting factors. Therapeutic perihepatic packing, using dry radio-opaque marked packs to tamponade the liver between the body wall and the diaphragmatic surface, is the safest, easiest and most effective emergency measure to halt the bleeding. Elective re-exploration is performed 48–72 hours later once resuscitation is complete, at which stage measures can be applied to stop any residual bleeding (Cue *et al.*, 1990; Krige *et al.*, 1992). Alternatively, hepatic vascular isolation can be achieved by controlling the inferior vena cava, both above the liver through a small pericardiodiaphragmatic incision and below it (Evans *et al.*, 1993), as well as cross-clamping the free edge of the lesser omentum with a vascular or soft bowel clamp, as proposed by Pringle (1908) (Fig. 71.3). With mobilization of the liver, the parenchymal and vascular injuries can then be repaired, particularly the vulnerable retrohepatic vessels. Vascular occlusion can safely be maintained for at least 45 min without long-term sequelae (Feliciano and Pachter, 1989; Evans *et al.*, 1993). This procedure is technically easier to perform in a child than an adult.

Although rare, complications may develop during the convalescent phase of non-operative management. Delayed rupture of a subcapsular haematoma may

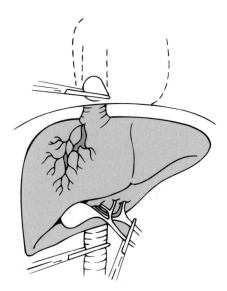

Fig. 71.3 Hepatic vascular isolation technique.

occur up to 2 weeks after injury, which can be monitored with ultrasonography and only occasionally requires open surgical drainage. An abscess may develop at or around the site of rupture (Scott *et al.*, 1988), which also requires drainage. A persistent biliary leak or bile peritonitis, confirmed by endoscopic retrograde cholangiopancreatography (ERCP), may be managed successfully with external drainage in most instances. If this fails distal decompression can be effected via a sphincterotomy or a temporary endoscopically placed biliary stent. If it is refractory, internal drainage may be successfully achieved by the placement of a Roux-en-Y loop on to the site of the bile leak (Hollands and Little, 1991; Martin *et al.*, 1992; Steiner *et al.*, 1994). Rarely, segmental hepatic resection may be necessary. Haemobilia, due to an intrahepatic false aneurysm, presents with upper gastrointestinal bleeding often associated with severe colic. The diagnosis is confirmed by endoscopy and arteriography. The aneurysm can be embolized at the same time (de Lagausie *et al.*, 1992). Rupture of the extrahepatic bile duct and/or the accompanying hepatic artery usually results from seat-belt injury and requires immediate surgical correction. The hepatic artery may be ligated without major sequelae to the liver.

(III) SPLEEN

Successful conservative management of the traumatized spleen has been the stimulus for the widespread application of non-operative management of the paediatric blunt trauma victim. The landmark paper of King and Schumaker (1952) emphasized the vital role played by the spleen in immune protection as evidenced by the increased mortality after splenectomy (0.5–3%) when compared to those with intact spleen. Singer (1983) and an American Academy of Pediatrics survey (Cogbill *et al.*, 1989) further emphasized this increased incidence of overwhelming postsplenectomy infection (OPSI) in the asplenic patient. This is due to the lack of surveillance of the spleen, particularly for encapsulated organisms, as well as failure of production of immunoglobulin M and tuftsin, which acts as an opsonic protein enhancing the bacteriocidal and phagocytic properties of neutrophils. The spleen is also a source of properdin, a vital component in the alternative complement activation pathway.

The application of conservative management is more successful in children than in adults (Delius *et al.*, 1989), for several reasons. The most important factor is a thickened splenic capsule containing functional smooth muscle and elastica, which undergoes fibroelastic replacement with ageing (Morgenstern and Uyeda, 1983). The increased incidence of indirect trauma together with a radial vascular pattern parallel to the tear, and a lower incidence of overlying rib fracture because of their increased elasticity, all contribute to decreased splenic injuries in children compared with adults (18%

vs 42.5%) (Delius *et al.*, 1989). The incidence of associated injuries, particularly to the intestine, is also lower (Oldham *et al.*, 1990).

The diagnosis may be suspected in patients with a left-sided chest injury, or with pain and tenderness in this region together with haemodynamic instability. Physical signs may be absent, although flank ecchymoses (Turner's sign) or periumbilical bruising (Cullen's sign) and tenderness on rectal examination are supporting evidence. A screening abdominal radiograph may show an elevated left hemidiaphragm, inferomedial stomach displacement or evidence of intraperitoneal fluid. The diagnosis can be confirmed on ultrasound, ^{99}technetium colloid scan, or CT, with its advantage of quantifying the severity as well as demonstrating any other visceral damage. Diagnostic peritoneal lavage will confirm a haemoperitoneum without localizing its origin.

Treatment is aimed at splenic preservation, with or without surgery. Conservative management includes resuscitation and intensive monitoring of the patient's condition for at least 48–72 hours while maintaining haemodynamic stability. If in the initial resuscitation period the blood volume transfused exceeds 40 ml/kg or there is suspicion of a mandatory laparotomy injury, urgent laparotomy should be performed. For those managed without surgery, bed rest should be continued until the tenderness resolves (usually 2–4 days), with discharge on day 7 and advice to restrict physical activity for 8–12 weeks. A follow-up scan to confirm complete healing should be performed at this stage. The incidence of successful conservative management ranges from 87 to 98% (King and Schumaker, 1952; Pearl *et al.*, 1989; Lakhoo *et al.*, 1991). Serial follow-up studies of the damaged spleen have confirmed significant improvement or return to normality within 20 weeks in the majority of cases (Bethel *et al.*, 1992).

One of the contraindications to conservative management is the risk of excessive blood transfusion (mortality 0.014%/unit) (Feliciano *et al.*, 1992), although isolated splenic injuries require a lower volume than if other viscera are also injured and a haemoglobin level of 7 g/100 dl blood has been shown to have adequate oxygen carrying capacity provided the intravascular volume is normal (Cosentino *et al.*, 1990). Delayed rupture is less common in children (Pearl *et al.*, 1989) than the reported 2–8% incidence in adults (Koury *et al.*, 1991; Farhat *et al.*, 1992). At operation, splenic salvage is the main aim, and full mobilization of the spleen with delivery into the operative field is necessary for adequate assessment. Measures to stop the haemorrhage include pressure, coagulation of bleeding sites, topical haemostatic agents such as Fibrin glue, splenorraphy with deep investing sutures, suture ligation of individual vessels, or partial splenectomy incorporating the segmental arterial blood supply and aiming to maintain at least 30–50% of the splenic tissue (Morgenstern and

Sequelae and outcome

Recent articles have emphasized the long-term sequelae that accompany survivors of paediatric trauma (Harris *et al.*, 1989; Wesson *et al.*, 1989). Both immediate and long-term effects impinge on the victim as well as his or her supporting family unit. More disturbing were the changes – emotional, scholastic and personality – in nearly half of their uninjured siblings and the finding that more than 60% of discharged patients had at least one impairment (Lescohier and Discala, 1993). The family unit composition was disturbed in 40% 1 year after the trauma, with financial implications being a major burden (Harris *et al.*, 1989).

The role of the paediatric surgeon must extend past the confines of the trauma unit. Child accident prevention units have evolved which aim to identify and improve areas where children are at risk, for example restraining car seats, and the geographical variation makes the paediatric surgeons' input vital. Motor vehicle accidents are a prime cause of paediatric trauma and an environmental approach, as well as targeting education at the vulnerable age group, has been shown to be effective (Roberts, 1993) in reducing the incidence.

The burden of the paediatric surgeon who cares for the victim of blunt abdominal trauma extends from the site of the trauma, via transport to the trauma centre, where there is a structured regimen of resuscitation and largely conservative management, and continues on through long-term rehabilitation. Only with his or her expertise being applied at all stages on this collision course to potential disability and even death can the surgeon hope to improve the patient's long-term outcome.

References

Abrahams, J.S. 1975: Editorial comment. *Journal of Trauma* **15**, 192.

Bass, D.H. and Lakhoo, K. 1991: Pancreatic injuries in children. *South African Journal of Surgery* **29**, 39–40.

Bass, D.H., Mann, M.D., Cremin, B.J. and Cywes, S. 1990: A comparison between scintigraphy and computed abdominal tomography in blunt liver and spleen injuries in children. *Pediatric Surgery International* **5**, 443–5.

Bass, D.H., Semple, P.L. and Cywes, S. 1991: Investigation and management of blunt renal injuries in children: a review of 11 years' experience. *Journal of Pediatric Surgery* **26**, 196–200.

Bass, J., Di Lorenzo, M., Desjardins, J.G., Grignon, A. and Ouimet, A. 1988: Blunt pancreatic injuries in children: the role of percutaneous external drainage in the treatment of pancreatic pseudocysts. *Journal of Pediatric Surgery* **23**, 721–4.

Baumann, L., Greenfield, S.P., Aker, J. *et al.* 1992: Non-operative management of major blunt renal trauma in children: in hospital morbidity and long-term follow-up. *Journal of Urology* **148**, 691–3.

Bethel, C.A., Touloukian, R.J., Seashore, J.H. and Rosenfield, N.S. 1992: Outcome of non-operative management of splenic injury with nuclear scanning. Clinical significance of persistent abnormalities. *American Journal of Diseases in Children* **146**, 198–200.

Brandt, M.L., Luks, F.I., Spigland, N.A., Di Lorenzo, M., Laberge, J.M. and Ouimet, A. 1992: Diaphragmatic injury in children. *Journal of Trauma* **32**, 298–301.

Brown, R.A., Bass, D.H., Grant, H.W. and Cywes, S. 1991: Blunt trauma causing diaphragmatic rupture in children. *Pediatric Surgery International* **61**, 345–7.

Brown, R.A., Bass, D.H., Rode, H., Millar, A.J.W. and Cywes, S. 1992: Gastrointestinal tract perforation in children due to blunt abdominal trauma. *British Journal of Surgery* **79**, 522–4.

Bulas, D.I., Taylor, G.A. and Eichelberger, M.R. 1989: The value of CT in detecting bowel perforation in children after blunt abdominal trauma. *American Journal of Radiology* **153**, 561–4.

Clark, D.E., Georgitis, J.W. and Ray, F.S. 1981: Renal artery injuries caused by blunt trauma. *Surgery* **90**, 87–96.

Cogbill, T.H., Moore, E.E., Jurkovich, G.J., Morris, J.A., Mucha, P. and Shackford, S.R. 1989: Non-operative management of blunt splenic trauma: a multicenter experience. *Journal of Trauma* **29**, 1312–17.

Cosentino, C.M., Luck, S.R., Barthel, M.J., Reynolds, M. and Raffensperger, J.G. 1990: Transfusion requirements in conservative non-operative management of blunt splenic and hepatic injuries during childhood. *Journal of Pediatric Surgery* **25**, 950–4.

Cue, J.I., Cryer, G., Miller, F.B., Richardson, J.D. and Polk, H.C. 1990: Packing and planned re-exploration for hepatic and retroperitoneal haemorrhage: critical refinements of a useful technique. *Journal of Trauma* **30**, 1007–13.

Cywes, S., Bass, D.H., Rode, H. and Millar, A.J.W. 1990a: Blunt abdominal trauma in children. *Pediatric Surgery International* **5**, 350–4.

Cywes, S., Kibel, S.M., Bass, D.H., Rode, H., Millar, A.J.W. and De Wet, J. 1990b: Paediatric trauma care. *South African Medical Journal* **78**, 413–18.

Cywes, S., Bass, D.H., Rode, H. and Millar, A.J.W. 1991: Blunt liver trauma in children. *Injury* **22**, 310–15.

Delius, R.E., Frankel, W. and Coran, A.G. 1989: A comparison between operative and non-operative management of blunt injuries to the liver and spleen in adult and pediatric patients. *Surgery* **106**, 788–93.

Dickinson, S.J., Shaw, A. and Santulli, T.V. 1970: Rupture of the gastro-intestinal tract in children by blunt trauma. *Surgery, Gynecology and Obstetrics* **131**, 655–7.

Drost, D.F., Rosemurgy, A.S., Kearney, R.E. and Roberts, P. 1991: Diagnostic peritoneal lavage. Limited indications due to evolving concepts in trauma care. *American Surgeon* **57**, 126–8.

Durham, R. 1990: Management of gastric injuries. *Surgical Clinics of North America* **70**, 517–27.

Eichelberger, M.R., Mangubat, E.A., Sacco, W.J., Bowman, L.M. and Lowenstein, A.D. 1988: Outcome analysis of blunt injury in children. *Journal of Trauma* **28**, 1109–17.

Eichelberger, M.R. and Randolph, J.G. 1985: Progress in pediatric trauma. *World Journal of Surgery* **9**, 222–35.

Enderson, B.L. and Maull, KI. 1991: Missed injuries. The trauma surgeon's nemesis. *Surgical Clinics of North America* **71**, 399–418.

Evans, S., Jackson, R.J. and Smith, S.A. 1993: Successful repair of major retrohepatic vascular injuries without the use of shunt or sternotomy. *Journal of Pediatric Surgery* **28**, 317–20.

Fabian, T.C., Mangiante, E.C., White, T.J., Patterson, C.R., Boldreghini, S. and Britt, L.G. 1986: A prospective study of 91 patients undergoing both computed tomography and peritoneal lavage following blunt abdominal trauma. *Journal of Trauma* **26**, 602–8.

Farhat, G.A., Abdu, R.A. and Vanek, V.W. 1992: Delayed splenic rupture: real or imaginary? *American Surgeon* **58**, 340–5.

Feliciano, D.V. 1990: Management of traumatic retroperitoneal haematoma. *Annals of Surgery* **211**, 109–22.

Feliciano, D.V. 1991: Diagnostic modalities in abdominal trauma. *Surgical Clinics of North America* **71**, 241–56.

Feliciano, D.V. and Pachter, H.L. 1989: Hepatic trauma revisited. *Current Problems in Surgery* **26**, 453–524.

Feliciano, P.D., Mullins, R.J., Trunkey, D.D., Crass, R.A., Beck, J.R. and Helfand, M. 1992: A decision analysis of traumatic splenic injuries. *Journal of Trauma* **33**, 340–7.

Fischer, R.P., Beverlin, B.C., Engrav, L.H., Benjamin, C.I. and Perry, J.F. 1978: Diagnostic peritoneal lavage. Fourteen years and 2,586 patients later. *American Journal of Surgery* **136**, 701–4.

Fischer, R.P., Miller Crotchett, P. and Reed, R.L. 1988: Gastrointestinal disruption: the hazard of non-operative management in adults with blunt abdominal injury. *Journal of Trauma* **28**, 1445–9.

Fiser, D.H. 1990: Intraosseous infusion. *New England Journal of Medicine* **322**, 1579–81.

Funnell, I.C., Bornman, P.C., Krige, J.E.J., Beningfield, S.J. and Terblance J. 1994: Endoscopic drainage of traumatic pancreatic pseudocyst. *British Journal of Surgery* **81**, 879–81.

Goins, W.A., Rodriguez, A., Lewis, J., Brathwaite, C.E.M. and James, E. 1992: Retroperitoneal haematoma after blunt trauma. *Surgery, Gynecology and Obstetrics* **174**, 281–90.

Gruessner, R., Mentges, B., Duber, C., Ruckert, K. and Rothmund, M. 1989: Sonography versus peritoneal lavage in blunt abdominal trauma. *Journal of Trauma* **29**, 242–4.

Guice, K., Oldham, K., Eide, B. and Johansen, K. 1983: Haematuria after blunt trauma: when is pyelography useful? *Journal of Trauma* **23**, 305–11.

Haller, J.A. 1983: Pediatric trauma. The no. 1 killer of children. *Journal of the American Medical Association* **249**, 47.

Hardacre, J.M., West, K.W., Rescorla, F.R., Vane, D.W. and Grosfield, J.L. 1990: Delayed onset of intestinal obstruction in children after unrecognised seat belt injury. *Journal of Pediatric Surgery* **25**, 967–9.

Harris, B.H., Schwaitzberg, S.D., Seman, T.M. and Hermann, C. 1989: The hidden morbidity of pediatric trauma. *Journal of Pediatric Surgery* **24**, 103–6.

Hendrickson, M., Matlak, M.E., Jaffe, R.B., Johnson, D.G. and Black, R.E. 1990: Treatment of traumatic pancreatic pseudocysts in children: the role of percutaneous catheter drainage. *Pediatric Surgery International* **5**, 347–9.

Hollands, M.J., Little, J.M. 1991: Post-traumatic bile fistulae. *Journal of Trauma* **31**, 117–20.

Hoy, G.A. and Cole, W.G. 1992: Concurrent paediatric seat belt injuries of the abdomen and spine. *Pediatric Surgery International* **7**, 376–9.

Jaffe, D. and Wesson, D. 1991: Emergency management of blunt trauma in children. *New England Journal of Medicine* **324**, 1477–82.

Kanter, R.K., Zimmerman, J.J., Strauss, R.H. and Stoeckel, K.A. 1986: Pediatric emergency intravenous access. Evaluation of a protocol. *American Journal of Diseases in Children* **140**, 132–4.

Karp, M.P., Jewett, T.C., Kuhn, J.P., Allen, J.E., Dokler, M.L. and Cooney, D.R. 1986: The impact of computed tomography scanning on the child with renal trauma. *Journal of Pediatric Surgery* **21**, 617–23.

King, H. and Schumaker, H.B. 1952: Splenic studies: I. Susceptibility to infection after splenectomy performed in infancy. *Annals of Surgery* **136**, 239–42.

Kirks, D.R., Caron, K.H. and Bisset, G.S. 1992: CT of blunt abdominal trauma in children: an anatomic 'snapshot in time'. *Radiology* **182**, 631–2.

Koury, H.I., Peschiera, J.L. and Welling, R.E. 1991: Non-operative management of blunt splenic trauma: a 10-year experience. *Injury* **22**, 349–52.

Krige, J.E.J., Bornman, P.C. and Terblance, J. 1992: Therapeutic periphepatic packing in complex liver trauma. *British Journal of Surgery* **79**, 43–6.

Lagausie, P. de, Pariente, D., Gauthier, F., Dreuzy, O. de and Valayer, J. 1992: Embolization of traumatic hemobilia in a child. *Pediatric Surgery International* **7**, 61–3.

Lakhoo, K., Bass, D.H. and Cywes, S. 1991: Blunt splenic trauma in children. *South African Journal of Surgery* **29**, 108–9.

Lescohier, I. and Discala, C. 1993: Blunt trauma in children: causes and outcome of head versus extracranial injury. *Pediatrics* **91**, 721–5.

Lobe, T.E. and Schropp, K. 1993: *Pediatric laparoscopy and thoracoscopy*. Philadelphia, PA: W.B. Saunders.

Long, J.A. and Philippart, A.I. 1990: Bowel injuries. In Coran, A.G. and Harris, B.H. (eds), *Pediatric trauma: Proceedings of the Third National Conference*. Philadelphia, PA: J.B. Lippincott, 118–20.

McAnish, J.W. 1992: Editorial comment. *Journal of Urology* **147**, 1336.

Martin, H.C.O., Liu, K.W. and Gaskin, K.J. 1992: Stricture of the common bile duct secondary to blunt abdominal trauma. *Pediatric Surgery International* **7**, 140–2.

Millar, A.J.W., Rode, H., Stunden, R.J. and Cywes, S. 1988: Management of pancreatic pseudocysts in children. *Journal of Pediatric Surgery* **23**, 122–7.

Morgenstern, L. and Shapiro, S.J. 1979: Techniques of splenic conservation. *Archives of Surgery* **114**, 449–54.

Morgenstern, L. and Uyeda, R.Y. 1983: Non-operative management of injuries of the spleen in adults. *Surgery, Gynecology and Obstetrics* **157**, 513–18.

Murphy, J.P. 1990: Genitourinary trauma. In Ashcraft, K.W. (ed.), *Pediatric urology*. Philadelphia, PA: W.B. Saunders.

Newman, K.D., Bowman, L.M., Eichelberger, M.R. *et al.* 1990: The lap belt complex: intestinal and lumbar spine injury in children. *Journal of Trauma* **30**, 1133–40.

Oldham, K.T. and Caty, M.G. 1990: Liver and spleen trauma in childhood. In Coran, A.G. and Harris, B.H. (eds), *Pediatric Trauma: Proceedings of the Third National Conference*. Philadelphia, PA: J.B. Lippincott, 89.

Oldham, K.T., Guice, K.S., Ryckman, F., Kaufman, R.A., Martin, L.W. and Noseworthy, J. 1986: Blunt liver injury in childhood: evolution of therapy and current perspective. *Surgery* **100**, 542–9.

Pagliarello, G. and Carter, J. 1992: Traumatic injury of the diaphragm: timely diagnosis and treatment. *Journal of Trauma* **33**, 194–7.

Paterson Brown, S. 1991: Strategies for reducing inappropriate laparotomy rate in the acute abdomen. *British Medical Journal* **303**, 1115–18.

Pearl, R.H., Wesson, D.E., Spence, L.J. *et al.*, 1989: Splenic injury: a 5-year update with improved results and changing criteria for conservative management. *Journal of Pediatric Surgery* **24**, 428–31.

Pokorny, W.J., Brandt, M.L. and Harberg, F.J. 1986: Major duodenal injuries in children: diagnosis, operative management and outcome. *Journal of Pediatric Surgery* **21**, 613–16.

Pringle, J.H. 1908: Notes on the arrest of hepatic haemorrhage due to trauma. *Annals of Surgery* **48**, 541–9.

Roberts, I.G. 1993: International trends in pedestrian injury mortality. *Archives of Disease in Childhood* **68**, 190–2.

Rodriguez-Morales, G., Rodriguez, A. and Shatney, C.H. 1986: Acute rupture of the diaphragm in blunt trauma: analysis of 60 cases. *Journal of Trauma* **26**, 438–44.

Sargent, J.C. and Marquardt, C.R. 1950: Renal injuries. *Journal of Urology* **63**, 1–8.

Scott, C.M., Grasberger, R.C., Heeran, T.F., Williams, L.F. and Hirsch, E.F. 1988: Intra-abdominal sepsis after hepatic trauma. *American Journal of Surgery* **55**, 284–8.

Shaw, J.H.F. and Print, C.G. 1989: Post-splenectomy sepsis. *British Journal of Surgery* **76**, 1074–81.

Singer, D.B. 1973: Post-splenectomy sepsis. In Rosenberg, H.S. and Bolande, R.P. (eds), *Perspectives in pediatric pathology*. Chicago, IL: Year Book, 285.

Sivit, C.J., Eichelberger, M.R., Taylor, G.A., Bulas, D.I., Gotschall, C.S. and Kushner, D.C. 1992: Blunt pancreatic trauma in children: CT diagnosis. *American Journal of Radiology* **158**, 1097–100.

Sivit, C.J., Taylor, G.A., Bulas, D.I., Kushner, D.C., Potter, B.M. and Eichelberger, M.R. 1992: Post-traumatic shock in children: CT findings associated with hemodynamic instability. *Radiology* **182**, 723–6.

Smith, S.D., Nakayama, D.K., Gantt, N., Lloyd, D. and Rowe, M.I. 1988: Pancreatic injuries in childhood due to blunt trauma. *Journal of Pediatric Surgery* **23**, 610–14.

Snyder, H. McC. and Caldamone, A.A. 1986: Genitourinary injuries. In Welch, K.J., Randolph, J.G., Ravitch, M.M., O'Neill, J.A. and Rowe, M.I. (eds), *Pediatric surgery*. Chicago, IL: Mosby Year Book, 179.

Steiner, Z., Brown, R.A., Jamieson, D.H., Millar, A.J.W. and Cywes, S. 1994: Management of haemobilia and persistent biliary fistula after blunt liver trauma. *Journal of Pediatric Surgery* **29**, 1575–7.

Taylor, G.A., Eichelberger, M.R., O'Donnell, R. and Bowman, L. 1991: Indications for computed tomography in children with blunt abdominal trauma. *Annals of Surgery* **213**, 212–18.

Teasdale, G. and Jennett, B. 1974: Assessment of coma and impaired consciousness: A practical scale. *Lancet* **ii**, 81–4.

Teigen, C.L., Venbrux, A.C., Quinlan, D.M. and Jeffs, R.D. 1992: Late massive haematuria as a complication of conservative management of blunt renal trauma in children. *Journal of Urology* **147**, 1333–6.

Templeton, J.M. 1993: Mechanism of injury: biomechanics. In Eichelberger, M.R. (ed.), *Pediatric trauma. Prevention, acute care, rehabilitation*. St. Louis, MO: Mosby Year Book, 27.

Tepas, J.J., Mollitt, D.L., Talbert, J.L. and Bryant, M. 1987: The pediatric trauma score as a predictor of injury severity in the injured child. *Journal of Pediatric Surgery* **22**, 14–18.

Tepas, J.J., Ramenofsky, M.L., Mollitt, D.L., Gans, B.M. and DiScala, C. 1988: The pediatric trauma score as a predictor of injury severity: an objective assessment. *Journal of Trauma* **28**, 425–9.

Touloukian, R.J. 1983: Protocol for the non-operative treatment of obstructing intramural duodenal haematoma during childhood. *American Journal of Surgery* **145**, 330–4.

Trunkey, D. and Federle, M.P. 1986: Computed tomography in perspective [Editorial]. *Journal of Trauma* **26**, 660–1.

Ward, R.E., Flynn, T.C. and Clark, W.P. 1981: Diaphragmatic disruption secondary to blunt abdominal trauma. *Journal of Trauma* **21**, 35–8.

Wesson, D.E., Ein, S.H. and Villamater, J. 1980: Intraoperative autotransfusion in blunt abdominal trauma. *Journal of Pediatric Surgery* **15**, 735–6.

Wesson, D.E., Williams, J.I., Spence, L.J., Filler, R.M., Armstrong, P.F. and Pearl, R.H. 1989: Functional outcome in pediatric trauma. *Journal of Trauma* **29**, 589–92.

Working Party of the British Committee for Standards in Haematology: Clinical Haematology Task Force 1996: Dysfunctional Spleen. *British Medical Journal* **312**, 430–3.

Zorludemir, U., Ergören, Y., Yucesan, S. and Olcay, I. 1988: Mortality due to trauma in childhood. *Journal of Trauma* **28**, 669–71.

CHAPTER 72

Rupture of the urethra

J.P. BLANDY

Introduction	Type I fractures with minimal displacement
Types of injury	Type II fractures with significant displacement
Continence and sexual function	Combined urethral and rectal injury
The management of ruptured urethra	References

Introduction

Strictures of the urethra are not common in children, and among these traumatic strictures are probably rarest of all (Pritchett *et al.*, 1993). They are all different, but it is possible to distinguish certain underlying principles.

Types of injury

ENDOSCOPIC INJURY

If the wall of the urethra is lacerated there is no displacement of the urethra, and if secondary tissue necrosis from extravasation of urine can be prevented scarring is minimal. Extensive sloughing of the wall of the urethra was formerly seen when urethral catheters were used in cardiac surgery in children: this could cause stenosis of the whole length of the urethra (Johnston *et al.*, 1991).

PERINEAL INJURY

In perineal injury the corpus spongiosum is pinched against the symphysis pubis but seldom transected. The ends of the urethra are splinted by the corpora cavernosa (Fig. 72.1). Unless extravasation of urine leads to soft tissue necrosis, the worst that can happen is for the injury to heal with a stricture, but it is always short and easy to treat.

COMPRESSION FRACTURES OF THE PELVIS

There are two main types of pelvic fracture associated with urethral injury. In either type, when seen in boys, not only may the membranous urethra be torn (as in adults) but sometimes the prostate and bladder neck as well.

In the common type of pelvic fracture a compressive force squeezes the pelvis until it snaps. The pelvic ring gives way in two places. Behind this, there is always more or less dislocation of the sacroiliac joints. In front, in an anteroposterior compressive injury the symphysis may burst apart, or the thin pubic and ischial rami may

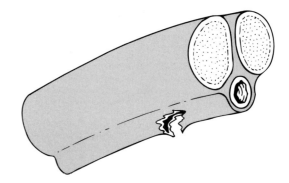

Fig. 72.1 The corpus spongiosum is splinted by the corpora cavernosa; even if completely severed, its ends cannot retract.

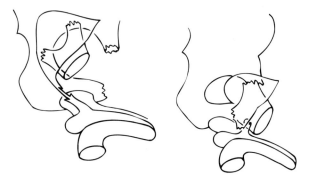

Fig. 72.2   The prostate and urethra are fixed to the pelvis above by the puboprostatic ligament, and below by the attachment of the corpora cavernosa to the ischial rami.

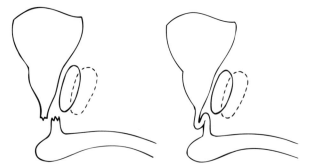

Fig. 72.3   In compression fractures of the pelvis the pelvic ring springs back nearly, but not completely, to its former shape.

break on either side of the symphysis (Jenkins *et al.*, 1992). The soft tissues, with or without a complete X-shaped segment of symphysis, are forced back with the prostate and bladder, which are firmly attached by the puboprostatic ligament. The bulbar urethra is fixed to the corpora cavernosa which are attached to the ischiopubic rami behind the fracture line. The urethra is stretched until it gives way – sometimes partially and sometimes completely (Fig. 72.2).

After the injury the ring of the pelvis springs back and the symphysis returns nearly, but not quite, to its previous position (Fig. 72.3). The upper end comes to lie just behind, or to one side of the lower end, i.e. if the urethra has not been completely severed it will be bent into an S-shape, whereas if it is torn right across the upper end will lie behind and to one side of the lower end.

Compression fractures can be recognized from both the history and the plain X-ray at the time of admission. They are completely different from shearing injuries, where there is displacement of one entire half of the pelvis.

SHEARING FRACTURES OF THE PELVIS WITH SEVERE DISPLACEMENT

In these fractures the compressing force is directed up the extended lower limb through the acetabulum, to force one half of the pelvis upwards (Fig. 72.4). Either the sacroiliac joint is dislocated or there is a fracture of the ilium or sacrum on either side of it. One half of the pelvis rides upwards with the bladder and prostate. If the opposite corpus cavernosum and bulbar urethra remain fixed to the other half of the pelvis, then the membranous urethra is stretched until it gives way (Jenkins *et al.*, 1992) (Fig. 72.4).

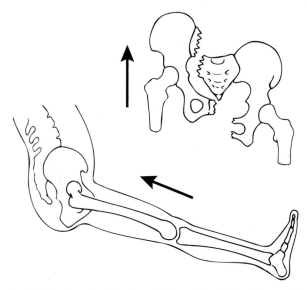

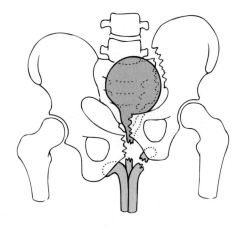

Fig. 72.4   Shearing fracture of the pelvis. Half of the pelvis is forced upwards. If the urinary tract remains attached to one half of the pelvis it will not be injured.

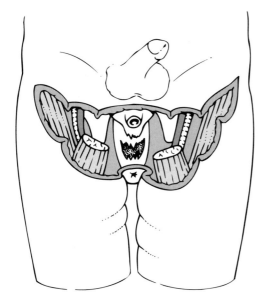

Fig. 72.5 Crushing or rolling injuries may avulse the adductors and split the rectum.

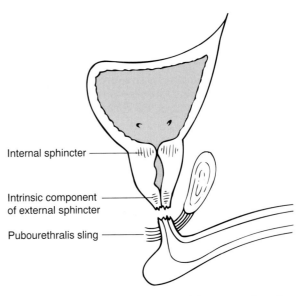

Fig. 72.6 The conventional view of the ruptured urethra imagines the external sphincter to be below the site of rupture. In fact the intrinsic component of the external sphincter (on which continence depends) is usually intact.

In this second kind of pelvic fracture the displaced parts do not spring back into place, and unless the bony dislocation can be reduced, a gap will remain between the ends of the urethra which is equal to the distance between the separated bones (Jenkins *et al.*, 1992).

COMBINED RECTAL INJURY

A crushing or rolling injury may fracture the pelvis, avulse the adductor muscles from the pelvis and split the anterior wall of the rectum (Fig. 72.5). There are always many other injuries (Blandy and Singh, 1972). After resuscitation the priority is to avoid gangrene by diverting faeces from the wound by a colostomy. (In several cases referred to the author secondary tissue loss from gas gangrene greatly exaggerated the original damage.) Just as in gunshot injuries of war the wound is debrided and on no account should any attempt be made at primary suture (Kudsk *et al.*, 1990).

Continence and sexual function

CONTINENCE

The conventional notion of the rupture of the membranous urethra, repeated from text to text, depicts the membranous urethra giving way above the 'sphincter'. The truth is far more interesting and complex. The urethral sphincter system has three distinct components. Firstly there is the bladder neck, a ring of α-adrenergic involuntary smooth muscle supplied by sympathetic nerves (Gosling *et al.*, 1982) (Fig. 72.6).

Secondly, below this lies the intrinsic urethral sphincter, downstream of the verumontanum, which is made up of an inner sleeve of smooth muscle and an outer sleeve of slow-twitch striated muscle, both of which are involuntary. This is the 'external sphincter' familiar to every urologist as the distal landmark in transurethral resection (Blandy and Notley, 1993).

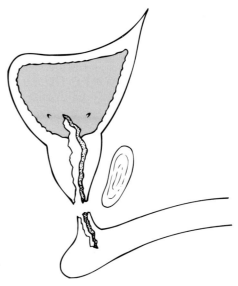

Fig. 72.7 In adults the urethra always tears below the intrinsic component of the external sphincter. In boys the tear may go right through the prostate and bladder neck.

Surrounding the intrinsic urethral sphincter is the fast-twitch striated muscle of the compressor urethrae, i.e. the pubourethralis component of the levator ani.

In micturition (Hald and Bradley, 1982) all three elements of the sphincter relax when the detrusor muscle contracts. There are four phases to this process: (1) when the bladder is empty, the striated levator ani contracts; (2) there is a slow contraction of the intrinsic sphincter which milks urine back from the prostatic urethra into the bladder; (3) the smooth muscle of the bladder neck contracts; and (4) the voluntary external sphincter relaxes, as it cannot keep up its contraction for more than a few minutes. Note that continence requires at least one of the two involuntary sphincters to be intact.

In adult males the urethra ruptures downstream of the intrinsic sphincter and verumontanum, and the bladder neck is usually intact. In prepubertal boys the tear may go up through the prostate and bladder neck (Fig. 72.7), rupturing both of the involuntary components of the sphincter. Fortunately, incontinence may not be permanent, perhaps through healing of the normal sphincter systems or from growth of the prostate in puberty.

In severe pelvic injuries the sympathetic nerves may be injured and the bladder neck may be paralysed. The bladder neck may also be injured by pressure necrosis from traction on a Foley balloon, a method formerly used in the management of urethral rupture.

SEXUAL FUNCTION

Erection

In erection the corpora cavernosa and spongiosum fill from the terminal branches of the internal iliac artery in response to parasympathetic stimuli (Tanagho and Lue, 1990). The parasympathetic fibres may be torn if the fracture line in the ilium runs through the lateral wall of the pelvis, which is the reason why erectile impotence is sometimes seen without any urethral injury. The penile arteries and the parasympathetic fibres run in a pair of neurovascular bundles which lie anterolateral to the prostate and lateral to the membranous urethra. Anything that stretches the membranous urethra must stretch these bundles. They may also be injured in surgical reconstruction of the urethra (Fig. 72.8).

Ejaculation

Sperm are stored in the vasa deferentia. On ejaculation they empty into the prostatic urethra and are then syringed out of the urethra by the seminal vesicles, the fluid from which makes up most of the ejaculate. The bladder neck contracts to prevent retrograde ejaculation. Contraction of the vesicles and closure of the bladder neck are both under α-adrenergic sympathetic control. A fracture of the sacrum may sever the presacral

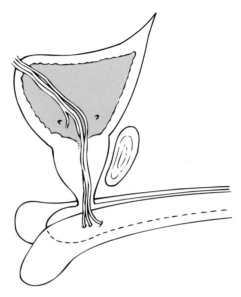

Fig. 72.8 The neurovascular bundles supplying the erectile tissue of the penis run alongside the prostate and membranous urethra.

sympathetic nerves and result in ejaculatory paralysis. Pressure necrosis of the bladder neck from traction on a Foley catheter may cause retrograde ejaculation.

The management of ruptured urethra

ENDOSCOPIC INJURY

Most periurethral injuries will heal without any stricture, provided the urine is diverted for a few days. In children a suprapubic cystostomy avoids further injury to the urethra. Extravasation of urine into the perineum calls for incision and drainage before it can cause soft tissue necrosis. The long multiple strictures seen after urethral catheterization for cardiac surgery pose some of the most difficult problems for urethroplasty, and are outside the scope of this chapter (Johnston *et al.*, 1991).

PERINEAL INJURY

A suprapubic cystostomy is performed as soon as possible. The perineum is frequently examined so that any collection of fluid can be promptly drained. The urethra should be left alone. After about 10 days a water-soluble urethrogram will usually show no extravasation and the suprapubic can be removed. Careful follow-up is needed since stricture may occur several years later, although at worst it will be short and will usually respond to urethrotomy or dilatation, and at the very worst it can be cured by excision and end-to-end anastomosis.

PELVIC FRACTURE

On admission few of these children are fit to undergo primary reconstruction, because of their other injuries. Urethral bleeding signifies some injury to the urethra. A glance at the X-ray of the pelvis shows whether there is likely to be major displacement of the urethra. A simple urethrogram with a water-soluble contrast medium can be taken at the time of the initial X-rays and any extravasation confirms that the urethra has been damaged and calls for a suprapubic cystostomy.

If the bladder can be felt with certainty, a trocar cystostomy is performed, making sure that a surplus length of catheter lies in the bladder. If the catheter is only just inside the bladder, it may be extruded later on when the pelvic haematoma resolves. Haematoma and bruising often make it difficult to palpate the bladder but an ultrasound will enable a tube to be placed correctly. If in doubt, it is safer to make a small suprapubic incision and make quite sure that the tube is in the bladder.

When laparotomy is indicated to rule out or treat injury to other viscera this will provide the opportunity to insert a catheter into the bladder under vision. It is tempting to proceed and attempt primary repair of a ruptured urethra but this should be resisted since it may provoke uncontrollable haemorrhage from pelvic veins.

Type I fractures with minimal displacement

Once a suprapubic tube has been inserted there is no urgency for subsequent treatment, although the best results are obtained by ensuring that the urethral lumen is patent, even if this requires urethroplasty, within the first 10–14 days, before the tissues have become rigid and fixed (Al-Rifaei *et al.*, 1991; Boone *et al.*, 1992).

When the child is fit, an up-and-down cystourethrogram, injecting contrast medium through the urethra and the suprapubic tube, will show whether the urethra is blocked or patent. If one of the new very small-calibre flexible endoscopes is available this will make it possible to confirm that the way into the bladder is clear and the urethra is obviously healing. In such a case nothing active needs to be done, but the examination should be repeated from time to time over the next few weeks because in some children the fracture may slip and lead to a more serious malalignment of the urethra.

EARLY OPERATION

If the lumen is completely blocked, it is necessary to operate to overcome the block. Ideal operating conditions are found in the first 10 days after the injury, when the haematoma will have already made the dissection. The urethra is exposed through a midline perineal incision and the bulb is mobilized off the corpora cavernosa

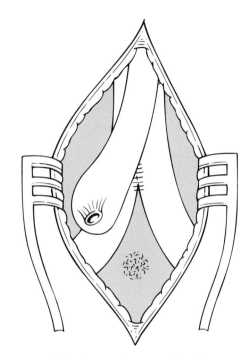

Fig. 72.9 The bulbar urethra is mobilized.

for about 5 cm (Fig. 72.9). Because of the haematoma, the proximal (upstream) urethra is easily found by passing a sound down through the suprapubic track (Fig. 72.10). The severed ends are anastomosed over a fine silicone tube using absorbable sutures (Fig. 72.11). The suprapubic tube is secured by a suprapubic button.

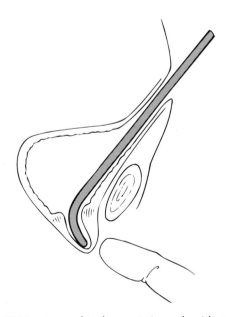

Fig. 72.10 A sound in the prostatic urethra identifies the upper severed end.

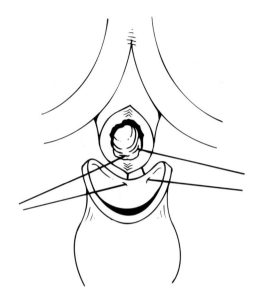

Fig. 72.11   End-to-end anastomosis of the urethra.

LATE OPERATION

Urethrotomy

Sometimes only a thin membrane separates the upper prostatic from the lower bulbar urethra. If a flexible cystoscope is passed down the suprapubic track, one may see and cut down on the glow of light, and re-establish continuity (Chiou *et al.*, 1989) (Fig. 72.12).

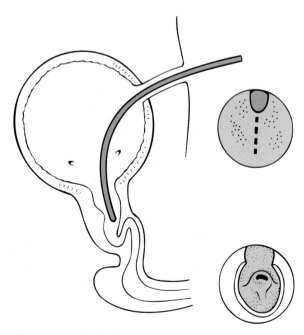

Fig. 72.12   The light of the flexible cystoscope passed down through the suprapubic track identifies the thin tissue separating the torn ends of the urethra.

The advantage of this method is that it avoids injury to the neurovascular bundles of the penis or the intrinsic part of the external sphincter.

Open end-to-end anastomosis

If the barrier of scar tissue between the prostatic and bulbar urethra is so thick that no glow of light can be seen, a formal end-to-end anastomosis is necessary. The dissection is similar to that described above, but more difficult because of the dense scar tissue. A flexible cystoscope passed down the suprapubic track may help to identify the proximal urethra.

Type II fractures with significant displacement

Once the suprapubic tube has been placed there is no urgency about repairing the urethra, and in practice other injuries usually enforce delay in repair of the urethra. In principle, the sooner the severed ends of the urethra are brought together again the better, and the key to successful reanastomosis of the ruptured urethra lies in accurate reduction and fixation of the pelvic fracture, because it is only by replacing the dislocated bones that the ends of the urethra can come together (Blandy, 1986) (Fig. 72.13).

Fortunately, the modern technique of external fixation of major pelvic fractures used to control haemorrhage has brought many advantages, not least the early approximation of the displaced ends of the urethra. The fixator should be placed after discussion with the urologist to allow access to the suprapubic tube and a Pfannenstiel incision.

As soon as blood loss has been corrected and the child's general condition is satisfactory, and ideally within the first 10 days of admission, an up-and-down cysto-urethrogram is performed. It is even better to examine the urethra directly with a narrow flexible endoscope. These investigations may show that the urethra is in continuity because the bulbar urethra is attached to the same half of the pelvis as the bladder and prostate. In such a case nothing further needs to be done.

EARLY REPAIR

If the urethra is completely blocked, and if the pelvic fracture has been well reduced, then the severed ends can be anastomosed through a midlife perineal incision, exactly as described above. In practice it can be very difficult to identify the upstream end of the urethra. Rather than risk further damage to the neurovascular bundles (Fig. 72.14) of the penis or the intrinsic component of the external sphincter by dissecting blindly, it is better to make a second Pfannenstiel incision and separate the bladder and prostate from the symphysis.

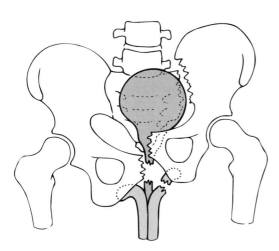
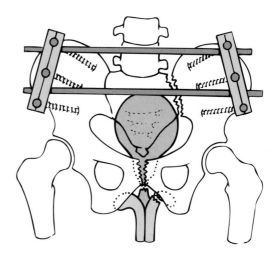

Fig. 72.13 In shearing injuries of the pelvis, replacing the dislocated bones brings the ends of the urethra together. In applying the fixator one should allow enough room to make a Pfannenstiel incision.

The prostate is sometimes found to be displaced sideways and the puboprostatic ligament may have to be divided on one side to correct this. Great care is taken to preserve at least one neurovascular bundle to the penis so as to safeguard potency.

Once the prostate has been mobilized the anastomosis is performed without tension, over a fine silicone tube.

LATE REPAIR

Unfortunately, most children with the aftermath of these injuries are referred late, sometimes because it was never possible to reduce the fracture or apply external fixation and sometimes because of other life-threatening injuries. More often the delay has been due to the outdated and erroneous doctrine that attempts at repair should be deliberately postponed for several months

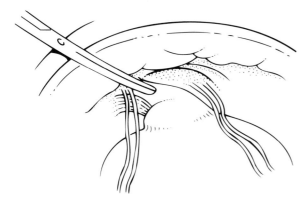

Fig. 72.14 The prostate may be found to be twisted round. In freeing it so as to align it with the urethra, care must be taken to avoid injuring the penile neurovascular bundle.

(Glass *et al.*, 1978). Whatever the cause of the delay, the child has an unreduced pelvic fracture, and between the ends of the urethra there is a solid block of scar tissue and callus.

An anteroposterior and lateral X-ray of the pelvis are needed to show the bony anatomy, and an up-and-down cystourethrogram will show the position of the prostatic and bulbar urethra. Whenever possible a flexible cystoscopy is performed through the suprapubic track. This will sometimes bring to light an unexpected trap. In patients in whom an attempt has been made to railroad a Foley catheter through the rupture the catheter is passed in a false passage in the trigone (Fig. 72.15). When the catheter is removed the patient at first passes urine but is incontinent. Within a few days the false passage shrinks and the patient develops retention. Dilatation of the false passage is carried out and the cycle of incontinence followed by retention is established. The up-and-down cystourethrogram may show a bizarre double 'bladder neck'. The flexible cystoscope will identify the real bladder neck with the catheter emerging through the trigone.

One symphysis may ride above the other, to form a wall of bone twice the normal depth, or may move up behind the other, so that the symphysis is twice its normal thickness (Fig. 72.16).

Resection of the entire pubis has been suggested as a method of overcoming the gap between the ends of the urethra. This should be avoided as the resultant defect in the ring of the pelvis allows the penis to sink back and give rise to a distressing deformity. Instability of the pelvic girdle makes it difficult for the child to run or jump.

The block of bone that separates the ends of the urethra can be removed without interrupting the pelvic ring, by cutting a window of bone from the inferior and posterior aspect of the malunited symphysis (Blandy, 1990).

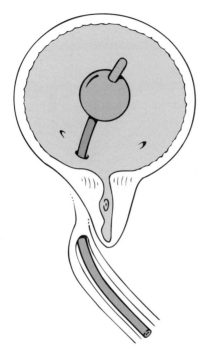

Fig. 72.15   The problem with the neglected shearing fracture. The ends of the urethra are separated by a block of scar and callus, and the Foley catheter may have been placed in a false passage into the trigone.

One should start with a perineal incision and mobilize the bulbar urethra. The corpora cavernosa diverge at this level and can be further separated by incising the septum between them. Retracting the corpora reveals the inferior edge of the malunited symphysis. The dorsal vein of the penis and the two dorsal arteries should be displaced to one side (Fig. 72.17).

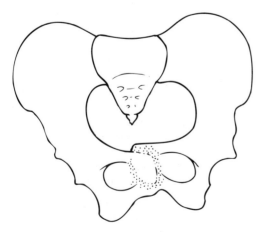

Fig. 72.16   The unreduced shearing fracture may give a symphysis that is twice as deep or twice as thick as it should be.

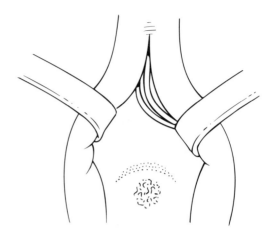

Fig. 72.17   By retracting the corpora the lower end of the malunited symphysis can be seen.

A generous window of bone and callus is then taken out using bone saw, rongeurs and osteotomes, until the inner periosteum of the symphysis is exposed (Fig. 72.18). One can feel the tip of a bougie passed down through the suprapubic track. Cutting down on the tip of the bougie opens the prostatic urethra which is spatulated and sutured to the mobilized bulbar urethra (Fig. 72.19).

If access is restricted and it is impossible to be certain of the whereabouts of the prostate, a Pfannenstiel incision should be made and the prostate dissected from the malunited symphysis. A gouge will help to remove more callus from the back of the malunited symphysis. This approach has the advantage that the anastomosis can be wrapped in omentum which is claimed to prevent late stenosis (Turner-Warwick, 1978).

Combined urethral and rectal injury

Primary care of these very severe injuries should have been limited to resuscitation, debridement, and diversion of faeces and urine. In boys, the injury may involve all of the sphincters, and a suprapubic cystostomy alone will not prevent urine leaking into the perineal wound to retard healing and make nursing very difficult. Rather than persevere with percutaneous nephrostomies it is better to make an ileal conduit diversion as soon as possible.

A good opportunity for the diversion may be taken when secondary suture of the pelvic injuries is planned. This provides an opportunity to inspect the injuries thoroughly and close the lacerations in the rectum and its sphincter.

Skin defects will usually require staged split skin and rotation grafts, as will the repair of the missing section of urethra (Blandy and Singh, 1972). When everything is

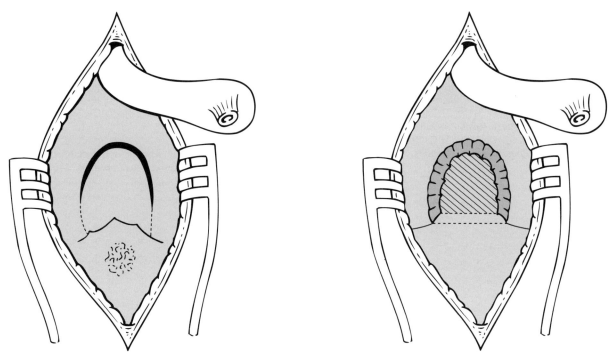

Fig. 72.18 A window of bone is removed from the inferior margin of the symphysis.

healed up, the colostomy can be closed and the ileal conduit joined back on to the bladder. The long-term outlook is guarded: some recover continence and few become potent. Those with a skin-lined urethra may develop calculi on the hairs and the skin graft may form a pouch. Urinary infections are commonly seen in the succeeding decade and may progress to form calculi. The follow-up requires constant vigilance (Rogers *et al.*, 1992).

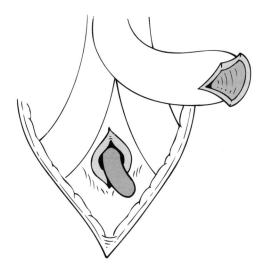

Fig. 72.19 The prostatic urethra is found by palpating the tip of a sound passed through the suprapubic track.

References

Al-Rifaei, M.A., Gaafar, S. and Abdel-Rahman, M. 1991: Management of posterior urethral strictures secondary to pelvic fractures in children. *Journal of Urology* **145**, 353–6.

Blandy, J.P. 1986: *Operative urology,* 2nd ed. Oxford: Blackwell Scientific, 215.

Blandy, J.P. 1990: Posterior urethroplasty after trauma. Part II. *AUA Update Series* **9** (28), 218–23.

Blandy, J.P. and Notley, R.G. 1993: *Transurethral resection,* 3rd ed. London: Butterworth.

Blandy, J.P. and Singh, M. 1972: Fistulae involving the adult male urethra. *British Journal of Urology* **44**, 632–43.

Boone, T.B., Wilson, W.T. and Husmann, D.A. 1992: Postpubertal genitourinary function following posterior urethral disruptions in children. *Journal of Urology* **148**, 232–4.

Chiou, R.K., Gonzalez, R., Ortlip, S and Fraley, E.E. 1989: Endoscopic treatment of posterior urethral obliteration: long-term follow-up and comparison with transpubic urethroplasty. *Journal of Urology* **140**, 508–11.

Glass, R.E., Flynn, J.T., King, J.B. and Blandy, J.P. 1978: Urethral injury and fractured pelvis. *British Journal of Urology* **50**, 578–82.

Gosling, J.A., Dixon, J.S. and Humpherson, J.R. 1982: *Functional anatomy of the urinary tract.* London: Maruzen/Gower Medical.

Hald, T. and Bradley, V.E. 1982: *The urinary bladder neurology and dynamics.* Baltimore, MD: Williams & Wilkins.

Jenkins, B.J., Badenoch, D.F., Fowler, C.G. and Blandy, J.P. 1992: Long-term results of treatment of urethral injuries in males caused by external trauma. *British Journal of Urology* **70**, 73–5.

Johnston, M.A., Hughes, D.A. and Asmy, A.F. 1991: Late complications of undetected urethral stricture after cardiac surgery in a child. *British Medical Journal* **303**, 772–3.

Kudsk, K.A., McQueen, M.A., Woeller, G.R., Fox, M.A., Mangiante, E.C. and Fabian, T.C. 1990: Management of complex perineal soft-tissue injuries. *Journal of Trauma* **30**, 1155–60.

Pritchett, T.R., Shapiro, R.A. and Hardy, B.E. 1993: Surgical management of traumatic posterior urethral strictures in children. *Urology* **42**, 59–62.

Rogers, J.S., McNicholas, T.A. and Blandy, J.P. 1992: Long-term results of one-stage scrotal patch urethroplasty. *British Journal of Urology* **9**, 621–8.

Tanagho, E.A. and Lue, T.F. 1990: Physiology of penile erection. In Chisholm, G.D. and Fair, W.R. (eds), *Scientific foundations of urology*, 3rd ed. Oxford: Heinemann, 420–6.

Turner-Warwick, R.T. 1978: The use of omental pedicle graft in urinary tract reconstruction. *Journal of Urology* **116**, 341–7.

CHAPTER 73

Thermal and chemical burns

P.L. LEVICK

Introduction
Classification of burns and scalds
Management
Burns at specific sites

Subsequent care of the burn patient to
achieve wound healing
Reconstructive surgery

Introduction

Burns and scalds in children have enormous economic and social consequences. Thermal injury is the second highest cause of death in children after road accidents, and the sequelae, both mental and physical, can remain with patients for the rest of their lives. There are two peaks of incidence of burns and scalds in children, the first being at 18 months when the toddler is exploring his or her environment. Children in this age group commonly pull hot fluids such as tea and coffee over themselves, giving the typical distribution of scalds to the face, dominant upper arm, neck and chest. Despite improvements in the home and general public awareness of the dangers of hanging kettle leads, this group of children remains the single largest group of burns victims and continues to rise in number every year. The second group of children comprises the youngsters, usually boys, who are exploring the laws of chemistry and physics. These children may sustain devastating burns from conflagrations of petrol or contact with high-voltage electricity. Each and every summer vacation the staff of burns units are saddened by the admission of children who have poured petrol on to bonfires or played games on the electrified railway. The common factor between these two groups is that neither of them knew the dangers of their actions. It behoves us all, therefore, actively to promote accident prevention in children. Young parents must be made aware of the dangers in the home and the school curriculum should include graphic warnings about inflammable liquids and electricity. Despite the increase in frequency of these tragic accidents it is astonishing how few of the parents of toddlers realize the damage that a cup of tea could do to their child.

Classification of burns and scalds

The majority of burns are caused by heat and if the burning agent is moist, such as hot water or steam, it is called a scald. The thermal burn is a wound in which there is coagulative necrosis of the skin which can be caused by direct heat or flames, actinic rays (sunburn), radiation, chemicals, electricity and friction. Coagulative necrosis can also be caused by cold (i.e. frostbite).

Management

FIRST AID AND IMMEDIATE CARE

The temperature of the burning agent must be reduced. This means removal of clothing in the case of a scald and with burns, the patient must be removed from the source of heat and any flames extinguished. The intense pain of the injury can then be reduced by the application of cold, clean water soaks, which require changing every few minutes. With electrical burns it is important to switch off the electrical supply first, then, if the victim is unconscious, cardiac arrest must be excluded and cardiopulmonary resuscitation applied if necessary. With chemical burns the affected areas must be irrigated with copious amounts of clean water. (The only exception to this is phenol, where water may accelerate absorption, and polyethylene glycol should be used.) With the more usual acids or alkalis, the areas should be irrigated with water until litmus paper placed on the skin no longer reacts. In some cases it is necessary to continue this irrigation for several hours. Any injured child should be taken immediately to the nearest accident and emergency department.

Prompt and effective initial management is essential because the increased capillary permeability of burn shock is most marked in the first 8 hours, gradually reducing over the next 48 hours. Burn shock is contributed to by the loss of circulating blood volume, which is greatest during the first 24 hours, through water, electrolyte and plasma protein loss in blister fluid, exudate, oedema and by evaporation. These losses are caused by vasodilatation and increased capillary permeability of the wound, mediated by the liberation of histamine, kinins, prostaglandins and fibrin degradation products. In addition the heat losses from a burned area may be considerable. The shock is also increased by the overwhelming intense pain.

SEVERITY OF THE INJURY

The factors that determine the severity of the injury include the extent and depth of the burn, and associated injuries.

Extent of body surface burned

Burned children require intravenous resuscitation if their injury exceeds 10% of their body surface area. Patients with smaller area burns may still require intravenous fluid, particularly if there are any other reasons for increased fluid loss such as diarrhoea. Small children have disproportionately large heads in relation to the rest of their body. The head and neck in a 1-year-old child is 18% of the body surface area and in a 5-year-old child it is 13%. 'Wallace's rule of nines' is therefore not appropriate for assessment of area in children. The patient's own palm area approximates to 1% of the body surface area and can be a useful guide for assessing the total of patchy burns.

Depth of burn and causative agent

Burns are either partial or full thickness depending on the depth of skin destruction. Partial thickness burns heal because remnants of epidermis in hair follicles and sweat glands spread over the wound surface. Wounds caused by burning clothing, electricity or hot metal are usually full thickness, whereas flash explosions or scalds are usually partial thickness. Children, however, have delicate skin and minor scalds may be still be full thickness depending on the agent's temperature and time of contact. Partial-thickness injury will usually appear moist, red and blistered, whereas a full thickness burn is usually white or brown, dry and firm to the touch. The appearance of the wound can be very deceptive, even to the most experienced eye, and it is important that the initial carers for an injured child do not give the parents any prediction of whether scarring will occur or not. A burn surgeon will often hear angry parents complain that, 'The first doctor told me there would be no scars'. The sterile pinprick test may be used to define full-thickness loss (in which the nerve endings are destroyed) but partial-thickness burns may also be anaesthetic and the test is generally unreliable in small children. It is therefore best in all but the most definite cases not to predict to the parents the depth of the wound and likelihood of permanent scarring.

Associated injuries or illnesses

Concurrent illness increases the mortality and the presence of any pre-existing renal, cardiovascular or metabolic disorders must be established. Any associated fractures should be treated by closed conservative methods and it must be remembered that these will increase the fluid requirements. Young children are often injured at a time when they are suffering from a viral infection which may have an adverse effect on their immunity (see later).

RESPIRATORY TRACT BURNS

Patients with suspected respiratory tract burns or smoke inhalation should receive humidified oxygen by mask and regular pulmonary physiotherapy. Crystalloid fluid administration should be restricted to that necessary to maintain hydration and renal function. Patients with oral or nasal burns who develop stridor and respiratory distress may have laryngeal oedema and endotracheal intubation should be considered before total obstruction occurs. Tracheostomy should only be carried out if intubation is impossible or prolonged. Lower respiratory tract burns cause oedema with bronchospasm and treatment may include the administration of aminophylline. Steroids are indicated if bronchospasm is not relieved by bronchodilators alone. Severe cases may develop respiratory failure manifested as increasing difficulty in breathing and deteriorating arterial blood gases, in which event mechanical ventilation is indicated.

IMMEDIATE EVALUATION AND TREATMENT

A burn is an open wound and therefore antitetanus toxoid should be given. Patients should be assessed in a closed, warm room as follows.

Emergency sedation

Patients must be reassured and treated in a quiet, confident manner. Full-thickness burns are relatively painless owing to the destruction of nerve endings. The pain of partial-thickness burns may be relieved by cold water compresses and dressings. Opiates may cause vomiting or respiratory depression, and therefore should be used with great caution in small intravenous doses. Trimeprazine tartrate (Vallergan) is the sedative of choice for children.

Fluid replacement therapy

Untreated patients can develop hypovolaemic shock because of losses from the burn wound and the formation of inflammatory oedema. The fluid loss is proportional to the area of the wound and the rate of loss is maximal immediately after burning, diminishing during the first 36 hours. The fluid loss resembles plasma and should be replaced with colloid solution such as human plasma protein fraction, human albumin 4.5%, or a synthetic plasma expander such as Dextran 110. Several formulae exist to calculate the rate of administration but the requirements must be adjusted according to the particular needs of each patient.

A practical guide for fluid replacement

Children

In the first 24 hours one plasma volume equivalent (40 ml/kg) will be required for every 15% of the body surface burned. Half of this volume is given in the first 8 hours and the other half in the next 16 hours. On the second day about half of these amounts will be required.

Another formula that can be used is to weigh the patient and estimate the area burned as:

$$\frac{\text{Weight in kg} \times \text{percentage burn}}{2}$$

= amount of fluid needed in first 4 hours

At the end of 4 hours the urinary output is assessed (this should be 50 ml/hour in an adult and 15 ml/hour in a baby) and the next 4-hour input adjusted accordingly. At the end of 8 hours, if urinary output is adequate, the same amount is given in the next 16 hours. Fluid requirements can be monitored by estimating the haematocrit.

Adults

During the first 24 hours between 1 and 1.5 litres of colloid will be required for every 10% of body surface burned. Half of this volume is given in the first 8 hours from the time of burning (not the time of admission) and the other half in the next 16 hours. On the second day about half these amounts will be required.

CLINICAL ASSESSMENT OF PROGRESS

Progress is assessed by examination of the patient's general clinical state with measurements of haematocrit and urine output. The clinical examination includes pulse rate, blood pressure, temperature, jugular and peripheral vein filling, and skin perfusion, colour and temperature. The haematocrit should approximate to the normal expected value for that patient and the urine output should be 0.5–1 ml/kg/hour at any age. For severe cases it may be necessary to measure the central venous pressure and continue fluid replacement for longer than 36 hours. Normal metabolic crystalloid requirements should be administered orally or intravenously in addition to the colloid of burned fluid replacement.

INITIAL BURN WOUND CARE

The majority of burn wounds require no cleansing but adherent clothing, dirt or foreign material should be removed by gentle rinsing with warm, sterile saline. It is not necessary to rupture clean blisters. If a full-thickness burn encircles the neck, trunk or limbs, escharotomies are required where the dead (anaesthetic) skin should be incised along axial lines to prevent the trapped oedema producing a tourniquet effect and eventual ischaemic contracture or gangrene. Partial thickness areas do not need incision. This procedure may cause haemorrhage, necessitating blood transfusion.

TETANUS PROPHYLAXIS AND ANTIBIOTIC THERAPY

Tetanus toxoid booster should be given in all cases. Patients with extensive burns should receive a 5-day course of penicillin or erythromycin. Broad-spectrum antibiotics should not be given unless there is evidence of systemic infection. Barrier nursing and laminar flow air may help to prevent secondary infection (but the latter may increase fluid losses).

NUTRITIONAL REQUIREMENTS

Patients with severe burns occasionally develop paralytic ileus, so for the first 12 hours the oral intake should be restricted to 1 ml/kg/hour. Thereafter the volume may be increased with half-strength milk, followed by a liquid diet. A nasogastric tube should be passed in severely burned patients to test initially for gastric ileus by hourly aspirations, and to provide a route for additional calories and proteins.

BURN DRESSINGS

Burn dressings may be either oily-based tulles or water-based creams. Tulles may contain agents such as nitrofurazone or chlorhexidine and promote drying of the wound, but tend to adhere and cause pain at dressing changes. Water-based creams are more comfortable for the patient but need to contain antibacterial agents, such as silver sulphadiazine, to reduce the emergence of Gram-negative organisms in the wet wound environment. *Pseudomonas* infection may be combatted using 0.5% silver nitrate compresses, applied once or twice daily. Synthetic membranes, human amnion, homograft and xenograft, may be used on clean superficial wounds, but these temporary skins should not be used on deep burns because they may encourage bacterial growth in necrotic tissue. Cadaver or donor skin, or amnion must not be used without confirmation that the source is HIV negative.

Burns at specific sites

HAND BURNS

Burned hands should be enclosed in polythene bags, elevated and actively exercised to reduce oedema and restore a full range of movement before digital joint capsule contracture has occurred.

BURNS OF THE FACE AND SCALP

The majority of facial burns heal spontaneously and should be treated by exposure with daily applications of Flamazine cream or betadine. The hair trapped in a burned scalp should be carefully trimmed to prevent matting which would encourage bacterial growth.

BURNS OF THE EYES AND EYELIDS

The eyes should be examined with fluoroscein for corneal damage as soon as possible (before oedema of the eyelids makes examination difficult), and burned eyelid skin grafted before significant ectropion has developed.

COLD INJURY

Frostbite may be associated with hypothermia. If the body core temperature falls below 32°C, the patient should be rewarmed slowly over a period of several hours and cardiac arrhythmias controlled with intravenous lignocaine. Oxygen should be administered together with intravenous 5% dextrose prewarmed to 38°C. Areas of frostbite should be thawed with tepid water (at 40°C) and then treated as thermal burns.

RADIATION BURNS

Acute radiation injury produces damage to the skin and local tissues resembling thermal burns but differs in that the necrosis evolves more slowly and deeply than the initial erythema suggested. Surgery is not indicated until the wound has passed into the subacute stage, characterized by the disappearance of the erythema and oedema. Subacute and chronic radiation injury should be treated as the wound appearances indicate, with healing by skin grafting or flap cover.

Subsequent care of the burn patient to achieve wound healing

BURN WOUND CARE AND SURGERY

Dressings

The majority of burns should be dressed on alternate days for the first three weeks to allow natural healing of the partial thickness areas. Bacteriological swabs should be taken at each dressing. The dressings of definitely superficial wounds may be left undisturbed for several days. Ketamine anaesthesia is useful for major burns dressing changes.

Skin grafting

Full-thickness burns heal slowly from the wound edges and significant areas therefore need skin grafting. Excision and grafting may be carried out at an early stage if the patient's general condition is satisfactory, but may be associated with significant haemorrhage. Careful bacteriological monitoring of the wound is carried out prior to the grafting to exclude the presence of *Streptococcus pyogenes*, which will destroy skin grafts and should be treated with flucloxacillin or erythromycin.

Skin grafts are taken from areas of normal skin with a free-hand or mechanical dermatome. The graft thickness should be 1/15 000 of an inch in adults and 1/10 000 of an inch in children. Areas to be grafted are cleaned with saline or aqueous chlorhexidine, and residual slough is excised with scissors. The graft should be fenestrated with a scalpel blade or mesh dermatome to prevent loss from haematoma, anchored with sutures or skin staples and dressed with tulle, covered by gauze and elasticated bandages. The first graft dressing should be carried out on the third postoperative day, and then at 2- or 3-day intervals until healing is complete. Exposed bone, joints or tendons may require cover with full-thickness flaps. The donor site dressing should be left undisturbed, if possible, until healing has occurred, which is usually 10 days.

Patients with extensive burns have limited areas for skin graft donor sites. Keratinocytes may be cultured *in vitro* to provide sheets of epidermis to assist wound healing. Cadaver or donor skin and a variety of synthetic membranes may be used as temporary skin cover provided that there is confirmation that the source is HIV negative.

NUTRITIONAL SUPPORT

Patients with burns exceeding 30% require a high protein and calorie diet, which is usually administered by a fine bore nasogastric tube, in addition to a normal diet. For children the calorie and protein intake should be at least equal to that which the child normally receives at his or her age and weight, remembering to correct any deficiencies caused by starvation before anaesthesia.

IMMUNOLOGY AND ANTIBIOTIC THERAPY

Septic complications are the major cause of death in burn patients, who are immunodepressed by the effects of their injury. Patients' immune reserves should be reinforced by the intermittent administration of fresh frozen plasma to provide antibodies and opsonins, and haemoglobin levels maintained by fresh blood transfusion. Small children have immature and inadequate immunity and may develop neutrophil (polymorphonuclear) leucopenia. This serious complication should be treated by fresh-frozen plasma or blood, together with an antibiotic if a pathogenic organism is present on the burn wound. Antibiotics should, in general, be used with caution because they may give rise to the emergence of resistant pathogenic organisms. Burns patients are also susceptible to viral and fungal infection. Isolation and barrier nursing are essential for the most severely burned cases.

PHYSIOTHERAPY

Regular pulmonary physiotherapy is essential for all patients with significant burns who should also be encouraged to exercise their main muscle groups and joints.

PSYCHOLOGICAL SUPPORT

Burn patients may become significantly depressed and require constant encouragement and positive reassurance to prevent them becoming lethargic and anorexic.

LATE COMPLICATIONS

These include protein losing enteropathy caused by hypoproteinaemia (oedema and delayed wound healing), chronic renal failure, immune deficiency and the consequences of chronic scarring and deficient temperature regulation.

Reconstructive surgery

Patients must be carefully encouraged to return to a normal life. Deep areas of burn, whether grafted or not, will invariably give rise to severe and permanent scars. These scars, termed hypertrophic, are particularly troublesome in children and are hard, red, raised, irregular and pruritic. The process of maturation, that is softening, flattening and the return of normal skin colour, takes many months or years to completion. During this period contraction of the scar tissue occurs, particularly over flexor creases. The fitting of pressure garments decreases the time of scar maturation and reduces the extent of contracture formation. These garments are constructed from tight-fitting elasticated material and should be worn day and night, with exception of removal for bathing and anointing of the scarred areas with moisturizing creams.

SURGICAL TECHNIQUES FOR CONTRACTURE RELEASE

Narrow bands of contracture can be released by the Y-V plasty technique, whereas broad bands are treated by incision and inlay skin grafting. Areas of scar may be removed by the transposition of local or microvascular free flaps. The range of local transposition flaps is increased by tissue expanders, consisting of inflatable balloons that are inserted under the normal skin adjacent to the area to be excised. The tissue expander is inflated over a period of several weeks or months by injections of saline and then removed to allow the expanded skin to be transposed.

CHAPTER 74

Non-accidental injury: physical

T. STEPHENSON

Introduction
Diagnosis of non-accidental injury
Subsequent management
Neurosurgery

Orthopaedic surgery
Plastic surgery
Munchausen syndrome by proxy
References

Introduction

Non-accidental injury should not be confused with injuries due to neglect. If the parenting is inadequate, small children can easily be injured in the home through genuine accidents, whereas non-accidental injury is the result of deliberate injury, either premeditated or in anger. Out of every 300 referrals to a children's casualty department, one will be suspected non-accidental injury (Somers and Molyneux, 1992), compared to 30 genuine head injuries, 30 fractures and 5 burns or scalds.

Diagnosis of non-accidental injury

The possibility of child abuse may already have been raised because the child is presented to the doctor by a social worker, perhaps following an anonymous allegation. The doctor should follow the written local procedure and his or her role is to advise social services whether there is medical evidence to support or refute the allegation. It should be emphasized here that the doctor rarely makes a definitive 'diagnosis'. The doctor's views must be taken in conjunction with statements of eye witnesses, social workers, the police, etc. A different set of circumstances arise when the doctor is the first person to consider the possibility of child abuse.

In arriving at an opinion, the doctor should take a full history and perform a full examination. In child abuse work, however, the history is likely to be at best economical with the truth and at worst may be a total fabrication. However, the adage that 'history is 95% of the diagnosis' still holds true, not because the history can be relied upon but for the opposite reason, that child abuse is often suspected because the history is patchy, inconsistent and not in keeping with the findings.

HISTORY

The history should be recorded verbatim. If it is not consistent with the injuries this is worrying. Common explanations that are offered and are not generally acceptable are given in Table 74.1. The same person

Table 74.1 Common explanations offered for non-accidental injuries

- 'It happened while I was dressing the child'
- 'The child fell out of bed or off the sofa'
- A friend or sibling did it
- 'It happened during rough and tumble play with an adult'
- 'He bruises easily'
- Scalds due to contact with radiators or domestic hot water

may give a different history on repeated questioning or a different history may be given by different observers. These different versions should be recorded in the notes without comment. Other clues in the history are delay in presentation (Fig. 74.1) and frequent previous attendances to casualty with unexplained injuries. The parents may volunteer that the child is accident prone and whilst there do seem to be some boisterous children, especially boys, who do have a run of genuine accidents, this should not be accepted automatically.

Whilst non-accidental injury clusters in families drawn from inner-city areas, similar social class gradients are seen in genuine accidents to children. For example, road traffic accidents are five times more common in children whose fathers come from social class V than in children from professional families (Sibert and Davies, 1992).

EXAMINATION

Very few physical findings are pathognomonic of non-accidental injury. However, some features are more common in non-accidental injury than in genuine accidents and these may be useful in a 'balance of probability' assessment. All prepubertal children should be undressed completely for the examination. The child's height, weight and head circumference should be plotted on a centile chart. There may be evidence of poor hygiene, dirty clothing, dirty nappy, extensive nappy rash or frank failure to thrive. The main clue to child abuse on physical examination is that there are multiple injuries in time and space. Ageing of soft tissue injuries is an inexact science but it may be very obvious that certain injuries are of very different ages (Wilson, 1977). Multiple injuries are rare in children unless they are involved in a motor vehicle accident or similar trauma.

The shape and site of injuries may also give a clue. Young children are very prone to have bruising to the lower legs, whereas children who have sustained non-accidental injury more commonly have soft tissue injuries to the head and neck area and the trunk (Fig. 74.2) (Roberton *et al.*, 1982). Accidental injuries are usually irregular in shape, whereas regular margins to an injury suggest that it has been caused by an object such as a shoe or belt buckle.

A few injuries are particularly suggestive of non-accidental injury. Multiple bruises, approximately 1 cm in diameter, which may be found on the cheeks, chest, back, arms or thighs, may be due to fingertip pressure. There are no genuine accidental injuries that can give multiple 1 cm circular bruises on different surfaces of the body. A black eye is not uncommon in children as a result of a genuine accident, but the presence of two black eyes is particularly worrying, unless the child has had a direct blow to the forehead, e.g. from a car dashboard, or a scalp injury or a skull fracture. A torn upper frenulum is almost always a non-accidental injury. Bite marks may occur from animals (in which cases the mark is usually U-shaped with puncture wounds from the canine teeth) but human bites should always cause concern. These are crescent shaped and the size of the mark may give a clue as to whether it was inflicted by an adult or a child. Toddlers certainly do bite but most parents would not allow their child to sustain multiple bites in this way. Linear bruising on the buttocks suggests beating with a cane or a strap. As with the history, the importance of accurate documentation of

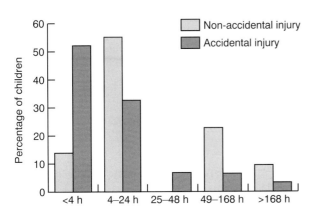

Fig. 74.1 Delay in presentation following accidental fractures (*n* = 502 children) and non-accidental fractures (*n* = 22 children).

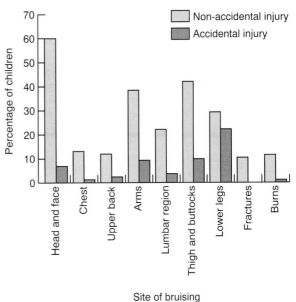

Fig. 74.2 Distribution of bruises in 400 normal children and 84 children with suspected or definite non-accidental injuries, aged 0–11 years (Roberton *et al.*, 1982).

injuries cannot be overestimated and casualty departments should provide a body chart (analogous to that used for burns) to allow even the least artistically inclined to record the injuries. This should be a contemporaneous record of the site, dimensions and colour of each injury. Vague hatching and shading should be avoided as this is virtually uninterpretable in court many months later. Few departments offer a 24-hour photographic service and therefore this diagram may be very important in any subsequent legal action.

INVESTIGATION

Investigations have only a small part to play in the diagnosis of non-accidental injury. It is our practice always to explain to the parents why a skeletal survey is being undertaken and such investigations should never be performed without telling the parents. Approximately 25% of children in Nottingham are investigated and only about one in 20 of these will show positive findings.

Investigations are indicated in the following circumstances.

1. The bruising looks unusually extensive or there is a very large scalp haematoma. A platelet count and clotting studies should be carried out to exclude idiopathic thrombocytopenic purpura and haemophilia.
2. If examination suggests the presence of an underlying fracture, then an X-ray of the appropriate part with corresponding views of the contralateral limb or joint should be obtained on medical grounds alone. If a fracture is found in any child in whom there is a possibility of non-accidental injury, a skeletal survey should be performed. This may show other old fractures. The finding of multiple rib fractures in the absence of any history of a major trauma such as a motor vehicle accident is virtually diagnostic of non-accidental injury (Worlock *et al.*, 1986). The different patterns of fractures seen in accidental and non-accidental injury are shown in Fig. 74.3. Radiological evidence of multiple injuries over time is very suggestive of child abuse (Chapman, 1992).

CONSENT TO EXAMINATION

When parents or legal guardians present a child to be seen by a doctor, there is implied consent that the doctor will examine as much of the child as he or she feels necessary. Indeed, failure to do so may subsequently be regarded as negligent. There is therefore no obligation to seek consent even if the examination is for suspected non-accidental injury. However, if an older child specifically refused to undress, there would be little to be gained by trying to pursue this forcibly. A court order does not allow a doctor to proceed against the informed

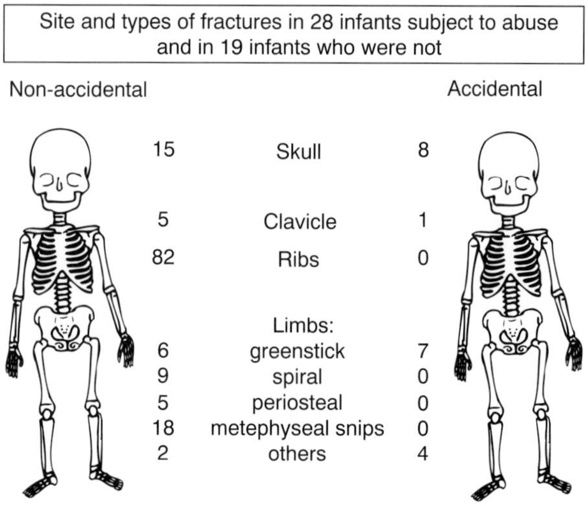

Site and types of fractures in 28 infants subject to abuse and in 19 infants who were not

	Non-accidental		Accidental
	15	Skull	8
	5	Clavicle	1
	82	Ribs	0
		Limbs:	
	6	greenstick	7
	9	spiral	0
	5	periosteal	0
	18	metephyseal snips	0
	2	others	4

Fig. 74.3 Site and type of fractures in 28 infants (i.e. less than 18 months old) subjected to abuse and in 19 infants who were not (after Worlock *et al.*, 1986).

wishes of a child who does not consent. Under an emergency protection order, parental presence or consent is not necessary. Finally, the rules of consent are not relevant in the case of a medical emergency: if a child is unconscious, disorientated or not thought to understand adequately the seriousness of his or her condition, the doctor should act in the best long-term interests of the child.

Children between 16 and 18 years of age are now considered to have the same capacity as an adult to consent to examination or treatment. A child under the age of 16 is able to consent provided he or she is sufficiently mature and intelligent to be able to understand what is involved in treatment ('Gillick competent'). Whether the child is competent to consent to treatment or surgery is left as a matter for the doctor to decide and this is a grey area (McCall Smith, 1992). The most difficult area is when a child under the age of 16 withholds consent to treatment or surgery even though he or she would be judged to have the capacity to give consent (Devereux *et al.*, 1993).

Subsequent management

IMMEDIATE ACTION

If a surgeon suspects non-accidental injury, it is then reasonable to involve the paediatric team. All previous hospital records should be obtained and an inquiry should be made into the local 'at-risk' register. If the surgeon is unwilling or unable to involve a paediatrician, the following approach is recommended. An adversarial situation should be avoided. The parents should never be accused and the doctor must not state unequivocally that the child has been abused but simply explain that the findings do not seem to be consistent with the explanation that was given and under these circumstances there is a procedure that must be followed. The doctor should explain that social services must be involved immediately. It is for social services to decide whether the police should be involved and this is not a role for the doctor. If the child requires further treatment, traction or surgery, then obviously he or she must be admitted. If no further treatment is necessary, it is for social services to decide whether it is safe for the child to return home. The doctor may be asked for his view on the causation and severity of the injuries.

CASE CONFERENCE

A case conference will be held, usually within 1 week of the incident. If the doctor is unable to attend, he or she must ensure that a written report is available. The report should state the doctor's name, qualifications, position and experience. The report should start with the facts, beginning with the history and including a verbatim record of the parents' explanation. Hearsay is allowed in case conferences, although a different view may be taken if the case proceeds to court. All photographs or charts should be included and the explanation should be graphic. 'A deep straight cut on the forearm about 1/4-inch deep' is more meaningful to lay people than 'a linear laceration on the volar surface of the distal upper limb'. The report should finish with an opinion of the mechanism of the injuries. This should be followed by an unequivocal conclusion as to whether the doctor thinks the injury is accidental or non-accidental. The doctor does not have to believe beyond reasonable doubt that the wound was due to a bread knife but merely on the balance of probability that this was so (Speight, 1987). Parents are now entitled to be present at case conferences.

APPEARING IN COURT

Although only about 3% of cases lead to criminal proceedings to punish the guilty perpetrator, many more cases lead to action in the civil courts. This can be very intimidating. The doctor may be called as a witness to fact (in his or her professional capacity as someone who has seen and treated the child) or as an expert witness to give opinion on the possible mechanisms and causation of injuries. It is extremely important that the doctor is seen to be impartial, irrespective of which side has called him or her to give evidence. It is wise for the witness to decide his or her opinions in advance and to speak clearly and in plain language. It is also wise to know the limits of one's expertise and to be willing to say 'I do not know' if that is the case. It is important that the witness emphasizes to the court that in child abuse work, the injuries must be taken in their entirety and the whole picture is more important that any single injury. Phrases such as 'consistent with non-accidental injury' should be avoided as the burden of proof in a civil court is balance of probability and this can be interpreted by asking oneself the question 'is it more likely than not that the injury amounts to ill-treatment?' (Taitz and King, 1986).

Neurosurgery

Accidental skull fractures are usually single and follow serious trauma. There is evidence that children who fall from heights up to 3 feet are extremely unlikely to sustain skull fractures (Helfer *et al.*, 1977; Nimityongskul and Anderson, 1987). Compound fractures, depressed fractures and multiple skull fractures are particularly uncommon. Skull fractures are rare in young children, particularly before the sutures have fused, and therefore a skull fracture in any infant without an adequate explanation, particularly one who is not mobile, is suspicious.

Intracranial bleeding can arise as a result of trauma (either accidental or non-accidental) or spontaneously (an aneurysm, arterio-venous malformation or coagulopathy). However, vascular anomalies within the brain are rare in childhood as a cause of intracranial haemorrhage. Acute subdural haematoma is the most common non-accidental head injury (Billmire and Myers, 1985). This requires significant trauma (unless the child has an underlying coagulopathy) but there is not always an associated skull fracture (30%) (Harwood-Nash, 1992) or loss of consciousness. Acute subdural haematoma may be the result of either an object striking the head or the child being shaken, tearing bridging meningeal veins. A common finding on a computed tomography (CT) scan is an interhemispheric (parafalcial) subdural haematoma (Zimmerman *et al.*, 1978). Detailed cranial ultrasonography may provide further clues (Jaspan *et al.*, 1992). The clinical picture following acute subdural haematoma is variable – there may be vomiting, seizures, impaired consciousness or irritability. It may go undetected and then progress to a chronic subdural haematoma. The development of a chronic subdural haematoma may be insidious and the diagnosis delayed, the child presenting with pallor, irritability, failure to thrive or an increase in skull size.

Orthopaedic surgery

One of the most common forms of physical abuse is non-accidental fracture (Fig. 74.3). Spiral fractures are particularly worrying as they imply twisting injuries and the presence of subperiosteal calcification is suggestive of child abuse. Periosteal calcification may not be visible for days to weeks after the injury and the films may therefore need to be repeated. However, a spiral fracture may occur in any setting in which there is rotational force on a bone such as when a leg is trapped under the rest of the body during a fall. Transverse fractures imply a direct blow to the bone or snapping of the bone over a fulcrum. Transverse fractures through the radius and ulna may occur as a result of a blow while the child is holding the arm up in defence. Fractures in a child who is not yet mobile should always cause concern. Firm restraint may be required to change the nappy of a writhing toddler, but this should not result in fractures. This simply emphasizes the very considerable forces that are required to cause fractures even in a young infant. One in eight fractures in children under 18 months may be non-accidental (Worlock *et al.*, 1986). Metaphyseal chip injury should also raise suspicion. Metaphyseal injuries occur when the limbs are subjected to pulling or torsional forces, causing fractures through newly forming bone. The most common site of these injuries is in the distal humerus and femur or the proximal tibia.

If any of the above observations suggest concern, a skeletal survey should be carried out. Genuine multiple fractures are only seen in young children in the context of severe trauma. Fractures of different ages (Table 74.2; Hobbs, 1989a) suggest multiple separate injuries (Chapman, 1992). Rib fractures are typically caused non-accidentally by squeezing of the child's thorax during shaking. The force required is far in excess of that involved in the normal rearing, dressing, feeding or restraining of children. Most parents quickly note the child's pain and loss of function following accidental fracture of a limb, which is particularly painful during manoeuvres such as dressing, whereas there is often alleged delay in recognition of non-accidental fractures (Fig. 74.1).

The suggestion is sometimes made that the child has a form of osteogenesis imperfecta. In a city of 500 000 people, the chance of encountering a child under 1 year old with osteogenesis imperfecta who shows no other features or family findings of the disease (skeletal deformity, blue sclerae, wormian bones, hypermobility of the joints, deafness, abnormal teeth in relatives) would be roughly one in a million. Therefore, there would be one case every 100 years, whereas the annual incidence

of fractures caused by non-accidental injury would be about 15 cases (Taitz, 1987; Ablin *et al.*, 1990). Several other conditions in young children (congenital syphilis, scurvy, copper deficiency, infantile cortical hyperostosis, and Menke's kinky hair syndrome) may render the bones more susceptible to injury but these are all very rare and have characteristic clinical or radiological appearances that should allow differentiation from non-accidental injury (Shaw, 1988; Carty, 1988). Only in children with the rare abnormalities discussed above, or with extreme osteoporosis or rickets, might cardiac massage or physiotherapy result in fracture.

Radiological changes may also be seen in the period shortly after birth. Fractures of the clavicles are not uncommon and skull fractures occur rarely with forceps delivery. These fractures are sometimes depressed. Periosteal changes in the diaphysis of the long bones may also be seen but are usually symmetrical and transient. Expert radiological dating of the abnormality and a careful obstetric history should allow distinction from non-accidental injury.

A pulled elbow typically occurs when a toddler trips and the adult holds on, pulling and twisting causing subluxation of the head of the radius. This injury is not indicative of abuse and some children will repeatedly dislocate the same elbow.

Plastic surgery

The most common type of non-accidental burn is a cigarette burn which leaves a circular red mark, sometimes with a blister if the injury is recent, but this is by no means diagnostic. However, if the injuries are multiple an accidental explanation becomes less tenable. Scalds are also fairly common and there may be characteristic shapes, e.g. the symmetrical stocking distribution seen on the child suspended in a bath of very hot water is rare but very characteristic. A genuine accidental scald from a hot bath leaves an irregular mark with splashes, usually affecting only one foot or hand. Domestic hot water supplies [the Child Accident Prevention Trust (1985) recommend no higher than 54°C] are capable of being heated to a temperature at which very severe burns can occur. Scalds often follow the contour of clothes and an assessment should be made of whether the explanation is consistent with the pattern and distribution of the injuries (Keen *et al.*, 1975; Hight *et al.*, 1979; Hobbs, 1986). If a child pulls a kettle or cup of hot water over themselves, the scald predominantly affects the shoulders, upper arms, upper trunk and chin, with sparing of the neck crease. Scalds from a hot drink thrown at a child produce a scattered splash effect.

Very well-demarcated or geometric regular burns are usually dry burns due to contact with hot objects such as a poker. In general, central heating radiators are not

Table 74.2 The dating of fractures (Hobbs, 1989a)

Event	Timescale
Resolution of soft tissue change	4–10 days
Periosteal new bone formation	10–14 days
Loss of fracture line definition	14–21 days
Soft callus	14–21 days
Hard callus	21–42 days
Remodelling	1 year

Table 74.3 Thermal injuries

Average bath temperature	40.5°C
Adult notices discomfort	43.0°C
Adult reaction time to withdraw	0.2 s

Duration of exposure (s)	Temperature (°C)	Thermal injury
10	50	Redness
10	60	Very superficial burn
10	70	Full thickness burn
1	>70	Partial thickness burn
60	55–65	Partial thickness burn

hot enough to cause severe burns and an older child will usually pull their hand away very quickly (Table 74.3 and Fig. 74.4). Some older radiators can be extremely hot (up to 80°C) and a young infant may be trapped against the surface for some time by the bedclothes or during sleep (Hobbs, 1989b).

Non-accidental burns more commonly affect the face and head, perineum, buttocks and genitalia than accidental burns. Hands commonly show burns to the dorsal surface in physical abuse whereas in genuine accidents the palm is usually affected. Sadly, the possibility of a burn being non-accidental because it appears too severe cannot be dismissed.

A detailed history should be taken of the duration of exposure and unusual areas of sparing of injuries should also be noted. The depth of a burn depends on the temperature, the duration of exposure and thickness of the skin (Fig. 74.4). Children, particularly infants, have considerably thinner skin than adults and the duration of exposure needs therefore to be shorter. Skin disorders can mimic burns (Table 74.4) (Bull and lawrence, 1989).

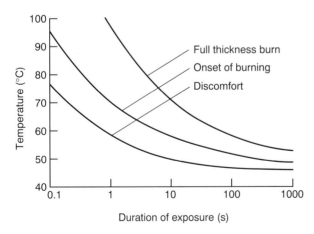

Fig. 74.4 Diagram of temperature and duration of exposure curves sufficient to cause discomfort or burns in adults (Bull and Lawrence, 1979).

Munchausen syndrome by proxy

This diagnosis may be applied to any parent who persistently fabricates symptoms on behalf of a child or induces symptoms in the child, so causing that child to be regarded as ill. Examples that may present to surgeons are the use of adult or animal blood to simulate urinary or rectal bleeding in the child, deliberate salt poisoning of the child leading to vomiting and diarrhoea, claims that the child has joint pains or an intermittent limp, and the induction of apnoeas by suffocation which may lead to referral to an ear, nose and throat surgeon to exclude congenital abnormality of the upper airway.

The diagnosis is usually first suspected because the symptoms or signs of disease are only noticed when one of the parents is present. There seems to be no unifying diagnosis, treatment of the condition is ineffective and symptoms only cease when the parents are excluded from contact. If a surgeon suspects that symptoms or signs are being fabricated, an experienced paediatric colleague should be involved early on. A period of covert surveillance may be necessary and eventually the perpetrator must be confronted by someone with previous experience of such cases. The

Table 74.4 Conditions that may be confused with non-accidental burns

Skin conditions which may mimic burns	Conditions associated with unusual accidental burns
Epidermolysis bullosa	Congenital insensitivity
Impetigo	to pain
Contact dermatitis	Syringomyelia
Severe nappy rash	Spina bifida
Toxic epidermal	Cerebral palsy
necrolysis	Mental retardation
	Epilepsy
	Peripheral neuropathy

important message is that once the surgeon considers the diagnosis, endless and exhaustive investigation and testing should not be pursued (Meadow, 1985, 1990; Stephenson, 1993).

ACKNOWLEDGEMENT

I am very grateful to Miss Fiona Bailie for advice on non-accidental burns.

References

Ablin, D.S., Greenspan, A., Reinhart, M. and Grix, A. 1990: Differentiation of child abuse from osteogenesis imperfecta. *American Journal of Radiology* **154**, 1035–46.

Billmire, M.E. and Myers, P.A. 1985: Serious head injury in infants: accidental or abuse? *Pediatrics* **75**, 340–2.

Bull, J.P. and Lawrence, J.C. 1979: Thermal conditions to produce skin burns. *Fire and Materials* **3**, 100–5.

Carty, H. 1988: Brittle or battered? *Archives of Disease in Childhood* **63**, 350–2.

Chapman, S. 1992: The radiological dating of injuries. *Archives of Disease in Childhood* **67**, 1063–5.

Child Accident Prevention Trust 1985: Scalds and recommendations for their prevention. In Report of a Working Party of the Child Accident Prevention Trust: *Burn and scald accidents in children*. London: Bedford Square Press, 37–41.

Devereuz, J.A., Jones, D.P.H. and Dickenson, D.L. 1993: Can children withhold consent to treatment? *British Medical Journal* **306**, 1459–61.

Harwood-Nash, D.C. 1992: Abuse to the paediatric central nervous system. *American Journal of Neuroradiology* **13**, 569–75.

Helfer, R.E., Slovis, T.L. and Black, M. 1977: Injuries resulting when small children fall out of bed. *Pediatrics* **60**, 533–5.

Hight, D.W., Bakalar, H.R. and Lloyd, J. 1979: Inflicted burns in children. *Journal of the American Medical Association* **242**, 517–20.

Hobbs, C.J. 1986: When are burns not accidental? *Archives of Disease in Childhood* **61**, 357–61.

Hobbs, C.J. 1989a: Fractures. *British Medical Journal* **298**, 1015–8.

Hobbs, C.J. 1989b: Burns and scalds. *British Medical Journal* **298**, 1302–5.

Jaspan, T., Narborough, G., Punt, J.A.G. and Lowe, W.E.J. 1992: Cerebrocontusional tears as a mark of child abuse – detection by cranial ultrasonography. *Paediatric Radiology* **22**, 237–45.

Keen, J.H., Lendrum, J. and Wolman, B. 1975: Inflicted burns and scalds in children. *British Medical Journal* **4**, 268–9.

McCall Smith, A. 1992: Consent to treatment in childhood. *Archives of Disease in Childhood* **67**, 1247–8.

Meadow, R. 1985: Management of Munchausen syndrome by proxy. *Archives of Disease in Childhood* **60**, 385–93.

Meadow, R. 1990: Suffocation, recurrent apnoea and sudden infant death. *Journal of Pediatrics* **117**, 351–7.

Nimityongskul, P. and Anderson, L.D. 1987: The likelihood of injuries when children fall out of bed. *Journal of Pediatric Orthopedics* **7**, 184–6.

Roberton, D., Barbor, P. and Hull, D. 1982: Unusual injury? Recent injury in normal children and children with suspected non-accidental injury. *British Medical Journal* **285**, 1399–401.

Shaw, J.C.L. 1988: Copper deficiency in non-accidental injury. *Archives of Disease in Childhood* **63**, 448–55.

Sibert, J. and Davies, P.A. 1992: Poisoning, accidents and sudden infant death syndrome. In Campbell, A.G.M. and McIntosh, N. (eds), *Forfar and Arneil's textbook of paediatrics*, 4th ed. Edinburgh: Churchill Livingstone, 1777–800.

Somers, C.L. and Molyneux, E.M. 1992: Suspected child abuse: cost in medical time and finance. *Archives of Disease in Childhood* **67**, 905–10.

Speight, N. 1987: Case conferences for child abuse. *Archives of Disease in Childhood* **62**, 1063–5.

Stephenson, T.J. 1993: Beyond belief – Munchausen syndrome by proxy. *Law Society Gazette* **90**, 28–9.

Taitz, L.S. 1987: Child abuse and osteogenesis imperfecta. *British Medical Journal* **295**, 1082–3.

Taitz, L.S. and King, J. 1986: Medical evidence in child abuse. *Archives of Disease in Childhood* **61**, 205–6.

Wilson, E.F. 1979: Estimation of the age of contusions in child abuse. *Pediatrics* **60**, 750–2.

Worlock, P., Stower, M. and Barbor, P. 1986: Patterns of fractures in accidental and non-accidental injury in children: a comparative study. *British Medical Journal* **293**, 100–2.

Zimmerman, R.A., Bilaniuk, L.T., Bruce, D., Schut, L., Uzzell, B. and Goldberg, H.I. 1978: Interhemispheric acute subdural haematoma: a computed tomographic manifestation. *Neuroradiology* **16**, 39–40.

CHAPTER 75

Non-accidental injury: sexual abuse

B.L. PRIESTLEY AND A. HEGER

Introduction
Clinical features
Appearances in abused versus
non-abused children

Acute sexual abuse
References
Further reading

Introduction

Child sexual abuse is the involvement of a child by an adult, or teenager – in activities which lead to the sexual gratification of the adult. Such activities include fondling, tickling, touching, rubbing, kissing, licking, sucking, mutual masturbation, penetration of the mouth, vagina or anus by tongue, finger or penis and the use of children in pornography.

Abusers are very commonly either related to the child or a member of the household, e.g. the mother's cohabitee. They may be otherwise known to the child, such as a teenage babysitter, neighbour, nursery attendant or care giver in a children's home. In only about 20% of cases is the abuser a total stranger to the child. In about one-third of cases of abuse, the perpetrator is a teenager.

Victims are often vulnerable children such as those living in a chaotic or fragmented family with little family support or children with multiple handicaps. It is being increasingly recognized that severe communication problems or learning difficulties place children at heightened risk of abuse.

Other risk factors include a past history of sexual abuse within the family – 'the best predictor of future behaviour is past behaviour', alcoholism in a male family member, depression or low intelligence in the mother, especially if associated with refusal of sexual relationships, and the presence of a stepfather figure in the household. Although sexual abuse occurs at all levels in society, it is most frequently recognized in association with deprivation.

Abuse often starts early in childhood, though it may not present until many years later. In one large series, 40% of victims were under the age of 5 years (Hobbs and Wynne, 1989). Abuse of boys accounts for about one-third of suspected cases. In younger children anal or anogenital abuse is common, whereas penetrative genital abuse is common in older prepubertal and post-pubertal girls.

Clinical features

Presentation of abuse occurs in various ways, some fairly clear and others leading only to a suspicion of the possibility of abuse. When the suspicion reaches a certain critical level a multidisciplinary assessment is essential. Concern may arise as a result of:

- a disclosure by the child or an incomplete partial allegation
- a statement by a parent, carer or witness of abuse
- behavioural changes in the child, e.g. anxiety, excessive clinginess, irritability, fear of men, eating and sleeping disturbance, recurrence of enuresis, constipation, soiling, compulsive masturbation or other sexualized behaviour. In the older child abuse may result in alteration in school performance, withdrawal and isolation and later running away, drug abuse, attempted suicide and prostitution
- onset of psychosomatic symptoms such as headaches, abdominal pain and frequency of micturition

- physical symptoms or signs such as anogenital soreness, inflammation, bruising, bleeding, multiple anal fissures, recurrent vaginal discharge, hymenal damage, anogenital warts, sexually transmitted infections and, in the postpubertal girl, pregnancy. Pregnancy in a teenager who conceals the identity of the father should prompt consideration of abuse.

Any professional coming into contact with children should be aware of the spectrum of ways in which abuse may manifest and also of the sometimes intense pressure upon the child to maintain secrecy. As indicated by Sgroi (1975), the diagnosis of sexual abuse is entirely dependent on the willingness of the individual to entertain the possibility that abuse may have occurred.

The paediatric surgical team may encounter abuse in any of the above guises. However, direct referral to the team is likely to occur:

- when a child presents in the accident and emergency department with anal or genital injury such as bruising, bleeding or tears and an assessment is needed as to the extent of the injury, whether a repair is required and whether the injury is likely to be accidental or non-accidental
- when a child presents with a history of anal pain and defecation problems. Anal fissures may be associated with bowel disturbances, with skin diseases such as anogenital lichen sclerosis and with abuse
- with a history of recent onset of micturition problems
- with recurrent vaginal discharge or soreness, raising the possibility of a vaginal foreign body
- during a routine consultation, when a parent or carer volunteers concern over possible abuse, often whilst the child was in another's care, or on an access visit.

INITIAL ASSESSMENT

The child and carer should, where possible, be seen in a friendly and comfortable environment. A detailed history is required and any spontaneous statements by the child should be accurately and fully documented. However, detailed questioning about an alleged abusive event should not be undertaken by those inexperienced or untrained in the field because of the need to avoid both repetitive interviews and prejudicial leading questions.

The examination should be conducted in the presence of a caring adult trusted by the child. This is usually the mother. The examiner should be experienced or should enlist the assistance of a senior experienced colleague. It is important to keep detailed records and to document fully both positive and negative findings.

Firstly, the child's demeanour is noted, whether cheerful and confident or withdrawn and unhappy. The ease and closeness of relationship with the parent(s) or carer are noted as is the ease with which the examiner can establish a friendly response from the child.

A full general examination is next undertaken leaving the specific problem area until the last. It is important to assess the child's nutrition and growth, documenting height, weight and head circumference percentiles and the developmental status of the child. Any areas of bruising, scratching, abrasions, burns or bites are carefully listed, since there is a well-established association between non-accidental injury and child sexual abuse. About 20% of children with non-accidental injury are also subjected to sexual abuse and 15% of sexually abused children show signs of physical injury. More specifically, love bites may be found around the neck or breasts and groups of finger tip bruises around the knees or on the upper thighs in children forcibly restrained for sexual abuse (Hobbs and Wynne, 1990).

GENITAL EXAMINATION

The genitalia are best examined with the child lying supine in the frog-legged position with the soles of the feet touching (Fig 75.1). In girls under the age of 3 years it may be more reassuring to the child to be held in this position on the mother's lap. It is customary to refer to a clock face to describe the position of findings, with 12 o'clock anterior and 6 o'clock posterior, i.e. closest to the anus, as shown on the diagram.

The prone knee–chest position may also be used. There is less experience in the UK in the interpretation of findings in this position, but the knee–chest position may be indicated when the supine examination does not allow the examiner to assess fully whether the posterior 180° of the hymen is free of any evidence of previous trauma. The prone position facilitates evaluation of the posterior rim of the hymen. The use of this position is more difficult for the child and it should be used only when necessary.

The external genitalia are inspected for redness, swelling, discoloration or other signs of injury. The labia are then separated and the vestibule is fully inspected, noting the urethral orifice and the approximate size of the hymenal orifice. It should be appreciated that external measurement of the hymenal orifice can only be an estimate. Labial traction is then applied, the examiner grasping the posterior parts of the labia majora between thumb and forefinger and gently pulling both posteriorly towards the couch and inferiorly towards the child's feet. This technique results in the maximal hymenal diameter in the horizontal direction. It gives a clearer view of the configuration and margin of the hymen and the presence of any abrasions, bruises, bumps, notches, clefts or tears. Any vaginal discharge is noted, along with any genital warts, which are usually small and sited within the labia.

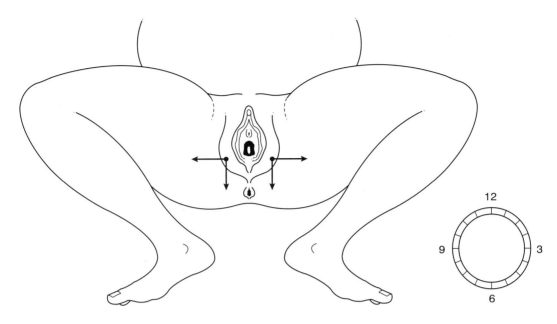

Examination position
Gentle traction between thumb and index finger at posterior
edge of labia majora to show hymen

Fig. 75.1 Position for genital examination. (After Royal College of Physicians Report, 1991.)

Increasingly in larger units or referral centres, the use of a colposcope has allowed for the photodocumentation of clinical findings. The major benefit of colposcopic documentation has been the potential for peer review, making further examinations of the child unnecessary. Although it is unlikely that colposcopy will reveal significant positive findings of abuse that would otherwise go undetected by a trained evaluator, it does allow less experienced examiners easy access to consultation with more experienced senior colleagues.

In a boy the penis and scrotum are inspected for superficial signs of injury which may include marks of a ligature, a tear of the frenulum of the prepuce, burns or bruising.

PERIANAL EXAMINATION

This is best carried out in the left lateral position with the child lying curled up. The buttocks are gently separated using the palms of the examiner's hands and held so for 30 s whilst the area is inspected carefully. Any inflammation, soreness, bruising or oedema is noted. Internal haemorrhoids are extremely rare in childhood and tend to occur at positions 4, 7 and 11 o'clock and usually in association with a positive family history. During the 30-s observation period, the external anal sphincter will often relax, allowing better visualization of the anal margin for a fissure, i.e. a break in the continuity of the stratified epithelium or the pale scar of a previous fissure.

On occasion, both external and internal anal sphincters slowly relax, allowing the anus to open up widely, thereby providing a clear view within. This is referred to as reflex anal dilatation. Its presence is influenced by anxiety, the degree of relaxation of the child, the presence of stool in the rectum, which may not always be visible through the dilated anus, and other features such as moderate to severe constipation. This is especially the case after the use of suppositories or enemata. Reflex anal dilatation may also be seen in children who are seriously ill for any reason and has been reported in Crohn's disease, in haemolytic uraemic syndrome and in sick children on ventilators. It may also be found in children with neuromuscular weakness, e.g. spina bifida, myotonic dystrophy and in some normal children. Anal dilatation is sometimes seen as part of post mortem changes.

Reflex anal dilatation (Fig. 75.2), has been found more commonly in abused than in non-abused children. If the anal dilatation is greater than 15 mm in the horizontal diameter and is a reproducible sign, it is of greater significance and should raise the suspicion of abuse. This is a 'soft' sign and in no way diagnostic.

It is important to note that there is a wide overlap in physical signs between abused and non-abused populations and it is very important not to make a diagnosis of abuse on signs of uncertain significance (Royal College of Physicians, 1997). It is equally important to note that there are no abnormal physical signs in one-half to two-thirds of abused children.

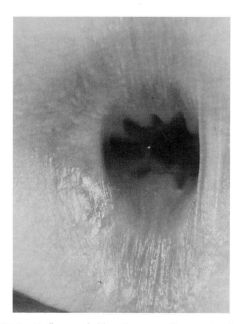

Fig. 75.2 Reflex anal dilatation revealing anal valves.

CHANGES IN FEMALE GENITALIA WITH AGE

Physical findings in abuse vary according to the type of abuse perpetrated and the age of the child, since genital appearances alter with age. In the newborn the labia, are thick and prominent, as is the hymen which often appears closed. The clitoris is turgid, under the influence of maternal hormones.

During the preschool and primary school years the labia majora are flat and the labia minora are delicate thin folds. The hymen is commonly a posterior rim variant, although annular and less commonly fimbriated types also occur. The hymenal orifice is occasionally septate or the hymen, rarely, cribriform. The hymen is thin and with a delicate margin during childhood. This changes in appearance as a result of oestrogenization, often becoming sleeve-like and fleshy during puberty.

Appearances in abused versus non-abused children

Signs found in both abused and non-abused populations include hymenal mounds (7–34% of normal girls), labial fusion (22–39%), mid-line avascular areas in the posterior fourchette (4–26%), and longitudinal intravaginal ridges (25–90% of normal) (McCann *et al.*, 1990; Berenson *et al.*, 1992).

Hymenal notches or clefts are found commonly in non-abused children in the 11 and 1 o'clock positions or in the mid-line anteriorly, and less commonly at 3 and 9 o'clock. Confirmation that these are within the normal range is provided by the finding of hymenal clefts in the newborn (Berenson *et al.*, 1991). It should be noted that

notches or clefts have not been found posteriorly, i.e. between 4 and 8 o'clock, in non-abused children. However, care should be taken in coming to the conclusion that notches between 4 and 8 o'clock are diagnostic of penetration. A frequent mistake of inexperienced physicians is to conclude that the normal space or depression lying between longitudinal ridges that extend out on to the hymenal edge at 4 and 8 o'clock is in fact a notch and therefore indicative of penetrative trauma.

The only diagnostic signs of abuse (in the absence of reasonable alternative explanation) are a laceration or scar in the hymen, marked attenuation of a portion or all of the hymen where the tissue has become worn away by friction leaving an enlarged, and often asymmetrical hymenal orifice and, with regard to the perineal area, a laceration of the lining of the anal canal, extending on to the perianal skin.

All other positive findings, whilst they may be used to support a child's story of abuse, can only be regarded as being consistent with abuse, but with possible alternative explanations. Thus, erythema or inflammation may result from the friction of intercrural intercourse but may also be found in association with threadworms, eczema, streptococcal or other skin infection, thrush, enuresis, poor hygiene and scratching.

Vulval and perianal inflammation and induration have been described in Crohn's disease and are also seen in anogenital lichen sclerosis. This is a skin condition of uncertain aetiology and more commonly found in older women. However with increased awareness of abuse, young girls with persistent vulval symptoms are now referred more frequently for specialist care and more cases of lichen sclerosis are being recognized. It has on occasion been misdiagnosed as sexual abuse, with distressing consequences.

Lichen sclerosis

This first appears as flat topped ivory papules which coalesce producing a pale sclerotic appearance with wrinkling. It is associated with markedly increased friability of the skin with easy superficial fissuring, bleeding and bruising. Purpuric patches are common, especially as a result of scratching and there is an increased susceptibility to superficial infection.

Involvement of the anogenital region often takes the form of a figure-of-eight with inflammation of the perianal region, spreading into the anal canal (Fig. 75.3). The lining epithelium of the anal canal may become soggy and fissured, causing painful defecation or severe constipation. The condition responds to potent topical steroids and moisturizing preparations but requires prolonged treatment, in contrast to the inflammation resulting from abuse which clears rapidly when the abuse ceases. Whilst lichen sclerosis and sexual abuse may co-exist, the vast majority of cases have no such association. It should be noted that the hymen

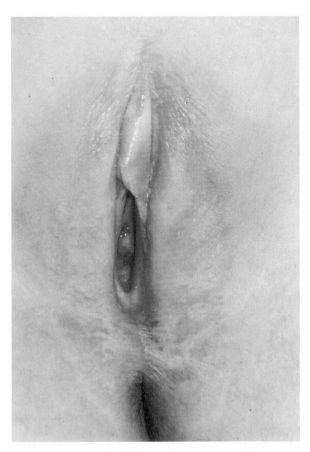

Fig. 75.3 Anogenital lichen sclerosis et atrophicus.

itself appears not to be involved in the changes of lichen sclerosis. Perianal lichen sclerosis has not been reported in boys.

Fusion of the labia minora

This condition is found frequently in infancy and is likely to resolve spontaneously over 1 or 2 years. These labial adhesions are usually transparent and delicate. It is known that labial adhesions may occur after any irritation such as local inflammation, nappy rashes, non-specific vaginitis or sexual abuse. It would be difficult to distinguish those labial adhesions associated with abuse from those which occur from other causes.

Size of the hymenal orifice

At one time this was regarded as highly significant in the context of abuse. The only truly reliable measurements of hymenal orifice size come from colposcopic photographs. Even with these precise measurements it is now appreciated that the hymenal orifice may be very variable in appearance and it is noted that an experienced examiner may achieve greater relaxation in the child and a greater dimension of the hymenal orifice. The hymen is elastic and the surrounding tissues are contractile, allowing marked variation with the degree of relaxation achieved and the examination technique used. Although the size of the orifice has been reported as less than 4 mm up to the age 5 years and 1 mm per year of age prepubertally, these measurements are at best only a guide. However, a hymenal orifice greater than 15 mm in a prepubertal child is abnormal and should raise suspicion of abuse.

Conversely, a hymenal orifice measuring only 5 mm can no longer be regarded as proof that nothing of larger diameter has entered the vagina. Whilst penile penetration is likely to leave signs of trauma in a prepubertal girl, this is probably not uniformly the case. Further, hymenal tears often heal rapidly so that a small contracted hymen, albeit scarred, may result from abuse.

Hymenal tears

In penile abuse tears are likely to be found in the posterior quadrant of the hymen with associated injury to the posterior fourchette at the attachment of the perineal body (Fig. 75.4A). Appearances may change rapidly with healing (Fig. 75.4B).

With digital penetration, any damage to the hymen depends on the age, development and size of the child. This damage may be anywhere on the hymen but anterior damage is difficult to assess since the majority of hymens are posterior rim, or crescentic, with an absence of hymen anteriorly. In addition, studies on normal girls and on the newborn have shown that there are congenital notches anteriorly, which must not be confused with abuse.

In the case of accidental injury the surrounding tissues, i.e. the labia or occasionally the vestibular fossa, are likely to be traumatized whilst the hymen itself remains intact (Fig 75.5).

Anogenital warts

These are a cause for concern in the context of sexual abuse. Over 70 types of human papilloma virus have been identified and a number of these carry an increased risk of neoplasia. The virus may be perinatally transmitted and may not be apparent for many months. Therefore warts appearing up to the age of 3 years are usually regarded as perinatally acquired. Views vary widely as to the relationship with abuse, some authorities believing that the majority are acquired in this way, with others suggesting only a minority results from abuse. There are as yet no clear guidelines but it seems likely that the presence of anogenital warts is significantly associated with abuse in a proportion of children and therefore warrants investigation.

Sexually transmitted disease (STD)

STD in a child is highly significant and requires explanation. Gonococcus, chlamydia and herpes simplex may all be acquired perinatally. Chlamydia acquired

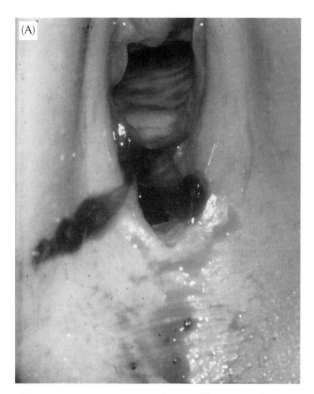 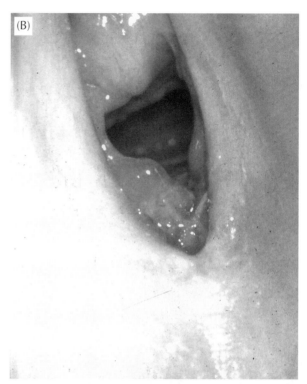

Fig. 75.4 (A) Acute rape with tear of hymen and posterior fourchette; (B) same child as in (A), 1 week later.

perinatally may be isolated on occasion during the first 3 years of life but the isolation of gonococcus in a child after the perinatal period makes a diagnosis of abuse almost certain. The case is less clear for chlamydia and herpes but is nevertheless a cause for concern. The association of STD with genital warts indicates abuse.

Vaginal discharge

Discharge in a young child requires appropriate cultures to be taken. Once STD has been excluded the condition is one that is seen quite commonly in both non-abused and abused children. Simple infections may be the cause, such as *Haemophilus influenzae* or *Streptococcus*. The isolation of *Gardnerella vaginalis* in a prepubertal girl has been regarded as suspicious, but a recent study (Ingram *et al.*, 1992) demonstrated that the incidence of this organism in the vagina is no higher in abused than in non-abused girls.

Vaginal foreign body

This is a very infrequent finding, although on occasion it results in a persistent offensive, sometimes blood-stained discharge. Examination under a general anaesthetic is required in this situation in order to exclude and/or remove a foreign body. The presence of a foreign body in the vagina, especially if repeated, should prompt an assessment for possible sexual abuse.

Acute sexual abuse

If a child is seen within 72 hours of an episode of sexual abuse, then it is important that appropriate forensic samples are collected under proper conditions and with the chain of evidence maintained (Royal College of Physicians, 1997). These samples may include saliva or gingivolabial swabs from the oral cavity, skin swabs from areas of possible semen deposition and both external and internal vaginal and anal swabs where feasible. Material for DNA analysis may be obtained from the vagina up to 7 days after the abuse making forensic evidence still important at this interval.

Swabs for culture for STD should usually be obtained at the same time, particularly in the case of an acute assault by a stranger. In the case of chronic abuse within the family the need for culture is less urgent. It is essential that the collection of both forensic samples and swabs for STD is expertly dealt with, hence the need to obtain advice or assistance from an experienced colleague.

It is important to examine any victim of abuse as soon as possible after the event in order to document the healing trauma of acute sexual assault (Fig. 75.4). It may take only 24–48 hours or up to 2 weeks for genital trauma to heal. Early examination may allow documentation of clinical evidence important in the prevention of further abuse.

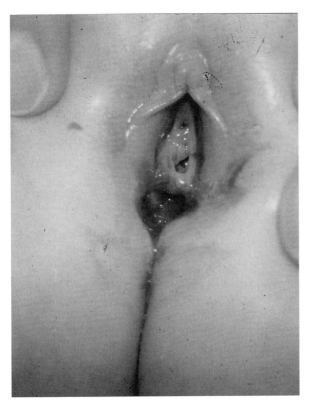

Fig. 75.5 Injury to vestibular fossa: child sat on toy duck in the bath.

A doctor who examines a child for abuse will need to be prepared to submit reports, attend a case conference and attend court if necessary. Appropriate expertise must be available at all stages when abuse is suspected. A senior colleague or paediatrician with an interest and specialist knowledge should therefore be consulted. Most health districts in the UK have a designated doctor for child protection who will provide practical advice and support or will indicate where this can be obtained.

The Children Act 1989 (UK) stipulates that the child's best interest is the paramount concern and that professionals should work in partnership with the child's parents. Informed consent is required, preferably from both parent and child, prior to examination. When the doctor's suspicion of abuse reaches a certain critical level and abuse is regarded as a real possibility then there must be full multidisciplinary consultation and assessment.

References

Hobbs, C.J. and Wynne, J.M. 1989: Sexual abuse of English boys and girls: the importance of anal examination. *Child Abuse and Neglect* **13**, 195–210.

Sgroi, S.M. 1975: Sexual molestation of children: the last frontier in child abuse. *Child Today* **4**, 18–21.

Hobbs, C.J. and Wynne, J.M. 1990: The sexually abused battered child. *Archives of Disease in Childhood* **65**, 423–7.

Royal College of Physicians 1991: *Physical signs of sexual abuse in children*. London: Royal College of Physicians (Revised ed. 1997).

Berenson, A., Heger, A., Hayes, J.M. *et al*. 1992: Appearance of the hymen in prepubertal girls. *Pediatrics* **89**, 387–94.

McCann, J., Wells, R., Simon, M. and Voris, J. 1990: Genital findings in pre-pubertal girls selected for non-abuse: a descriptive study. *Pediatrics* **86**, 428–39.

Berenson, A., Heger, A. and Andrews, S. 1991: Appearance of the hymen in newborns. *Pediatrics* **87**, 158–65.

Ingram, D.L., White, S.T., Lyna, P.R., Crews, V.F., Schmid, J.E., Everett, V.D. and Koch, G.G. 1992: *Child Abuse and Neglect* **16**, 847–53.

Further reading

Emans, S.J. and Heger, A. 1992: *Evaluation of the sexually abused child. A medical textbook and photographic atlas*. Oxford: Oxford University Press.

Working together, under the Children Act 1989. London: HMSO, 1991.

Child protection: medical responsibilities. London: Department of Health, 1993.

CHAPTER 76

Causes and prevention of accidents in children

A. MACKELLAR

Introduction	Development of injury prevention programmes
Causes of injury	Summary
Injury surveillance	References

Introduction

After the first birthday, accidental injury is the leading cause of death in childhood in all countries that publish mortality statistics and results in as many deaths as all other causes added together (Fig. 76.1) (O'Connor, 1982; Rodriguez, 1990; Cywes, 1990; Francescutti *et al.*, 1991; Sibert, 1991; Wilson *et al.*, 1991). For every death, between 35 and 40 children are admitted to hospital and a further 4500 attend hospital emergency departments (EDs) for treatment of injuries. Accidental injury is a major cause of ill health in childhood and has been aptly described as 'The neglected disease of modern society' (Cywes, 1990). In the USA, C. Everett Koop described injury thus: 'If a disease were killing our children in the proportion that accidents are, people would be outraged and demand that this killer be stopped' (Feely and Bahatia, 1993).

As public health measures have reduced the impact of the common infectious diseases, injury has become increasingly important (Fig. 76.1), yet the notion has persisted that injuries are to a large extent accidental and unavoidable. Nothing could be further from the truth. Injuries are both predictable and preventable and require the same approach to management as other diseases. Traditionally, injury events have been described as 'accidents', a term some would prefer to avoid because of the concept that they could not have been reasonably prevented. People are now aware that there are many ways to create a safer environment for children and thus reduce the likelihood of injury.

Injuries most commonly present for treatment in the late afternoon or evening, on weekends and on public and school holidays (MacKellar, 1988). They are, for the most part, treated by family doctors, junior medical staff in hospital EDs or surgical specialists in training, with only a few receiving attention from senior

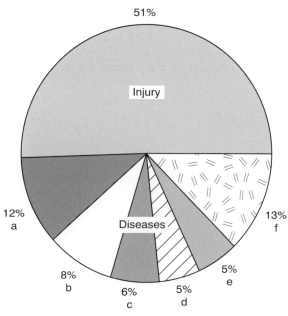

Fig. 76.1 Causes of death in children over 1 year of age.

consultants. This may explain why injury has not been recognized by many surgeons as a serious child health issue and few studies have been reported on how the injuries might have been prevented. The situation has much in common with wound infection which, in the 1960s was a frequent occurrence in hospitals, despite the availability of antibiotics, and surgeons had a similar attitude to it. The introduction of an epidemiological approach to management gradually revealed the extent of the problem and enabled it to be solved. Injury requires that the same meticulous epidemiological methods be used if we are to achieve its control.

Causes of injury

Energy is the cause of most injuries. It is commonly associated with motion or with physical, chemical or electrical agents. The disease (injury) results when the host (the child) and the agent interact in an environment that permits it. Changes involving the host, the agent or the environment can be brought about to reduce the risk of injury. Haddon's matrix (Table 76.1) (Haddon, 1980) provides an ideal starting point from which to examine the wide variety of causal factors and how they may be countered by different intervention strategies. The matrix can be used for all types of injury. Drowning, traffic accidents and playground injuries have been selected to show how appropriate strategies may be used as injury prevention measures at different phases of the event.

AGE AND GENDER

Data from different countries show remarkable similarity as regards age and gender. The first peak in injury occur-

rence in early childhood lies between 1 and 3 years and the second as children enter adolescence from 13 years onwards (Haddon, 1980). These peaks indicate the important roles of growth and development which, although they affect all children, are more significant in these age groups when mobility and behavioural changes are most marked. Overall, three boys are injured for every two girls, but this difference varies with age, associated with the tendency to more risk taking by older boys.

SOCIOECONOMIC FACTORS

Socioeconomic status has frequently been cited as playing a major role in injury occurrence (Wilson and Baker, 1987). Lack of supervision of children in single parent homes and circumstances where both carers are working allows greater opportunity for injury. Poor housing conditions and lack of suitable play areas contribute to an increased frequency of burns and pedestrian injuries in disadvantaged areas. Limited education and financial hardship lead to failure to use or acquire basic safety items for the home. Injury, however, is also a disease affecting the affluent, as demonstrated by the increasing number of immersion accidents in backyard swimming pools and trampoline, skateboard and roller blade injuries.

GEOGRAPHICAL LOCATION

Injury mortality statistics from the USA, the UK, Australia and southern Africa show the importance of geographical location with different injury patterns and incidence from rural and urban areas, from hot and cold climates and from other geographical factors, which highlight the need for local as well as national data

Table 76.1 Haddon's matrix

	Host	Agent	Environment
Pre-event			
Drowning	Swimming lessons	Pool cover	Isolation fencing
Motor vehicle injuries	Driver training	Seat belt	Road design
Playground	Separation of ages	Equipment height	Equipment siting
Event			
Drowning	Wearing safety vest	Pool alarm	Parental supervision
Motor vehicle injuries	Using seat belt	Air cushion	Crash barriers
Playground	Children's behaviour	Type of equipment	Undersurface of playground
Post-event			
Drowning	Cardiopulmonary Resuscitation	Inspection of pool	Rapid transit to emergency department
Motor vehicle injuries	Rehabilitation	Review of safety equipment	Rapid transit to emergency department
Playground	Effective treatment	Inspection of playground	Rapid transit to emergency department

(Waller *et al.*, 1989). Burn injuries are more common in cold climates, while drowning is a greater problem in warm climates, where there are more backyard swimming pools. Children in rural areas appear to be at greater risk of injury than those living in cities, despite the higher incidence of pedestrian injuries in urban areas.

ENVIRONMENT

Environmental factors play an important role in injury causation. The home is the most frequent location for accidents involving children, 67% in children under 5 years, 57% in the 5–9 year-old age group and 47% in 10–14 year olds (MacKellar, 1988). The living and sleeping areas are most commonly involved, as they are the rooms in which young children spend most of their time. Falls are the most common cause and head injuries the most frequent outcome. Although the kitchen, bathroom and laundry produce fewer injuries, they tend to be more serious, for example burns and poisoning, and are more likely to require hospital attendance or admission for treatment. As children grow older, more time is spent in the backyard or area immediately adjacent to the home, which then becomes an important site of injury.

Children spend much of their time playing, so play areas and playgrounds, play equipment and toys are regularly documented as contributing to injuries (Tinsworth and Kramer, 1989). Where no suitable play facilities are available, children will improvise using whatever space and materials are at hand, sometimes with unfortunate outcomes. At an early age children have to learn to cope with the natural and artificial hazards of their own environment. Part of this learning comes from parental or other instruction and guidance and part by experience of trial and error. Parents and the community must accept responsibility for providing as safe an environment as possible, allowing children the opportunity for risk taking with minimal chance of injury.

Transportation is an essential element of modern life, whether on foot, by bicycle or in motor or other vehicles. Children are at risk whenever they are involved in this activity and motor vehicle accidents are the most common cause of accidental death in childhood (Mortality statistics, 1989). Pedestrian, bicycle and passenger accidents vary in frequency in different communities, at different times of year and in different climatic conditions. Pedestrian injuries are more common in urban areas, and bicycle-related injuries in the summer months. More than 1000 children every year are admitted to hospital in the UK after bicycle accidents (Avery and Jackson, 1993). The number of child passenger injuries has increased with greater car ownership by parents, often of old vehicles not fitted with appropriate restraints. Children are regularly transported by buses, very few of which have seat restraints and most of which have been on the road for many years.

SPORTS AND LEISURE ACCIDENTS

Sports injuries have become more common, with increased attention being given to participation in sport and games being played at a higher level of intensity. The sports responsible vary according to social class and geographical location. In England, football (soccer) carries the greatest risk for boys and hockey for girls. In Wales and Scotland rugby is more often responsible for male injuries. In the USA, American football, baseball and basketball are the principal culprits, and in Canada, ice hockey (Wilson *et al.*, 1991; Avery and Jackson, 1993). Many of these injuries can be prevented.

CONSUMER PRODUCTS

Faulty or unsafe products or packaging of these products can lead to injury or poisoning. Small parts of toys may become detached and be accidentally inhaled by toddlers or poisonous substances may be marketed in unsuitable containers and easily accessible to small children. Medicinal substances in many countries are now distributed in containers with childproof lids or strip packaging, but household cleaning and garden products, which can be dangerous to children, are still sold without safety caps and stored in unlocked cupboards. Arrows and sling-like toys have been linked with eye injuries (Bremner, 1993).

DROWNING

As a cause of death, drowning ranks high, either second or third according to the country or state. In the UK and the eastern seaboard of the United States, it occupies third place after motor vehicles and burns, but in Australia and California the order is changed, with drowning in second place (Sibert, 1991; Wilson *et al.*, 1991). Infants have drowned in as little as 5 cm of water in baths or buckets in their own homes. For toddlers in the 1–5-year age group, the backyard swimming pool is the greatest danger, while older children are more likely to drown in natural or artificial hazards in the countryside, e.g. canals, dams, rivers, lakes or the sea.

ANIMALS

Each year, almost 2% of all children in the USA require medical treatment of an animal bite or sting (Fife *et al.*, 1984), the most common being dog bites. Recent media attention has focused on pit bull terriers, which have been rated especially dangerous (Lockwood, 1986). Horseback riding is another activity with a high injury rate, greater for girls than boys because of increased exposure (Barber, 1973; Bixby-Hammet and Brooks, 1990). Head injuries and fractures are the common types of injury.

Injury surveillance

The first vital step towards injury control is the development of injury surveillance, which comprises the routine collection of data about injuries and includes information about the age and gender of the victim, the nature and outcome of injury and the body part injured, how and where the injury occurred, product involvement and whether or not safety measures were used at the time of the accident. Surveillance also embraces analysis of the data collected to determine injury trends and the effectiveness or otherwise of injury prevention programmes (Moller and Vimpani, 1985; Vimpani, 1991).

Injury mortality data are now available from most westernized countries and provide the principal source of information. Hospital inpatient statistics have been collected in some countries since the 1970s, but seldom include enough information about the mechanism of injury or product involvement to be useful in planning or evaluating prevention programmes. Neither mortality nor inpatient hospital data becomes available until at least a year after the event, and therefore they are not sufficiently timely for monitoring purposes. Hospital EDs have recently become computerized in some centres, which has provided an excellent opportunity for more timely and detailed injury data collection. In general, many sources, each with an interest in a particular cause or type of injury, have provided the data. Many agencies collect information about traffic accidents, but not nearly so much data is available about home and leisure accidents. The Home Accident Surveillance System (MASS) and the Leisure Accident Surveillance System (LASS) in the UK and the Consumer Safety Institute in The Netherlands collect some data, but no country has, as yet, introduced a uniform national hospital surveillance system. In Australia, a National Injury Surveillance and Prevention Program (NISPP) commenced in 1986 and operated through the EDs of most children's and some adult hospitals (Vimpani, 1991). A similar system is now operating in Canada. NISPP provided valuable, timely information about injuries, but was not acceptable to busy major adult EDs because of the extra workload associated with the completion of a special form. An attempt is now being made to introduce a simpler version which can be completed by trained clerical staff at the time of the first ED attendance. It was named Basic Routine Injury Surveillance (BRIS) (Harrison and Tyson, 1993), but has now been changed to Minimum Data Set for Injury Surveillance. If successful, this surveillance system will be a major advance in the accurate and timely documentation of injury, which will assist the planning, implementation and evaluation of injury prevention programmes with which surveillance must be closely linked.

Development of injury prevention programmes

Injury is a much more complex health issue than other diseases. Its prevention requires the co-operation of many different disciplines and organizations. Health professionals, especially surgeons, play a major role in treatment and must accept that their knowledge of injury, gained from personal experience, should be used to publicize its importance as a child health issue. Other professionals such as nurses, engineers, architects, teachers, designers and traffic police are essential members of any team brought together to reduce injuries. The need for the development of such a team approach has been recognized by the establishment of the Child Accident Prevention Trust in the UK, the National Safe Kids Campaign in the USA and Child Accident Prevention Foundations in Australia, New Zealand and southern Africa. These organizations have the common aims of increasing community awareness of the seriousness of childhood injury as a health issue and of developing a wide variety of strategies to deal with it. Injury is a local as well as a national problem and the variations in the pattern of injury in different regions emphasize the need for data collection to take place in all hospital EDs. Parents and other community members pay much more attention to statistics that are directly relevant to their children, and communities will be willing to take an active role in projects when there is regular feedback on their progress.

A wide variety of intervention strategies has a place in injury prevention programmes. They may be either active or passive or a mixture of both. They may be aimed at legislative, behavioural or environmental change. They may be carried out at local, state or national government level. Most programmes will include a variety of approaches and all require multidisciplinary co-operation. In general, effective passive strategies are more attractive than those requiring individual action, e.g. airbags that inflate automatically in a road crash are theoretically more desirable than seat restraints, although they are more expensive to install. Ideally, both should be available.

ROAD SAFETY

Returning to Haddon's matrix, it can be appreciated how different strategies can be used to prevent injuries in the same situation. Legislation to install seat restraints in motor vehicles cannot be passed until politicians have been persuaded that it will be acceptable to their electorate. It is a passive measure and is of no value unless accompanied by the active measures of buckling up by the occupant and enforcement by the police. The value of seat restraints in motor vehicles is now well established but not yet universally accepted by some communities (Ruta *et al.*, 1993). There is a need for greater publicity to be given to the benefits and for greater support for their use to be provided by health care workers and their professional organizations. Infants and young children require special seat restraints, appropriate to their age and stage of development. These are now widely available in most countries. Hire facilities, which extend their use to economically disadvantaged parents, are a valuable community service.

BICYCLE HELMETS

The severe head injuries sometimes sustained by bicyclists can be reduced by the wearing of helmets (Wood and Milne, 1988; Thompson *et al.*, 1989). The state of Victoria in Australia passed the first bicycle helmet legislation in 1991. Since that measure was introduced there has been a considerable fall in the number of deaths and hospital admissions of children with head injuries following bicycle accidents (Vulcan *et al.*, 1993). Other Australian states have now followed the Victorian example and enacted similar legislation. This outcome could not have been achieved without the support of the data provided by the NISPP and the extensive efforts of the Road Trauma Committee of the Royal Australasian College of Surgeons, the Accident Research Centre at Monash University in Melbourne and the Child Accident Prevention Foundation of Australia, an excellent example of teamwork.

PEDESTRIAN SAFETY

Many children die or are severely injured as pedestrians (Campbell, 1981). The problem is most serious in urban areas where traffic is congested and playgrounds are almost non-existent. If possible, traffic should be diverted from urban areas using bypasses, vehicle speed reduced by a variety of traffic-calming devices in residential areas and suitable play areas provided for children. Town planners should site schools away from main traffic routes and provide safe crossings where busy roads have to be crossed by children on their way to or from school. Buses transporting children should have special warning lights and should not be passed by other vehicles when the lights are flashing and children alighting. Parents must recognize that children under 7 years of age should not be expected to be able to cope with traffic on their own because of their size and difficulties with assessing the speed and intentions of motorists (Rivara, 1988).

HOME ACCIDENTS

As 57% of all accidents to children take place in or around the home, it appears logical to make every effort to improve the safety of the home environment. The first essential is to raise the level of awareness of parents and other caregivers to the potential injury hazards that exist in all homes and show how they can be reduced or eliminated (Eichelberger *et al.*, 1990). Child safety centres can provide this information to the community (MacKellar, 1991). Safety demonstration homes (Kidsafe homes) have now been established in all mainland states in Australia and are being planned in England, Northern Ireland, South Africa, Canada and New Zealand. These homes illustrate the dangers to which children are exposed in the different rooms of a house and how they may be overcome. Examples are fire and stoveguards to prevent burns and scalds, smoke alarms to alert occupants to fires, suitable flooring material to reduce the impact of falls, installation of barriers to prevent access to dangerous areas and to eliminate falls down steps, storage of household detergents and cleaners in childproof locked cupboards and thermal valves to control the temperature of hot water from taps. When new homes are designed or old homes altered, architects should be encouraged to remember the safety needs of children and the elderly, who may live in the house. Community health nurses and doctors should provide parents and other caregivers with the facts about injuries and how they may be prevented. City and local councils should be encouraged to develop programmes to produce a safer home environment for children. Legislation to install earth linkage circuit breakers, smoke detectors and thermal valves in new or renovated homes should be enacted.

PLAYGROUND SAFETY

Many playgrounds are still dangerous places for children (Avery and Jackson, 1993). Equipment may be inappropriate and the surfacing unsuitable, with no arrangement in place for separation of different age groups. The toddler and the older child should have different areas with equipment appropriate to their growth and development. The height of apparatus from the ground, e.g. monkeybars, must be monitored to avoid fractures of the upper limb resulting from falls. The material selected for playground surfaces is important as it should absorb as much impact as possible.

WATER SAFETY

As drowning is such a prominent cause of death in childhood, it is important that parents and children should be aware of the water dangers in their home and neighbourhood (Sibert, 1991). Parental supervision and early introduction of swimming lessons at the age of 4 years are helpful measures. Backyard swimming pools, which have become increasingly popular in warm climates, should be separated from houses by a special childproof isolation fence with a self-closing gate. Owners of pools should be familiar with cardiopulmonary resuscitation measures.

SPORTS INJURIES

In recent years sport has become more competitive and played at a higher level of intensity. Emphasis should be placed on adequate training and warm-up exercises before taking part in sport and the use of appropriate safeguards, e.g. shinpads, mouthguards and headgear, during the activity emphasized.

COMMUNITY INTERVENTIONS

Swedish experience has highlighted the important role that communities may play in injury prevention programmes, and demonstrated how a team approach at the local level can achieve a reduction in the number of accidents (Schelp, 1987). The hypothesis on which their programmes have been based is that the feedback of local data to the community about the seriousness of injury as a health issue stimulates community interest and leads to changes in attitude, behaviour and the environment which reduce the injury rate. Community leaders have played a vital part in the success of these projects in rural areas. The same level of success has not been achieved in an urban setting, where leaders are more likely to change and the community is less cohesive (Bjaras, 1987).

Summary

Accidental injury presents the greatest health risk to children after their first birthday. The creation of a safer environment in which children may grow up free from the danger of serious injury should be the aim of all adults responsible for child care and is a major challenge to the wide range of health and other professionals who plan, create and work or live in that environment (Sibert, 1991). Not all accidents can be prevented, but when an accident occurs people should ensure that every possible measure has been taken to minimize the injury that may follow. The surgeons and others who treat children's injuries must encourage the collection of the data necessary to develop and evaluate the injury prevention programmes, which are essential to control the injury epidemic that afflicts our children.

References

Avery, J.G. and Jackson, R.H. (eds) 1993: *Children and their accidents.* London: Edward Arnold.

Barber, H.M. 1973: Horseplay; survey of accidents with horses. *British Medical Journal* **3**, 532–4.

Bixby-Hammett, D.M. and Brooks, W.H. 1990: Common injuries in horseback riding: a review. *Sports Medicine* **9**, 36–47.

Bjaras, G. 1987: Experiences in local activities in Sweden. The Sollentuna Project. In Berfenstam, R., Jackson, H. and Erikson, B. (eds), *The healthy community. Child safety as a part of health promotion activities,* vol. 3. Stockholm: Folksam, Vetenskap and Forskning, 167–73.

Bremner, M.H. 1993: Kids play the safe way. *Medical Journal of Australia* **158**, 646.

Campbell, B.J. 1981: *The young child in pedestrian accidents.* Chapel Hill, NC: University of North Carolina Highway Research Centre.

Cywes, S. 1990: The neglected disease of modern society and the Child Accident Prevention Foundation of Southern Africa. *South African Medical Journal* **6**, 381.

Eichelberger, M.R., Gotschall, C.S., Feely, H.B. *et al.* 1990: Parental attitudes and knowledge of child safety. *American Journal of Diseases of Children* **144**, 714–20.

Feely, H.B. and Bahatia, E. 1993: National Safe Kids Campaign. Cure for the disease. In Eichelberger, M.R. (ed.), *Pediatric trauma.* Baltimore, MD: Mosby Year Book 671–82.

Fife, D., Barancik, J.L. and Chatterjee, B.F. 1984: North Eastern Ohio Trauma Study: 11. Injury rates by age, sex and cause. *American Journal of Public Health* **74**, 473–8.

Francescutti, L.H., Saunders, L.D. and Hamilton, S.M. 1991: Why are there so many accidents? Why aren't we stopping them? *Canadian Medical Association Journal* **144**, 57–8, 60–1.

Haddon, W. Jr 1980: Advances in the epidemiology of injuries as a basis for public policy (Landmarks in American Epidemiology). *Public Health Reports* **95**, 411–21.

Harrison, J. and Tyson, D. 1993: Injury surveillance in Australia. *Acta Paediatrica Japonica* **35**, in press.

Lockwood, R. 1986: Vicious dogs: communities, humane societies and owners struggle with a growing problem. *Humane Society News* Winter.

MacKellar, A. 1988: Annual Report of the Western Australian Childhood Injury Surveillance System for 1987. Perth: Child Accident Prevention Foundation of Australia.

MacKellar, A. 1991: Child safety and demonstration homes. *Medical Journal of Australia* **154**, 575–6.

Moller, J.N. and Vimpani, G.V. 1985: *Child Injury Surveillance System: a feasibility study for Australia.* Melbourne: Child Accident Prevention Foundation of Australia.

Mortality Statistics, Cause, 1989. *Office of Population Census and Surveys 1990.* London: HMSO.

O'Connor, P.J. 1982: *An analysis of Australian child accident statistics.* Melbourne: Child Accident Foundation of Australia.

Rivara, F.P. 1988: *Strategies for preventing child pedestrian injuries,* Position paper. Seattle, WA: Harborview Injury Prevention and Research Centre.

Rodriguez, J.G. 1990: Childhood injuries in the United States. A priority issue. *American Journal of Diseases of Children* **6**, 625–6.

Ruta, D., Beattie, T. and Narayau, V. 1993: A prospective study of non-fatal road traffic accidents: what can seat restraints achieve? *Journal of Public Health Medicine* **15**, 88–92.

Schelp, L. 1987: Epidemiology as a basis for evaluating a community intervention program on accidents. Sundyberg: Karolinska Institute.

Sibert, J.R. 1991: Accidents to children: the doctor's role. Educational or environmental change. *Archives of Disease in Childhood* **66**, 890–3.

Thompson, R.S. *et al.* 1989: A case control study of the effectiveness of bicycle safety helmets. *New England Journal of Medicine* **320**, 1361–7.

Tinsworth, D.K., and Kramer, J.T. 1989: *Playground equipment related injuries involving falls to the surface.* Washington DC: Consumer Product Safety Commission.

Vimpani, G.V. 1991: *National injury surveillance and prevention project: final report.* Canberra: Australian Institute of Health, Australian Government Publishing Service.

Vulcan, A.P., Cameron, M.H. and Finch, C.P. 1993: Effect of the mandatory bicycle helmet wearing law in Victoria, Australia – the first two years. Paper presented at the Second World Conference on Injury Control, Atlanta, May 1993.

Waller, A.E., Baker, S.P. and Szocka, A. 1989: Childhood injury deaths: national analysis and geographic variations. *American Journal of Public Health* **79**, 310–15.

Wilson, M.H. and Baker, S.P. 1987: Structural approach to injury control. *Journal of Social Issues* **43**, 73–86.

Wilson, M.H., Baker, S.P., Teret, S.P. *et al.* 1991: *Saving children – A guide to injury prevention.* New York: Oxford University Press.

Wood, T. and Milne, P. 1988: Head injuries to pedal cyclists and the promotion of helmet use in Victoria, Australia. *Accidents Analysis and Prevention* **20**, 177–85.

PART VI

Miscellaneous

CHAPTER 77

Principles of transplantation

M.T. CORBALLY

Introduction	Pancreas transplantation
Organization of transplant services: UKTSSA	Intestinal transplantation
and regional retrieval	Heart and heart–lung transplantation
Immunosuppression	The future
Liver transplantation	References
Renal transplantation	Further reading

Introduction

Transplantation for end-stage organ failure is now well-established therapy. Regarded in the 1960s as experimental surgery, transplantation has evolved to its current level primarily because of improved immunosuppression and organ preservation fluids. In addition, improvements in surgical and anaesthetic techniques, proper patient selection and control of infection following transplantation have increased 2-year survival to 80% or better for most recipients. Notwithstanding the technical demands, paediatric transplantation represents a special challenge to transplant surgeons. Children manifest altered drug metabolism, ongoing growth and development needs and heightened immunoresponsiveness, and are often nutritionally depleted at presentation. Successful transplantation in the paediatric population facilitates a return to normal growth and development and removes the social limitations of chronic illness and, in renal disease, the restrictions of life on dialysis.

The global acceptance of transplantation is such that over 50 000 solid organ transplants are now performed annually, with over 2000 in the UK alone (Table 77.1). Increased transplant activity has contributed to improved overall survival in end-stage renal, liver, heart, heart–lung and intestinal failure but in itself has generated a significant shortage of donor organs. This is particularly true in rarer blood groups and in the paediatric population, particularly for smaller organs.

Appropriate size matching is an important consideration for heart and heart–lung recipients but is less important in renal and, recently, liver transplantation.

This chapter will address the typical indications for transplantation, the relevant recipient work-up, management of the donor and organ procurement, basic principles of transplant immunology, current immunosuppression and outcome following transplantation. The subject is clearly vast and therefore the liver will be chosen as the clinical model for purposes of clarity. However, aspects for kidney, pancreas, heart, heart–lung and small intestine that are relevant to paediatric surgery will also be discussed.

Table 77.1 UK transplant activity April 1995–March 1996

	1994	1995
Kidney	1728	1768
Live related kidney	136	152
Kidney and pancreas	21	29
Pancreas	3	16
Heart	307	311
Domino heart	23	27
Heart and lung	52	58
Lung	116	113
Liver	644	687

From UKTSSA Annual Report (1996).

Organization of transplant services: UKTSSA and regional retrieval

The co-ordination and management of a large number of donor organs from different centres would be extremely complex and potentially wasteful without the input of the UK Transplant Support Service Authority (UKTSSA), now an independent authority within the National Health Service (NHS). This centralized government body acts to monitor all transplant activity within the UK and provides an objective and unbiased forum for organ sharing. Similar agencies are available in other European countries and the USA. In addition, information on donor blood group and suitability of the donor is passed from the central UKTSSA source to the various transplant centres. Information on recipient and graft outcome is prospectively acquired. UKTSSA does not determine priority for any organ. This is determined using prearranged criteria between the various transplant centres. Priority for organ usage is based on the following sequence:

1. NHS-eligible patients, registered as superurgent in a designated transplant centre (agreement to list as superurgent follows discussion between the various transplant centres and implies acute, life-threatening deterioration in liver function, in a patient without prior chronic liver disease and within a specified time from the development of jaundice to the onset of encephalopathy).
2. NHS-eligible patients registered in an NHS designated centre.
3. NHS-eligible patients registered in a non-designated centre.
4. Non-eligible patients in a designated centre.
5. Non-eligible patients in a non-designated centre.

A similar arrangement operates for cardiac and renal grafts and ensures effective co-operation between different centres and equal distribution of organs. The eight transplant centres in the UK and the Republic of Ireland have agreed to retrieve on the basis of their own geographical regions but will refer the organ in the event of a superurgent patient in another region. Excellent communication and co-operation between centres is clearly vital.

BRAIN DEATH

The majority of organ grafts are retrieved from heart-beating but brain-dead patients. Brain death is said to be present when there is no evidence on serial testing of any cerebral or brainstem activity. The introduction of this concept has greatly influenced the quality and number of grafts obtained, as the donor is brought to the operating theatre with a diagnosis of brain death but with the heart still beating (circulatory support often necessary) and respiratory function maintained by artificial ventilation. Complications related to prolonged supportive care or delay in the diagnosis of brain death reduce the availability of essential grafts and contribute to morbidity following engraftment. A rapid, but accurate diagnosis facilitates organ retrieval and graft utilization. A period of at least 24 hours without neurological change is recommended before the diagnosis of brain death is made, especially in children under 5 years of age. The following criteria must be confirmed before brain death can be diagnosed and the organs considered for transplantation:

- The cause of death must be known.
- The potential donor should be normothermic and not exposed to alcohol or other central nervous system depressant drugs (barbiturates may be used to reduce intracranial pressure but the level should be less than 1 mg%).
- Tests of brain death should be made by experienced medical personnel, e.g. consultant anaesthetist with no direct ties to the transplant programme.
- Absence of brain function is indicated by:
  – no cough, light, or corneal reflex
  – no motor response to pain
  – no eye movement on caloric testing
  – no efforts to breathe independently from the ventilator.

Preoxygenation with 100% oxygen and continuous endotracheal oxygen is used by some units to minimize the risk of hypoxaemia or haemodynamic deterioration during tests of brain death. These tests of brain death should be repeated after an interval of 30 min by another independent physician of equal experience. In some situations, especially small infants, an electroencephalogram (EEG) may also be performed but cerebral angiography is rarely required. If performed, angiography will demonstrate a complete absence of brain flow. Cardiac angiography is sometimes performed if there is any doubt about the quality of a potential cardiac donor.

LIVING RELATED TRANSPLANTATION

Increased competition for organs has resulted in a renewed interest in living related transplantation. Although common in renal transplantation, especially in North America (50% of paediatric renal transplants are living related), living related liver and small bowel transplantation have only recently been accepted into clinical practice. In theory, living related transplantation confers many distinct advantages:

- fewer immunological differences and therefore better graft survival
- less immunosuppression needed, with fewer immunosuppressive complications
- shorter cold ischaemic time with better earlier graft function

- elective planning of the transplant procedure
- no competition with the cadaveric donor/recipient pool.

However, there remains a reluctance to utilize living related organs and this derives from the previously reported morbidity and mortality, although small, in most reported series. Clearly, donation of a left lateral hepatic segment is potentially more hazardous than a left nephrectomy or isolated ileal segment. To date there has been one donor death in over 800 living related liver transplants. It is accepted that living related transplantation should be reserved for centres with a significant transplant experience.

MAINTENANCE OF THE POTENTIAL DONOR

Following the offer of a potential organ the recipient centre will establish suitability of the donor by determining the following: cause of death, liver, renal and cardiac function. Details of age, gender, blood group and body size and weight are also obtained. Previous medical history is important, e.g. congenital heart disease would preclude utilization of the heart but not the liver or kidneys. Prolonged hospital and/or intensive care unit (ICU) stay has a negative effect on the quality of most organs but the use of inotropes (< 15 µg/kg/min of dopamine or low doses of adrenaline or noradrenaline) does not preclude organ utilization. Higher doses are likely to compromise hepatic and splanchnic blood flow and may result in graft refusal. Other contraindications to graft utilization include untreated septicaemia but not chest or meningeal infection. Excess liver fat is usually apparent at laparotomy or after graft perfusion but biopsy may be required to quantify the amount of fatty change. Fatty livers in excess of 50–60% are rarely used because of the risk of primary non-function. However, because of the increased numbers of centres offering transplantation and the increasing demand for organs it is likely that livers more usually discarded will be utilized. Most renal grafts are utilized. Strict criteria for cardiac utilization, including on-table pressure studies, may be performed prior to cardiac retrieval.

Given the above information it should be possible to determine the suitability of the organ and the most suitable recipient. Before the graft is finally accepted it is important to evaluate the viral status of the donor. Donors seropositive for human immunodeficiency virus (HIV) or hepatitis A, B, or C are not utilized. Cytomegalovirus (CMV)-seropositive donors are accepted but CMV-mismatch patients must receive ganciclovir following transplant. Minor abnormalities of liver enzymes may not preclude organ acceptance, especially if this is due to a short period of haemodynamic instability that has been subsequently stabilized.

Most units have established protocols for the maintenance of donor stability prior to organ retrieval. In brief, it is important to recognize and treat early any sign of haemodynamic instability and to prevent the complications of prolonged ventilation and give supportive care. In general, the nursing care of the donor is that of the unconscious patient and includes care of pressure areas, bladder and gastric drainage, etc. Antibiotics are given for established infection or for prophylaxis.

DONOR PROCEDURE AND ORGAN PRESERVATION

Most organs are retrieved as part of a multiorgan procedure. This involves the participation and co-operation of a number of different transplant teams. A midline incision is placed from the suprasternal notch to the symphysis. The liver is inspected and the chest opened in the midline. The colon, small intestine and pelvic structures are inspected. The cardiac and renal/pancreatic teams usually inspect the heart and kidneys and pancreas, respectively, at this time. The ligamentous attachments of the liver are divided and the common bile duct is identified in the free edge of the lesser omentum, encircled, ligated and divided. The gastroduodenal artery is ligated and divided, exposing the portal vein. A thorough search for variant arterial branches is now performed to exclude a right hepatic artery from the superior mesenteric artery and a left hepatic artery from the left gastric artery. Damage to either vessel may compromise subsequent transplantation or require complex reconstruction. The inferior vena cava (IVC) is then encircled with a vessel loop above the renal veins and the infradiaphragmatic aorta encircled with tape. The infrarenal aorta and superior mesenteric vein are encircled in preparation for perfusion. The cardiac and renal teams usually complete their dissection at this time. Following cannulation of the infrarenal aorta (heparin is given at this time) and superior mesenteric vein and clamping of the infradiaphragmatic aorta, the donor IVC is opened in the chest and perfusion of the liver begun using cold University of Wisconsin (UW) solution through the portal vein and Marshall's solution or UW through the aorta. The completed arrangement for *in situ* cold perfusion is shown in Fig. 77.1. For paediatric retrieval 50 ml/kg of UW solution is used. Approximately half of the perfusate is given on the table and the remainder given on the back table. The heart is rapidly removed following intra-aortic cardioplegia. Liver and renal perfusion continues for 20–30 min or until the venous effluent begins to clear. During perfusion the gallbladder is opened and drained of bile. The biliary system is subsequently irrigated further through the divided common bile duct. The portal vein is divided at the level of the splenic vein and the coeliac artery taken with a cuff of aorta. The liver is removed to the back table for further perfusion. The

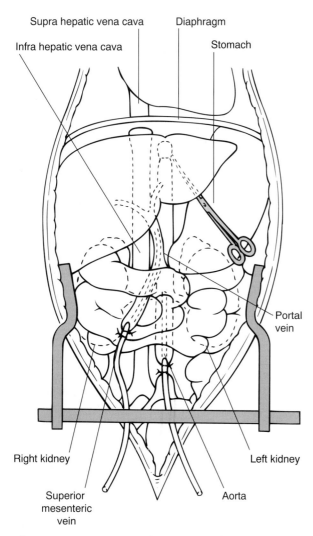

Supra hepatic vena cava

Infra hepatic vena cava

Diaphragm

Stomach

Portal vein

Right kidney

Left kidney

Superior mesenteric vein

Aorta

Fig. 77.1 Donor set up, showing cannulae in the portal vein (via the superior mesenteric vein) and in the distal aorta for perfusion. (Reprinted with permission from Williams *et al.*, 1995.)

iliac arteries and veins are removed as trouser grafts for possible conduit construction at the transplant procedure. The renal team remove the kidneys, usually as the last part of the multiorgan procedure, *en bloc* with the aorta and IVC. The kidneys are separated with their respective arteries and veins on the back table. The liver is placed within three bags and packed in an ice chest for transport to the recipient centre.

Modifications to this technique are necessary if the pancreas is also to be retrieved. In this procedure the splenic and left gastric arteries are not ligated but perfused with UW solution. Portal perfusion is obtained through the superior mesenteric vein (SMV) up to the portal vein. A shorter portal vein is usually left with the liver and the hepatic artery may be divided just distal to the gastroduodenal artery.

TRANSPLANT IMMUNOBIOLOGY

The cells of every organism carry antigens that enable the host to recognize self from non-self. These antigens (major histocompatability antigens, minor histocompatability antigens and blood group antigens) are different from individual to individual and play a major role in the acceptance or rejection of a transplanted organ. In general, the greater the antigenic differences between the recipient and donor the greater the risk of graft rejection. Although these reactions may be controlled with appropriate immunosuppressive drugs it is usual clinical practice to achieve as close a match as possible. In the case of well-vascularized grafts such as heart and liver it is sufficient to transplant on the basis of a blood group match only, whereas renal and pancreatic grafts are transplanted on the basis of the closest possible antigenic match.

There are several major histocompatibility complex (MHC) antigens, encoded on chromosome 6. These antigens are also called human leucocyte antigens (HLA). The most significant are those described at loci A, B, and C for class I antigens and DR, DQ, DP for class II antigens (there are structural differences between the two groups). Their function was probably not meant to be the distinction of self from non-self but that of assisting in the elimination of virally infected cells or neoplastic cells with abnormal cell surface antigens. Routinely, HLA matching is determined by serotyping. In renal transplants the presence of circulating cytotoxic antibody is also determined by incubating serum from potential recipients with lymphocytes of potential donors. Lymphocyte lysis indicates a significant risk of hyperacute rejection (aggressive rejection occurring within 10–30 min of graft reperfusion) and is a contraindication to that transplant. HLA matching is not normally performed in cardiac or liver patients unless there is a possibility of prior sensitization or in an emergent situation. However, cardiac graft survival has been shown to correlate with HLA matching with 83% as compared to 71% 3-year survival with improved matching. Overall antibody reactivity to common HLA antigens may be determined using a mixed panel of lymphocyte donors. A high lysis rate (percentage panel reactive antibody) indicates a greater potential for graft loss and suggests that it may be difficult to obtain a well-matched donor.

Graft survival following transplantation is dependent on an adequate blood supply and the prevention and treatment of rejection. Immunosuppressive therapy aims to prevent rejection, yet preserve the host's ability to fight infection. The process of recognition of antigen begins by the presentation of an antigen to an antigen-presenting cell such as a macrophage or dendritic cell. The antigen is processed and ultimately presented to the T helper cell (TH-bearing cell determinant CD4). This process stimulates the production of interleukin 1 (IL-1), which stimulates the proliferation and development of

T helper cells. In turn, activated T helper cells release interleukin 2 (IL-2) and interferon-γ(INF-γ) which lead to the further differentiation of T killer cells. These cells react with and destroy the antigen and its bearing cell. If unchecked, this process would lead to rejection and graft loss.

REJECTION

Although by definition acute rejection is said to occur in the initial weeks following transplantation and at day 5–7, it may occur at any time. Acute rejection occurs in up to 70% of all liver recipients and is diagnosed by the finding of a lymphocytic cellular characterised by the transient elevations in transaminases, glutathione S-transferase and bilirubin but less marked increases in γ-glutamyltransferase and alkaline phosphatase. There may be mild left upper quadrant tenderness and a mild elevation in temperature. Acute rejection is seen in the initial weeks following transplantation and is reversible with appropriate therapy. Graft biopsy is usually necessary to diagnose rejection but may be misleading in small intestinal transplantation. Treatment is usually with pulsed, bolus steroids.

Chronic rejection typically occurs between 3 and 12 months post-transplant although it may occur in the immediate post-transplant period. The frequency varies but may be as high as 22% in some series, being more common in children and HLA-mismatched grafts, and following CMV infection. The presentation is that of progressive jaundice with histological evidence of an arteriopathy (foam cells and an obliterative arteriopathy) and loss of bile ducts (vanishing bile duct syndrome). Random percutaneous biopsy may not be adequate to confirm the diagnosis, which may be aided by angiography. A peripheral pruning of the smaller arteries along with a beaded arterial tree appearance are diagnostic. Although FK506 has been shown to rescue some patients with chronic rejection the usual outcome is retransplantation. If there is a clinical suspicion of CMV infection this should also be treated.

Immunosuppression

Prior to cyclosporine most patients were managed using a combination of azathioprine and prednisolone. Today most centres use a cyclosporine-based immunosuppressive regimen including azathioprine and low-dose steroids.

Cyclosporine is a fat-soluble extract derived from fungi imperfecta. It is a potent immunosuppressive agent that blocks the secretion of IL-2 and thus inhibits the proliferation of T killer cells. It is metabolized by the cytochrome P-450 system in the liver and drug interactions must be considered when other drugs are used, e.g. erythromycin may increase its effect and rifampicin may reduce its levels and result in rejection. There are many side-effects, including gingival hyperplasia, nephrotoxicity, hepatotoxicity, hirsutism, hypertension, fluid retention, Raynauds phenomenon, breast fibroadenoma and tremor. It is usual to monitor drug and serum creatinine levels regularly. Drug levels depend on an adequate bile flow for absorption. A newer preparation of cyclosporine, 'Neoral', does not depend on bile for absorption.

FK506 is a macrolide antibiotic derived from *Streptomyces tsukubaensis*. It has a similar effect to cyclosporine but is considerably more potent, with similar side-effects to cyclosporine. Initially used as a salvage agent in severe liver rejection, it has demonstrated value in first-line therapy in liver grafts, chronic liver rejection and intestinal transplantation. FK506 blocks IL-2 production and expression.

Azathioprine is a purine analogue that inhibits both RNA and DNA synthesis. It has been the backbone of immunosuppressive therapy and is still used in combination therapy. Bone marrow suppression is a common complication and must be monitored by regular whole blood counts.

Steroids (prednisolone) are used routinely with cyclosporine and azathioprine. They block the action of IL-1 and also have an anti-inflammatory effect. Long-term side-effects include a cushingoid appearance, hypertension and growth suppression. Although complete weaning from steroids is desirable it is not always achieved and alternate-day steroid regimens have demonstrated improved growth in comparison with standard protocols.

Biological agents are antibodies directed against a variety of cell surface antigens and differ in their degree of specificity. Antilymphocyte globulin is a heterologous antiserum directed against lymphocytes and leucocytes. OKT3 is a more specific monoclonal antibody directed against the CD3 receptor and hence it affects all T lymphocytes. It is effective in steroid-resistant rejection but may cause bronchospasm and anaphylaxis unless pretreatment with methylprednisolone is given. Other monoclonal antibodies include anti-CD4, anti-IL-2 receptor and anti-ICAM.

Liver transplantation

INDICATIONS

In general, transplantation is considered when life is endangered or when the quality of life is unacceptably poor. The general indications for liver transplantation are shown in Table 77.2.

In children, biliary atresia remains the most frequent indication for OLTx. Increasingly, OLTx is performed for metabolic diseases such as α_1-antitrypsin deficiency, Wilson's disease, tyrosinaemia, cystic fibrosis (which may also require a heart or heart–lung transplant), Byler disease and Crigler–Najjar syndrome. Although a Kasai portoenterostomy may be initially successful in 40–50% of patients it is becoming increasingly clear that the majority of patients will require OLTx after 10 years to preserve a good quality of life. In a recent multicentre review from Japan, only 15% of patients were alive without transplantation at 10 years and only 7.8% were in excellent health. Any organ transplant is contraindicated when there is active infection, widespread malignancy or a serious risk of patient non-compliance. The common indications for liver transplantation are shown in Table 77.3.

PREOPERATIVE EVALUATION OF POTENTIAL RECIPIENTS

The main purpose of the evaluation is to determine the suitability of the recipient and to confirm the diagnosis and urgency of transplantation. The patient is screened for medical and nutritional fitness and assessed for any potential technical problems. Malnutrition is common in children with both cholestatic and non-cholestatic liver diseases. These patients are often anorexic and hypercatabolic and have significant steatorrhoea as a result of deficient bile secretion. An accurate assessment of nutritional status is important and aggressive nutritional therapy is instituted prior to transplantation. The evaluation should be performed by a multidisciplinary team consisting of the surgeon, hepatologist, anaesthetist, pathologist and radiologist. Further advice is often sought from the nutritionist, psychologist, social worker, immunologist, microbiologist, haematologist and transplant nurse specialist and co-ordinator. The decision to list the patient for transplantation is made at the completion of the assessment. Occasionally, the decision will be deferred and the patient placed on a pending list.

From a surgical aspect there are several important variables that are considered in each patient. These are the patient's general state, the presence or absence of coagulopathy, the nature and type of previous surgery and, in particular, any upper abdominal surgery which may complicate the transplant procedure and, in the presence of severe portal hypertension make it hazardous. A Doppler ultrasound is part of the routine work-up of all transplant patients to detect any abnormalities of the portal vein. Although portal vein thrombosis itself does not preclude a transplant it should be documented to facilitate appropriate surgical strategies, such as a venous jump graft from the superior mesenteric vein to the donor portal vein. An aortoportogram is performed if the ultrasound is inconclusive or shows portal vein thrombosis. Visceral anomalies associated with biliary atresia such as abdominal situs inversus and the polysplenia syndrome are not a contraindication to transplantation.

It is also important to document any active infection that may preclude transplantation and also any latent infection that may be reactivated by immunosuppressive therapy. An active infection is a contraindication to transplantation but controlled sepsis in an afebrile patient is not. Potential recipients are screened for serological evidence of latent viral infection such as CMV, Epstein–Barr virus (EBV), varicella-zoster, HIV, and hepatitis B and C. CMV infection may be primary or represent reactivation. Seronegative patients are susceptible to serious CMV if the donor was seropositive. Prophylactic treatment with hyperimmune serum is indicated in this situation and treatment with ganciclovir may also be necessary.

RECIPIENT PROCEDURE

Extended preservation times are now possible using UW solution and by keeping the organ in cold UW storage. However, most would prefer to avoid extended preservation times beyond 14 hours for the liver because of the increased risk of late biliary strictures. The recipient operation proceeds through three separate phases: recipient hepatectomy, engraftment and perfusion, and completion haemostasis and wound closure.

Recipient hepatectomy

The abdomen is entered through a bilateral subcostal incision with a possible vertical extension. Troublesome bleeding requires suture ligation. There are often major varices in the falciform ligament and this is divided

Table 77.2 General indications for liver transplantation

- Intractable ascites
- Bacterial peritonitis
- Intractable pruritus
- Bilirubin > 100
- Worsening liver synthetic function (coagulopathy, hypoalbuminaemia)
- Encephalopathy
- Failure to thrive despite optimal nutritional support

Table 77.3 Specific indications for liver transplantation

- Biliary atresia
- α_1-Antitrypsin deficiency
- Tyrosinaemia
- Wilson's disease
- Acute fulminant liver failure
- Hepatoblastoma
- Drug-induced liver failure
- Hepatitis
- Neonatal haemochromatosis
- Neonatal giant cell hepatitis

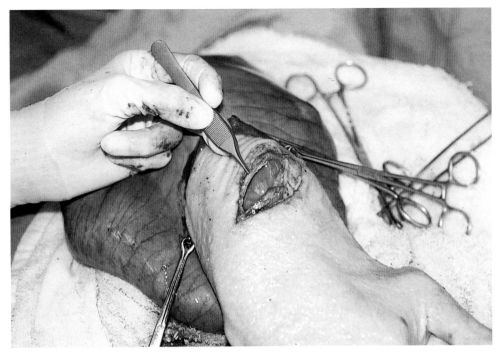

Plate 1 Late creation of a diaphragmatic hernia in a fetal lamb (*c.* 120 days).

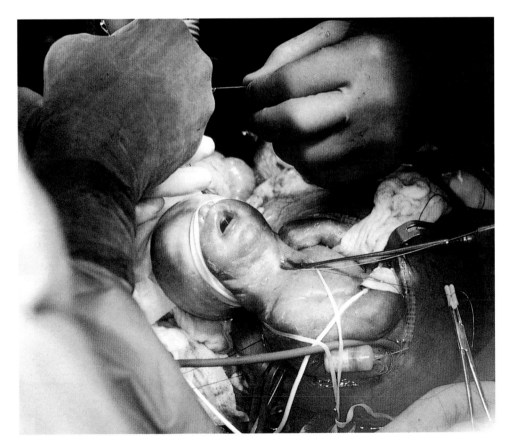

Plate 2 Human fetal PLUG for congenital diaphragmatic hernia (by kind permission of Professor Michael Harrison).

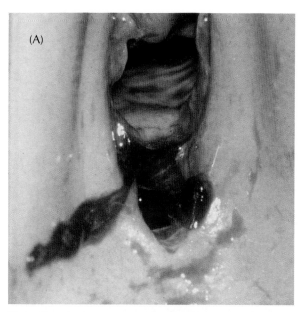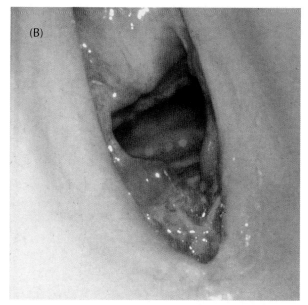

Plate 15 (A) Acute rape with tear of hymen and posterior fourchette; (B) same child as in (A), 1 week later.

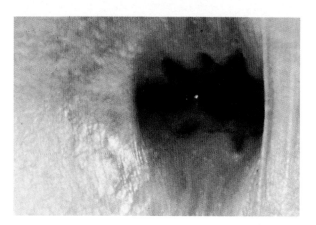

Plate 16 Reflex anal dilatation revealing anal valves.

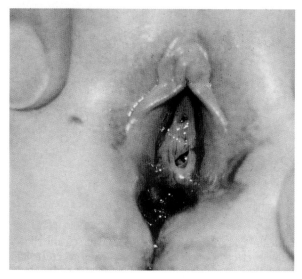

Plate 17 Injury to vestibular fossa: child sat on toy duck in the bath.

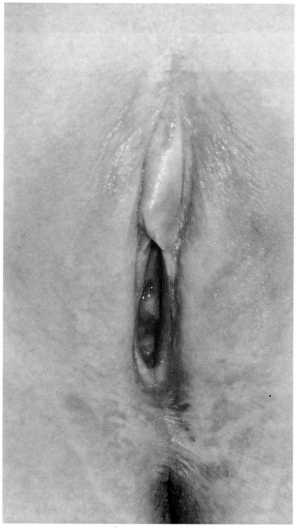

Plate 18 Anogenital lichen sclerosus et atrophicus.

between clamps. A self-retaining abdominal wall retractor (Thompson, Surgical Instruments, IL, USA) is invaluable in exposing the suprahepatic space. The recipient hepatectomy may be exceedingly difficult owing to dense vascular adhesions from previous surgery and if there is significant portal hypertension. An associated coagulopathy may further complicate the dissection.

The common bile duct (if present) and the hepatic artery are identified, ligated and divided. Arterial variations are present in as many as 25–30% of patients, the most common being a right hepatic artery arising from the superior mesenteric artery (SMA) and a left hepatic artery from the left gastric artery. The portal vein is cleared of all adherent tissue and ligated when the donor liver is ready for implantation. The native liver is removed by ligation of the portal vein, ligation and division of the right adrenal vein, and division of the superior and inferior vena cava between heavy vascular clamps. A rapid check for retrocaval bleeding is performed and the area sutured if required. Children tolerate IVC clamping well and venovenous bypass is rarely used.

Engraftment and perfusion

Following completion of the bench dissection the donor liver is brought to the table and the suprahepatic and infrahepatic caval anastomoses are performed. Before completion of the anterior wall of the infrahepatic caval anastomosis the liver is perfused through the portal vein with 500 ml of cold saline. This washes out residual UW solution which would otherwise produce dangerous hyperkalaemia on reperfusion. The portal vein anastomosis is now performed. It is important to ensure that the portal vein is not excessively long and tortuous. A growth factor of 20–30% is usually incorporated in the portal venous anastomosis. A venous jump graft to the superior mesenteric vein is required if portal blood flow is inadequate (previous thrombus) or if the vein is absent (biliary atresia/polysplenia syndrome). Alternatively, the recipient SMV or its confluence with the splenic vein may be exposed by extended mobilization of the head of the pancreas anterior to the portal vein for direct anastomosis. The arterial anastomosis is performed next, using either a continuous or an interrupted 6/0 Maxon suture (Fig. 77.2). In 20% of adults and 40% of children an infrarenal arterial conduit is constructed using donor iliac arteries. A conduit is usually performed for retransplantation or if the recipient common hepatic/coeliac artery is small or of poor quality. In children, the donor aorta may be used as an intact conduit with the coeliac artery in continuity.

Once haemostasis has been established the biliary anastomosis may be constructed. A direct duct-to-duct anastomosis using 5/0 or 6/0 PDS suture is usually possible. A Roux-en-Y choledochojejunostomy is performed for all cases of biliary atresia, in neonatal recipients and whenever the recipient bile is considered inadequate. The usual length of the Roux loop is 40 cm or longer from the choledochoenterostomy to the enteroenterostomy, which in turn is approximately 15–20 cm from the duodenojejunal flexure.

Haemostasis and abdominal closure

Complete haemostasis should be secured before closure. The liver should be lifted forward and the retrohepatic areas and all anastomoses closely examined. Irrigation with saline is useful in identifying bleeding points. In addition, selective packing of all areas around the liver allows further identification of bleeding sites. Additional sutures may be needed to secure haemostasis. The abdomen is irrigated with 1 litre of normal saline containing 1.5 g/l of cefuroxime (amphotericin 50 mg/l, in retransplantation or fulminant liver failure) and closed leaving two drains *in situ*. Primary wound closure is usually performed, but skin closure or siliastic closure may be required in small infants even when a left lateral segment graft has been used. Delayed fascial closure should be possible after 7–10 days.

Modifications to the technique described above may be necessary if the liver is too large, or the donor vena cava is much smaller than that of the recipient. In the former, the donor liver can be reduced to fit the recipient's hepatic fossa. Using current reduction techniques it is possible to transplant the right lobe across a body

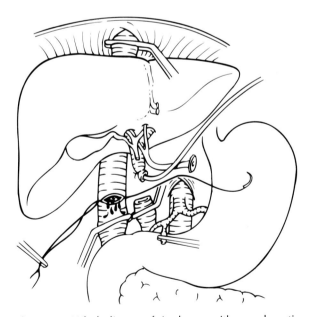

Fig. 77.2 Whole liver graft is shown with suprahepatic and infrahepatic IVC anastomosis nearly complete. The lower IVC anastomosis is completed after flushing out excess UW solution. The portal, arterial and biliary anastomosis are completed in that sequence. (Reprinted with permission from Williams *et al.*, 1995.)

weight ratio of 1.5:1, a left lobe across 3–4:1 or a left lateral segment across 10:1, e.g. a 40-kg donor's left lateral segment could be transplanted to a 4-kg recipient. For donor caval size discrepancy (where the donor vein is considerably smaller than the native IVC) the recipient vena cava may be retained and the caval anastomosis performed face-to-face or end-to-side. Because this technique is wasteful of the remaining liver the technique of split liver grafts has been perfected. This involves dividing the liver into two separate transplantable portions, usually a right lobe with retained IVC and hepatic artery and a left lateral segment with left hepatic artery and left portal vein (Fig. 77.3). Venous outflow is via the hepatic vein orifice which is anastomosed end to side to the IVC in a triangulation technique. Most livers are suitable for splitting but 25% may have such complex arterial anatomy as to make this impracticable. Both livers may be transplanted sequentially in the same centre, usually to an adult and paediatric recipient.

IMMEDIATE POST-TRANSPLANT COURSE

Management following liver transplantation involves intense support with particular attention to cardiovascular, respiratory, renal and clotting function. The procedure is often prolonged and associated with at least one blood volume loss and significant fluid shifts. Inotropic support, fresh frozen plasma, platelets and blood are used liberally as required. Ventilation may be necessary for several days and early extubation or reintubation should be avoided because of the risk of fungal sepsis. Graft function is monitored by the patient's well-being and level of consciousness, and the normalization of liver function. Transaminase levels are expected to have fallen considerably on day 1 owing to dilution during the transplant procedure, but should continue to decrease by 50% on each successive day. Serum bilirubin may take longer to normalize. Serum glutathione S-transferase provides a useful indicator of graft function which may be more sensitive than serum transaminase estimation. Enteral feeding may be recommended on day 2–3 if intestinal function is restored. Feeding may be delayed in the presence of a Roux-en-Y biliary reconstruction.

OUTCOME

The overall survival in children following OLTx is 75–85%, with an expected return to normal growth and development (Fig. 77.4). Surgical morbidity is greatest in the first 3 months post-OLTx and continues to be a problem in the very small child, the nutritionally depleted child and the child undergoing retransplantation for whatever reason. With current techniques, improved immunosuppression and organ preservation, overall survival of 80–85% is expected in children over 1 year of age but infants less than 1 year and 10 kg continue to sustain more complications following OLTx. Current survival in small infants is 65%. Children with fulminant liver failure continue to have survival rates of 50% following OLTx, partly due to technical factors but importantly due to a delay in referral to a transplant centre. However, with successful engraftment and survival an excellent quality of life can be anticipated.

After rejection, the most serious complications following transplantation are primary non-function, vascular thrombosis and infection. The cause of both primary non-function and vascular occlusion remains obscure but both are indications for urgent retransplantation. As many as two-thirds of patients following liver trans-

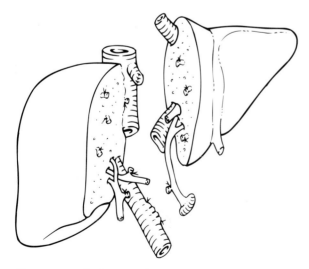

Fig. 77.3 Split liver graft. (Reprinted with permission from Williams *et al.*, 1995.)

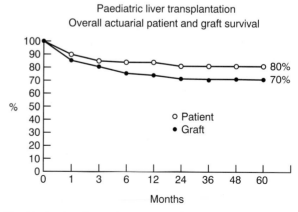

Fig. 77.4 Paediatric liver survival curve (King's College Hospital). (Reproduced by kind permission of Mr Nigel Heaton, King's College Hospital, London.)

plantation experience at least one significant infection, and it remains one of the most important causes of morbidity and mortality following transplantation. For reasons that are unclear, infection is more common after liver transplantation than after any other organ transplant. Infection may be derived from the patient, the graft or the environment and hence can be fungal, viral or bacterial. Bacterial infections tend to predominate in the initial 4–6 weeks post-transplant and cause wound, pulmonary or systemic sepsis. They may be associated with technical problems in the graft such as hepatic artery thrombosis, bile duct anastomotic complications or primary dysfunction or non-function. Opportunistic infections dominate later and comprise reactivation of latent infection, e.g. herpes simplex, CMV and EBV infections. EBV infection is associated with late lymphoproliferative disease [post-transplant lymphoproliferative disease (PTLD)], which occurs in 4–10% of patients post-transplantation and is related to overimmunosuppression. Immunosuppressive reduction or chemotherapy (as per lymphoma protocols) may be required. Long-term cancer surveillance is important in transplant survivors as such patients are at risk of developing a neoplastic process, especially squamous carcinoma of the skin which is usually aggressive. Other opportunistic infections such as *Pneumocystis carinii* and *Aspergillus* present as lung infections which require immediate investigation and treatment as they can progress rapidly.

Graft dysfunction occurs in approximately 5% of patients and may be severe enough (primary non-function) to warrant urgent retransplantation. Although the causes of primary non-function and dysfunction are not clear, it is more common where grafts of marginal quality have been used. While technical factors may relate to vessel thrombosis it is more common in small recipients and where the native hepatic artery has been used. Reduced sized grafts and infra-aortic iliac conduits have a lower incidence of graft thrombosis. Hepatic artery thrombosis may present as rapidly fulminant liver failure, bacterial sepsis, bile duct anastomotic problems, intrahepatic biliary strictures, intrahepatic abscess or a mild elevation in liver function tests. The diagnosis is confirmed by colour Doppler ultrasound and/or hepatic angiography. A minority with mild graft dysfunction may be managed expectantly by serial monitoring but most require re-exploration or retransplantation. Portal vein thrombosis occurs in 2% of patients and produces severe deterioration in liver function with gastrointestinal bleeding and ascites. Thrombectomy may be successful but retransplantation is usually required in the acute presentation.

Bile duct complications include bile leaks and biliary strictures, and may occur in 10–15% of patients. Arterial integrity must be confirmed in all biliary complications. Late biliary strictures can be treated by transhepatic balloon dilatation.

Renal transplantation

There is no doubt about the appropriateness of transplantation for end-stage renal disease in children. Although renal dialysis is an effective means of controlling uraemia, the problems of venous access, osteodystrophy and growth retardation, despite growth hormone, in the growing child combine to make it unattractive in the long term. Indeed, early transplantation is increasingly considered an option before any of the complications of dialysis have developed. In addition, dialysis is disruptive to school attendance and social development. Renal transplantation ensures a return to normal activities and, although complete normalization of growth is not usual, there is an accelerated growth phase following successful engraftment. Nevertheless, children under 5 years old constitute the most difficult group to transplant, with poorer overall results following transplantation. The main indications for kidney transplantation in children are shown in Table 77.4.

The optimal age for paediatric renal recipients is 6 years with an expected 2-year patient survival in excess of 90%. Cadaveric transplantation in children under 6 years is 75% or less. However, programmes offering living related renal transplantation report a 2- and 5-year recipient survival of 90 and 80%, respectively, in children under 2 years at the time of transplantation. This offers stark contrast to the recipient 2- and 5-year survival for cadaveric transplantation in this age group of 50 and 40%, respectively. In the absence of a living related renal transplant programme most children with end-stage renal disease are managed by peritoneal dialysis until their weight reaches at least 10 kg. To maximize growth and development while on dialysis, such patients undergo careful nutritional management, nasogastric feeds where required, control of bone disease using vitamin D, phosphate binders and correction of anaemia using recombinant human erythropoietin.

The recipient bladder function is determined before transplantation by contrast cystography and urodynamics. The small disused bladder may be regularly distended but if unsuccessful then ileal conduit diversion should

Table 77.4 Indications for renal transplantation

- Hypoplasia
- Obstructive uropathy
- Glomerulonephritis (membranous, IgA nephropathy, mesangiocapillary)
- Polycystic kidneys
- Medullary cystic disease
- Severe bilateral reflux nephropathy
- Postbilateral Wilm's nephrectomy
- Haemolytic uraemic syndrome
- Renal dysplasia

be performed at least 8 weeks before the transplant procedure. The vascular anastomoses are performed intraperitoneally to the distal aorta and the inferior vena cava. A bilateral nephrectomy is readily performed at the time of transplantation. Problems with using a large kidney are avoided by increasing recipient central venous pressure (CVP) at the time of reperfusion to improve graft perfusion and minimize graft thrombosis, and judicious use of bicarbonate to avoid acidosis from limb ischaemia during partial or complete aortic occlusion. However, graft perfusion may be sluggish initially when an adult kidney is used. In addition, the graft is usually warmed with saline before releasing the clamps to avoid hypothermia. The ureter is implanted into the bladder using a Leadbetter–Politano technique if the bladder has been shown previously to function normally. If not then an ileal conduit may be required. Postoperative management requires meticulous attention to maintenance of an adequate blood volume, tissue perfusion and graft function. Diuretic therapy is given if urinary output is poor despite an adequate intravascular volume. A prolonged ileus is not uncommon.

Complications include rejection, infection and vessel thrombosis. It is imperative to take a biopsy sample to confirm rejection before increasing immunosuppressive therapy. Very young recipients do not tolerate over-aggressive treatment of a chronically failing graft or infection in the presence of escalating immunosuppressive regimens.

Pancreas transplantation

To date, more than 3000 pancreas transplants have been performed world-wide, with a primary goal of euglycaemia in patients with diabetes. The most usual indication is the diabetic patient with renal failure. Such patients receive a combined kidney–pancreas graft. Since these patients would require immunosuppression for the renal graft there is no added immunosuppressive risk to control pancreatic rejection.

Most pancreatic grafts are obtained from a cadaveric donor, although living related pancreas transplantation is performed in some centres. HLA matching is performed on all potential donors. The recipient operation varies in the amount of pancreas used, the site of vascular anastomoses and the management of the duct. The graft is placed intraperitoneally and revascularized either to the external iliac artery and vein or to the portal system. The duct may be ligated with subsequent necrosis of the exocrine pancreas or drainage may be secured into the intestine or bladder.

Postoperative insulin is required for a variable period as hyperglycaemia may damage the islet cells. Complications include pancreatitis, rejection, vessel thrombosis (15%) and ascites. Overall 1-year patient and graft survival is 90 and 70%, respectively. Although regres-

sion of diabetic nephropathy may occur following successful pancreas transplant, there is no resolution of retinopathy or neuropathy. This may alter as earlier pancreas–renal transplants are performed before the onset of retinal or neural microangiopathy.

Intestinal transplantation

While home total parenteral nutrition has contributed to survival and growth in a large number of patients with intestinal failure, intestinal transplantation becomes an option when vascular access is compromised or when liver disease develops. Although confined to a few specialized centres and still regarded by many as experimental, small bowel transplantation is an effective therapy for intestinal failure in properly selected patients. There are as yet many problems to overcome, chiefly the shortage of suitable donor organs, the problems of rejection and immunosuppression, and CMV enteritis. Prolonged ischaemic times during surgery, inclusion of colonic segments with the graft, high immunosuppressive levels and the use of organs from a CMV-positive donor are associated with a poor outcome following small bowel transplantation. The most common indications for small bowel transplantation in children are shown in Table 77.5.

Most intestinal grafts develop at least one episode of rejection. Diagnosis of rejection may be difficult and requires twice-weekly endoscopic or stoma biopsies. Because rejection may be patchy and non-uniform it is advisable to perform multiple biopsies. Additional tests of graft function such as D-xylose absorption may be useful correlates of graft health and immunological acceptance.

Patient survival following small bowel transplantation has improved dramatically since the recognition that over-immunosuppression is harmful, that CMV infection and enteritis is a significantly morbid event and may contribute to chronic rejection, and that inclusion of colon with the small bowel graft is not necessary and may have been harmful. There is not sufficient long-term information on the outcome of small bowel grafts and while the initial results have been poor there have been several recent reports of improved survival

Table 77.5 Indications for small bowel transplantation

- Intestinal neuromyopathy
- Extensive intestinal loss following resection for NEC
- Small bowel Hirchsprung's disease
- Multiple ileal atresias
- Intestinal loss following midgut volvulus
- Microvillus disease
- TPN-induced liver failure (combined liver/small intestine)

and early restoration of intestinal function with adherence to the above. Recent reports suggest a 63% 1-year survival for composite liver and small bowel grafts and a 85% 2-year survival for isolated small bowel transplants (Langnas, A., Transplant Unit, Omaha, NE, USA, Presented at the IVth International Symposium on Small Bowel Transplantation, Pittsburg, 1995). Clearly, the total numbers transplanted to date have been small and follow-up therefore has been limited. However, the results are consistently encouraging and small bowel transplantation should no longer be considered an experimental procedure. The complexity of post-transplant management indicates that the procedure should only be performed in selected centres with extensive experience in immunosuppressive therapy.

Heart and heart–lung transplantation

HEART TRANSPLANTATION

As with liver transplantation the early results from cardiac transplantation were poor. The introduction of cyclosporine and the perfection of graft procurement from outside the transplanting centre has produced a dramatic improvement in survival. As with any other organ graft, appropriate selection remains important. The most frequent indications for cardiac transplantation are shown in Table 77.6.

Generally, cardiac transplantation is indicated when life expectancy is no greater than 6–12 months. There should be no other serious illness such as systemic malignancy, sepsis, liver or renal failure. Correctable prerenal renal failure or liver congestion with altered liver function is not an absolute contraindication for cardiac transplantation. Conventional medical and surgical therapy should have been tried. In addition to the normal transplant work-up, potential cardiac recipients must undergo cardiac catheterization with an assessment of pulmonary vascular resistance (PVR). If PVR is raised (> 8 Wood units) and not responsive to nitroprusside or prostaglandin E_1 then cardiac transplantation is not an option because of the high risk of mortality following engraftment. Mild elevations of PVR may warrant a slightly larger graft to provide an adequate muscle mass to overcome the high PVR.

Table 77.6 Indications for cardiac transplantation

- Major congenital cardiac anomalies not treatable or responsive to standard surgery
- Hypoplastic left heart syndrome
- Cardiomyopathy
- Myocarditis

Preoperative management of the potential recipient can be difficult, especially since infants may spend up to 6 months on the waiting list. Duct-dependent infants are maintained on prostaglandin E_1 with duct stenting or septostomy if saturations drop. Saturations of 70% are generally acceptable. Pulmonary artery banding may be required if pulmonary artery flow is high. Cardiac failure may require inotropic or ventilatory support and cyanotic infants may require systemic–pulmonary artery shunting. Multiple previous cardiac operations are not a contraindication to transplantation.

As in other organ transplant fields cardiac transplantation is limited by the availability of suitable donors. Donor matching is performed on the basis of ABO compatability and HLA matching is not usually performed. Donors weighing up to three times the recipient weight and receiving inotropic support are acceptable.

Significant acute rejection occurs in 70% of cardiac patients and, while initially mild and seen on endomyocardial biopsy (performed via the transjugular route), will progress to haemodynamic instability in the absence of appropriate therapy. Pulsed steroids followed by monoclonal treatment are required for persistent rejection. Infection is common following cardiac transplantation and requires aggressive treatment. Chronic rejection is the most important late complication and manifests as an aggressive distal atherosclerosis. Current 1-year survival is greater than 80%.

HEART–LUNG TRANSPLANTATION

As in heart transplantation proper patient selection is critical. The indications for heart–lung transplantation are shown in Table 77.7. Bacterial colonization is common in patients with cystic fibrosis and is not a contraindication to heart–lung transplantation. However, active sepsis, previous major posterolateral thoracotomy and sternotomy are contraindications.

Patients should be severely limited by their disease and be unable to pursue normal childhood activities such as school or play. Donors are selected on the basis of a normal chest X-ray, satisfactory gas exchange, normal lung compliance and an appropriate size match. Although weight is important, height is a better indicator of relative lung size.

Complications following transplantation include rejection and infection. Overall 1-year survival is greater than 70%.

Table 77.7 Indications for heart–lung transplantation

- Primary pulmonary hypertension
- Eisenmenger's syndrome
- Cystic fibrosis

The future

Despite the widespread acceptance of organ transplantation, the rates of organ donation are insufficient to meet all demands. Although waiting list mortality has been significantly reduced by innovations such as reduced graft transplantation, living related transplantation and split liver transplantation, patients continue to spend prolonged periods on transplant waiting lists with attendant morbidity. Organ shortage continues to be the major factor limiting progress in transplantation. The problem of organ shortage is most significant in children under 2 years and is aggravated by a continued reluctance to allow organ donation after death with many organs not being utilized. Efforts to increase organ donation rates have included live donor registers in the UK and compulsory donation in other European countries. Persistent organ needs have resulted in other novel approaches to the problems of organ shortage. These have included artificial systems for liver 'dialysis', mechanical auxiliary cardiac pumps and xenotransplantation. The improvements in immunosuppression and the more recent development of 'syngeneic' animal donors (zenograft) may well alter the current state of transplantation. However, the single, most important contribution that physicians can make is to encourage organ donation and to promote public awareness of the problems of organ shortage.

References

Corbally, M.T., Rela, M., Heaton, N.D. and Tan, K.C. 1995: Standard orthotopic operation, retransplantation and piggybacking. In Williams, R., Portmann, B. and Tan, K.C. (eds), *The practice of liver transplantation*. Edinburgh: Churchill Livingstone.

Cosimi, A.B. 1994: Clinical small-bowel transplantation. In Morris and Malt (eds), *Oxford textbook of surgery*. Oxford: Oxford Medical Publications.

Harmon, W.E. 1991: Opportunistic infections in children following renal transplantation. *Pediatric Nephrology* **5**, 118–25.

Heaton, N.D., Corbally, M.T., Rela, M. and Tan, K.C. 1995: Surgical techniques of segmental reduction, split and auxiliary liver transplantation. In Williams, R., Portmann, B. and Tan, K.C. (eds), *The practice of liver transplantation*. Edinburgh: Churchill Livingstone.

Najarian, J.S, , Frey, D.J., Matas, A.J. *et al.* Renal transplantation in infants. *Annals of Surgery* **212**, 353–65.

Opelz, G. and Wujciak, T. (for the Collaborative Transplant Study) 1994: The influence of HLA compatability on graft survival after heart transplantation. *New England Journal of Medicine* **330**, 816–19.

Otte, J.B., Yandza, T., de Ville de Goyet, J. *et al.* 1988: Pediatric liver transplantation: report on 52 patients with a 2-year survival of 86%. *Journal of Pediatric Surgery* **23**, 250–3.

Sager, S. and Ettenger, R.B. 1993: Kidney transplantation in children. *Seminars in Pediatric Surgery* **2**, 235–47.

Shaw, B.W., Gordon, R.D., Iwatsuki, S. and Starzl, T.E. 1985: Retransplantation of the liver. *Seminars in Liver Disease* **5**, 394–401.

Shaw, B.W., Jr, Wood, R.P., Stratta, R.J., Pillen, T.J. and Langnas, A.N. 1989: Stratify the causes of death in liver transplant recipients: an approach to improving survival. *Archives of Surgery* **124**, 895–900.

Sheldon, C.A., Churchill, B.M., McLorie, G.A. and Arbus, G.S. 1992: Evaluation of factors contributing to mortality in paediatric renal transplant recipients. *Journal of Pediatric Surgery* **27**, 629–633.

Starzl, T.E., Shaw, B.W., Griffith, B.P. and Bahnson, H.T. 1984. A flexible procedure for multiple cadaveric organ procurement. *Surgery, Gynaecology and Obstetrics* **165**, 223–30.

Stewart, S.M., Uauy, R., Kennard, B.D., Waller, D.A., Benser, M. and Andrews, W.S. 1988: Mental development and growth in children with chronic liver disease of early and late onset. *Paediatrics* **82**, 167–72.

Wajszczuk, C.P., Dummer, J.S., Ho, M. *et al.* Fungal infections in liver transplant recipients. *Transplantation* **40**, 347–53.

Further reading

Williams, R., Portmann, B. and Tan, K.C. (eds) 1995: *The practice of liver transplantation*. Edinburgh: Churchill Livingstone.

CHAPTER 78

Congenital heart disease: principles of management – medical

B.R. KEETON

Introduction
Incidence and aetiology
Clinical features
Diagnosis and investigations
Terminology: the segmental approach
in complex lesions

Preparation for surgery
Interventional cardiology
Care of the patient after surgery
Specific lesions
Further reading

Introduction

Major advances have been achieved since the 1960s in the medical and surgical management of congenital heart disease. Improvements in outcome have resulted from better understanding of the anatomy and physiology, advances in diagnostic techniques, particularly cardiac ultrasound and Doppler, and novel interventional catheter and surgical procedures combined with improved preoperative, intraoperative and postoperative care. A major contribution has been the liaison between the paediatric cardiologist and the paediatric cardiac surgeon, enabling a team approach to the patient's management which is crucial to a successful surgical programme.

Incidence and aetiology

Congenital cardiac defects occur in 6–8 per 1000 live births, and are more common if stillbirths and spontaneous abortions are included. This excludes simple bicuspid aortic valve, found in 1 in 80 of the population, and mitral valve prolapse which may be detected in up to 5% of young adults. Approximately 3.5 per 1000 live born infants present with critical congenital heart disease requiring intervention in the first year of life.

Factors recognized in the aetiology of congenital cardiac defects include chromosomal disorders, single gene disorders and various environmental factors, particularly maternal illnesses, drugs and infections. Recent research has identified chromosomal markers for certain syndromes involving congenital heart disease. Partial deletion of the long arm of chromosome 22 is found in the DiGeorge syndrome, CHARGE association, velocardiofacial syndrome and in some patients with isolated conotruncal heart defect. An abnormality of chromosome 7 has been identified in William's syndrome. It is likely that with further research new genetic markers will be identified for other congenital heart lesions.

Disorders affecting other systems occur in 15% of patients with congenital heart disease and these may be relevant in the patient's management. In 85% the heart lesion is an isolated defect and successful correction will leave an essentially normal child.

Antenatal diagnosis using cardiac ultrasound at 18–20 weeks gestation is possible for the majority of major abnormalities and is making an impact on the spectrum of disease presentation. Most obstetric departments undertake routine four-chamber view screening of all fetuses and paediatric cardiac units offer more detailed screening for at-risk pregnancies or for suspected abnormality.

Unless the disorder is a single gene disorder or there are other identifiable risk factors, the recurrence risk for most forms of congenital heart disease is around 4–5% for siblings and slightly higher for offspring of affected patients. Some lesions (e.g. atrioventricular septal defect) carry a higher risk of recurrence.

Clinical features

PRESENTING FEATURES

Children with congenital heart disease present with one or more of the following features: heart murmur, cardiac failure, cyanosis, shock/low cardiac output, rhythm disturbance, syncope and failure to thrive.

Murmurs

Innocent heart murmurs may be found in 50% of normal children. They have characteristic clinical features enabling them to be distinguished from pathological murmurs. Chest radiography, electrocardiogram and echocardiography may be used to confirm the structural and functional normality of the heart.

Cardiac failure

The term cardiac failure tends to be used in paediatric cardiology to include situations where ventricular contractility may be normal or even hyperactive but the patient is symptomatic because of increased pulmonary blood flow or pulmonary venous congestion resulting in tachypnoea, recession and feeding difficulty. The patient may also show fluid retention and systemic venous congestion giving hepatic enlargement and abdominal distension, occasionally with generalized oedema. Children with cardiac failure often fail to thrive because of diminished calorie intake or increased metabolic demand. They may exhibit features of low cardiac output with sweatiness, particularly of the head, cool peripheries and poor volume pulses.

Cyanosis

Cyanosis is detectable when there is 5 g/dl or more of reduced haemoglobin in the systemic capillary blood; thus its detection depends on the arterial oxygen saturation and on the haemoglobin. Considerable desaturation may exist without clinically detectable cyanosis.

The hyperoxia or nitrogen washout test (measurement of the arterial PO_2 after 10 min breathing in or ventilation with 100% oxygen) is helpful in diagnosing cyanotic congenital heart disease where there is generally little increase in PO_2 ($PO_2 < 20$ kPa) in response to oxygen breathing. Infants with severe lung disease or with persistent fetal circulation may show sufficient arterial hypoxia in 100% oxygen to mimic cyanotic heart disease. The absolute level of the arterial PO_2 may help in the clinical diagnosis. Patients with a very low PO_2 of the order of 2–3 kPa in 100% oxygen are likely to have transposition of the great arteries or very severe obstruction to pulmonary blood flow (these two alternatives being readily distinguishable on the plain chest X-ray). Infants with higher PO_2s of the order of 7–10 kPa in 100% oxygen are more likely to have a common mixing situation with mixing at atrial, ventricular or great artery level.

HAEMODYNAMIC FACTORS INFLUENCING PRESENTATION

Several important factors influence the timing and nature of presentation of congenital heart disease, particularly in the infant age group. Congenital heart disease is not a static condition as haemodynamic changes occur with time which modify the child's clinical status.

Pulmonary vascular resistance

In the full-term newborn pulmonary vascular resistance is high and the normal postnatal fall is delayed in the presence of an intracardiac communication. This postpones the onset of symptomatic cardiac failure in infants with dependent shunts, i.e. shunts which depend on pulmonary vascular resistance (ventricular septal defect, persistent ductus arteriosus or aortopulmonary window). It is unusual for such patients to present with cardiac failure in the first week of life and they may not develop significant symptoms until 4–6 weeks of age.

Untreated, patients with large left-to-right shunts and elevated pulmonary artery pressure are at risk of developing pulmonary vascular obstructive disease which, in time, becomes irreversible and results in shunt reversal (Eisenmenger reaction) thus precluding successful operation. Such patients must be followed closely and surgical intervention carried out before these changes occur. If the pulmonary artery pressure is two-thirds of the systemic pressure or greater then primary repair of the defect or, for more complex lesions, palliative pulmonary artery banding will be required in the early months of life. Irreversible pulmonary vascular changes are rare in the first 6 months of life.

In the premature infant, there is little muscle in the pulmonary arteriolar wall before 36 weeks' gestation, so the pulmonary vascular resistance falls more rapidly and left-to-right shunting may cause cardiac failure earlier, often in the first few days.

In obligatory shunting, i.e. shunt not dependent on pulmonary resistance, as in arteriovenous malformation (e.g. intracerebral or 'vein of Galen aneurysm') or ventriculoatrial shunting in the atrioventricular septal defect, cardiac failure occurs early.

Patency of ductus arteriosus

Spontaneous closure of the arterial duct will precipitate the presentation of patients whose pulmonary or systemic blood flow is duct dependent, e.g. in hypoplastic left heart syndrome, interruption of the aortic arch or severe coarctation of the aorta. Systemic blood flow depends on ductal patency and in pulmonary atresia or severe right heart outflow obstruction the pulmonary blood flow is compromised as the duct closes. Alprostadil (prostaglandin E_1) by intravenous infusion maintains the patency of the closing ductus and has revolutionized the management of such patients, allowing them to be resuscitated and kept in good condition pending further intervention. Alprostadil may cause apnoea, particularly at the higher dose regimes, so facilities for intubation and ventilation should always be available, particularly during the transportation of sick infants. Other side-effects include hyperpyrexia, bradycardia, seizures, hypotension, tachycardia and diarrhoea.

The prostaglandin synthetase inhibitor indomethacin is widely used in the premature neonate to induce closure of a patent ductus arteriosus. It is successful in around 90% of patients weighing over 1500 g but ductal reopening or failure to respond is more commonly seen in smaller infants. It is contraindicated in patients with renal dysfunction, clotting abnormalities (particularly thrombocytopenia) or necrotizing enterocolitis when surgery is the safer option. Careful echo and Doppler assessment of the duct is advisable prior to surgery.

Progression of obstructive lesions

Obstructive lesions may progress by thickening or inadequate growth of a valve or as a result of muscular hypertrophy of the heart. For example, in tetralogy of Fallot increasing infundibular obstruction to right ventricular outflow leads to cyanosis or hypoxic spells. In patients with a univentricular atrioventricular connection, spontaneous closure of the ventricular septal defect will produce obstruction to systemic or pulmonary outflow depending on which great vessel arises from the rudimentary ventricle.

Diagnosis and investigations

Accurate and complete diagnosis is essential for successful medical or surgical management of congenital heart defects. High-resolution cross-sectional cardiac ultrasound imaging with pulsed and continuous wave Doppler and colour flow mapping allows detailed diagnosis in virtually all cases, particularly in infancy where echocardiographic windows allow satisfactory images to be achieved in multiple planes. This obviates the need for cardiac catheterization in many patients. The surgeon must fully understand the anatomy and physiology of the lesion to be treated and with the paediatric cardiologist become skilled in the interpretation of echo images. Some patients will require cardiac catheterization and angiography for haemodynamic assessment or to elucidate certain aspects of the anatomy of the heart which cannot be gleaned from echo. This particularly applies to peripheral pulmonary artery anatomy. Other modalities of investigation, including magnetic resonance imaging, transoesophageal echocardiography, nuclear cardiac imaging, 24-hour monitoring for arrhythmias and stress testing, also play an important role in the preoperative and postoperative evaluation of certain patients.

Terminology: the segmental approach in complex lesions

It is important that the physician, surgeon and other members of the team communicate clearly and understandably. In the patient with complex congenital heart disease sequential segmental analysis permits a logical approach to the anatomical diagnosis of the defect which can be applied to all hearts no matter how abnormal. This is often preferable to alphanumeric shorthand classifications of defects. This step-by-step sequential analysis of the heart is a fundamental principle in the clinical and echocardiographic assessment and involves the following steps.

(1) DEFINE THE ATRIAL ARRANGEMENT (SITUS)

The situs is ascertained from the radiographic appearances of the visceral and bronchial arrangement, from the venous connections as defined on echo and from the morphology of the atrial appendages. It may be normal (situs solitus), mirror image (situs inversus) or ambiguous [bilateral left atria (left isomerism) or bilateral right atria (right isomerism)].

(2) DEFINE THE TYPE AND MODE OF ATRIOVENTRICULAR CONNECTION

The type of connection denotes the way in which the atria connect to the ventricle, whilst the mode of connection defines the morphology of the valve or valves at the atrioventricular junction.

The type of connection may be concordant (normal), discordant (left atrium connected to right ventricle, right atrium connected to left ventricle), ambiguous (atrial isomerism with two ventricles) or univentricular (both atria connect to one ventricular chamber – either double inlet or with absence of right or left connection, the morphology of the dominant ventricular chamber being left ventricular with an anterior rudimentary right ventricle, right ventricular with a posterior rudimentary left ventricle or indeterminate).

The mode of connection may be by two separate atrioventricular valves, by a straddling valve or by a common atrioventricular valve.

(3) DEFINE THE VENTRICULOARTERIAL CONNECTION

This may be concordant (normal), discordant (aorta from right ventricle, pulmonary artery from left ventricle), double outlet (both vessels from the same ventricle) or single outlet (one vessel with aortic atresia, pulmonary atresia or truncus arteriosus).

(4) DESCRIBE (LIST) ALL OF THE ASSOCIATED ANOMALIES

This will include a description of any abnormality of spatial relationships, anomalies of pulmonary and systemic venous return, details of septal defects, their number, size and position and their relationship with other structures, atrioventricular and semilunar valve, subvalve or supravalvular anomalies and any arterial abnormalities. Details of haemodynamic parameters such as shunts, pressures, gradients and resistance calculations should be included.

Preparation for surgery

THE ACUTELY ILL CHILD

Many infants presenting with symptomatic congenital heart disease will be in poor condition. Initial resuscitation will require attention to fluid balance, temperature control and biochemistry particularly blood sugar, calcium and pH. Intubation and ventilation, together with correction of metabolic acidosis by the administration of sodium bicarbonate (4.2%) or tris(hydroxymethyl)aminomethane (THAM) may be required. Alprostadil (prostaglandin E_1) will reopen a recently closed or closing duct to restore systemic or pulmonary blood flow in patients with duct-dependent circulation. It also reduces pulmonary resistance, which can be helpful in increasing pulmonary blood flow and hence intracardiac mixing in transposition. Administration of inotropes, particularly dobutamine which may be given initially via a peripheral line, will improve myocardial contractility and cardiac output, whilst dopamine infused via a central line will aid renal perfusion. It is usually advisable to establish central venous access to enable drug administration and monitoring of filling pressure as early as possible in the resuscitation of the critically ill cardiac infant.

Management of rhythm disturbances in the collapsed infant has to be handled with care since most anti-arrhythmic drugs depress myocardial function. Intravenous adenosine can usually be safely given to interrupt re-entrant tachycardia involving the atrioventricular node and also to aid in the diagnosis of ectopic tachycardia by transiently blocking atrioventricular conduction. Digoxin for supraventricular tachycardia should be used with care in the presence of hypokalaemia or renal impairment and it takes several hours to work. Direct-current countershock cardioversion should be considered at an early stage for arrhythmias associated with low cardiac output. Junctional tachycardia, which is incessant and often resistant to treatment, is the most common arrhythmia seen in the collapsed child presenting with structural heart disease. It is best controlled by cooling the paralysed and ventilated child to 32–34°C on a cooling blanket. Intravenous infusion of amiodarone has also been successful.

In spite of full resuscitative procedures some children will not improve until the defect has been palliated or corrected. In others one might attain a moderate improvement, giving a window of opportunity to intervene whilst the patient is in a reasonable state. The paediatric cardiac surgeon must be prepared to operate urgently on certain patients, particularly for emergency repair of symptomatic coarctation of the aorta, critical aortic stenosis, obstructed total anomalous pulmonary venous drainage in the young infant or for a systemic–pulmonary shunt.

THE STABLE CHILD

The patient's condition should be optimized prior to surgery, treating cardiac failure with diuretics and angiotensin converting enzyme inhibitors where appropriate.

Baseline biochemistry, haematology and coagulation, blood group and antibody screening, particularly for antibodies reacting at low temperature, should be undertaken, as well as recording an electrocardiogram (ECG) and taking a chest radiograph.

The importance of careful explanation to the child in simple terms that he or she can understand about what is to happen and in more detail to parents about the objectives, risks and benefits of the procedures to be undertaken should not be overlooked.

Interventional cardiology

A number of percutaneous transluminal catheter interventional cardiological procedures has been introduced in recent years as replacements for or adjuncts to surgery. Some, such as balloon dilatation of the pulmonary valve for pulmonary stenosis and of recoarctation of the aorta, transcatheter occlusion of the ductus using an umbrella device or embolization coils have become rapidly established as the treatment of choice, are very successful and associated with low risk. Other procedures, such as intravascular stenting, are very promising but have yet to be proven in the longer term. Controversy exists over some procedures, e.g. balloon dilatation for native coarctation and for aortic valve stenosis. Improvements in equipment design, e.g. lower profile balloons on smaller shaft sizes, have resulted in better outcomes with fewer complications. These procedures should have comparable or reduced morbidity and mortality to conventional surgical procedures and the outcomes must be carefully monitored in both the short-term and long-term follow-up.

Decisions on the preferred method of treatment should be taken jointly between the paediatric cardiologist and paediatric cardiac surgeon, bearing in mind the results of existing methods of treatment and the lessons learned over the years. The surgeon may be required to stand by for surgical intervention in the event of failure or the occurrence of a complication of a catheter procedure.

Care of the patient after surgery

Few operations for congenital heart disease are totally corrective and careful long-term follow-up will be required as the child grows. Operations such as atrial or ventricular septal defect closure, or persistent ductus arteriosus ligation have favourable long-term outcomes. In many instances, however, e.g. correction of tetralogy of Fallot, truncus arteriosus and pulmonary atresia, residual lesions such as pulmonary regurgitation remain or there may be a requirement for further surgery to replace homograft valves. Aortic valvotomy can only be regarded as palliative since virtually all patients will require later valve replacement. Endocarditis remains a risk after most operations and antibiotic prophylaxis for dental and surgical procedures is advised. Some patients require limitations to be placed on their physical activities. Following Mustard and Fontan operations late problems, particularly arrhythmias and ventricular failure, are common.

Adolescents and adult survivors of congenital heart disease, a growing group, need special provision for their long-term medical and psychosocial care, including advice on employability, insurability, contraception and reproductive capacity.

Specific lesions

ABNORMALITIES OF SYSTEMIC VENOUS CONNECTION

Persistence of the left superior vena cava (SVC) draining to the coronary sinus is commonly associated with congenital cardiac defects and should be recognized preoperatively since it may cause difficulty in venous cannulation for bypass. Rarely, it may drain directly to the left atrium causing cyanosis.

Bilateral superior caval veins are often seen in isomerism and absence of the abdominal portion of the inferior vena cava (IVC) with azygos continuation to the SVC is a hallmark of left isomerism.

ABNORMALITIES OF PULMONARY VENOUS CONNECTION

In total anomalous pulmonary venous connection (TAPVC) the pulmonary veins drain to a common channel lying behind the left atrium which drains via an ascending vein to the innominate vein and SVC (supracardiac), or directly to the heart most commonly to the coronary sinus (cardiac), or via a descending vein traversing the diaphragm to the portal venous system, thence into the IVC (infracardiac). Postoperatively there is a risk of pulmonary hypertensive crises, particularly when there has been obstruction (invariably found in infracardiac TAPVD). Nitric oxide via the ventilator and intravenous epoprostenol (prostacycline) may be necessary and monitoring of pulmonary artery pressure is helpful.

Partial anomalous pulmonary venous drainage may involve the whole of one lung or merely a segment of lung.

In the Scimitar syndrome, so called because of the characteristic X-ray appearance of the anomalous pulmonary vein, the lower part of the right lung drains to the inferior vena cava and there is usually a systemic arterial supply to and bronchial sequestration of that segment of the lung.

Anomalous connection of the right upper pulmonary veins to the SVC is often seen in sinus venosus atrial septal defect.

DEFECTS OF THE ATRIAL SEPTUM (ASD)

These may lie at the site of the fossa ovalis (secundum ASD), near the entrance of the SVC or IVC (sinus venosus ASD) or in the lower part of the septum (ostium primum ASD or partial atrioventricular septal defect). The latter is a defect of the atrioventricular septum and associated with abnormality of the atrioventricular valve, resulting in varying degrees of mitral regurgitation.

Small secundum defects may close spontaneously and are usually observed for the first few years of life. Right heart failure and atrial fibrillation resulting from right heart volume overload, paradoxical embolus and pulmonary hypertension may occur late, and therefore closure of all atrial septal defects associated with right heart dilatation after the age of about 5 years is recommended. Open heart surgery is the only option for the primum and sinus venosus defects but secundum defects can be closed using new transcatheter devices. It is likely that, with further refinement of such techniques, large numbers of children will avoid surgical intervention but the surgeon will be required to offer surgical stand-by in case of unsatisfactory deployment or displacement of the device.

DEFECTS OF THE ATRIOVENTRICULAR JUNCTION

These defects may be classified into partial (ostium primum defect, see above), complete (common atrioventricular valve with ventricular defect) and intermediate forms. The atrioventricular valve has an anterior and a posterior bridging leaflet which shows variations in its attachments to the interventricular septum and in the arrangement of the papillary muscles. The complete atrioventricular septal defect is common in Down's syndrome and pulmonary hypertension necessitates early repair. Echocardiography permits detailed identification of the atrioventricular valve and papillary muscle morphology, allowing the surgeon to plan the repair. This lesion may be associated with an unequal partitioning of the atrioventricular orifice with unbalanced ventricles leading to surgical difficulties. Abnormality of the left or right ventricular outflow tract may coexist.

ATRIOVENTRICULAR VALVE ABNORMALITIES

Tricuspid atresia

This is a form of univentricular atrioventricular connection where the tricuspid valve is atretic and the right atrium is separated from the ventricular mass by thick sulcus tissue. Systemic venous blood crosses the atrial septum to the left atrium. The aorta usually arises from the left ventricle and the pulmonary artery from the rudimentary right ventricle (concordant ventriculoarterial connection) but the arteries may be transposed. The atrial communication may become restrictive and atrial septostomy by balloon or blade may be required. The degree of cyanosis depends on the size of the intraventricular communication which governs the magnitude of pulmonary blood flow. In those with restrictive pulmonary blood flow a preliminary shunt – Modified Blalock–Taussig or in the older infant modified Glenn shunt (bidirectional superior cavopulmonary anastomosis) – will be required. In those with unrestrictive pulmonary flow pulmonary artery banding is needed to prevent pulmonary vascular disease prior to consideration of a Fontan or total cavopulmonary connection operation.

Other atrioventricular valve abnormalities

Congenital tricuspid valve abnormalities include congenital regurgitation with valvular dysplasia or Ebstein's anomaly. Hypoplasia of the tricuspid is usually associated with pulmonary atresia and intact ventricular septum. Congenital mitral valve anomalies (stenosis, hypoplasia and atresia) are often associated with other left heart defects including hypoplastic left heart syndrome, aortic stenosis and coarctation of the aorta.

DEFECTS OF THE INTRAVENTRICULAR SEPTUM

Ventricular septal defect (VSD) is the most common congenital cardiac defect, occurring in 50% of children with congenital heart disease as an isolated lesion or as part of a more complex abnormality. The defects are classified as perimembranous (abutting on the central fibrous body) or muscular and described according to their position in the inlet, trabecular or outlet portion of the septum. They may be single or multiple. Most VSDs tend to become smaller with age (30–40% will close spontaneously, particularly the smaller defects). Patients are usually managed medically in the first instance. Indications for surgical closure are cardiac failure unresponsive to medication, failure to thrive, pulmonary hypertension (two-thirds of systemic or greater) or rising pulmonary vascular resistance, and large shunt (pulmonary:systemic flow ratio > 2.5:1) associated with cardiomegaly. Irreversible pulmonary vascular changes may occur in the first 6–12 months of life and surgical closure is mandatory in those with pulmonary hypertension to prevent the Eisenmenger reaction. A small minority of defects can be closed using a transcatheter device. If the defect is close to the aortic valve, aortic regurgitation may develop and surgical repair may prevent its progression.

There is a small risk of endocarditis in patients followed medically and although substantially reduced following surgical repair it is not totally eradicated.

If the VSD is part of a more complex lesion such as double-outlet right ventricle or double-inlet ventricle, diminution in size of the defect will restrict the outlet from one ventricle. Surgical enlargement may be required.

The surgeon must know the disposition of the atrioventricular conduction bundle in relation to the various types of ventricular septal defect so that surgically induced heart block can be avoided.

DISORDERS OF VENTRICULOARTERIAL CONNECTION AND OUTFLOW TRACTS

Transposition of the great arteries (TGA)

Severe cyanosis is usually evident in the newborn period but if there is a large atrial or ventricular septal defect diagnosis may be delayed for a few weeks. Initial management is with alprostadil (prostaglandin E_1) infusion to maintain ductal patency. A balloon atrial septostomy (Rashkind procedure) will enable intracardiac mixing and stabilize the child until surgical repair is undertaken. Cardiac catheterization is seldom required for diagnosis since the anatomy can be demonstrated on echocardiography. The origins and course of the proximal coronary arteries can usually be ascertained, although this may be difficult, but abnormal coronary anatomy does not preclude successful anatomical correction.

Tetralogy of Fallot

The anatomical hallmark is leftward and anterior displacement of the infundibular septum resulting in overriding of the aorta across a large unrestrictive ventricular septal defect and infundibular pulmonary stenosis with associated right ventricular hypertrophy. The pulmonary valve ring is often narrowed and there may be supravalvular and pulmonary artery narrowing. Less common but surgically important associated lesions include the presence of multiple ventricular septal defects and anomalous origin of the left anterior descending coronary artery from the right coronary.

Most children present in the first year of life. Cardiac catheterization is not mandatory but is still preferred by some units to demonstrate the anatomy of the peripheral pulmonary arteries and thus exclude arborization and coronary artery abnormality. Hypercyanotic spells may be life threatening and require urgent treatment including the administration of oxygen, morphine, sodium bicarbonate, intravenous propanolol to reduce infundibular muscle spasm or noradrenaline to increase systemic resistance. Severe spells indicate the need for surgical intervention.

PULMONARY ATRESIA

Pulmonary atresia with ventricular septal defect may have central pulmonary arteries supplied by the ductus or these may be very hypoplastic with a multifocal pulmonary blood supply via systemic–pulmonary collateral arteries.

In pulmonary atresia with intact ventricular septum there are varying degrees of hypoplasia of the three parts of the right ventricle (inlet, trabecular and outlet parts) and of the tricuspid valve.

AORTIC STENOSIS

Critical aortic valve stenosis presents in infancy with collapse and low cardiac output requiring urgent treatment. The optimal treatment remains controversial, with some advocating transcatheter balloon dilatation and others (the present author included) regarding surgery as safer and having improved long-term results. Milder forms of stenosis may be followed medically but when pressure gradients reach 70 mmHg and there is left ventricular hypertrophy intervention is recommended to avoid the risk of sudden death.

Subvalve stenosis is usually an acquired and progressive lesion requiring surgery because of increasing gradient, symptoms and the development of aortic regurgitation. Supravalve stenosis is either of the hourglass type just above the valve or a tubular hypoplasia.

PULMONARY VALVE STENOSIS

Intervention is usually recommended if the right ventricular pressure is two-thirds or greater than the systemic pressure. Most patients respond to percutaneous balloon dilatation but surgery is sometimes required for dysplastic valves. This may be associated with Noonan's syndrome.

COARCTATION OF THE AORTA

Symptomatic patients usually present in early infancy. The child's condition can usually be improved by reopening the ductus with alprostadil infusion prior to urgent surgical repair. Balloon dilatation of native coarctation remains controversial but is generally accepted as the treatment of first choice for recoarctation.

Further reading

Emmanoilides, G.C., Riemenschneider, T.A., Allen, H.D. *et al.* (eds) 1995: *Heart disease in infants, children and adolescents.* Baltimore, MD: Williams & Wilkins.

Garson, A., Bricker, J.T. and McNamara, D.G. (eds) 1990: *The science and practice of pediatric cardiology.* Philadelphia, PA: Lea & Febiger.

CHAPTER 79

Congenital heart disease: principles of management – surgical

J.L. MONRO

History	**Palliative procedures**
Perfusion	**Operations for specific defects**
Surgical approach	**References**

History

Cardiac surgery is a relatively new speciality. In 1938 Gross tied the persistent ductus arteriosus of a child with endocarditis (Gross and Hubbard, 1939). In 1945 Blalock anastomosed the subclavian artery to the pulmonary artery in a child with Fallot's tetralogy to increase the blood supply to the lungs and thus make her pinker, and in the same year Crafoord resected a coarctation of the aorta. In 1954 Gibbon closed an atrial septal defect using cardiopulmonary bypass.

The success of these early pioneers stimulated an upsurge of interest in treating previously untreatable congenital cardiac conditions, and within the next few years most conditions had been corrected, though initially with a rather high mortality.

The early cardiopulmonary bypass machinery and oxygenators were somewhat cumbersome and damaging to blood. During the 1960s the technology improved markedly and by the 1970s disposable oxygenators were being used routinely with much improved results. In the late 1970s the general introduction of cardioplegia to help with myocardial preservation during longer and more difficult operations requiring a still heart, allowed a range of procedures to be developed for treating even the most complicated lesions, including transplantation.

The improvement in diagnostic methods (as described in the previous chapter) and postoperative management since the 1970s has made a major contribution to the advances that have been made in congenital cardiac surgery.

Perfusion

It is necessary to provide a still, relatively bloodless field in which the defects inside the heart can be repaired. Blood is therefore drained from the heart into a reservoir from which the desaturated blood is pumped via a plastic tube that goes through a roller pump and to the oxygenator (Fig. 79.1). The most common oxygenator now used in paediatric practice is a membrane oxygenator. Oxygen diffuses into the desaturated blood returning from the patient and the saturated blood is pumped through a filter back into the ascending aorta.

Previously, bubble oxygenators were usually used and oxygen was bubbled through the returning desaturated blood which became saturated, but needed to pass through a defoamer before being pumped back into the body. These oxygenators cause more haemolysis, particularly during longer procedures. When the heart is open any unwanted blood is sucked back to the reservoir so that it is not wasted.

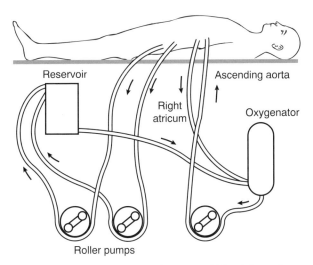

Fig. 79.1 Perfusion circuit: desaturated blood flows from the right atrium to the oxygenator, where it is oxygenated. The oxygenator also incorporates a heat exchanger to maintain the temperature of the blood returning to the patient. Oxygenated blood is pumped from the oxygenator back to the ascending aorta of the patient. Blood can also be sucked from the heart via tubes to a reservoir, from where it returns via the oxygenator to the patient.

In larger children the pump circuit can be primed with Hartman's solution or some other clear fluid. However, in smaller children this would result in too much dilution and the circuit is usually primed with one or two units of blood. The patient must of course be heparinized to prevent clotting, and after bypass this is discontinued. After the cannulae have been removed protamine is given to reverse the effects of the heparin.

An arterial cannula is inserted into the aorta for the return of saturated blood to the heart and this can be quite difficult in small neonates. It is usual to insert two venous cannulae and pass them into each vena cava. A snare can be placed around each vena cava and these are tightened on to the cannulae so as to produce an airtight fit, thus allowing the right atrium to be opened and a good, bloodless view to be obtained of the inside of the heart (Monro and Shore, 1984).

Once bypass is commenced and full flow achieved, the aorta is cross-clamped and myocardial protection achieved by infusing a potassium-rich 'cardioplegic' solution into the ascending aorta. This stops the heart and reduces damage to the ischaemic myocardium. The dose can be repeated at 25–30-min intervals. The heart can then be opened and the defect repaired. Care must be taken to remove all air from the heart by filling it with blood before finally closing the incision. In addition, it is usual to have a sucking vent in the aorta so that any residual bubbles of air will be sucked out, rather than cause a cerebral air embolus which could be fatal.

The running of the cardiopulmonary bypass machine is usually managed by a dedicated perfusionist who is also responsible for ensuring that the blood gases and potassium remain satisfactory during the period of bypass. He or she must also co-operate with the anaesthetist who will need to ensure that the patient is adequately sedated and paralysed before bypass commences. Any further anaesthetic is added to the bypass reservoir.

It is usual to cool the patient with a heat exchanger incorporated in the circuit to about 28°C as this gives extra protection should it be necessary to stop the pump for a short period. In small infants where the venous cannulae and any venous return to the heart can get in the way, deep hypothermia can be used. The baby can be surface cooled to about 32°C and then the chest opened, bypass instituted and the patient cooled to 18°C, at which temperature the circulation can be stopped for up to 40 min and then the patient rewarmed on bypass. An alternative which is more commonly used now is to cool down from normal temperature to 18°C entirely on bypass and then following correction to rewarm in the same manner. This method is more expeditious but care must be taken to obtain even cooling, and a longer period of cooling bypass is required.

Surgical approach

For all operations requiring cardiopulmonary bypass it is usual to use a midline incision, the sternum being divided longitudinally with a mechanical saw. The sternum is separated fairly widely by a self-retaining retractor (Finocietto). For 'closed' operations such as repair of coarctation of the aorta or ligation of a persistent ductus arteriosus a left thoracotomy through the fourth intercostal space is used.

Wound closure is achieved with heavy sutures to approximate the sternum or ribs and a drain is inserted to allow any persisting blood loss to drain into an underwater seal drain on suction.

Palliative procedures

It is not always possible or prudent to correct a lesion and a palliative or temporary procedure may be performed to either to increase the arterial saturation in a cyanosed child or to reduce the flow of blood to the lungs, which are in danger of flooding.

THE MODIFIED BLALOCK–TAUSSIG SHUNT

The Blalock–Taussig shunt has been superseded by the modified Blalock–Taussig shunt in which a short length of Goretex tubing (usually 4 or 5 mm in diameter) is inserted between the subclavian artery (usually right) and the pulmonary artery. A direct anastomosis between the ascending aorta and pulmonary artery (Waterston, 1962) can be made but it is difficult to judge the size exactly and this procedure is now rarely performed.

PULMONARY ARTERY BANDING

If there is a large ventricular septal defect (VSD) or uni-ventricular heart with no pulmonary stenosis, the lungs will be flooded and in time pulmonary vascular disease may develop. The large pulmonary blood flow can be reduced by banding the pulmonary artery. A piece of tape is tied around the pulmonary artery to narrow it considerably so that the flow to the lungs is much reduced. When the child is larger the defect can be repaired and the band removed. This procedure is now usually reserved for multiple VSD and univentricular hearts.

POSTOPERATIVE CARE

This is a very important factor in the successful outcome following cardiac surgery. It is usual for the patient to be transferred to the intensive care unit and to be ventilated until the cardiac output is satisfactory, the patient is awake and there is no bleeding. This may be for a few hours or even several days in sick neonates. Careful monitoring is needed, with arterial and venous pressure lines (a left atrial pressure line may be needed as well as a right). The urine output and peripheral temperatures give a good guide to the cardiac output. Small babies require an overhead heater to help them to stay warm.

If the cardiac output is inadequate, it is important to determine and correct a cause if possible and echocardiography is very helpful. If it is due to a poorly functioning left ventricle, inotropic supporting drugs such as dobutamine and adrenaline may be used.

The congenital disorders of the heart have been described in the previous chapter and set out in a logical order progressing anatomically through the various levels of the heart. Therefore the various conditions to be treated surgically will be described in the same order.

Operations for specific defects

ATRIUM

Secundum atrial septal defect (ASD)

This is one of the most common defects and many patients are completely asymptomatic despite a left-to-right shunt of 2 or 3:1. However, closure is advisable, usually before the age of starting school as patients run the risk of developing arrhythmias later in life. In addition, paroxysmal embolus is an important risk, particularly in pregnancy.

Surgery requires bypass, clamping of the ascending aorta and cardioplegia, with opening of the right atrium. In young children it is usually possible to close the defect by direct suture. If the suture is started inferiorly air can be expelled from the left atrium as the upper part of the defect is closed, and then the suture run down again to close the defect more safely with a double layer. The aortic clamp is removed and the heart starts to beat while the right atrium is closed. Bypass can then be easily discontinued, the cannulae removed and the chest closed.

In older patients or those with a large defect it may be necessary to close the defect with a patch, and autologous pericardium, taken as the chest is opened, is very satisfactory.

Sinus venosus atrial septal defect

This defect is high in the atrial septum and at least some pulmonary veins usually drain directly into the lower superior vena cava (SVC). All of the blood from the lungs must be directed into the left atrium and a patch (e.g. of pericardium) is needed for this. Care must be taken to avoid narrowing the lower end of the SVC or damaging the sinoatrial node.

The risks of atrial septal defect closure are extremely low, although care must be taken to avoid air embolus. Tension in closure must be avoided (with a patch if necessary) to prevent recurrence.

Total anomalous pulmonary venous drainage (TAPVD)

Patients with TAPVD present early in infancy and may be extremely ill, particularly if the veins are obstructed. Surgery is usually required on an emergency or urgent basis. The common pulmonary venous channel must be connected to the left atrium and the connection to the venous system and atrial septal defect closed. The operation is best performed with deep hypothermia and total circulatory arrest. The venous cannula can be removed and a dry field helps to provide unobstructed operating conditions in these neonates.

Supracardiac TAPVD

This is the most common type of TAPVD, in which the right atrium is opened and an instrument placed through the atrial septal defect to demonstrate the part of the left atrium that approximates to the common venous channel. Matching incisions are made and the anastomosis is performed with fine monofilament sutures. It may help future growth if some interrupted sutures are used anteriorly. The atrial septal defect is closed, taking care to remove air from the left side of the heart, the right atrium closed and the ascending vein ligated. Bypass is recommenced and the baby rewarmed before bypass is stopped.

Intracardiac TAPVD

Here the pulmonary veins drain into the coronary sinus. Therefore all that is necessary is to cut back into the coronary sinus to widen its entry and to close the atrial septal defect with a patch of pericardium so as to include the coronary sinus which drains into the left atrium.

Infracardiac TAPVD

This is the rarest form of TAPVD, in which the pulmonary veins drain into a descending vein which passes through the diaphragm into the liver from where drainage occurs into the inferior vena cava (IVC). It is necessary to anastomose the descending vein to the back of the left atrium and tie off the descending vein below the lowest pulmonary vein as it passes through the diaphragm.

TAPVD can be of mixed type and although enough information can usually be obtained by echocardiography without cardiac catheterization, the surgeon needs to check the anatomy at operation. Providing the anastomosis is satisfactory and grows, the child should have no further problems.

The overall early mortality is between 10% and 20% but the fatalities tend to occur among those with obstructed veins referred late.

ATRIOVENTRICULAR JUNCTION

Repair of these defects is performed on bypass through the right atrium.

Partial atrioventricular septal defect (ostium primum defect)

The defect is low in the atrial septum, abutting the atrioventricular valves. The anterior leaflet of the mitral valve is cleft and there may be considerable mitral regurgitation. However, the mitral valve can be tested and if not regurgitant the cleft can be left unsutured. The defect is closed with a patch of pericardium which is sutured to the base of the tricuspid valve leaflets, around the area of the atrio-ventricular node and back along the edge of the defect so as not to interfere with the conducting mechanism. Air must be removed from the left side of the heart and the right atrium closed.

The early mortality is low and depends on the competence of the mitral valve. Late mitral regurgitation can increase, leading to further mitral valve repair or replacement.

Complete atrioventricular septal defect

Because these patients have a large pulmonary artery blood flow, they are prone to develop pulmonary vascular disease if left even beyond a few months and therefore operation should be performed in the first 3–4 months of life. Many of these patients have Down's syndrome.

In addition to the atrial component, there is a ventricular septal defect so that the atrioventricular valve leaflets are left floating in the middle of the defect. The anterior mitral and tricuspid leaflets combine to form a common anterior bridging leaflet, and the posterior likewise.

The approach is again through the atrium and it is easier to close the ventricular component of the defect with a separate patch such as Goretex or Dacron, taking care to place the sutures on the right side of the septum so as to avoid the conducting mechanism. The pericardial patch used to close the atrial component is sutured to the atrioventricular leaflets at the same time as the ventricular patch, taking care to attach the valve leaflets at the correct height so as to avoid distorting the valves, which might lead to incompetence. Again, the cleft formed by the central approximation of the anterior and posterior bridging leaflets can be sutured if the mitral valve leaks.

The early mortality for this condition is relatively high (10–25%), mainly because of mitral valve deficiency and heart block problems. The tissue of the mitral valve is quite friable in infants less than 3 months of age and great care must be taken not to allow sutures to cut out.

The mitral valve can also be congenitally stenosed, sometimes with all the chordae attached to one papillary muscle (parachute valve). This can be difficult to repair, although some relief can be obtained by splitting down the papillary muscle. The mitral valve is also prone to stenosis following rheumatic fever, which though now fortunately rare in western society is still very common in developing countries. Fortunately, it usually responds well to valvotomy, whether performed open (on bypass) or closed with a dilator.

Mitral regurgitation should be treated by repair, but if this is not possible valve replacement can be performed, even in infants. With growth, repeated valve replacement will be required and the child must receive anticoagulants.

VENTRICULAR SEPTUM

Ventricular septal defect

As described in the previous chapter there are different types of defect, which may be multiple. The most common is the perimembranous and the principles of closure apply to the other types (although the high subpulmonary or outlet defect can more easily be closed through the pulmonary valve). Traditionally, these VSD were closed through a right ventriculotomy but since the 1970s it has been usual to close most VSD through the right atrium.

The right atrium is opened as for closure of an ASD. The septal leaflet of the tricuspid valve is retracted with everting stay sutures to reveal the VSD. This is closed with a patch of Goretex or Dacron using either continuous or interrupted sutures. Care must be taken to avoid the bundle of His, which runs just below the margin of a perimembranous defect on the left side, so the sutures should be placed on the right side of the septum. Air must be removed from the ventricle and then the right atrium closed.

Muscular defects are further from the tricuspid valve, and can be multiple. Multiple defects can be difficult to close from the right side as they are concealed by the trabeculae. It may even be necessary to open the left ventricle, where a clear view of the defects can be obtained, but this should be avoided if possible because it leads to left ventricular damage. In small babies with multiple VSD, pulmonary artery banding is probably a better initial line of approach.

Infants with a large VSD tend to go into failure in the first month of life and fail to thrive. Their VSD needs to be closed and because they are so small the operation is more difficult and the risks, e.g. of heart block, are somewhat higher. However, VSD closure should have an early mortality of less than 5% and it should be the definitive operation. Residual VSD are very rare.

VENTRICULOARTERIAL CONNECTION

Transposition of the great arteries

This is a lethal condition, but the introduction of the balloon septostomy markedly improved the immediate management. Between 1965 and 1985 the standard management in most units would be to perform a balloon septostomy on presentation and provided the saturation was adequate, to leave the child until about 6–12 months of age and perform an atrial baffle repair (Senning, 1959; Mustard, 1964). This resulted in about 90% of children surviving, compared with the natural history of 90% dying before the age of 1-year. The Mustard procedure involves excising the atrial septum and inserting a U-shaped patch of pericardium to direct the systemic venous blood behind it into the left ventricle. The returning pulmonary venous blood comes over the patch through the tricuspid valve, into the right ventricle and thence to the aorta. Although this operation results in red blood going to the aorta and blue blood to the lungs, late complications such as right ventricular failure, tricuspid regurgitation, baffle obstruction and arrhythmias have resulted in a significant late mortality and morbidity. The Senning operation may reduce baffle obstruction but still requires the right ventricle to act as the systemic ventricle.

To overcome these problems the anatomical correction or switch procedure was introduced in the late 1970s (Jatene *et al.*, 1976) and has become the treatment of choice. This involves transecting the great vessels, suturing the distal aorta to the proximal pulmonary artery (which arises from the left ventricle) and suturing the distal pulmonary artery to the proximal aorta. It is necessary to reposition the coronary arteries by cutting them out on a small button which can then be sutured into the posteriorly placed pulmonary artery. The early mortality for this procedure was initially very high but with experience has fallen to 5% or less in many centres. Some late problems can occur, such as the development of a stenosis in the pulmonary artery at the site of the anastomosis. This can be easily dealt with by a subsequent patch. However, the long-term results are otherwise very good, and the prospect of a lifetime with a left ventricle pumping the systemic circulation has to be better than in the Mustard procedure.

It is important to perform the switch procedure in the first 2 weeks or so of life while the left ventricle is still hypertrophied. When the pulmonary resistance falls the left ventricle becomes thin-walled and unable to sustain systemic pressures.

Patients with transposition may also have a VSD. This usually causes a persistence of systemic pressure in the left ventricle, allowing the switch procedure to be performed a few months later. However, the operation must not be postponed for too long, or pulmonary vascular disease may develop.

TETRALOGY OF FALLOT

Correction involves closure of the VSD and widening the right ventricular outflow tract. The severity of the outflow tract obstruction usually determines how soon the child requires surgery. The infundibular muscle can be very contractile, causing blue spells, which can be reduced by propranolol. However, those infants with hypoplastic pulmonary valve rings are likely to require surgery in infancy. Correction is obviously the treatment of choice, but in the 1960s correction in infancy carried a high mortality in most centres and therefore the usual approach was two-stage. A shunt procedure (such as a Blalock shunt) would be performed and then the child corrected a few years later. Some surgeons, particularly using deep hypothermia (Barratt-Boyes *et al.*, 1970) achieved better results with correction in infancy and this has been the author's preference. Other surgeons continue to use a two-stage approach, and controversy still exists as to which is safer and produces less long-term morbidity.

Traditionally, the VSD is closed through a right ventriculotomy, and if there is hypoplasia of the pulmonary valve ring, the incision is continued upwards and a transannular patch inserted. This inevitably results in pulmonary regurgitation and the compromise must be reached, to relieve adequately the outflow tract obstruction, but not to cause too much pulmonary regurgitation, which in turn can cause late problems.

In order to prevent damage to the right ventricle the transatrial approach has been used in the last few years, even in infants. The VSD is closed as usual and the obstructing infundibular muscle can be cut out through the tricuspid valve. It will still be necessary to insert a transannular patch if the annulus is small.

Surgeons are tending to correct patients with this condition at a younger and younger age. If the mortality is low and the eventual incidence of pulmonary regurgitation is no higher it would seem sensible to perform the operation at about 1 year of age, even if the child is not severely cyanotic.

The early mortality for correction over the age of 1 year should be less than 5%. In infancy it is likely to be slightly higher, but if over 10% a two-stage approach should be considered. Late pulmonary regurgitation is usually very well tolerated and the great majority of these patients leads a completely normal life following repair.

AORTIC STENOSIS

Valve stenosis

This is the most common left ventricular outflow tract obstruction. The valve is most commonly bicuspid and if the stenosis is mild the patient may present quite late on, perhaps not requiring valve surgery until adult life. Many children with moderate stenosis can cope well for years, with limitation of their activities, but when operation is needed, it is best to perform valve repair. A valvotomy where the fused commissures are split out to the valve ring can increase valve opening and improve the cross-sectional area greatly. However, if it is a bicuspid valve where the two fused cusps have no support, division of these cusps would result in severe regurgitation. Valvotomy may allow the child to grow into adulthood, when a full-size valve can be inserted. If the valve is so disordered that no repair is possible without causing severe regurgitation, then valve replacement will be needed and this can be performed even in small children, particularly using techniques to widen the aortic root. However, if a mechanical valve is used anticoagulants will be necessary and so replacement is best avoided.

Infants may present with aortic stenosis, which is a lethal condition. Urgent surgery is necessary and the outcome should be successful provided endomyocardial fibroelastasis is not present. In this early age group, aortic stenosis can be part of the hypoplastic left heart syndrome. If this is the case there is a hypoplastic left ventricle and the outcome is very much worse. In any case, even in the event of a successful valvotomy, further surgery will be necessary and the parents should be warned of this.

Valvotomy is performed using cardiopulmonary bypass and one venous cannula, as there is no need to open the right side of the heart. After cross-clamping the aorta and giving cardioplegic fluid into the ascending aorta, the aorta is opened and a narrow sucker placed through the aortic valve (in very small babies the orifice may be as small as 2 mm). This gives time to split the appropriate cusps and close the aorta before releasing the aortic clamp. It is better not to insert a direct left ventricular vent, so preserving left ventricular function.

Subvalve stenosis

Usually this takes the form of a fibrous membrane a few millimetres below the aortic valve. It can be demonstrated very clearly by echocardiography and operation is indicated when the gradient is more than about 60 mmHg.

At operation the aorta is opened and the aortic valve carefully retracted to expose the membrane, which can normally be shelled out all the way round. Some help with a knife may be necessary and care should be taken anteriorly where the membrane lies across the bundle of His. The early results are very good, although the obstruction can occasionally recur.

A much more severe type of tubular subaortic obstruction can occur, particularly in patients who have had previous operations such as closure of VSD. This is much more difficult to deal with and may involve operations to widen the aortic root.

Supravalvular aortic stenosis

This is often associated with William's syndrome and usually takes the form of a pinching-in of the aorta at the level of the top of the cusps. The aortic valve cusps may be pulled in to such an extent that they can almost occlude the coronary ostia and also cause regurgitation.

Surgical intervention involves incising the aorta right down into the non-coronary sinus and inserting a patch of Dacron, Goretex or suitable material to widen the aorta.

Pulmonary stenosis

Most stenoses of the pulmonary valve are now dealt with by the interventional cardiologist. However, some very dysplastic valves cannot be split by a balloon and surgery has to be performed.

The pulmonary valve is exposed on bypass by incising the pulmonary artery and looking down on the valve. Ideally, the fused commissures are divided, but if the valve is very dysplastic, it may be necessary to excise the valve or insert a transannular patch.

Persistent ductus arteriosus (PDA)

This is a fairly common condition and even patients who are asymptomatic should have their ducts closed.

Children above 1 year of age usually have their ducts closed by the interventional cardiologists with an umbrella-like device. Premature babies, who may weigh as little as 600 g, are often dependent on ventilators and their ducts should be closed surgically. A left thoracotomy through the fourth intercostal space gives good exposure, and the duct is dissected out and doubly ligated or clipped. It is usually possible to close the chest without a drain, but care must be taken not to leave a pneumothorax.

It is usually possible to extubate the infants immediately following duct closure. The early mortality is very low, but depends on the condition of the child and associated problems.

Coarctation of the aorta

The typical localized narrowing beyond the left subclavian artery causes delay in the flow of blood to the lower part of the body and hypertension in the upper. Patients may present desperately ill in the first few days of life or be discovered at routine examination as adults.

In infancy, the condition of the patient may be improved preoperatively with prostaglandin, which keeps the duct open and allows more blood supply to the lower body, including the kidneys. Although there have been reports of success with ballooning, this has severe complications and a significant recurrence rate.

In infancy the diagnosis can usually be established satisfactorily with echocardiography alone. In older patients angiography is useful to establish the site and severity of the obstruction and also the presence and adequacy of collateral vessels. In an infant, particularly if some moderate cooling of the patient is used, aortic cross-clamping should be safe for the time needed to undertake the repair. In older patients, if there are inadequate collateral vessels, even a short period of aortic clamping could be damaging. In particular, the blood supply to the spinal cord can be compromised, causing paraplegia. Although this complication is extremely rare, parents should be warned of its possibility and every care taken to prevent it.

The standard method of repair is to open the chest through the left fourth intercostal space, and having exposed the aorta to cross-clamp above and below the coarctation. The coarcted segment is excised and the ends joined together. This would not be safe if the collaterals were not adequate, in which case a different technique involving some bypass to allow flow to the descending aorta should be used.

In infants (particularly less than 3 months old) it has been found that if the coarctation was resected and an end-to-end anastomosis performed, there was a worrying incidence of recoarctation, so the technique of subclavian flap repair was introduced (Waldhausen and Nahrwold, 1966). This involves division of the subclavian artery at the level of the take-off of the vertebral artery, and incising the subclavian artery down and on through the coarctation and well beyond. The flap of artery thus formed is then sutured down to widen the aorta. The ridge of narrowing forming the coarctation should be left *in situ*, as excision can cause weakening of the aorta and possibly later aneurysm formation. This operation is quick and simple and the results are very good. Furthermore, there seems to be little effect from dividing the subclavian artery.

Despite a good repair, late recoarctation can occur and therefore patients should be followed at appropriate intervals throughout life.

References

Barratt-Boyes, B.G., Simpson, M.M. and Neutze, J.M. 1970: Intracardiac surgery in neonates and infants using deep hypothermia. *Circulation* **62** (Suppl. III), 73.

Blalock, A. and Taussig, H. 1945: The surgical treatment of malformations of the heart. *Journal of the American Medical Association* **132**, 189–202.

Crafoord, C. and Nylin, G. 1945: Congenital coarctation of the aorta and its surgical treatment. *Journal of Thoracic Surgery* **14**, 347–61.

Gibbon, J.H. 1954: Application of a mechanical heart and lung apparatus to cardiac surgery. *Minnesota Medicine* **37**, 171.

Gross, R.E. and Hubbard, J.P. 1939: Surgical ligation of a patent ductus arteriosus. *Journal of the American Medical Association* **112**, 729.

Jatene, A.D., Fontes, V.F., Paulista, P.P. *et al.*, 1976: Anatomic correction of transposition of the great vessels. *Journal of Thoracic and Cardiovascular Surgery* **72**, 364–70.

Monro, J.L. and Shore, G. 1984: *A colour atlas of cardiac surgery – congenital heart disease.* London: Wolfe Medical, 17–29.

Mustard, W.T. 1964: Successful two-stage correction of transposition of the great vessels. *Surgery* **55**, 469–72.

Senning, A. 1959: Surgical correction of transposition of the great vessels. *Surgery* **45**, 966–80.

Waldhausen, J.A. and Nahrwold, D.L. 1966: Repair of coarctation of the aorta with a subclavian flap. *Journal of Thoracic Cardiovascular Surgery* **51**, 532–3.

Waterston, D.J. 1962: Treatment of Fallot's tetralogy in children under one year of age. *Rozhledy V Chirurgh* **41**, 181–3.

CHAPTER 80

Solid tumours of childhood

F.J. RESCORLA AND J.L. GROSFELD

Introduction
Neuroblastoma: Wilms' tumour
Neuroblastoma

Hepatoblastoma
Rhabdomyosarcoma
References

Introduction

Childhood cancer represents the leading disease causing death in children between the ages of 1 and 15 years of age (Young *et al.*, 1986). Central nervous system tumours are the most common of the solid tumours, followed by neuroblastoma, Wilms' tumour, rhabdomyosarcoma and hepatoblastoma. These four tumours are of significant importance for paediatric surgeons and will be the focus of this chapter.

Nephroblastoma: Wilms' tumour

First described in 1898 by Max Wilms, Wilms' tumour (nephroblastoma) represents one of the more common paediatric solid malignancies. Significant improvement in the survival for Wilms' tumour has occurred by refinement of combined programmes of multidisciplinary therapy in co-operative group studies. These multi-institutional programmes have also allowed collection of tumour specimens for numerous studies concerning the molecular genetics of Wilms' tumour. Wilms' tumour can occur as a result of genetic changes, although the exact frequency of these alterations is not known. The Wilms' tumour suppressor gene (WT1) located on the short arm of chromosome 11 (11p13) was identified in 1990 (Call *et al.*, 1990; Gessler *et al.*, 1990). WT1 is required for normal renal development and mutations at this position are responsible for

some sporadic cases of Wilms' tumour. It has also been noted to be present in nearly all patients with the Denys–Drash syndrome (pseudohermaphrodism, genito-urinary anomalies and Wilms' tumour) and many with sporadic aniridia.

A second Wilms' tumour gene (WT2) has also been identified on chromosome 11 (11p15) in association with the Beckwith–Wiedemann syndrome (Koufos *et al.*, 1989). Recent studies have also identified abnormalities on chromosome 16 in patients with Wilms' tumour (Kondo *et al.*, 1984). The significance of these findings is unclear at the present time, but they may lead to studies that allow prognostic evaluation based on the tumour chromosomal pattern. Wilms' tumour is also more common in patients with Pearlman's syndrome, hemihypertrophy, aniridia and nephroblastomatosis.

CLINICAL PRESENTATIONS AND EVALUATION

The most frequent clinical presentation of **Wilms'** tumour is an asymptomatic abdominal mass. **Hypertension** may be present in one-quarter of children. Haematuria may be observed in 10–15% of cases. Initial evaluation in the USA currently includes a computed tomography (CT) scan of the abdomen with oral and intravenous contrast to assess the involved kidney, lymph nodes, liver and the contralateral kidney (Fig. 80.1). An abdominal ultrasound examination is performed initially by some to discern between a cystic

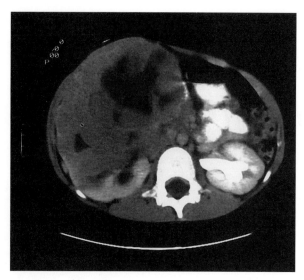

Fig. 80.1 Abdominal CT scan demonstrating a large right-sided Wilms' tumour.

lesion and a solid intra-abdominal mass. An ultrasound study of the ipsilateral renal vein and inferior vena cava (IVC) is routinely performed at the author's institution to evaluate for tumour thrombus. Although a radiograph of the chest is always performed to evaluate for the presence of lung metastases, the role of diagnostic chest CT scans is controversial. A report from the Third National Wilms' Tumor Study (NWTS-3), evaluating patients with normal chest radiographs and lung nodules detected by CT only, noted no difference in survival if the patients were treated with less intensive therapy (based on the abdominal stage) without lung irradiation compared with more intensive therapy with lung irradiation (Green *et al.*, 1991; D'Angio *et al.*, 1993). Unfortunately, these data were accrued from a relatively small group of patients (32 in NWTS III). Another small series from St Jude Children's Hospital noted an increased relapse rate in those children with normal chest radiographs and positive CT findings who were treated ignoring the CT findings (Williams *et al.*, 1988). Chest CT is believed to be the most accurate means to define extra-abdominal disease and therefore this study is routinely performed preoperatively (Cohen, 1994). The exact treatment necessary for infants and children with positive CT findings only is unclear.

OPERATIVE MANAGEMENT

In the USA, using the NWTS protocols, Wilms' tumour has generally been treated by initial operative resection. Exceptions include some cases of preoperative rupture, extremely large tumours (that may not be safely resected) or tumours with associated intracaval disease. A transperitoneal exploration is performed through a generous supraumbilical transverse abdominal incision.

Complete abdominal exploration is performed to evaluate for possible metastatic disease. If convenient, the contralateral kidney is explored first. Gerota's fascia is incised and the kidney evaluated by visual inspection and palpation of the anterior and posterior surfaces. Biopsies are obtained from any suspicious lesions. The ipsilateral tumour-bearing kidney is then approached by initially mobilizing the overlying colon attachments. For right-sided lesions the duodenum is mobilized and occasionally the attachments of the liver must be incised and mobilized to allow adequate exposure and safe mobilization of large upper pole renal lesions. For tumours on the left side, reflection of the spleen and pancreas medially will permit excision of large tumours arising in the upper pole.

If the renal artery and vein are easily accessible they should be ligated prior to mobilization of the tumour, but in some instances this is not possible. The renal vessels are doubly ligated and divided. The renal vein and vena cava should be palpated for tumour not identified by preoperative assessment and if present the tumour should be entirely removed. A plane of dissection is established outside Gerota's fascia and the tumour is gently mobilized. The adrenal gland may be left in place if it is not adherent to the tumour but is almost always removed with upper pole tumours. Because of the risk of urothelial spread, the ureter is divided low in the pelvis. Tumours that have grown into surrounding structures should be removed in continuity when possible if complete removal of all tumour can be safely performed. Removal of adjacent structures is rarely necessary. Careful note should be made of preoperative tumour rupture. The resection must be carried out gently to avoid intraoperative tumour spill, which may adversely affect outcome. Perirenal and para-aortic lymph nodes should be removed for staging purposes, but a formal radical lymph node dissection is not recommended.

STAGING

The current staging system for Wilms' tumour used in NWTS-5 (National Wilms' Tumor Study, 1986) is listed in Table 80.1. Accurate staging is dependent on observations by the paediatric surgeon at the time of abdominal exploration and removal of the tumour.

HISTOLOGY

Wilms' tumours are generally classified as having favourable (FH) or unfavourable histology (UH). Ninety per cent of Wilms' tumours have FH. Anaplasia (UH) is present in approximately 4.5–10% of tumours and is uncommon in children less than 2 years of age. Most patients with anaplasia have a worse prognosis, with the exception of stage I UH lesions which do well when treated similarly to stage I FH.

Table 80.1 Current staging of Wilms' tumour for NWTS-5

Stage	Description
I	Tumour limited to kidney and completely excised. (intact capsule, no rupture, no residual)
II	Tumour extends beyond the kidney but is completely excised (penetration through capsule, tumour in vessels outside kidney, local spill)
III	Residual non-haematogenous tumour confined to abdomen (lymph nodes: hilar, periaortic), diffuse peritoneal spill, tumour growth through peritoneal surface, peritoneal implants, gross or microscopic residual, incomplete resection due to infiltration of vital structures)
IV	Haematogenous metastases (lung, liver, bone, brain)
V	Bilateral renal involvement (attempt to stage each side by above criteria prior to biopsy)

Other renal neoplasms that have an unfavourable histology but are distinct from Wilms' tumour, including instances of clear cell sarcoma of the kidney (CCSK) and rhabdoid tumour of the kidney. CCSK is treated as a high-risk Wilms' tumour and rhabdoid tumours are not being treated on current Wilms' tumour protocols.

TREATMENT

The modern-day treatment of Wilms' tumour has evolved as a result of carefully performed co-operative group studies in the USA and Europe. The NWTS started in 1969 with NWTS-1 and is currently completing NWTS-4, which started in 1986. In Europe the International Society of Paediatric Oncology (SIOP) has conducted several co-operative Wilms' tumour trials. The following represents a summary of the treatment outcome of the National Wilms' Tumour Studies.

NWTS-1 (conducted between 1969 and 1974) demonstrated that radiation therapy was not necessary for stage I patients less than 2 years of age, and two-drug therapy with actinomycin-D and vincristine was superior to either drug alone for stage II disease.

NWTS-2 (conducted between 1974 and 1980) showed that local irradiation could be eliminated for all patients with stage I disease and that 6 months of vincristine and actinomycin-D was as effective as 15 months for stage I patients. The addition of adriamycin was effective for patients with stage IV disease and UH.

The results of NWTS-3 (1981–1985) showed that: (1) 10 weeks of actinomycin D and vincristine was adequate therapy for stageI/FH, (2) actinomycin D and vincristine without radiotherapy was adequate for stage II/FH, (3) three-drug therapy (actinomycin-D, vincristine and adriamycin) was better for stage III/FH

(allowing a decrease in radiation dose to 1000 cGy with doxorubicin or alternatively using 2000 cGy and avoiding doxorubicin), (4) adding cyclophosphamide as a fourth drug was not effective for stage IV disease; and (5) doxorubicin improved survival for CCSK, and stage I/anaplastic tumours could be treated similarly to stage I/FH (D'Angio, 1993).

NWTS-4 was started in 1986 and was completed in September 1994. The current treatment schema for NWTS-4 is listed in Fig. 80.2.

The basic question posed in NWTS-4 is: can the results in NWTS-3 be improved by using actinomycin-D in a pulsed intensive fashion over a shorter treatment period? Although the final results are pending, preliminary data indicate that the results of NWTS-4 duplicate those of NWTS-3 (Table 80.2) (D'Angio, 1993).

NWTS-5, which opened in July 1995, will attempt to refine therapy further. Selected stage I patients (age < 2 years and tumour weight < 550 g; Cassady stage I) do not receive adjuvant therapy (Green *et al.*, 1993). A study by Larsen *et al.* (1990) reported eight patients in this favourable subgroup who survived with surgery alone. NWTS-5 will further attempt to define tumour markers, variations of biological activity and improved treatment regimens for patients in relapse.

PREOPERATIVE CHEMOTHERAPY

In the USA preoperative chemotherapy has usually been reserved for: (1) bilateral Wilms' tumours; (2) presence of intravascular tumour in the inferior vena cava; (3) tumours found to be inoperable at exploration or (4) cases where excision of other visceral organs would be required to remove the tumour completely at initial exploration (Ritchey *et al.*, 1993). In Europe,

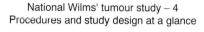

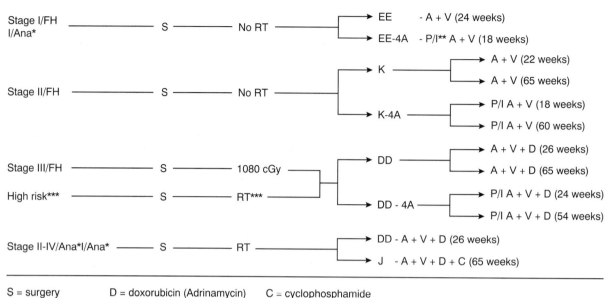

S = surgery   D = doxorubicin (Adrinamycin)   C = cyclophosphamide
A = actinomycin D   V = vincristine

  * Ana = anaplastic tumours
 ** P/I = pulsed, intensive
*** High risk = clear cell carcinoma of kidney (CCSK) (all stages) and stage IV/FH. CCSK patient receive XRT (1080 cGy),
     and stage IV/FH patients relieve XRT (1080 cGy) if the primary tumour would qualify as stage III were there no metastages.

Fig. 80.2   Schema for NWTS-4.

however, the use of preoperative chemotherapy has been much more popular. Several SIOP studies have demonstrated that preoperative chemotherapy decreases tumour size and the rupture rate at delayed excision, although survival data do not significantly differ from the NWTS data (Tournade *et al.*, 1993). There is also a risk of ambiguity in staging when preoperative chemotherapy is employed (Zuppan *et al.*, 1991). If tumour thrombus is identified in the IVC, preoperative

Table 80.2   Preliminary 4-year comparison of NWTS-4 vs NWTS-3 data

Stage/histology	Relapse-free survival NWTS-4/NWTS3 (%)	Survival NWTS-4/NWTS3 (%)
I/FH[a]	90/90	98/97
I/Ana[b]	90/87	90/87
II/FH	82/88	95/92
III/FH	90/79	94/84
IV/FH	71/76	82/83
CCSK[c]	67/65	88/76
Totals	86/85	94/91

[a]FH, favourable histology; [b]Ana, anaplasia; [c]CCSK, clear cell sarcoma of the kidney.

chemotherapy with delayed nephrectomy is probably safer (Ritchey *et al.*, 1988; Crombleholme *et al.*, 1994). Increased morbidity and mortality have been noted in NWTS-3 after operative removal of intracaval or intra-atrial tumour, and complications include haemorrhage and tumour embolization with cardiac decompensation.

There has also been interest in nephron-sparing surgery attempting partial nephrectomy after cytoreductive chemotherapy. The potential advantage of partial nephrectomy is to preserve maximal renal function and lessen the chance of renal loss due to trauma, infection, chemotoxicity and hyperperfusion, as well as from the occurrence of a metachronous bilateral Wilms' tumour. The disadvantages include theoretical increased risk of local recurrence, increased operative time and the inability to administer postoperative local irradiation. Partial nephrectomy is most suited for small polar lesions and is applicable in only a small proportion of unilateral Wilms' tumours (Williams *et al.*, 1991; Greenberg *et al.*, 1991; Gentil-Martins, 1993).

BILATERAL WILMS' TUMOURS

Bilateral Wilms' tumours are noted in 5–7% of the cases of Wilms' tumour and are often associated with intra-lobar nephrogenic rests. The current strategy with bilateral tumours is to preserve adequate renal parenchyma and function. Initial management includes bilateral biopsy followed by two-drug (vincristine and actinomycin-D) chemotherapy. An attempt should be made to stage each side independently. Most of the lesions have FH and only 4% of the cases have discordant histology. Subsequent second-look exploration is performed when there is evidence of significant decrease in tumour size to allow a partial nephrectomy on at least one side. Occasionally, a third- or fourth-look procedure may be necessary. This has led to a lower nephrectomy rate in NWTS-4 than in earlier studies, and has also been reflected in a lower incidence of renal failure in bilateral Wilms' in NWTS-4 (6.6%) than in NWTS-3 (9.9%).

The survival for this group of patients is still quite good, with children with FH having an 84% 3-year survival. However, those with UH have only a 16% survival (D'Angio *et al.*, 1989). The 3-year survival for those cases in which the most advanced lesion was a stage I tumour was 92% compared with 75% for those with stage III as the most advanced side (Blute *et al.*, 1987). Instances of bilateral tumours unresponsive to treatment and requiring bilateral nephrectomy are treated with chemotherapy and dialysis for at least 1 year before being considered for renal transplantation.

METASTATIC DISEASE AND RELAPSE

Although the current overall survival for patients with Wilms' tumour in all groups is very good (> 85%), children with metastases still have a more guarded outcome (Table 80.2). As noted in the NWTS treatment scheme, patients with stage IV and lung metastases have the primary tumour excised and initially receive chemotherapy and irradiation to the lung fields. If the lung lesions persist then surgical removal is considered. This approach was determined by a NTWS study which demonstrated that there was no difference in outcome following surgery and chemotherapy and/or radiation compared with chemotherapy and initial irradiation alone.

Tumour relapse remains a very serious problem that is associated with significant mortality. Survival after relapse remains less than 50%, indicating the need for newer therapies (Grundy *et al.*, 1989). Children initially treated with two-drug therapy are candidates for adriamycin-containing regimens. Several agents, including ifosfamide, etoposide, cisplatinum and carboplatinum, have demonstrated some effectiveness. In addition, intensive chemotherapy and autologous bone marrow transplant is undergoing evaluation as a phase II study for retrieval therapy in children with recurrent or unresponsive Wilms' tumours.

LATE EFFECTS OF TREATMENT

Late effects observed in NWTS-1 and NWTS-2 data indicate a 1% incidence of a second malignant neoplasm and a 7% incidence of benign tumours (Breslow *et al.*, 1988). A decreased incidence of second tumours in the treatment port and scoliosis has been observed in patients not receiving irradiation (Evans *et al.*, 1991). A recent report by Kovalic *et al.* (1991) described four patients with hepatocellular carcinoma occurring 9–16 years after successful treatment of right-sided Wilms' tumour that included chemotherapy and irradiation.

The potential occurrence of a hyperfiltration injury in the remaining kidney has been of some concern after unilateral nephrectomy but has not proved to be a significant long-term problem. A study evaluating 12 long-term survivors noted no evidence of significant renal alterations when compared with controls (Bhisitkul *et al.*, 1991).

Neuroblastoma

Neuroblastoma is the most common solid tumour of infancy and childhood, exceeded only by brain tumours. Despite collection of a large clinical database and significant research efforts, the prognosis for advanced cases remains quite dismal. Neuroblastoma arises in the neural crest cells located in the sympathetic nervous system. Approximately 50% of cases are located in the adrenal medulla, 24% in other abdominal sympathetic ganglia sites and the remainder in the mediastinum (20%), pelvis (3%) and neck (3%) (Grosfeld, 1987). Neuroblastoma has been noted in children with other neural crest disorders including Hirschsprung's disease, Klippel–Feil Syndrome and Waardenburg's syndrome, as well as cases of Beckwith–Wiedemann syndrome. Neuroblastoma has also been observed in the fetal alcohol syndrome and in mothers with seizure disorders requiring phenylhydantoin treatment.

CLINICAL PRESENTATION AND EVALUATION

Neuroblastoma occurs more frequently in boys (2:1) and has a reported incidence of 8.5 cases per million. Neuroblastoma most commonly presents as an abdominal mass. Mediastinal cases occasionally present with respiratory distress when a very large space-occupying tumour compresses and displaces the lungs and the tracheobronchial tree (Fig. 80.3). Up to 30% of posterior mediastinal neuroblastomas are noted as an unsuspected finding on chest radiographs obtained for other conditions.

The presence of Horner's syndrome (ptosis, meiosis, anhidrosis and heterochromia) may lead one to suspect a tumour affecting the stellate ganglia. Proptosis or bilateral orbital ecchymosis ('panda eyes') is indicative of metastases to the orbit. Leg pain may indicate the presence of long bone metastases. Hypertension may occur in up to 25% of cases owing to release of

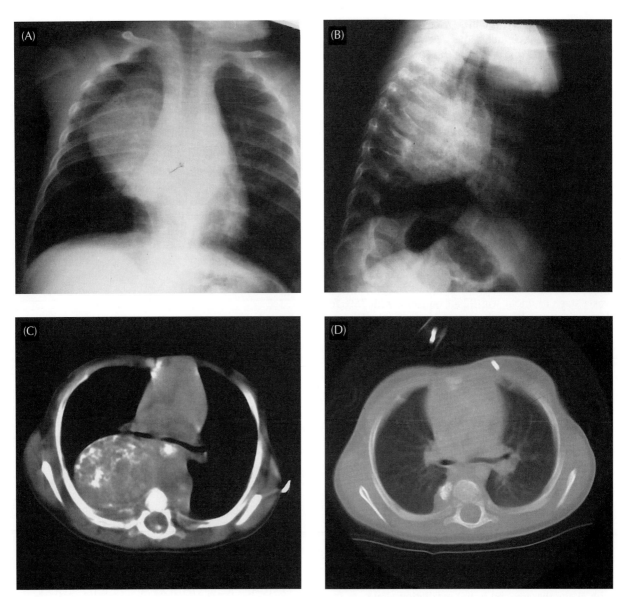

Fig. 80.3 (A, B) Chest radiographs demonstrating a posterior mediastinal neuroblastoma in a 6-month-old child who presented with respiratory distress. (C) CT scan demonstrating mass. The mass protrudes between the intercostal spaces and was biopsed through a small posterior incision. (D) CT scan demonstrating decrease in tumour size after chemotherapy.

catacholamines by the tumour. Systemic signs in advanced cases may include anaemia, weight loss and malnutrition. Extension of the tumour through the intervertebral foramina into the extradural space may lead to a symptomatic spinal cord compression or cauda equina syndrome. Neuroblastoma may also occur with ataxia associated with opsoclonus and polymyoclonus, also known as the 'dancing eye–feet syndrome' which is probably related to antigen–antibody complexes. Another unusual manifestation of neuroblastoma includes hypokalaemic watery diarrhoea syndrome associated with release of vasoactive intestinal polypeptide (VIP) from the tumour. Rare parasympathetic

neuroblastomas have been reported, which secrete acetylcholine. Some neonates and infants will present with hepatomegaly and subcutaneous nodules (stage IV-S) and may develop respiratory distress from the enlarged liver.

Plain radiographs of the mass will show stippled calcifications in approximately 50% of cases. Computed tomography (CT) with intravenous contrast allows evaluation of the relationship of the tumour to the major blood vessels and other structures and will also demonstrate calcifications in the tumour in approximately 80% of cases. The CT study usually allows differentiaton between a Wilms' tumour and neuroblastoma, as neuroblastoma generally displaces the kidney inferiorly and laterally without distortion of the collecting system. Magnetic resonance imaging (MRI) is the most accurate method of assessing extradural tumour extension and is useful in selected cases. A ^{99m}Tc pertechnetate bone scan is performed to detect bony metastases. ^{123}I-labelled metaiodobenzylguanidine (MIBG) is also useful in identifying bony metastases and also localizes in the primary tumour. Bone marrow aspirates are performed to evaluate for the presence of tumour cells. Urine is collected for a 12- or 24-hour period to evaluate catecholamine degradation products [vanillyemandelic acid (VMA) and homovanillic acid (HVA)], which are useful tumour markers. It is useful to acquire preoperative serum neuron specific enolase and serum ferritin levels, which may be of prognostic value.

MASS SCREENING

The Japanese have initiated mass screening programmes evaluating urinary levels of VMA and HVA in infants at 6 months of age (Sawad *et al.*, 1984). This has uncovered a large number of infants with neuroblastoma with an exceptional survival compared to that of patients who present with clinical disease (Sawada 1986). One report of 170 cases detected by screening reported survival in 165 (97%) (Sawada, 1989). Screening programmes have doubled the detected incidence of neuroblastomas noted in young infants, but have not decreased the number of cases in older children (V = Bessho *et al.*, 1991). Many of the cases detected by early screening probably represent tumours that spontaneously regress in patients who do not present with clinical disease (Sawada, 1991; Ishimoto *et al.*, 1990; Bessho *et al.*, 1991). The majority of tumours detected by screening do not have N-myc amplification. In addition, mass screening may be negative at 6 months in some children who later present with advanced disease. Ishimoto *et al.* (1990) reported six patients with false-negative urine tests at 6 months who later presented with advanced disease (one stage III and five stage IV), and recommended repeat screening at 18 months of age.

OPERATIVE MANAGEMENT

The goal of surgical management is complete removal of the tumour, but this is often not possible at the time of presentation. Small neck, mediastinal and pelvic tumours may be removed initially but many abdominal tumours are very large and often unresectable. Although some authors report improved survival following extensive resections, the evidence is not compelling and its safety has not been confirmed (Haase *et al.*, 1991; Shamberger *et al.*, 1991). In patients with very large abdominal tumours most paediatric surgeons perform an initial biopsy and then perform a second-look procedure after cytoreductive chemotherapy. At the second procedure complete resection is attempted, which often involves an extensive dissection of the major intra-abdominal vessels and kidney.

PATHOLOGY AND TUMOUR CHARACTERISTICS

In 1984, Shimada *et al.* proposed a classification system of neuroblastoma based on histological features which is used in the Children's Cancer Group (CCG) protocols. Tumours are divided into stroma-rich and stroma-poor categories. Stroma-rich tumours represent a favourable pattern with Schwann-like spindle cells. Stroma-poor tumours are divided into favourable and unfavourable tumours based on the age at diagnosis, neuroblastoma differentiation and the mitotic karyorrhexis index (MKI). Joshi *et al.* (1992), of the Pediatric Oncology Group (POG), have developed an alternative histologic system based on tumour grade and patient age.

A number of biological variables has been investigated in neuroblastoma (Table 80.3). Neuroblastomas have

Table 80.3 Characteristics of favourable and unfavourable neuroblastomas

	Favourable	Unfavourable
Age (years)	< 1	> 1
Stage	I, II, IV-S	III, IV
Location	Neck, mediastinum, pelvis	Abdomen
Serum markers	Vasoactive intestinal polypeptide	Serum ferritin
		Neuron-specific enolase
Urine		HVA:VMA elevation
Tumour markers		
N-myc oncogene	Low	High
trk	High	Low
DNA flow		
Cytometry	Aneuploid	Diploid
Chromosomal		
abnormality	Absent	1p36 deletion

been characterized cytogenetically with loss of heterozygosity (deletion) at the lp36 chromosomal position (Brodeur *et al.*, 1981; Brodeur and Fong, 1989; Fong *et al.*, 1989). Work by Brodeur and associates suggests that a suppressor gene is located in this area and that loss of this gene contributes to the development of neuroblastoma or disease progression. DNA flow cytometry studies are also of significance, indicating that aneuploid tumours have a more favourable clinical outcome. Look *et al.* (1991) have also noted that aneuploid tumours in children less than 1 year of age had a better response to chemotherapy than those in older children. Diploid tumours are more often associated with unfavourable clinical stage, older patients, unfavourable histology and poor outcome.

Many patients with advanced stages of neuroblastoma may express amplification of the N-myc oncogene (Brodeur *et al.*, 1984; Brodeur, 1990). N-myc amplification (<10 copies) is noted most frequently in stage III and IV and less frequently in low-stage or stage IVS patients. N-myc amplification is associated with tumour progression and poor outcome regardless of the stage and is frequently observed in those stage II, III and IV patients who remain ill (Seeger *et al.*, 1985).

Brodeur and colleagues have demonstrated that the trk proto-oncogene, a component of the high-affinity nerve growth factor receptor, is important in the regression and/or differentiation of immature sympathetic neuroblasts (Nakagawara *et al.*, 1993). N-myc and trk have an inverse relationship. High levels of expression of trk are predictive of a favourable outcome and are most often seen in infants under 1 year of age with stage I, II and IV-S tumours.

Table 80.4 Evan's staging system (CCG) for neuroblastoma

Stage	Description
I	Tumour confined to organ of origin
II	Tumour extends beyond organ of origin but does not cross the midline; unilateral lymph nodes may be involved
III	Tumour extends beyond midline; bilateral lymph nodes may be involved
IV	Distant metastases (skeletal, other organs, soft tissues, distant lymph nodes)
IV-S	Would be stage I or II except for remote disease confined to liver, subcutaneous tissues and bone marrow, but without evidence of bone cortex involvement

Table 80.5 Pediatric Oncology Group staging for neuroblastoma

Stage	Description
A	Complete resection of primary tumour, with or without microscopic residual. Intracavitary lymph nodes, not adherent to and removed with primary tumour, negative. Liver negative
B	Grossly unresected primary tumour. Nodes and liver negative
C	Complete or incomplete resection of primary tumour. Intracavitary nodes, not adherent to primary tumour, positive. Liver negative
D	Any dissemination of disease beyond intracavitary nodes, i.e. extracavitary nodes, liver, skin, bone marrow, bone
D (S)	Would be Evan's stage I or II except for metastatic tumour in liver, bone marrow or skin

The expression of class I major histocompatibility complex (MHC) antigen within the tumours has been evaluated by Squire *et al.* (1990) and is highest in stage IV-S patients and lowest in stage IV disease.

STAGING

Several staging systems exist for neuroblastoma. In the USA the Children's Cancer Group uses the Evan's staging system (Table 80.4), (Evans *et al.*, 1971) and the Pediatric Oncology Group (Table 80.5) (Nitschke *et al.*, 1988) and St. Jude (Table 80.6) (Hayes *et al.*, 1983) each have their own staging systems. Although all of

Table 80.6 St Jude staging system for neuroblastoma

Stage	Description
I	Localized tumour completely resected
IIA	Localized tumour resected with microscopic residual
IIB	Localized unresectable or partially resected tumour
IIIA	Disseminated metastases to liver, lymph node, or skin disease with no bone or bone marrow involvement
IIIB	Disseminated disease with one localized bone lesion but no bone marrow involvement
IIIC	Disseminated disease with bone marrow and/or generalized bone involvement

Table 80.7 International neuroblastoma staging system

Stage	Description
1	Localized tumour confined to area of origin; complete excision, with or without microscopic residual; ipsilateral and contralateral lymph nodes negative
2A	Unilateral tumour with incomplete excision; ipsilateral and contralateral lymph nodes negative
2B	Unilateral tumour with complete or incomplete excision; positive ipsilateral regional lymph nodes; contralateral lymph nodes negative
3	Tumour infiltrating across the midline or without lymph node involvement, or unilateral tumour with contralateral lymph node involvement, or midline tumour with bilateral lymph node involvement
4	Dissemination of tumour to distant lymph nodes, bone, bone marrow, liver and/or other organs
4-S	Localized primary tumour as defined for stage 1 or 2 with dissemination limited to liver, skin and/or bone marrow

the staging systems are in agreement about localized tumours and disseminated tumours, as well as the infants with Evan's stage IV-S disease, there are significant differences concerning the role of the midline and adherent or non-adherent lymph nodes in the other stages. The European International Union Contra Cancer uses the TNM system, where T refers to tumour size, N to nodal status and M to presence or absence of metastases (Harner, 1982). A new international staging system has been devised in order to develop a common set of criteria that can be evaluated world-wide (Table 80.7) (Brodeur *et al.*, 1988). All of the staging systems are somewhat imperfect as they fail to include the biological activity of the various tumours and the primary tumour site, which may significantly affect outcome.

TREATMENT AND PROGNOSTIC GROUPING

Infants and children with neuroblastoma can be classified into various prognostic groups based on stage and biological markers. Low-risk neuroblastomas would include those with localized disease (Evans stage I and stage II with single-copy N-myc) and most stage IV-S patients. This group has an expected survival of over 90% and is treated with surgery alone for stage I and II and usually observation for stage IVS. Patients with the unusual presentation of 'dancing-eye syndrome' and those with VIP secretion tend to have more mature tumours with a 90% survival. An intermediate group

consists of those patients with stage III tumours with favourable histopathology, N-myc < 10 copies and normal serum ferritin levels, and stage IV infants (< 1 year) with < 10 copies of N-myc. These patients are treated with multimodal chemotherapy [cisplatinum, etoposide (VP-16), doxorubcin and cyclophosphamide] and radiation therapy. These patients have a survival of approximately 70%. The high-risk group unfortunately represents the vast majority of cases, including unfavourable stage II patients with N-myc amplification and the remainder of the stage III and IV patients. Despite aggressive therapy including autologous bone marrow transplantation, these high-risk patients have a survival between 10% and 30%. The ability to attain complete tumour resection in these patients is of prognostic significance and should be attempted in all cases. Current protocols are evaluating the effect of intensive chemotherapy alone or in combination with autologous bone marrow transplant.

Hepatoblastoma

CLINICAL PRESENTATION AND EVALUATION

Hepatic malignancies remain the fourth most common solid organ tumour in childhood. Hepatoblastoma and hepatocellular cancer are the two most common types of tumour. Hepatoblastoma is the more common, occurring in approximately 70% of cases and generally presenting at a younger age (<18 months) (Gauthier *et al.*, 1986). Approximately 90% of infants with hepatoblastoma have elevation of the serum α-fetoprotein level. Hepatocellular carcinoma, representing 20–30% of cases, generally occurs in an older age group (6–10 years). The differential diagnosis at the time of initial presentation includes a number of benign hepatic neoplasms such as mesenchymal hamartoma, haemangioendothelioma, adenoma and focal nodular hyperplasia, as well as the more frequently occurring, retroperitoneal tumours, neuroblastoma and Wilms' tumour.

There is an increased risk of hepatoblastoma in patients with tyrosinaemia, type 1 glycogen storage disease, Beckwith–Wiedemann syndrome, Fanconi's disease and hemihypertrophy. There is also a relationship between hepatitis B virus and hepatocellular cancer. Hepatic carcinoma has also occurred in children with cirrhosis of the liver due to a variety of causes [e.g. biliary cirrhosis following total parenteral nutrition (TPN), in children with biliary atresia, histiocytosis] and following hepatic irradiation. Liver tumours may be associated with a loss of heterozygosity on the long arm of the fifth chromosome (5q). Hepatoblastoma has been observed in the offspring of patients with the familial adenomatous polyposis gene which also resides on the fifth chromosome.

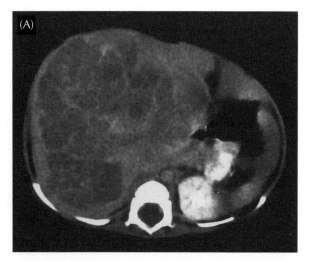
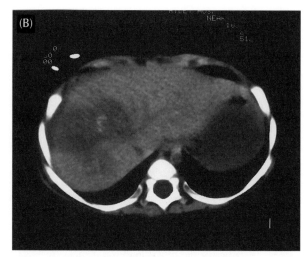

Fig. 80.4 (A) CT scan of an 18-month-old male with a large hepatoblastoma involving right and left lobes of the liver. (B) After chemotherapy, showing reduction of the tumour primarily to right lobe. Completely resected with a right trisegmentectomy.

The histologic variants among hepatocellular carcinoma include the fibrolamellar type, which may have a more favourable outcome than other forms of hepatocellular carcinoma. In instances of hepatoblastoma, cases with fetal histology have a more favourable outcome (especially when it presents as a stage I tumour) compared with embryonal, macrotubular or anaplastic histology (Haas *et al.*, 1989).

The initial evaluation of a patient with a liver tumour includes obtaining serum α-fetoprotein (which is elevated in more than 90% of cases) and serum ferritin levels, as well as an abdominal CT scan with contrast (Fig. 80.4). A chest radiograph and bone marrow aspirate are also obtained. MRI scans have been occasionally useful to detect the relationship between the tumour and the major vessels. More recently, however, helical (spiral) CT with three-dimensional (3D) reconstruction has been the most effective study to evaluate this relationship and tumour resectability.

OPERATIVE MANAGEMENT

The best (and usually the only) chance for cure is complete surgical resection of the tumour, whether at initial presentation or as a delayed procedure. Tumours localized in one lobe can be resected at the time of diagnosis with a formal hepatic lobectomy. Larger lesions with extension into the hepatic segments of the opposite anatomical lobe may occasionally be resected with an extended right or left hepatectomy (trisegmentectomy). If a primary resection cannot be accomplished, a biopsy of the tumour is performed followed by courses of chemotherapy and subsequent delayed hepatic resection. The biopsy may be performed with an open technique, but in some cases, when the preoperative

imaging indicates extension of tumour to the opposite lobe or evidence of multifocal disease, a percutaneous biopsy may be performed to confirm the diagnosis. The disadvantage of this approach is that an occasional patient may have a lesion based in one lobe only which compresses the contralateral lobe and could be amenable to initial resection.

After cytoreductive chemotherapy every attempt should be made to perform a complete resection of the tumour. Extended hepatic resections are frequently required and the patient must be adequately monitored and prepared with venous access through two large-bore upper-extremity catheters for prompt blood replacement if necessary. These procedures should be performed by experienced paediatric surgeons who are knowledgeable about the anatomy and techniques of liver resection. In

Table 80.8 Staging for hepatoblastoma (CCG)

Stage	Description
I	Confined to the liver and completely removed by surgery
II	Confined to liver and further subdivided into stages IIA and IIB. Stage IIA is defined as microscopic residual disease at the margin of resection after surgery. Stage IIB is defined by the presence of regional disease
III	Macroscopic residual tumour remains after surgery. This stage includes tumours that have been ruptured or with nodal involvement
IV	Metastatic disease

some cases hepatic vascular exclusion, which involves occlusion of the IVC above and below the liver with portal triad clamping, may be useful. Although the use of lasers and ultrasonic dissection have been suggested by some authors we have not found these adjuncts necessary to perform hepatic resection.

STAGING

The staging system used in the CCG is listed in Table 80.8.

TREATMENT

The current treatment for hepatoblastoma has been evolving since the 1960s. Several studies have demonstrated the effectiveness of preoperative chemotherapy in shrinking tumours that were initially considered unresectable, allowing complete resection at a subsequent second-look procedure (Fig. 80.4) (Weinblatt *et al.*, 1982; Filler *et al.*, 1991; Black *et al.*, 1991; Reynolds *et al.*, 1992). Before 1986, long-term survival was only possible in stage I patients, who had survival as high as 85%. In contrast, patients with stages II, III and IV disease had a dismal prognosis.

In 1986, CCG embarked on a single-arm pilot study using continuous infusion of adriamycin and *cis*-platinum. Patients with stage I tumours were excluded from the study. Thirty-one per cent of patients with hepatoblastoma were treated with primary resection and 69% with initial biopsy. Four of 22 patients (18%) had progressive disease but 17 of 22 (77%) responded to preoperative chemotherapy and had a second-look resection of the tumour (Ortega *et al.*, 1991; King, 1993). If a complete resection was performed 63% survived, but only 7% survived following a partial resection. For the entire group survival by stage was 70% in stage II, 48% in stage III and 18% in stage IV. The survival for hepatocellular carcinoma was a disappointing 13%. The next study was an intergroup study (CCG–POG) evaluating different chemotherapy protocols using *cis*-platinum and adriamycin vs *cis*-platinum, 5-fluorouracil and vincristine. This was based on a St Jude pilot study which showed a significant response with *cis*-platinum and vincristine in four out of five patients and a partial response in 13 of 13 patients treated with the combination of *cis*-platinum, vincristine and 5-fluorouracil (Champion *et al.*, 1982). The study was completed between 1989–1992. There were no differences in survival in patients receiving *cis*-platinum–adriamycin and those receiving cisplatin–vincristine and 5-fluorouracil, but the toxicity of the former regimen was significantly greater. Eight adriamycin–*cis*-platinum patients had toxicity related deaths. Patients receiving adriamycin–*cis*-platinum also experienced an increased rate of life-threatening events, a longer hospital stay and required TPN support for two and a half times greater duration. The 3-year survival for hepatoblastoma

is approximately 70% and that for hepatocellular carcinoma is 25%. Based on these observations, our current treatment protocol therefore includes *cis*-platinum, vincristine and 5-fluorouracil. Sporadic reports describe the resolution of pulmonary metastases following chemotherapy in a number of patients.

Unfortunately, some children with liver cancer have unresectable tumours even after administration of chemotherapy. Treatment options for this group include tumour chemoembolization or liver transplantation. Tagge *et al.* (1992) reported survival in five of six children with hepatoblastoma and three of seven with hepatocellular carcinoma following liver transplantation. Koneru *et al.* (1991) reported the results of 12 children who underwent liver transplantation for hepatoblastoma and noted survival in six cases. Children with anaplastic histology, multifocal lesions and vascular invasion had recurrence and are considered poor transplant candidates. The current role of liver transplantation in hepatoblastoma and hepatocellular carcinoma is unclear but may it may be feasible in highly selected cases.

Rhabdomyosarcoma

Rhabdomyosarcoma (RMS) is the most common soft-tissue tumour in children. This is a highly malignant tumour which invades local structures early and eventually spreads by lymphatic and haematogenous routes to distant sites. The incidence is approximately eight per million children less than 15 years of age. RMS patients have an increased incidence of genitourinary and central nervous system anomalies including the Arnold–Chiari malformation. RMS has also been observed in the fetal alcohol syndrome and in families with the Li–Fraumeni familial cancer syndrome associated with breast cancer, lung cancer and glioblastoma. These cases are probably associated with a germ-line mutant p53 suppressor gene. We have seen one patient with RMS who has the Beckwith–Weidemann syndrome.

Considerable improvement in survival has occurred since the 1970s as a result of combined multidisciplinary treatment programmes using operative resection, radiotherapy and multiagent chemotherapy. The Intergroup Rhabdomyosarcoma Study (IRS) began in 1972 and has accrued large numbers of patients which have since led to refinement in therapy.

CLINICAL PRESENTATION AND EVALUATION

RMS is more common in boys than girls (3:2). It has a peak incidence between 2 and 5 years of age with a second surge noted between 12 and 18 years of age (Grosfeld *et al.*, 1985). Rhabdomyosarcoma may occur in a variety of sites including the head and neck (including the orbit), trunk, retroperitoneum, genitourinary tract, perineum and extremities, as well as unusual locations

Table 80.9 IRS clinical grouping classification

Group	Description
I	Localized disease that is completely resected: (a) tumour confined to organ or muscle or origin (b) contiguous involvement: infiltration outside the muscle or organ of origin with regional nodes uninvolved
II	Grossly resected tumour with (a) microscopic residual disease and negative lymph nodes (b regional disease completely resected but positive lymph nodes (c) regional disease with positive nodes grossly resected but with microscopic residual disease
III	Incomplete resection of tumour or biopsy with gross residual disease present
IV	Metastatic disease at diagnosis (lung, brain, liver, distant lymph nodes, bone marrow)

such as the common bile duct, bronchus, anterior abdominal wall, buttocks and paraspinal area. In infancy the most common areas are head and neck, bladder, prostate and vagina, whereas older children have a wider distribution of sites with a predication for the trunk and extremities. The diagnostic tests obtained are dependent on the specific primary site of the tumour, but may include ultrasound, CT or MRI. Additional diagnostic tests would include a chest radiograph, radioisotopic bone scan and bone marrow aspirate in an attempt to identify metastatic disease. Unfortunately, there are no specific tumour markers for RMS.

STAGING

The current clinical staging system used by the IRS is listed in Table 80.9 (Maurer *et al.*, 1988). The clinical group is related to the amount of residual tumour after surgery and the status of regional lymph nodes. The clinical group can be altered by the extent of surgery. If a biopsy only is performed the patient is classified as clinical group III, whereas if the same tumour was resected, the tumour could be classified as group I or II. The extent of resection is also influenced by the location of the primary tumour because of specific anatomical limitations (head and neck, bile duct, etc.).

PATHOLOGY

RMS have been classified histologically as favourable or unfavourable tumours. Favourable tumours include embryonal lesions (including the botryoid variant), extraosseous Ewing's sarcoma, undifferentiated and mixed tumour types, while unfavourable histological types include alveolar, anaplastic and monomorphous round cell tumours (Newton *et al.*, 1988).

The embryonal type is most frequently noted in the head, neck and genitourinary tract. It is the most common histology in infants and small children and is associated with a more favourable prognosis. The botryoid variant (grape-like appearance) occurs in submucosal locations and often protrudes into the lumen of structures such as the bladder, vagina, uterus, nasopharynx and occasionally the common bile duct.

Alveolar RMS account for approximately 20% of cases, occurring most commonly in the extremities and trunk, although they also have been noted at other sites. Alveolar tumours have a poor prognosis and are associated with the highest rate of regional lymph node involvement, local tumour recurrence, bone marrow involvement and distant spread.

OPERATIVE MANAGEMENT

The overall goal of treatment is complete extirpation of the tumour. Unfortunately, this is not always possible and in some patients cytoreductive chemotherapy may allow tumour shrinkage and a subsequent complete resection with excellent survival (Fig. 80.5). In view of this each site will be covered individually.

HEAD AND NECK

Head and neck tumours can be divided into the orbit, non-parameningeal (cheek, neck, temple, scalp, parotid, oropharynx and larynx) and cranial parameningeal lesions (nasopharynx, middle ear, nasal cavity, mastoid region, pterygopalatine and infratemporal fossa).

Tumours of the orbit can usually be treated with multimodal chemotherapy and radiation after a diagnostic biopsy, avoiding the need for orbital exenteration in most cases. Survival in this group is 89% (Grosfeld *et al.*, 1985; Maurer *et al.*, 1988).

Non-parameningeal sites should be treated with excision if possible, but this is usually possible only in superficial tumours. In most cases biopsy followed by chemotherapy and irradiation followed by a secondary surgical procedure yields good results (55% survival) (Maurer *et al.*, 1988).

Children with RMS in parameningeal sites have a lower survival (47%) owing to meningeal involvement and toxicity of intrathecal therapy in these cases (Maurer *et al.*, 1988).

EXTREMITY AND TRUNK SITES

RMS of the extremity occurred in 23% of patients in the IRS (Maurer *et al.*, 1988). The incidence of alveolar

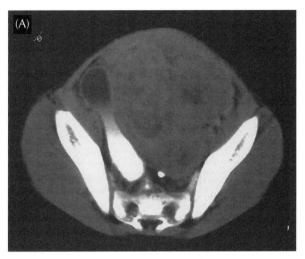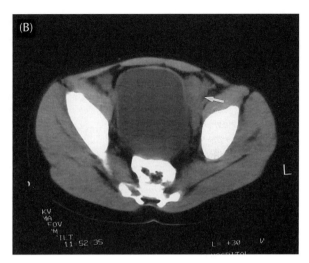

Fig. 80.5 (a) CT scan demonstrating a large pelvic mass in a 7-year-old boy. Biopsy revealed a rhabdomyosarcoma. (b) After chemotherapy, a small residual tumour on the left side of the bladder (arrow) was successfully resected with bladder salvage.

histology is higher in this group. The management of extremity lesions has varied, but the current recommendations include: (1) total gross resection of the tumour, even if a more disabling procedure is required; (2) regional lymph node biopsy or dissection; and (3) early primary re-excision of those cases with histological documentation of positive margins of resection following the initial operation (Lawrence *et al.*, 1988). Hays *et al.* (1989) demonstrated that re-excision of the primary site improved survival and decreased the local recurrence rate of extremity tumours.

BLADDER/PROSTATE

Primary RMS of the bladder often present with a mass, haematuria, difficulty voiding or occasional urinary tract obstruction. The therapy for pelvic RMS in boys has been controversial. In the late 1960s and early 1970s extensive surgery (anterior exenteration) combined with chemotherapy and irradiation provided excellent survival (91%). However, the adverse effects of the surgery (e.g. permanent urinary diversion) led to primary chemotherapy trials and more limited surgery (Grosfeld *et al.*, 1969). Unfortunately, this was associated with a significantly decreased disease-free survival (46%) (Raney *et al.*, 1990). Early attempts at bladder salvage were associated with a disappointing 25% success rate. Modifications of treatment in IRS-2 and -3, however indicate that intensive chemotherapy combined with early irradiation therapy (not less than 4000 rad) and conservative surgery resulted in survival with a functional bladder at 3 years in 65% of boys. In addition, youngsters with primary tumours involving the dome of the bladder fared well with partial cystectomy. Boys with primary tumours of the prostate fared less well than those with bladder primaries.

VAGINAL/UTERINE

Most vaginal tumours occur in infants and young children and are often the botryoid type of embryonal tumours. The tumour will occasionally prolapse from the vagina and may be associated with vaginal discharge or bleeding. In girls with vaginal tumours, excellent survival (> 90%) can be achieved with primary chemotherapy after an initial biopsy, allowing preservation of all major pelvic organs in most cases (Hays *et al.*, 1988). Primary tumours of the lower two-thirds of the vagina usually can be locally excised (partial vaginectomy) after chemotherapy. Primary tumours located near the cervix, however, will usually require a hysterectomy. Irradiation to these lesions can effectively be administered with brachytherapy.

Uterine RMS usually presents in older girls as a prolapsing mass through the cervix or an infiltrative intramural mass. Biopsy of a prolapsed polypoid tumour can be performed transvaginally or after dilatation and curettage of the cervix in infiltrative cases. Some girls with polypoid tumours improve after simple polypectomy and chemotherapy, whereas those with infiltrative tumours remain ill even after hysterectomy. The overall survival for this group is 50–60% (Hays *et al.*, 1988).

PARATESTICULAR TUMOURS

Most paratesticular tumours are embryonal tumours. Operative management is through an inguinal approach with early high ligation of the cord structures and orchiectomy.

The role of retroperitoneal lymph node sampling has been debated. A study by Weiner *et al.* (1994) from IRS-3 noted that 14% of boys with a negative clinical evaluation by CT scan had positive lymph nodes on

Table 80.10 TNM pretreatment staging classification for rhabdomyosarcoma

Stage	Site	TNM status
I	Orbit, genitourinary (non-bladder/non-prostate), head and neck (non-parameningeal)	T1 or T2, A or B, N0 or N1, M0
II	Genitourinary/bladder–prostate, extremity, parameningeal, other	T1 or T2, A, N0, M0
III	Genitourinary/bladder–prostate, extremity, parameningeal, other	T1 or T2, A or B, N0 or N1, M0
IV	Any site	T1 or T2, A or B, N0 or N1, M1

A, < 5 cm; B, > 5 cm.
T1, confined to site of origin; T2, extension or fixation to surrounding tissue.

pathological examination. Overall, 27% of those who presented with non-metastatic disease had positive retroperitoneal lymph nodes. Patients with stage I disease or those with negative retroperitoneal lymph nodes can avoid irradiation. The overall survival in this group is excellent (93%).

OTHER SITES

RMS may also present in other less common sites. It may occur as a polypoid mass within the common hepatic or common bile ducts resulting in obstructive jaundice. Unfortunately, widespread disease at presentation is common in these cases (Ruymann *et al.*, 1985). In view of the poor survival, recent reports recommend aggressive surgery including pancreaticoduodenectomy, chemotherapy and irradiation (Martinez-Fernandez *et al.*, 1982).

RMS can also occur in the anterior abdominal wall, retroperitoneum, chest wall, perianal region and perineum, and the buttocks. Surgical resection remains the mainstay of therapy in these unusual cases. Survival is related to histology and stage of disease at presentation but rarely exceeds 50% at these sites.

METASTATIC DISEASE

Patients presenting with metastatic disease have a very poor prognosis with a 10-year survival of 20% (Maurer

et al., 1988). Metastases occur through both lymphatic and haematogenous routes and involve lymph nodes, bone, bone marrow, liver and brain.

Local recurrence is an ominous finding and emphasizes the need for adequate surgical margins and new second-line chemotherapy agents.

RESULTS

Survival, as noted above, is dependent on site, group and histology. Long-term results from IRS-2 indicate 10-year survival as follows: group I, 83%: group II, 70%: group III, 52%; and group IV, 20% (Maurer *et al.*, 1988). Survival according to histology from IRS-2 was: botryoid, 85%: extraosseous and embryonal, 60–65%: indeterminate, alveolar and unclassified, 40% Newton *et al.*, 1988). The overall 5-year survival from IRS-1 was 53%, IRS-2 was 63% and IRS-3 was 71%.

CURRENT TREATMENT SCHEMA

The current IRS-4 utilizes a TNM-based pretreatment staging (Table 80.10) for randomization of the treatment arm for chemotherapy and radiation therapy (Table 80.11). The basic questions are to evaluate efficacy of the various agents as well as to evaluate conventional vs hyperfractionated radiotherapy for those with gross residual disease after surgery (clinical group III).

Table 80.11 Treatment schema for IRS-4 based on TNM stage and group

Stage	Chemotherapy	Radiotherapy		
		Group I	Group II	Group III
1	VAC vs VAI vs VIE	No RT	Std RT	Hyperfx RT vs Std RT
2	VAC vs VAI vs VIE	No RT	Std RT	Hyperfx RT vs Std RT
3	VAC vs VAI vs VIE	Std RT	Std RT	Hyperfx RT vs Std RT
4	VM vs IE followed by VAC, Std RT			

V, vincrintine; A, actinomycin D; C, cyclophosphamide; I, ifosfamide, E, etoposide; M, melphalan.
Std RT – standard radiotherapy; Hyperfx, RT, hyperfractionated radiotherapy.

References

Bessho, F., Hashizume, K., Nakajo, T. *et al.* 1991: Mass screening in Japan increased the detection of infants with neuroblastoma without a decrease in cases in older children. *Journal of Pediatrics* **119**, 237–41.

Bhisitkul, D.M., Morgan, E.R., Vozar, M.A. and Langman, C.B. 1991: Renal functional reserve in long-term survivors of unilateral Wilms' tumor. *Journal of Pediatrics* **118**, 698–702.

Black, C.T., Cangir, A., Choroszy, M. and Andrassy, R.J. 1991: Marked response to preoperative high-dose cisplatinum in children with unresectable hepatoblastoma. *Journal of Pediatric Surgery* **26**, 1070–3.

Blute, M.L., Kelalis, P.P., Offord, K.P. *et al.* 1987: Bilateral Wilms' tumor. *Journal of Urology* **138**, 968–73.

Breslow, N.E., Norkool, P.A., Olshan, A. *et al.* 1988: Second malignant neoplasms in survivors of Wilms' tumor: a report from the National Wilms' Tumor Study. *Journal of the National Cancer Institute* **80**, 592–5.

Brodeur, G.M. 1990: Neuroblastoma: clinical significance of genetic abnormalities. *Cancer Surveys* **9**, 673–88.

Brodeur, G.M. and Fong, C.T. 1989: Molecular biology and genetics of human neuroblastoma. *Cancer Genetics and Cytogenetics* **41**, 153–74.

Brodeur, G.M., Green, A.A., Hayes, F.A. *et al.* 1981: Cytogenetic features of human neuroblastomas and cell lines. *Cancer Research* **41**, 4678–86.

Brodeur, G.M., Seeger, R.C., Barrett, A. *et al.* 1988: International criteria for diagnosis, staging and response to treatment in patients with neuroblastoma. *Journal of Clinical Oncology* **6**, 1874–81.

Brodeur, G.M., Seeger, R.C., Schwab, M., Varmus, H.E. and Bishop, J.M. 1984: Amplification of N-myc in untreated human neuroblastomas correlates with advanced disease stage. *Science* **224**, 1121–4.

Call, K.M., Glaser, T., Ito, C.Y. *et al.* 1990: Isolation and characterization of a zinc finger polypeptide gene at the human chromosome 11 Wilms' tumor locus. *Cell* **60**, 509–20.

Champion, J., Green, A.A. and Pratt, C.B. 1982: Cisplatin (DDP): an effective therapy for unresectable or recurrent hepatoblastoma [Abstract]. *Proceedings of the American Society of Clinical Oncologists* **671**, 173.

Cohen, M.D. 1994: Current controversy: Is CT scan of the chest needed in patients with Wilms' tumor? *American Journal of Pediatric Hematology and Oncology* **16**, 191–3.

Crombleholme, T.M., Jacir, N.N., Rosenfield, C.G., *et al.* 1994: Preoperative chemotherapy in the management of intracaval extension of Wilms' tumor. *Journal of Pediatric Surgery* **29**, 229–31.

D'Angio, G.J. 1993: An overview of NWTS 4 and prospective for NWTS 5. Presented at the Progress and Controversies in Pediatric Surgical Oncology Meeting, October, San Francisco, CA.

D'Angio, G.J., Breslow, N., Beckwith, J.B. *et al.* 1989: The treatment of Wilms' tumor: results of the Third National Wilms' Tumor Study. *Cancer* **64**, 349–60.

D'Angio, G.J., Roseberg, H., Sharples, K. *et al.* 1993: Position paper: Imaging methods for primary renal tumors of childhood: costs versus benefits. *Medical Pediatric Oncology* **21**, 205–12.

Evans, A., Norkool, P., Evans, I., Breslow, N. and D'Angio, G.J. 1991: Late effects of treatment for Wilms' tumor: a report from the National Wilms' Tumor Study Group. *Cancer* **67**, 331–6.

Evans, A.E., D'Angio, G.J. and Randolph, J.G. 1971: A proposed staging for children with neuroblastoma. *Cancer* **27**, 374–8.

Filler, R.M., Ehrlich, P.F., Greenberg, M.L. and Babyn, P.S. 1991: Preoperative chemotherapy in hepatoblastoma. *Surgery* **110**, 591–7.

Fong, C.T., Dracopoli, N.C., White, P.S. *et al.* 1989: Loss of heterozygosity for the short arm of chromosome 1 in human neuroblastomas: correlation with N-myc amplification. *Proceedings of the National Academy of Science, USA* **86**, 3753–7.

Gauthier, F., Valayer, J., Thai, B.L., Sinico, M. and Kalifa, C. 1986: Hepatoblastoma and hepatocarcinoma in children: analysis of a series of 29 cases. *Journal of Pediatric Surgery* **21**, 424–29.

Gentil-Martins, A. 1993: Nephron sparing surgery for Wilms' tumor. Presented at Progress and Controversies in Pediatric Surgical Oncology Meeting, October, San Francisco, CA.

Gessler, M., Poustka, A., Cavenee, W. *et al.* 1990: Homozygous deletion in Wilms' tumors of a zinc-finger gene identified by chromosome jumping. *Nature* **343**, 774–8.

Green, D.M., Breslow, N.E., Beckwith, J.B. *et al.* 1993: Treatment outcomes in patients less than 2 years of age with small, stage I, favourable-histology Wilms' tumors: a report from the National Wilms' Tumor Study. *Journal of Clinical Oncology* **11**, 91–5.

Green, D.M., Fernbach, D.J., Norkool, P., Kollia, G. and D'Angio, G.J. 1991: The treatment of Wilms' tumor patients with pulmonary metastases detected only with computed tomography: a report from the National Wilms' Tumor Study. *Journal of Clinical Oncology* **9**, 1776–81.

Greenberg, M., Burnweit, C., Filler, R. *et al.* 1991: Preoperative chemotherapy for children with Wilms' tumor. *Journal of Pediatric Surgery* **26**, 949–56.

Grosfeld, J.L. 1987: Neuroblastoma: current concepts of management. *Surgical Rounds* **10**, 47–60.

Grosfeld, J.L., Clatworthy, H.W., Jr and Newton, W.A. Jr 1969: Combined therapy in childhood rhabdomyosarcoma: an analysis of 42 cases. *Journal of Pediatric Surgery* **4**, 637–45.

Grosfeld, J.L., Weber, T.R., Weetman, R.M. *et al.* 1985: Rhabdomyosarcoma in childhood: analysis of survival in 98 cases. *Journal of Pediatric Surgery* **18**, 141–5.

Grundy, P., Breslow, N., Green, D.M. *et al.* 1989: Prognostic factors for children with recurrent Wilms' tumor: results from the second and third National Wilms' Tumor Study. *Journal of Clinical Oncology* **7**, 638–47.

Haas, J.E., Muczynski, K.A., Krailo, M. *et al.* 1989: Histopathology and prognosis in childhood hepatoblastoma and hepatocarcinoma. *Cancer* **64**, 1082–95.

Haase, G.M., O'Leary, M.C., Ramsay, N.K.C. *et al.* 1991: Aggressive surgery combined with intensive chemotherapy improves survival in poor-risk neuroblastoma. *Journal of Pediatric Surgery* **26**, 1119–24.

Harner, M.H. (ed.) 1982: *International union against cancer (UICC): TNM classification of pediatric tumors.* Geneva: UICC, 18–22.

Hayes, F.A., Green, A.A., Hustu, H.O. *et al.* 1989: Surgico-pathologic staging of neuroblastoma: prognostic significance of regional lymph node metastases. *Journal of Pediatrics* **102**, 59–62.

Hays, D.M., Lawrence, W., Jr, Wharam, M. *et al.* 1989: Primary re-excision for patients with 'microscopic residual' tumor following initial excision of sarcomas of trunk and extremity sites. *Journal of Pediatric Surgery* **24**, 5–10.

Hays, D.M., Shimada, H., Raney, R.B. *et al.* 1988: Clinical staging and treatment results in rhabdomyosarcoma of the female genital tract among children and adolescents. *Cancer* **61**, 1893–903.

Ishimoto, K., Kiyokawa, N., Fujita, H. *et al.* 1990: Problems of mass screening for neuroblastoma: analysis of false negative cases. *Journal of Pediatric Surgery* **25**, 398–401.

Joshi, W., Cantor, A.B., Altshuler, G. *et al.* 1992: Age-linked prognostic categorization based on a new histologic grading system of neuroblastomas. *Cancer* **69**, 2197–2211.

King, D. 1993: Update on recent US intergroup hepatic tumor studies. Presented at Progress and Controversy in Pediatric Surgical Oncology Meeting, October, San Francisco, CA.

Kondo, K., Chilcote, R.R., Maurer, H.S. *et al.* 1984: Chromosome abnormalities in tumor cells from patients with sporadic Wilms' tumor. *Cancer Research* **44**, 5376–81.

Koneru, B., Flye, M.W., Busuttil, R.W. *et al.* 1991: Liver transplantation for hepatoblastoma: the American experience. *Annals of Surgery* **213**, 118–21.

Koufos, A., Grundy, P., Morgan, K. *et al.* 1989: Familial Wiedemann–Beckwith syndrome and a second Wilms' tumor locus both map to 11p15.5. *American Journal of Human Genetics* **44**, 711–19.

Kovalic, J.J., Thomas, P.R.M., Beckwith, J.B., Feusner, J.H. and Norkool, P.A. 1991: Hepatocellular carcinoma as second malignant neoplasms in successfully treated Wilms' tumor patients. *Cancer* **67**, 342–4.

Larsen, E., Perez-Atayde, A., Green, D.M. *et al.* 1990: Surgery only for the treatment of patients with stage I (Cassady) Wilms' tumor. *Cancer* **66**, 264–6.

Lawrence, W., Jr, Hays, D.M., Heyn, R. *et al.* 1988: Surgical lessons from the Intergroup Rhabdomyosarcoma Study (IRS) pertaining to extremity tumors. *World Journal of Surgery* **12**, 676–84.

Look, A.T., Hayes, F.A., Shuster, J.J. *et al.* 1991: Clinical relevance of tumor cell ploidy and N-myc gene amplification in childhood neuroblastoma: a Pediatric Oncology Group Study. *Journal of Clinical Oncology* **9**, 581–91.

Martinez-Fernandez, L.A., Haase, G.M., Koep, L.J. and Ajers, D.R. 1982: Rhabdomyosarcoma of the biliary tree: the case for aggressive surgery. *Journal of Pediatric Surgery* **17**, 508–11.

Maurer, H.M., Beltangady, M., Gehan, E.A. *et al.* 1988: The Intergroup Rhabdomyosarcoma Study I: a final report. *Cancer* **61**, 209–20.

Nakagawara, A., Arima-Nakagawara, M., Scavarda, N.J. *et al.* 1993: Association between high levels of expression of the TRK gene and favourable outcome in human neuroblastoma. *New England Journal of Medicine* **328**, 847–854.

National Wilms' Tumor Study 4, Protocol, 1986.

Newton, W.A., Jr, Soule, E., Hamoudi, A. *et al.* 1988: Histopathology of childhood sarcomas, Intergroup Rhabdomyosarcoma studies I and II: clinicopathologic correlation. *Journal of Clinical Oncology* **6**, 67–75.

Nitschke, R., Smith, E.I., Shochat, S. *et al.* 1988: Localized neuroblastoma treated by surgery. A Pediatric Oncology Group Study. *Journal of Clinical Oncology* **61**, 1271–9.

Ortega, J.A., Krailo, M.D., Haas, J.E. *et al.* 1991: Effective treatment of unresectable or metastatic hepatoblastoma with cisplatin and continuous infusion doxorubicin chemotherapy. A report from the Children's Cancer Study Group. *Journal of Clinical Oncology* **9**, 2167–76.

Raney, R.B., Jr, Gehan, E.A., Hays, D.M. *et al.* 1990: Primary chemotherapy with or without radiation therapy and/or surgery for children with localized sarcoma of the bladder, prostate, vagina, uterus, and cervix: a comparison of the results in Intergroup Rhabdomyosarcoma Studies I and II. *Cancer* **66**, 2072–81.

Reynolds, M., Finegold, D.M., Cantor, A. and Glicksman, A. 1992: Chemotherapy can convert unresectable hepatoblastoma. *Journal of Pediatric Surgery* **27**, 1080–4.

Ritchey, M.L., Kelalis, P.P., Breslow, N. *et al.* Intracaval and atrial involvement with nephroblastoma: review of national Wilms' tumor study III. *Journal of Urology* **140**, 1113–18.

Ritchey, M.L., Kelalis, P.P., Haase, G.M. *et al.* 1993: Preoperative therapy for intracaval and atrial extension of Wilms' tumor. *Cancer* **71**, 4104–10.

Ruymann, F.B., Raney, R.B., Crist, W.M. *et al.* 1985: Rhabdomyosarcoma of the biliary tree in childhood. *Cancer* **56**, 575–81.

Sawada, T. 1986: Outcome of 25 neuroblastomas revealed by screening in Japan. *Lancet* **i**, 377.

Sawada, T. 1989: Present status of mass screening for neuroblastoma. *Pediatric Reviews* **22**, 336–56.

Sawada, T., Kidowaki, T. and Sakamoto, I. 1984: Neuroblastoma: mass screening for early detection and its prognosis. *Cancer* **53**, 2731–5.

Seeger, R.C., Brodeur, G.M., Sather, H. *et al.* 1985: Association of multiple copies of the N-myc oncogene with rapid progression of neuroblastomas. *New England Journal of Medicine* **313**, 111–16.

Shamberger, R.C., Allarde-Segundo, A., Kozakewich, H.P.W. and Grier, H.E. 1991: Surgical management of stage III and IV neuroblastoma: resection before or after chemotherapy? *Journal of Pediatric Surgery* **26**, 1113–18.

Shimada, H., Chatten, J., Newton, W.H., Jr *et al.* 1984: Histopathologic prognostic factors in neuroblastoma: definition of subtypes of ganglioneuroblastoma and an age-linked classification of neuroblastoma. *Journal of the National Cancer Institute* **73**, 405–16.

Squire, R., Fowler, C.L., Brooks, S.P., Rich, G.A. and Cooney, D.R. 1990: The relationship of class I MHC antigen expression to Stage IV-S disease and survival in neuroblastoma. *Journal of Pediatric Surgery* **25**, 381–6.

Tagge, E.P., Tagge, D.U., Reyes, J. *et al.* 1992: Resection, including transplantation, for hepatoblastoma and hepatocellular carcinoma: impact on survival. *Journal of Pediatric Surgery* **27**, 292–7.

Tournade, M.F., Com-Nougue, C., Voute, P.A. *et al.* 1993: Results of the Sixth International Society of Pediatric

Oncology Wilms' Tumor Trial and Study: a risk-adapted therapeutic approach in Wilms' tumor. *Journal of Clinical Oncology* **11**, 1014–23.

Weinblatt, M.E., Siegel, S.E., Siegel, M.M., Stanley, P. and Weitzman, J.J. 1982: Preoperative chemotherapy for unresectable primary hepatic malignancies in children. *Cancer* **50**, 1061–4.

Wiener, E.S., Lawrence, W., Hays, D. *et al.* 1994: Retroperitoneal node biopsy in paratesticular rhabdomyosarcoma. *Journal of Pediatric Surgery* **29**, 171–8.

Wilimas, J.A., Douglass, E.C., Magill, L., Fitch, S. and Sustu, H.O. 1988: Significance of pulmonary computed tomography at diagnosis in Wilms' tumor. *Journal of Clinical Oncology* **6**, 1144–6.

Wilimas, J.A., Magill, L., Parham, D.M., Kumar, M. and Douglass, E.C. 1991: The potential for renal salvage in nonmetastatic unilateral Wilms' tumor. *American Journal of Pediatric Hematology and Oncology* **13**, 342–4.

Wilms, M. 1898*: Die mischgeschwulste der Nieren*. Leipzig: Arthur Georgi, 1–90.

Young, J.L., Jr, Ries, L.G., Silverberg, E., Horm, J.W. and Miller, R.W. 1986: Cancer incidence, survival, and mortality for children younger than age 15 years. *Cancer* **2**, 598–602.

Zuppan, C.W., Beckwith, B., Weeks, D.A., Luckey, D.W. and Pringle, K.C. 1991: The effect of preoperative therapy on the histologic features of Wilms' tumor. *Cancer* **68**, 385–94.

CHAPTER 81

General principles of plastic surgery

B. MORGAN

Wound healing
Skin cover techniques
Flaps
Skin expansion
Birthmarks

Cleft lip and palate
Deformities of the ear
References
Further reading

Wound healing

The process of wound healing is no different in children than in adults. However, there is a tendency for children to form hypertrophic scarring in situations which in adults or in the elderly would heal in a fine line and a soft pale scar. Conventional histology is not able to differentiate between hypertrophic scarring and keloid scarring but clinically a hypertrophic scar will appear very soon after the wound has healed, it will increase in size, be red and irritate for about 3 months and then very slowly mature so that at 3–4 years the child will be left with a pale broad scar which is symptomless and usually soft but has an irregular surface. Keloid scars, in contrast, occur in scars that have already healed, maybe for some months or even years and then begin to grow, itch and are painful. The growth is noted to extend outside the confines of the original scarring. It is not understood quite why they should be more common in children. If, however, a wound heals by secondary intention and there is delay it is more likely to develop a hypertrophic scar (Rockwell *et al.*, 1989).

Treatment measures either to prevent or to speed the resolution of hypertrophic scarring are as follows:

1. Continuous pressure. This is provided, particularly in burns patients, by a specially measured and fitted pressure garment such as a sleeve or a vest. Steroids may be applied to the surface as haelan tape or topical ointment. Injections of triamcinolone (10 mg/1 ml)

into the scar is effective but not a measure that is easily accomplished in children since it is painful and care has to be taken that the steroid does not leak into the surrounding tissues, in which case an area of atrophy may develop.

3. Silicone sheeting. A special preparation of silicone sheeting can be applied for some hours by the parent to the hypertrophic scar. It may produce some irritation while it is applied and is sometimes not well tolerated but perseverance is rewarding in speeding the resolution of the scar.

4. Scar excision and resuture. It is likely that hypertrophic scars, if excised, will recur and there is a high risk of this happening with keloid scars. If the history is of a slow healing by secondary intention of a wound then it is more likely that a scar excision with a primary closure will avoid recurrence of the hypertrophic scar.

PRIMARY CLOSURE OF A WOUND

The management of a traumatic laceration in childhood can be taxing. This is because of the emotion engendered in the parent, a tearful and uncooperative child and the difficulties of administering local anaesthetic. There is a tendency for the surgeon to be less than thorough so that the wound is not properly cleansed, debrided, cleaned of road dirt and properly explored for deeper damage to nerves and tendons. Sutureless repairs using steristrips or a tissue adhesive should only be carried out in the most superficial wounds, which are not dirty or ragged. Synthetic and absorbable materials have the advantage of avoiding suture removal but may produce more scarring. Intracutaneous prolene can be removed easily in a child by just pulling on one end but is difficult to insert if there is an irregular edge. Z-plasty to improve the direction of the scar is definitely not recommended as a primary procedure, except for the most experienced plastic surgeon.

SKIN COVER

Skin defects in childhood occur from congenital deformities such as meningomyocele, aplasia cutis congenita of the scalp, following excision of large hairy naevi and in conjoint twins. The majority of problems of skin cover in childhood, however, result from trauma such as burns (dealt with elsewhere), road accidents, particularly where the child is a pedestrian and is run over, bites and fingertip injuries. A few are iatrogenic, for instance, extravasation injuries. It is important to note, however, that if an extravasation injury is seen at an early stage, skin necrosis can be prevented by copious irrigation with saline under the skin and suction (Gault, 1993): 'if in doubt, get it out'.

Skin cover techniques

In some areas in neonates wound contracture and healing by secondary intention proceeds rapidly and without excessive scarring, and examples of this are seen in treatment of some spinal defects and exomphalos. Extravasation injuries in neonates can be allowed to heal by secondary intention with the proviso that when the child is older release and skin graft may be necessary. Another situation in childhood where provision of skin cover may not be necessary is fingertip injuries, provided there is minimal skin loss and no bone exposed.

DIRECT CLOSURE

If the skin loss is small and the surrounding skin mobile the skin can be undermined in the subcutaneous plane and rearranged to close the defect. This should be done without tension and it is advisable to use two layers with an absorbable material subcutaneously and a continuous nylon or prolene intradermally. Interrupted suturing is best if there is an irregular or serpiginous edge and is preferable if there is oozing from the skin edge as it will assist haemostasis. A skin approximation device is available for use in the operating theatre (Hirshowitz *et al.*, 1993), under general anaesthesia, which stretches the skin slowly so that the edges can be brought together and sutured, but the process may take an hour.

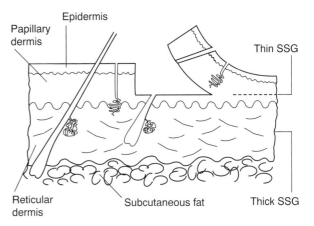

Fig. 81.1 Section of skin showing the levels for taking thin and thick split skin grafts.

SPLIT SKIN GRAFTING

This is the simplest method of skin cover but cannot be used over bare cortical bone, tendon or cartilage, because the skin graft needs to adhere to a well-vascularized bed (Fig. 81.1). A split skin graft initially survives for the first 36 hours from the plasma exuding from the surface. Capillaries then grow out from the granulation tissue or other tissues in the bed and grow into the skin graft so that at between 36 and 48 hours the skin grafts will have become vascularized, and this is shown by developing a 'capillary return' on release of pressure. Anything that prevents this ingrowth of capillaries will result in failure of the skin graft so that haematoma, seroma, infection or movement of the skin graft over the surface will prevent take.

Harvesting of a skin graft is usually done with a skin graft knife. This consists of a disposable blade which fits into a handle with a roller and is gently moved back and forth over the donor area by the operator at an angle of about 30°. It is essential to keep the skin firm and under tension, and this is difficult in babies. The usual donor sites are the thighs, and the inside of the thigh is preferable but also the inside of the upper arm can also be used. Many parents ask for the buttocks to be used so the slight blemish that results will be hidden under clothing, but this is a difficult site from which to take a skin graft and should only be done by a trained surgeon. When taking a skin graft from the thigh the assistant should grasp the back of the thigh with the left hand and, using a skin graft board, tension the skin away from the operator. The operator's left hand also has a skin board which draws away from the knife, thereby feeding the skin into the blade as this is moved gently to and fro (Fig. 81.2).

Once the skin has been taken it leaves the lower layers of the dermis, with hair follicles, sweat glands and sebaceous glands. The epithelium grows across from

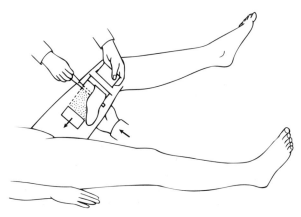

Fig. 81.2 Split skin graft from the thigh. The surgeon holds the skin graft knife with the right hand but flattens and pulls a board in front of the knife edge with the left hand and cuts uphill. The assistant (not shown) flattens and tensions the thigh from behind and with a board pulls down and away from the donor area.

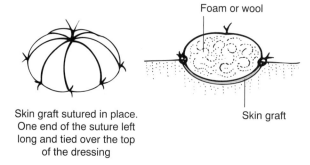

Skin graft sutured in place. One end of the suture left long and tied over the top of the dressing

Fig. 81.3 Method of suturing and dressing a skin graft to maintain a uniform pressure.

these structures and covers the raw area in approximately 10 days. Many different types of dressing can be used but it is important to use something that will not stick and will absorb the blood and exudate that comes from the surface. Whitehead's varnish and Jelonet make a better dressing for skin graft donor sites than Jelonet alone (Stanley *et al.*, 1988).

The area will be painful postoperatively and on discussion with anaesthetists it is recommended that a weak solution of Marcain is allowed to soak into the dressing as it is applied. The dressing should be left undisturbed for at least 1 week, and 10 days is preferable. It should then be soaked off in the bath, which will be less painful for the child. However, contamination with urine in donor areas on the thigh of the child is not unusual and, although urine does not adversely affect the healing, a wet dressing will quickly become colonized with *Pseudomonas aeruginosa*, causing delay and problems with healing. Most areas will leave a slight colour change that is just perceptible at 1 year. However, hypertrophic or frank keloid scarring may occur at a donor site.

The skin graft is spread on Vaseline gauze dressing with the raw surface upmost. It is placed on the wound (raw surface down) and held by a variety of fixation techniques. The area can be sutured, held with skin staples, or glued in place with cyanacrelate or fibrin glue, and sometimes no fixation is necessary. A pressure dressing is applied to prevent seroma or haematoma under the skin graft. On limbs this can consist of foam or gauze firmly bandaged into place. On the head and neck it is customary to use tie-over dressings where one end of the fixation suture is left long and tied over a bolus dressing of foam, flavine wool or saline-soaked cotton wool to a similar suture on the other side, thus

creating a parcel (Fig. 81.3). In co-operative patients and in large areas on the trunk the skin graft can be left exposed and it is possible to delay the application of the skin graft for 24–48 hours after the operation. This can be done in the ward by experienced medical or nursing staff. It is not painful but does necessitate the patient remaining in a position that does not displace the graft or rub on it. The skin can be stored for up to 3 weeks in a domestic refrigerator at approximately 4°C. It should be wrapped in a saline-soaked gauze but not immersed in saline.

Many mechanical aids to skin grafting are available. A skin graft dermatome is electrically or pneumatically driven to take large sheets of even-depth skin. The Paget or drum dermatome, which is now rarely used, has a cylinder which is glued to difficult sites for taking skin grafts such as the anterior abdominal wall and will take a thick split skin graft of a large area. Meshing the skin can be helpful in two ways: firstly, the skin can be expanded to cover a larger area; and secondly, the multiple holes in the skin graft allow egress of seroma and haematoma, there is usually a better take and it is particularly pertinent for burns grafts. The meshed appearance of the grafts can be seen many years later and for some surgeons this would be a contraindication to the technique (Fig. 81.4).

Skin grafts contract: thin grafts contract the most and thick split skin grafts the least. This can cause problems with grafts that are used over joints and may cause deformities in the neck around the mouth, eyes and breasts. They are also hairless, and have a colour that is rarely the same as the surrounding skin and a texture that does not look or feel like normal skin.

FULL-THICKNESS GRAFTS

These have advantages over split skin graft in that they shrink little and their colour and texture are usually a better match for the surrounding skin. However, they leave a donor area that needs to be closed directly so they cannot be very large and they do not take as easily

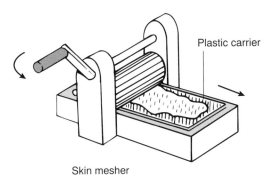

Skin mesher

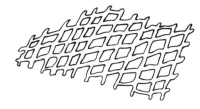

Meshed and expanded split skin graft

Fig. 81.4 A skin mesher machine for obtaining a meshed and expanded split skin graft.

as split skin graft. For the face, defects can be filled with skin taken from behind the ear or just in front of the ear with minimal scarring resulting. However, if hairs are included in the graft they will probably persist. Grafts taken from behind the ear are known as post-auricular Wolfe grafts (PAWG). When reconstructing the nostril margin for a bite injury, a small piece of cartilage can be included from the ear, which is known as a composite graft.

Flaps

Skin flaps contain a functioning arterial and venous system of vessels, and therefore they are not reliant on the vascularity of the bed where they are placed. They are therefore used to cover areas that have no, or poor, blood supply, such as open joints, bare cortical bone over tendons, exposed metal work and prostheses, on irradiated tissue and where a normal skin texture and bulky tissue are required.

Skin receives its blood supply from the underlying fascia and muscles with vessels that course in a perpendicular direction to the skin. However, there are some important systems in the body where large vessels run horizontally, such as the pectoral vessels, which branch from the internal mammary artery, pierce the chest wall just lateral to the sternum and then run laterally. This arrangement of vascular supply to the skin is the basis of the current classification of flaps.

RANDOM PATTERN FLAPS

A flap of skin and subcutaneous tissues is raised from the deep fascia and the blood supply enters the flap through a base or pedicle (Fig. 81.5). The arrangement of this base or pedicle is not aligned to any special vascular supply. A number of different shapes can be used such as a rectangular transposition flap, rotation flap, Z-plasty and a trapezoid or Limberg flap. There is a limitation to the size and dimensions of a random pattern flap and a useful rule is never to make the length of the flap longer than the width of the base. However, this rule only applies with relatively small flaps as the volume of tissue that has to be supplied by the vessels in the base will increase by the square. Most of the random pattern flaps are transferred from adjacent tissue and are therefore called local flaps. It is possible to transfer a random pattern flap from a distance, using either jump flaps or tube pedicles. This technique is rarely used now as it takes many months to make a distant transfer and with microsurgery the transfer can be made in one procedure.

AXIAL PATTERN FLAPS

In this instance the flap is arranged so that the artery and vein run axially down its length, meaning that a much longer flap can be raised. An example of this is the forehead flap where the whole of the skin of the forehead could be raised on one superficial temporal artery, and this was a useful way of carrying out intraoral reconstructions some years ago. However, this flap is rarely used now because of the poor appearance of the scarring on the forehead.

Deltopectoral flap

This flap, raised with the sternal margin as a base, contains the first three perforating vessels branching from the internal mammary artery and vein running axially to the shoulder. It was used extensively for head and neck reconstruction.

Groin flap

The superficial circumflex iliac artery branching from the femoral is the axial vessel in this flap, the base of which lies just lateral to the femoral artery (Fig. 81.6). A long, safe flap extends over the iliac crest. This is a useful flap for resurfacing skin loss of the hand from trauma.

MUSCLE FLAPS

Most muscles have a significant blood supply coming from one source. The skin overlying the muscle can survive by the flow in the vessels from the muscle to fascia and then directly vertically to the skin. A myocutaneous flap can be raised on a narrow pedicle. The best

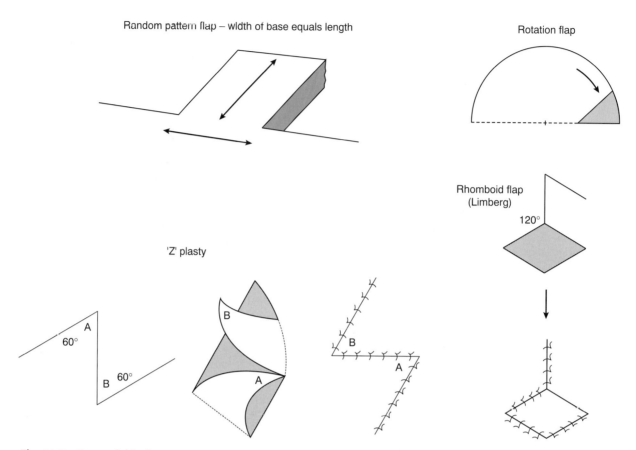

Random pattern flap – width of base equals length

Rotation flap

Rhomboid flap
(Limberg)
120°

'Z' plasty

A
60°

B 60°

B

A

Fig. 81.5 Types of skin flap.

example of this is the latissimus dorsi flap. The main blood flow to the muscle is from the lateral thoracic artery. The muscle, with a significant amount of overlying skin, can be raised and moved, usually forwards over the chest wall or on to the arm, shoulder, neck and lower part of the face. Many other useful myocutaneous flaps are available. It is not always necessary to take the overlying skin but merely to raise the muscle and, when it has been transferred to the new site, to apply a skin graft to the surface. In this technique some of the undesirable bulk is avoided.

FASCIAL FLAPS

Most fascial layers in the body are rich in blood vessels. Three techniques use fascia as a source of blood supply:

- fascia with the overlying skin attached, the best example being the flap in the lower leg which contains in the fascia the long saphenous vein and is particularly resilient in an area where flaps often do not work particularly well
- fascia covered with a skin graft

- fascia used without any covering: wound contraction and epithelialization can occur rapidly, so that both fascial and muscle flaps can be placed without a covering of skin.

OMENTUM

The omentum has an excellent blood supply and it can usually be narrowed down to one main vessel, which is the pedicle. Techniques are available to lengthen the omentum and yet keep an excellent blood supply, and it can be brought out of the abdominal cavity and covered with a skin graft which takes extremely well on this vascular material. It is usually used for chest reconstructions but can stretch an enormous distance. Because of the small size of omentum in childhood it is unlikely to be a useful source of skin cover in children.

FREE FLAP TRANSFER

Any of the above flaps, apart from the random pattern, can be transferred as free flaps. That means that the axial or main artery and vein are divided and anastomosed to a recipient artery and vein at the new site. The

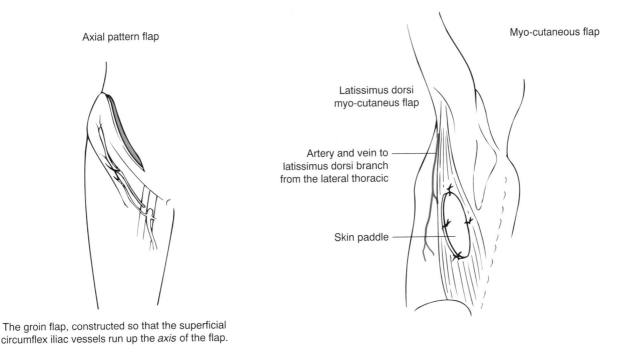

Axial pattern flap

Myo-cutaneous flap

Latissimus dorsi
myo-cutaneus flap

Artery and vein to
latissimus dorsi branch
from the lateral thoracic

Skin paddle

The groin flap, constructed so that the superficial
circumflex iliac vessels run up the *axis* of the flap.
A long flap with a narrow base

Fig. 81.6   Axial pattern groin flap and a myocutaneous flap using the latissimus dorsi muscle.

small size of these vessels necessitates the use of magnification, preferably with an operating microscope. Flaps with larger vessels are more reliable and have become the workhorse of the plastic and microvascular surgeon. The two most common flaps used are the latissimus dorsi muscle, or muscle and skin flap, and the radial artery fascial and skin flap.

COMPOSITE FLAPS

The excellent blood supply in many of the above flaps allows them to include bone, nerve tendon and even joint in the transfer. In congenital hand deformities it is possible to sacrifice a toe or part of a toe and transfer it by microvascular means to produce an essential opposition function. In this context one should remember that traumatically amputated parts are nothing more than rather complex composite flaps, so that parts of digits, a significant part of a limb, scalp and parts of the face may be replanted if arteries and veins are available and the tissue is not too mangled.

Skin expansion

As in a pregnancy, the skin is able to be stretched considerably and this stretched skin can be used to close a defect (Fig. 81.7). The technique uses a silicone bag, of which many different sizes and shapes are available from the manufacturers. Attached to this bag is a tube

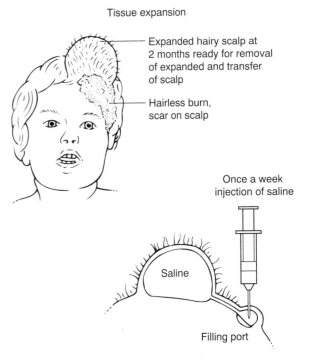

Tissue expansion

Expanded hairy scalp at
2 months ready for removal
of expanded and transfer
of scalp

Hairless burn,
scar on scalp

Once a week
injection of saline

Saline

Filling port

Fig. 81.7   Method of expanding the skin and subcutaneous tissue by regular injections of saline into a tissue expander.

and port. The port consists of a silicone dome over a metal circle. At the first operation an incision is made through the skin and the skin undermined adjacent to a site of future skin defect. The skin is undermined, the bag inserted, together with the port, and then the wound closed. It is then possible to fill the bag slowly over several weeks by injecting saline into the port through the skin. As the bag enlarges, so the skin is stretched and there is some recruitment of skin from the surrounding areas (Sharpe and Burd, 1989). When several hundred millilitres of saline have filled the expander a second operation is performed, the expander removed, and the loose and baggy skin transposed or rotated into the defect.

This technique is particularly useful for areas of alopecia and scarring on the scalp in children, but can also be used with caution in other areas.

Birthmarks

These originate from vascular, pigment-forming or neural tissue. They can be trivial lesions that merely need parental reassurance, but some may have serious consequences and lead to life-threatening situations.

VASCULAR MALFORMATIONS

Salmon patch

As the name indicates, this is a pale pink colour in otherwise normal skin, usually over the occiput or back of the neck, but can occur in other places. It is noted at birth but will have disappeared by 1 year.

Strawberry naevus or capilliary haemangioma

At birth there is usually nothing to show, although in some instances a very small red patch is seen. Within the first 2 or 3 weeks of life the red patch grows out from the surface quite rapidly to look, as its name implies, like a strawberry. It may continue growing at quite an alarming rate or stop at a diameter of approximately 1 cm. It stops growing at 3–6 months and the natural history of this lesion is for grey patches to develop very slowly on the surface. These spread and the lesion will shrink, so that by the time the child is aged 5 or 6 years it will have become pale, the same colour as the surrounding skin, and flat. However, the skin that has been stretched may never become quite normal and sometimes there is a baggy and wrinkled texture to it, which may need surgery to improve the area cosmetically. It is usually recommended that this natural resolution be allowed to proceed because attempts at excision or sclerosing these lesions usually end up with more scarring than would occur by natural resolution. However, the parents of the child with a strawberry naevus will need constant reassurance and

support, and it is useful to show photographs of children, before and after. They also worry about ulceration and bleeding. Ulceration may be a problem in the buttocks or perineal region, whereas bleeding is easily controlled by surface pressure. Small areas can usefully be excised with minimal scarring. Strawberry naevi can, however, have serious and even lethal complications.

A large strawberry naevus situated in the vicinity of the eye can obstruct vision and an eye with no vision in the first few months of life becomes blind. Urgent measures to shrink these lesions in the vicinity of the eye are therefore necessary. Various regimes using steroids have been described, and either short bursts of systemic steroids or interlesional injections are helpful.

Kasabach–Merritt syndrome

In this condition an existing haemangioma suddenly becomes larger and is associated with systemic changes of fibrinogenaemia and severe haemorrhage elsewhere. This is due to pooling of platelets in the haemangioma and is best treated by oral steroids.

Port wine stain (naevus flammeus)

This is a patch of discoloured skin on any part of the body, although it is somewhat more common in the head and neck, and may vary in size from 1 to 20 cm or even larger. The colour in childhood is usually a pale pink but becomes redder or possibly even takes on a purplish hue in adulthood. It never regresses but in adulthood will develop an uneven surface, even to producing papillomata. A rarer association is the Sturge–Weber syndrome, with skin changes on the face but also vascular malformation of the meninges and possibly epileptic fits.

Treatment of the port wine stain is a much easier proposition since the introduction of suitable lasers. It is important that the correct wavelength is used. The energy and time of the exposure are critical to prevent scarring and a large naevus may need many treatment sessions.

Vascular malformations

The old terminology of cavernous haemangioma is not used now. Vascular malformations consist of large venous spaces in a subcutaneous situation, may also vary in size from less than 1 cm to several centimetres in diameter and involve all tissues including bone. They can occur in any part of the body and sometimes are multiple. Most of them are low flow, where there is no direct arterial input into the malformation. The high-flow situation occurs when there is a feeding artery into the malformation, thus forming an arteriovenous fistula. The former lesions are unsightly, are in the way because of their large volume and their size is often positional so that they may appear quite small on the head and neck in the upright position but enlarge grossly when the head is put down. The small ones can be excised. The large ones, particularly if they involve many different tissues, are difficult to deal with surgically and embolization of these low-flow lesions is not recommended. The high-flow lesions with an arteriovenous fistula require surgical treatment. They are recognized by the presence of a bruit and confirmed by an arteriogram. Embolization, just prior to surgery, is a very useful technique to prevent uncontrollable haemorrhage. It can be repeated by a skilled radiologist but is not a permanent cure. Ligation of the feeding vessels is definitely contraindicated as this prevents the possibility of control with embolization and the vascular malformation would usually gain a significant source of blood flow from elsewhere. These large high-flow vascular malformations can produce a life-threatening situation (Erdman *et al.*, 1995).

A little known technique of intralesional suturing, described by Popescu, is also worth considering in this situation.

Cystic hygroma

The developmental abnormality of lymphatics can present anywhere in the body but most commonly it is seen in the neck and lower face. It appears in babyhood as a large multicystic swelling which involves all tissues including muscles and nerves. The size and situation of these can produce significant airway problems. Complete surgical excision is often not possible because the tissues that are involved are very vascular, which is an added problem. If there is no airway problem then surgery can be delayed and in a few instances the cystic hygroma will reduce in size over some years, but recurrent infections and associated swelling may indicate surgical excision.

Pigmented lesions

Melanocytes start life in the neural crest and migrate to lie in the basal layer of the epidermis. Congregations of melanocytes occur in this situation and are called moles or naevi. If the collection of melanocytes is situated at the junction of the epidermis and dermis they are appropriately called junctional naevi. There is a tendency for the collection of naevi to move down into the dermis, in which case they are called intradermal naevi. If a mole has melanocytes in both situations then they are compound naevi (Fig. 81.8).

Junctional naevi appear as flat brown patches never larger than 0.5 cm. Compound naevi are raised from the surface and may be pink or brown and become hairy. They often have a rather warty surface.

Intradermal naevi are raised above the surface of the surrounding skin, usually brown in colour and quite often hairy. Both the compound and intradermal naevi may be quite large in surface area and are often called congenital naevi, as they are present from or shortly after birth. Some congenital hairy naevi can be very large and the classic description is of a naevus around the waist, buttocks and upper thighs, aptly called a bathing trunk naevus.

Malignant melanoma is rare in childhood but it will usually present in these congenital hairy naevi. There is evidence to show that sunburn in childhood can predispose to malignant melanoma in adult life and parents should be advised to protect their children from ultraviolet light.

Dysplastic naevi are seen in adolescents, they may be familial and there is an incidence of multiple melanomas occurring in adults with this syndrome. These dysplastic naevi can be recognized as being multiple and irregular, with an ill-defined edge and uneven pigmentation. They are usually raised from the surface of the surrounding skin.

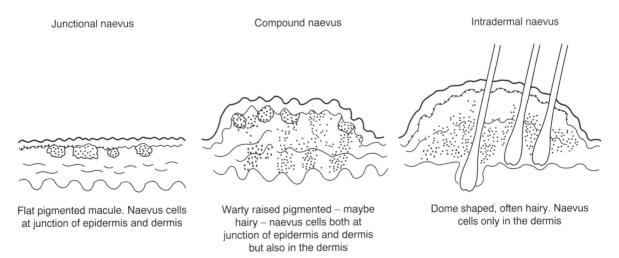

Junctional naevus	Compound naevus	Intradermal naevus
Flat pigmented macule. Naevus cells at junction of epidermis and dermis	Warty raised pigmented – maybe hairy – naevus cells both at junction of epidermis and dermis but also in the dermis	Dome shaped, often hairy. Naevus cells only in the dermis

Fig. 81.8 Cross-sections to show the pathological anatomy of a junctional naevus, a compound naevus and an intradermal naevus.

Blue naevus occur anywhere in the body but chiefly on the backs of the hands and dorsum of the feet, are never larger than 1 cm in diameter, and are often dome shaped and have a slate-blue colour. They consist of melanocytes, which are deeply situated in the dermis, hence the slate-blue colour. They are benign.

Excision biopsy of moles in childhood should be carried out through small elliptical excisions, placing the ellipse in the lines of election, that is the crease lines. On the back it is preferable to take merely a circular incision and either close it with a purse-string suture or interrupted sutures as a straight line. An ellipse on the back always spreads to a rather ugly scar.

It is difficult to estimate the risk of melanoma in the giant hairy naevi and published papers show an incidence varying from less than 10% to over 30%. Excision requires skin grafting and ugly scarring commonly results.

Dermabrasion or shaving of the giant hairy naevi within 2 months of birth succeeds in lightening the dark-brown colour of these naevi but dark hairs may still produce a significant blemish and it is not clear whether this treatment provides any prophylaxis against malignant change.

A raised circular lesion (spitz naevus) may occur in the skin of children and adolescents, on the cheeks. This is a benign tumour but the histology can be confusing and have feature of a melanoma.

Cleft lip and palate

The incidence of cleft lip and palate in the UK is approximately 1 in 1000 live births. Embryologically, there is a failure of fusion or breakdown in the fusion between the median frontonasal process and the two maxillary processes. This results in a cleft, either to the right or to the left of the midline or sometimes on both sides, thus one has a unilateral cleft or a bilateral cleft lip. The cleft may extend back through the alveolus to the incisive foramen (Fig. 81.9).

The cleft of the palate occurs as a result of failure of fusion of the palatal shelves. In a submucous cleft the soft palate has no union of the muscle across the midline, but the mucosa is intact and usually the uvula is bifid. A cleft of the soft palate has muscle and mucosa but the bony hard palate is intact. The defect can occur through the palatal bone to join up with the cleft of the lip, resulting in unilateral or bilateral cleft lip, which extends right the way through to involve the midline of the palate.

A cleft lip is a cosmetic deformity which may involve the nose to a considerable extent. The cleft of the palate is a functional deformity which affects sucking and speech because it is impossible for the child to close the nose off from the mouth (nasopharyngeal incompetence).

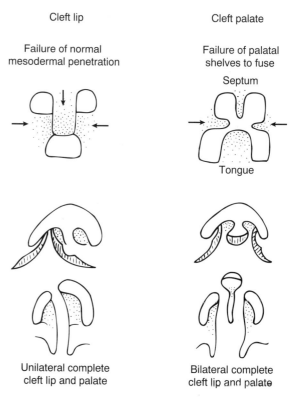

Fig. 81.9 Diagrams to show the anatomy of complete and incomplete unilateral and bilateral cleft lip and palate.

Any treatment of patients with cleft lip and palate must involve a team, usually consisting of a plastic surgeon, an oral and maxillofacial surgeon, orthodontists, an ear, nose and throat surgeon, speech therapists, paediatric nurses and counsellors. The first important part of the treatment is to establish adequate feeding, and special teats are available that can obstruct the leak into the nose as the baby sucks. Alternatively, a teat with a large hole in it or even spoon feeding may be recommended.

The lip is repaired first. With adequate facilities and experienced staff this can be completed in the neonatal period, otherwise the cleft lip is repaired at 3 months of age. In the neonatal period a simple lip adhesion is performed, whereas at 3 months a rotation advancement technique is recommended (Fig. 81.10) (Millard, 1994).

The cleft of the palate is repaired at about 1 year of age and the present fashion is to use the Von Langenbeck technique. It is important to have a functioning soft palate as the child begins to phonate, otherwise permanent speech defects may result. However, extensive dissection in the region of the hard palate results in maxillary hypoplasia, which is evident in teenagers and may necessitate extensive maxillary surgery later. Clefts of the lip and palate will usually need an alveolar bone graft at the time of the appearance of permanent denti-

Repair of cleft lip and palate

Millard rotation
advancement of lip

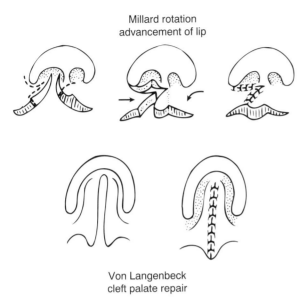

Von Langenbeck
cleft palate repair

Fig. 81.10 Repair of cleft lip and palate.

tion, at about the age of 10 years. Three operations may be all that is necessary. However, there can be problems with nasopharyngeal incompetence and poor speech, which necessitate a pharyngoplasty. There can be deficiency of soft tissue of the upper lip in which an Abbe flap, swinging tissue from the lower lip to the upper lip, and finally nasal obstruction and cosmetic deformity will necessitate corrective rhinoplasty in the late teens.

Deformities of the ear

ACCESSORY AURICLES

These are common and need to be removed surgically as there is often a spur of cartilage extending quite deeply, alongside which is a prominent artery. A local anaesthetic excision in outpatients is hazardous.

PITS AND SINUSES

A pit at the root of the helix extends down, usually for 1.5–2 cm in front of the cartilage of the ear. Cysts and recurrent infections are commonly associated with these disturbances. Careful exploration with magnification is needed to ensure that no epithelial remnants remain. Cysts and recurrent infections commonly associated with sinuses in the lower part of the ear may extend between branches of the facial nerve and very careful exploration is necessary.

BAT EAR CORRECTION

It is best to leave this surgery until the child is 6 years old and preferably has some say in whether he or she wishes for it to be done. The operation is performed under a general anaesthetic as a day case. Firstly, an ellipse of skin is excised from the back of the ear and then the cartilage is incised along the antihelix fold from the pins and affixed in the mastoid as an osteo-integrated implant. Alternatively, costal cartilage is carved to the shape of the ear and inserted underneath the skin. Some months after this initial operation, the cartilage graft is brought out from the side of the head and skin graft applied behind the ear. At the same time a lobe can be constructed from neck skin and a third operation can produce a conchal fossa. An acceptable cosmetic appearance can be achieved with this technique and it is the preferred option for most children and parents. The first alternative is sometimes chosen to avoid secondary scarring and to limit the surgical procedure to two interventions.

References

Erdman, M.W.H., Davies, D.M., Jackson, J.E. and Allison, D.J. 1995: Multidisciplinary approach to the management of head and neck arteriovenous malformations. *Annals of the Royal College of Surgeons of England* **77**, 53–9.

Gault, D. 1993: Extravasation injuries. *British Journal of Plastic Surgery* **46**, 91–6.

Hirshowitz, B., Lindenbaum, E. and Har-Shaiy 1993: A skin-stretching device for the harnessing of the viscoelastic properties of skin. *Plastic Reconstructive Surgery* **92**, 260.

Millard, D.R., Jr 1994: Embryonic rationale for the primary correction of classical congenital clefts of the lip and palate. *Annals of the Royal College of Surgeons of England* **76**, 150–60.

Rockwell, Cohen and Ehrilch 1989: Keloids and hypertrophic scars. *Plastic and Reconstructive Surgery* **84**, 827–37.

Sharpe, D.T. and Burd, R.M. 1989: Tissue expansion in perspective. *Annals of the Royal College of Surgeons of England* **71**, 175–80.

Stanley, D., Emerson, D.J.M. and Daley, J.C. 1988: Whitehead's varnish and jelonet – a better dressing for skin graft donor sites than jelonet alone. *Annals of the Royal College of Surgeons of England* **70**, 369–71.

Further reading

McGregor, A. and McGregor, I.A. 1995: *Fundamental techniques of plastic surgery*, 9th ed. Edinburgh: Churchill Livingstone.

CHAPTER 82

Orthopaedic surgery

G.R. TAYLOR AND N.M.P. CLARKE

Introduction	References
General orthopaedic pathology	Further reading
Regional orthopaedics	

Introduction

Nicholas Andre published *L'Orthopedie* in Paris in 1741. This text described the correction of musculo-skeletal deformities in children and from its title he is credited with the neologism 'orthopaedic', which he derived from the Greek *orthos* (straight) and *paideia* (rearing of children). This term, along with his illustration of a staff used to straighten a young tree, have become synonymous with the specialty. It now embraces a far wider scope of disease and treatments, encompassing trauma, musculoskeletal oncology and occupational disease.

Paediatric orthopaedics is now a recognized subspeciality in its own right, although the majority of the workload is still performed by generalists with an interest in the field. The outcome of treatment for childhood orthopaedic conditions is better in experienced hands. There are many rare associations with multisystem anomalies and disease, which must be recognized if the child is to be properly managed. This requires a close working relationship with other medical specialties, principally, paediatricians, paediatric surgeons, oncologists and paediatric radiologists. With the prospects of genetic and fetal interventions becoming more common, the speciality is likely to grow even more distanced from its parent.

This chapter is aimed at the paediatric, rather than the orthopaedic surgeon and has therefore been slanted towards conditions that present to both specialties or require combined management. For this reason and lim-itations of space, some areas such as trauma, metabolic disorders, neoplasia and operative techniques are only outlined. Congenital anomalies, especially where they form part of a wider paediatric syndrome, are briefly reviewed, although the generalized skeletal dysplasias are not included. The time-honoured approach of dealing with general musculoskeletal disease processes followed by a regional overview has been adopted. In each regional section the focus has been on the causes of pain in that part of the body and specific common conditions, with deformity and pain being the usual causes of referral to both paediatricians and orthopaedic surgeons.

General orthopaedic pathology

MUSCULOSKELETAL INFECTION

Osteomyelitis and septic arthritis have become relatively unusual in developed countries with improvements in social conditions, nutrition and the availability of antibiotics. It remains a huge problem in the developing world and carries a significant mortality, as well as the morbidity of chronic osteomyelitis and prematurely degenerating joints. Recent reports have quoted an incidence of as few as 20 cases of osteomyelitis and 10 septic arthritis per year in large units serving populations of between 300 000 and 500 000 in the western world (Cole *et al.*, 1972; Mollan and Piggot, 1977). The clinical presentation has changed in the west over the last few decades to a less florid, subacute condition (Jones *et al.*, 1969).

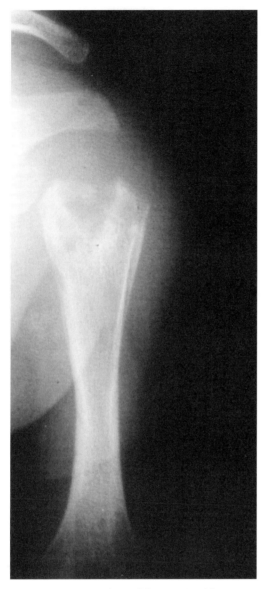

Figure 82.1 Osteomyelitis of the proximal humerus in a young child showing patchy loss of trabecular pattern, density and a double line at the cortical surface due to periosteal bone formation.

The pathology is generally believed to be due to a haematogenous seeding of the metaphysis with opportunist pathogens. Direct inoculation may occur from trauma, iatrogenic causes and spread from adjacent visceral abscess, but these constitute a minority of cases. The source of the organism is commonly the respiratory tract, middle ear or urinary tract (as well as the umbilicus in neonates). The causative organism varies with the age group, with staphylococcus, streptococcus and haemophilus being the most likely, the latter particularly in children under 2 years old.

The infection has a predilection for the metaphysis and this is thought to relate to the microvascular anatomy. In the infant perforating vessels may cross the growth plate to the cartilaginous epiphysis, but early in childhood this route ceases to exist. The capsules of hip, knee and elbow contain part of the metaphysis and allow direct spread of infection into the joint. This is the likely sequence in the development of septic arthritis, but direct infection of the synovium may occur. If left untreated, the infection produces a subperiosteal abscess, which progressively strips that structure and devascularizes the cortex. Rupture of the periosteum leads to the formation of a soft tissue collection that may become large, clinically apparent and visible on ultrasound. Medullary spread further injures the vascular supply and a large section of bone can die and give rise to a sequestrum, which harbours organisms and creates the conditions for chronic osteomyelitis. Approximately 10 days into this process radiographs may show little other than rarefaction of the medulla and early new bone formation initiated by the activated periosteum. If allowed to continue the periosteum will form a sleeve of bone (involucrum) around the sequestrum and an equilibrium may develop between quiescence and repeatedly discharging sinuses.

The above description is almost never seen in the developed world. The pattern varies through the variable systemic illness that accompanies the local pathological changes. Dissemination and multifocal infection is a serious, life-threatening complication with a 10–20% mortality. This produces an endocardial shock with circulatory, respiratory and renal complications. Immunocompromised patients are at risk, including the neonate who becomes septic with no early localizing features. In most instances medical intervention alters the course of events. If treatment with antibiotics is started with the first clinical signs, then it is possible to abort the infection before any significant damage occurs in the bone.

Septic arthritis is a surgical emergency, since irreversible destructive changes have been observed in pus-filled joints within 24 hours. The bacterial toxins, along with the enzymes released by neutrophils, rapidly degrade hyaline cartilage. Aspiration is not always reliable and arthrotomy must be considered when there is strong clinical suspicion and a negative aspiration. There is considerable controversy in this area and good results have been reported with aspiration and antibiotics as the mainstay of treatment. A large series has been reported which concluded that the worst results followed a delay in surgical lavage and suggested that open drainage was the safest course (Patterson, 1970).

Most cases of osteomyelitis in the West are low grade and not always easily recognized. Tenderness and mild pyrexia, with or without changes in the blood indices, ought to arouse suspicion. The diagnosis of septic arthritis is essentially a clinical one, but osteomyelitis carries a little less urgency and it is often possible to investigate with isotope scans or magnetic resonance imaging (MRI). Erythrocyte sedimentation rate (ESR) and C-reactive protein (CRP) are useful to monitor progress, but are not diagnostic in themselves.

The treatment depends on identification of the infecting organism. When cultures are negative, it may be advisable to start antibiotic therapy. Splintage of the affected part relieves pain and may, in itself, have a therapeutic role. The role of surgery remains controversial, but all authors agree that infected joints require urgent drainage, whatever the method.

Unusual organisms occasionally complicate the clinical picture. Tuberculosis still presents with low-grade malaise and pain, particularly in the spine. Causes of pain in the musculoskeletal system are considered in each regional section. It must be remembered that infection is protean in its clinical manifestation, but almost invariably causes pain. In children it is a more common diagnosis than that of psychogenic symptoms and must always be excluded in the diagnostically difficult case.

NEOPLASIA

Musculoskeletal neoplasia in children is rare. The treatment is specialized and it is perilous for the inexperienced surgeon to dabble in its management. A confident diagnosis is essential, since the radiographic findings may not distinguish between benign and malignant lesions. With the increasing use of MR scanning, radiologists have been in a stronger position to make this distinction, but a histological diagnosis is required to plan treatment. Biopsy is hazardous, since it may lead to tissue seeding and metastasis. If an unusual radiographic lesion is found in a child presenting with a swelling or pain it is essential to pursue the diagnosis initially non-invasively and refer the case if there is doubt or a lack of local expertise. If an open biopsy is to be taken, this should be performed by the surgeon who will carry out any definitive excision.

The principal objectives of treatment are to save the child, to save the limb if possible and to preserve function. The histological examination of tumour tissue is complex and therefore a regional service has been developed in the UK. This approach was adopted in Sweden years ago and this has led to the use of 'safe' fine-needle biopsies to confirm the diagnosis (Akerman, *et al.*, 1985). Each type of tumour has a spectrum of subtypes with variable behaviour and aggressiveness. This has been helpful in designing management programmes which make use of chemotherapy, radiotherapy and surgery.

Children may present with local symptoms or following the incidental discovery of a lesion on an X-ray. A range of benign cysts and lesions of bone exists (Table 82.1) and may cause difficulty in diagnosis,

Table 82.1 Benign bone lesions

Type of lesion	Radiographic features
Non-ossifying fibroma	Oval radiolucent area with thin sclerotic shell bone, eccentric in cortex
Fibrous dysplasia	Radiolucent areas with hazy, ground-glass appearance. Bone may deform
Compact exostosis	Sessile, dense enlagement of cortex, especially skull
Osteochondroma	Defined exostosis from metaphysis, may have tip surrounded by flecks of calcification
Chondroblastoma	Rounded, demarcated radiolucency in epiphysis
Enchondroma	Defined margin, central radiolucency at junction of metaphysis and diaphysis. Common in hands and feet
Osteoblastoma	Osteolytic lesion with flecks of calcification and surrounding sclerosis. Flat bones and vertebrae
Osteoid osteoma	Small radiolucent nidus, surrounded by sclerosis in diaphysis. High uptake on isotope scan
Bone cyst	Demarcated radiolucency in metaphysis, especially humerus and femur. Thin cortex, may be expanded: 'fallen fragment sign'
Aneurysmal cyst	Eccentric, trabeculated cyst in metaphysis
Giant cell tumour	Eccentric, radiolucent area in 'epiphysis', bounded by subchondral bone plate

Table 82.2 Malignant bone tumours in childhood

Type of tumour	Radiographic features
Osteosarcoma	Metaphyses of long bones. Destruction of cortex with Codman's triangles, sunburst spicules
Ewing's sarcoma	Diaphysis of long bones. Periosteal reaction, 'onion skin' layering, Codman's triangles
Fibrosarcoma	Bone destruction
Malignant fibrous histioctioma	Bone destruction
Chordoma	Radiolucency and soft tissue mass at sacrum

especially if there has been an infection, or a fracture in relation to a benign lesion. Myositis ossificans, stress fractures and old haematomata may also lead to difficulties in diagnosis. The bone tumours most commonly seen in children are listed, with a brief indication of the radiological features, in Table 82.2. The mortality for malignancy has steadily improved since the 1970s. A series of 205 children treated for bone malignancy, between 1978 and 1988, was reported by Mercuri *et al.* (1991), which consisted of osteosarcoma, Ewing's tumour, fibrosarcoma and malignant fibrous histiocytoma. Sixty-three per cent underwent surgical excision and 98% chemotherapy. At 30 months 65% were alive and disease free. Few amputations were required in this group (the main treatment before the advances in chemotherapy since the mid-1970s), but there was a disparity in functional results between those in whom joints could be preserved and the worse outcome when arthrodesis was unavoidable.

Preservation of limbs is now possible despite extensive resections. Many of these tumours remain confined to a limb compartment by the fascial planes until a relatively late stage. Surgical excision is planned using MRI and/or computed tomography (CT) imaging and compartmectomy is carried out, sometimes with removal of the entire long bone. This necessitates the use of custom-made prostheses, and in young children, a growing prosthesis, which may be lengthened as the child grows. The golden rules of resection include isolating and ligating the draining vessels and lymphatics prior to disturbance of the tumour, thus reducing the risk of seedling metastases.

EWING'S SARCOMA

This is believed to arise from endothelial, marrow cells, usually in tubular bones, particularly the tibia, fibula and clavicle. It is most often encountered in the 10–20-year-old age group, presenting with pain and often mild malaise. The ESR may be raised and the radiographic appearance may show diaphyseal new bone formation (classically a layered 'onion skin' appearance). It may be confused with osteomyelitis, but imaging will reveal local soft tissue extension, with or without calcification. Treatment is based on chemotherapy and a 5-year survival of approximately 50% would be typical. Surgery and radiotherapy have a role in combination with chemotherapy, but they do not significantly improve overall survival.

OSTEOSARCOMA

This aggressive tumour comprises a range of histological variants, but all carry a poor prognosis. It is relatively common in the young, although there is a second 'peak' later in life. The presentation is usually with pain at long bone metaphysis. Radiographs show variable destruction of the bone with extension into the soft tissues (sunburst spicules and Codman's triangle). Further imaging is useful and biopsy is necessary to plan treatment. The management of this malignancy involves radical resection and chemotherapy. Cases occur in inoperable sites or at an advanced stage and may only be palliated with radiotherapy.

SKELETAL TRAUMA IN CHILDHOOD

Children's skeletons differ from adults' in a number of respects which have a bearing on the pattern of skeletal injury that is seen and its results. Their proportions and overall mass differ, with a relatively large head in relation to the body. The skeleton is more flexible and the long bones have a thicker, more resilient periosteum, which may reduce the displacement of fractures. The most significant feature is the presence of the unossified growth plate (physis). This is an area of relative weakness. A range of injuries to the physis (Salter–Harris classification) is encountered which has implications for future growth and may lead to deformity or limb length discrepancies. It is essential to recognize injury to these regions, accurately to reduce and ensure that the treatment itself does not lead to further damage or deformity.

The relative elasticity of the young bone, its altered length to width ratio and the thicker periosteum permit buckling injury (torus fracture), greenstick fractures (one cortex broken) and plastic deformity (bowing). These bony injuries are more stable than those of adult bone. Fractures in the very young are not immediately obvious and radiographs a week later may reveal a periosteal reaction that confirms the injury. A further difficulty to those not used to dealing with children is the recognition of the normal epiphyses and physeal lines, and differentiating these from a fracture.

Table 82.3 Types of osteogenesis imperfecta

Type	Defect	Clinical features
I	Decreased type I collagen	Blue sclerae, normal stature. Hearing loss in 50%
II	Abnormal alpha I and alpha II chains	Lethal perinatally. Small, fractured, partially mineralized skeleton
III	Abnormal alpha I and alpha II chains	Bluish sclerae, progressive deformities, short stature
IV	Abnormal alpha I and alpha II chains	Short stature, mild deformity, dentinogenesis common. Minority with hearing loss

OSTEOGENESIS IMPERFECTA

Osteogenesis imperfecta (OI) is a group of clinically related metabolic disorders of genetic origin, which result in abnormalities of type I collagen. This is the principal fibrillar collagen in bone and forms long, cross-linked chains that give bone its resilience. OI occurs in approximately 1 in 20 000 births and four types are recognized (Table 82.3).

Type II and III were called osteogenesis congenita because fractures were seen at birth and the others osteogenesis tarda as the appearance of fractures may be delayed. Type II is lethal short-limbed dwarfism and the diagnosis is made by a pathologist. Type III patients have short stature, spinal deformities and progressive limb deformity. They require orthopaedic attention for the above, but are usually wheelchair bound. Intra-

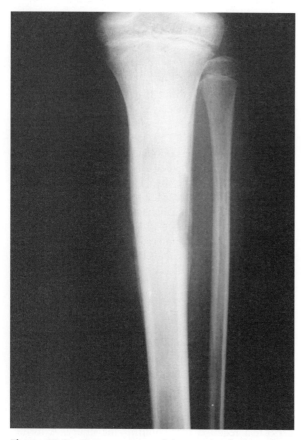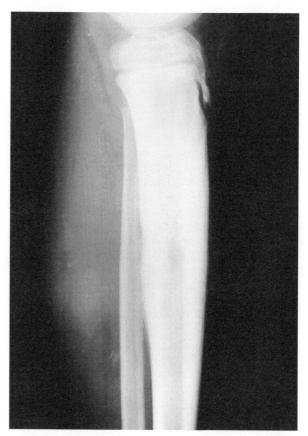

Figure 82.2 Osteosarcoma of the proximal tibia. The anterior and lateral views show that the texture of the bone is extensively altered and the trabecular pattern destroyed. The cortex is eroded and there are multiple layers of periosteal new bone formation.

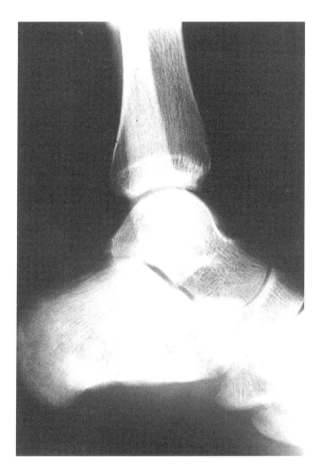

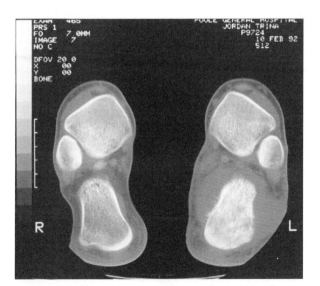

Figure 82.3 Ewing's sarcoma of the calcaneum. The radiograph shows loss of the trabecular pattern in the lower half of the bone. The CT scan vividly depicts the extent of soft tissue involvement.

medullary rods and spinal fusions may be used to correct or limit deformity. Type IV is intermediate between I and III and treatment is applied to each problem as and when it occurs.

Type I is the child who may present with a fracture and an unconvincing story of minimal trauma. Radiographs sometimes reveal older fractures and a suspicion of non-accidental injury (NAI) raises anxiety. Extraskeletal features, which include blue sclerae, hypermobility, easy bruising, deafness aortic valve problems and dentinogenesis, may aid the diagnosis. There is often a family history, but spontaneous mutations occur. A skull X-ray showing Wormian bones is helpful, but in doubtful cases fibroblast culture and biochemical analysis of collagen synthesis are needed.

NEUROMUSCULAR CONDITIONS

These comprise a large range of disorders, which produce problems that may benefit from orthopaedic intervention from early childhood onwards (Table 82.4). None is curable and so the treatments are aimed at preventing progressive loss of function, or compensatory measures designed to improve function and so reduce disability. The orthopaedic aspects of these conditions may be divided into categories (Table 82.5).

The orthopaedic approach to children with complex limb dysfunction has been suboptimal, as there has been a tendency to focus on isolated joint problems rather than the overall function. Gait analysis has pioneered the concept of observing the integration of pathological changes in function and secondary compensatory mechanisms. The latter may look abnormal, but may well be a response to improve limb efficiency rather than a problem requiring correction. An understanding of the natural history of neuromuscular disease is an essential part of the orthopaedic assessment. It enables a management plan to be formulated and the advisability or timing of a surgical procedure decided. A combined approach with the advice of paediatricians and a paediatric neurologist is a necessary component in the management of these patients.

Table 82.4 Neuromuscular disorders in childhood

Diagnosis
• Cerebral palsy
• Spina bifida
• Friedreich's ataxia
• Brachial plexus injuries
• Hereditary peripral neuropathies
• Poliomyelitis
• Spinal cord lesions
• Muscular dystrophies

Table 82.5 Causation and results of neuromuscular imbalance and sensory loss

Causation	Result
Joint deformity	Muscular imbalance
	Spasticity
	Contracture
	Subluxation of joints
Muscle weakness	Postural control
	Balance
	Limb function
	Gait
	Scoliosis
Sensory disturbance	Skin and joint damage
	Incoordination

CEREBRAL PALSY

Cerebral palsy is a result of brain damage in the neonatal period. It is associated with prematurity, anoxia and kernicterus. It is non-progressive, although its effects become more apparent with development. The approximate incidence is of 1 in 2000 births and there are four main types:

- Spastic (60%): increased tone of muscles which 'gives' with passive stretch. Graded according to limb involvement:
  – monoplegia (5%): one limb affected
  – hemiplegia (40%): one side of body affected
  – diplegia (30%): lower limbs only affected
  – tetraplegia or triplegia (25%): four or three limbs affected
- Athetoid (rare): uncontrollable, writhing movements (tongue)
- Ataxic (rare): incoordination, tremor
- Rigid, constant hypertonic muscles.

The essential limb pathology is thought to be a shortening of the muscle–tendon unit, which fails to keep pace with the growth of the bones and therefore allows contractures to develop. If left untreated this leads to secondary joint problems and a decrease in function. Animal experiments support this theory, as in the normal mouse muscle sarcomeres are added at the musculotendinous junction as a response to stretch. In genetically spastic mice this process does not occur (Ziv *et al.*, 1984).

The child may show little other than a delay in normal developmental milestones, but some have early postural problems. With increasing muscle imbalance the growth of the long bones may be distorted with torsional deformity of femur and tibia, misalignments and length discrepancy. Treatment options include physiotherapy, neurosurgical rhizotomy of posterior nerve roots and orthopaedic bone or soft tissue procedures. Contractures may be released or tendons lengthened. Tendon transfers help to rebalance antagonist groups and osteotomy is used to correct deformity.

SPINAL MUSCULAR ATROPHY

This is an autosomal recessive condition, occurring in 1 in 20 000 live births. The anterior horn cells degenerate with subsequent muscle weakness. There are three main types. The severe infantile form (type I) leads to early death. Type II children will probably not walk, but will survive and type III may walk with aids. These children all develop scoliosis, which often requires surgical treatment.

FRIEDREICH'S ATAXIA

This is an autosomal recessive ataxia with an incidence of live births of 1 in 50 000. It is caused by a degeneration of the spinocerebellar tracts, posterior columns and cerebellum. The affected child becomes clumsy and develops an unbalanced gait from 5 years of age. The mean age of onset in two large series was 11 and 12 years (Harding, 1981; Filla *et al.*, 1990). Deformities such as pes cavus and scoliosis occur, with the child becoming wheelchair bound by the early 20s. The diagnosis is suggested by the triad of ataxia, areflexia and an extensor planter reflex. Death is usually brought about by an associated cardiomyopathy in the 50s.

HEREDITARY MOTOR SENSORY NEUROPATHIES

The best known of these rare conditions is Charcot–Marie–Tooth disease. A variety of orthopaedic problems is seen in children affected by these neuropathies, such as pes cavus, 'cock-up' toes, hip dysplasia and scoliosis (10%). Treatment depends on the severity of the orthopaedic problems.

MUSCULAR DYSTROPHIES

These distressing conditions produce progressive muscle weakness, with alteration of the postural muscles and ultimately respiratory difficulties. Duchenne muscular dystrophy is an X-linked recessive disease and is often apparent in the toddler. There may be delay in walking and poor balance. Muscular pseudohypertrophy is frequent and the weakening child adopts tactics to compensate, such as climbing up his or her legs to a standing position (Gower's sign). The progression to a wheelchair and scoliosis with poor head control may only take until the early teens. Death from cardiorespiratory complications usually occurs in the second decade. Blood tests for creatinine kinase and aldase, electromyographic (EMG) studies and muscle biopsy will confirm the diagnosis.

Table 82.6 Orthopaedic operations for neuromuscular disorders

Site	Operative procedure	
Growth plate	Fusion	Epiphyseodesis (staple or bone graft across physis, ablation by curettage and drilling)
	Distraction	Chondrodiastasis
Long bone operations	Osteotomy	Varus, valgus, multiplanar, rotational
	Lengthening	Callostasis (with angular correction, hemicallostasis)
Joints	Opening	Arthrotomy
	Fusion	Arthrodesis
	Excision	Excision arthroplasty or excision hemiarthroplasty
	Replacement	Arthroplasty or hemiarthroplasty
Tendons	Transfer	
	Lengthening	Z-lengthening
	Division	Tenotomy

ORTHOPAEDIC OPERATIONS

Orthopaedic surgery's primary role is to restore or enhance function (Table 82.6). Many operations are designed to relieve pain and this allows use of a limb that was previously inhibited. The musculoskeletal system can only function if forces can be generated and produce a resultant movement. Clearly, this relies on working joints and a stable skeleton. Soft tissue surgery is a major part of orthopaedics, but the speciality is best known for its 'carpentry' with bone.

Regional orthopaedics

THE NECK

Problems with the cervical spine are not a common cause for referral in paediatric orthopaedic practice. Torticollis, is the most frequently seen complaint, and the remainder consist of rare congenital or post-traumatic conditions, which are often asymptomatic.

Odontoid anomalies

There is a range of developmental abnormalities which affect the odontoid peg (dens). Most are harmless, incidental findings on radiographs, but others may predispose to atlanto-axial instability. The dens at birth is separated from the body of the axis by a cartilaginous growth plate. This is below the base of the peg and has usually fused by the age of 6 years, but may be mistaken for a fracture by the inexperienced practitioner. Three persistent ossification anomalies are recognized: aplasia, hypoplasia and os odontoideum. The first is very rare, while with the second there is a short peg and the third a separated ossified tip connected by cartilage.

The last may give the appearance of a non-ununited fracture. The first two tend to lead to instability with pain and/or neurological symptoms in late childhood or as young adults and may require surgical stabilization. Certain childhood syndromes ought to alert the clinician, especially following trauma, and these include Down's, Morquio's and Klippel–Feil syndromes. In 15% of 404 Down's children, approximately 2% required surgery for atlanto-axial instability (Pueschel and Scola, 1987).

Atlanto-axial instability

This occurs owing to both congenital and acquired causes, such as trauma or infection. The severe traumatic case is often fatal because of cord injury. Insufficiency of the ligaments stabilizing the dens to the arch of the first vertebra permits abnormal motion of the peg, which may injure the cord progressively. Lateral radiographs may show an abnormally enlarged interval between the odontoid and C_1 ($\leq$ 3 mm in the child), which may increase with flexion. Tomography is helpful, although not always diagnostic, unless dynamic scans are obtained by rotating the head (Phillips *et al.*, 1989).

The child may present with torticollis, pain in the neck and unwillingness to move the head. The degree of neurological compromise depends on the mode of onset and its duration. Conservative treatment may be successful in the mild case using halter traction. Surgical fusion is advisable in the unstable congenital or severe acquired forms.

Klippel–Feil syndrome (cervical vertebral synostosis)

Klippel and Feil described the condition that bears their name in 1912, following post-mortem examina-

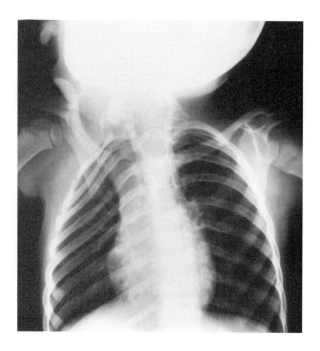
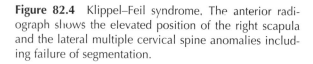
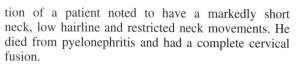
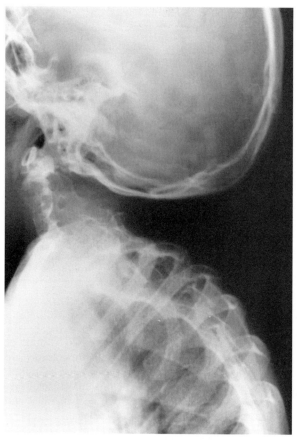

Figure 82.4 Klippel–Feil syndrome. The anterior radiograph shows the elevated position of the right scapula and the lateral multiple cervical spine anomalies including failure of segmentation.

tion of a patient noted to have a markedly short neck, low hairline and restricted neck movements. He died from pyelonephritis and had a complete cervical fusion.

Subsequently, all patients with a varying number of congenitally fused cervical vertebrae have been ascribed the eponym, although not all will have the three clinical signs. The condition is caused by a failure of embryological segmentation and may be inherited. Associated abnormalities are shown in Table 82.7, and it is important to note the high incidence of spinal anomalies (Hensinger, 1991).

Investigations and treatment are geared towards the particular problem. Segmental instability above or below the fused segment may cause pain or neurological symptoms requiring surgical treatment.

THE BACK

Back pain in children (Table 82.8)

Back pain in children is far less common than in adults. If persistent for more than a week or two it merits investigation. A study of 100 children with back pain of more than 2 months' duration showed that 84 had clear evidence of underlying skeletal pathology (Hensinger,

1993). The ill-defined musculoligamentous complaints of adults are unusual in children. Careful history and examination will need to be supplemented by radiographic and blood investigations.

Congenital abnormalities of the spine are often pain free. With diastematomyelia the spinal cord may be tethered and lead to pain. The usual presentation is with either orthopaedic problems, e.g. wasting, pes cavus or disturbance of bladder function.

The majority of causes of back pain manifest in later childhood or adolescence and result from insult or developmental disorders (Thompson, 1993).

Infection

Primary osteomyelitis or tuberculosis of the spine is now rare in the developed world. Presentation with pain, with or without systemic and radiographic signs of infection, does not exclude the diagnosis. Standard investigations include a full blood count, ESR and CRP. Isotope scans are helpful in localizing the problem before the plain radiographs show rarefaction of the vertebral body and later changes of sclerosis and new bone formation. The treatment is conservative, involving rest, with or without a body cast, and antibiotics appropriate to the organism. The most likely bacterium

Table 82.7 Features and associations with Klippel–Feil syndrome

System	Incidence (%)	Type of anomaly
Hearing impairment	30	
Genitourinary	30	Unilateral kidney, horseshoe kidney, duplex ureter, pelviureteric obstruction
Cardiopulmonary		Ventricular septal defect, patent ductus arteriosus
Neurological	20	Synkinesia (involuntary paired movements of hands and arms)
Spinal deformity	60	Scoliosis
Facial asymmetry	20	
Sprengel's deformity	25–35	
Upper limb malformations		Supernumary digits, syndactyly, hypoplastic thumb

is *Staphylococcus aureus*, but unusual organisms such as *Salmonella* and *Brucella* may occur. If there is doubt and a failure to respond, CT-guided needle aspiration may be used to make a culture.

Resolution usually occurs within 3 months. A cast or brace may be required, depending on the radiographic appearance. The worst scenario is that of bony collapse,

Table 82.8 Causes of back pain in children

Cause	Result/anomaly
Congenital	Vertebral anomalies Diastematomyelia
Developmental	Scoliosis Kyphosis
Trauma	Acute Stress fracture Osteogenesis imperfecta Non-accidental injury
Mechanical	Instability Disc prolapse Overload Spondylolysis/spondylolisthesis
Infection	Discitis Osteomyelitis
Rheumatic	Juvenile rheumatoid arthritis Ankylosing spondylitis
Metabolic	Juvenile osteoporosis Storage diseases
Neoplastic	Benign Malignant
Psychogenic	

which may lead to a kyphotic deformity. Pressure on the spinal cord is rare but would require surgical decompression.

Discitis

Discitis is a condition which presents similarly to the infections described above, except that systemic symptoms are absent or muted. In this instance the disc space itself is affected. together with the adjacent vertebral endplates. There is debate as to whether this is a primary disc infection, an endplate infection or even an infection at all. One theory is that it is a sterile inflammatory response to trauma.

It usually affects the lumbar spine of children under 10 years of age. Isotope imaging reveals high uptake centred in the disc space and radiographs may show loss of disc height and changes in the endplate. MR is also sensitive to changes in the early stages. Treatment consists of symptomatic measures, as above, and antibiotics. Antibiotic treatment ought to be reserved for those cases with positive culture or to those that fail to respond to symptomatic measures. Treatment lasts for about 3 months and long-term sequelae are unusual.

Trauma

The resultant effect of trauma on the spine depends on the transfer of energy and the ability of the spinal column to absorb it. Therefore abnormalities in its structure such as fused segments and deformity predispose to injury. Likewise, the bone composition affects the outcome, for instance weakness due to osteogenesis imperfecta or storage diseases.

Spondylolysis/spondylolisthesis

Present in 6% of the population, spondylolysis refers to a defect in the bony neural arch, whereas spondylolis-

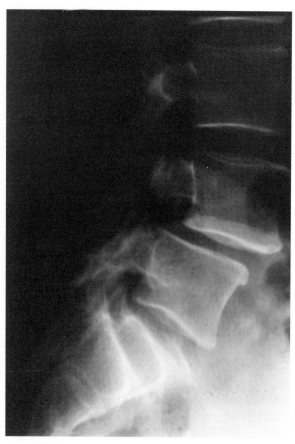

Figure 82.5 Spondylolisthesis: the lateral view of the spine shows a forward translation of the fourth lumbar vertebra upon the fifth of approximately 25% of the vertebral body width.

thesis is the forward displacement of one vertebral body on its lower neighbour. Not surprisingly, the former may lead to the latter, but this is by no means always the case, neither are these conditions invariably symptomatic or require treatment.

An accepted classification is (Wiltse *et al.*, 1976):

- group I: dysplastic (20%)
- group II: isthmic (50%)
- group III: degenerative (25%)
- group IV: traumatic (rare)
- group V: pathological (rare).

The first two groups occur in children and will be discussed. The true traumatic spondylolisthesis is exceptionally rare, as are those caused by metabolic disorders, and will not be discussed.

Pathology

Older texts have described this as a congenital anomaly, but in a review of the literature by Hensinger (1989) only one case report of an infant with spondylolysis was found. There is a familial risk (Wynne-Davies and Scott, 1979). First-degree relatives of patients with the dysplastic form (group I) were found to have an increased risk of having the isthmic type (group II). It is unusual to see it on the radiographs of children under 5 years old and the frequency then rises until the early 20s. The dysplastic group accounts for a minority. In these children there is a malformation of the lumbosacral facet joints, which are unstable and permit a slow forward slip. This may be severe, leading to almost complete translation (spondyloptosis). Related abnormalities, e.g. spina bifida occulta, are often present (94%). The isthmic group has a lytic area in one or both pars interarticularis, most frequently at the lumbosacral junction or the level above (L4/5). This area is believed to be caused by repeated stresses through the weakest part of the neural arch. There is epidemiological evidence to support this as it is more common amongst athletes, notably gymnasts and fast bowlers, who place excessive extension stress on the lumbar spine (Hardcastle *et al.*, 1992). The spondylolysis may elongate, leading to spondylolisthesis. Attempts at repair may generate a mass of tissue around the lesion.

It is more common in boys, but girls often have the severe forms of the disease. The reason for this is unknown.

Clinical presentation

Many adults are seen who have never had symptoms. It is believed that overload from sports, work or trauma initiates symptoms. Symptoms often present at the time of the pubertal growth spurt. Children may be referred with low backache radiating to the back of the thighs with a postural deformity (increased lumbar lordosis). Alteration of the gait due to tight hamstrings is another presenting feature. Only a minority of affected children become symptomatic but will present in early adulthood.

Neurological symptoms are exceptional even with a pronounced spondylolisthesis. There may be muscle spasm with restriction of straight leg raising. Radiographs may show a lytic area (best seen on oblique views) with or without a slip. The degree of slip is graded from 1 to 4 as a percentage of vertebral body width on the lateral radiograph. CT scanning or MRI may be used if there is any doubt about the diagnosis, or if neurological symptoms are present.

Treatment of spondylolysis

A bone isotope scan is helpful in localizing the lytic area if there is an active repair process, and to differentiate from other pathological lesions such as a discitis or osteomyelitis. The majority of painful spondylolytic lesions in children will settle with rest. In severe cases it may be necessary to operate and bone graft the lysis, with or without internal stabilization.

Treatment of spondylolisthesis

Progressive dysplastic forms will require stabilization and grafting. The isthmic variety may be observed unless it progresses beyond a 50% slip or is symptomatic in spite of conservative treatment.

Scoliosis

Scoliosis presents as a deformity noticed by the parents or through school screening programmes. Usually pain free, the diagnosis follows observation of the deformity.

Pathology

The pathology is unknown, although the mechanics and natural history of the deformity have been extensively studied. The curves have been shown to occur in a triplanar deformity, with a significant rotational component (Dickson and Leatherman, 1990). The rotation distorts the ribs and gives rise to the ugly rib hump. This and the lateral curvature tend to reduce the capacity of the thorax asymmetrically, compromising one lung more than the other with a reduction in vital capacity. In severe deformities pulmonary vascular resistance is increased with the risk of developing cor pulmonare.

Classification

The curves are thoracic, thoracolumbar or lumbar and may be single or double, balanced or unbalanced. Full-length standing posteroanterior films are required to show the deformity, with a similar lateral to reveal any sagittal deformity.

Scoliosis is either postural or structural. Postural scoliosis is a mobile deformity which may occur as a result of muscle imbalance. Postural scoliosis may be abolished by sitting the patient or lying them prone.

Structural scoliosis is not correctable using the above manoeuvres. The principal types are:

- congenital (birth)
- infantile idiopathic (< 3 years; more boys than girls)
- juvenile idiopathic (3–10 years)
- adolescent idiopathic (> l0 years; 90% girls)
- neuromuscular.

The idiopathic type accounts for 80% of patients. The incidence in the population is 1.2% (Kostuik, 1990). The majority are minor curves that require no treatment, but about 2–3 per 1000 children will need some formal treatment.

Congenital: hemivertebrae, fused vertebrae and rib anomalies may lead to scoliosis. Initially there may be no obvious deformity, but as the child grows a deformity may become apparent.

Infantile idiopathic: 90% will spontaneously resolve or remain mild. When prone nursing of infants became popular it was associated with a decreased incidence of idiopathic infantile scoliosis. Recent concerns over the sudden infant death syndrome may reverse this trend. A trial of serial plaster jackets applied under general anaesthetic may produce a satisfactory result, but, those that progress often require surgery.

Juvenile idiopathic: this group has a poor prognosis and bracing or spinal fusion is required to arrest the deformity.

Adolescent idiopathic: this is the largest category and many may be observed or braced. Follow-up to skeletal maturity is important as there is a significant risk at puberty as a proportion progress at a late stage. Adult progression is rare and unpredictable.

Neuromuscular: the following conditions are associated with scoliosis: poliomyelitis, cerebral palsy, syringomyelia, Friedreich's ataxia and other muscular dystrophies, neurofibromatosis and spina bifida. The prognosis and treatment depend on the causation of the scoliosis, but severe cases will require a spinal fusion.

Kyphosis

Kyphotic deformity in childhood may be caused by a number of conditions:

- poor posture
- neuromuscular weakness
- congenital vertebral anomalies
- collapse of one or more vertebral bodies: infection, neoplasia, eosinophilic granuloma, juvenile osteoporosis, osteogenesis imperfecta, collagen disorders
- Scheuermann's disease.

Scheuermann's disease

This is a growth disorder of unknown aetiology which Scheuermann described in 1920. It principally affects the developing thoracic vertebrae leading to a structural kyphotic deformity, which by definition must show at least three adjacent vertebral bodies wedged anteriorly by 5°.

Pathology

The aetiology is unknown. A number of observations have been made of the affected patients, who are taller than average and have an advanced skeletal age. Girls are affected twice as often as boys. Levels of growth hormone are increased. A familial factor occurs, as well as an association with hypovitaminosis and a low calcium diet. Histological examination of the endplates has shown non-specific abnormalities in the bone architecture. No hypothesis has been able to correlate these findings, but the pathology is not a simple growth failure of the vertebral body ring apophysis (Lowe, 1990).

The wedging affects a varying number of vertebrae and Schmorl's nodes may be visible on lateral radiographs (small herniations of the disc through the endplate).

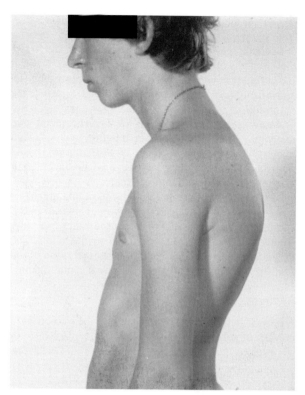

Figure 82.6 Scheuermann's disease: the resulting thoracic kyphosis producing a round shouldered posture.

Clinical presentation

The deformity begins in adolescence, often with the parents first noticing a round-shouldered posture and development of back pain related to activity. Symptoms settle after growth has finished, but severe kyphosis will result in long-term pain from secondary degenerative changes. On examination, the hump may be associated with a mild scoliosis (30%).

Treatment

Minor curves which are asymptomatic simply require review. Symptomatic Scheuermann's is treated empirically with rest from provocative activities, physiotherapy and braces if persistently painful. When curvature exceeds 45° many surgeons would advocate the use of extension braces to prevent deterioration. Surgical fusion and/or correction is occasionally necessary in adolescence for severe curves exceeding 70°.

THE UPPER LIMB

Children present with a variety of uncommon congenital upper limb deformities (Table 82.9), but relatively few require orthopaedic treatment. Most of the deformities are exceptionally rare and will not be discussed in any detail.

Sprengel's shoulder

Sprengel described congenital elevation of the scapula in 1891. The scapula is hypoplastic and misshapen, and lies in an elevated position. In about one-third the scapula articulates superiorly with the cervical spine. It is often associated with Klippel–Feil abnormalities of the cervical spine and ribs.

Initially the deformity does not cause any symptoms, but as the child grows the shoulder movements are restricted. There is a wide spectrum and the mild cases require no treatment, but the more severe cases cause a cosmetic problem and have a functional deficit.

Surgical treatment to bring the scapula down to a more normal position involves extensive muscle releases and reattachments, which should only be performed when the child is more than about 3 years old.

Congenital dislocation of the head of the radius

This may not be apparent until the child is a few years old and it is noticed that there is restriction of forearm rotation. Radiographs show a dislocated radial head with an abnormally long shaft and a bowed ulnar. The condition may be familial. Despite the deformity the child adapts with little functional disability and surgical treatment is to be avoided.

Congenital radioulnar synostosis

This is a bony connection between the proximal ends of the radius and ulnar which usually fixes the forearm in a pronated position. There are different forms with varying abnormalities in the shape of the bones, and there may be associated anomalies of the digits. Surgery is of dubious efficacy and if left untreated function may be satisfactory.

Table 82.9 Congenital anomalies of the upper limb

Site	Anomaly
Shoulder	Sprengel's shoulder (Klippel–Feil) Pseudoarthrosis of clavicle
Elbow	Dislocation of radial head Radioulnar synostosis
Forearm and wrist	Radial club hand Madelung's deformity Ulnar club hand Distal ulnar dysplasia Carpal abnormalities or fusions Ulnar dimelia
Hand	Congenital amputations Finger abnormalities Supernumery digits Hypoplastic digits Lobster claw hand Syndactyly

Congenital pseudoarthrosis

This rare condition may occur in any of the upper limb long bones and is associated with neurofibromatosis. The bone has a radiolucent area and may lead to progressive deformity. Internal fixation with bone grafting is required.

Radial club hand

This is now included under the heading of radial dysplasia, since it is the worst of a range of congenital anomalies resulting from degrees of hypoplasia of the preaxial border of the forearm, including the radius, carpal bones and the thumb. Part or all of these bones may be absent. True radial club hand occurs 1 in 30 000, is bilateral in 50% and is obvious at birth. The hand is held in marked radial deviation and the thumb is absent. It is found in association with the Holt–Oram, Fanconi, Vater and thrombocytopenia–radial–dysplasia syndromes. The treatment is difficult. The child may adapt surprisingly well without treatment and obtain good function.

ULNAR CLUB HAND

This is the mirror image condition of radial club hand, with the postaxial elements of the forearm affected. The principal problems relate to the wide variety of hand deformities that are part of the condition and dictate the role of surgery. It is associated with the Cornelia de Lange and Pillay syndromes, mesomelic dwarfism and Weyer's oligodactyly.

MADELUNG'S DEFORMITY

This deformity is a volar and ulnar subluxation of the carpus on the wrist. It may be congenital or acquired:

- congenital:
  idiopathic (autosomal dominant 50% penetrance)
  Leri–Weill syndrome
  Turner's syndrome
  multiple epiphyseal dysplasia
  achondroplasia
  mucopolysaccharidoses
- acquired:
  post-traumatic
  Ollier's disease
  infection
  multiple exostoses.

Surgical correction of the deformity is reserved for severe cases, or those with pain. Any pre-existing cause is treated initially, followed by osteotomy or excision of the distal ulnar and wrist arthrodesis.

Ulnar dimelia

In this anomaly the thumb is missing and there are accessory fingers which are duplicated, hence the term mirror hand. The forearm contains two ulnae and no radius. Wrist arthrodesis may be required.

THE HIP AND PELVIS

Of all joints in the child, the hip appears to suffer more pathology than any other. It is by no means clear what the developmental, anatomical and mechanical conditions are that render it so vulnerable, but the consequences are that not only does it constitute a significant proportion of the workload in children's orthopaedics, but it probably generates a large part of the adult osteoarthritic population (Solomon, 1976). This section deals initially with developmental dysplasia of the hip and then concentrates on painful hip conditions and their differential diagnosis.

Developmental dysplasia of the hip

Developmental dysplasia of the hip (DDH) is increasingly replacing the former term congenital dislocation of the hip (CDH), following the observation that hips which are clinically reduced in the newborn may later present dislocated. The term DDH is widely used, since it was argued that part of the disease spectrum evolved in childhood rather than being apparent at birth (Klisic, 1989). This refers to the dysplastic hip that never dislocates, but may cause symptoms early in life, due to instability and early degenerative changes. The exact cause is unknown but it is probably multifactorial. This is supported by many associated risk factors (Table 82.10).

Early detection and treatment is essential in order to minimize the resultant dysplasia. The aim is to bring about a stable, concentric reduction of the femoral head in the acetabulum as soon as possible, since this will

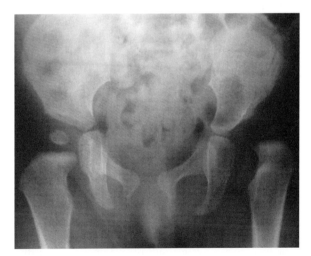

Figure 82.7 Pelvic radiograph of a 'late presenting' dislocation of the left hip in a thirteen month old child. The ossific nucleus on the affected side is delayed and the femur displaced cephalad and laterally. The acetabulum is significantly underdeveloped compared to the right.

Table 82.10 Risk factors associated with developmental dysplasia of the hip

- First-born child (50% of cases)
- Female (75% of cases)
- Family history
- Twins
- Racial differences (rare in Negroes)
- Breech birth
- Oligohydramnios
- Pre-eclampsia
- Foot deformity
- Spinal deformity
- Plagiocephaly
- Caesarian section
- Neonatal special care

influence the development of both the femoral head and the acetabulum. Although this has been understood for many years, the relationship is unclear and has led to the introduction of screening programmes.

Pathology

The hip may appear morphologically normal at birth. Those that are subluxed or dislocated may have a lax capsule, an infolded limbus and an hypertrophied ligamentum teres. If untreated, during infancy adaptive changes begin to occur due to the abnormal mechanics of the unstable or dislocated joint. The femoral head dislocates posteriorly and is pulled into a superolateral position by muscle action. The capsule elongates and may develop an hour-glass constriction, which prevents closed reduction. The femoral head may remain normal early in life, apart from delay in appearance of the ossification centre. The acetabulum remains shallow and is anteverted. If the child is not treated prior to weightbearing these changes consolidate and a false acetabulum develops. The hip abductors shorten and are unable to function normally. This may permit the child to walk, although there may be delay and an altered gait. In the long term, the false joint suffers a premature degeneration with pain and disability from the third decade onwards.

Clinical presentation

Developmental dysplasia of the hip may present at four different periods: newborn, infancy, early walking and adult. In the newborn the diagnosis may be made as a result of the standard birth examination or neonatal screening. The infant may later present following the 3-month check or as a result of maternal concern that the hip fails to abduct as far as the other when changing nappies or is 'clicky'. There may be asymmetric skin creases in the thigh or a delay in walking. These signs are less obvious in the child with bilateral DDH. Once walking, the gait is abnormal owing to a discrepancy in leg length or altered abductor function. This may not be noticed until the child is 2 or more years old. Later, problems manifest in adult life secondary to degenerative changes which cause pain.

Screening

DDH is one of the more common deformities at birth and potentially crippling. In all but the rare teratologic forms, there is a clear window of opportunity to treat it successfully if diagnosed in the first few months of life. Screening was instigated to achieve an early diagnosis and has now been widely adopted. This is based on a clinical examination in which the flexed hip is abducted and felt to reduce (Ortolani's test) or the flexed femur is held and gently pistoned in and out of the acetabulum (Barlow's test) (Ortolani, 1937; Klisic, 1989). Criticisms of this approach concern the inaccuracy of the examination and that injudicious examination might harm an unstable hip. Radiographs are not a satisfactory alternative as the normal femoral head ossific nucleus does not appear until the child is 6–9 months old (Lowett and Morse 1892). In recent years the use of ultrasound has been widely investigated because of its sensitivity and ability to demonstrate the dynamics of the abnormal hip (Graf, 1984; Clarke *et al.*, 1985).

Attempts have been made to develop targeted screening of at-risk children using ultrasound (Table 82.10), which may amount to some 10% of the population. Screening programmes, though, have not eliminated the tragic few children who inexplicably present late on walking (Boeree and Clarke, 1994). A further difficulty is that the sensitivity of ultrasound in detecting mild dysplasia and instability leads to overdiagnosis and treatment of hips that might have spontaneously resolved. This is supported by the marked variation in treatment rates between similar populations in different centres (from 4 per 1000 to more than 20 per 1000). This may be reduced by delaying the examination until the baby is 2–3 weeks old. It has not yet been convincingly proven that ultrasound screening programmes are significantly superior to clinically based ones (Catterall, 1994).

Treatment

The aim of treatment is to bring about a stable, concentric reduction of the affected hip as early in the child's life as possible in order to maximize the potential for normal morphological development. Set against this is the risk of avascular necrosis of the femoral head. Surgical treatment is related to the age of the child. Neonates noted to have unstable or frankly dislocating hips are initially treated by double nappies in order to promote abduction, which is the posture most likely to maintain reduction of the hip. A certain number will stabilize spontaneously in the first few weeks. One explanation is that there is increased laxity at birth due to the effects of maternal relaxin, which then resolves.

In the first month these children are assessed by a biplanar, dynamic ultrasound in order to assess the position of the femoral head, stability and the depth of the acetabulum. Unstable or dysplastic hips are treated in a Pavlik harness, which abducts, flexes and externally rotates the hips.

A small proportion of cases either never reduce or fail to stabilize. In these children a dynamic arthrogram is performed to see whether the hip is reducible. In some a closed reduction is possible, following traction and adductor release, and to maintain the position in a plaster spica followed by abduction splints. Where a concentric closed reduction is not possible then an open reduction and capsular reefing using an anterior approach is performed, followed by plaster splintage. The results are satisfactory in over two-thirds of patients. In some the acetabulum will fail to develop or subluxation recurs. In these cases a stabilizing procedure, such as a Salter pelvic osteotomy, is required to reorientate the acetabulum (Salter, 1961).

Acetabular dysplasia

The acetabulum forms from the ilium, the pubis and the ischium. This conjunction is the triradiate cartilage which lies in its floor. This complex arrangement has to develop in a co-ordinated fashion in order to fit the femoral epiphysis. This congruence is known to be influenced by both the juxtaposition of the femoral head and mechanical factors acting on the joint. Dysplasia occurs when the relationship of the femoral head and the acetabulum is disturbed by malposition, incongruence or insufficiency. The most common causes are congenital dislocations or subluxations. A second group of patients exists with dysplasia who present in late childhood or early in adult life.

Failure of acetabular–femoral congruence may be caused by acquired conditions such as avascular necrosis as well as genetic and developmental disorders. It is classified into aspherical congruence (e.g. Perthes'), aspherical incongruence (e.g. late Perthes', avascular necrosis) and spherical incongruence (e.g. neuromuscular disease) (Staheli, 1990). When surgery is planned it is important to determine which type of dysplasia is present. Arthrography is indicated, which has the advantage of providing a dynamic visualization of the abnormal joint mechanics. Different types of pelvic osteotomies have been described to correct acetabular dysplasia.

The painful hip in childhood

Children often present with pain in the hip or a limp without a history of trauma. In the majority no specific cause will be identified (Table 82.11) and the diagnosis

Table 82.11   Causes of a painful hip in children

Cause	Differential diagnosis
Infection	Septic arthritis Osteomyelitis of femur and pelvis
Rheumatic disease	Juvenile rhematoid arthritis Seronegative arthropathy Viral arthralgia, e.g varicella, measles Idiopathic chondrolysis
Trauma	Fracture Soft tissue, e.g. avulsion rectus femoris Non-accidental injury
Slipped femoral epiphysis	
Neoplasia	Benign: bone cysts, fibrous dysplasia, osteoid osteoma, granuloma, eosinophilic granuloma Malignant: Ewing's sarcoma, metastasis
Dysplasia	Instability Neuromuscular subluxation
Avascular necrosis	Perthes' disease Sickle-cell disease
Haemophilia	
Irritable hip	

of irritable hip (transient synovitis) will be made. It is essential to exclude septic arthritis, osteomyelitis or a slipped epiphysis.

Pain from hip pathology may be referred to the knee. Toddlers are often unable to localize their pain and can be difficult to examine. A careful examination from foot to abdomen usually reveals the affected part by a combination of local tenderness or restriction of joint movement compared with the unaffected side. The abdomen must be palpated since movement of the hip may irritate inflamed pelvic peritoneum and cause groin pain. Inguinal herniae and lymphadenopathy in the groin may masquerade as hip pain. Investigations such as radiographs of the limb (two plane views for the hip) and blood tests, e.g. ESR and FBC, act as a baseline screen before undertaking specific imaging and serological investigations. Isotope scans are particularly helpful in the young limping child whose history and examination are inconclusive.

Irritable hip

Irritable hip is a diagnosis of exclusion first recognized in 1892 (Lovett and Morse, 1892). It represents a group of pathologies which evade specific diagnosis, but by definition have a good outcome. There have been two long-term follow-up studies which have reported an incidence of late, mild coxa magna, but neither related this to pathological consequences (de Valderrama, 1963; Nachemson and Scheller, 1969). Several other series have described this condition (Hauesien *et al.*, 1986; Taylor and Clarke, 1994).

Clinical presentation

There is an acute history of pain and limp which increases in severity over 2–4 days. Occasionally the child may wake up with severe symptoms and refuses to walk. There is muscle spasm with loss of internal rotation and abduction, and fixed flexion in the more severe cases. Over one-third will have a low-grade pyrexia and a raised ESR. Tenderness over the hip joint or the adjacent pelvis should be sought, as the latter may be the only physical sign of osteomyelitis in the pelvis. The clinical features in an audit of 509 consecutive admissions are shown in Table 82.12 (Taylor and Clarke, 1994).

Table 82.12   Features of irritable hip

Male:female ratio	2.25:1
Mean age	5.8 years
Side affected	Equal
Duration of symptoms	4.1 days
Prior to presentation	
Recurrence rate	14.8%

Pathology

Ultrasound studies have shown that two-thirds of children with an irritable hip have an effusion. Aspirations of the effusions have not shown organisms or specific biochemical markers of disease, only non-specific inflammatory exudate and synovium (Wingstrand, 1986). The effusion probably causes the pain (Erken and Katz, 1990). The capsule is in its most lax position when the hip is flexed and externally rotated, and this is the way children prefer to lie. Isotope imaging of consecutive patients has produced consistent patterns of isotope uptake, including generalized synovitis, occult ischaemic segments in the epiphysis, extracapsular damage and normal images (Wingstrand, 1986).

Treatment

The patient may require admission for investigation and treatment of symptoms. It is essential to exclude sepsis which, in the severe case of irritable hip, may need emergency aspiration or capsulotomy. This is an unusual situation, but is a course which must be pursued, since the results of septic arthritis are rapid and devastating. In the majority, simple bed rest with or without traction and anti-inflammatory drugs for a few days is are all that is needed.

Although it has been suggested that irritable hip may precede Perthes' disease, or the effusion may even give rise to this condition, there is no real evidence for this, even in children who have experienced more than one episode of irritable hip (Taylor and Clarke, 1995). Different series have quoted an incidence of Perthes' disease following irritable hip, ranging from 1% to 17% (Jacobs, 1971; Hauesien *et al.*, 1986; Taylor and Clarke, 1994).

Legg–Calvé–Perthes' disease

Perthes' disease is an uncommon condition in which one or both femoral epiphyses undergo a varying degree of avascular necrosis. The end result depends on the extent to which the femoral head is involved and the age at presentation. Epidemiological studies have shown an incidence of between 1 and 1.5 in 10 000 (Wynne-Davies and Gormley, 1978). Genetic and environmental factors play an aetiological role and are shown in Table 82.13. There is no predictive investigation or treatment available. The genetic component has been the subject of conflicting reports, but recently a multifactorial inheritance pattern for Perthes' disease has been reported (Jacobs, 1971; Hall, 1985).

Pathology

The pathological changes may be divided into three stages:

* ischaemia: radiographically normal or widened joint space

- revascularization: sclerosis and fragmentation, metaphyseal resorption
- remodelling: coxa magna/coxa plana.

The causes of the ischaemic change are unknown, but the inflammatory reaction affects the whole joint, with thickening and oedema of the synovium, capsule and ligamentum teres. An effusion is common. In the weeks following infarction revascularization occurs with the deposition of new bone and patchy resorption, which explains the radiographic changes of sclerosis and fragmentation. Hyperaemia of the metaphysis may lead to rarefaction, resulting in metaphyseal cysts. Deformation and remodelling may distort the epiphysis in the worst cases to produce the flattened, extruded coxa plana deformity, whereas mild cases may heal with normal anatomy, save a degree of coxa magna (Wenger *et al.*, 1991).

Clinical presentation

Children usually present between 4 and 8 years of age with a history of limp and low-grade pain in the hip or knee. A comparison of children presenting with Perthes' disease against those with irritable hip showed that the mean duration of symptoms prior to admission was 3.4 months compared to 4 days (Taylor and Clarke, 1994). On examination there may be spasm, but seldom tenderness. The diagnosis is confirmed by radiographs.

The portion of bone that dies is variable in size. Isotope scans of children with painful hips have revealed a small population who show an ischaemic segment but do not progress to bone death and the radiological

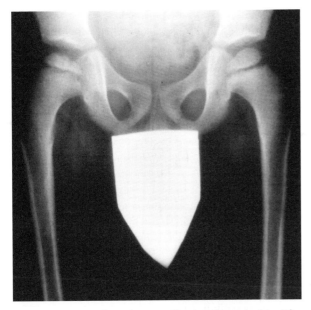

Figure 82.8 Perthes' disease affecting the right hip. The ossific nucleus is flattened and irregular with a sclerotic appearance and apparent widening of the joint space.

Table 82.13 Factors associated with Perthes' disease

Factor	
Male:female ratio	4:1 (7:1 in bilateral)
Racial	Rare in Negroes and Chinese
Geographical	More common in urban population
Environmental	More common in lower socio-economic groups
Low birth weight	
Genetic	Evidence of delayed bone age Herniae and genitourinary abnormalities (4%) Disproportionate growth, small feet and trunk

characteristics of Perthes' disease (Royle and Galasko, 1992), suggesting that there may be a proportion of children who are subclinically affected.

Grading

The severity of the epiphyseal involvement is related to the outcome (Catterall, 1971). The reliability of these signs is open to question (Christensen *et al.*, 1986) as some cases may change grade in the course of the disease. Additional head-at-risk signs have been described in order to improve prognostic accuracy, and include:

Clinical:	progressive loss of movement adduction contracture obesity
Radiological:	Gage's sign lateral epiphyseal calcification diffuse metaphyseal change subluxation (break in Shenton's line) horizontal growth plate.

Treatment

The natural history of Perthes' disease has shown that without treatment a large proportion of patients will only have minimal symptoms until the fifth or sixth decades (McAndrew and Weinstein, 1984), but some experience pain and disability as young adults (Clarke and Harrison, 1983). Age at presentation is a significant prognostic indicator, with onset of disease before prior to 6 years being favourable.

As 60% of affected patients will do well without medical intervention, the decision on whether, and how to treat any given child is a problem. The management of Perthes disease involves:

- diagnosis
- symptomatic treatment
- clinical review ('supervised neglect')
- containment: orthotic/operative
- late surgery.

Symptomatic treatment in the acute presentation involves bed rest with or without traction and analgesia. Pain generally settles within days and the child may be mobilized.

'Supervised neglect' is a widely used term to describe the regular radiological and clinical review of children until the Perthes' lesion is healed, thus determining patients with minimal deformity of the cartilaginous anlage. 'Containment' means ensuring that the epiphysis is maximally centred within the acetabulum, thus minimizing deformity. The position that achieves this is abduction and internal rotation. This may be achieved by plaster splintage or an Atlanta brace. This is well tolerated and the child remains active and weightbearing. Recumbency and traction have failed to alter the course of the disease.

An operative means of containment is used if the brace fails or as an alternative method of treatment. The femoral head is contained by a proximal femoral varus osteotomy, or the acetabulum is realigned to achieve the same end by an inominate osteotomy. The results of these differing approaches are not easily comparable, but the general opinion is that containment treatment influences the outcome; however, no method has been established as superior at the present time (Herring, 1994).

Late surgery includes removal of loose bodies and osteotomy to correct hinge abduction. Once osteoarthritis is established the patient must be managed symptomatically until such time as arthroplasty is indicated.

Slipped epiphysis

Slipped capital femoral epiphysis (SCFE) is a displacement of the femoral epiphysis with respect to the metaphysis through the hypertrophic zone of the growth plate (physis). The aetiology is unknown. The largest study in the literature was published from Sweden in 1984 (Hansson *et al.*, 1984), detailing 532 cases between 1910 and 1982 (Table 82.14).

Pathology

The pathological term for SCFE is epiphysiolysis. The result is that the metaphysis externally rotates and translates anteriorly with respect to the epiphysis, which remains in the acetabulum. There is evidence that the mechanical changes may be initiated by hormonal or metabolic anomalies affecting the physis. This distortion of the anatomy may affect the anterior retinacular vessels leading to avascular necrosis. Another complication is that of chondrolysis, with thinning

Table 82.14   Factors associated with a slipped femoral epiphysis

Factor	
Mean age	Boys: 14.4
(years)	Girls: 12.2
Genetics	More common in first-degree relatives (10%)
Hip	Left more commonly affected than right
Anatomy	Decreased angle femoral anteversion
	Obesity
Bilateral	30–50%
Hormonal	Pituitary and thyroid abnormalities

and degeneration of the articular cartilage. This predisposes to early arthritis. When the slip arrests, premature epiphyseal fusion and remodelling occurs and may lead to secondary mechanical problems. A study of osteoarthritic femoral heads removed during arthroplasty suggests that small, clinically occult slips are not uncommon and may cause early osteoarthritis (Solomon, 1976).

Classification

Traditionally, 'slips' have been divided into acute, chronic, and acute on chronic. This is an arbitrary division since it is derived from the history of the patient's symptoms. Whether the mechanical events are proportional to the symptoms has not been established. A preslip state has been proposed in which the child complains of a painful hip in the absence of other pathology.

Clinical presentation

The characteristic clinical picture is of either sudden onset, or intermittent hip or knee pain in an overweight pubertal child. The child limps and may recall an episode of trauma. On examination there is spasm, shortening and external rotation. The diagnosis is confirmed by radiographs.

Treatment

The primary aim of treatment is to prevent any further displacement and preserve the blood supply to the epiphysis. Restoration of the anatomy is a complex problem, since attempts to do so run a high risk of damaging the vascular supply. The safe course is to fix the hip *in situ*, however severe the problem, and then to tackle any subsequent problems after the growth plate has closed. Slips may be divided into:

- mild: less than one-third of the epiphysis on anterior–posteria (AP) view; ≤ 20° tilt on lateral view

- moderate: between one and two-thirds epiphysis on AP view; 20–40° tilt on lateral view
- severe: at least two-thirds epiphysis on AP view; ≥ 40° tilt on lateral view.

In general, the treatment strategy adopted must depend on the degree of the slip, the state of the growth plate and the expertise of the surgeon. The main options are:

- *early surgery:*
  pin the affected side *in situ*
  closed reduction and fixation
  open reduction and fixation
  plaster immobilization *in situ*
  closed reduction and immobilization
- *late surgery:*
  femoral neck osteotomy
  proximal femoral osteotomy
  excision of anterosuperior boss.

Closed reduction has a poor reputation, except possibly in the rare acute traumatic slip, because of the risks of avascular necrosis. Plaster spica immobilization has really been superseded by simple percutaneous methods of pinning. Early open reduction and high cervical osteotomy remain controversial and should be reserved for severe slips treated by the few surgeons who have sufficient experience of the technique. Percutaneous fixation for the mild and moderate slips *in situ* using a single-threaded screw across the physis is the treatment of choice. This must be performed under fluoroscopic guidance. Severe slips are treated by an epiphyseodesis using a bone block placed across the physis, combined with excision of the anterosuperior part of the metaphysis (Heyman *et al.*, 1957). Cervical osteotomy has led to an avascular necrosis rate of 5–20%. This complication may prove disastrous and is almost unknown in untreated severe cases.

The opposite hip

There is a risk of slipped epiphysis in the contralateral hip in 60% of children (Haggland *et al.*, 1988). This event is often separated by months or even years and has led to debate on whether the opposite epiphysis ought to be treated simultaneously or kept under radiographic review, or whether symptons should be relied upon to declare the problem.

THE KNEE

Unlike the hip, the knee causes relatively few problems in early childhood. In adolescence referrals increase with anterior knee pain, which comprises a mixed group of diagnoses. Ligament and meniscal pathology is far less common than in adults. Proximal tibial deformity will be discussed in this section, since such problems present as knock knees or bow legs and are perceived as a knee complaint.

The painful knee in children

With the exception of traumatic events, pain in the knee in the young child is referred pain from the hip until proven otherwise. Normal hip movement and radiographs are required to exclude pathology, unless there are clear signs of knee pathology. The knee is easier to examine than the hip and signs of tenderness and effusion need to be carefully elicited. The differential diagnosis of knee pathology is listed in Table 82.15 (Stanitski, 1993; Jackson, 1994).

Table 82.15 Causes of a painful knee in children

Infection	
Trauma	Ligamentous
	Meniscal
	Fracture
	Osteochondritis dissecans
Rheumatological disease	Juvenile rheumatoid arthritis, Henoch–Schönlein
Neoplasia	
Patellar conditions	Bipartate patellar
	Overuse syndromes (jumper's knee, Sinding–Larsen–Johansson)
	Patellar tracking abnormalities
Osgood–Schlatter apophysitis	
Reflex sympathetic dystrophy	
Plica syndrome	
Haemophilia	
Idiopathic anterior knee pain	

Infection, neoplasia and rheumatological disorders will generally declare themselves following radiographs and standard blood investigations in conjunction with the clinical findings. Further investigations include MRI, diagnostic arthroscopy and isotope scans.

Osgood–Schlatter disease

Pain is localized at the tibial tubercle, which may be enlarged and tender. It occurs in adolescent boys more often than in girls and may be bilateral. The pain is exacerbated by activity. The disease is probably caused by repetitive strain and minor injury to the tubercle. Radiographs sometimes show enlargement and fragmentation of the apophysis. The treatment comprises reassurance and rest from physical activity.

Sinding–Larsen–Johansson disease

In this condition pain and tenderness are located at the unossified junction of the patella and its ligament. It is related to activity and resolves with rest and maturity.

Jumper's knee

This completes the triad of adolescent overload syndromes around the patella. The location of the pain is at the proximal insertion of the quadriceps mechanism into the superior pole of the patella. The treatment is rest.

Multipartite patella

Radiographs of the patella may show a bipartite or multipartite patella due to separate ossification centres that have failed to coalesce. These have been classified by Saupe, with the most frequent form being a lateral segment (75%). Modification of activities is usually sufficient to relieve symptoms. Excision may be successful in the persistent case.

Osteochondritis dissecans of the distal femur

The dissecans lesion is usually a hemispherical segment of the medial femoral condylar surface, which may loosen and become detached. The current view is that it is a stress fracture. MRI reveals an avascular change in the surrounding bone, before it detaches. Clinically there is local tenderness on the condyle (best examined in flexion) and pain on straightening the flexed, medially rotated knee.

The presentation varies from chronic intermittent episodes of pain, to true locking and effusions. The osteocartilaginous segment may remain attached but loose and cause pain that may be relieved by fixation *in situ*. Loose bodies are removed arthroscopically. Large lesions can predispose to secondary degenerative changes in the knee.

Discoid meniscus

Meniscal lesions are uncommon in children. Occasionally, symptoms of clunking and pain may occur suggesting an intra-articular lesion. Meniscal tears may occur in the adolescent and should be treated by arthroscopic repair or excision as appropriate. A discoid lateral meniscus is sometimes found and is believed to be an embryological abnormality. This may require a partial, arthroscopic excision, depending on the symptoms (Dickhaut and DeLee, 1982).

Tibia vara (Blount's disease)

Tibia vara, as the name suggests, is a developmental condition in which the tibia grows into a varus angulation as a result of a growth disturbance at the proximal physis. Bow legs, described by Blount in 1937, are often given his name, as Blount's disease produces a bow-leg deformity. The normal adult knee has a valgus angulation of 5–7°, but this is reached through childhood from an early varus position. Studies of normal development have indicated that the infant varus has usually reversed to a peak valgus position at about 14 months and later reaches the adult position. A range of conditions may give rise to both varus and excessive valgus angulation, with the eponymous Blount's disease reserved for the spontaneous infantile form with otherwise normal bone metabolism. Table 82.16 lists a number of causes of abnormal knee angulation in childhood (Greene, 1993).

This condition is most commonly seen in obese, Negro girls who walk early. A familial trait has been observed. It appears in early childhood and causes considerable parental concern. Histological changes have been found in the medial portion of the proximal tibial physis and in some cases a bridging fibrocartilaginous bar is present. A radiographic classification is described based on a large series and this is widely used to guide treatment (Langenskiold and Riska, 1964). Treatment is required with either a brace in children under 3 years old or proximal osteotomy in older children.

THE FOOT

The foot accounts for a large proportion of the paediatric orthopaedic workload. The common deformities at birth are congenital talipes equinovarus, metatarsus adductus and curly fifth toes. Rarer abnormalities include accessory digits, cleft foot, macrodactyly and hallux varus. These latter anomalies will not be discussed and this section will focus on the more common problems and causes of foot pain. The differential diagnosis for foot pain is seen in Table 82.17 (de Rosa, 1992).

Congenital talipes equinovarus

Congenital talipes equinovarus (CTEV), commonly referred to as club foot, is a congenital deformity of the

Table 82.16 Causes of abnormal knee angulation in children

Trauma	Injury to growth plate
	Bone bar across growth plate
	Ligamentous insufficiency
	Malunited fracture
Metabolic	Rickets
	Osteogenesis imperfecta
Skeletal dysplasia	
Blount's disease	
Focal proximal tibial deficiency	
Multiple exostoses	
Metaphyseal chondroplasia	

foot affecting approximately 1 in 1000 live births. Males are affected two to three times as often as females and 50% are bilateral. There is a spectrum of severity, related to the degree of joint laxity present (Barlow and Clarke, 1994).

Aetiology

Several theories have been proposed which implicate both genetic and intrauterine factors. Intrauterine compression is thought to account for some postural cases, which usually resolve with conservative measures. In others, anatomical variations within the soft tissues or neuromuscular dysfunction contribute. The idea that the

Table 82.17 Causes of painful feet in children

Associated with deformity	Spasmodic flat foot: tarsal coalition
	Flexible flat foot: foot strain
	Pes cavus (metatarsalgia)
	Adolescent bunion
Trauma	Stress fracture
	Foreign body
Inflammatory conditions	Juvenile rheumatoid
	Osteochondritis
	(e.g. Köhler's disease)
	Sever's disease
Infection	
Neoplasia	

bones of the tarsus develop abnormally owing to a primary germ plasm defect and the associated changes in muscles and ligaments are adaptive, is currently popular. A paper in which 16 club feet and 27 normal feet in aborted fetuses were examined histologically demonstrated that the earliest discernible changes occurred in the ligaments, rather than bone (Fukuhara *et al.*, 1994). Talipes may be postural, typical or atypical, the latter occurring with arthrogryposis and myelodysplasia and often proving resistant to treatment.

Pathology

Pathological changes have been identified in both the bones of the tarsus and the soft tissues, including the muscles of the calf. The talus displays a variety of abnormalities, both in its shape and its relationship with the calcaneum. Soft tissue contractures vary in severity and include the posteromedial ligaments, tendons and joint capsules.

Clinical deformities

The entire foot and calf are usually smaller than the unaffected side, with hindfoot equinus and varus. The forefoot is adducted and supinated. Postural cases may be gently corrected on examination, but the remainder exhibit a varying degree of flexibility.

Treatment

The rationale of management is to try to bring about correction of the deformity early in life and permit as normal a development of the skeleton as possible. Initially, manual stretching and strapping may prove adequate, but subsequent manoeuvres may evolve into serial casting, soft tissue releases and finally bony surgery.

Flat foot

Flat feet (pes planus) cause considerable parental anxiety and account for many referrals to orthopaedic clinics. The principal causes are:

- congenital vertical talus
- physiological flat foot
- spasmodic flat foot
- neuromuscular
- collagen disorders.

Congenital vertical talus

Congenital vertical talus is usually identified at birth, whereas other types of flat feet are not apparent until the child begins to walk. The deformity is severe, with the talus abnormal in both its shape and its relationships with the other bones of the hindfoot. The dislocated head of the talus is palpable as a rounded prominence in the medial plantar aspect of the foot. Both it and the calcaneum assume an equinus position and the forefoot dorsiflexes at the mid-tarsus, hence the term 'rocker-bottom foot'. If left untreated secondary changes occur with growth and the resultant foot is deformed, rigid and uncomfortable with weight borne on the middle of the sole. The treatment is surgical since it cannot be corrected conservatively and any gains from non-operative measures are usually lost as deformity recurs with growth.

Physiological flat foot

Physiological flat foot is common and causes the child no specific problem. The toddler's foot is flexible and plump, so that on weightbearing the medial arch collapses. Clinically, the arch may be restored by passively dorsiflexing the big toe or asking the child to stand on tiptoe. These manoeuvres demonstrate that the 'deformity' is mobile and correctable.

Spasmodic flat foot

This category encompasses a variety of painful conditions, usually affecting the older child or adolescent, in which the foot adopts an everted position with a valgus heel, due to peroneal spasm, rather than a true flattening of the arch. Causes include tarsal coalitions, other anatomical abnormalities and inflammatory conditions. Tarsal coalitions may be complete or incomplete. Some have a fibrous component and where radiographs fail to establish the diagnosis MRI may be helpful. Talonavicular and talocalcaneal bars are the most common. In most cases a period of splintage may bring relief, but occasionally surgical excision of the bar is necessary.

Metatarsus adductus (primary metatarsus varus)

This is one of the most common foot deformities. The forefoot is adducted and generally sufficiently flexible to be manually correctable, while the hindfoot is normal. The mild case may be left and the parents reassured that normal shoewear and growth will prevent any progression and probably lead to improvement. The more severe case may be treated by gentle stretching and strapping, serial plaster casts and rarely surgery.

Pes cavus

Pes cavus (cavo-varus) describes a foot with a higher than normal arch and instep and is usually associated with clawing of the toes. The aetiology may be divided into three types: neurological, idiopathic and post talipes. In the first category, recognizable conditions such as Charcot–Marie–Tooth and Friedreich's ataxia create a muscular imbalance that results in the deformity. It is important to be sure that there is no identifiable lesion such as a spinal tumour in children who suddenly present with a progressive cavus deformity. The idiopathic group shows abnormal EMG patterns, but they cannot be identified as part of any syndrome. Some patients have a family history suggesting a genetic predisposition. The final group includes patients with residual or relapsing deformity following treatment for CTEV.

Unless treated, cavo-varus tends to progress and the plantar fascia and small muscles of the foot develop secondary contractures. Progressive clawing of the toes leads to increased metatarsal head loading with migration of the fibrofatty pad, subsequent metatarsalgia and painful callosities on the dorsum of the proximal interphalangeal joints. The calcaneum assumes a varus position. In the young child the joints will be flexible, and muscle–tendon rebalancing and plantar release may improve foot posture and retard progression of deformity. Later bony surgery may be required to reshape the tarsus and realign the calcaneum into valgus (Coleman, 1992).

Curly toes

Curly toes are widespread in children and often lead to a consultation. Parents should be reassured that they rarely cause problems and are best left alone. Where there is undue deformity, flexor tenotomy is a safe and useful procedure (Ross and Menelaus, 1984). In situations where the fifth toe overrides then it may be necessary to advise early surgery. The toe may be repositioned by a soft tissue procedure (e.g. V-Y-plasty of the fifth toe) and will then develop in normal alignment.

Hallux valgus

Predisposition to this deformity may be apparent in the school-age child with a broad foot due to metatarsus primum varus. It is unusual to perform a corrective osteotomy of the first metatarsal in this age group. Reassurance and broad-fitting shoes should manage the immediate problem and surgery is postponed until adulthood.

Köhler's disease (osteochondritis of the navicular bone)

This condition presents as a painful foot. There is tenderness and thickening over the instep and radiographs reveal a collapsed and dense navicular bone. The symptoms are controlled by rest and sometimes splintage is necessary. The osteochondritis usually recovers. The clinical end result is good, although the radiographs remain abnormal.

References

Akerman, M., Rydholm, A. and Persson, B.M. 1985: Aspiration cytology of soft-tissue tumors. The 10-year experience at an Orthopaedic Oncology Center. *Acta Orthopedica Scandinavica* **56**, 407–21.

Barlow, I.W. and Clarke, N.M.P. 1994: Congenital talipes equinovarus. *Surgery* **11**, 211–15.

Barlow, T.G. 1962: Early diagnosis and treatment of congenital dislocation of the hip. *Journal of Bone and Joint Surgery* **44B**, 292–301.

Boeree, N.R. and Clarke, N.M.P. 1994: Ultrasound imaging and secondary screening for congenital dislocation of the hip. *Journal of Bone and Joint Surgery* **76B**, 525–33.

Catterall, A. 1971: The natural history of Perthes' disease. *Journal of Bone and Joint Surgery* **53B**, 37–53.

Catterall, A. 1994: The early diagnosis of congenital dislocation of the hip [Editorial]. *Journal of Bone and Joint Surgery* **76B**, 515–16.

Christensen, F., Soballe, K., Ejested, R. and Luxhoj, T. 1986: The Catterall classification of Perthes' disease: an assessment of reliability. *Journal of Bone and Joint Surgery* **68B**, 614–15.

Clarke, N.M.P. and Harrison, M.H.M. 1983: Painful sequelae of coxa plana. *Journal of Bone and Joint Surgery* **65A**, 13–18.

Clarke, N.M.P., Harcke, H.T., McHugh, P. *et al.* 1985: Real-time ultrasound in the diagnosis of congenital dislocation and dysplasia of the hip. *Journal of Bone and Joint Surgery* **67B**, 406–12.

Cole, W.G., Dalziel, R.E. and Leith, S. 1972: Treatment of acute osteomyelitis in childhood. *Journal of Bone and Joint Surgery* **64B**, 218–23.

Coleman, S.S. 1992: Pes cavus. *Current Orthopaedics* **6**, 81–7.

Dickhaut, S.C. and DeLee, J.C. 1982: The discoid lateral meniscus syndrome. *Journal of Bone and Joint Surgery* **64-A**, 1068–73.

Dickson, R.A. and Leatherman, K.D. 1990: *Spinal deformities*. In Dickson, R.A. (ed.), *Spinal surgery: science and practice*. London: Butterworths, 388–99.

Erken, E.H.W. and Katz, K. 1990: Irritable hip and Perthes' disease. *Journal of Pediatric Orthopaedics* **10**, 322–6.

Filla, A., DeMichele, G., Caruso, G. *et al.* 1990: Genetic data and natural history of Friedreich's disease; a study of 80 Italian patients. *Journal of Neurology* **237**, 345–51.

Fukuhara, K., Schmollmeier, G. and Uhthoff, H.K. 1994: The pathogenesis of club foot. *Journal of Bone and Joint Surgery* **76B**, 450–7.

Graf, R. 1984: Fundamentals of sonographic diagnosis of infant hip dysplasia. *Journal of Pediatric Orthopaedics* **4**, 735–40.

Greene, W.B. 1993: Infantile tibia vara. *Journal of Bone and Joint Surgery* **75A**, 130–43.

Hagglund, G., Hansson, L.I., Ordeberg, G. and Sandstrom, S. 1988: Bilaterality in slipped upper femoral epiphysis. *Journal of Bone and Joint Surgery* **70B**, 179–81.

Hall, D.J. 1985: Genetic aspects of Perthes' disease: a critical review. *Clinical Orthopaedics* **209**, 100–14.

Hansson, L.I., Hagglund, G. and Ordeberg, G. 1984: Slipped capital femoral epiphysis in southern Sweden 1910–1982. *Clinical Orthopaedics* **191**, 82–94.

Hardcastle, P., Annear, P., Forster, D.H. *et al.* 1992: Spinal abnormalities in young fast bowlers. *Journal of Bone and Joint Surgery* **74B**, 421–5.

Harding, A.E. 1981: Friedreich's ataxia: a clinical and genetic study of 90 families with an analysis of early diagnostic criteria and intrafamilial clustering of clinical features. *Brain* **104**, 598–620.

Hauesien, D.C., Weiner, D.S. and Weiner, S.D. 1986: The characterisation of 'transient synovitis of the hip' in children. *Journal of Paediatric Orthopaedics* **6**, 11–17.

Hensinger, R.N. 1985: Back pain in children. In Bradford, D.S. and Hensinger, R.N. (eds), *The pediatric spine*. New York: Thieme, 41–60.

Hensinger, R.N. 1985: Congenital abnormalities of the cervical spine. *Clinical Orthopaedics* **264**, 16–38.

Hensinger, R.N. 1989: Current concepts review: spondylolysis and spondylolisthesis in children and adolescents. *Journal of Bone and Joint Surgery* **71A**, 1098–107.

Herring, J.A. 1994: Current concepts review: the treatment of Legg–Calvé–Perthes' disease. *Journal of Bone and Joint Surgery* **76A**, 448–58.

Heyman, C.H., Herndon, C.H. and Strong, J.M. 1957: Slipped femoral epiphysis with severe displacement. *Journal of Bone and Joint Surgery* **39A**, 293–303.

Jackson, A.M. 1994: Anterior knee pain. *Current Orthopaedics* **8**, 83–93.

Jacobs, B.W. 1971: Synovitis of the hip in children and its significance. *Pediatrics* **47**, 558–66.

Jones, N.S., Anderson, D.J. and Stiles, P.J. 1969: Osteomyelitis in a general hospital: a five-year study showing an increase in subacute osteomyelitis. *Journal of Bone and Joint Surgery* **69B**, 779–83.

Klisic, P.J. 1989: Congenital dislocation of the hip: a misleading term. *Journal of Bone and Joint Surgery* **71B**, 136.

Kostuik, J.P. 1990: Current concepts review: operative treatment of idiopathic scoliosis. *Journal of Bone and Joint Surgery* **72A**, 1108–13.

Langenskiold, A. and Riska, E.B. 1964: Tibia vara (osteochondrosis deformans tibiae): a survey of 71 cases. *Journal of Bone and Joint Surgery* **46A**, 1405–20.

Lovett, R.W. and Morse, J.L. 1892: A transient or ephemeral form of hip disease, with a report of cases. *Boston Medical Surgery Journal* **127**, 161.

Lowe, T.G. 1990: Current concepts review: Scheuermann disease. *Journal of Bone and Joint Surgery* **72A**, 940–5.

McAndrew, M.P. and Weinstein, S.L. 1984: A long-term follow-up of Legg–Calvé–Perthes' disease. *Journal of Bone and Joint Surgery* **66A**, 860–9.

Mercuri, M., Capanna, R., Manfrini, M. *et al.* 1991: The management of malignant bone tumors in children and adolescents. *Clinical Orthopaedics* **264**, 156–8.

Mollan, R.A.B. and Piggot, J. 1977: Acute osteomyelitis in children. *Journal of Bone and Joint Surgery* **59B**, 2–7.

Nachemson, A. and Scheller, S. 1969: A clinical and radiological follow-up study of transient synovitis of the hip. *Acta Orthopedica Scandinavica* **40**, 478–500.

Ortolani, M. 1937: Un sego poco e sua importanza per la diagnosi precore di prelussazione conenita del'anca. *Pediatrica* **45**, 129–36.

Patterson, D.C. 1970: Acute suppurative arthritis in infancy and childhood. *Journal of Bone and Joint Surgery* **52B**, 474–82.

Petterson, H. and Theander, G. 1978: Ossification of the femoral head in infancy. *Acta Radiologica Diagnosis* **20**, 170–8.

Phillips, W.A., Hensinger, R.N. and Arbor, A. 1989: The management of rotatory atlanto-axial subluxation in children. *Journal of Bone and Joint Surgery* **71A**, 664–8.

Pueschel, S.M. and Scola, F.H. 1987: Atlanto-axial instability in individuals with Down's syndrome: epidemiologic, radiographic and clinical studies. *Pediatrics* **80**, 555–60.

Rosa, P. de 1992: Pain in the foot in childhood. *Current Orthopaedics* **6**, 88–97.

Ross, E.R.S. and Menelaus, M.B. 1984: Open flexor tenotomy for hammer toes and curly toes in childhood. *Journal of Bone and Joint Surgery* **66B**, 770–1.

Royle, S.G. and Galasko, C.S.B. 1992: The irritable hip. Scintigraphy in 192 children. *Acta Orthopedica Scandinavica* **63**, 25–8.

Salter, R.B. 1961: Innominate osteotomy in the treatment of congenital dislocation and subluxation of the hip. *Journal of Bone and Joint Surgery* **43B**, 518–39.

Solomon, L. 1976: Patterns of osteoarthritis of the hip. *Journal of Bone and Joint Surgery* **58B**, 176–83.

Staheli, L.T. 1990: Surgical management of acetabular dysplasia. *Clinical Orthopaedics* **264**, 111–21.

Stanitski, C.L. 1993: Anterior knee pain in the adolescent. *Journal of Bone and Joint Surgery* **75A**, 1407–16.

Taylor, G.R. and Clarke, N.M.P. 1994: Management of irritable hip: a review of hospital admission policy. *Archives of Disease in Childhood* **71**, 59–63.

Taylor, G.R. and Clarke, N.M.P. 1995: Recurrent irritable hip in childhood. *Journal of Bone and Joint Surgery* **77B**, 748–51.

Thompson, G.H. 1993: Back pain in children. *Journal of Bone and Joint Surgery* **75A**, 928–38.

Valderrama, J.A. de 1963: The 'observation hip' syndrome and its late sequelae. *Journal of Bone and Joint Surgery* **45B**, 462–70.

Wenger, D.R., Ward, T. and Herring, J.A. 1991: Current concepts review: Legg–Calve–Perthes' disease. *Journal of Bone and Joint Surgery* **73A**, 778–88.

Wiltse, L.L., Newman, P.H. and McNab, I. 1976: Classification of spondylosis and spondylolisthesis. *Clinical Orthopaedics* **117**, 23–9.

Wingstrand, H. 1986: Transient synovitis of the hip in the child. *Acta Orthopedica Scandinavica* **57** (Suppl. 219), 5–61.

Wynne-Davies, R. and Gormley, J. 1978: The aetiology of Perthes' disease. Genetic, epidemiological and growth factors in 310 Edinburgh and Glasgow patients. *Journal of Bone and Joint Surgery* **60B**, 6–14.

Wynne-Davies, R. and Scott, J.H.S. 1979: Inheritance and spondylolisthesis: a radiographic family survey. *Journal of Bone and Joint Surgery* **61B**, 301–5.

Ziv, I., Blackburn, N., Rang, M. and Korerska, J. 1984: Muscle growth in normal and spastic mice. *Developmental Medicin and Child Neurology* **26**, 94–9.

Further reading

Apley, A.G. and Solomon, L. 1993: *System of orthopaedics and fractures*, 7th ed. London: Butterworth Heinneman.

Bennett, G.C. 1987: *Paediatric hip disorders*. Oxford: Blackwell.

CHAPTER 83

Paediatric laparoscopic surgery

H.L. TAN

Introduction
Anatomical differences
Physiological differences
Laparoscopic trocar techniques
The ergonomics of laparoscopic surgery

Operative laparoscopy
Other laparascopic procedures
Minimally invasive paediatric urology
Conclusions
Further reading

Introduction

Laparoscopy in paediatric surgery is not new. In 1970 Drs Stephen Gans and George Berci evaluated endoscopy in children with the development of the Hopkins rod lenses and found it to be useful for diagnosis and simple procedures such as tissue biopsies. However, that year also saw the introduction by EMI of the computerized tomography (CT) scanner. This, together with the development of ultrasound imaging, and later magnetic resonance imaging (MRI), made it possible to diagnose intracoelomic pathology by non-invasive means, hence laparoscopy did not find a useful role except in the diagnosis of intra-abdominal testes until relatively recently.

The parallel development of technology such as the development of extremely bright light sources, for example xenon or metal halide lamps, high-resolution video monitors and miniature charged coupled device (CCD) video cameras allowed a miniature high-resolution camera to be attached to the eyepiece which could be now be held by an assistant to transmit very high-quality endoscopic images onto a video monitor. This advance led to endoscopic performance of complex operative procedures.

Kurt Semm from Keil was the first to describe complex laparoscopic procedures such as appendicectomy and hysterectomy. Dr Phillip Mouret led the revolution in adult general surgery when he described laparoscopic cholecystectomy in 1987. Laparoscopic cholecystectomy was subsequently popularized by Drs Dubois, Perissat, Olsen and Reddick and although there was initial resistance and concern, it has become universally accepted today by 'adult' general surgeons as the treatment of choice for cholelithiasis.

Paediatric surgeons were more reluctant to embrace laparoscopic surgery until relatively recently and for very good reasons. The use of a blind Veress needle for insufflation is potentially hazardous, especially in infants. The incidence of complications from the use of Veress needle in children has been reported at between 3% and 10%, which is unacceptably high. However, the adoption of the open laparoscopy or Hasson technique for the introduction of the cannula has virtually eliminated the risk of inadvertent visceral injuries, and has made laparoscopy in infants much safer bringing about greater acceptance of laparoscopic surgery.

The size of the laparoscopic instrumentation has also been a problem. Adult laparoscopic instruments are generally too long for infants and this with the fact that many instruments required 10 mm diameter instrument cannulae meant that they were largely unsuitable for use in small infants. It is senseless to make several 10 mm incisions for laparoscopy in infants when many paediatric procedures are performed through incisions that are often not much more than 2–3 cm long.

These problems have since been resolved by the availability of shorter paediatric laparoscopic instruments and appropriately smaller diameter trocars. The recent introduction of the microlaparoscopy, with instrument diameters of 2–3 mm will see further adaptation of this to paediatric laparoscopic surgery, as these newer instruments can even be introduced through intravenous cannulae, further minimizing the trauma of surgical access.

Although paediatric laparoscopic surgery is safe, there are significant anatomical and physiological differences which have to be taken into account when attempting laparoscopy in children.

Anatomical differences

THE UMBILICUS

In a neonate, the two umbilical arteries (lateral umbilical ligaments) and the umbilical vein (ligamentum teres) are not obliterated for several weeks and there is a potential risk of gas embolism if CO_2 is insufflated into one of these patent vessels by a blind puncture technique. This is attached to the umbilical cicatrix in an infant. Owing to these anatomical features, it is generally wiser to establish the primary trocar in the supraumbilical region in infants. In older children, this difference is less obvious.

THE BLADDER

The neonate bladder is an intra-abdominal organ. This presents special problems, as the bladder is more liable to inadvertent perforation in infants. The peritoneum is also lax in the lower abdomen, allowing the parietal peritoneum to tent away from the advancing trocar, making the introduction of suprapubic and lower abdominal trocars difficult.

The inferior epigastric arteries are especially prominent in young children and is the most common vessel injury reported in both paediatric and adult laparoscopy. Care must be taken to avoid damaging this vessel.

THE UPPER ABDOMEN

The falciform ligament and the umbilical vein (ligamentum teres) form a very prominent fold in infants and children. It is easy to become 'lost' within this fold, when performing a Hasson open laparoscopy using a midline incision in the linea alba. It is therefore easier to make a transverse incision in the linea alba to gain entry into the abdominal cavity.

THE VISCERA

The neonatal and infant liver lies below the costal margin and reaches the umbilicus in neonates. The inferior vena cava and aorta are barely 1 cm away from the ante-rior abdominal wall and can be at substantial risk from perforation by blind trocars techniques even with the so-called safety shielded trocars. It is therefore recommended that all instrument trocars be introduced by direct internal video inspection to avoid visceral damage.

Physiological differences

RESPIRATION

Infant breathing is predominantly diaphragmatic and the increased intra-abdominal pressure from insufflation will splint the diaphragm leading to increased ventilatory requirements. This can be witnessed as an immediate rise in end tidal CO_2 of about 10 mmHg when the abdomen has been insufflated. This is correctable by the anaesthetist but becomes increasingly difficult if the intra-abdominal pressure is high. It is best to use no more than 10 mmHg pressure for abdominal insufflation in infants below 10 kg, higher pressures can be used with relative safety in children over this weight. Lower insufflation pressures in the infant will result in less splinting of the diaphragm, but under 10 mmHg the introduction of secondary trocars and cannulae becomes extremely difficult and hazardous.

HYPOTHERMIA

There is a substantial risk of children developing hypothermia when undergoing laparoscopic surgery. Maintaining the pneumoperitoneum by using high flow insufflation in particular, is fraught with hazard as the insufflated CO_2 is cold, and substantial heat loss can occur. The answer is to minimize gas leakage by using the smallest diameter cannulae possible and ensuring that all cannulae and instruments have adequate and sound gas seals.

There is an additional safety concern with high flow insufflators as most manufacturers have a default setting of 1 litre of CO_2/min, and do not allow insufflation at less than this rate. Given that a neonatal abdomen can only hold 500 ml of CO_2 when fully inflated, using high flow insufflation can cause the abdomen to distend too rapidly, and possibly result in arrythmias.

Notwithstanding all these potential limitations, many advances have now been made in paediatric laparoscopic surgery, and sufficient experience has been gained to establish an increasing role for laparoscopic surgery in paediatric surgery.

Laparoscopic trocar techniques

THE HASSON TECHNIQUE

Open laparoscopy or the Hasson method for the introduction of the primary trocar is safe and does not take any more time than using a blind Veress needle. While it is accepted that there are many variations in the technique, the technique used by the author will be described as it has been shown to be quick, easy and safe.

A full thickness supraumbilical semicircumferential incision is made in the skinfold down to the level of the linea alba. The plane between the subcutaneous fat and linea alba should be developed sufficiently to allow two pairs of haemostats or Kocher's forceps to be placed on the linea alba to lift the linea alba into the wound. A transverse incision is then made in the linea alba between the two instruments, whereupon the underlying round ligament in an infant or the translucent parietal peritoneum will drop away from the linea alba. The peritoneum is then held between two mosquito haemostats and a small incision made to gain access into the abdominal cavity. It should be immediately obvious that you are in the abdominal cavity as lifting the linea alba allows room air to fill the abdominal cavity, and you should immediately recognize normal viscera, usually omentum, underneath. If you are not sure, then in all probability you are still extraperitoneal.

In a small infant, it is easiest to hook the umbilical vein through the linea alba drawing the peritoneum with it. The peritoneum is then opened beside the falciform ligament, gaining access into the abdomen. A purse string should be placed in the linea alba *before* inserting in the primary trocar. This purse string is then tightened around the trocar with a single throw to stabilize the trocar and thus prevent gas leakage. The same suture can be used to close the defect by tightening the purse string at completion of the laparoscopic procedure. We have not to date witnessed any trocar injuries in any patient using this method.

SECONDARY TROCAR PLACEMENT

While it is easiest to introduce instrument trocars in older children by a direct puncture technique, in children we recommend that a small full-thickness skin incision be made which is wide enough to accommodate the cannula as this is the most difficult layer to penetrate. In neonates and infants, this incision is extended as a full thickness stab with a 11 scalpel blade under direct vision, and the stab is then widened sufficiently by spreading a pair of straight mosquito forceps along the tract so that a blunt trocar can be introduced in an atraumatic manner.

The ergonomics of laparoscopic surgery

Unlike conventional surgery, laparoscopic surgery is not intuitive. The general principles so often used to plan patient positioning, exposure and the floor plan (position of the surgeon, assistant and scrub nurse) in open surgery, if applied to laparoscopic surgery may be completely inappropriate. Many factors which are not considered important such as gravitational effects on internal organs can play an important role in the planning of laparoscopic surgery and are critical to the success or otherwise of laparoscopic surgery.

EYE–HAND CO-ORDINATION AND PARADOXICAL MOVEMENT

Laparoscopic instruments have to be inserted through an instrument port and work around a fulcrum. Hence instruments moved in one direction by the surgeon will be seen to move in the opposite direction both horizontally *and* vertically. This is first-order paradoxical movement and one can get used to this in a few minutes, as it is no different from rowing a boat. This however only applies in the situation where the endocamera is pointing straight ahead, and the video monitor is placed *directly in front of the surgeon.*

If on the other hand, the endocamera is pointing towards to surgeon, a left to right movement by the surgeon will also be seen as a left to right movement on the video monitor, that is the sideways movements is *not* paradoxical and yet the vertical movement continues to be. In other words, the horizontal axis is now reversed, and a second degree of paradox is introduced, and much like driving using the rear view mirror, many simple tasks then become much more difficult and sometimes impossible if this second-order paradox is introduced into laparoscopic surgery.

This problem of displaced visual co-ordination has been studied by Kohler in 1939 where he and other experimental subjects wore reversing prisms on spectacles for long periods of time. They reported 'days or weeks were spent in correcting movements disturbed by the reversal, some of which were incorrectly repeated hundreds of times'. In cases where left and right were reversed, someone trying to walk along a straight path would lurch from side to side like a drunk.

Most surgeons in fact intuitively recognize this and place themselves in an optimum position, so that they are correctly aligned with the camera and video. This however, is not the case with surgical assistants as it is commonplace to witness the assistant or theatre nurse on the other side facing the surgeon, working from a second video monitor. The assistant is now forced to work with second-order paradoxical movement and the only way he or she can control the instruments is by deliberately thinking about the movements each time, this is a potentially dangerous particularly if quick or fine movements are required, for example in controlling bleeding or endosuturing. It is impossible to suture let alone cut a suture in this position.

Ergonomic rule:
Surgeon assistant and scrub nurse must be on the same side.
The video monitor must be straight ahead, and camera pointing towards the monitor.
Do not use more than one video monitor.

The natural instinct is for surgeons to place instrument and cannulae as close to the operative field as possible, but this is impractical in laparoscopic surgery, as placing instrument and telescopic ports too close to the operative field will only restrict the ability to manipulate instruments around the fulcrum. As a general rule it is best to place trocars and cannulae about half the working length of your telescope and instruments away from the operative field.

There is much more to the ergonomics of laparoscopic surgery which cannot be effectively covered in this general chapter, but this gives an indication on the differences between open surgery and laparoscopic surgery.

Operative laparoscopy

DIAGNOSTIC LAPAROSCOPY

Contrary to expectations, diagnostic laparoscopy is not performed as often as one would expect. The availability of CT scanning, ultrasound and MRI has permitted an accurate and non-invasive means of delineating intracoelomic pathology, so that there is rarely a need to perform laparoscopy. It has been useful in three areas, namely for impalpable testes, in childhood malignancies and for the diagnosis of chronic inflammatory bowel disease.

LAPAROSCOPY FOR UNDESCENDED TESTES

Although undescended testes remain one of the most common paediatric surgical conditions, the majority of undescended testes are in the superficial inguinal pouch or within the inguinal canal, and only 1–3% of undescended testes are truly intra-abdominal and require laparoscopy. Laparoscopy is only indicated rarely and only in the patient in whom neither the cord nor the testis can be felt in the inguinal canal. If either of these structures can be felt, one should proceed to conventional inguinal exploration to bring an emergent testis down or to remove an atrophic testis.

Technique

The patient is positioned close to the foot of the table with a video monitor placed in the midline between the assistant and the surgeon. The patient should be positioned head down and the bladder emptied immediately prior to surgery. The surgeon should stand on the contralateral side to the testis being explored.

A 5 mm Hasson cannula is inserted by the method already described, and general laparoscopy performed. It is necessary to insert two 5 mm instrument ports, one in the contralateral iliac fossa, and the other on the ipsilateral side in the same line as the internal ring but above the umbilicus, as this will facilitate instrumentation. The internal inguinal ring is easily identifiable by following the external iliac vessels to where it meets the inferior epigastric vessels.

If an indirect hernia is present, the telescope is advanced into the inguinal canal and a testis if present, will be easily seen. If there is no hernia sac, it may be possible to identify the gubernaculum and, then follow it proximally to the intra-abdominal testis which is sometimes hidden behind the caecum or the sigmoid colon.

Another alternative is to locate the vas deferens behind the bladder and follow it either to its blind ending, or to the testis.

An atrophic testis can be easily removed using the 'Tan' bipolar forceps, specially designed to coagulate and cut at the same time.

If a testis is found in close proximity to a sac, try to relocate the testis into the inguinal canal. If you can easily do this laparoscopically, then convert to conventional orchidopexy, as it should be possible to bring this emergent testis into the scrotum. If on the other hand, the testis is truly well away from the internal ring, then one should attempt a staged Fowler–Stephens procedure. There are many ways to divide the internal spermatic vessels including the use of titanium clips, and the use of extra or intracorporeal suturing. In reality, it is just as easy and considerably less expensive to coagulate the vessels with the 'Tan' bipolar forceps, dividing the vessels in the process.

A second-look laparoscopy should be performed 6 months later and orchidopexy performed entirely laparoscopically by mobilizing the testis with its vas and vessels on a cuff of peritoneum. The inguinal canal will be absent in this instance, but one can be created by pushing a laparoscopic dissector from the internal ring lateral to the inferior epigastric vessels, into the scrotum where a sub-dartos pouch is created. A straight haemostat is then introduced up this tract created to grab the intra-abdominal testis to bring it into the scrotum.

LAPAROSCOPY IN CHILDHOOD MALIGNANCY

This may yet prove to be an important indication for diagnostic and therapeutic laparoscopy. While percutaneous needle biopsies have been useful for histological diagnosis of childhood malignancies, the need for larger tissue samples for cell culture has led to the increasing use of laparoscopic sampling of nodes and malignant tissue.

It is possible to obtain a large sample of neuroblastoma tissue for *n-myc* oncogene studies, but bleeding can be extremely difficult to control unless one performs the biopsy through the mesentery of the bowel. This allows the mesenteric defect to be sutured over to tamponade any likely bleeding in the retroperitoneum.

We have also staged tumours laparoscopically and this is especially useful in pelvic sarcomas where it can be difficult to tell on conventional organ imaging if there is local spread. If pelvic radiotherapy is required, it is an easy exercise to perform bilateral oopheropexy by suturing the ovaries to the side wall of the abdominal wall.

One of the most useful indications for laparoscopy is the child on chemotherapy with an acute abdomen. There is generally a great reluctance to perform exploratory laparotomy on these children who are generally neutropenic, with associated clotting disorders and poor wound healing. Laparoscopy is a most useful diagnostic tool and, contrary to most beliefs, the presence of a coagulation disorder is not a contra-indication. We have performed appendicectomies in such children for appendicitis without peri-operative problems.

CHRONIC INFLAMMATORY BOWEL DISEASE

The role of laparoscopy in chronic inflammatory bowel disease is being evaluated. While Crohn's disease is usually diagnosed on colonoscopic biopsies, laparoscopy has been used to diagnose Crohn's disease in patients where the gastroscopy and colonoscopy have not been conclusive. It is easy to identify the typical features of Crohn's disease laparoscopically, and to document accurately the length of the lesion and whether there are skip lesions. Laparoscopy should have a useful place in the management of chronic inflammatory bowel disease.

Other laparoscopic procedures

CHOLECYSTECTOMY

Cholelithiasis is a relatively uncommon condition in children, but it is now accepted that laparoscopic cholecystectomy is the procedure of choice.

We have not found it necessary to perform intraoperative cholangiography if the patient has normal liver function and a normal preoperative ultrasound demonstrates non-dilated bile ducts.

APPENDICECTOMY

In many European institutions, laparoscopic appendicectomy has become the most common procedure performed in children. Most patients can be discharged within 24 hours of laparoscopic appendicectomy, except for when there is accompanying peritonitis, or if the appendix is perforated or associated with an appendix abscess.

Contrary to most beliefs, it is possible to perform a thorough debridement and lavage of the entire

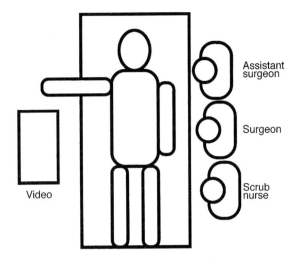

Fig. 83.1   Theatre layout of lap appendectomy.

peritoneal cavity, pelvis and subphrenic spaces at a laparoscopic appendicectomy.

Figure 83.1 illustrates a suitable theatre layout for an laparoscopic appendicectomy and Fig. 83.2 shows the port positions for this procedure. The stages of the laparoscopic appendicectomy are shown in Fig. 83.3.

The procedure is performed using one 10 mm umbilical Hasson trocar, and two other instrument ports, one in the midline in the suprapubic skin crease and the other in the right upper quadrant of the abdomen about 10 cm above the caecum.

There are many ways of controlling the mesoappendix including the use of an extracorporeal endoloop suture to ligate the mesoappendix *en masse*, and the use of titanium clips or Endo-GIA to divide the appendiceal artery, our method of choice is to skeletonize the appendix using the bipolar 'strip-tease' technique. While it is possible to use monopolar diathermy to control the mesoappendix, this is potentially hazardous in

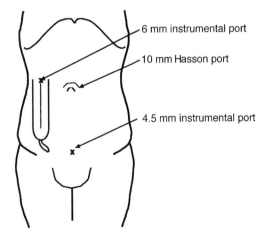

Fig. 83.2   Port positions for laparoscopic appendectomy.

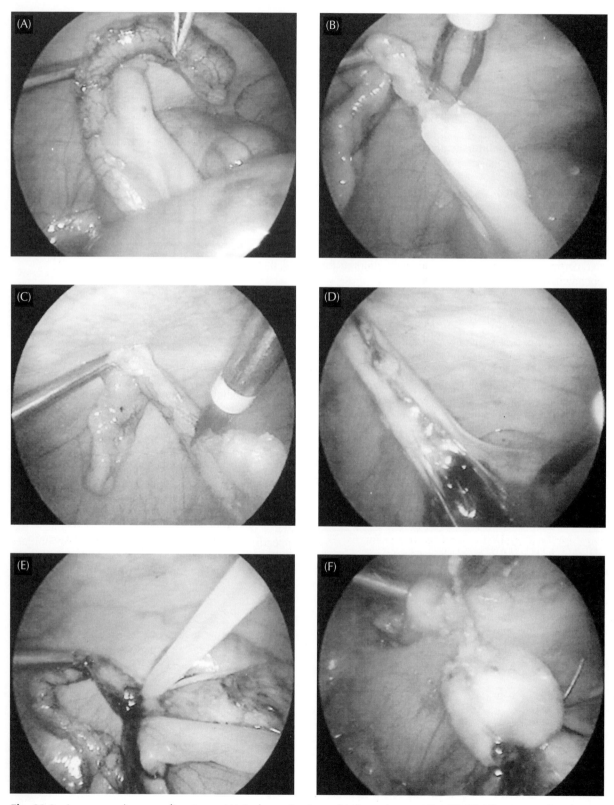

Fig. 83.3 Laparoscopic appendicectomy: (A) Endoscopic view of inflamed appendix. (B) Dividing appendiceal artery with Tan Bipolar forceps. (C) Skeletonizing appendix. (D) Appendix skeletonized to base. (E) Base ligated with Endoloop™. (F) Appendix being divided.

appendicectomy, as the return path for the current is through the base of the appendix, and caecal perforation has been reported using a monopolar technique. The stump of the appendix can be ligated with two endoloops, and there is generally no need to perform a purse-string suture to bury the stump.

FUNDOPLICATION

Laparoscopic fundoplication appears to be the most common laparoscopic procedure performed in North America, where the experience with gastro-oesophageal reflux appears to be different from the European counterparts, and successful laparoscopic fundoplication has been reported in infants as young as 4 weeks old.

This is not an operation to be performed by the novice laparoscopist as it requires dexterity and skills in intracorporeal suturing. There are also inherent dangers of breeching the mediastinal pleura when dissecting the crura resulting in a left tension pneumothorax, and there have been reported cases of injury to the aorta at laparoscopic fundoplication. In the hands of the skilled laparoscopic surgeon it is a relatively easy operation and may reduce operative morbidity.

We have not found it necessary to divide the short gastric vessels in performing laparoscopic fundoplication, and the left lobe of the liver can be retracted upwards away from the hiatus without a need to mobilize it.

LAPAROSCOPIC PYLOROMYOTOMY

Laparoscopic pyloromyotomy remained contentious for a while, as it appeared to make hard work of a relatively simple open operation. However it has now been demonstrated by many centres to be a safe procedure with minimal morbidity and is being increasingly accepted as the operation of choice for infantile hypertrophic pyloric stenosis. The results have been shown to be at least as good as conventional pyloromyotomy.

Technique

There are three ways to perform laparoscopic pyloromyotomy, these are Alain's, the author's and Rothenberg's but only the author's technique will be described.

Figure 83.4 illustrates a suitable theatre layout for laparoscopic pyloromyotomy and Fig. 83.5 shows the Ramstedt's port positions for this procedure. The stages of the laparoscopic pyloromyotomy are shown in Fig. 83.6.

The stomach must be emptied with an oro gastric tube. The patient is positioned at the foot of the operating table, and the surgeon sits at the end, with an assistant surgeon on the right of the surgeon. The video monitor is placed on the left-hand side of the operating table at the head end so that it is in the same visual line to facilitate eye–hand co-ordination. The patient should be tilted into about 15° head up position. This allows the transverse colon to fall away from the pylorus under gravity.

A direct viewing (0°) 4 mm telescope is inserted through an umbilical Hasson cannula using the technique already described. Under direct video-endoscopy, one 4 mm secondary port is inserted in the line of the nipple just below the costal margin on the left side. A second much smaller abdominal puncture is made on the right side to introduce the duodenal grabber. It is not necessary to insert an additional instrument port on the right because there is no interchange of instruments necessary on this side. Care must be taken not to damage the underlying liver when inserting the ports or interchanging instruments.

Two atraumatic graspers are inserted and the stomach and olive readily identified. It may be necessary to lift the falciform ligament with the right sided grasper to visualize the pylorus. The first part of the duodenum is stabilized just distal to the vein of Mayo by this instrument and is retracted inferiorly downwards and laterally, away from the overhanging neonatal liver,

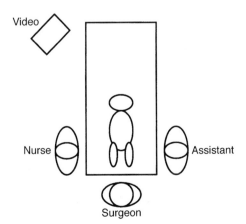

Fig. 83.4 Lap pyloromyotomy layout.

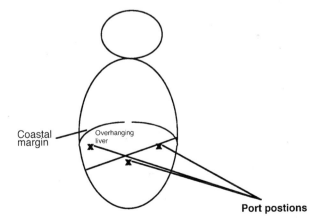

Fig. 83.5 Port position for laparoscopic Ramstedt's.

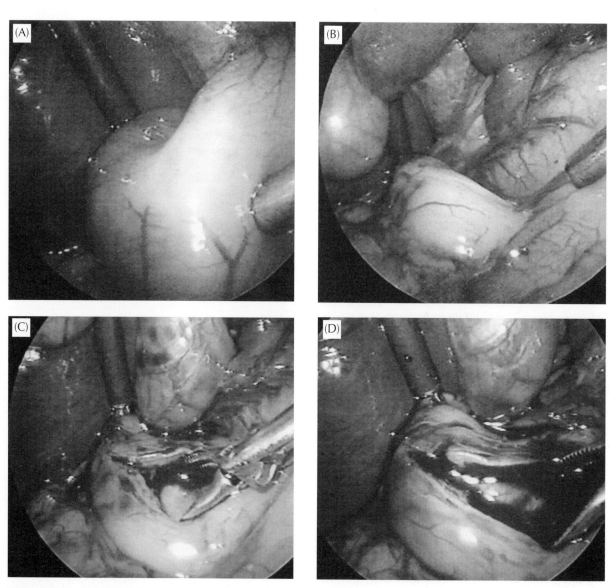

Fig. 83.6 Laparoscopic pyloromyotomy: (A) Typical endoscopic view of pyloric tumour. Note: duodenum stabilized by atraumatic grasper and antral limit of olivebeing 'palpated'. (B) Making deep incision in olive with 'Tan' endotome. (C) Spreading tumour. (D) Checking for mucosal perforation.

otherwise it will be difficult to perform the pyloromyotomy. This also serves to stabilize the pylorus.

The Tan endotome is then passed through the left-upper quadrant port, and a sero-muscular incision made, beginning at the duodenal end, cutting towards the antrum. This incision should be deep into the olive otherwise difficulty will be encountered with the spreader. There is no need to extend the incision beyond the olive.

The endotome is exchanged for the Tan pyloric spreader which should be thrust through the seromuscular incision until slight resistance of the intact mucosa is felt. The tumour is then spread by opening its jaws.

The mucosa is inspected at this point in time. On completion of spreading, 30–50 ml of air is insufflated into the stomach by the anaesthetist, causing the mucosa to bulge, when it should be reinspected to exclude inadvertent perforation. It is not necessary to divide the last few fibres at the duodenal end, as this is the potential site for perforation.

The abdomen is then deflated, and steristrips are used to close the instrument ports except for the umbilical incision which is closed by tightening the purse string.

Although this is a technically easy laparoscopic procedure to perform taking less than 15 min to complete, attention to detail is required to achieve low morbidity. We have now performed 70 laparoscopic pyloromyotomy using this technique without a single case of recurrence or mucosal perforation.

Minimally invasive paediatric urology

URINARY CALCULI

Interest in minimally invasive paediatric urology began with the evaluation of the role of extracorporeal shockwave lithotrypsy (ESWL) and percutaneous nephrolithotripsy (PCNL) for the management of urinary calculi. Unlike the experience with adults however, ESWL has been successful in treating only 26% of paediatric calculi in the author's series of 60 patients. This is a reflection of the aetiology of paediatric urinary calculi, as 40% of stones were infective, 23% were metabolic, and 12% had pre-existing renal tract abnormalities. These differences in aetiology makes ESWL unsuitable for the majority of stones in children, and as a result, we have relied on percutaneous or endoscopic means to manage our upper tract stones, and to retrieve broken or migrated double pig tailed stents, of which there were seven.

It has been demonstrated that percutaneous nephroscopy can be performed safely in children, the youngest to-date being a 16-week-old infant with an incomplete cystine staghorn. However there are special considerations in children that one has to address including the risks of hypothermia, the small size of the collecting system, and measures to minimize blood loss. We have developed a single staged dilator to perform safe PCNL in children. Most endourological procedures including PCNL can now be performed through a 14 or 16 Fr Amplatz operating sheath via a direct renal puncture technique. A 9.5 or 11 Fr operating cystoscope with an offset lens serves as an ideal infant nephroscope, as the 5 Fr operating channel will accommodate the small ultrasonic or lithoclast probe.

LAPAROSCOPIC NEPHRECTOMY/PARTIAL NEPHRECTOMY

The role of laparoscopic nephrectomy is still evolving. We have now performed 36 laparoscopic nephrectomies including 12 partial nephrectomies for duplex systems. There has not been any conversion to open nephrectomy, and no laparoscopic-related complications. One patient with a non-functioning kidney impacted with calculi developed postoperative sepsis, and two patients had intraoperative bleeding from renal vessel injuries which were controlled laparoscopically, but all children have done well.

It is now being reported that retroperitoneal nephrectomies are being performed but the author continues to perform nephrectomies via the transperitoneal route, as there is minimal mobilization of intraperitoneal structures, and the risk of adhesions after laparoscopic surgery has been shown to be minimal.

PUJ OBSTRUCTION

PUJ obstruction is the commonest obstructive uropathy in children. In spite of the various minimally invasive techniques available to treat PUJ obstruction, conventional open pyeloplasty until now, remains the gold standard with a success rate of over 90%.

Endopyelotomy has been used successfully in children, but the success of this technique in our series is only about 80%, which is similar to that achieved in adult series. Likewise, the published results of retrograde balloon dilatation in the author's series is inferior to that of open dismembered pyeloplasty.

Dismembered pyeloplasties remains the gold standard, but this remains a challenging operation to perform laparoscopically, as only very few attempts have been reported. However, the author has developed and refined the technique for laparoscopic transperitoneal dismembered pyeloplasty and a total of 16 pyeloplasties have now been performed by the author, the youngest being three months old. All uretero-pelvic anastomoses were completed by intracorporeal hand suturing. The refinements achieved has reduced the operating time from 160 min to less than 90 min for the last ten cases. This is the same as the time taken for conventional open surgery. Our preliminary results show that the success rate is 86%, fast approaching that of conventional open pyeloplasty.

VATS DECORTICATION

An increasing number of authors have reported successful thoracoscopic decortication of loculated empyema, and our results certainly show that there is considerable benefit to the child if a thoracotomy can be avoided.

Thoracoscopic decortication however, is a painstaking operation, as it can be extremely laborious to remove the peel from the lung and visceral pleura.

ADHESIOLYSIS

We have now managed 27 patients laparoscopically with suspected or established small bowel obstruction, with the need to convert to laparotomy in only one child. Diagnostic laparoscopy is an extremely useful tool in patients presenting with severe recurrent abdominal pains after open surgery, as it is possible to either exclude adhesion obstruction with certainty, or else deal with the adhesions entirely laparoscopically.

Acute and sub-acute small bowel obstruction can also be managed laparoscopically provided the abdomen is not too distended.

Conclusions

It is still too early to draw conclusions about the relative merit or otherwise of laparoscopic versus open operations. The question that needs to be asked is whether it is necessary for the results of laparoscopic procedures to be better than open operation? The important consideration is that it be safe. If it can be demonstrated that a laparoscopic procedure is as safe as its open counterpart and offers equivalent results then it is reasonable to offer the minimally invasive procedure as an alternative. This is still clearly an evolving and rapidly developing field.

Many of the problems encountered with laparoscopic surgery have been that it is a new technique, and unlike conventional surgery is not intuitive, requiring all surgeons to relearn new technical skills. However, with increasing experience and dexterity most surgeons are now finding it increasingly easier to perform laparoscopic procedures and in the same time as it would take them to perform a conventional open procedure. This leads to acceptance of the technique.

The benefits of pain reduction and decreased scarring are of primary concern to patients, therefore as in adult surgical practice, laparoscopic surgery offers a satisfactory alternative to open surgery in skilled hands.

Further reading

Alain, J.L., Grousseau, D. and Terrier, G. 1991: Extramucosal pyloromyotomy by laparoscopy. *Journal of Pediatric Surgery* **26**, 1191–2.

Dubois, F., Berthelots, G. and Levard, H. 1989: Cholecystectomy par coeliosoopie. *Presse Med* **18**, 980–9.

Dubois, F. and Card, P. 1990: Coelioscopic cholecystectomy: A preliminary report of 36 cases. *Annals of Surgery* **211**, 60–2.

Gans, S.L. and Berci, G. 1973: Peritoneoscopy in infants and children. *Journal of Pediatric Surgery* **6**, 399–405.

Gans, S.L. and Berci, G. 1971: Adyanoes in endoscopy of infants and children. *Journal of Pediatric Surgery* **6**, 199–233.

Kohler, I.: Quoted by Smith, K.U. and Smith, W.M. 1966: Perception and motion, in Vernon, M.D. (ed.) *Experiments in visual perception*. Penguin. Excerpted from Smith, K.U. and Smith, W.M.: *Perception and motion*. Philadelphia, PA: W.B. Saunders, 1962, Chapter 5.

Patkin, M. 1967: Ergonomic aspects of surgical dexterity. *Medical Journal of Australia* **2**, 775–7.

Perissat, J., Collet, D. and Belliard, R. 1990: Gallstones: laparoscopic treatment – cholecystectomy, cholecystostomy, and lithotripsy. *Surgery Endoscopy* **4**, 1–5.

Reddick, E.J. 1988: Laparoscopic laser cholecystectomy. *Clinical Laser Monthly* **6**(10), 400–1.

Reddick, E.J. and Olsen, D.O. 1989: Laparoscopic laser cholecystectomy: A comparison with minilap cholecystectomy. *Surgery Endoscopy* **3**, 181–3.

Rothenberg, S. 1997: Laparoscopic pyloromyotomy: the slice and pull technique. *Pediatric endosurgery and innovative techniques*, Vol. 1, No. 1. Mary Ann Liebert.

Semm, K. 1983: Endoscopic appendectomy. *Endoscopy* **15**, 50–64.

Tan, H.L. and Najmaldin, A. 1993: Laparoscopic pyloromyotomy for infantile hypertrupic pyloric stenosis. *Pediatric Surgery International* **8**, 376–8.

Tan, H.L., Segawa, O. and Stein, J.E. 1995: Laparoscopic bipolar strip-tease appendicectomy. *Surgery Endoscopy* **9**, 1301–3.

Index

Abcess
  intra-abdominal 411
  perianal 379
Abdomen
  acute 240
  blunt trauma to 696–708
  development of 130, 146
  examination 404
  laparoscopic surgery and 825
  recurrent pain 240
  ultrasound examination of 60–1
  wall defects 96
    fetal 14
Abdominal
  injury 674
  mass 501, 628
  pain
    acute 378, 402–15
    recurrent 426–21, 423
Abuse 46
  sexual 379, 382, 731–7
  see also non-accidental injury
Accident and emergency departments 43
Accidental injury 738–44
Acetyl cholinesterase 207
AChE, *see* acetyl cholinesterase
Acidosis, metabolic 494, 503, 515
Acid–base
  imbalance 118, 494, 503
  status 108
Actinomycosis 3
Admission 44–6, 54
Adolescence 46
Adrenal gland, ultrasound examination of 62
Aerocele, traumatic 688

AFP screening, *see* alpha feto protein screening
Aganglionosis
  total colonic 207
  total intestinal 207
Air insufflation 358
Airway
  anomalies 170–86
  management 670–1
  obstruction 172
  problems during transfer 75
Alpha feto protein screening 12–13, 14, 15
Alveolar–arterial oxygen tension difference 159
Amino acids 118
Amniocentesis 13, 14, 15, 32
Amputations 3
Anaemia 594–5
  Fanconi's 36
  implications for anaesthesia 90
Anaesthesia 86–101
  day patients 82, 84–5, 96–8
  equipment for 92–3
  induction 91–2, 94
  monitoring 92–4
  neonatal 94–5
Anal fissures 377, 438
Analgesia
  postoperative 95, 98
Anastomotic stricture 192
Anatomical dolls 52
Androgen
  biosynthesis and metabolism 295–6
    defects in 297–9
  insensitivity syndrome 298
Aneurysms, traumatic 689
Animal bites 740

Animal models 21–22
Anorectal
    acquired conditions 376–9
    anomalies 213–25
        optimal age for operation 222–3
    defects 593
    embryology 214–16
    manometry 209, 648
Antegrade pressure recording 620
Antenatal diagnosis 11–19
    of bladder exstrophy 594
    of congenital diaphragmatic hernia 155, 159
    of exomphalos 147–8
    of gastroschsis 147–8
    of posterior urethral valves 629
    of renal tract abnormalities 500
    of spina bifida cystica 284–5
Anterior wall defects 145–52
Anti-Müllerian hormone 290, 293, 294
Antibiotic therapy 721, 723
Antibiotics 222
Antidepressants 640
Antidiuretics 640
Aorta, coarctation of 765, 772
Aortic
    injuries 695
    stenosis 765, 771–2
Appendicitis 413, 414–15
    acute 407–9
Appendix
    removal at time of laparotomy 361
ARF (acute renal failure), *see* renal failure
Arnold–Chiari malformation 279, 284
Arterial septum, defects of 763, 768
Arteriography 699–700
Ascaris lumbricoides 427
Ascites 445, 451
Assessment of trauma patient
    primary 670–3
    secondary 673–4
Asphyxia, traumatic 694
Associations 5–6
    see also CHARGE association, VATER association
Asthma
    implications for anaesthesia 90
    medication, effects of 365
ATN (acute tubular necrosis), *see* tubular necrosis
Atrioventricular
    junction, defects of 764, 769
    valve, defects of 764
Atrium, defects of 768–9, *see also* arterial septum
Audit 137–42
    comparative 138
Autoimmunity deficiency disease 3
Autosomal
    dominant inheritance 34–5
Auxology 516

Back
    infection 808–9
    pain 809–12
Balanitis 322
Barium enema 208, 233, 234
Basal metabolic rate 117
Bile duct
    perforation 423–4
    rhabdomyosarcoma 424
Biliary
    atresia 241–50
    system, ultrasound examination of 62
Biofeedback 439
Birth defects 3
    classification of 4–10
Birthmarks 796–8
Bishop–Koop ileostomy 204–5
Bladder
    diverticula 552
    epispadias 527, 590–602
    exstrophy 3, 527, 590–602
    function 276, 571, 599, 637
    injury 705
    laparoscopic surgery and 826
    neuropathic 481
    stones 663
    unstable 481
Blalock–Taussig shunt 767–8
Blind loop syndrome 201
Blood
    gases 159
    loss 672
BMR, *see* basal metabolic rate
Body proportion, changes in 124–5
Bow legs, *see* genu varum
Bowel
    development of large and small 131
    function in cloacal exstrophy 599–600
    injury 704–5
    washout 222
    see also inflammatory bowel disease
Brain
    neonate, ultrasound examination of 60
Brain damage 685
Brain death 748
Branchial anomalies 464–5
Breath hydrogen 231
Breathing 671
Bronchi
    development of 130
Bronchogenic cyst 170, 182–3
Bronchomalacia 170, 176
Budd–Chiari syndrome 444
Burns 719–723

CAM, *see* cystic adenomatoid malformation
Carbohydrate malabsorption 228

Carbohydrates 117
Carcinoma 3
Cardiac
 failure 760
 scanning 761
  fetal 15
Cardiology, interventional 762–3
Cardiovascular system 87
 development of 132
Care units 678
Care-by-parent schemes 52
Caroticocavernous fistula 689
Carriers 33, 37
Case conferences 727
Case selection
 fetal surgery 26–7
Catheters
 central venous 121
Caudal regression syndrome 6–7
CCAM, *see* congenital cystic adenomatoid malformation of
 lung
CDH, *see* congenital diaphragmatic hernia
Cellular retinoic acid binding protein 8
Central nervous system 87–8, 103, 133–6, 280
Centres of health information and promotion 51
Cerebral circulation 682
Cerebral palsy 806
Cerebral perfusion pressure 683
Cerebrospinal fluid 135, 260–9, 279, 683, 688
CHARGE association 6, 170, 188
 charts 511, 512–13
 effect of renal failure on 509–18
Chemotherapy 775
Chest
 drains 163
 funnel, *see* pectus excavatum
 pigeon, *see* pectus carinatum
 radiological changes 127, 128, 129
 ultrasound examination of 60
 wall deformaties 455–60
Child
 care 49–53
  historical 50
  in hospital 39–48, 49–53
 consent 46
 centred care 43–4
 see also abuse
Child Protection Committee 47
Children First 40–1
Children's Act 46, 47, 737
CHIP
 see Centres of health information and promotion
Choanal
 atresia 170–1
 stenosis 170–1
Cholangitis 248
Cholecystitis 412, 422–3

Choledochal cyst 241, 250–5
Cholelithiasis 423
Chromosome
 21: 6, 32, 200, 201
 abnormality 31–3, 281, 293–301, 519, 520, 521–2, 523,
  580
 X-linked conditions 35
 Y-linked conditions 327
Chylothorax 170, 184
Circulation 672
Circumcision 320–6
CLE, *see* congenital lobar emphysema
Cleft palate and lip 3, 36, 798–9
 see also Van de Woode syndrome
Cloacal
 anomalies 223
 exstrophy 593, 594, 596, 597
Clostridia 228
Clostridium butyricum 228
Clostridium difficile 209
CNS, *see* central nervous system
Cold injury 722
Collateral circulation 444
Colorectal obstruction 199
Colostomy 218–19, 440–1
Community, role in care 50, 54–8, 743
Computed tomography 171, 358, 406, 424, 575, 673, 684,
 685, 686, 687, 699, 773–4, 778, 782, 786
Congenital anomalies 4–10
 antenatal diagnosis of 11–19
 gross 5
Congenital cystic adenomatoid malformation of lung 158,
 170, 178–81
Congenital diaphragmatic hernia 95
 fetal 14–15, 21, 22, 23–4
Congenital lobar emphysema 170, 176–8
Congestive cardiac failure 500
Conscious level 686
Consent
 of child 46
 of parent/guardian 46
Constipation 412, 418, 435–41
Constriction rings 3
Consumer products in accidental injury 740
Continence 436–7, 711
 criteria of clinical continence 223–4
 radiological assessment of continence 224
Conus
 medullaris 275
 tethering 275
Counselling
 genetic 31–8
Court Report 40, 54
CRABP, *see* cellular retinoic acid binding protein
CRABPI gene 8
Cranialfacial anomalies 170, 172
Craniofacial repair 688

Criminal proceedings, for non-accidental injury 727
Critical incident reporting 138
Crohn's disease 380, 381–6, 390
Croup 98–9
CSF, *see* cerebrospinal fluid
CT, *see* computed tomography
Culture 47
CVC, *see* central venous catheters
Cyanosis 760
Cyst
    bronchogenic 170, 182–3
Cystic adenomatoid malformation 24–5
Cystic fibrosis 3, 33–4, 359
Cystic hygroma 461–2
Cystinuria 662
Cystography 69, 478, 479
Cystoscopy 647
    damage 379
    stenosis 322

Day care standards 83–5
Day surgery for children 80–5
Day units for children 43
Defecation 437
Deformation, definition of 6
Denaturing gradient gel electrophoresis 208
Department of Health 40, 41
Dermoid cysts 3, 274, 466–7
Development, disordered 3
DGCE, *see* denaturing gradient gel electrophoresis
Diabetes 3, 638
    diagnosis using 15
Diagnostic peritoneal lavage 699
Dialysis 506–7, *see also* haemodialysis
Diaphragm 154
    eventration 165–6
    see also congenital diaphragmatic hernia
Diastematomyelia 275
Diet, implication in disease 381, 387
DiGeorge syndrome 8, 15
Discitis 413, 809
Disease
    causes of 3
        genetic 3
        intrauterine environmental factors 3
Disruption, definition of 7
DMSA, *see* ^{99m}Tc-DMSA
Donor procedure 749–50
Doppler principle, use in ultrasound 60
    Colour Doppler 60, 64, 65
Down's syndrome 3, 5, 15, 32
DPL, *see* diagnostic peritoneal lavage
Drowning 740, 742
Drug administration 88–9, 90–1
Dry-bed training 642
Ductus arteriosus, patency of 761
Duodenal atresia 32, 198, 200–1

fetal 15
Duodenal stenosis 200–1
Dymorphisms 5
Duplex pelvicalyccal collecting system 523–4
Dysplasia
    definition of 7–8

Ear deformities 799
ECG, *see* electrocardiogram
ECMO *see* extracorporeal membrane oxygenation
EDN-3 gene 208
EDNRB gene 208
Education
    Act 46, 53
    in hospital 45–6, 52
Effective renal plasma flow, calculation of 68
Electrocardiogram 75, 672
Electrocardiography, *see* ECG
Electrolyte
    imbalance 118, 493–4, 515
    infusion 108
    management 105–6
Embryonic tumours 3
Embryos 5, 6–7,8
    see also fctus, fetal
Emergency medical service 677–80
Emotional stress
    of hospitals 44
EMS, *see* emergency medical service
End-stage renal failure 498, 505
Endopyelotomy in pelviureteric junctional hydronephrosis 623
Endoscopic variceal ligation 450
Endoscopy 348, 350, 384, 446
Endothelin-B receptor gene, *see* EDNRB gene
Endotracheal
    intubation 670
    tube sizes 130
Enemas 440
    in Crohn's disease 385
    in intussusception 358, 360
    Malone antegrade continence 440
    in ulcerative colitis 387
Enteral feeds 228–9
Enteric nervous system 206–7
Enterocolitis 208, 209
Enterostomy 233
Enuresis 500
    alarms 641
    nocturnal 636–43
Environmental factors in accidental injury 740
Epididymal anomalies 331
Epiglottitis 98–9
Epilepsy, post-traumatic 689
Epileptic seizures
    implications for anaesthesia 90

Epulis, congenital 467
Erb's palsy 174
ESRF, *see* end-stage renal failure
Ethical issues
    of fetal surgery 21
    genetic counselling and 37
Ethnic groups 47
Ewing's sarcoma 803
Exomphalos 147, 148–9
Extracorporeal membrane oxygenation 15, 155, 162–3, 164
Extracranial haematomas 683
Extradural
    fibrous bands 273
    lipomata 274
    squamous epithelial tubes 273–4
Extrahepatic anomalies 243–4

Facial
    injury 671
    vein, common 109
Facio-auriculo-vertebral spectrum 8
Faecaloma 438–9
Family
    effect of a handicapped child in 288
    information centres 51
    problems, abdominal pains caused by 419
    ureteric reflux 548
    support 190, 505
Family-centred care 43–4, 50–53
Fat 117
Feed
    postoperative regimens 350–1
    reintroduction of 233
    treatment in gastro-oesophageal reflux 370
Female
    genitalia, *see* genitalia, female
    infertility 411
    virilized 300–2, 303
Femoral vein 110
Fertility in exstrophy/epispadias patients 600
Fetal
    abnormality 11–19, 20–21
    cardiac interventions 26
    death
        protocol for autopsy 5
    immune tolerance 28
    laser ablation 26
    material, histopathological examination of
        5
    monitoring 26
    pleural effusions
    polcystic kidney disease 575, 577
    scanning, 11–18,
    surgery 20–30
    ureteric reflux 547
    ventriculomegaly 26
First aid 719

Fistulae 610, 612
Flail chest 694
Fluid
    infusion 108
    management 105–6, 489, 493–4
        in intussusception 359
    replacement 673, 721
    requirements 108
    restriction 639
    therapy 94–5
Folic acid 3, 36, 281
Foot anomalies 820–3
Foreign body
    removal of 98
Foreskin, *see* prepuce
Fowler–Stephens technique 335
Fractures 727–8
Fraenum 467
Free radicals 227
Fusion failure 3

Gallbladder 422–4
Gangrene 358
Gastric
    emptying
        delayed 366–7
        study 368
    varices 448
Gastro-oesophageal reflux 364–75
Gastroduodenal duplications 398–9
Gastroenteritis 412
Gastrointestinal
    causes of recurrent abdominal pain 419
    complications 150
    duplication 396–401
    system 130
    tract
        ultrasound examination 61
        water loss from 107
Gastroschisis 36, 145–52
    fetal 28
    transfer in 76, 77
Gender assessment 303
General Medical Council 47
General practitioner 54, 56, 57
Genetic
    counselling 31–8, 207
    factors
        in enuresis 637
        in polycystic kidneys 574, 576
        in pyloric stenosis 345–6
        in spina bifida 281
        in urological anomalies 519–28
    mutation 208
    sex
        determination 291–3
        differentiation 293–6

Genitalia
  ambiguous 290–306
  examination of 732–3
  female
    acquired conditions 379
    defects 592
    development of 131
  male
    defects 592
    development of 131–2, 327–9, 338
  tumours of 785
  see also abuse, circumcision, genetic sex determination,
    prepuce, sex development, torsion, undervirilized male,
    warts
Genitourinary system
  development of 131
Genu varum 133
Geographic location in accidental injury 739
Glasgow Coma Score 77, 670, 673, 679, 686
Glomerular filtration rate 68
Glomerulonephritis 487
Glucose 117
  intolerance 119
Goldenhar syndrome, *see* facio-auriculo-vertebral spectrum
GP, *see* general practitioner
Graft 506, *see also* transplant
Grob technique 149
Gross operation 148–9
Growth 124–6
Gynaecological causes of recurrent abdominal pain 419

'H' fistula, *see* tracheo-oesophageal fistula
Haddon's matrix 739
Haemangioma 170, 174
Haematology 88
Haematuria 500
Haemodialysis 496, 497
Haemofiltration 496, 497
Haemolytic uraemic syndrome 487
Haemophilia 3
Haemorrhage per rectum 378
Haemorrhoidal veins 439
Haemothorax 693
Handicapped child
  looking after 288
Hashimoto's disease 3
Hasson technique in laparoscopic surgery 826–7
Head 461–9
  injuries 681–91
  see also tumours
Health authorities 41
Health care delivery systems 140
Heart
  congenital disease 759–65, 766–72
  fetal defects 14, 759–60
  –lung transplantation 757
  murmurs 760

  implications for anaesthesia 90
  progression of obstructive lesions 761
  sequential analysis of 761
  transplantation 757
Height velocity 511
Helicobacter pylori 418
Henoch–Schönlein purpura 358, 377, 378, 413, 488, 501
Hepatic
  system 88
  tumours 781–3
Hepatitis
  neonatal 241
  viral 412
Hepatobiliary injury 702
Hernia 309–19
  epigastric 317
  femoral 316
  inguinal 151, 309–16, 413
    incarcerated 311
  paraumbilical 316
  sliding 314
  transfer of patient with 77
  umbilical 317, 318
  ventral 151
  see also congenital diaphragmatic hernia, hydroceles
Hip disorders 813–19
^{131}I-Hippurate 68, 72, 72
Hirschsprung's disease 3, 36, 199, 206–12, 437
HMD, *see* hyaline membrane disease
Home
  postoperative care 83, 85
Home accidents 742
Homeostasis 102–115
Hormonal response
  neonate 102, 103–4
  surgery and 103–4
Hormones 332, 516
Hospital
  admission 44–6, 54, 686
  attitudes to different ethnic groups 47
  discharge 56–7
  facilities 41–3
  liasion with general practitioner 56
  primary assessment on arrival 670
  preadmission programmes 51
  preparation for 50–1
  receiving
    transfer patients 78
    trauma patients 669–75
  service level 41, 42
  see also day units, day surgery, operating theatres,
    recovery area
HUS, *see* haemolytic uraemic syndrome
Hyaline membrane disease 194
Hydramnios 281
Hydroceles 316
Hydrocephalus 260–9, 279, 285–6

Hydronephrosis
  contralateral 571
  fetal 15–16
Hydrops 422
Hymen
  imperforate 379
  size of oriface 735
  tears in 735
Hyperbilirubinaemia 245
Hypercalcaemia 661
Hypercalciuria 661
Hyperkalaemia 494
Hyperoxaluria 661
Hyperphosphataemia 494
Hypersplenism 445, 451
Hypertension 500, 569
Hyperuricaemia 662
Hypnosis in enuresis 642
Hypocalcaemia 495
Hypoglycaemia 428
Hypospadias 322, 603–16
  repair 605–10
Hypothalamo-pituitary–gonadal axis 329
Hypothermia, risk in laparoscopic surgery
  826
Hypovolaemia 127, 129, 485, 488

ICP, *see* intracranial pressure
Idiopathic intestinal obstruction 199
Immunobiology 750
Immunology after burns 723
Immunosuppression 751
In utero surgery, *see* fetal surgery
Incontinence 644–57
Induction, *see* anaesthesia induction
Indwelling catheters 109
Infants
  anaesthesia 96
  electrolyte management 105–6
  fluid management 105–8
  handling of 189
  oesophageal atresia in 188, 189, 190
  oxygen consumption 188–9
  transporting 189
  urinary infection in 480
Infections 3, 150
  bacterial 3
  parasitic 3
  viral 3
Inflammatory bowel disease 379, 380–95, 418
  injuries 695
  motility study 369
  pH monitoring 368
Injury
  prevention programmes 741–3
  surveillance 741
Inner ear 135

Intestinal
  abnormalities
    fetal 15
  colonization 227
  obstruction 197–205
  tract, development of 197–8
  transplantation 756–7
Intra-abdominal cystic duplication 399
Intracranial
  lesions 683
  pressure 683
Intracranial pressure 135, 261
Intradural lipoma 275
Intrahepatic obstruction 444
Intralipid 117, 119
Intraosseous infusion 111–13
Intraspinal anomalies 271–5
Intrauterine intervention 3
Intravascular access 111
  see also intraosseous infusion
Intravenous
  pyelogram 217
  urograms 63, 479, 618, 647
Intraventricular septum, defects of 764
Intrinsic acute renal failure 485–6, 493
Intussusception 77, 356–63
Iodine 67
Islet cell adenomas 429
Isotope studies 618–19, 647
IVP
  see intravenous pyelogram
IVU
  see intravenous urogram

Jejunoileal atresias 3, 199
Jost paradigm 290
Jugular vein 109

Kidney
  cake, *see* lumbar
  contralateral 571
  horsehoe 522, 584
  injury 700
  lumbar 585
  multicystic dysplastic 565–72
  polycystic 573–81
  see also renal
Klippel–Feil syndrome 809
Knee, painful 819–20
Knock knee
  see valgum
Kyphoscoliosis 283, 284
Kyphosis 283, 284, 811

Labial adhesions 379, 735
Ladd's band 201
Laminar arch defects 272

Laparoscopic surgery 406, 700,
825–34
appendicetomy 411, 829–31
fundoplication 831
pyeloplasty 624
pyloromyotomy 350, 351, 831–3
Laparotomy 233
Laryngeal
cleft 170, 174
mask airway 92, 93
nerve palsy 195
obstruction 174
Laryngomalacia 170, 173
Laryngospasm 365
Laryngotracheobronchitis, *see* croup
Larynx anomalies 170, 173–4
Leg
normal development 133
see also genu, varum, valgum
Leucocytosis 405
Leukaemia 36
Lichen sclerosis 734
Limb
abnormalities of lower 276
abnormalities of upper 812–13
Liver
transplantation 751–5
ultrasound examination of 62
LMA, *see* laryngeal mask airway
Lumboperitoneal shunt 264
Lung 130
agenesis 176
anomalies 170–86
development 153–4
hypoplasia 154, 157
–thorax transverse ratio 159

MACE, *see* Malone antegrade continence enema
Macroglossia 170, 172
Magnetic resonance imaging 135, 270, 278, 406, 424,
648
MAGPI operation 609
Maingot keel operation 150, 151
Male
genitalia, *see* genitalia, male
undervirilized 296, 304
Malformation
definition of 6
Malnutrition
due to Crohn's disease 385
due to gastro-oesophageal reflux 366
Malrotation 201–2, 418
Manual evacuation 439
MAP, *see* mean airway pressure
Maternal morbidity
in fetal surgery 23, 27
MCD, *see* Multicystic dysplastic kidney

MCU, *see* micturating cysto-urethrogram
Mean airway pressure 160
Meatal stenosis 321, 323
Meckel's diverticulum 198, 199, 240, 310, 358,
412
Meconium 208
ileus 3, 199
Megaureters 526
Megaureters 555–64
Meiotic division
disorder 6
Mendelian inheritance risks 33–5, 36
Meningocele 282
Meningomyelocele 282
Mesenteric adenitis 412
Metabolic response
neonate 102, 104–5
surgery and 104–5
Micturating cysto-urethrogram 474, 479
Middle ear 135
Midline skin fusion defect 467
Minerals 118
Minimal access techniques 27–8
Minority groups 47
Morgagni hernia 154, 165
MRI, *see* magnetic resonance imaging
Mucosal
blood flow 229
ectropion 612
Munchausen syndrome by proxy 729–30
MURCS 6
Muscular dystrophies 806
Musculoskeletal system
defects 592
development of 133, 134
infection 800–2
neoplasia 802–3
ultrasound examination of 64
Myelocele 282–3
Myelodyspasia 3
Myelomeningoceles 279
see also meningomyelocele

Naevus, sebaceous 467
Nasal obstruction 170, 171–2
National Association for the Welfare of Children in Hospital,
see NAWCH
National Health Service 40, 41, 138–9
NAWCH 40, 50
NEC, *see* necrotizing enterocolitis
Neck 461–9
abnormalities 807–8
radiological changes 127
see also tumours
Necrotizing enterocolitis 96, 226–37
transfering patients with 76
Neonatal intensive care units 226

Neonate
anaesthesia 94–6
bleeding 376–7
electrolyte management 105–6
emergencies 95–6
fluid management 105–6
hepatitis 241
hormonal response 104
intestinal obstruction 197–205
intestine 227
metabolic response 102, 104–5
necrotizing enterocolitis 376
pelviureteric junctional hydronephrosis 620
polcystic kidney disease 575, 577
renal failure 487, 488
spinal abnormalities 275
ultrasound examination of brain 60
urinary infection 480
ventilation 189
Neoplasia
abdominal pain caused by 419
testicular 331
Nephroblastoma, *see* Wilms' tumour
Nephroblastomatosis 522
Nephrolithotomy 664
Nephrotic syndrome 500
Nephroureterectomy 563
Nerve biopsy 136
Nesidioblastosis 428
Neural tube defects
fetal 14
Neuroblastoma 62–3, 777–81
Neurocristopathies 8
Neurofibromatosis 3
Neurogenic bowel 439–41
Neurological dysfunction 284
Neuromuscular disorders 805–7, *see also* cerebral palsy
Neurosurgical unit 687
Neurosurgery 727
NICU, *see* neonatal intensive care units
Nissen fundoplication 371–5
Non-accidental injury 724–30, 731–7
Nutritional 116–17, 515, 517
requirements for patients with severe burns 721, 723
see also malnutrition

Obstetric issues 148
Obstruction, intestinal 96
Occurrence screening 138
Oesophageal
Oesophageal atresia 175, 187–96
fetal 15
long-gap 192–3
transfering patients with 76
without fistula 192–4
Oesophagogastric manometry 369
Oesophagoscopy 369

Oesophagus
development of 130
anastomotic leakage 191
diverticulum 192
motility 192
shelf 192
OI, *see* oxygenation index
Omental disease 412
Omphalocele 145–52
Operating table position 222, 829, 831
Operating theatres 81, 829, 831
Oral medication 440
Orchidopexy 332–5, 336
Organ preservation 749–50
orientation 332
Ortho-iodo hippurate, *see* ^{131}I-hippurate
Orthopaedic surgery 727–8, 800–24
Ossification 133
Osteogenesis imperfecta 804
Osteosarcoma 803
Outflow tract obstruction 545
Outpatients facilities 42, 84
Ovarian pathology 413
Ovaries
development of 131
OVI, *see* oxygenation ventilation index
Oxygen therapy 189
Oxygenation index 160
Oxygenation ventilation index 160

Paediatric
community nursing 54–7
intensive care units 43, 73
transport 73–9
trauma score 696, 697
Pain measurement scales 52
Palliative procedures for heart disease 767
Pancreas 424–31
annular 425
divisum 425–6
transplantation 756
Pancreatic
cysts 429
injury 704
lesions 430
trauma 430
Pancreatitis
acute 426–7
chronic 427–8
Paraphimosis 321–2, 323
Paraureteric diverticulum 525, 552–4
Parental
attitude to enuresis 637
counselling 147
beliefs 322
roles 52

Parenteral nutrition 116–21
  preparation of feed 119
  long-term 119, 120–1
  metabolic complications 119
  monitoring 119
  total 119, 120
Parotid gland 465–6
Patent processus vaginalis 331
Patient-controlled analgesia 52
PCA, *see* patient-controlled analgesia
Pectus
  excavatum 455–7
  carinatum 457–8
Pelvis
  disorders of 813–19
  fracture of 709–10
  ultrasound examination of 64
Pelviureteric junction
  obstruction 622
  hydronephrosis 526, 527, 617–25,
    622
Peptic ulcer disease 418
Performance indicators 140–1
Perfusion 766–7
Perianal examination 733
Pericardial tamponade 693
Perineum
  acquired conditions of 376–9
  trauma to, *see* straddle injuries
Periodic syndrome 413
Peritoneal drainage 232–3
Peroperative haemostasis 615
Persistent fetal circulation 155
Persistent pulmonary hypertension of the newborn
    155
Perthes' disease 815, 816–18
PFC, *see* persistent fetal circulation
Phimosis 321, 322
Phrenic nerve palsy, *see* Erb's palsy
Pierre Robin syndrome 170, 172
Pilomatrixoma 467
Pituitary gonadal axis 516
Plastic surgery 728–9, 790–9
Platt Report 39, 40, 50, 54
Play 45, 52
  specialists 45
Playground safety 742
Pleura
  development of 129
PLUG procedure 27
Pneumothorax, open 694
Poisoning 3
Poland syndrome 459
Polyhydramnios 155, 159
  maternal 187, 195
Polyuria 638, 646
Portal hypertension 248–9, 442–54

Portoenterostomy 245–7
Posterior urethral valves 16–17
Posthitis 322
Postnatal
  diagnosis of congenital diaphragmatic hernia 155
Postoperative
  analgesia 94, 96
  apnoea
  complications 411
  fetal surgery management 23
  pain management 52
Postrenal acute renal failure 487, 497
Posture 189
Potassium 107–8, 494
PPHN, *see* persistent pulmonary hypertension of the
    newborn
Pre-TRF, *see* preterminal renal failure
Preauricular sinus 466
Pregnancy
  termination 14, 147–8, 160
Prehepatic obstruction 443–4
Prematurity 150
  oesophageal atresia and 190, 194
  tracheo-oesophageal fistula and 195
Premedication 90 1
Prenatal, *see* antenatal
Preoperative
  assessment of neonates 94
  starvation 89
Prepuce 320–6
Preputial plasty 323
Prerenal acute renal failure 484–5, 493
Preterminal renal failure 498, 501–5
Primary Health Care Team 55–7
Prophylaxis
  to prevent urinary tract reinfection 480
Prophylaxis 231
Prune belly syndrome 335, 559
Pseudo-tuberculosis 3
Psychological issues
  abdominal pain and 417–18
  anaethesthetic 89, 96
  burn patients 96
  circumcision 325
  exstrophy/epispadias 600
  genetic counselling and 37
  growth related 516
  preterminal renal failure and 505
Puberty 511, 514
PUJ, *see* pelviureteric junction
Pulmonary
  artery pressure 160
  contusion 694
  hypoplasia 628
  sequestration 170, 181–2
  vasoconstriction 161
  vascular resistance 760

Pulmonary atresia 765
Pulmonary physiotherapy 723
Pulmonary venous connection, abnormality of 763
Pulomonary valve stenosis 765
Pyloric stenosis 3, 36, 96
   infantile hypertrophic 344–55

Radiation burns 722
Radiology 405
Radionuclides 67, 406
Radiopaque dye studies 217
Radiopharmaceuticals 68
Raised intraluminal pressure 229
Rapid eye movement 87
   recessive inheritance 33–4
Reconstructive surgery after burns 723
Recovery area 82
Rectal
   biopsy 648
   injury 711, 716
   polyps 377–8, 439
   prolapse 378, 438
Rectal duplication 400
Recti, divarication of 317
Refluo technique 335
Regional perinatal medical centres 13–14
Regional service for spinal bifida 284, 286
Regional trauma units 676–80
Rehabilitation
   after head injury 689
   after transplant 506
Religion 47
REM, *see* rapid eye movement
Renal
   abnormalities 3, 72, 487, 488, 520–8
   agenesis 520, 582–89
   calculi 658–63
   cystic disease 520, 573–81
   development 531–2, 565
   dysplasia 520, 565–72
   ectopia 522, 582–8, 585–8
   failure 484–508, 599
     acute 484–97
     chronic 497–506
   function 106, 547
   fusion 582–8
   mass lesions 72
   osteodystrophy 504, 516
   parenchymal imaging, *see* static renography
   pelvic 583–4
   replacement therapy 495
   scarring 481, 546
   system 88
   thoracic 583
   tract
     anomalies in association with spinal defects 283, 285

ultrasound examination of 63–4
   transplant 634, 755–6
     evaluation of 72
   trauma 72
   venous thrombsis, *see* thrombosis
Renogram 68, 69, 70
Renography
   dynamic 68–9
   isotope 67–72
   static 68
   replacement 194
   varices 444, 446
Respiration during laparoscopic surgery 826
Respiratory
   distress 692–3
   tract burns 720
Respiratory system 86–7
   development of 129
   distress 160
   failure 150
Resuscitation 669–75
Retroperitoneal haematoma 705
Rhabdomyosarcoma 783–6
Ribs, congenital abscence of 459
Road safety 741–2
RRT, *see* renal replacement therapy
Rubella 3
RVT (renal venous thrombosis), *see* thrombosis

Sacral
   agenesis 646
   anomalies 217
Sacrococcygeal teratoma
   fetal 26
Salivary gland 466
Sarcoma 3
Scalds, *see* burns
Scalp injuries 688
Scanning, *see* ultrasound
SCFA, *see* short-chain fatty acids
Scheuermann's disease 811–12
Scintiscan 699
   pulmonary 369
Sclerotherapy 448, 449, 452, 461
Scoliosis 811
Scrotal inflammation 411
SCT, *see* sacrococcygeal teratoma
Sedation, emergency 721
Separation of child from parents 44
Sepsis 110, 118, 119, 121, 122, 323
Sequence
   definition of 7
Serum alpha-fetoprotein screening, *see* AFP screening
Sex
   determination 293–4
   development 291–3
   differentiation 294–6

Sexual function
    after urethral rupture 712
    in exstrophy/epispadias patients 600
Sexually transmitted disease 735–6
Shandling tube 440
Shock 672–3
Short stature 500, *see also* growth
Short-chain fatty acids 228
Shunts
    portosystemic 450
        angiography 451
Shunts, *see* lumboperitoneal shunt, ventriculoatrial shunt,
        ventriculoperitoneal shunt
SIDS, *see* sudden infant death syndrome
Silastic bag 150
Silo 150
Single strand conformation polymorphism 208
Skeletal
    abnormalities 276
        in spina bifida 286
    general development 133
    maturation 511
    trauma 803
Skin
    cover 791
    expansion 795–6
    flaps 793
    grafting 791–3
Skull
    radiological changes 126, 127
Skull fractures 683
Skull fractures 688, 689
SLE, *see* systemic lupus erythematosus
Small stomach 192
Socioeconomic factors in accidental injury 739
Sodium
    levels in sweat 199
    requirements 107
Solvito 119
Spermatogenesis 331
Sphrintzen syndrome, *see* velocardiofacial syndrome
Spina bifida 3, 36, 279–89
Spinal
    anomalies 217
    cord 133–5
    dysraphism 3, 270–8, 281
    radiography 277
    trauma 809
    see also back pain
Spinous process defects 272
Spleen injury 703–4
Splenectomy 451
Spondylolisthesis 809–11
Spondylolysis 809–11
Sports and leisure accidents 740, 742, 743
SSCP, *see* single strand conformation polymorphism
Staffing 41, 42, 43, 54–7, 74–5, 84

Staging systems for tumours 774. 775, 780–1, 783, 784, 786
Staphylococcus albus 228
STD, *see* sexually transmitted disease
Sternum
    congenital cleft 458–9
    congenital fissure, *see* congenital cleft sternum
Stillbirth
    protocol for autopsy 5
Stomach
    development of 130
Stool-reducing substances 231
Straddle injuries 379
Stress
    of carers 288
    in enuresis 637
Subclavian vein 109
Subglottic stenosis 170, 174
Sucrulphate scan 384
Suction biopsy 209
Sudden infant death syndrome 95, 365
Suppositories 440
Supra-hepatic obstruction 444
Surface stigma in spinal dysraphism 283
Syndrome of inappropriate antidiuretic hormone secretion
        (SIADH) 232
Syndromes
    definition of 5
Syphilis 3
Systemic lupus erythematosus 488
Systemic venous connection, abnormality of 763

^{99m}Tc dimercapto-succinic acid 479
^{99m}Tc-diethylenetriaminepenta-acetic acid,
        see ^{99m}Tc-DTPA
^{99m}Tc-dimercaptosuccinic acid, *see* ^{99m}Tc-DMSA
^{99m}Tc-DMSA 68, 72
^{99m}Tc-DTPA 68, 69, 558
^{99m}Tc-MAG-3: 68, 69, 72, 558
^{99m}Tc-mercaptoacetyltriglycine, *see* ^{99m}Tc-MAG-3
Technetium 67
Temperature
    monitoring 94
    regulation 88
Tension pneumothorax 671, 693
Teratomas 462
Terminal care 57
Testes
    ascending 331
    cryptorchid 329
    development of 131–2
    torsion 338–43
    undescended 151, 327–37, 828
        iatrogenic 331
Testicular dysgenesis 296–7
Tetanus prophylaxis 721
Tethering of conus 274
Tetralogy of Fallot 765, 770–1

Thermal injury 728–9, *see also* burns
Thoracic
   duplication 397
   injuries 692–5
Thymic remnants 467
Thyroglossal cysts 464
Thyroid gland 463
Thrombosis
   renal venous 487
Tocolytic agents
   in fetal surgery 24, 26
TOF, *see* tracheo-oesophageal fistula
Torsion
   of spermatic chord 338–43
Torticollis 466
Toxoplasmosis 3
TPN, *see* total parenteral nutrition
Trace elements 118
Trachea, development of 130
Tracheal
   agenesis 174–5
   stenosis 174–5
Tracheo-oesophageal fistula 77, 95, 175, 187–96
   recurrent 192
Tracheomalacia 170, 175
Transfer of patients 77–8, 674, 689
   equipment 75–6
   predeparture checklist 75
   preparation 73
   transport vehicle 74
Transplantation 747–57
   liver 751–5
   living related 748–9
   rejection 751
   renal 506, 634
   see also donor procedure, graft, organ preservation
Transport, *see* transfer
Trauma 3, 322
   blunt to abdomen 671, 674, 696–708
   chemical 3
   cold injury 3
   electrical 3
   iatrogenic 325
   injury
      direct 3
      indirect 3
   paediatric centre 678
   perineum, *see* straddle injury
   radiation 3
   regional units 676–80
   team in hospital 668, 669
   thermal 3
Treacher–Collins syndrome 8
Trisomy
   13: 155
   18: 155
   21, *see* chromosome 21

Tuberculosis 3
Tubular duplication 399
Tubular necrosis 484, 486
Tubulointerstitial disease 486, 499
   tumour 569
   ultrasound 190
   vascular disease 71–2
   water requirements 107
   see also end-stage renal failure, growth, intrinsic acute
      renal failure, neonate renal failure, prerenal acute renal
      failure, preterminal renal failure, postrenal acute renal
      failure, urine
Tumours 773–89
   head 170, 172, 784
   neck 170, 172, 784
   see also Ewing's sarcoma, musculoskeletal system,
      neuroblastoma, osteosarcoma, rhabdomyosarcoma,
      Wilms' tumour

Ulcerative colitis 380, 386–90
Ultrasound 11–12, 13, 14, 15, 59–66, 110, 135, 147, 155,
   190, 218, 230, 285, 347–8, 358, 405–6, 423, 424, 479,
   500, 542, 575, 618, 646, 674, 699, 761
United Nations Convention on the Rights of the Child
   40, 49
Upper air passages
   development of 129–30
Upper respiratory tract infections
   implications for anaesthesia 90
Ureter
   double 531–43
   ectopic 534–8
   obstruction 556
Ureteroceles 538–43, 612
   ectopic 527
Ureteroscopy 664
Urethral
   obstruction 628
   plate 604
   rupture 709–18
   stenosis 612
   valves 527
      posterior 626–35
Urethrotomy 714
Urinary D-lactate 231
Urinary immunoreactive thromboxane 231
Urinary tract
   anomalies 332, 531–43
   fetal congenital abnormalities 14–15, 25–6,
      531–2
   infections 71, 322, 411, 473–83, 500, 545–6, 637–8
      complicating surgery 481
   lower
      dysfunction of 556
   see also ureters
Urine
   analysis 405, 493

drainage 615
flow 555–6
samples, collection and handling 475–6
Urolithiasis 3, 658–666
Urological anomalies 519–30
Uropathy 418
obstructive 70
Uterus
development of 131

VACTERL 6
VACTERL, *see* VATER
Vaginal
discharge 736
foreign body 736
Valgum 133
Van der Woode syndrome 36
Variceal
bleeding 448
haemorrhage 446
Varices 444, 446, 448, 450, 451
Varicoceles 340–1
Vas
injury 334
'long loop' 335
Vasal anomalies 331
Vascular
access 121–2
venal 108, 132
arterial 132–3
imaging, using ultrasound 64–5
ring 175
thrombosis 110
Vasopressin 447
VATER 6, 36, 188, 217
Velocardiofacial syndrome 8
Ventilation index 159
Ventricular
septal defect 769–70
system 135
Ventriculoarterial disorders 764–5, 770

Ventriculoatrial shunt 264, 279
Ventriculoperitoneal shunt 264–9, 279
Vertebral bodies anomalies 272–3
Vesicoureteric reflux 71, 480–1, 524–5, 532, 533–4, 544–51, 552, 556, 623, 659
Videourodynamics 647
Viral infections
in intussusception 358
in spina bifida 281
Vitalipid 119
Vitamin D 247
Vitamins 3, 118
deficiency 281
Vitellointestinal duct 238–40
embryology 238
Vocal cord palsy 170, 173–4
Voiding
cystourethrography 618
dysfunctional 549
symptoms 628
Volvulus
of midgut 377
neonatorum 201
VUR, *see* vesicoureteric reflux

Waardenburg 6
Warts, anogenital 735
Water
imbalance 515
loss 106
Water safety 742
Welfare of Children and Young People in Hospital 40, 47
White cell count 405
Wilms' tumour 3, 63, 523, 569, 773–7
Wolffian system 556
Wound
healing 790
infection 351, 410

Zollinger–Ellison syndrome 429
Zuelzer–Wilson disease 207